Health Assessment & Physical Examination

Fourth Edition

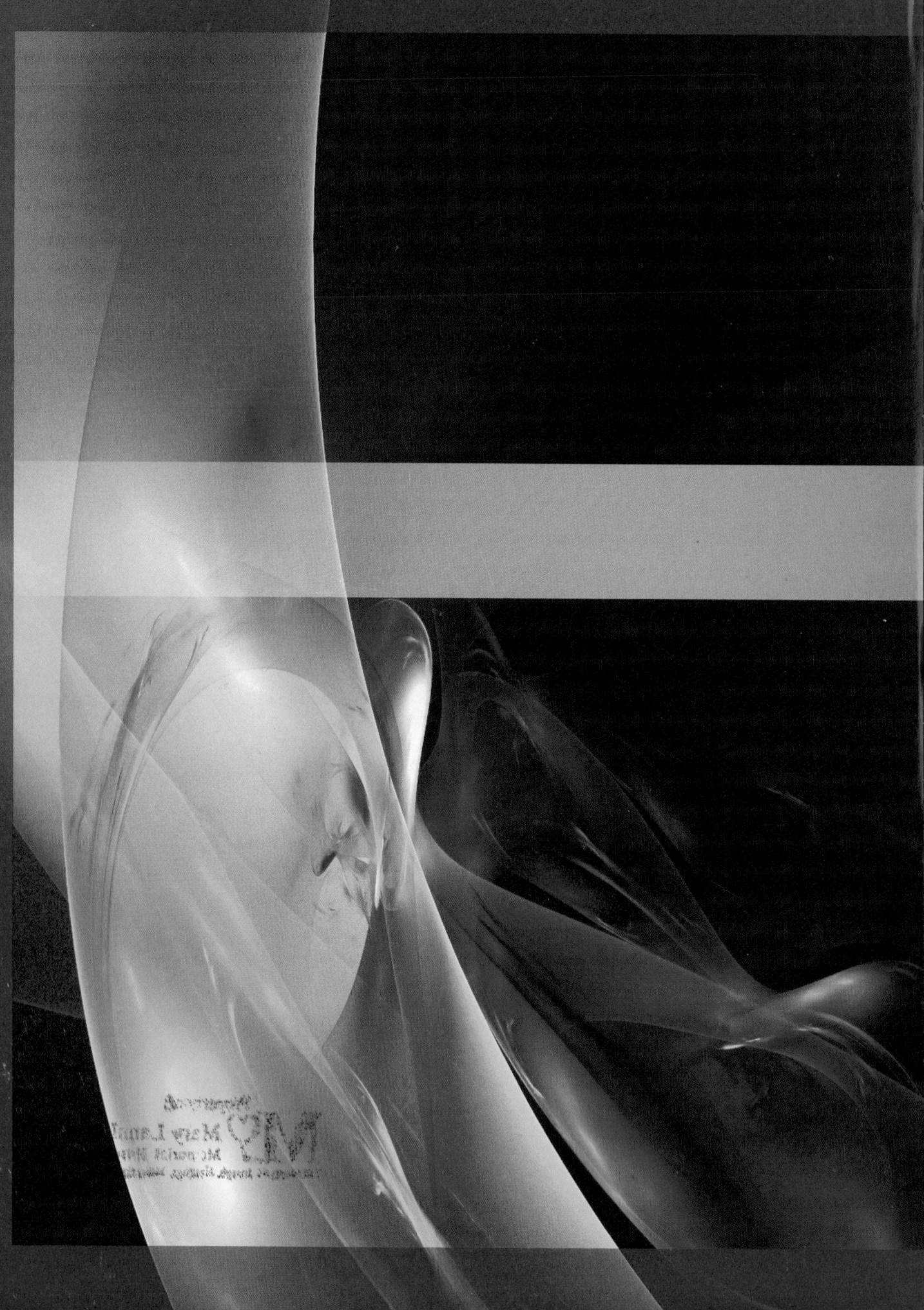

Health Assessment & Physical Examination

Fourth Edition

Mary Ellen Zator Estes,
RN, MSN, FNP-BC, NP-C

Family Nurse Practitioner in Internal Medicine
Fairfax, Virginia
and
Nursing Consultant
Vienna, Virginia

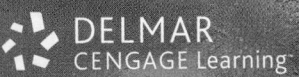

DELMAR
CENGAGE Learning

Australia • Brazil • Japan • Korea • Mexico • Singapore • Spain • United Kingdom • United States

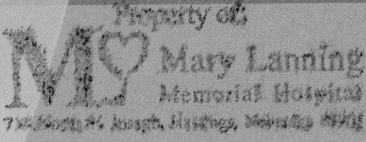

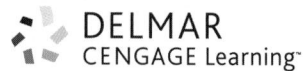

Health Assessment & Physical Examination, Fourth Edition

Mary Ellen Zator Estes

Vice President, Career and Professional Editorial: Dave Garza

Director of Learning Solutions: Matthew Kane

Executive Editor: Stephen Helba

Managing Editor: Marah Bellegarde

Senior Product Manager: Elisabeth Williams

Editorial Assistant: Samantha Miller

Vice President, Career and Professional Marketing: Jennifer McAvey

Marketing Director: Wendy Mapstone

Senior Marketing Manager: Michelle McTighe

Marketing Coordinator: Scott Chrysler

Production Director: Carolyn Miller

Production Manager: Andrew Crouth

Senior Content Project Manager: Stacey Lamodi

Senior Art Director: Jack Pendleton

Technology Project Manager: Benjamin Knapp

Production Service: Elm Street Publishing Services

Compositor: Integra Software Services Pvt. Ltd.

For product information and technology assistance, contact us at
Cengage Learning Customer & Sales Support, 1-800-354-9706
For permission to use material from this text or product, submit all requests online at **www.cengage.com/permissions.**
Further permissions questions can be e-mailed to
permissionrequest@cengage.com

Library of Congress Control Number: 2008932912

ISBN-13: 978-1-4354-2756-3

ISBN-10: 1-4354-2756-4

Delmar
5 Maxwell Drive
Clifton Park, NY 12065-2919
USA

Cengage Learning is a leading provider of customized learning solutions with office locations around the globe, including Singapore, the United Kingdom, Australia, Mexico, Brazil, and Japan. Locate your local office at: **international.cengage.com/region**

Cengage Learning products are represented in Canada by Nelson Education, Ltd.

To learn more about Delmar, visit **www.cengage.com/delmar**

Purchase any of our products at your local college store or at our preferred online store **www.ichapters.com**

Notice to the Reader
Publisher does not warrant or guarantee any of the products described herein or perform any independent analysis in connection with any of the product information contained herein. Publisher does not assume, and expressly disclaims, any obligation to obtain and include information other than that provided to it by the manufacturer. The reader is expressly warned to consider and adopt all safety precautions that might be indicated by the activities described herein and to avoid all potential hazards. By following the instructions contained herein, the reader willingly assumes all risks in connection with such instructions. The publisher makes no representations or warranties of any kind, including but not limited to, the warranties of fitness for particular purpose or merchantability, nor are any such representations implied with respect to the material set forth herein, and the publisher takes no responsibility with respect to such material. The publisher shall not be liable for any special, consequential, or exemplary damages resulting, in whole or part, from the readers' use of, or reliance upon, this material.

Printed in the United States of America
1 2 3 4 5 6 7 13 12 11 10 09

To all those who strive for higher education.

Most especially, for Katie and Andrew . . . reach

for the stars!

CONTENTS

UNIT 1

LAYING THE FOUNDATION / 1

CHAPTER 1 CRITICAL THINKING AND THE NURSING PROCESS / 3

CHAPTER 2 THE PATIENT INTERVIEW / 17

UNIT 2

SPECIAL ASSESSMENTS / 87

CHAPTER 4 DEVELOPMENTAL
ASSESSMENT / 89

CHAPTER 5 CULTURAL
ASSESSMENT / 121

CHAPTER 6 SPIRITUAL
ASSESSMENT / 155

CHAPTER 7 NUTRITIONAL
ASSESSMENT / 195

UNIT 3

PHYSICAL EXAMINATION / 243

CHAPTER 8 PHYSICAL ASSESSMENT TECHNIQUES / 245

CHAPTER 9 GENERAL SURVEY, VITAL SIGNS, AND PAIN / 261

CHAPTER 10 SKIN, HAIR, AND NAILS / 289

CHAPTER 11 HEAD, NECK, AND REGIONAL LYMPHATICS / 341

CHAPTER 12 EYES / 367

UNIT 5

PUTTING IT ALL TOGETHER / 991

CHAPTER 26 THE COMPLETE HEALTH HISTORY AND PHYSICAL EXAMINATION / 993

CONTRIBUTORS

Patricia Connor Ballard, ACNS-BC, PhD
Director, Inova Learning Network
Inova Health System
Falls Church, Virginia
   Chapter 18: Musculoskeletal System

Beverly Bayer, RN, MS, FNP
Family Nurse Practitioner, Internal Medicine
Fairfax, Virginia
and
FNP Clinical Preceptor
Georgetown University
Washington, DC
   Chapter 19: Mental Status and Neurological Techniques

Mitzi Boilanger, MS, RNC
Clinical Nurse Specialist
Riley Hospital for Children, Clarian Health
Indianapolis, Indiana
   Chapter 23: The Pregnant Patient

Tamera D. Cauthorne-Burnette, RN, MSN, FNP, CS
Family Nurse Practitioner
Montpelier Family Practice
Montpelier, Virginia
and
Family Nurse Practitioner
James E. Jones, Jr., MD and Associates
Obstetrics and Gynecology
Richmond, Virginia
and
Graduate Clinical Faculty
Medical College of Virginia

Virginia Commonwealth University
School of Nursing
Richmond, Virginia
   Chapter 10: Skin, Hair, and Nails
   Chapter 14: Breasts and Regional Nodes
   Chapter 20: Female Genitalia

Catherine Wilson Cox, RN, PhD, CCRN, CEN, CCNS
Assistant Professor
The University of North Carolina at Wilmington
School of Nursing
Wilmington, North Carolina
and
CAPT, NC, USN (Reserve Component)
Camp Lejeune, North Carolina
   Chapter 16: Heart and Peripheral Vasculature

Deirdre M. Carolan Doerflinger, CRNP, PhD
Clinical Nurse Specialist, Geriatrics
Inova Fairfax Hospital
Falls Church, Virginia
and
Adjunct Assistant Professor of Psychiatry
and Behavioral Sciences
George Washington University
School of Medicine and Behavioral Sciences
Washington, DC
and
Adjunct Faculty
College of Health and Human Services
George Mason University
Fairfax, Virginia
   Chapter 25: The Elderly Patient

Jane L. Echols, PhD
Professor of Nursing, Retired
Asheville, North Carolina
> *Chapter 4: Developmental Assessment*
> *Chapter 5: Cultural Assessment*

Barbara Springer Edwards, RN, BSN, MTS
Former Director of Nursing Care
Cardiac Surgical Unit
Alexandria Hospital
Alexandria, Virginia
> *Chapter 6: Spiritual Assessment*

Kathryn K. Ellis, RN, MSN, FNP, ANP
Assistant Professor and Director FNP Program
School of Nursing and Health Studies
Georgetown University
Washington, DC
> *Chapter 13: Ears, Nose, Mouth, and Throat*

Randie R. McLaughlin, RN, MSN, ANP
Adult Nurse Practitioner
Frederick, Maryland
> *Chapter 21: Male Genitalia*
> *Chapter 22: Anus, Rectum, and Prostate*

Kathy Murphy, MSN, RN, PNP-BC
Clinical Nurse Specialist/Pediatric Nurse Practitioner
Children's Healthcare of Atlanta–Egleston
Atlanta, Georgia
> *Chapter 24: The Pediatric Patient*

Susan Abbott Rogge, RN, NP
Department of Obstetrics and Gynecology
University of California, Davis
Sacramento, California
and
Private Practice
Sacramento, California
> *Chapter 23: The Pregnant Patient*

REVIEWERS

Marianne Adam, RN, MSN, CRNP
Assistant Professor, BSN Program
Moravian College
Bethlehem, Pennsylvania

Cynthia A. Blum, RN, PhD(c)
Assistant Professor, Nursing
Florida Atlantic University
Boca Raton, Florida

Shirley K. Comer, RN, MSN, JD
Lecturer, Department of Nursing
College of Health Professions
Governors State University
University Park, Illinois

Kim Cooper
Indiana State University
Terre Haute, Indiana

Dorcas Fitzgerald, RN, CNS, DNSc
Professor, Nursing
Coordinator, RN-BSN Completion Program
Youngstown State University
Youngstown, Ohio

Janice Hausauer, MS, FNP
Adjunct Assistant Professor
Montana State University College of Nursing
Bozeman, Montana

Karen Hessler, RN, FNP, PhD(c)
Assistant Professor of Nursing
University of Northern Colorado
Greeley, Colorado

Patricia McLean Hoyson, RN, PhD, CNS, CDE
Chairperson and Associate Professor
Department of Nursing
Youngstown State University
Youngstown, Ohio

Leeanne L. Humiston, RN, MSN
Nursing Faculty
Southeastern Community College
Keokuk, Iowa

Robin Johns, MSN
Assistant Professor and Coordinator of the
School of Nursing at Athens
Medical College of Georgia
Athens, Georgia

James Johnson, MD
Professor
School of Nursing
Canyon College
Nashville, Tennessee

Cathy R. Kessenich, DSN, ARNP
Director of the MSN Program
Professor of Nursing
University of Tampa
Tampa, Florida

Catherine Lazo-Miller, RN, MSN
Nursing Lecturer, School of Nursing
Full-Time Faculty
Indiana University Northwest
Gary, Indiana

PREFACE

Health assessment forms the foundation of all nursing care. Assessment is an ongoing process that evaluates the whole person as a physical, psychosocial, and functional being, whether the patient is young or old, well or ill. *Health Assessment & Physical Examination,* fourth edition, provides a well-illustrated approach to the process of holistic assessment, including physical assessment skills, clinical examination techniques, and patient teaching guidelines.

Readers will welcome the text's clear presentation as they learn the basic skills of health assessment. Practicing nurses will find the book helpful as a review of the pathophysiological basis for abnormal findings to update their health assessment knowledge base.

CONCEPTUAL APPROACH

This text is designed to teach readers to assess a patient's physical, psychological, social, and spiritual dimensions of health as a foundation of nursing care. The skills of interviewing, inspection, percussion, palpation, auscultation, and documentation are refined to teach readers to make clinical judgments and promote healthy patient outcomes.

The concept for *Health Assessment & Physical Examination,* fourth edition, arose from a need for straightforward, well-organized assessment information that could be easily read and assimilated. The goals that form the foundation of this text are empowering readers as educated decision makers, developing their skills of analysis and critical thinking, and encouraging excellent clinical and nursing skills.

Health Assessment & Physical Examination, fourth edition, embraces a dual focus based on nursing as the art and science of caring. Strong emphasis on science encompasses all the technical aspects of anatomy, physiology, and assessment, while highlighting clinically relevant information. Emphasis on caring is displayed through themes of assessment of the whole person: cultural, spiritual, familial, and environmental considerations; patient dignity; and health promotion. Such an approach encourages nurses to think about and care for themselves as well as their patients.

Health Assessment & Physical Examination, fourth edition, offers a user-friendly approach that delivers a wealth of information. The consistent, easy-to-follow format with recurring pedagogical features is based on two frameworks:

1. The **IPPA** method of examination (**I**nspection, **P**alpation, **P**ercussion, **A**uscultation) is consistently applied to body systems for a complete, detailed physical assessment.
2. The **ENAP** format (**E**xamination, **N**ormal Findings, **A**bnormal Findings, **P**athophysiology) is followed for every IPPA technique, providing a useful and valuable collection of information. Pathophysiology is included for each abnormal finding, acknowledging that nurses' clinical decisions need to be based on scientific rationale. It also enables the reader to study the content specifically relevant to her or his own practice.

Readers of *Health Assessment & Physical Examination,* fourth edition, will need an understanding of anatomy and physiology, as well as a familiarity with basic nursing skills and the nursing process.

ORGANIZATION

Health Assessment & Physical Examination, fourth edition, consists of 26 chapters organized into five units. **Unit 1** lays the foundation for the entire assessment process by guiding the reader through the nursing process, the critical thinking process, the patient interview, and the health history. Specific tips on professionalism, approaching patients, and discussing sensitive topics help the reader understand the importance of the nurse-patient partnership in the assessment process.

Unit 2 highlights developmental, cultural, spiritual, and nutritional areas of assessment, emphasizing the holistic nature of the assessment process. These chapters are key in encouraging the reader to be aware of personal feelings and biases and how they may affect interactions with patients and coworkers.

Unit 3 opens with a description of fundamental assessment techniques, including measuring vital signs and assessing pain, and then details assessment procedures and findings for specific body systems. The format used for all applicable physical assessment chapters in this unit includes:

1. Anatomy and physiology
2. Health history
3. Equipment
4. Physical assessment
   a. Inspection
   b. Palpation
   c. Percussion
   d. Auscultation
5. Case study

The examination techniques presented are described for adult patients. Because assessment techniques and findings may differ in pregnant women, children, and the elderly, these populations are discussed in separate chapters in **Unit 4.** The chapter on the pregnant patient includes variations in examination techniques and special techniques used only on pregnant patients, as well as normal and abnormal findings related to pregnancy. The chapter on the pediatric patient presents physical differences in the examination and explains special techniques used only with children. In addition, *Health Assessment & Physical Examination,* fourth edition, provides a new chapter, "The Elderly Patient." This separate chapter on the older adult highlights the psychological, developmental, cognitive, and physical assessments that are appropriate for this population.

Unit 5 helps the reader assimilate and synthesize the wealth of information presented in the text in order to perform a thorough, accurate, and efficient health assessment and physical examination. Specific guidelines and reminders on gaining patients' cooperation, being sensitive

to legal and ethical considerations, and documenting accurately make this unit a complete health assessment resource tool.

NEW TO THIS EDITION

- All-new multicultural patient profiles (case studies) humanize the material and help readers apply the critical thinking concepts that they have learned in the chapters.
- More than 150 new photographs and illustrations have been added.
- New review questions have been added at the end of each chapter.

Chapter-specific enhancements are also highlighted in this new edition:

- **Chapter 1,** *Critical Thinking and the Nursing Process,* includes descriptions of two additional nursing documentation systems, the Minimum Data Set and OASIS-B1.
- **Chapter 2,** *The Patient Interview,* introduces the technique of motivational interviewing.
- **Chapter 3,** *The Complete Health History Including Documentation,* contains an expanded health history section. In addition, it addresses the timely issues of Internet addiction, genetic testing, ethnicity and pharmacology, and dangerous sexual practices.
- **Chapter 4,** *Developmental Assessment,* introduces Duvall's family life cycle theory.
- **Chapter 5,** *Cultural Assessment,* has updated, extensive references and provides a comprehensive cultural assessment case study.
- **Chapter 6,** *Spiritual Assessment,* introduces the parish nursing movement. The chapter also highlights a new spiritual assessment tool.
- **Chapter 7,** *Nutritional Assessment,* has been updated to include criteria for the metabolic syndrome. In addition, sections on glycosylated hemoglobin and vitamin D have been added to represent current trends in nutritional assessment.
- **Chapter 8,** *Physical Examination Techniques,* updates the CDC elements of Standard Precautions.
- **Chapter 9,** *General Survey, Vital Signs, and Pain,* contains information on the Joint Commission's mandate for a comprehensive pain assessment.
- **Chapter 10,** *Skin, Hair, and Nails,* depicts many new pathological conditions. The timely topic of MRSA infections is discussed.
- **Chapter 11,** *Head, Neck, and Regional Lymphatics,* provides comprehensive tables outlining the signs and symptoms of hypo- and hyperthyroidism as well as hypo- and hyperparathyroidism.

- Chapter 12, *Eyes*, now has risk factors for cataracts, glaucoma, and macular degeneration.
- Chapter 13, *Ears, Nose, Mouth, and Throat*, includes information on the tooth numbering system and nasal septum perforation.
- Chapter 14, *Breasts and Regional Nodes*, has updated breast cancer risk factors. Red flags for breast cancer are highlighted as are the five types of breast cancer.
- Chapter 15, *Thorax and Lungs*, provides information on the increasing prevalence of drug-resistant tuberculosis. The SARS epidemic and avian flu are highlighted.
- Chapter 16, *Heart and Peripheral Vasculature*, includes the advanced technique of assessing the ankle-brachial index. In addition, the new classification system for myocardial infarction is described.
- Chapter 17, *Abdomen*, details risk factors for urinary tract infections. Updated guidelines for the early detection of colon and rectal cancers are also included. In addition, the Bristol Stool Scale is described.
- Chapter 18, *Musculoskeletal System*, provides DEXA screening criteria. In addition, risk factors for sports injuries and the female athlete triad are presented.
- Chapter 19, *Mental Status and Neurological Techniques*, now has the signs and symptoms of Lyme disease and postconcussive syndrome.
- Chapter 20, *Female Genitalia*, discusses the new human papillomavirus vaccine. Cervical cancer screening guidelines are updated.
- Chapter 21, *Male Genitalia*, includes the timely topics of male sexual assault and risk factors for HIV infection.
- Chapter 22, *Anus, Rectum, and Prostate*, provides guidelines for the early detection of prostate cancer. The chapter also includes when and how an anal Pap should be performed.
- Chapter 23, *The Pregnant Patient*, now lists the various drug safety categories for pregnant women.
- Chapter 24, *The Pediatric Patient*, has a thorough description of color vision screening.
- Chapter 25, *The Elderly Patient*, is an entirely new chapter. Enjoy!
- Chapter 26, *The Complete Health History and Physical Examination*, provides a comprehensive and new patient case study. Electronic medical records and the Speak Up™ campaign are discussed.

SPECIAL FEATURES

Many successful features from the previous editions of *Health Assessment & Physical Examination* have been retained in this new edition. These features stimulate critical thinking and self-reflection, develop technical expertise, and encourage readers to synthesize and apply the information presented in the text.

- **Reflective Thinking** boxes introduce ethical controversies and clinical situations readers are likely to encounter, stimulating critical thinking, effective decision making, and active problem solving. They also promote self-examination on particular issues so readers can understand the varying viewpoints possibly held by patients and coworkers. These boxes encourage reflection on issues in a personal context, raise awareness of the diversity of opinions, and foster empowerment.
- **Life 360°** boxes help readers examine their feelings and emotional behavior about learning how to be comfortable with diverse types of patients, as well as learning how to make their patients comfortable.
- **Nursing Checklists** offer an organizing framework for the assessment of each body system or for approaching a given task. Certain **Nursing Checklists** outline specific questions or points to consider when caring for patients with assistive devices.
- **Nursing Tips** help the reader to apply basic knowledge to real-life situations and offer hints and shortcuts useful to both new and experienced nurses.
- **Nursing Alerts** highlight serious or life-threatening signs or critical assessment findings that need immediate attention.
- The **ENAP** format (examination, normal findings, abnormal findings, pathophysiology) allows the reader to study the content that is specifically relevant to her or his own practice. The **IPPA** format (inspection, percussion, palpation, and auscultation) is applied consistently to each assessment skill.
- **Health Histories** outline all areas of assessment related to each body system. The standard format used throughout the text teaches the importance of consistency and organization when discussing topics with patients during the health history interview.
- **Case Studies** humanize the material and help readers apply critical thinking concepts. They present realistic scenarios and offer readers an opportunity to apply the chapter material, thereby encouraging extrapolation and intuitive thinking. These case studies list normal and abnormal assessment findings in the context of a clinical scenario. Each case study includes a sample patient history, physical assessment findings, and, when appropriate, laboratory data in documentation format, emphasizing the nurse's responsibilities for correct charting. Most case studies are written in abbreviated format to simulate real clinical documentation, but they deliberately have different charting styles to reflect the wide variety of norms in actual clinical practice.

PEDAGOGICAL FEATURES

Health Assessment & Physical Examination, fourth edition, also includes many pedagogical features that promote learning and accessibility of information. This text guides the novice as well as the advanced practice nurse in the art and science of conducting a comprehensive health history, health assessment, and physical examination.

- **Competencies** open each chapter and introduce the main areas targeted for mastery in each chapter. They also provide a checkpoint for study and tie in to crucial assessment skills.
- **Outstanding photographs and illustrations** highlight assessment techniques and procedures, anatomy and physiology, and normal and abnormal findings. The photo program is expanded and updated, especially in the area of the older adult.
- **Key Terms** are highlighted and defined in the text the first time they are used.
- **Assessment in Brief** at the end of chapters offer a conceptual framework for chapter review, highlighting main points.
- **Review Questions** offer readers an opportunity to assess their understanding of the content and better define areas needing additional study. All chapters include self-quizzes on key information to test knowledge. Many chapters also include short scenarios with related questions.
- **References** and a **Bibliography** document the theoretical basis of each chapter and provide additional resources for continued study.
- **Web Site** boxes at the end of each chapter direct the reader to additional online resources.
- The **Glossary** at the end of the book defines all key terms used in the text and serves as a comprehensive resource for study and review.
- The **Index** facilitates access to material and includes special entries for tables and illustrations.
- A list of **Abbreviations and Symbols** inside the back text cover includes common abbreviations used in charting, along with their definitions, for quick reference.

EXTENSIVE TEACHING AND LEARNING PACKAGE

A complete supplements package was developed to achieve two goals:

1. To assist readers in learning the essential skills and information needed to secure a career in the nursing profession.
2. To assist instructors in planning and implementing their programs for the most efficient use of time and other resources.

BACK-OF-BOOK STUDYWARE CD

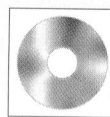

Complimentary to users of this book, the back-of-book CD is an interactive tool to help users assess and increase their knowledge. Elements include: an audio glossary, a Spanish glossary, video skills, image labeling exercises and animations, heart and lung sound simulations, case studies with questions, and study questions for every chapter.

CLINICAL COMPANION

ISBN 1-4354-2758-0

The *Clinical Companion to Accompany Health Assessment & Physical Examination,* fourth edition, is a pocket-sized clinical guide. The content mirrors that of the main text, focusing on easy access and rapid retrieval of information.

STUDENT LAB MANUAL

ISBN 1-4354-2757-2

The *Student Lab Manual to Accompany Health Assessment & Physical Examination,* fourth edition, provides a guide for laboratory activities and a means of exploring and applying concepts presented in the core text. Features include:

- A list of key terms in each chapter to facilitate learning of terminology
- An in-depth review of each body system
- Physical examination skills checklists for readers to note their findings
- Self-assessment quizzes for every chapter
- A list of abbreviations

INSTRUCTOR RESOURCES CD

ISBN 1-4354-2759-9

Free to all instructors who adopt *Health Assessment & Physical Examination,* fourth edition, in their courses, this comprehensive resource includes the following:

Instructor's Guide

- **Key Terms** list provides the key terms for each chapter alphabetically with corresponding definitions.
- **Helpful Hints and Exercises** offer tips for laboratory exercises, clinical skill building, small group work, and classroom discussion.
- **Skills Checklists** outline physical assessment techniques to be evaluated for each body system and comprehensive head-to-toe assessment outlines.
- **Care Plans** correspond to the case studies presented in the text.

Computerized Test Bank

The computerized test bank includes multiple choice questions for each chapter and can be used to generate custom tests. A rationale, text reference, and Bloom's taxonomy level are indicated for each question.

Lecture Slides in PowerPoint®

A vital resource for instructors, presentations created in PowerPoint for each chapter parallel the content in the textbook, serving as a foundation on which instructors may customize their own presentations.

Image Library

The Image Library is a software tool that includes an organized digital library of hundreds of illustrations and photographs from the text. Copy and save any of the images on the CD to facilitate classroom presentations. You can also easily paste images into a Microsoft PowerPoint presentation.

WebTutor Advantage Courses

Offered in both Blackboard (ISBN 1-4354-2760-2) and WebCT (ISBN 1-4354-2761-0) formats, these online resources offer value as standard components to any comprehensive assessment course. Correlated to the text, each format contains chapter summaries, PowerPoint slides, frequently asked questions, Web site listings, and more. To assist in study and skill building, these online courses also include a bank of study questions in various formats: fill-in, matching, multiple choice, and true/false.

Online Companion

ISBN 1-4354-2762-9

Visit the Estes online companion resource at
www.delmar.cengage.com
for additional content and study aids.
Click on Online Companions and then select
the Nursing discipline.

Delmar offers a series of Online Companions™. The *Estes Online Companion*™ enables users of *Health Assessment & Physical Examination,* fourth edition, to access a wealth of information designed to enhance the book. Included in the Online Companion are:

- Expanded glossary
- Web links with annotations
- Frequently asked questions
- Microsoft PowerPoint presentations
- Chapter summaries
- Discussion questions

To access the site for *Health Assessment & Physical Examination,* fourth edition, simply point your browser to http://www.delmar.cengage.com/companions. Select the nursing discipline.

HOW TO USE THIS TEXT

These pages offer suggestions for how you can use the features of this text to gain competence and confidence in your assessment and nursing skills.

NURSING**TIP**

Use of Gloves

Use gloves for palpation of the skin only if there is any probability of contact with body fluids or if the patient is in isolation.

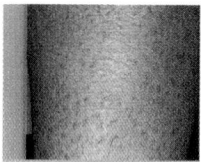

FIGURE 10-14 Ichthyosis Vulgaris.
Courtesy of Robert A. Silverman, M.D., Clinical Associate Professor, Department of Pediatrics, Georgetown University.

PALPATION OF THE SKIN

Moisture

E Palpate all nonmucous membrane skin surfaces for moisture using the dorsal surfaces of the hands and fingers.

N Normally, the skin is dry with a minimum of perspiration. Moisture on the skin will vary from one body area to another, with perspiration normally present on the hands, axilla, face, and in between the skin folds. Moisture also varies with changes in environment, muscular activity, body temperature, stress, and activity levels. Body temperature is regulated by the skin's production of perspiration, which evaporates to cool the body.

A Excessive dryness of the skin, **xerosis**, as evidenced by flaking of the stratum corneum and associated pruritus, is abnormal.

P Hypothyroidism and exposure to extreme cold and dry climates can lead to xerosis.

A Very dry, large scales that are light colored or brown are abnormal (Figure 10-14).

P Ichthyosis vulgaris is a skin abnormality originating from a keratin disorder. It can be associated with atopic dermatitis.

A Diaphoresis is the profuse production of perspiration.

P Causes include hyperthyroidism, increased metabolic rate, sepsis, anxiety, or pain.

Temperature

E Palpate all nonmucosal skin surfaces for temperature using the dorsal surfaces of the hands and fingers.

N Skin surface temperature should be warm and equal bilaterally. Hands and feet may be slightly cooler than the rest of the body.

A Hypothermia is a cooling of the skin and may be generalized or localized.

P Generalized hypothermia is indicative of shock or some other type of central circulatory dysfunction. Localized hypothermia is indicative of arterial insufficiency in t...

A Generalized hyperther... be generalized or localiz...

P Generalized hypertherm... roidism, or increased m... hyperthermia may be ca...

Tenderness

E Palpate skin surfaces for... and fingers.

N Skin surfaces should be...

A Tenderness over the s... generalized.

P Discrete tenderness ma... and generalized tender... phoma or allergic reacti...

E Examination   **N** Normal Findings   **A** Abnormal...

ENAP FORMAT: In order for the assessment process to become "instinctual" for you, we have highlighted each step of the ENAP process:

Examination sequences show you the step-by-step process of performing an assessment.

Normal Findings, highlighted in blue, describe what you will find in a normal assessment.

Abnormal Findings outline the variations from normal you may see in pathological states.

Pathophysiology explains the scientific rationale for abnormal conditions; many are illustrated.

ENAP reminder boxes repeat on assessment pages for easy reference.

REFLECTIVE THINKING

Painful Stimuli Application

In the neurosurgical intensive care unit you assess your patient. You note that she has ecchymotic areas on her sternum and subungal hematomas on the right hand.

- What does this information mean to you?
- Is there any additional information that you need to gather?
- What action would you take in this situation?

REFLECTIVE THINKING helps you develop sensitivity to ethical and moral issues and guides you to think critically in clinical situations and become an active problem solver. You may want to read each one and explore the issues *before* reading the chapter. Then as you read the chapter, evaluate your original thoughts. If you read the boxes as you go through the chapter, you may want to write down your thoughts, then go back and look at them later.

LIFE 360°

Prioritizing Care

The home health nurse is meeting with Mr. S. for the first time. Mr. S. is a 44-year-old male with acute cardiomyopathy waiting for a heart transplantation. The nurse performs a health and physical assessment on Mr. S., then discusses the plan of care with him. Mr. S. and the nurse disagree on the current priorities of care.

- What nursing interventions would you implement in this situation?
- Is there additional information that you would attempt to elicit from the patient?
- How can you align nursing priorities with patient priorities to deliver efficient and necessary care?

LIFE 360° boxes explore situations throughout the lifespan. Page through and read each one *before* reading the chapter. Then challenge yourself to evaluate your own opinions after reading all of the chapter content.

The heart's primary function is to pump blood to all parts of the body. The circulating blood not only brings oxygen and nutrients to the body's tissues but also helps to take away the body's waste products. The body's activities determine the amount of blood that is pumped. The heart will beat faster or slower and the blood vessels will expand or relax in order to properly distribute the blood that the body demands.

ANATOMY AND PHYSIOLOGY

HEART

In a resting, healthy adult, the heart contracts 60 to 100 times while pumping 4 to 5 liters of blood per minute. An individual's heart is about the size of a clenched fist. The human heart is remarkably efficient considering its size in relation to the rest of the body.

The heart is located in the thoracic cavity between the lungs and above the diaphragm in an area known as the mediastinum (Figure 16-1). The base of the heart is the uppermost portion, which includes the left and right atria as well as the aorta, pulmonary arteries, and the superior and inferior venae cavae. These structures lie behind the upper portion of the sternum. The apex, or lower portion of the heart, extends into the left thoracic cavity, causing the heart to appear as if it is lying on its right ventricle.

Pericardium

The heart and roots of the great vessels lie within a sac called the pericardium, which is composed of fibrous and serous layers. The fibrous layer is the outermost

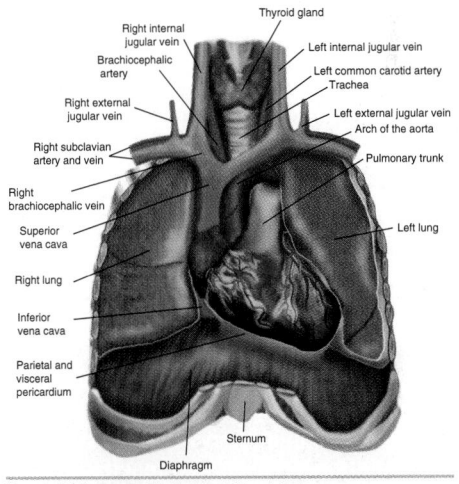

FIGURE 16-1 Position of the Heart in the Thoracic Cavity

ANATOMY AND PHYSIOLOGY: Understanding the functions of the body systems is an important component of completing an accurate assessment. The information necessary for a complete and accurate assessment is highlighted, and detailed illustrations help you visualize anatomy in the context of an actual patient.

NURSING CHECKLIST
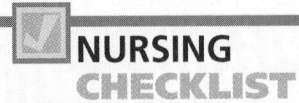

Assessment of Cognitive Function

You should have on hand:
- Preprinted lists of objects, phrases, and numbers for patient recall and explanation
- Answers to long-term memory questions to accurately assess recall
- Alternate tests prepared for patients with language barriers, aphasia, deafness, blindness, etc.
- Paper and pencils for patient to use to respond

NURSING TIPS: The wide variety of helpful hints, tips, and strategies presented here will help you as you work toward professional advancement. Study, share, and discuss them with your colleagues.

NURSING CHECKLISTS outline important points for you to consider for an assessment. Checklists also serve as a reference guide to reviewing procedural steps and summarizing the assessment process.

NURSING**TIP**

PMI versus Apical Impulse

The term *PMI* has fallen out of favor because it can be a misnomer if cardiac pathology causes a stronger impulse in a different region. Any movement other than the apical impulse is abnormal and should be described in terms of type, location, and timing in relation to the cardiac cycle.

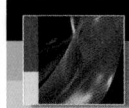

HEALTH HISTORY

The musculoskeletal health history provides insight into the link between a patient's life and lifestyle and musculoskeletal information and pathology.

PATIENT PROFILE

Diseases that are age-, gender-, and race-specific for the musculoskeletal system are listed.

Age

Osteosarcoma (10–20 and 50–60)
Ankylosing spondylitis (20–40)
Bursitis (20–40)
Rheumatoid arthritis (onset 20–40 unless juvenile form of the disease)
Systemic lupus erythematosus (SLE) (25–35)
Low back pain (30–50)
Gout (onset over 30, postmenopausal female)
Osteoporosis (menopausal female)
Carpal tunnel syndrome (pregnant or menopausal female)
Degenerative joint disease or osteoarthritis (onset after 55 in the female and before 45 in the male)
Multiple myeloma (50–70)
Paget's disease (50–70)
Fibromyalgia (40–75)

Gender

Female   Osteoporosis, rheumatoid arthritis, scoliosis, SLE, postmenopausal gout, polymyalgia r myasthenia gravis, multiple sclerosis (MS), sen

Male   Ankylosing spondylitis, gout, Paget's disease, Reite contracture, psoriatic arthritis, muscular dystro lateral sclerosis (ALS), low back pain

Race

Caucasian   Rheumatoid arthritis, primary osteoarthritis, osteoporosis, Paget's disease, Dupuytren's con spondylitis

African American   SLE, rheumatoid arthritis

CHIEF COMPLAINT   *Common chief complaints for the musculoskeletal syste on the characteristics of each sign or symptom is provide*

1. Pain   The subjective sense of discomfort in the axial or

Location   Muscle, bone, tendon, ligament, or joint

Quantity   Degree of interruption in the patient's usual activ (changes in ambulation, bathing, dressing, food p transfer to a sitting or standing position, climbing pulling)

Associated Manifestations   Inflammation, skin abrasion, laceration, bruis deformity, muscle spasm, paresthesia, decreased

---

HEALTH HISTORIES teach you an organized, thoughtful, and consistent approach to patient care, and guide your interview through each body system. This enables you to link health history clues to the patient's history and clinical status.

CASE STUDY

The Patient with Musculoskeletal Trauma

This case study illustrates the application and objective documentation of the musculoskeletal assessment. Milton was hit by a car while crossing the street and presents to the Emergency Department for evaluation and treatment.

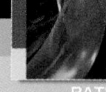

HEALTH HISTORY

PATIENT PROFILE   38 yo MBM

CHIEF COMPLAINT   "Everything hurts!"

HISTORY OF PRESENT ILLNESS   Patient transported to the ER 15 min ago following an MVA. While crossing a busy street against the cross signal, pt was hit by an SUV going approximately 35 mph. Upon impact, pt was thrown into the air, landing 20 ft away onto the street. Brief loss of consciousness at the scene as reported by EMS. EMS reports admission VS are HR 120 regular, BP 110/80 mm Hg from the Ⓛ thigh, RR 32 and labored, axillary temp 98.2 °F. 2+/3+ femoral pulses, EMS reports from transport: PERRLA, S1 and S2 present s̄ MGR; airway is patent s̄ tracheal deviation, breath sounds are ↓ over the Ⓛ lung fields. O2 saturation by pulse oximetry is 95% using a partial non-rebreather mask. No facial pallor or lip cyanosis. New ecchymosis is seen over most of the body, especially the Ⓛ side of the chest. Bleeding lacerations/abrasions are noted on the Ⓡ upper arm and over the Ⓡ thigh. 18-gauge IV in Ⓡ forearm and 18-gauge IV in Ⓡ dorsal foot vein, both inserted by EMS prior to ER transport. IV fluid of normal saline is infusing at wide-open rate via both IVs (total of 375 cc normal saline infused upon ER admission).

PAST HEALTH HISTORY

Medical History   Seasonal allergic rhinitis during the summer mos, as manifested by nasal congestion and sneezing
Nondisplaced complete fx of the Ⓡ humerus at age 14 due to a playground jungle gym fall. Treated by manual reduction under sedation/narcotic analgesia and casting. No complications or long-term adverse effects of injury

Surgical History   Dental removal of 4 impacted wisdom teeth under local anesthesia/conscious sedation at age 17. No complications or adverse effects of procedure
Appendectomy under general anesthesia at age 22. No complications or adverse effects of procedure

Allergies   SAR as above requiring OTC medication. No comprehensive allergy testing or desensitizing tx performed
Shellfish, had torso hives and facial angioedema following consumption of lobster at age 24; does not have Epi Pen

continues

CASE STUDIES in each body system chapter help you practice performing a complete health history and physical examination with an actual patient. Documentation-style entries teach you correct charting, and the variations in styles reflect real-life situations you will ultimately encounter in practice.

NURSING**ALERT**

Center of Balance during Pregnancy

Warn the pregnant woman that she is more vulnerable to falls and accidents because of the change in her center of balance. Pregnant women should exercise caution when changing position, moving over uneven surfaces, ascending and descending stairs, and participating in activities such as riding a bicycle.

NURSING ALERTS help you identify and respond efficiently and effectively to critical situations to ensure the health and safety of your patients.

ADVANCED TECHNIQUE

Forced Expiratory Time

Forced expiratory time is a gross measurement of the forced expiratory volume (FEV).

To perform this assessment:

E
1. Place your stethoscope over the patient's trachea.

2. Instruct the patient to inhale as deeply as possible and then exhale forcefully through the mouth (as if blowing out a candle).

3. Time the exhalation phase.

N Normal exhalation occurs in less than 4 seconds.

A The forced expiratory time is abnormal if it is greater than 4 seconds.

P Patients with COPD have a prolonged forced expiratory time and FEV because of the air trapping in the lungs. A complete exhalation is difficult to achieve.

ADVANCED TECHNIQUES help you identify examination sequences that are performed in selected clinical scenarios based on a patient's clinical presentation and history.

REVIEW QUESTIONS

1. Which of the following patients has the highest risk of contracting tuberculosis?
   a. A 19-year-old anorexic patient who spends a lot of time with her grandmother in a nursing home
   b. A 48-year-old patient who grows corn and milks cows who presents with a cough
   c. A 75-year-old patient with pneumonia and shingles
   d. A 33-year-old patient with a history of alcoholism who recently moved to the United States from Sicily
   The correct answer is (a).

2. Which of the following clinical assessment findings indicates that a patient may be experiencing immediate respiratory distress?
   a. A respiratory rate of 19
   b. Use of sternocleidomastoid muscles to breathe
   c. The presence of dilated superficial veins on the chest
   d. A costal angle of 110°
   The correct answer is (b).

3. A patient reports that he was climbing Mount Hood and noted an increase in the depth of his respirations. This physical assessment finding is called:
   a. Biot's respirations   c. Hyperpnea
   b. Apneustic respirations   d. Air trapping
   The correct answer is (c).

4. Kussmaul's respirations are respirations that:
   a. Have an increased depth and slow rate
   b. Are the body's attempt to raise its $PaCO_2$ level
   c. Are regularly irregular
   d. Are tachypneic and hyperpneic
   The correct answer is (d).

5. The nurse suctions the patient's endotracheal tube and notes that the secretions are rust colored. What is a possible etiology of this patient's pathology?
   a. Asthma
   b. Pulmonary edema
   c. Viral infection
   d. Pneumococcal pneumonia
   The correct answer is (d).

6. While performing diaphragmatic excursion, you measure a distance of 1.5 cm. This finding suggests:
   a. A normal distance   c. Hypoventilation
   b. Pneumonectomy   d. High diaphragm level
   The correct answer is (c).

7. A breath sound that is high in pitch, loud in intensity, has a blowing quality, and has a longer expiratory than inspiratory phase is called:
   a. Vesicular   c. Bronchovesicular
   b. Bronchial   d. Adventitious
   The correct answer is (b).

8. During inspection of a patient's thorax, you note that the patient's ribs attach to the sternum at a 45° angle. This patient has:
   a. A normal finding   c. Cystic fibrosis
   b. Pleural effusion   d. Chronic bronchitis
   The correct answer is (a).

9. You auscultate abnormal breath sounds on the patient's right chest at the fifth rib in the midclavicular line. In which lobe of the lung are you auscultating this sound?
   a. Right upper lobe   c. Right lower lobe
   b. Right middle lobe   d. Right oblique fissure
   The correct answer is (b).

10. In which condition might you expect to see a barrel chest, clubbing, a rib angle greater than 45°, tachypnea, decreased tactile fremitus, and decreased voice sounds?
    a. Pneumothorax   c. Pulmonary edema
    b. Emphysema   d. Atelectasis
    The correct answer is (b).

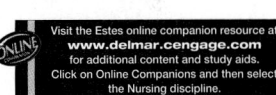
Visit the Estes online companion resource at **www.delmar.cengage.com** for additional content and study aids. Click on Online Companions and then select the Nursing discipline.

REVIEW QUESTIONS at the end of each chapter present questions to assist you with the learning process and help you assimilate the information presented in the text. Many chapters contain short case scenarios with related questions, which help you apply the information you have learned to actual clinical cases.

ASSESSMENT IN BRIEF

Thorax and Lung Assessment
Inspection
- Shape of thorax
- Symmetry of chest wall
- Presence of superficial veins
- Costal angle
- Angle of the ribs
- Intercostal spaces
- Muscles of respiration
- Respirations
  – Rate
  – Pattern
  – Depth
  – Symmetry
  – Audibility
  – Patient position
  – Mode of breathing
- Sputum

Palpation
- General palpation
  – Pulsations
  – Masses
  – Thoracic tenderness
  – Crepitus
- Thoracic expansion
- Tactile fremitus
- Tracheal position

Percussion
- General percussion
- Diaphragmatic excursion

Auscultation
- Breath sounds
- Adventitious sounds
- Voice sounds

Advanced Techniques
- Locating the site of a fractured rib
- Forced expiratory time

Assistive Devices
- Oxygen
- Incentive spirometer
- Endotracheal tube
- Tracheostomy tube
- Mechanical ventilation
- Pulse oximeter
- Peak flow meter

ASSESSMENT IN BRIEF cards show the steps for performing each type of assessment and physical examination. These are printed on perforated heavy paper stock so you can use them as a resource while studying or in clinical situations.

ACKNOWLEDGMENTS

For any text to survive to the fourth edition is a testament to its readability, accuracy, and timeliness. I am pleased to have the honor of updating this text, which boasts an art package that is second to none, with over 1,000 photos and illustrations. If a picture states a thousand words, then this is the most informational text of its kind on the market!

Many individuals have assisted in the process to see this fourth edition to market. I want to especially thank the following individuals:

- Contributors, old and new, who thoughtfully revised their chapters to ensure that current research and national guidelines are included. I appreciate their candid use of actual patients in their case studies, which provide a wealth of knowledge and diversity. Truth can be stranger than fiction!
- The reviewers who provided feedback on each chapter. The geographical distribution of the reviewers is always a plus as we learn that there is more than one way to accomplish the same goals.
- The many people who graciously agreed to assist with the pictures for this edition: Hytham Ahmed, Frances Alexander, Beverly Bayer, John Coffey, Kevin Coffey, Jennifer Dingus, Barbara Edwards, Andrew Estes, Katie Estes, Daphne Estill, Kely Green, Cheryl Healy, Nick Healy, Anna Hitcho, Mary Hitcho, Susan Hottman, Dolly Lakhie, Mary Beth Mabalot, Israa Mohamed, Morgan Radice, Katie Rubinger, Tracy Ryan, Cami Thompson, and Jay Tyroler.
- Dr. Robert A. Silverman and Dr. Daniel D. Rooney, who once again were able to provide photographs of pathological conditions. Also, thank you to Dr. Terrace Waggoner for permission to use the color vision charts.
- The various individuals and organizations who granted permission to use copyrighted material.
- The medical illustrators at Argosy Publishing, who produced top-notch re-creations of normal and pathological states.
- Debbie Meyer, Project Editor at Elm Street Publishing Services, who helped keep the production of the text on track.
- My family and friends, who are always there to encourage me. Most especially, my husband, Matt, who helped me through the ever changing world of technology.
- The Delmar Cengage Learning team, who once again proved their ability to produce fantastic, state-of-the-art textbooks to meet the challenges of the 21st century. My thanks go especially to Stacey Lamodi, Benjamin Knapp, and Steve Helba. And once again, thank you to Beth Williams, who was the rock around which this project revolved. After 15 years, it continues to be a pleasure to work with you.

Mary Ellen Zator Estes

ABOUT THE AUTHOR

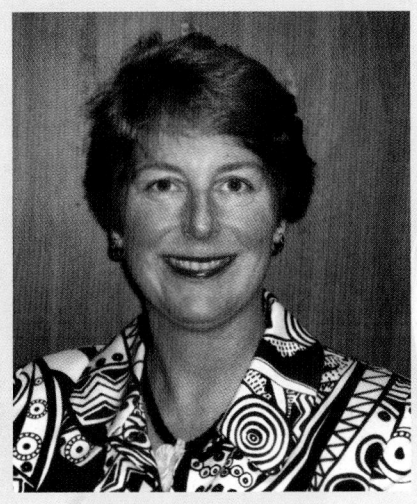

Mary Ellen Zator Estes obtained her baccalaureate and Master's degrees in nursing and her Family Nurse Practitioner certificate from the University of Virginia. She has taught at the University of Virginia, Marymount University, Northern Virginia Community College, and The George Washington University Medical Center. She has also served as Clinical Faculty for Ball State University.

With over 25 years' experience as a clinician and academician, Ms. Estes has taught health assessment and physical examination courses to nurses and nursing students from a variety of backgrounds. Her hands-on approach in the classroom, clinical laboratory, and health care setting has consistently led to positive learning experiences for her students.

Ms. Estes's professional development is well demonstrated at the local, regional, and national levels. She has delivered numerous presentations throughout the country. She has been an active member of the Virginia Council of Nurse Practitioners, the American Academy of Nurse Practitioners, Sigma Theta Tau, American Association of Critical Care Nurses, American Nurses Association, and Virginia Nurses Association.

Ms. Estes has been listed in *Who's Who in American Nursing* and *Who's Who in American Education.* She is currently a nurse practitioner at an internal medicine practice in Fairfax, Virginia, and a Nursing Consultant.

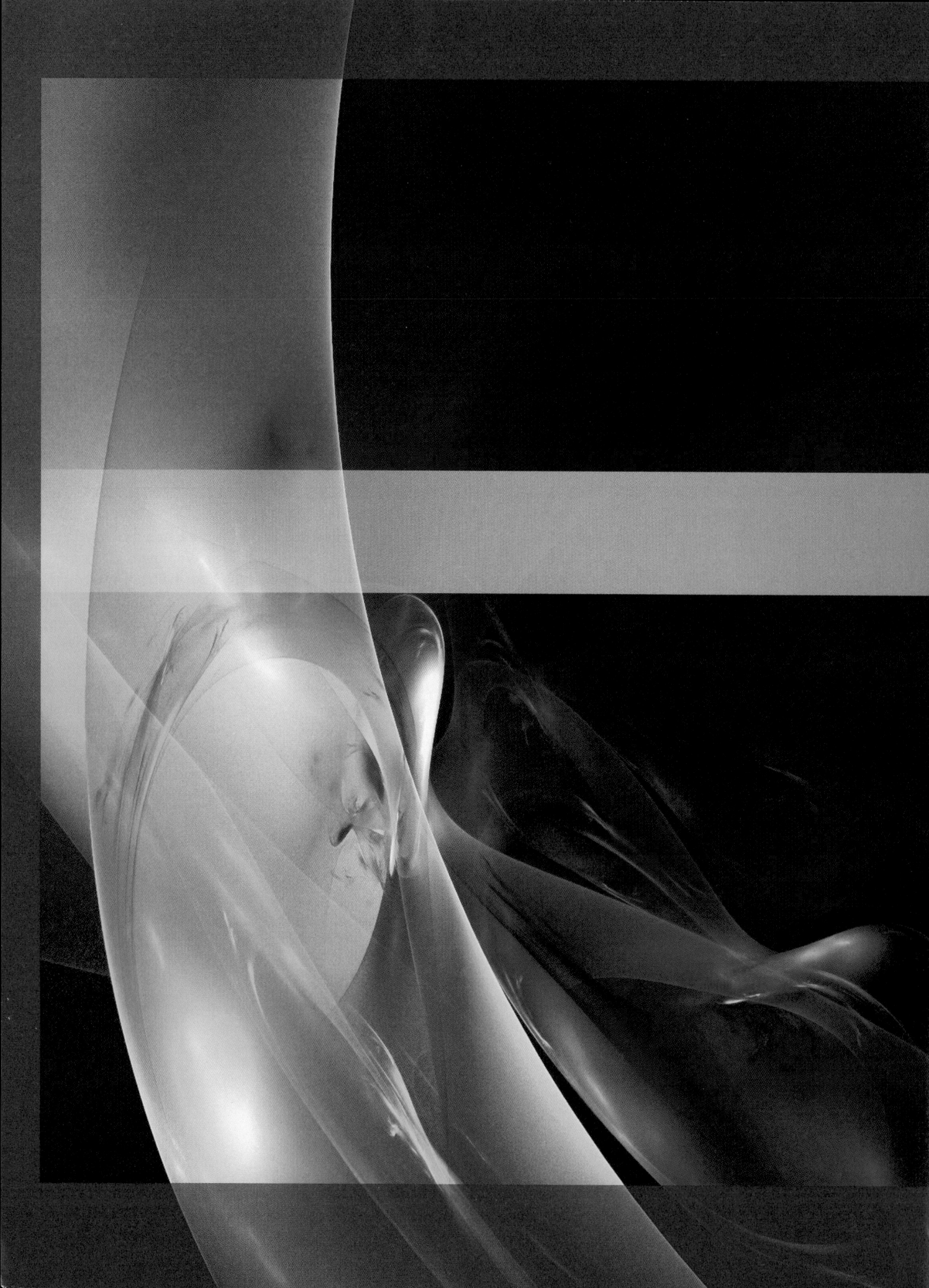

UNIT 1 Laying the Foundation

But I do say these [people] had the true nurse-calling—the good of their sick first.

—Florence Nightingale

CHAPTER 1

Critical Thinking and the Nursing Process

COMPETENCIES

1. Describe how nursing is both an art and a science.

2. Discuss the components of critical thinking.

3. Apply the Universal Intellectual Standards to the critical thinking process.

4. Define the nursing process.

5. Describe the six steps of the nursing process.

6. Explain the distinction among actual, risk, and wellness nursing diagnoses.

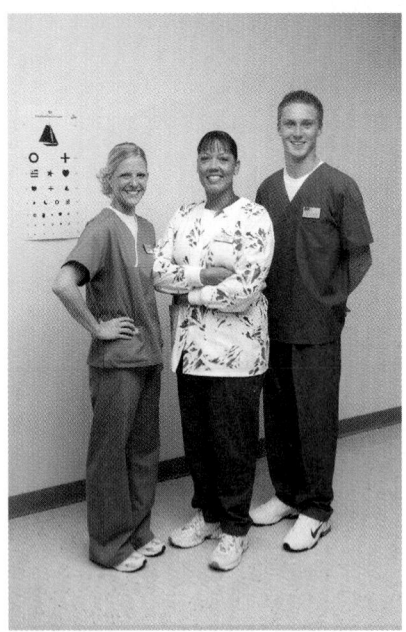

FIGURE 1-1 **Nurses possess a wide variety of experiences that they take into each patient encounter.**

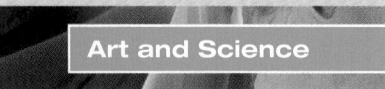

REFLECTIVE THINKING

Art and Science

It is often said, "Medicine is curing, but nursing is caring." Do you agree? Support your response.

Nursing is a blend of art and science. The art of nursing allows nurses to incorporate aspects of caring and sharing into their practice. Over time nurses build repertoires of professional experiences that serve as a clinical portfolio of responses to various patient situations (Figure 1-1). Experienced nurses make intuitive links that are not made by novice nurses because experienced nurses can delve into their professional portfolio of experiences and select strategies that have been successful in the past. Professional intuition develops over time as nurses begin to link certain patterns or events to specific outcomes. Experienced nurses seem to do this with little conscious effort. The novice, on the other hand, may need guidance to perceive links intuitively recognized by the experienced nurse.

For example, a critical care nurse may feel that his or her patient is "going down the tubes" despite the fact that the patient's vital signs are stable. The experienced nurse has a "feel" for the patient and the situation. A few hours later the patient goes into cardiopulmonary arrest. How did the experienced nurse know this? That is part of the art of nursing.

The science of nursing involves the use of analytical thinking. In analytical thinking, the nature of information is studied, the information is broken into its constituent parts, and relationships and patterns are identified. Causation, key factors, and possible outcomes to a situation may all be identified. The science of nursing is based on scientific principles and research data. For example, with knowledge of lung physiology, pathophysiology of asthma, and environmental triggers, the nurse can analyze why the asthmatic patient is having an acute attack in a room filled with cigarette smokers and a wood burning fire. Analytical thinking skills can be learned and are developed as clinical experience is gained.

Both the art and science of nursing are used when conducting health assessments and physical examinations. Critical thinking and clinical reasoning are essential elements of this process.

CRITICAL THINKING AND CLINICAL REASONING

Critical thinking is a purposeful, goal-directed thinking process that strives to problem solve patient care issues through the use of clinical reasoning. It combines logic, intuition, and creativity. **Clinical reasoning** is a disciplined, creative, and reflective approach used together with critical thinking; its purpose is to establish potential strategies to assist patients in reaching their desired health goals. Critical thinking and clinical reasoning skills are essential to every nurse's clinical practice. For example, a patient in the cardiac care unit complains of chest pain after eating dinner and immediately lies down for a nap. Your critical thinking skills lead you to assess all aspects of the patient's condition in an effort to determine the etiology of the pain and treat it accordingly. You recognize that, in addition to the patient's diagnosis of angina, the patient also has a history of gastroesophageal reflux disease (GERD) and a hiatal hernia. The patient takes omeprazole 40 mg every morning. You pursue a line of questioning that teases out more information about the patient's pain. You use clinical reasoning skills to determine that the patient's pain is most likely gastrointestinal in nature because the pain is located in the epigastric area, whereas recent chest pain was located in the substernal region. In addition, the patient had no EKG changes with the pain, and the pain was relieved when the patient sat up.

There are eight guidelines outlined by the Foundation for Critical Thinking that address some of the key elements of reasoning (Table 1-1). Knowing and understanding these guidelines help both the novice and the experienced nurse master the reasoning process. The time frame in which this mastery occurs differs for every person. Like many skills, the more clinical reasoning is practiced, the more natural it becomes.

TABLE 1-1 Key Elements of Clinical Reasoning

- All reasoning has a purpose.
- All reasoning is an attempt to figure something out, to settle some question, or to solve some problem.
- All reasoning is based on assumptions.
- All reasoning is done from some point of view.
- All reasoning is based on data, information, and evidence.
- All reasoning is expressed through, and shaped by, concepts and ideas.
- All reasoning contains inferences by which we draw conclusions and give meaning to data.
- All reasoning leads somewhere, and has implications and consequences.

From *Helping Students Assess Their Thinking,* by R. Paul and L. Elder, 1997. Retrieved January 17, 2008, from http://www.criticalthinking.org.

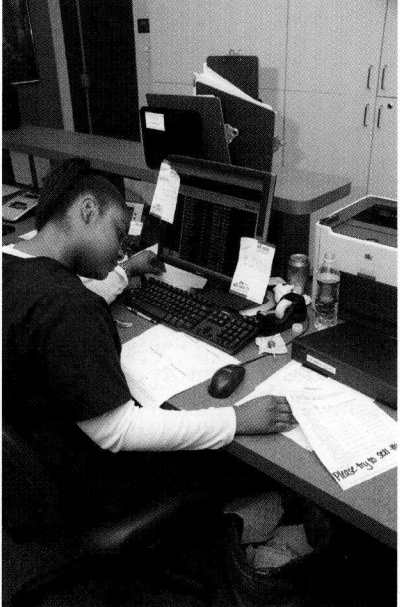

FIGURE 1-2 Critical thinking involves analysis in which the nurse examines patient data available from a variety of sources.

COMPONENTS OF CRITICAL THINKING

According to Pesut and Herman (1999), critical thinking encompasses many skills, including interpretation, analysis, inference, explanation, evaluation, and self-regulation. These skills will be discussed to show their relationship with health assessment and physical examination.

Interpretation of situations requires the nurse to decode hidden messages, clarify the meaning of the information, and categorize the information. For example, a patient may claim to be seeking health care for a bad cough and cold, but actually may be concerned about whether the cough is a sign of lung cancer. Accurate interpretation implies that the nurse is clinically competent and professionally capable of obtaining the information.

During analysis, the nurse examines the ideas and data that were presented, identifies any discrepancies, and reflects on the reason for the discrepancies. The nurse can then begin to frame the main points of the patient's story (Figure 1-2). For instance, a patient may complain of insomnia but upon questioning reveals that he or she sleeps 6 hours at night and takes a 2-hour nap each afternoon. Often discrepancies lead to a clearer picture of the patient's overall situation.

Inference speculates, derives, or reasons a specific premise based on information and assumptions obtained from the patient. Inference can be a challenging skill for the novice nurse because a certain level of knowledge and experience must be possessed in order to draw conclusions and provide alternatives in any given scenario. If a patient complains of an exacerbation of asthma every morning, the nurse can inquire about a history of heartburn or GERD. An experienced nurse would make the association between these causative factors.

Explanation requires that the conclusions drawn from the inferences are correct and can be justified. The use of scientific and nursing literature constitutes the basis for clinical justification. To continue with the example in the preceding paragraph, GERD as a contributing factor of asthma is well documented in the literature; there is a documented scientific link between GERD and asthma.

The evaluation process examines the validity of the information and hypothesis. This leads to a final conclusion that can be implemented. For example, the nurse assesses a 5-year-old child with cystic fibrosis who is experiencing labored breathing and wheezing. Based on the findings, the nurse implements a nebulizer treatment, postural drainage, and chest physiotherapy. The nurse reassesses the patient after treatment and finds that there is no wheezing and the respiratory rate is within normal limits.

Self-regulation is a key component to the critical thinking process. During this process, the nurse reflects on the critical thinking skills that were employed and then determines which techniques were effective and which were problematic. After interviewing a patient, the nurse reflects on whether leading, biased, or judgmental questions were posed to the patient. The nurse might also reflect on the use of open-ended questions and effectiveness of an interpreter. The recognition of both positive and negative outcomes is crucial to developing higher-level thinking skills and professional expertise.

UNIVERSAL INTELLECTUAL STANDARDS FOR CRITICAL THINKING

The quality of critical thinking can be evaluated by applying the seven Universal Intellectual Standards (UIS) proposed by Elder and Paul (1996). These standards are clarity, accuracy, precision, relevance, depth, breadth, and logic.

Clarity, simply stated, asks whether the message or information is clear. For example, an alcoholic patient may report a substance abuse problem. The nurse, using critical thinking skills, would need to clarify the substance abuse specifically as an alcohol problem versus a problem with other substances.

The second key element of the UIS is accuracy. Have the thinking process and information been accurate? For example, thinking that an alcoholic patient drinks to excess every day may be an inaccurate fact. The patient may be more of a binge alcoholic, drinking heavily only on certain occasions. The nurse would need to ask questions to ensure accurate understanding of information.

Precision is the third UIS. To state that a patient "drinks excessively" is judgmental and not precise. How much is excessive? Precision in thinking and data collection is essential. The statement, "The patient reports drinking a fifth of whiskey every day" is precise.

Has the thinking been relevant? If the alcoholic patient presents with the need for rehabilitation secondary to alcohol withdrawal and delirium tremens, then the information that the patient's grandfather died at age 82 of renal failure is not relevant at this time. This latter statement may be a true statement, but it does not connect to the central issue of alcoholic rehabilitation.

The UIS of depth can be a challenging standard for novice nurses to achieve because they may not possess the appropriate knowledge base to know when to delve deeper into a given problem for related data. For instance, perhaps the nurse did not ascertain that the patient has four relatives who are also alcoholics, or that the patient recently had a child die and was fired from a job, which led to an exacerbation of the drinking.

The sixth UIS is breadth. Does the alcoholic patient's story have more to it than was relayed to the nurse? Is there a need to consider the views of another person such as a spouse, relative, friend, or significant other? Are there additional data that need to be obtained in order to gain an accurate impression of the patient's situation?

Finally, the UIS of logic needs to be applied to clinical reasoning. Does the patient's or significant other's story seem logical? If the patient stated that her only child recently died and that caused her to drink heavily, and then later this child comes to visit her mother, what does this imply? Another way to think logically is attributing signs and symptoms to disease entities. The patient experiences tremors—is this due to alcohol withdrawal or Parkinson's disease? Logical thinking would seem to point to the former etiology.

Consistent application of these standards to critical thinking leads to sophistication of clinically useful skills.

CRITICAL THINKING AND THE NURSING PROCESS

There are many frameworks for critical thinking in the health care professions. Medicine frequently uses the scientific method of recognizing cues, formulating hypotheses, gathering data, and evaluating hypotheses to frame its critical thinking. The nursing profession has developed its own unique tool to frame critical thinking, the nursing process.

The nursing process is the framework on which the American Nurses Association developed the Nursing Scope and Standards of Practice (ANA, 2004). These standards give the profession broad guidelines to which nurses can be held accountable in their practice. These nursing standards are the tenets on which the entire health assessments and physical examinations of the patient are conducted. Table 1-2 contains the ANA Nursing Scope and Standards of Practice.

The **nursing process** includes six phases: assessment, nursing diagnosis, outcomes identification, planning, implementation, and evaluation. It is a dynamic

TABLE 1-2 ANA Nursing Scope and Standards of Practice

Standard 1. Assessment
The registered nurse collects comprehensive data pertinent to the patient's health or the situation.

Standard 2. Diagnosis
The registered nurse analyzes the assessment data to determine the diagnoses or issues.

Standard 3. Outcomes Identification
The registered nurse identifies expected outcomes for a plan individualized to the patient or the situation.

Standard 4. Planning
The registered nurse develops a plan that prescribes strategies and alternatives to attain expected outcomes.

Standard 5. Implementation
The registered nurse implements the identified plan.

Standard 5A: Coordination of Care
The registered nurse coordinates care delivery.

Standard 5B: Health Teaching and Health Promotion
The registered nurse employs strategies to promote health and a safe environment.

Standard 5C: Consultation
The advanced practice registered nurse and the nursing role specialist provide consultation to influence the identified plan, enhance the abilities of others, and effect change.

Standard 5D: Prescriptive Authority and Treatment
The advanced practice registered nurse uses prescriptive authority, procedures, referrals, treatments, and therapies in accordance with state and federal laws and regulations.

Standard 6. Evaluation
The registered nurse evaluates progress toward attainment of outcomes.

Reprinted with permission from American Nurses Association, *Nursing Scope and Standards of Practice,* © 2004, nursesbooks.org, Silver Spring, MD.

process that uses information in a meaningful way through problem-solving strategies to place the patient, family, or community in an optimal health state. The primary focus of this text is assessment. The physical, emotional, mental, developmental, spiritual, and cultural assessments provide the foundation for the other steps of the nursing process.

ASSESSMENT

Assessment is the first step of the nursing process. It is the orderly collection of information concerning the patient's health status. The assessment process aims to identify the patient's current health status, actual and potential health problems, and areas for health promotion. The sources of information for the assessment include the health history, the physical assessment, and diagnostic and laboratory data. Collectively, these data constitute the nursing database from which the nurse will develop a plan of care for the patient, and they serve as a baseline against which future comparisons can be made (Figure 1-3).

Health History

The health history interview is a means of gathering **subjective data**, usually from the patient. These data are subjective in that they cannot always be verified by an independent observer. Subjective data include what the patient says and what the patient thinks. It includes attitudes and beliefs of the patient. In some instances,

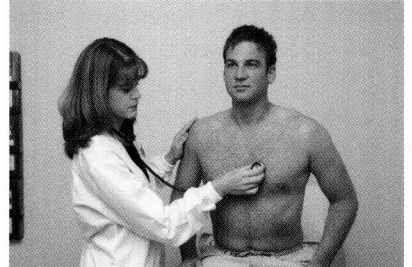

FIGURE 1-3 Physical assessment is one component of the nursing database.

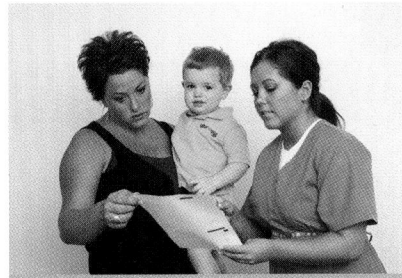

FIGURE 1-4 The health history can be gathered from many sources. In the case of a child, the health history is usually provided by a parent or caregiver.

however, this information can be validated during the physical assessment; for instance, the existence of a patient-reported breast lump can be confirmed through palpation.

The health history can also be obtained from sources other than the patient. Relatives, neighbors, and friends of the patient can provide insightful data for the health history (Figure 1-4). In some instances, total strangers may be the only source of information, as in the case of a severe accident in which the patient is rendered unconscious. The patient's old charts or medical records are additional sources of information, as are health care colleagues. The nurse can and should use every available medium to gather as much information about the patient as possible. The health history is further discussed in Chapter 3.

Physical Assessment Findings

Physical assessment findings constitute a second source of information that is used in the assessment phase of the nursing process. Physical assessment findings constitute **objective data**, or information that is observable and measurable, and can be verified by more than one person. These data are obtained using the senses of smell, touch, vision, and hearing. This text describes the systematic and comprehensive physical examination techniques that will elicit these data (see Chapters 8–25).

The physical assessment data can be obtained in a body system or head-to-toe approach. Table 1-3 lists the body systems that are assessed. Another approach to physical assessment is the use of Gordon's Functional Health Patterns, which group human behaviors into 11 patterns that facilitate nursing care (Gordon, 2006). Table 1-4 lists the **Functional Health Patterns**. This text uses the head-to-toe approach for physical assessment.

Diagnostic and Laboratory Data

The final element that contributes to the gathering of information in the assessment phase of the nursing process is diagnostic and laboratory data. Results of blood and urine studies, cultures, X-rays, and diagnostic procedures constitute objective data about the patient's status.

It is imperative that the nurse documents all assessment findings. The written record is a legal tool used to chart the patient's current health status. Chapter 26 discusses documentation and covers the legal issues of the written patient record. The documented patient assessment also serves as a means of communicating information to other health care colleagues.

Remember that the assessment phase of the nursing process is dynamic. The nurse is continuously adding information to the database, validating the data, and interpreting the data. With these data the nurse is ready to progress to the second phase of the nursing process, the nursing diagnosis.

NURSING DIAGNOSIS

The National Conference Group for Classification of Nursing Diagnoses convened in 1973 to establish a nomenclature to describe conditions treated by nurses. Since that time this group has met biannually. In 1982 the organization changed its name to the North American Nursing Diagnosis Association (**NANDA**). Later, in 2002, NANDA expanded globally and was renamed NANDA-I, or NANDA International. NANDA-I is the recognized leader in the formulation, classification, and testing of nursing diagnoses. NANDA-I (2009, p. 419) defines a **nursing diagnosis** as "a clinical judgment about individual, family, or community responses to actual or potential health problems/life processes. A nursing diagnosis provides the basis for selection of nursing interventions to achieve outcomes for which the nurse is accountable."

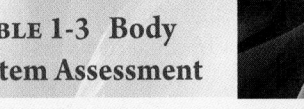

TABLE 1-3 Body System Assessment

1. General survey, vital signs, and pain
2. Skin, hair, and nails
3. Head, neck, and regional lymphatics
4. Eyes
5. Ears, nose, mouth, and throat
6. Breasts and regional nodes
7. Thorax and lungs
8. Heart and peripheral vasculature
9. Abdomen
10. Musculoskeletal system
11. Mental status and neurological techniques
12. Female or male genitalia
13. Anus, rectum, and prostate

REFLECTIVE THINKING

Are Nursing and Medicine Distinct?

Florence Nightingale stated over 100 years ago: "Nursing and medicine must never be mixed . . . it spoils both." Do you think this statement reflects your philosophy on the use of nursing diagnoses?

Nursing diagnoses are holistic in nature. Nurses diagnose and treat "human responses to actual or potential health problems" (ANA, 1995, p. 9). Nurses are licensed to treat patients based on nursing diagnoses and by virtue of their educational and clinical preparation. Nursing diagnoses increase nurses' accountability for the services they render.

Nursing Diagnosis Formulation

The nursing diagnosis is formulated after the assessment data are analyzed. The process involves four steps as identified by Gordon (2006): collecting information, interpreting information, clustering information, and naming a cluster or problem formulation. Collecting information refers to the data collected in the assessment phase of the nursing process. This process is a continuous means to gain as much information about the patient as possible.

In step 2, the data are interpreted. The nurse collects data for the purpose of positively impacting the patient's health status. The information is not collected to just fill a chart. The diagnostic importance of the information becomes relevant in the interpretation of it. The data, or cues, are evaluated against the standards for a patient population. Using inferential reasoning, the nurse begins to see patterns or clusters of data.

Clustering of the information is performed in the third step of nursing diagnosis development. The data are sorted into meaningful groups, usually according to Gordon's Functional Health Patterns or NANDA-I's **Human Response Patterns.** All of the accepted NANDA-I nursing diagnoses can be organized under either of these two patterns to create nursing diagnosis **taxonomies,** or classification systems. User preference usually dictates the choice of clustering information pattern and taxonomy.

Naming the cluster is the final step in the formulation of the nursing diagnosis. This is the phase when the actual NANDA-I diagnostic label (NANDA-I approved nursing diagnosis) is used. Patterns can surface that lead to the development of more than one nursing diagnosis. Conversely, the cues may seem unrelated and no nursing diagnosis is derived from the data. In this case, the nurse needs to review the accuracy of the data. Refer to Appendix A for a listing of NANDA-I nursing diagnoses.

Types of Nursing Diagnoses

There are three types of nursing diagnoses: actual, risk, and wellness. **Actual nursing diagnoses** are typically problem oriented and describe human responses that have been validated by the nurse, such as *Disturbed sleep pattern* and *Impaired memory.* The second type of diagnosis is the **risk nursing diagnosis.** NANDA-I (2009, p. 419) defines the risk nursing diagnosis as "human responses to health conditions/life processes that may develop in a vulnerable individual, family, or community. It is supported by risk factors that contribute to increased vulnerability." Examples of risk nursing diagnoses include *Risk for suicide* and *Risk for falls.* The **wellness nursing diagnosis** represents the patient's striving for a higher level of health and wellness. It focuses on the strengths of a patient. *Readiness for enhanced spiritual well-being* and *Readiness for enhanced family processes* are two examples of wellness nursing diagnoses.

Some patient problems are not completely within the domain of the nurse's scope of practice and require the nurse to look beyond the nursing diagnosis. For instance, the patient experiencing cardiac tamponade (medical diagnosis) with decreased cardiac output and anxiety (nursing diagnoses) needs immediate nursing and medical attention. The nurse is not ethically or legally permitted to do all that the situation requires to alleviate the tamponade; the nurse, physician, and

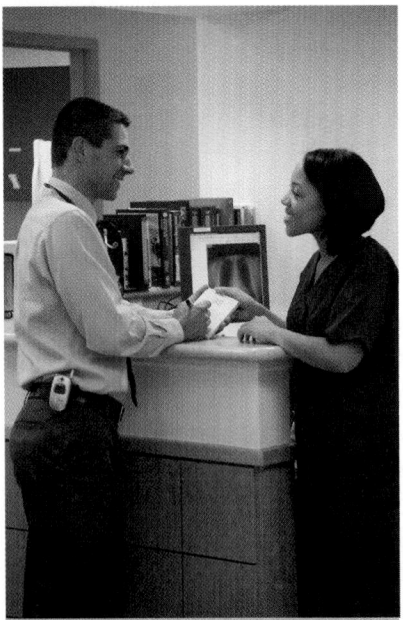

FIGURE 1-5 Nurses may collaborate with social workers, physicians, and other members of the health care team to maximize patient care.

health care team will work collaboratively to relieve the problem. Thus, a **collaborative problem** is a patient problem that requires the nurse to work jointly with the physician and other health care workers in monitoring, planning, and implementing the patient care (Figure 1-5).

Writing the Nursing Diagnosis

A nursing diagnosis can have up to four components: the descriptor, the label or human response, the related factors, and the defining characteristics, or risk factors. The **descriptor** or **qualifier** is an adjective that describes or qualifies the human response. Examples of NANDA-I approved descriptors are *impaired, ineffective,* and *readiness for enhanced.*

The label or human response is the actual or potential health problem or wellness factors that the nurse has synthesized from the clustered data. The NANDA-I approved nursing diagnostic labels are the human responses that form the basis for the complete nursing diagnosis. Examples of human responses are hypothermia, acute pain, and social isolation. The human responses are amenable to nursing interventions.

Related factors are the third component of the nursing diagnosis. They are the "factors that appear to show some type of patterned relationship with the nursing diagnosis" (NANDA-I, 2009, p. 420). They are the origin of the patient's health problem and can be changed with nursing interventions. In the nursing diagnosis, the human response and related factors are joined by the phrase "related to." Examples include *Ineffective breathing pattern related to pain* and *Impaired oral mucous membrane related to ineffective oral hygiene.* Frequently, the related factors are secondary to another condition, and this is noted in the nursing diagnosis; for example, *Fatigue related to anemia secondary to pregnancy.*

Defining characteristics and *risk factors* are the final components of a nursing diagnosis. Defining characteristics are signs, symptoms, and statements made by the patient that validate the existence of the actual or wellness nursing diagnosis. In the nursing diagnosis, the related factors and defining characteristics are joined by the phrase "as evidenced by." Examples are *Social isolation related to perception of inability to engage in satisfying personal relationships as evidenced by sad dull affect, no eye contact, and expresses feelings of aloneness imposed by others;* and *Anxiety related to threat of death as evidenced by expressed concerns due to change in life events, shakiness, and voice quivering.* Risk factors are "environmental factors and physiological, psychological, genetic, or chemical elements that increase the vulnerability of an individual, family, or community to an unhealthful event" (NANDA-I, 2007, p. 333). In the nursing diagnosis *Risk for powerlessness,* some risk factors might be chronic illness, aging, dying, and poor body image.

Another approach to writing a nursing diagnosis is the **PES method.** In this practical approach, *P* is the problem, *E* is the etiology, and *S* is the signs and symptoms. The PES method of writing nursing diagnoses arrives at the same nursing diagnosis as in the above theoretical approach.

Writing a correct nursing diagnosis is a skill that requires knowledge and practice. Even experienced nurses need to refer to expert sources to validate information. The Nursing Tip on the next page describes common errors made when writing nursing diagnoses.

OUTCOMES IDENTIFICATION

Outcomes identification represents the third step in the nursing process. After the nursing diagnoses have been formulated, patient goals are established. The **patient goal** is directed toward the removal of related factors or patient response

NURSING**TIP**

Common Errors in Writing Nursing Diagnoses

1. Writing in legally inadvisable terms.
   Incorrect: *Impaired skin integrity related to decreased turning*
   Correct: *Impaired skin integrity related to shearing forces*
2. Using value judgments.
   Incorrect: *Caregiver role strain related to laziness*
   Correct: *Caregiver role strain related to complexity of activities*
3. Using medical diagnoses.
   Incorrect: *Guillain-Barré syndrome*
   Correct: *Dressing/grooming self-care deficit related to neuromuscular impairment*
4. Formulating a nursing diagnosis based on insufficient data.
   A 2-year-old presents to the ER for the first time with a broken tibia.
   Incorrect: *Risk for other-directed violence related to child abuse*
   Discussion: The nurse may suspect child abuse but further assessment is warranted. One admission for a traumatic injury does not necessarily constitute child abuse. If the child had presented frequently to the ER with accidental injuries, the nursing diagnosis may be accurate, but the nurse would need to gather additional data to validate the diagnosis.
5. Formulating a nursing diagnosis based on incorrect data.
   The nurse walks into a patient's room and observes that the breastfeeding mother is unable to latch-on her newborn.
   Incorrect: *Ineffective breastfeeding related to maternal anxiety as evidenced by unsatisfactory breastfeeding process*
   Discussion: If the nurse formulates this nursing diagnosis after this brief patient encounter, it would be erroneous. The baby had difficulty with latch-on because it was just fed a bottle in the nursery. The nurse needs to assess all data prior to formulating nursing diagnoses.

to an adverse condition. Goals are broad statements that are not measurable. For example, if a nursing diagnosis is *Anxiety related to change in health status,* the patient goal might be the following: The patient will experience a reduction in anxiety.

A **patient outcome** is a statement of the expected change in patient behavior denoting progress toward resolution of the altered human response over a specific period of time. These are written after the patient goals. Patient outcomes indicate the progression toward goal achievement. Realistic and measurable patient outcomes are written by the nurse to ensure continuity in the patient's care. Adjectives such as *more, less, increased,* and *decreased,* and verbs such as *know* and *understand* are avoided because they are subjective and not measurable. Quantitative phrases such as "walk 15 feet" and "lose 8 pounds" are used as appropriate objective outcomes. Measurable verbs such as *state, identify,* and *list* are used.

Every patient outcome must include a time frame that designates the time by which the patient outcome should be met. The time frame can be short or long term. **Short-term outcomes** denote a time frame over a relatively short period of time, such as 1 hour, 1 day, or 1 week. **Long-term outcomes** usually extend over weeks or months. Each nursing diagnosis can have more than one patient outcome. The complexity of the patient's problem and the type of problem dictate the number of patient outcomes required to develop a comprehensive plan of care.

Patient outcomes need to be evaluated consistently to determine the effect of the nursing care. The Nursing Outcomes Classification (NOC) taxonomy has developed 385 patient outcomes (Moorhead, Johnson, Maas, & Swanson, 2008). The nurse can now define patient outcomes using standardized language and refer to a set of indicators with a measurement scale to evaluate these outcomes. The NOC outcomes were developed to complement NANDA-I nursing diagnoses and can be used in nursing practice, nursing education, and nursing research.

PLANNING

Planning is the fourth step in the nursing process. It involves the prioritization of nursing diagnoses and care and the selection of nursing interventions.

Prioritization

The nurse formulates all of the nursing diagnoses that are derived from the clustering of data. When there is more than one nursing diagnosis, the nurse must determine which problem(s) are the most vital to the patient's well-being at that particular time. It is necessary to **prioritize,** or rank, the importance of each nursing diagnosis. When possible, the patient should assist the nurse with the prioritization of needs. Patients who are actively involved with the decision-making process are more likely to be amenable to nursing care, to assist with their care, and to be agreeable to the plan of care.

A theoretical framework that can be used to prioritize nursing diagnoses is Maslow's Hierarchy of Needs (Figure 1-6). According to Maslow, basic needs such as food and oxygen take priority over all other issues. For example, the patient experiencing a myocardial infarction must have her physiological needs met before safety needs are attended to. In some instances, though, patients' needs may not follow Maslow's hierarchy, or they may change over time, requiring reprioritization of nursing diagnoses. The terminal breast cancer patient may be more concerned with playing with her children than staying well hydrated. Some nursing diagnoses are equally important and can be prioritized together at the same level. The nurse, in conjunction with the patient and family, is continually reevaluating and revising the priority of the nursing diagnoses.

LIFE 360°

Prioritizing Care

The home health nurse is meeting with Mr. S. for the first time. Mr. S. is a 44-year-old male with acute cardiomyopathy waiting for a heart transplantation. The nurse performs a health and physical assessment on Mr. S., then discusses the plan of care with him. Mr. S. and the nurse disagree on the current priorities of care.

- What nursing interventions would you implement in this situation?
- Is there additional information that you would attempt to elicit from the patient?
- How can you align nursing priorities with patient priorities to deliver efficient and necessary care?

Intervention Selection

Interventions are planned strategies, based on scientific rationale, devised by the nurse to assist the patient in meeting the patient outcomes. When appropriate, the patient, family, and significant others can assist in planning the interventions. As with nursing diagnosis prioritization, patients are more likely to be motivated and follow the interventions if they have been involved in the decision-making process.

Every patient outcome has its own nursing interventions. When appropriate, a frequency is included in each intervention, such as "turn every 2 hours." The number of interventions per patient outcome varies. What is essential is that the plan of care is comprehensive to ensure that the patient can meet the outcome. The interventions can be independent and collaborative nursing actions. **Independent nursing interventions** are those that the nurse is legally capable of implementing on the basis of education and experience. **Collaborative interventions** are physician prescribed and nurse implemented. With all interventions, sound nursing judgment is required. The critically ill hypertensive patient in an intensive care unit on a sodium nitroprusside infusion, with a blood pressure of 74/49, needs immediate nursing action. The nurse, using sound judgment, turns the infusion off and consults with the physician about a new plan of care. The nurse may also have standing orders indicating the parameters of treatment that lead to the discontinuing of the infusion.

The Nursing Interventions Classification (NIC) complements the taxonomies of NANDA-I and NOC by devising research-based nursing interventions (Bulechek, Butcher, & Dochterman, 2008). More than 542 independent and collaborative interventions for nursing care delivered to individual patients, families, and communities have evolved. These interventions encompass both physiological and psychological realms.

Evidence-Based Practice

There is a growing trend in health care toward **evidence-based practice.** No longer are health care practices being done "because they have always been done that way," nor are they being done intuitively. Rather, evidence-based practice uses the outcomes of well-designed and executed scientific studies to guide clinical decision making and clinical care. For example, the use of hormone replacement therapy (HRT) for postmenopausal women has changed dramatically as a result of the Heart and Estrogen/Progestin Replacement Study (HERS) and the HRT arm of the Women's Health Initiative (WHI). The ultimate goal of evidence-based practice is to assist the patient's quality of life by improving outcomes. Through the use of computer research, clinical conferences, and expert testimony, nurses are able to incorporate evidence-based practice into their professional lives.

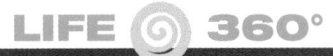

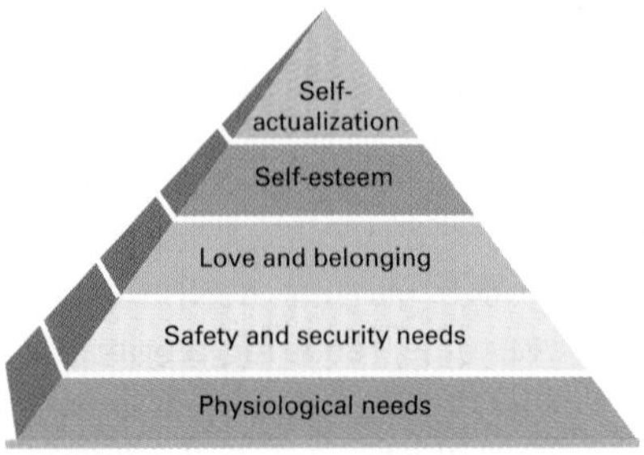

FIGURE 1-6 Maslow's Hierarchy of Needs. *Adaptation based on Maslow's Hierarchy of Needs.*

IMPLEMENTATION

The fifth step in the nursing process is **implementation.** In this phase, the nurse executes the interventions that were devised during the planning stage to help the patient meet predetermined outcomes. The time frame of the implementation phase varies from patient to patient and from nursing diagnosis to nursing diagnosis. Remember that the nurse usually simultaneously implements the interventions from multiple nursing diagnoses for a patient at any given time. The patient may achieve the outcome for one nursing diagnosis while progressing toward the outcome for another.

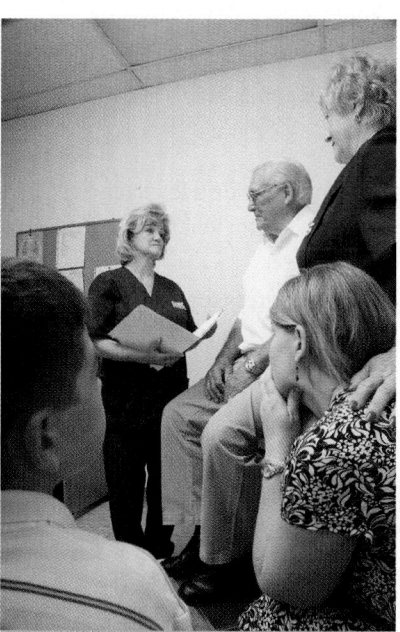

FIGURE 1-7 The patient and his family meet with the nurse to discuss progress on the patient care plan.

Implementation is a dynamic process. The nurse is continually interacting with the patient, the family, and other health care colleagues, obtaining new data and making new judgments (Figure 1-7). Plans of care can be changed or eliminated altogether based on the continuous flow of information.

EVALUATION

Evaluation is the final phase of the nursing process. During evaluation, the patient's progress in achieving the outcomes is determined. Even before the time frame for assessing outcomes is reached, the nurse is continually assessing the patient's progress toward the outcomes, making evaluation a continual and dynamic process.

The nurse, in conjunction with the patient and the family, evaluates the status of the plan of care. One of two of the following conclusions can be made about the patient outcome: It was met, or it was not met. When the patient outcome has been met, the nurse documents this information and then periodically reevaluates the patient's need for knowledge on the health matter.

If the outcome was not met, this should be documented. Some factors to consider are as follows: Was the diagnosis appropriate? Was the time frame adequate? Were the interventions accurate and comprehensive? Was the patient outcome accurate? Had the patient's condition changed sufficiently that the outcome was no longer appropriate? Did the patient understand his or her role in the process? After considering these factors, the nurse and the patient can decide to revise the patient outcome and nursing interventions or to eliminate them. Based on the ongoing assessment and evaluation, new nursing diagnoses may be formulated that warrant nursing intervention. These will be added to the patient's plan of care.

Each outcome is evaluated separately. A frequent mistake is the practice of evaluating the interventions rather than the outcomes; the outcome should be evaluated, not the mechanics of achieving it.

CRITICAL PATHWAYS

In the United States, managed care via case management is being introduced and used as a cost-effective, high-quality patient care delivery system in many institutions across the country. Critical pathways are at the core of the case management approach. **Critical pathways** or maps show the outcome of predetermined patient goals over a period of time; that is, they state what activity the patient should be capable of performing daily, on the basis of the patient's Diagnostic-Related Grouping (DRG). The critical incidents, or most crucial nursing interventions for each step of the pathway, are delineated.

One of the advantages of critical pathways is the early recognition of variances from the path. Once the variance is identified, the nurse, in collaboration with other members of the health care team, plans and implements specific interventions to deal with the variance. Evaluation is performed on a daily basis by the case manager, the primary nurse, or other designee.

Although the terminology is different, critical pathways incorporate the assessment, planning, implementation, and evaluation phases of the nursing process. Nursing diagnoses are not usually incorporated into critical pathways. Mention is made of this managed care delivery system due to its increasing popularity in inpatient, outpatient, and community settings, where critical pathways are replacing the nursing care plan as a documentation tool.

DOCUMENTING THE NURSING PROCESS

There are many methods that nurses use to document the nursing process, including the progress note and the nursing care plan. The progress note documents the patient's progress toward achieving stated outcomes. There are many different progress note charting systems in use:

SOAPIER: Subjective data, objective data, analysis of data stated as a nursing diagnosis, plan, intervention/implementation, evaluation, revision

PIO: Problem, intervention, outcome

CBE: Charting by exception

Focus® charting

DAR: Data, action, response/revision

PIE: Problem, intervention, evaluation

MDS: Minimum data set; federal regulations require this form to be completed in long-term facilities at varying intervals, depending on whether the patient needs intermediate care or skilled care

OASIS-B1: Outcome and assessment information set; to be used in home health care from the Center for Health Services and Policy Research

Each charting method has advantages and disadvantages. The nurse should verify institutional policy on charting directives.

The **nursing care plan** combines the elements of the nursing process to document the progress of patient care in a standardized fashion. Nursing care plans serve as a means of communicating patient progress with other health care colleagues and ensuring continuity of care among the nursing staff.

ASSESSMENT IN BRIEF

Critical Thinking and Nursing Process Review

1. Critical thinking and clinical reasoning are incorporated into all aspects of patient care.

2. The quality of critical thinking can be evaluated by applying the seven UIS.

3. Nurses frame their critical thinking by using the nursing process.

4. Apply all six phases of the nursing process to address different patient problems.

5. Begin with a thorough assessment of the patient, using a health history, physical assessment, and laboratory data and diagnostic procedures. Document findings.

6. Formulate and prioritize nursing diagnoses according to the patient's status. Record on the patient's clinical record.

7. Work with the patient to develop mutually agreeable and achievable outcomes and interventions.

8. Implement actions in conjunction with other members of the health care team.

9. Evaluate the patient's progress toward achieving outcomes.

10. Continually reassess and reprioritize diagnoses and outcomes as the patient's status changes in order to provide the best patient care.

11. Document the patient's progress toward outcomes.

REVIEW QUESTIONS

1. Why are experienced nurses more likely to make intuitive links that are not made by novice nurses?
   a. Experienced nurses have more years of education than novice nurses.
   b. The novice nurse possesses less goal-directed thinking processes.
   c. The experienced nurse can delve into a professional portfolio of clinical experiences.
   d. The novice nurse is less capable of analyzing causative factors and possible outcomes.

   The correct answer is (c).

2. Which critical thinking component examines the validity of information and hypotheses?
   a. Inference
   b. Evaluation
   c. Interpretation
   d. Self-regulation
   The correct answer is (b).

3. Using Elder and Paul's Universal Intellectual Standards for critical thinking, which standard is exemplified in the following statement:
   The patient experienced chest pain this afternoon and one of the patient's favorite hobbies is reading murder mysteries.
   a. Clarity
   b. Accuracy
   c. Logic
   d. Relevance
   The correct answer is (d).

4. The ANA Standard of Practice "Assessment" refers to the nurse:
   a. Collecting comprehensive data pertinent to the patient's health
   b. Analyzing the assessment data to determine the diagnoses
   c. Identifying expected outcomes for an individualized plan of care
   d. Employing strategies to promote health and a safe environment
   The correct answer is (a).

5. Which of the following constitutes objective data?
   a. The patient is experiencing fatigue.
   b. The patient has burning back pain.
   c. The patient is complaining of shortness of breath.
   d. The patient has muscle atrophy.
   The correct answer is (d).

6. What type of nursing diagnosis is defined as "human responses to health conditions/life processes that may develop in a vulnerable individual, family, or community"?
   a. Actual nursing diagnosis
   b. Risk nursing diagnosis
   c. Wellness nursing diagnosis
   d. Collaborative nursing diagnosis
   The correct answer is (b).

7. What error was made in this nursing diagnosis: Patient unable to perform ADLs due to laziness.
   a. Writing in legally inadvisable terms
   b. Using value judgments
   c. Formulating a diagnosis based on incorrect data
   d. Making a diagnosis based on insufficient data
   The correct answer is (b).

8. Starting at the base of Maslow's Hierarchy of Needs, which of the following sequences ascends in the correct progression?
   a. Safety and security needs, self-esteem, physiological needs, love and belonging, and self-actualization
   b. Physiological needs, safety and security needs, love and belonging, self-esteem, and self-actualization
   c. Love and belonging, self-esteem, safety and security needs, physiological needs, and self-actualization
   d. Self-actualization, self-esteem, love and belonging, safety and security needs, and physiological needs
   The correct answer is (b).

9. In the nursing diagnosis, "Impaired skin integrity related to prolonged immobilization as evidenced by pallor to the left buttock," which component is the descriptor?
   a. Impaired
   b. Skin integrity
   c. Prolonged immobilization
   d. Pallor to the left buttock
   The correct answer is (a).

10. Documenting physical examination findings in sleep-rest or activity-exercise sections is using which assessment model?
    a. Body system assessment
    b. Functional Health Patterns
    c. NANDA-I taxonomy
    d. Maslow's hierarchy
    The correct answer is (b).

REFERENCES

American Nurses Association. (1995). *Nursing: A social policy statement.* Kansas City, MO: Author.

American Nurses Association. (2004). *Nursing: Scope and standards of practice.* Washington, DC: Author.

Bulechek, G. M., Butcher, H. K., & Dochterman, J. M. (Eds.). (2008). *Nursing Interventions Classification (NIC)* (5th ed.). St. Louis, MO: Mosby.

Elder, L., & Paul, R. (1996). Universal intellectual standards. Retrieved January 17, 2008, from http://www.criticalthinking.org

Gordon, M. (2006). *Manual of nursing diagnosis* (11th ed.). Sudbury, MA: Jones and Bartlett.

Moorhead, S., Johnson, M., Maas, M., & Swanson, E. (Eds.). (2008). *Nursing outcomes classification (NOC)* (4th ed.). St. Louis, MO: Mosby.

NANDA International (2009). *NANDA-I Nursing diagnoses: Definitions & classifications 2009–2011.* West Sussex, United Kingdom: John Wiley & Sons, Ltd.

Paul, R., & Elder, L. (1997, March 1). Helping students assess their thinking. Retrieved January 17, 2008, from http://www.criticalthinking.org

Pesut, D. J., & Herman, J. (1999). *Clinical reasoning: The art and science of critical and creative thinking.* Clifton Park, NY: Thomson Delmar Learning.

BIBLIOGRAPHY

Ackley, B. J., & Ladwig, G. B. (2008). *Nursing diagnosis handbook: An evidence-based guide to planning care* (8th ed.). St. Louis, MO: Mosby.

Alfaro-LeFevre, R. (2005). *Applying nursing process: A tool for critical thinking* (6th ed.). Philadelphia: Lippincott Williams & Wilkins.

Broyles, B. (2006). *Clinical decision making: Case studies in pediatrics.* Clifton Park, NY: Delmar Cengage Learning.

Carpenito-Moyet, L. J. (2007). *Nursing diagnosis: Application to clinical practice* (12th ed.). Philadelphia: Lippincott.

Comer, S. R. (2005). *Delmar's geriatric nursing care plans.* Clifton Park, NY: Delmar Cengage Learning.

Craig, J. (2007). *The evidence-based practice manual for nurses* (2nd ed.). Oxford, UK: Churchill Livingstone.

DeLaune, S. C., & Ladner, P. K. (2006). *Fundamentals of nursing, standards and practice* (3rd ed.). Clifton Park, NY: Delmar Cengage Learning.

Doenges, M. E., Moorhouse, M. F., & Murr, A. (2006). *Nursing care plans: Guidelines for individualizing client care across the life span* (8th ed.). Philadelphia: F. A. Davis.

Gebbie, K. M., & Lavin, M. A. (1975). *Classification of nursing diagnoses. Proceedings of the First National Conference.* St. Louis, MO: Mosby.

Gordon, M. (2008). *Assess notes: Assessment and diagnostic reasoning.* Philadelphia: F.A. Davis.

Gregory, D. S. (2006). *Clinical decision making: Case studies in maternity and women's health.* Clifton Park, NY: Delmar Cengage Learning.

Gutierrez, K. (2008). *Pharmacotherapeutics: Clinical reasoning in primary care* (2nd ed.). Philadelphia: Saunders.

Ignatavicius, D. D., & Workman, L. (2006). *Medical-surgical nursing: Critical thinking for collaborative care* (5th ed.). Philadelphia: Saunders.

Levin, R. F., & Feldman, H. R. (Ed.). (2006). *Teaching evidence-based practice in nursing. A guide for academic and clinical settings.* New York: Springer.

Nightingale, F. (1859). *Notes on nursing: What it is, and what it is not.* Philadelphia: Lippincott.

Richardson, B. K. (2007). *Clinical decision making: Case studies in psychiatric nursing.* Clifton Park, NY: Delmar Cengage Learning.

Rodgers, S. (2008). *Thomson Delmar Learning's Medical-surgical nursing care plans.* Clifton Park, NY: Delmar Cengage Learning.

Schuster, P. M. (2008). *Concept mapping: A critical thinking approach to care planning* (2nd ed.). Philadelphia: F. A. Davis.

Scudder, L. (2006). Using evidence-based information. *The Journal for Nurse Practitioners, 2,* 180–185.

Seaback, W. W. (2006). *Nursing process, concepts and application* (2nd ed.). Clifton Park, NY: Delmar Cengage Learning.

Shieh, C. (2006). Practice-based evidence: How one nurse turned her day-to-day experiences into research. *AWHONN, 10*(5), 375–378.

Wilkinson, J. M. (2007). *Nursing process and critical thinking* (4th ed.). Upper Saddle River, NJ: Pearson Prentice Hall.

WEB SITES

Best BETS (Best Evidence Topics):
http://www.bestbets.org

The Cochrane Collection:
http://www.cochrane.org

National Guideline Clearinghouse:
http://www.guideline.gov

NANDA-I:
http://www.nanda.org

Network for Language in Nursing Knowledge Systems:
http://www.nlinks.org

American Nurses Association:
http://www.nursingworld.org

CHAPTER 2
The Patient Interview

COMPETENCIES

1. Prepare an appropriate setting for the nurse-patient interview.

2. Recognize personal perceptions that facilitate or hinder the interview process.

3. Define effective interviewing techniques.

4. Describe problematic interviewing behaviors.

5. Demonstrate how to transform problematic interviewing behaviors into more effective ones.

6. Adapt the interview process for the patient with special needs.

The nursing health assessment interview is a purposeful, time-limited verbal interaction between the nurse and the patient. It is initiated to collect specific information regarding the patient and the patient's health status. Other purposes include validating appropriate health and illness information presented by the patient or found in the patient's record, and identifying the patient's knowledge of personal health and illness status. Accurate and complete information about the patient serves as a foundation for subsequent nurse-patient interactions and for medical and nursing interventions. The nurse-patient interaction requires skill in interviewing techniques, which the nurse can learn and refine.

THE PATIENT INTERVIEW

The nursing assessment interview can be differentiated from the more traditional medically oriented interview. The medical interview typically focuses on the patient's physical or emotional state, while the nursing interview is more holistic in nature and includes comprehensive information about the total patient. The nursing interview includes an assessment of physical, mental, emotional, developmental, social, cultural, and spiritual aspects of the patient. Data are collected concerning the patient's present and past states of health, including the patient's family status and relationships, cultural background, lifestyle preferences, and developmental level. Other factors considered in data collection are the patient's self-concept, religious affiliation, social supports, burden of care, sexuality, and reproductive processes.

THE ROLE OF THE NURSE

The nurse is often the first person from the health care team to interact with the patient. The nurse frequently assumes the role of intermediary for the patient to the larger health care system. A critical role of the nurse is to assist the patient in effectively utilizing the system. The climate and tone of the initial patient interview may influence all future interactions the patient has in the health care setting (Figure 2-1). The nurse's attitude and expectations, both positive and negative, set the stage for the interview and can affect its outcome.

First impressions of individuals are important and imprint long-lasting thoughts and feelings. The personal appearances of both the patient and the nurse contribute significantly to the formation of first impressions. In American culture, health care providers who present a professional appearance that is appropriate for the particular setting in which they work are more readily accepted. Likewise, the manner in which the patient physically presents to the nurse may influence the nurse's perceptions of the patient.

The nurse is the facilitator of the interview and thus collaborates with the patient in establishing a mutually respectful dialogue. Encouraging the patient to speak freely and expressing concern for the patient are essential in this process. For example, if the patient thinks that no one in the health care setting listens to his or her concerns and feelings, the patient will likely say very little. Because accurate data

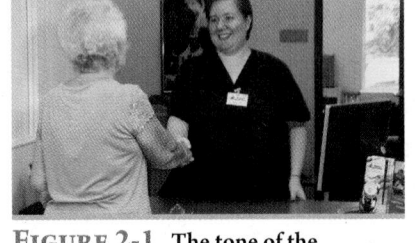

FIGURE 2-1 The tone of the nurse-patient introduction sets the stage for the patient interview and patient care.

REFLECTIVE THINKING

Assessing Personal Biases

Affirmative action laws promote nondiscrimination in the workplace. Assess your personal feelings or biases toward treating or working with an individual who is lesbian, gay, bisexual, or transgender (LGBT). How can you create a welcoming environment for all patients? Would you treat an LGBT colleague different from a non-LGBT colleague?

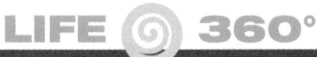

LIFE 360°

Initial Patient Impression

A 19-year-old mother with her 14-month-old child come to the emergency department. You are the nurse assigned to care for them. You note that their clothes are dirty, malodorous, and in ill repair. What might your initial perception of the mother and child be? How might this affect the patient interview?

collection is the primary purpose of the interview, the patient must feel comfortable and safe enough to provide information, to ask questions, and to express fears or concerns. The nurse can foster an atmosphere of safety and comfort by approaching each patient with an accepting, respectful, and nonjudgmental attitude.

THE ROLE OF THE PATIENT

The patient is an active and equal participant in the interview process and should feel free to openly communicate thoughts, feelings, perceptions, and factual information. Most patients possess previous knowledge of or experience with the health care system that influences their current perceptions and behavior. Understanding how patients see their role in this system is vital to the successful completion of any health interview. In some cultures, passivity is the norm in health care matters (see Chapter 5). However, powerlessness is contrary to the active participation required of the patient in the interview process.

In today's health care arena, patients are taking a more active role in both their own health care and in health care decisions (Figure 2-2). Patients are much more apt to question health care providers, to treat themselves, and to demand a role in decision making. Frequently, patients actively seek health care providers who possess clinical competence as well as a willingness to provide individualized attention in a genuine, caring relationship.

MOTIVATIONAL INTERVIEWING

When interviewing the patient, the nurse can also assume the role of motivational interviewer. This technique was originally developed to work with patients using addictive substances. Motivational interviewing can also be used to positively impact a patient's life by changing long-term behavior that is deleterious to a person's health (e.g., smoking, unhealthy diets). Through the use of empathy the nurse can gain a patient's trust to use this technique. First, the patient must be able to identify that a situation exists that needs to be altered in his or her life. In addition, the patient must be willing to acknowledge that a change in his or her behavior is needed to reach a better health state, and the patient must be ready to accept assistance. The nurse, in conjunction with the patient, must jointly set realistic goals for the patient. It is the responsibility of the nurse to motivate the patient to become independent and self-motivated as the behavior change process begins. Verbal encouragement at visits, reviewing behavior diaries at visits, phone calls, e-mailing, providing appropriate reading material and resources, and community self-help groups (if indicated) are all ways that the patient can sustain his or her motivation to change the deleterious behavior. Thus, in order to have the highest chance of success, the nurse should meet with the patient on a regular basis (the interval depends on the patient's individual situation and can vary from daily to weekly). The nurse must also recognize that the patient may "backslide" during the intervention period; this too can be a normal part of the motivational process.

FACTORS INFLUENCING THE INTERVIEW

Factors that can affect the patient's comfort level and, therefore, the effectiveness of the interview are discussed in the following sections.

APPROACH

Prior to approaching the patient, gather all available patient information; admission data and past medical records are often available and may significantly reduce the time needed for the interview.

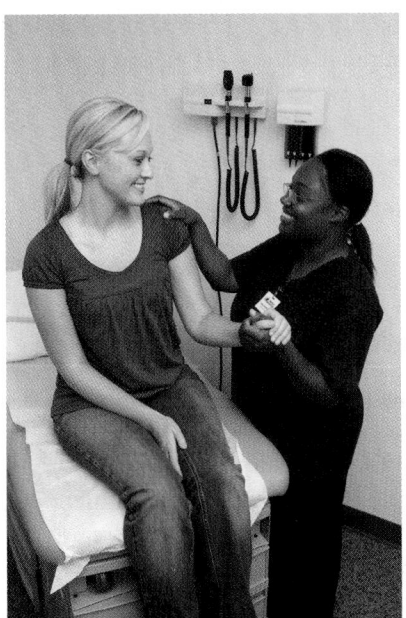

FIGURE 2-2 Patients are encouraged to take an active role in their health care.

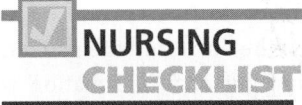

REFLECTIVE THINKING

Using Motivational Interviewing

How would you employ motivational interviewing with a patient who has smoked two packs of cigarettes daily for 40 years?

☑ NURSING CHECKLIST

Preparing for the Interview

1. Gather all available patient information.
2. Seek out an appropriate setting for the interview.
3. Set aside a block of time for the interview.
4. Assess yourself for possible problematic thoughts or feelings.
5. Begin the interview with a friendly introduction.
   - Introduce yourself by name and title.
   - Call the patient by formal name, for example, "Mr." or "Mrs. Adams."

REFLECTIVE THINKING

Breaking Confidentiality

Your emergency room female patient reveals that her extensive physical injuries are the result of a beating administered by her husband rather than the result of a fall as she had initially stated. She asks you not to share this information with anyone because she is fearful of her husband's reaction. What is your immediate reaction to this disclosure? What is your institution's policy concerning confidentiality? What are your responsibilities in this situation? Is a report mandated by law in your state for this action?

LIFE 360°

Patient Interview Environment

Look at Figure 2-3. What are the pros and cons of conducting a patient interview in this setting? How could you maximize the interview in this location?

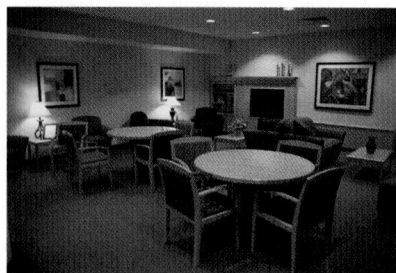

FIGURE 2-3

Begin the interview with an introduction, including your name and title. Initially call the patient by his or her formal name and ask how the patient prefers to be addressed. Simple communication utilizing appropriate names is respectful and helps identify patients as unique persons at a time when they may be feeling quite anxious. Giving recognition helps to lower patient anxiety and increase patient comfort level.

Examples of approaches you can use:

"Good morning, Mrs. Harris."
"Hello, Mr. Carpenter, it has been a long time since you were last here."

Providing the patient with an explanation of what is to follow and an approximate time frame for the interview helps in establishing trust. This information also helps to increase the patient's feeling of control. The more effective you are in establishing trust, the easier it will be to obtain information from the patient, for example: "Good morning, Mr. Rapt, my name is Marielle Pereira. I'm a registered nurse. I'd like to ask you some questions about why you are here today."

ENVIRONMENT

The setting for the interview has a direct influence on the amount and quality of information gathered. Time and effort spent in seeking out an appropriate setting for the interview indicate concern for the patient and for the quality and quantity of information collected. Whenever possible, the interview should be conducted in a private room with controlled lighting and temperature. When a private setting is impossible, control the environment to minimize distractions and interruptions and to increase the comfort level of the patient. Utilize any physical barriers available in the room to provide as much privacy as possible. When all efforts to ensure even minimal privacy fail, conduct a shortened interview to gather only immediately pertinent information. Defer the complete interview until a later time when privacy can be ensured.

CONFIDENTIALITY

Confidentiality is essential in developing trust between the nurse and the patient. The patient's willingness to communicate private and personal information is predicated on the assumption that this information will be used with discretion and for the benefit of the patient (see Figure 2-4). Your verbal assurance of confidentiality often eases the patient's concerns and fosters trust in the relationship. In practice, there are certain exceptions to absolute confidentiality. For example, in a teaching institution where a team approach is used, information must be shared. Another important reason for sharing confidential information is when the patient is a danger to self or others. Nurses need to be familiar with institutional policy as well as legal statutes on patient confidentiality and the consequences of not adhering to them. It is essential to inform the patient prior to the interview when information will be shared with others. Frequently, patients may have friends or family members with them. To ensure patient comfort and confidentiality, ask the patient whether these people should remain in the room for the interview.

HIPAA

Mandatory compliance with the Privacy Rule of the Health Insurance Portability and Accountability Act (HIPAA) came into force on April 14, 2003. This regulation affects all health care providers as well as service organizations, information system vendors, and universities. The goal of HIPAA is to safeguard the

Observing HIPAA Regulations

The advice nurse in a primary care office receives a phone call from a patient's wife inquiring as to her husband's laboratory results. The patient's chart is consulted and the patient does not have his wife listed as someone who can receive confidential information about him. What action should be taken? What are the ramifications of this decision?

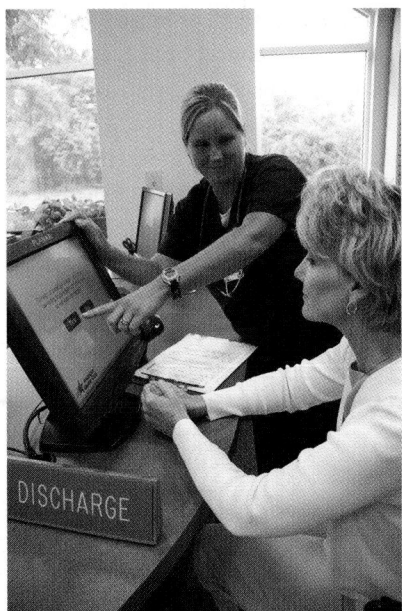

FIGURE 2-4 Sharing patient information with colleagues is an important nursing role. Confidentiality must be observed at all times.

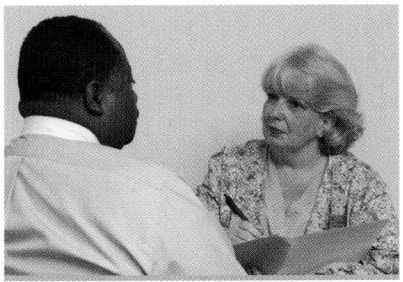

FIGURE 2-5 The patient interview often requires note taking. Maintain rapport and eye contact as much as possible.

confidentiality of all patient information, as well as to provide security for this information, whether it is in electronic or another form. In addition, HIPAA states that individuals have a right to access their medical records and to be informed of who else has been granted permission to view them. Inappropriate use and release of confidential patient information is now punishable by law. The extent to which HIPAA regulations have made an impact on the health care system varies greatly across the country.

NOTE TAKING

Although it is advisable to jot down information during the interview, the simple act of writing down what the patient says may cause some patient discomfort (Figure 2-5). Early in the interview, explain the necessity of jotting down pertinent information and show the patient the form you will be using. You will become adept in skills that expedite charting information. Frequently, the patient will lead the interview or discuss sensitive issues. When this occurs, give full attention to the patient and defer formal recording of information. Jot down short phrases, words, and dates that can be used to complete formal data recording following the interview.

TIME, LENGTH, DURATION

To become fully involved with the patient, enough time must be set aside for the interview. When scheduling an interview for the hospitalized patient, look at the patient's daily activities, then select a block of time for the interview that does not conflict with the patient's mealtime or other planned activities. Do not hesitate to ask the patient what interview times would be least disruptive to daily routine, and try to accommodate the patient's request.

BIASES AND PRECONCEPTIONS

Personal belief and value systems, attitudes, biases, and preconceptions of both the nurse and the patient influence the sending and receiving of messages. The cultural and family contexts of each serve as a lens for interpreting societal views on ethnicity, gender, and health care. Nurses' and patients' views of themselves as cultured and gendered beings are highly influential in how they think and feel about health and illness and have an impact on how they respond to different clinical situations; for example, the nurse may unintentionally treat male and female patients differently, even in something as simple as addressing the patient (e.g., "Mr. Johnson" versus "Becky"). The nurse must be sensitive to personal as well as patient contexts in order to treat all patients fairly and respectfully.

The nurse's subjective impressions of the patient may lead to faulty assumptions about patient abilities or illnesses. For example, a patient who appears thin and frail may be viewed by the nurse as seriously ill or unable to participate in activities

REFLECTIVE THINKING

Decreasing Anxiety in the Interview

Remember the last time that you were anxious. How did you demonstrate that anxiety (behaviorally, physically, etc.)? What did you do that helped you to calm down? Identify some specific actions you might take to decrease a patient's anxiety during the joining stage of the interview process.

of daily living when, in fact, this patient may not be seriously ill or incapacitated in any way. To counter faulty assumptions, biases, and preconceptions, continually validate information and personal impressions through the use of careful data gathering and effective interviewing techniques.

Generally, the nurse's subjective feelings during the interview are an indication of the climate of the interview and can be used to provide additional assessment information. For example, the nurse's feelings of anxiety during an interview may be an indication or a reflection of the patient's feelings of fear, anxiety, or anger. Careful attention to these feelings may direct you to change the interview format (to lower patient anxiety) or to refocus the questions (to gather specific data).

STAGES OF THE INTERVIEW PROCESS

There are three stages in the interview process: the introduction or the joining stage, the working stage, and the termination stage.

STAGE I

The **joining stage** is the introduction or first stage of the interview process, during which the nurse and the patient establish trust and get to know one another. Work with the patient to define the relationship and establish goals for this and any subsequent interactions.

STAGE II

The **working stage** of the interview process is the time during which the bulk of the patient data is collected. It is a nursing responsibility to keep the interview goal directed, including refocusing the patient and redefining the goals established in the joining stage.

STAGE III

The **termination stage** is the last stage of the interview process, during which information is summarized and validated. During this stage, give the patient an indication of the amount of time left in the interview, and allow the patient the opportunity to give additional information and make comments or statements. For example, "We have about 5 minutes more, Mr. Nguyen, is there anything else you would like to add or mention?" Other important steps in the termination stage are summarizing and validating information and planning for future interviews.

FACTORS AFFECTING COMMUNICATION

Elements that can affect the sending and receiving of messages are discussed in the following sections.

LISTENING

Active listening, or the act of perceiving what is said both verbally and nonverbally, is a critical factor in conducting a successful health assessment interview. According to Bradley and Edinberg (1990), the primary goal of active listening is to decode patient messages in order to understand the situation or problem as the other person sees it. Pay careful attention to all sensory data to better understand the patient's message and formulate an appropriate response. Be aware of how personal characteristics, choice of communication techniques, and the manner and timing of their use can affect communication.

REFLECTIVE THINKING

Encouraging Active Listening

Remember the last time that you attempted to talk with someone who didn't appear to be listening. How did that make you feel? What kind of things did you do to get your message across? How many times have you listened to patients with "half an ear"? What might cause you to do this? Identify some specific actions that you might take to ensure that your patients feel heard.

REFLECTIVE THINKING

Assessing Nonverbal Communication

Record an audiovisual representation of yourself eliciting a health history from a classmate. Review the media by yourself. What nonverbal communication did you identify in yourself? Your classmate? Review the media with your classmate and have him or her identify the nonverbal communication. What were the positive and negative nonverbal actions?

REFLECTIVE THINKING

Nonverbal Communication

Look at the nurse-patient encounters in Figures 2-6 and 2-7. Describe the nonverbal communication that you see in each.

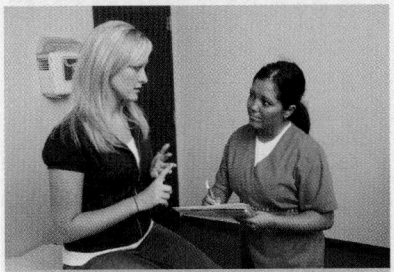

FIGURE 2-6

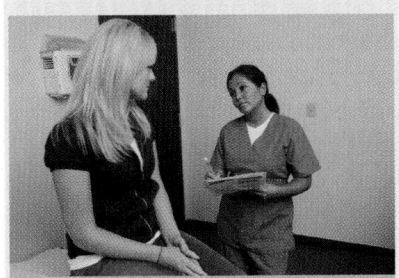

FIGURE 2-7

NONVERBAL CUES

Nonverbal communication is communicating a message without words. Nonverbal behaviors effectively supplement the spoken word and provide information about both nurse and patient. These behaviors can provide insight into the patient's cultural expectations, current physical and emotional states, and perceived self-image. Nonverbal cues such as body position, nervous repetitive movements of the hands or legs, rapid blinking, lack of eye contact, yawning, fidgeting, excessive smiling or frowning, and repetitive clearing of the throat may be indications of the patient's health and feelings that the patient may not be comfortable expressing verbally.

Health care settings often evoke a great deal of anxiety, uncertainty, or fear in patients. Loss of personal control is a major obstacle confronting patients in health care settings, whether they are seriously ill or not. In an attempt to maintain some control in unfamiliar circumstances and to decrease anxiety, patients frequently look to nurses for cues on how to behave or how to respond to questions. Nonverbal acts by the nurse can indicate empathy and attention or indifference and inattention. Such behaviors powerfully influence patient comfort levels, feelings of control, and willingness to share information. Because of this, nurses need to continuously monitor their own nonverbal behaviors.

DISTANCE

The amount of space a person considers appropriate for interaction is a significant factor in the interview process and is determined in part by cultural influences. In the United States, distances are generally categorized as follows:

- Intimate distance is from the patient to approximately 1.5 feet.
- Personal distance is approximately 1.5 to 4 feet.
- Social distance is approximately 4 to 12 feet.
- Public distance is approximately 12 feet or more.

Intimate distance is the closest and involves some touching or physical contact. Personal distance may also involve some touching or physical contact, and it may provide for ease of communication such as in cases of hearing impairment. In some cases, personal distance may be threatening or invasive to the patient. Social distance is considered appropriate for the interview process because it allows for good eye contact and for ease in hearing and in seeing the patient's nonverbal cues. Public distance is usually used in formal settings such as in a classroom where the teacher stands in front of the class. It is not considered appropriate for an interview.

PERSONAL SPACE

Personal space can be defined as the space over which a person claims ownership. In an inpatient health care agency, the patient's hospital room and bathroom are

NURSING**TIP**

The Use of Touch in the Patient Interview

You must be mindful of the use of touch during the patient interview. While a caring touch, a pat on the hand, or other gesture may send a message of empathy to a crying individual, it may not be appropriate in all situations. The patient's cultural background may dictate what is or is not appropriate (see Chapter 5). Also, if a patient has a history of physical abuse or neglect or is recovering from a skin disorder, such as a burn, a well-meaning touch may be interpreted in a hostile manner.

considered the patient's personal space. The patient may be very protective of this space and consider unauthorized use of it as an invasion of privacy.

EFFECTIVE INTERVIEWING TECHNIQUES

Effective interviewing techniques facilitate or support interactions between the nurse and the patient and foster their continuation. These techniques encompass both verbal and nonverbal approaches. The more skilled you can become in understanding the communication process, the more effectively you can use it in a purposeful, goal-directed manner to meet your needs for information and the patient's need for attention to health concerns or problems. Because individuals who come to a health care provider are frequently anxious, effectively communicating your interest and concern greatly enhances the effectiveness of the interview and interaction.

Certain specific verbal communication techniques are available to help you facilitate this interaction. The effectiveness of these techniques will vary from individual to individual. At first, these techniques may feel awkward, stilted, or forced; keep in mind that communicating effectively is a learned skill (similar to other nursing skills) and, as such, improves with practice.

USING OPEN-ENDED QUESTIONS

Open-ended questions encourage the patient to provide general rather than more focused information. Beginning the health assessment interview with open-ended questions provides the patient with a sense of control, leaving the choice of what to say, how much to say, and how to say it up to the patient. These questions indicate respect for the patient's ability to articulate important or pressing health concerns and, therefore, to help set priorities.

Examples of open-ended questions:

"What are some of your concerns about caring for your mother at home?"
"How do you typically deal with an asthma attack?"

Open-ended questions that begin with the words *how, what, where, when,* and *who* are usually more effective in eliciting the maximum amount of information than those that begin with the word *why.* "Why" questions can cause patients to become defensive and feel the need to somehow explain or defend their ideas and behaviors, thus setting up an adversarial relationship between nurse and patient. While open-ended questions are quite helpful in the health assessment interview, they can be time consuming and may not be appropriate in situations requiring rapid access to information and rapid response by health care providers. Overuse of this type of question, especially with the patient who is confused, vague in his or her responses, or extremely talkative, can cause the nurse to miss important information.

In certain situations, perhaps because of anxiety or unfamiliarity with the health care system, patients may attempt to ascertain what answers the nurse wants and what areas the nurse seems to feel are important. The patient will then focus on those, rather than on areas that are most important to the patient. With open-ended questions, you can encourage the patient to define what is important. When eliciting the health history, it is usually best to let the patient speak uninterrupted. After the patient completes an answer, you can proceed with questions or clarification.

USING CLOSED QUESTIONS

Closed questions are those that regulate or restrict patient response. They can frequently be answered with a "yes" or a "no." Closed questions can be used to focus the interview, pinpoint specific areas of concern, and elicit valuable information quickly and efficiently.

Examples of effective closed questions:

"Are you thinking of hurting yourself?"
"Has this type of allergic reaction ever happened to you before?"

However, if used too frequently, closed questions can disrupt communication because they limit patient responses and interaction. Even well-directed closed questions may take the initiative away from the patient, giving him or her the impression that the nurse is in charge of the interview, does most of the work, often knows the answer to the question asked, and is directing the patient's response.

Examples of ineffective closed questions:

"Do you still feel sad and depressed?"
"Are you afraid to tell your parents that you are sexually active?"

FACILITATING

Once the health assessment interview has started, there may be periods when patients stop talking because of anxiety, uncertainty, or embarrassment. You can use a variety of both verbal and nonverbal means to encourage patients to continue talking. Phrases such as "go on" or "uh-huh," the simple repetition of key words the patient has spoken, or even head nods or a touch on the hand prompt the patient to resume speaking and also indicate your continued interest and attention.

USING SILENCE

Silence, too, has its place in the assessment interview. Understood and used effectively by the nurse, periods of silence can help structure and pace the interview, convey respect and acceptance, and, in many cases, prompt additional patient data. Silence on the part of the patient may indicate feelings of anxiety, confusion, or embarrassment, or simply a lack of understanding about the question asked or an inability to speak English. Nonverbal data such as these are often lost if the nurse is a persistent talker. Conversely, if overused, silence can contribute to an awkward, disjointed interview providing minimal structure or direction for the patient and little helpful data for the nurse.

Using silence effectively may seem like a difficult skill to master. Frequently, silences seem longer than they actually are. When silences occur, you may feel discomfort and pressure to speak in order to be actually "doing" something therapeutic; instead, handle silences by being quiet and observing the patient's behavior for what is not being said verbally.

GROUPING COMMUNICATION TECHNIQUES

Communication techniques often seem mechanical and artificial to the beginning nurse; one way to make them less so is to group or cluster them according to their primary purposes. Grouping communication strategies on the basis of purpose helps to clarify the intent of each communication response (Cormier & Cormier, 1991) and indicate when in the assessment interview its use might be helpful. One simple way to group interview techniques is to divide them into two groups: listening responses and action responses.

Listening Responses

Listening responses are attempts made by the nurse to accurately receive, process, and then respond to patient messages. They provide one way for the nurse to

Recall your last experience as a patient in a hospital or other health care facility. Did you feel any sense of control regarding what was happening to you? Did you want any control in this situation? When you feel out of control, how do you behave? When you feel out of control, what do you do to alleviate this feeling? What behaviors do you think patients use to help them feel more in control when they are sick?

communicate empathy, concern, and attentiveness. Patients "need to know that the interviewer has heard what they have been saying, seen their point of view, and felt their world as they experience it" (Ivey, 1994, p. 99). In order to "listen" to what the patient says, the nurse must not only process the words spoken by the patient but also understand the context of the patient's experience.

Listening responses provide the nurse with a vehicle for understanding the patient's perspective. Patients will realize that they are heard and that you are working for and with them to elicit and clarify health concerns. Listening responses include making observations, restating, reflecting, clarifying, interpreting, sequencing, encouraging comparisons, and summarizing.

MAKING OBSERVATIONS. When making observations, the nurse verbalizes perceptions about the patient's behavior, then shares them with the patient. Calling to attention personal behavior about which the patient might be unaware may prove insightful and help increase the patient's conscious awareness of his or her behavior. Sharing observations is also a way to validate patient competency and sense of control in an environment or situation where a patient often feels out of control, uncertain, or overwhelmed.

Examples of making observations:

"Speaking about these symptoms seems to make you tense. I notice that you are clenching your fists and grimacing."
"I notice that each time you've been confronted with that particular problem, you've known how to handle it appropriately."

RESTATING. Restating involves repeating or rephrasing the main idea expressed by the patient and lets the patient know that you are paying attention. It promotes further dialogue and provides the patient with an opportunity to explain or elaborate on an issue or concern.

Examples of restating:

Patient: I don't sleep well anymore. I find myself waking up frequently at night.
Nurse: You're having difficulty sleeping? **or**
Nurse: You don't sleep well?

REFLECTING. Reflecting is another listening response; it focuses on the content of the patient's message as well as the patient's feelings. In reflecting, the nurse directs the patient's own questions, feelings, and ideas back to the patient and provides an opportunity for the patient to reconsider or expand on what was just said (Figure 2-8). The patient's point of view is given value, and the nurse, although indicating an interest in what the patient has to say, refrains from giving advice, passing judgment, or assuming responsibility for the patient's thoughts or feelings.

Examples of reflecting:

Patient: Do you think I should tell the doctor I stopped taking my medication?
Nurse: What do you think about that?
Patient: Well, yes, I think that I probably should. Not taking my medication could be one of the reasons I'm feeling so run-down. But that medication just makes me so teary and agitated.
Nurse: You sound a bit agitated now. It seems as if you've been thinking about this a lot.
Patient: I told that young doctor that I had problems with this medication and he just didn't listen.
Nurse: Sounds as if you are pretty angry with him.

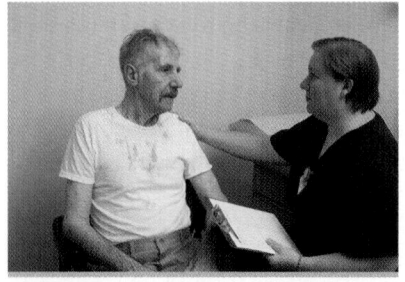

FIGURE 2-8 The nurse assists the patient in reflecting on his feelings.

CLARIFYING. Clarifying is a communication technique used by the nurse to make clear something the patient says or to pinpoint the message when the patient's words and nonverbal behavior do not agree. Be sure you understand exactly what the patient means before continuing, because communication may stop if the patient feels misunderstood or not heard. Distortions or misunderstandings about patient data can occur if the nurse interprets patient statements using only personal experiences and perceptions. Even more crucial is the fact that making assumptions may cause the interviewer to proceed from a faulty database.

Example of a clarifying response:

Patient: During certain activities, I have the most awful pain in my back.
Nurse: Tell me what you mean by awful. **or**
Nurse: I'm not sure that I follow you—when does this pain occur?

Example of a problematic response, involving an assumption:

Patient: We hardly have any time for exercise in our family. We are so busy.
Nurse: I know what you mean!

INTERPRETING. With interpreting you have the opportunity to share your inferences or conclusions gathered from the patient's interview. Although there is always the risk that your interpretation of the facts is incorrect, you are well poised to link events that perhaps the patient was not able to piece together.

Examples of interpreting:

Nurse: Your headaches seem to occur every time you eat nuts and chocolate. **or**
Patient: My stomach pains seem to occur only from late summer to midspring.
Nurse: From what you have just told me, could it be the stress of your teaching job (patient works from September to May) that is causing your pain?

SEQUENCING. To effectively assess patient needs, the nurse often requires knowledge of a time frame within which symptoms or problems developed or occurred. One way of getting at this information involves asking the patient to place a symptom, a problem, or an event in its proper sequence. Sequencing also helps both patient and nurse become aware of any patterns in the patient's behavior that might indicate recurring themes. They can relate to feelings (depression or anxiety), behavior (refusal to take appropriate medications, consistently putting self in risky situations), or experiences (being beaten, being hurt, being misunderstood by health care providers). Pattern identification provides the nurse with clues for further focus.

Examples of sequencing:

Nurse: Did this sharp pain occur each time you had sexual intercourse or only when you didn't empty your bladder first? **or**
Nurse: What specific events led you to feel overwhelmed and suicidal?

ENCOURAGING COMPARISONS. Encouraging comparisons is a technique that enables both participants in the health assessment interview to become more aware of patterns, themes, or specific symptomatology in the patient's life. It also helps the patient to deal more effectively with unfamiliar situations by placing the symptoms or problems in the context of something else that is familiar and, therefore, more comfortable to the patient. Often an awareness of successful prior dealings with similar situations increases patient confidence levels and self-care potentials.

REFLECTIVE THINKING

Practice Sequencing

You have interviewed a Mexican American man who has just returned from visiting his family in rural Mexico. The patient has been experiencing nausea, vomiting, diarrhea, anorexia, fever, and hematochezia. In addition, he has been on antibiotics for rhinosinusitis and received the live nasal vaccine for influenza. Devise a set of questions to clarify this patient's health history and to determine the sequence of events.

Examples of encouraging comparisons:

Nurse: Have you had similar experiences? **or**
In what way was this allergy attack different from or the same as your previous ones? **or**
In what way was your reaction to this medication similar to or different from your reaction to other antibiotics you've taken?

SUMMARIZING. Summarizing helps patients to organize their thinking. Because of this, summarizing is a communication technique that is especially useful at the end of the health assessment interview. A brief, concise review of the important points covered helps the patient identify anything that has been left out and provides the nurse with an opportunity to make sure that what he or she understood the patient to say is actually what was said. In addition, summarizing indicates interest and concern that the patient feels heard as well as finished.

Example of summarizing:

Nurse: During this past hour, you have shared with me several health concerns of which the most vexing to you is your difficulty in losing weight. Is that correct?

Summarizing also provides a means of smoothly transitioning to a new topic or section of the health assessment.

Example of transitioning:

Nurse: You talked about your past experience with diabetes and what happened to you yesterday; now let's talk about why you came in today.

Action Responses

Action responses are the second group of effective interviewing techniques. These responses stimulate patients to make some change in their thinking and behavior. Action responses include such communication techniques as focusing, exploring, presenting reality, confronting, informing, collaborating, limit setting, and normalizing.

FOCUSING. Focusing allows the nurse to concentrate on or "track" a specific point the patient has made. This technique is particularly useful with patients whose heightened anxiety level causes increased confusion, altered concentration, or jumping from topic to topic. With the nurse's assistance in focusing, the patient is able to proceed with the health history in a clearer, more organized, thoughtful, thorough manner.

Examples of focusing:

"Tell me more about the chest pain you experience when you begin to exercise." **or**

"You've mentioned several times that your wife is concerned about your smoking. Let's go back to that."

EXPLORING. In exploring, the nurse is attempting to develop, in more detail, a specific area of content or patient concern. The purpose of exploring is to identify patterns or themes in symptom presentation or in the way patients handle problems or health concerns.

Examples of exploring:

"Tell me more about how you feel when you do not take your medication."

"Could you describe for me how you handle those periods in your life when you feel out of control?"

PRESENTING REALITY. This technique, while typically used with patients with psychiatric issues or patients who are confused, is also useful in the health assessment interview when the nurse is confronted with a patient who exaggerates or makes grandiose statements. Presenting reality, when done in a nonargumentative way, encourages the patient to rethink a statement and perhaps modify it.

Example of presenting reality:

Patient: I can never get an appointment at this clinic.

Nurse: But Mr. Jasper, I've seen you several times in the past 4 months.

Patient: Well, yes, but I can never get an appointment at a time that is convenient for me.

CONFRONTING. Confronting is a verbal response that the nurse makes to some perceived discrepancy or incongruency in the patient's thoughts, feelings, or behaviors. Gently challenging an incongruency can help the patient reframe a situation in order to see things differently. Confrontation can be used to focus the patient's attention on some aspect of personal perception or behavior that, if changed, could lead to more effective or adaptive functioning (Cormier & Cormier, 1991). When confronting is used in a caring, empathetic manner, rather than in a critical or accusatory one, patients feel encouraged to see themselves as competent and effective individuals.

Example of confronting:

Patient: I have been working on lowering my risk for a heart attack. I take my atorvastatin daily and have been watching my diet.

Nurse: You say that you are working on reducing your cardiovascular risk, yet you continue to smoke two packs of cigarettes every day and your triglyceride level has doubled in the past 3 months. Let's review your heart-healthy care plan and see where you need assistance.

INFORMING. Providing the patient with needed information, such as explaining the nature of or the reasons for any necessary tests or procedures, is a nursing action that can help build trust and decrease patient anxiety. In addition to providing patients with needed facts or details, information giving is appropriate when trying to help patients become aware of possible choices and then evaluate those choices correctly.

Example of informing:

Patient: Dr. Jones told me that I need to have my gallbladder taken out.

Nurse: Did you understand what Dr. Jones told you about your gallbladder surgery?

Patient: No, I didn't understand what he said about the new technique. He said something about a tube.

REFLECTIVE THINKING

Using the Action Response of Confronting

You are reviewing lab results with a 49-year-old patient with type 2 diabetes. He tells you that he has been taking his medications as directed, is exercising regularly, and is following his diet. You show the patient that his HbA1c has increased from 8.0 to 10.2 over the past 9 months. What would you say to this patient?

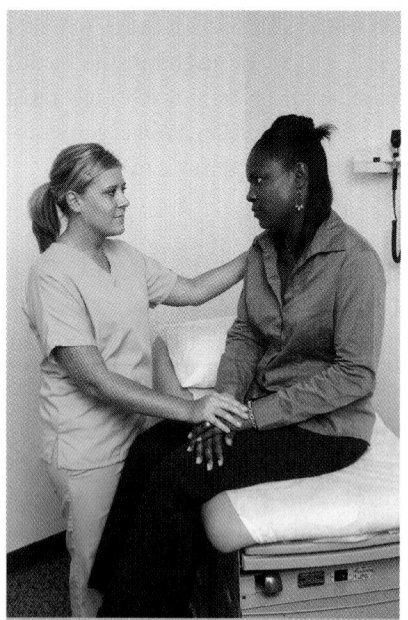

FIGURE 2-9 **In the communication technique of collaborating, the nurse sends the message that the patient and nurse can work together to achieve health goals.**

Nurse: There is a new technique where the surgeon inserts a tube in your abdomen to remove the gallbladder rather than making a large incision, which is the older procedure.

Patient: Yes, that was it, please tell me more about that.

COLLABORATING. In collaborating, the patient is offered a relationship in which both nurse and patient work together rather than one in which the nurse is in total control of the interaction. Use of this technique conveys the message that the patient has important personal knowledge and information to share (Figure 2-9). Collaborating provides a respectful way for the nurse to encourage patients' active involvement in their own health care, in setting goals, in gathering information, and in problem solving.

Example of collaborating:

Nurse: Perhaps you and I can talk further about your asthma and discover what specifically is making you so anxious.

LIMIT SETTING. During the interview with a seductive, hostile, or talkative patient, the nurse may find it necessary to set specific limits on patient behavior. If, for example, the patient persists in asking the nurse personal questions or rambles despite frequent attempts by the nurse to focus, it will be difficult to obtain information needed for task completion. This patient behavior may be a manifestation of stress produced by the interview situation itself or simply a characteristic specific to that particular patient. In such situations, patients may require some direction as to how to behave; provide guidance by calmly, clearly, and respectfully telling the patient what behavior is expected. Limit only the behavior that is problematic or detrimental to the purpose of the interview and avoid making a "big issue" of whatever it is that the patient is doing. When limit setting, do not argue or use empty threats or promises, but do offer the patient alternatives.

Example of ineffective limit setting:

"If you don't start answering my questions, we'll never finish, and you'll never get to see the nurse practitioner."

Example of appropriate limit setting:

Nurse: You know, it seems that you are feeling pretty unsure of how to behave now.

Patient: What do you mean?

NURSINGTIP

Answering Personal Questions

You bring a lifetime of experiences and emotions to each patient encounter. Your patient is in a similar position. It is only natural for the patient to be curious about you as the health care provider. Sharing personal experiences makes you a real person to the patient and helps to develop a respectful nurse-patient interaction. You need to be certain, however, that the information you divulge to the patient remains generic so that you do not cross the professional boundary to a more social interaction. Also, remember that the patient may ask personal questions in order to divert the interview to avoid uncomfortable or sensitive issues.

Nurse: Well, you're asking me a lot of personal questions and generally making it difficult for me to find out what is bothering you. The reason you are here is because you have some health concerns. How can I help you more clearly tell me what brought you to the clinic?

NORMALIZING. Very often, individuals faced with unexpected or life-threatening illnesses, or possible surgeries, respond in ways that seem extreme or out of the ordinary (e.g., becoming depressed or overly tearful). Normalizing allows the nurse to offer appropriate reassurance that their response may be quite common for this situation. This helps to decrease patients' anxiety and encourages patients to share thoughts and feelings they might otherwise keep to themselves for fear of being judged or misunderstood. However, if used inappropriately or out of context, normalizing may give false reassurance.

Example of normalizing:

"It is no wonder that you've been feeling shocked and overwhelmed since you first found that lump in your breast. Most women who have that experience react in a similar way."

NONTHERAPEUTIC INTERVIEWING TECHNIQUES

Just as there are certain communication techniques that facilitate communication between nurse and patient, there are also some interviewing techniques that change, distort, or block communication and should be avoided. Verbal and nonverbal behaviors that involve inattentiveness, imposition of values, judgment, lack of interest, or an "I know what's best for you" attitude hinder communication by creating distance rather than connection. Patients on the receiving end of these behaviors can feel angry, defensive, or incompetent and may refuse to actively participate. Such ineffective techniques include requesting an explanation, probing, offering false reassurance, giving approval or disapproval, defending, and advising.

REQUESTING AN EXPLANATION

Questions that begin with "why" are often perceived by the patient as challenging or threatening. Such questions ask the patient to provide a reason or justification for personal beliefs, feelings, thoughts, and behaviors and imply criticism. If patients are unable to provide these answers, either from lack of sufficient knowledge or because the answer is not known to the patient, he or she can feel inadequate, defensive, or angry; some questions are really unanswerable in that individuals are frequently unaware of why they do things. Asking the patient to describe the beliefs, feelings, or behaviors is preferable to asking why. Providing a description about what happened often helps the patient elaborate. Enlarging the context provides opportunities for the patient to increase self-awareness and for the nurse to increase the store of relevant information.

Example 1 of requesting an explanation:

Patient: I guess I drink two or three six-packs of beer a weekend.
Nurse: Why do you drink that much?
Patient: That's not very much; every one of my friends drinks the same amount.

A more appropriate response in the preceding example might be:

Nurse: It sounds as if you might be concerned about the amount of beer you drink. (reflecting)

Example 2 of requesting an explanation:

Patient: I'm not sure why I came to the clinic today; I just feel miserable. I don't want to see anyone. I just want to stay in bed with the covers pulled over my head.

Nurse: Why do you feel that way?

Patient: I don't know.

A more effective response would be:

Nurse: "What happened that caused you to feel so miserable?" (clarifying) or "It sounds as if you are feeling rather overwhelmed today." (reflecting)

PROBING

Repeated or persistent questioning of the patient about a statement or a behavior increases patient anxiety and can cause confusion, hostility, and a tendency to withdraw from the interaction. This patient withdrawal and the increasing periods of silence resulting from it can escalate the nurse's anxiety. Anxious nurses tend to become more active and more directive in the interview. The patient's unwillingness or hesitancy to discuss a certain event or health concern may indicate patient misunderstanding, misinformation, or a major problem area that needs further clarification or exploration.

A helpful rule of thumb for nurses to use in identifying probing is to pay particular attention to their own behavior and feelings. If in attempting to gather information, nurses feel frustrated or irritated, feel that they are pursuing the patient, or have become involved in a verbal tug of war with the patient, then they are most likely probing. More useful responses may include going on to the next part of the health assessment interview, asking the patient's permission to return to this subject later if it seems likely that more information will be needed, or just sitting quietly until the patient begins to speak.

Example 1 of probing:

Nurse: What makes you drink a six-pack of beer after dinner each night?

Patient: I'm not sure.

Nurse: Well, are there things going on in your life right now that would cause you to drink that much?

Patient: Not really.

Nurse: I don't really think that you would drink that much if things weren't happening in your life right now.

Example 2 of probing:

Nurse: What makes you think that you have arthritis?

Patient: I'm not sure, I just think I do. It just seems like I have the same health problems as my mother and she had arthritis.

Nurse: Well, do you have pain?

Patient: Yes. (pause)

Nurse: Why do you think the pain is arthritis pain?

If nurses can be patient, identify and manage their own anxiety, and allow silences, useful discussion usually ensues.

OFFERING FALSE REASSURANCE

False reassurances are vague and simplistic responses that question the patient's judgment, devalue and block patient feelings, and communicate a lack of understanding and sensitivity on the part of the nurse. The impulse to provide false reassurance

Consider the following example of false reassurance.

Mr. and Mrs. Quinn are awaiting results of diagnostic testing that will confirm or deny a diagnosis of fetal neurological impairment. Mrs. Quinn says to the nurse, "It's taking so long to get the results, I'm sure that there must be something wrong with the baby." The nurse replies, "Oh, no, you don't need to worry. Everything will be just fine!"

- What do you believe motivated the nurse's response?
- What impact will the nurse's response have on the Quinns?

typically originates in the nurse's own feelings of helplessness. Giving false reassurance is an attempt by the nurse to take care of herself or himself rather than the patient and to relieve personal feelings of anxiety. This behavior often increases patient anxiety. A more valuable nursing response would be to first acknowledge personal feelings of anxiety and then to acknowledge the patient's feelings.

Examples of false reassurance:

"Everything will be fine."
"I wouldn't worry about that."

Example of an appropriate response:

"It must be frightening to think about the possibility of surgery."

GIVING APPROVAL OR DISAPPROVAL

During the health assessment interview, nurses can feel pressured to comment judgmentally on a patient's statements, feelings, or behaviors, especially if these contradict the nurse's personal beliefs or feelings. Telling a patient what's right or wrong is moralizing. This may limit the patient's freedom to verbalize or behave in certain ways that might not please the nurse. Comments such as "What a good idea," "You shouldn't feel that way," or "That is bad" hinder the nurse's attempts to establish rapport, support patient competence, and facilitate communication. When there is concern that the patient's expressed beliefs or personal behaviors are ill-informed, harmful, or destructive, the nurse might more effectively explore the source of the belief or the impact of the patient's behavior on others.

Examples of effective responses:

"What made you come to that conclusion?"
"What do you think the consequences will be if you continue to keep your illness from your wife?"

DEFENDING

Occasionally, patients who have had previous stressful or unpleasant experiences with physicians, hospitals, or other agents of the health care system will engage in criticism or verbal attack. It is not helpful for the nurse to defend the object of the attack. Defending implies that the patient has neither the right to hold such opinions or feelings nor the right to express them, especially if they are hostile or angry. The nurse will not be able to change the patient's opinions or feelings by defending the individual or the object attacked. Rather, deflection or criticism of patient feelings more often either blocks expression of these feelings or reinforces them. Defending is not therapeutic because it requires the nurse to speak not just for herself or himself, but for others, something that nurses truthfully and realistically are not able to do.

Examples of inappropriate responses:

"This hospital has an excellent reputation. I'm sure that if you were kept waiting as long as you say, there was a good reason."
"No one here would lie to you."

It is more respectful and more useful to accept and support patients' rights to feel as they do and to express those feelings. The nurse can do this without agreeing with the expressed feelings. This empathetic behavior defuses any antagonism and minimizes patient resistance to the continued interaction.

Examples of appropriate responses:

Nurse: You sound pretty angry about your previous experiences in this hospital.

Patient: Of course I am. Wouldn't you be upset if no one ever told you what was going on and no one answered your call bell?

Nurse: I guess I'd be pretty upset if I thought people were not treating me respectfully.

ADVISING

Consistently telling a patient what to do does not foster competence. Advising encourages patients to look to others for answers, deprives them of the opportunity to learn from past mistakes, and discourages independent judgment. Because some patients may resort to dependent, passive behavior when faced with illness, it is important that the nurse not reinforce such dependence, but rather support the patient's healthy functioning as much as possible.

Example of ineffective responses:

Patient: Do you think that I should have an abortion?

Nurse: Well, if I were you, I'd certainly think long and hard before I'd have another child. You are having difficulty feeding the one you have now. **or**

Nurse: No, I think you should continue the pregnancy. Abortion is never the answer.

A more helpful response would be for the nurse to support the patient's own problem-solving ability through the use of therapeutic communication techniques such as exploring or reflection.

Examples of exploring:

"Tell me more about what made you consider an abortion."
"What other alternatives have you considered?"

Examples of reflection:

"Do you think you should?"
"How would you feel about having the abortion?"

USING PROBLEMATIC QUESTIONING TECHNIQUES

Experienced nurses as well as neophyte interviewers will find themselves occasionally feeling nervous and perhaps unsure of how to proceed during the health assessment interview. This anxiety can lead to the use of questioning techniques and interviewing responses that, although not specifically identified as nontherapeutic, are potentially problematic. Such techniques increase patient anxiety, decrease the flow of needed information, and have the potential to provide the nurse with irrelevant data. The following are several examples of problematic interviewing techniques.

Posing Leading Questions

Leading questions may indicate to the patient that the nurse already has a certain answer in mind. Their use can be intimidating to the patient and curtail further communication. This is especially true if these leading questions concern topics that the patient perceives as sensitive or possible sources of anxiety.

Examples of leading questions:

> "You've never had any type of sexually transmitted diseases, have you, Miss Jenkins?" **or**
>
> "Of course, you've told your daughter that her smoking really bothers you, Mr. Talbott, isn't that correct?"

Interrupting the Patient

Changing the subject or interrupting the patient prevents completion of a thought or idea and introduces a new focus. Such behavior may ease the nurse's discomfort, but it shows a lack of respect and often just confuses or irritates the patient. Questions should focus on one particular topic until all relevant data have been collected and the patient feels finished. Changing the subject or interrupting cuts off the flow of ideas and communicates the message that whatever the patient was addressing is not as important as what the nurse wants to discuss next.

Neglecting to Ask Pertinent Questions

It is easy to become complacent when conducting patient interviews. Do not let patients' outward physical appearances, personalities, or social standing distract you from ascertaining pertinent information. Do not make the assumption that because a patient is well dressed and discusses a luxury car that he or she is well off. Likewise, do not presume that a poorly dressed and ill-mannered person is poor and uneducated. All patients deserve to be treated respectfully during the patient interview.

Engaging in Talkativeness

Extreme talkativeness may indicate nervousness and uncertainty on the part of the interviewer. Attempts to maintain control of the interview and ease personal anxiety can cause the nurse to talk more than necessary. Increased verbal activity minimizes patient spontaneity and can increase patient passivity, causing the nurse to work even harder at obtaining necessary information. The message to the patient is that what the nurse thinks is more important than what the patient thinks and feels.

Using Multiple Questions

Nurses may confuse their patients by asking several questions at once. Too many questions may put patients on the defensive, minimizing patient participation and impeding the flow of necessary information.

Using Medical Jargon

The use of medical jargon or slang can be quite anxiety provoking for the patient. Nurses who belong to the larger health care system, which has its own culture and language, frequently use medical jargon; patients who may feel frightened and powerless in this unfamiliar environment are further disadvantaged by any perceived language barrier. The use of medical jargon can be seen by the patient as unwillingness to share or attempts to hide information, or it can give the impression that the nurse feels superior to the patient and is unwilling to engage in collaboration or mutual problem solving. Conduct the health assessment interview in a language that is common to both participants and check periodically with the patient as to clarity; this will indicate an interest in the patient's perspective and a desire to work collaboratively.

REFLECTIVE THINKING

Asking Essential Information

A 17-year-old female presents to the emergency department with acute abdominal pain. You are asked by the nurse manager to conduct the patient interview with the patient and her parents. Later you discover that the patient is experiencing a miscarriage. You tell your nurse manager that you never inquired about the patient's sexual activity. What variables in this scenario do you think led you to neglect this part of the interview?

Being Authoritative

The use of authority as a health care professional can be a problematic technique. It reinforces a patriarchal nurse-patient relationship and can in effect limit the cooperation of the patient.

Example of negative use of authority:

Nurse: I've been a nurse, Mr. Haddad, for over 10 years, and I think I know what is best for you.

In a few situations, the use of authority can be an effective communication technique.

Example of positive use of authority:

Nurse: As your health care provider, knowing about your previous heart attack, history of high blood pressure, and family history of stroke, I would suggest you consider stopping smoking.

Having Hidden Agendas

Frequently, patients seek health care for one problem but actually are concerned about other problems. The patient may believe that the overriding concern is embarrassing, private, or insignificant. Once in the presence of a health care provider, the patient may open up and discuss concerns. For example, a patient may seek care for a sore throat, then ask for blood work to test for HIV. The nurse should deal with the patient's concerns in the best way possible, then follow up when indicated.

INTERVIEWING THE PATIENT WITH SPECIAL NEEDS

Patients with special needs offer a particular challenge to the nurse during the interview. Although the goal of the interview and specific interviewing techniques remain the same, the process differs according to the patient's impairment. Conducting a successful assessment interview with the patient with special needs may require more time and effort than usual and often requires the help of an intermediary such as a family member or a friend of the patient. Remember that HIPAA laws require patient consent when an interpreter or other assistive individual is used.

THE PATIENT WITH IMPAIRED HEARING

Often, patients with impaired hearing will read lips, so it is important to remain within sight of the patient and face the patient when talking. When working with such a patient, ensure that the hearing aid is in working order and turned on. Background noise should be at a minimum because noise can be very distracting to the patient with a hearing aid. Even if an **intermediary**, or an individual who is a liaison between the patient and a member of the health care team, is with the patient to assist in communication, always face the patient and direct all communication to the patient (Figure 2-10). It is common for those speaking to a patient with impaired hearing to speak loudly or slowly; however, though well intentioned, such acts detract from the patient's ability to read lips. Tone and inflection of voice are lost to the patient with impaired hearing. However, other nonverbal cues such as facial expression and body movements can be used to convey the meaning of what is said.

Patients who have never had the ability to hear and those who have not heard for a long time may have speech that is difficult to understand. Often, the best approach to interviewing these patients is to allow additional time with them and to use a written form for gathering data. When communicating through writing, always remain with the patient to clarify questions and answers. Information can be reinforced with written instructions.

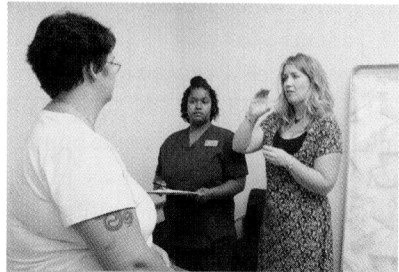

FIGURE 2-10 When working with a patient with impaired hearing, the interpreter needs to direct questions to the patient.

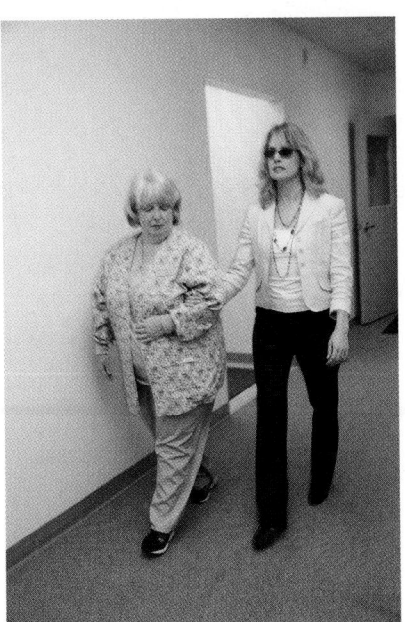

Figure 2-11 The nurse needs to inform the patient with impaired vision when a touch is to occur and ask permission.

The Patient with Impaired Vision

When interviewing a patient with a visual impairment, always look directly at the patient as if the patient were sighted. Because they cannot rely on visual cues, voice intonation, volume, and inflection are important to the visually impaired. It is common for those speaking to a visually impaired patient to speak loudly; this is insulting and can hinder communication.

Touch is especially important to the visually impaired; however, an unanticipated touch can be frightening. Before touching the patient, be certain to inform the patient and ask permission to touch (Figure 2-11). Advise the patient when you are entering or leaving the room and orient the patient to the immediate environment. Use clock hours to indicate position of items in relation to the patient. Those patients who are partially sighted may cling to the independence that their limited vision allows; offer assistance to the partially sighted and follow their cues or responses.

The Patient with Impaired Speech or Aphasia

When interviewing the patient who is speech impaired, ask simple questions that require "yes" and "no" answers and allow additional time for patient responses. Using this technique, it is often necessary to convert open-ended questions such as "How are you today?" to closed questions such as "Are you feeling well now?" You may need to repeat or rephrase the question if the patient did not understand. If you are unable to understand the patient's responses, use a written interview format, letter boards, or "yes" or "no" cards.

Even when all questions in the interview are asked and answered using closed questions, allow the patient the opportunity to contribute to the information gathering; for example, "I have asked all the questions I have to ask you for now. Would you like to tell me anything related to any of the questions I have asked?" then continue with, "Would you like to say anything else before we conclude the interview?"

When someone else is speaking for the patient, the nurse should speak and direct questions to the patient, not to the intermediary. If you ask the aphasic patient to complete a written format of the interview, remain with the patient to clarify questions and to explain data requirements.

The Patient Who Is Non-English-Speaking

Interviewing patients who do not speak English may require the assistance of an interpreter. Most health care agencies have a register of interpreters available. Sometimes the patient will bring a translator to the interview. The nurse should not

NURSING**TIP**

Caring for the Illiterate Patient

The illiterate patient is unable to complete or verify written assessment data. Therefore, alternative strategies are used when caring for the illiterate patient to ensure that education on treatment and follow-up is simple and clear. Some strategies to use include:

- Illustrated charts to describe procedures and treatments
- A picture of a clock to illustrate time
- Color-coded medications
- Patient recall on instructions to double-check accuracy
- Follow-up with home health care agency when indicated to ensure appropriate care

---

NURSING**TIP**

How to Use an Interpreter

1. Use a trained medical interpreter whenever possible.
2. When possible, allow the interpreter and patient a few minutes to converse before initiating the interview.
3. Instruct the interpreter to translate the patient's replies sentence by sentence, thus avoiding summarization. This will ensure that important information is not omitted.
4. Keep your questions brief. Inform the interpreter what information you are trying to obtain.
5. Maintain eye contact with the patient, not the interpreter, during the questioning and translating.
6. Observe the patient's nonverbal communication, being sensitive to cultural influences.
7. Be patient! Extra time needs to be allotted for this interview exchange.
8. When available, use preprinted questions and health care instructions in the patient's native language.

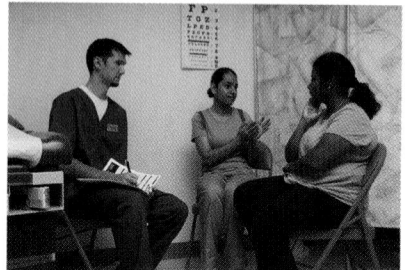

FIGURE 2-12 When using an interpreter, the nurse should pose questions directly to the patient, not to the interpreter.

assume that the translator can answer questions for the patient. It is important to direct interview questions to the patient and not to the interpreter (Figure 2-12).

Remember that pure translation from one language to another does not take into account dialects or **colloquialisms** (words and phrases particular to a community), which have the potential to offend someone. For example, the question "Are you pregnant?" when translated without taking into account colloquialisms may mean "Do you have intercourse outside of marriage?"

Pay special attention to nonverbal cues, especially facial expressions and body movements. Often, information that is lost in the translation to English can be gained through nonverbal cues. The use of signs, such as pointing, can be helpful in an emergency situation; however, a more complete interview should be deferred until an interpreter is present.

THE PATIENT WHO HAS A LOW LEVEL OF UNDERSTANDING

Interviewing the patient with a low IQ requires time and patience because the patient may require time to process questions and to formulate answers and may need clarification of the meaning or intent of questions. Hurrying may cause the patient to become confused, lose concentration, or to refuse to answer. It may be necessary to interview the patient's family or caregiver for supplemental information. Request permission from the patient to speak to someone else and respect the patient's right to be present during all phases of the interview. Always direct interview questions to the patient and allow the patient to request assistance from family members or the caregiver. Observe the interaction between the patient and the family or caregivers because nonverbal communication can provide valuable information about the patient's present health or illness state as well as about the relationship between the patient and the family member or primary caregiver.

THE PATIENT WHO IS CRYING

Patients may cry during the interview. On some occasions crying can be anticipated, such as when parents relate events that led to their child's death. Other times a patient may cry unexpectedly. The latter example affords an opportunity for you to gain information about something of importance to the patient by gently asking what is causing the emotional response. It is very important to show empathy and to allow the patient to cry. Offering tissues indicates to the patient that it is OK to cry and conveys a message of thoughtfulness. When the patient has regained composure, proceed with the interview.

The Patient Who Is Anxious and Angry

Patients and those who are speaking for patients in health care settings are frequently emotionally upset. For example, the parent of a sick child may be overwhelmed by events that led to the child's hospitalization. Emotional outbursts and crying are often the result of such stress. Allow the patient, family member, or significant other to express emotions. If it is obvious that the person being interviewed is holding back tears, give permission to express emotion with a simple statement such as, "I can see that you are upset; it's OK to cry."

When interviewing an obviously angry person, recognize and acknowledge the emotion. A natural instinct is to personalize the anger and become angry in return; instead, recognize the emotion and bring it to the patient's attention. "You appear very angry about something. Before we continue with the interview, please tell me about your feelings." Avoid statements such as "Take a moment to get hold of yourself," because this directive implies that the patient's feelings are not appropriate and should not be expressed. Acknowledging patients' emotions and giving them permission to express feelings will convey respect and enhance genuine communication.

The Patient Who Is Hostile

Before you begin the interview, review any documentation that might alert you to potential problems. Be especially cautious of those patients with a past history of violence or poor impulse control. Keep in mind that patients use hostile behavior because it gets them what they want. Hostility tends to be contagious. Do not reciprocate with anger and hostility.

You can minimize the risk of aggression through nonthreatening interventions such as limit setting and refocusing. Position yourself near an easily accessible exit. Do not turn your back on the patient and never allow the patient to walk behind you or come between you and the exit. Watch for signs of increasing tension in the patient (e.g., clenched fists, loud voice, angry tone of voice, narrowed eyes). Consider leaving the door to the room open to some degree to deter a potentially hostile patient.

Alert a colleague and security if the patient makes you nervous or anxious. Trust your instincts and remove yourself from potentially threatening and dangerous situations when necessary.

The Patient Who Is Sexually Aggressive

A sexually aggressive patient may act out during the interview. For example, the patient may stand very close to the nurse and say, "You have been so nice to me, I would like the chance to be nice to you." The nurse may counter this behavior by defining appropriate boundaries, sharing personal reactions, and refocusing the patient, for example, stating, "It makes me feel very uncomfortable when you stand this close to me. Let's get back to getting information to assist in your health care needs." It is important to set limits and to focus on tasks when dealing with sexually aggressive patients.

The Patient Who Is Under the Influence of Alcohol or Drugs

The patient who is under the influence of alcohol or drugs presents a unique challenge to the nurse. Depending on the quantity of alcohol consumed and the type of drugs ingested, the patient can have central nervous system (CNS) depression or the patient can be very disruptive with CNS stimulation. The patient's judgment may be impaired, which can lead to physical harm to those in the immediate environment. For this reason, when you have a violent or agitated patient, security personnel should be alerted and stationed nearby.

Patients under the influence of some drugs have been known to have superhuman strength and are capable of inflicting serious physical harm on themselves and others. To care for this person, place yourself at a safe distance, remain calm, and provide care in a nonthreatening manner.

THE PATIENT WHO IS VERY ILL

Patients who are very sick may not have the strength or ability to go through the entire interview process. Collect pertinent data from the patient and defer the remainder of the interview until later. If a patient is very sick, it may be necessary to interview a family member or significant other. Show respect for the patient by asking permission to do this and by allowing the patient to be present during the interview. Allow the patient to participate as much as possible in answering questions and giving information.

THE OLDER ADULT

Interviewing the older person may require additional time for question interpretation and patient responses. It may be necessary to schedule more than one interview for older patients because they may have multisystem changes or complaints, a weakened physical condition, or a cognitive impairment. It may be necessary to interview an older patient's family member or caregiver to assess the patient's past and present health or illness status. As in any interview situation, when the patient is assisted by another individual, include the patient and assess the quality of interaction between the two.

ASSESSMENT IN BRIEF

Effective Interviewing

- Be aware of personal beliefs and how these were acquired. Avoid imposing your beliefs on those you interview.
- Listen and observe. Attend to verbal and affective content as well as to nonverbal cues.
- Keep your attention focused on the patient. Do not listen with "half an ear." Do not think about other things when you are interviewing.
- Maintain eye contact with the patient as is appropriate for the patient's culture.
- Notice the patient's speech patterns and any recurring themes. Note any extra emphasis that the patient places on certain words or topics.

- Do not assume that you understand the meaning of all patient communications. Clarify frequently.
- Paraphrase and summarize occasionally to help patients organize their thinking, clarify issues, and begin to explore specific concerns more deeply.
- Allow for periods of silence.
- Remember that attitudes and feelings may be conveyed nonverbally.
- Consistently monitor your reactions to the patient's verbal and nonverbal messages.
- Avoid being judgmental or critical. Avoid preaching.
- Avoid the use of nontherapeutic interviewing techniques.

REVIEW QUESTIONS

1. Which of the following situations is an appropriate use of motivational interviewing?
   a. Encouraging a patient to get blood drawn to check critical lab values
   b. Tapering a patient's Dilantin dose so he or she can be free of medication
   c. Demonstrating to a patient how to check his pulse
   d. Counseling an obese patient on weight loss
   The correct answer is (d).

2. The goal of the Privacy Rule of the HIPAA is to:
   a. Ensure that the patient's insurance company has access to the patient's medical record
   b. Guarantee the patient the right to his or her medical record
   c. Protect the patient's medical record from collaborators in university settings
   d. Safeguard e-mail communications the patient has with an employer regarding health care matters

   The correct answer is (b).

3. At which stage of the interview process does the nurse-patient relationship get established?
   a. Joining stage
   b. Working stage
   c. Termination stage
   d. Reflective stage

   The correct answer is (a).

4. Which distance is the most appropriate to use when a certified diabetic nurse educator teaches dietary principles to 30 newly diagnosed diabetics in a classroom setting?
   a. Intimate   c. Social
   b. Personal   d. Public

   The correct answer is (d).

5. A patient is telling you about her fifth miscarriage at her fertility clinic visit. She becomes silent and starts to cry. You touch her hand, nod to her, and say "uh-huh." You have used the communication technique of:
   a. Making observations   c. Facilitating
   b. Clarifying   d. Interpreting

   The correct answer is (c).

6. The nurse tells the patient, "Let's look at the environment in which you are located when you have an asthma attack and see if we can identify your triggers." This statement exemplifies the communication technique of:
   a. Confronting   c. Collaborating
   b. Informing   d. Presenting reality

   The correct answer is (c).

7. The nursing assessment interview is:
   a. More problem focused than the medical interview
   b. Involves the patient as the only source of health care information
   c. A purposeful, time-limited verbal interaction between the nurse and the patient
   d. Performed only on the patient's initial visit to a health care facility

   The correct answer is (c).

8. With which of the following patients should the nurse use mostly closed questions?
   a. Patient with impaired hearing
   b. Patient with impaired vision
   c. Non-English-speaking patient
   d. Aphasic patient

   The correct answer is (d).

9. Which communication techniques are attempts made by the nurse to accurately receive, process, and respond to patient messages?
   a. Listening responses   c. Verbal responses
   b. Action responses   d. Active listening

   The correct answer is (a).

10. The nurse tells the patient who was just diagnosed with colon cancer, "It's OK to cry. Most people who are given that diagnosis react in a similar fashion." The nurse used the communication technique of:
    a. Presenting reality   c. Offering false reassurance
    b. Normalizing   d. Advising

    The correct answer is (b).

Visit the Estes online companion resource at
www.delmar.cengage.com
for additional content and study aids.
Click on Online Companions, then select
the Nursing discipline.

REFERENCES

Bradley, J. C., & Edinberg, M. A. (1990). *Communication in the nursing context* (3rd ed.). East Norwalk, CT: Appleton & Lange.

Cormier, W. H., & Cormier, L. S. (1991). *Interviewing strategies for helpers: Fundamental skills and cognitive behavioral interventions* (3rd ed.). Pacific Grove, CA: Brooks/Cole.

Ivey, A. (1994). *Intentional interviewing and counseling: Facilitating client development in a multicultural society* (3rd ed.). Pacific Grove, CA: Brooks/Cole.

Northouse, P. G., & Northouse, L. L. (1992). *Health communication: Strategies for professionals* (2nd ed.). Stamford, CT: Appleton & Lange.

BIBLIOGRAPHY

Antai-Otong, D. (2007). *Nurse-client communication: A life span approach.* Sudbury, MA: Jones & Bartlett.

Arnold, E. C., & Boggs, K. U. (2007). *Interpersonal relationships: Professional communication skills for nurses* (5th ed.). Philadelphia: Saunders.

Beckham, N. (2007). Motivational interviewing with hazardous drinkers. *Journal of the American Academy of Nurse Practitioners, 19*(2), 103–110.

Berry, J. A., & Stewart, A. J. (2006). Communicating with the deaf during the health examination visit. *The Journal for Nurse Practitioners, 2*(8), 509–515.

Colon-Emeric, C. S., Ammarell, N., Bailey, D., Corazzini, K., Utley-Smith, Q., Lekan-Rutledge, D., et al. (2006). Patterns of medical and nursing staff communications in nursing homes: Implications and insights from complexity science. *Qualitative Health Research, 16*(2), 173–188.

Davis, T. C., Wolf, M. S., Bass, P. F., Thompson, B. A., Tilson, H. H., Neuberger, M., et al. (2006). Literacy and misunderstanding prescription drug labels. *Annals of Internal Medicine, 145*(12), 887–894.

Herdener, M., & Vezeu, T. (2005). Low literacy in patients: Implications for the nurse practitioner. *The American Journal for Nurse Practitioners, 9*(9), 21–35.

Huffman, M. (2007). Health coaching: A new and exciting technique to enhance patient self-management and improve outcomes. *Home Healthcare Nurse, 25*(4), 271–274.

Joint Commission Resources, Inc. (2006). *The Joint Commission guide to improving staff communication.* Oakbrook Terrace, IL: Author.

Lieu, C. C., Sadler, G. R., Fullerton, J. T., & Stohlmann, P. D. (2007). Communication strategies for nurses interacting with deaf patients. *MEDSURG Nursing, 16*(4), 239–245.

Makoul, G., Zick, A., & Green, M. (2007). An evidence-based perspective on greetings in medical encounters. *Archives of Internal Medicine, 167*(11), 1172–1176.

Marquardt, P., & Vezeau, T. (2007). Motivational interviewing: The link between healthy choices and healthy patients. *The American Journal for Nurse Practitioners, 11*(8), 21–31.

McManus, A. J. (2008). Creating an LGBT-friendly practice: Practical implications for NPs. *The American Journal for Nurse Practitioners, 12*(4), 29–38.

Miller, W. R., & Rollnick, S. (2002). *Motivational interviewing: Preparing people to change addictive behavior* (2nd ed.). New York: Guilford Press.

Nelson, J. E., Mercado, A. F., Camhi, S. L., Tandon, N., Wallenstein, S., August, G. I., et al. (2007). Communication about chronic critical illness. *Archives of Internal Medicine, 167*(22), 2509–2515.

Riley, J. B. (2007). *Communication in nursing* (6th ed.). St. Louis: Mosby.

Tamparo, C. D., & Lindh, W. Q. (2008). *Therapeutic communication for health care.* Clifton Park, NY: Delmar Cengage Learning.

Wall, R. J., Curtis, J. R., & Engelberg, R. A. (2007). Family satisfaction in the ICU: Difference between families of survivors and nonsurvivors. *Chest, 132*(5), 1425–1433.

Wright, L., & Leahey, M. (2005). *Nurses and families: A guide to family assessment and intervention* (4th ed.). Philadelphia: F. A. Davis.

WEB SITES

Free Translation:
http://www.freetranslation.com

Gay, Lesbian, Bisexual, and Transgender Health Access Project:
http://www.glbthealth.org

I Love Languages:
http://www.ilovelanguages.com

National Coalition for LGBT Health:
http://www.lgbthealth.net

Registry of Interpreters for the Deaf:
http://www.rid.org

Language Translation Services:
http://www.worldlingo.com

CHAPTER 3

The Complete Health History Including Documentation

COMPETENCIES

1. State the purpose of the four different types of health history and provide an example of when each is used.

2. Identify the components of the complete health history.

3. Describe how to assess the 10 characteristics of a chief complaint.

4. Diagram a patient's genogram correctly.

5. Demonstrate sensitivity to patients of different races, religions, ethnic backgrounds, sexual orientations, and socioeconomic status when conducting a health history.

6. Conduct a complete health history on ill and well patients, and record the data.

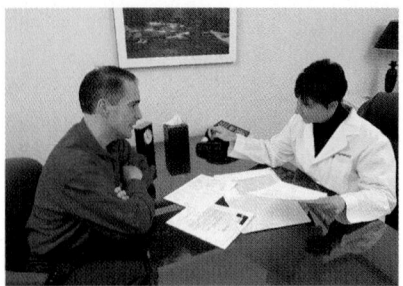

FIGURE 3-1 **The nurse conducts the health history as the first step in the nursing assessment.**

The health history is usually the first step of patient assessment (Figure 3-1). It is the collection of subjective information on the patient's health status from the well or ill patient and from other sources. The health history can provide information on a patient's health status as well as social, emotional, physical, cultural, developmental, and spiritual identities. Patient strengths and areas of need can be identified. This information is combined with the physical assessment findings to guide the nurse in formulating nursing diagnoses, which serve as the foundation for the plan of care for the patient.

The health history interview provides the mutual opportunity for the nurse and patient to become more comfortable with each other. The patient usually feels more at ease with the collection of health history data than with the physical contact necessary for the assessment. For this reason, the health history is usually performed prior to the physical assessment. The health history can be broadly or narrowly focused depending on the patient's needs and physical condition. The health history can also take different foci depending on whether it is conducted by a generalist or a specialist. Analysis of the information from the patient in the health history provides the basis for planning the health care education needed by the patient and indicates areas needing attention in the physical assessment. The written health history also serves as part of the legal documentation of the patient's health status and is a means of communicating information to other health care team members. It also serves as a mechanism on which insurance claims are accepted or denied.

Refer to Chapter 2 for communication techniques and strategies for dealing with patients who have special needs.

TYPES OF HEALTH HISTORY

There are four types of health history: complete, episodic, interval or follow-up, and emergency. The **complete health history**, described in this text, is a comprehensive history of the patient's past and present health status and covers many facets of a patient's life. It is usually gathered during a patient's initial visit to a health care facility on a nonemergency basis and upon admission to the hospital. The **episodic health history** is shorter and is specific to the patient's current reason for seeking health care. For example, the patient who seeks care for a sore throat and fever would have an episodic health history taken. The **interval** or **follow-up health history** builds on a preceding visit to a health care facility. It documents the patient's recovery from illness, such as the sore throat and fever, or progress from a prior visit. Finally, the **emergency health history** is elicited from

REFLECTIVE THINKING

Problems Encountered during History Taking

- What would you do if you were conducting a complete health history and the patient stated, "I don't feel like talking right now"?
- What would you do if the patient said, "These questions are all too personal! Why are you asking me all of this?"
- The young teenager seeking birth control tells you, "I hope you won't tell my mother about the abortion I had." How would you respond to this patient?

the patient and other sources in an emergency situation. Only information that is required immediately to treat the emergent need of the patient is gathered; after the life-threatening condition is no longer present, the nurse may elicit a more comprehensive history from the patient.

PREPARING FOR THE HEALTH HISTORY

Taking a complete health history with a patient may require 30 to 60 minutes; inform the patient before the interview starts of the amount of time that will be required. If the health history is not completed within the allotted time, it may be best to continue it later to avoid fatiguing the patient. If the patient will be spending some time in the health care facility, then additional information can be obtained during routine nursing tasks such as bathing or assessing vital signs. Some health care agencies request that the literate patient complete detailed health history forms prior to the interview; in this instance, the nurse can validate the responses during the health history and save valuable time. In addition, information can often be obtained from prior medical records, and then updated during the interview.

COMPUTERIZED HEALTH HISTORY

Some health care facilities use computerized health histories. These can be of two types: patient generated and health care provider generated. In patient-generated health histories, the patient responds on the computer to various questions, and then reviews information with the nurse for completeness. This type of computerized health history favors patients who may be embarrassed to verbally report specific information or those who "freeze" when asked for detailed information. When using a health care provider-generated health history, the nurse completes the information on screen after the patient interview. Frequently, these programs are user-friendly and time saving.

NURSING**TIP**

Legal Documents

At the initial patient interview in the inpatient as well as the outpatient setting, it is important to ask the patient whether he or she has a living will, an advance medical directive, and durable power of attorney for health care. These documents should be obtained from the patient at the outset and incorporated into the health care record.

NURSING**TIP**

Eliciting Information from Reluctant Patients

Some patients may seem reluctant to answer your questions regarding birthplace. Undocumented immigrants may fear deportation if they are identified in the health care system, especially if they are seriously ill. Remind these patients that you are there solely to assist them with their health care needs, and encourage them to provide accurate information to assist you in appropriate diagnosis and treatment because many diseases are specific to geographic locations.

NURSING**CHECKLIST**

General Approach to the Health History

1. Present with a professional appearance. Avoid extremes in dress so that your appearance does not become a hindrance to information gathering.
2. Ensure an appropriate environment, for example, good lighting, comfortable temperature, lack of noise and distractions, and adequate privacy. Refer to Chapter 2 for additional information.
3. Sit facing the patient at eye level, with the patient in a chair or on a bed. Ensure that the patient is as comfortable as possible because obtaining the health history can be a lengthy process.
4. Ask the patient whether there are any questions about the interview before it is started.
5. Avoid the use of medical jargon. Use terms the patient can understand.
6. Reserve asking intimate and personal questions for when rapport is established.
7. Remain flexible in obtaining the health history. It does not have to be obtained in the exact order it is presented in this chapter or on institutional forms.
8. Remind the patient that all information will be treated confidentially.

IDENTIFYING INFORMATION

The patient usually completes the identifying information prior to the actual physical examination.

TODAY'S DATE

Record the month, day, year, and time that the health history is recorded. If the health history is not written immediately, document the time that the health history was taken and the time when it is recorded.

BIOGRAPHICAL DATA

The following biographical data are usually requested for the patient record:

Patient name	Work address
Address	Work phone number
Phone number	Insurance
Date of birth	Usual source of health care
Birthplace	Source of referral
Social security number or other identifying number	Emergency contact
Occupation	

THE COMPLETE HEALTH HISTORY ASSESSMENT TOOL

All elements of a complete health history are outlined in the following pages. Two examples of the complete health history are given, one for the well patient and one for the ill patient.

SOURCE AND RELIABILITY OF INFORMATION

Usually the adult patient is the historian (Figure 3-2). However, in some instances, such as trauma, the historian may be someone other than the patient. Note the name of the historian as well as the relationship between the historian and the patient.

In addition, assess the reliability of the historian. Consider the mental state of the historian because emotions and certain medical conditions can influence the retelling of events. For example, the information provided by a patient with severe Alzheimer's disease may not be accurate. Note if an interpreter was used.

PATIENT PROFILE

The **patient profile** provides demographics that may be linked to health status. Note the patient's age, gender, and race because many diseases are linked to these characteristics. Also note the patient's marital status, as this may provide clues to support systems.

REASON FOR SEEKING HEALTH CARE AND CHIEF COMPLAINT

The **reason for seeking health care** is the reason for the patient's visit and is usually focused on health promotion. The **chief complaint** (CC) is the **sign** (objective finding) or **symptom** (subjective finding) that causes the patient to seek health care. The patient may present with multiple chief complaints for a single

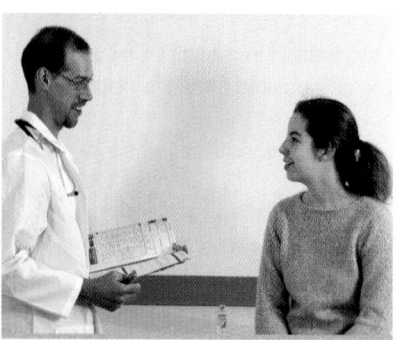

FIGURE 3-2 The nurse needs to note the source of the patient health history. When working with adult patients, the patient is usually the historian.

visit. The reason for seeking health care and the CC should be recorded as direct quotes from the patient.

"What concern(s) bring you here today?" **or**
"What caused you to seek health care today?"
"How long has this condition been concerning you?"

PRESENT HEALTH AND HISTORY OF THE PRESENT ILLNESS

If the patient is seeking health promotion, the present health states the patient's current health status.

The **history of the present illness** (HPI) is a chronological account of the patient's CC and the events surrounding it. The chronology can be taken in one of two ways: from the current state of the problem back to its origin (reverse chronology), or from the origin of the symptom leading to the current status (forward chronology). Either approach is acceptable as long as it is consistent with subsequent documentation of chronological events. Usually the patient describes one or two signs or symptoms that are abnormal and their progression. Allow the patient to give the detailed HPI without interruption, and then ask questions if information is incomplete.

"Describe the condition that you are experiencing from the earliest time that it occurred to the present." (forward chronology)

Ten characteristics of each CC can be ascertained for a complete HPI:

1. Location
2. Radiation
3. Quality
4. Quantity
5. Associated manifestations
6. Aggravating factors
7. Alleviating factors
8. Setting
9. Timing
10. Meaning and impact

Note that some CCs may not have all 10 qualifiers; hoarseness, for example, may not be characterized by quantity. The CC of headache will be used to demonstrate the use of these 10 characteristics.

Location

Location refers to the primary area where the symptom occurs or originates.

"Where does your head hurt? Can you point to the location of the pain?"
"Is it in one location in your head or spread out (diffuse or localized)?"
"Have you ever experienced this type of headache before? When?"
"Does this current headache differ from headaches you have had in the past?"

Radiation

Radiation is the spreading of the symptom or other CC from its original location to another part of the body. The areas of radiation can be diagnostic for specific pathologies.

"Does the headache move to another part of your head or body? If so, where?"
"Is the pain presently radiating?"
"Describe how the pain feels in the area to which it radiated."

Quality

The quality of the CC describes the way it feels to the patient. Use the patient's own terms to describe the quality of the CC. If the patient is having difficulty describing

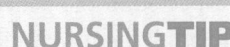

pain, for example, suggest some quality terms such as *gnawing, pounding, burning, stabbing, pinching, aching, throbbing,* and *crushing.*

"What does the headache feel like?"
"What word would you use to describe it?"
"Is the pain deep or closer to the skin (superficial)?"

Quantity

Quantity depicts the severity, volume, number, or extent of the CC. The patient may refer to the CC with such terms as *minor, moderate,* or *severe,* and *small, medium,* or *large.* While this terminology is important to the HPI, this information is subjective and is, therefore, difficult to quantify. If the patient consistently uses the same terms, then a relative scale can be used to assess whether the CC is improving or becoming worse as reported by the patient.

Another mechanism that can be used to assess the quantity of pain is a numerical scale, known as the **Visual Analog Scale**, which rates pain from 0 (*no pain*) to 10 (*worst pain possible*). Refer to Chapter 9 for additional pain intensity scales.

"Using a scale of 0 to 10, where 0 represents no pain and 10 is the worst pain that you can imagine, rate the pain that you are having now."
"When was the last time that your headache was at this level?"
"Has the severity of the headache changed? In what way?"
"Has the headache interfered with your normal daily activities? How?"

Associated Manifestations

The signs and symptoms that accompany the CC are termed **associated manifestations**. Rarely does a CC occur without affecting other components of the involved system or another body system. Positive findings are those associated manifestations that the patient has experienced along with the CC. Negative findings, also called **pertinent negatives**, are those manifestations expected in the patient with a suspected pathology but which are denied by the patient. If the patient does not mention specific signs or symptoms that might be present with a given illness, ask whether they are present. Document both positive findings and pertinent negatives because both give clues to the patient's condition. For example, a patient with headaches may have nausea, vomiting, and diaphoresis as positive associated manifestations. Photophobia and phonophobia are pertinent negatives because they might be present in a patient with headaches but are absent in this patient at this time; lack of these associated manifestations may lead to a different diagnosis.

"Besides your headache, are you experiencing any additional symptoms? What are they?"
"Have these symptoms occurred before? Do they always occur when you have a headache?"

Aggravating Factors

Those factors that worsen the severity of the CC are the **aggravating factors.**

"Have you done anything that makes your headache worse? What?"
"When you stopped this activity, did the pain lessen?"

Alleviating Factors

Alleviating factors are events that decrease the severity of the CC.

"Have you done anything that decreases the severity of the headache? What?"
"Has this worked in the past?"
"When you stopped this activity, did your headache become more severe?"

Setting

The setting in which the CC occurs can provide valuable information about the course of the HPI. The setting can be the actual physical environment in which the patient is located, the mental state of the patient, or some activity in which the patient was involved. The patient may or may not be aware of any link between the setting and the occurrence of the CC. For instance, the odor of some chemicals can induce headaches in some individuals.

"What were you doing when the headache started? Where were you?"
"Has this activity precipitated the headache on other occasions?"
"Has the headache occurred before in that setting? How many times?"
"What were you thinking about when the headache occurred?"
"Has the headache occurred before when you were feeling this way?"

Timing

The timing used to describe a CC has three elements: onset, duration, and frequency. Onset refers to the time at which the CC begins and is usually described as gradual or sudden. Duration depicts the amount of time in which the CC is present. *Continuous* and *intermittent* are terms that can be used to describe the duration of a CC. When possible, the duration of the CC should be stated in specific time increments, such as minutes, hours, or days. Frequency describes the number of times the CC occurs and how often it develops (e.g., number of times per day, season of year).

"When did the headache first start? How long did the headache last?"
"Did the headache come on suddenly or gradually?"
"Is the pain continuous or intermittent? If intermittent, how much time elapsed between episodes?"
"When was the last time you experienced a headache? Is the pain different in any way from the first time that you experienced it?"
"How often does the headache occur in a week? In a month?"
"Have you detected a pattern to the headache's occurrence?"

Meaning and Impact

The last two pieces of information needed in the HPI are the meaning or significance of the CC to the patient and the impact that the CC has on the patient. For example, the patient may be concerned because his or her father started having headaches at his or her age, and he was diagnosed with a brain tumor.

Second, the impact that the CC has on the patient's lifestyle should be investigated. For example, consider the elderly patient who complains of minor headache but admits to canceling routine activities; in this case, the condition is presented as mild, but its effects are serious.

"What does it mean to you to have these headaches?"
"How do you see the headaches affecting your lifestyle?"

PAST HEALTH HISTORY

The **past health history** (PHH) or past medical history (PMH) provides information on the patient's health status from birth to the present. The patient may think you are ignoring the reason for seeking health care. The following statements can ease the transition:

"I will get back to the reason for your visit today in a few minutes. Now I would like to ask some questions related to your health in the past."
"Sometimes the reason for an illness is connected with your past health. For this reason, let's discuss your past health."

Medical History

The medical history comprises all medical problems that the patient has experienced during adulthood and their **sequelae**, or aftermath. Chronic illnesses as well as serious episodic illnesses are included. Forward or reverse chronology can be used to describe the medical history as long as the approach is consistent with the chronological format in the HPI. If the patient denies medical illnesses, rephrase your questions. Some patients may discount "a little high blood pressure" as being insignificant.

"Are you presently under the supervision of a health care provider for any medical illness?" **or**

"Have you ever been diagnosed as having an illness? What was it?"

"When was the illness diagnosed?"

"Who diagnosed this problem?"

"What is the current treatment for this problem?"

"Do you follow the prescribed treatment? Do you have any difficulty following the prescribed treatment?"

"Have you ever been hospitalized for this illness? Where? When? For what period of time? What was the treatment? What was your condition after the treatment?"

"Have you ever experienced any complications (sequelae) from this disease? What were they? How were they treated?"

Surgical History

Record a complete account of each surgical procedure, both major and minor, including the year performed, hospital, physician, and sequelae, if known.

"Have you ever had surgery? What type?"

"Who was your physician at the time?"

"When, where, and by whom was the surgery performed?"

"Were you hospitalized? For what period of time?"

"Were there any complications? How were they treated?"

"Are you currently receiving any treatment related to this surgery?"

"Have you ever had an adverse effect from anesthesia?"

Allergies

Carefully explore all patient allergies, which may include medications, animals, insect bites, foods, and environmental allergens. Allergies are usually written in a conspicuous location in red ink on the patient's chart in order to stand out.

"Are you allergic to any medications? Animals? Foods? Insect bites? Bee stings?"

"Are you allergic to anything in the environment?"

"Are you allergic to anything that you touch?"

"What symptoms do you get when you are exposed to this substance?"

"What treatment do you use? Is it effective?"

"Have you experienced any complications from the allergies? Which?"

"Have you ever seen an allergist for this problem? What happened?"

"Do you carry an EpiPen with you?" (for patients with life-threatening allergies, such as bee stings)

Medications

Past and present consumption of medications, both prescription and over the counter (OTC), can affect the patient's current health status.

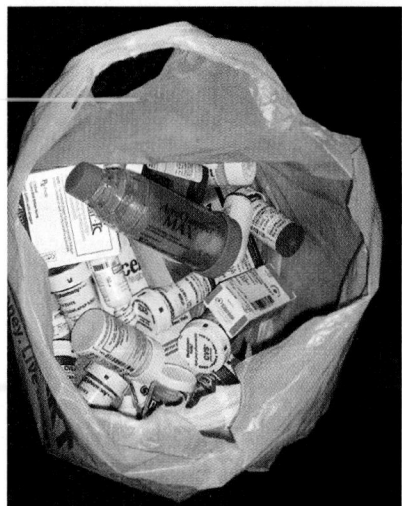

FIGURE 3-3 **Patients should be encouraged to bring to their health care visit all the substances that they take, both prescription and OTC agents.**

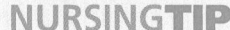

NURSING**TIP**

Obtaining an Accurate Medication History

Frequently, the patient discounts OTC medications such as aspirin, acetaminophen, ibuprofen, vitamins, cathartics, enemas, douches, cold remedies, and antacids. Ask the patient whether such products are used, because they can adversely interact with prescribed medications and with one another. Also, women frequently overlook birth control pills; keep this in mind when interviewing women of childbearing age.

The outcome of the medication history may point to a need for patient teaching. If contact is made with the patient prior to the health care visit, ask the patient to bring in all medications currently being taken (Figure 3-3).

PRESCRIPTION MEDICATION.

"What prescription medications are you currently taking? Who prescribed them?" **and**

"What prescription medications have you taken in the past? Who prescribed them?"

"What is the dose? How often do you take this medication?"

"How do you take this medication (e.g., pills, liquid, suppository, drops, inhaler, cream, ointment, injection)?"

"How long have you been taking this medication?"

"Have you ever experienced any side effects with this medication?"

"Have you ever had an allergic reaction to this medication? What happened?"

"Tell me the purpose of these medications."

OVER-THE-COUNTER MEDICATION.

"Do you currently take any over-the-counter medications? Which ones?"

"Why do you take this medication?"

"Do you take any home remedies? Which ones? For what purpose?"

Repeat all but the first and last questions from the *Prescription Medication* section.

"Do you ever take aspirin, acetaminophen, ibuprofen, antacids, calcium supplements, nutritional or herbal supplements, vitamins, or laxatives? Do you douche? Administer enemas? Do you take allergy pills or cold medications?" (If yes, repeat all but the first and last questions of the previous section.)

"Do you consume any probiotics? Which? How much? How often?"

GENERAL QUESTIONS.

"How long do you save unused drugs?"

"How do you dispose of unused drugs?"

"Where do you keep or store your medications?"

"Do you ever share medications or needles with another person? Who? For what reason? What drug do you share?"

"Do you have any questions concerning your medications?"

"Do you ever take more than the prescribed or recommended amount of prescription or OTC medication?"

Communicable Diseases

Communicable diseases can have a grave impact on the individual as well as on society. Some communicable diseases generate enough of a concern to the community that they are reportable to the public health department. The most talked

LIFE 360°

Over-the-Counter Products

The surgical nurse is conducting a preoperative history on a patient. The patient takes medication for hypertension, diabetes, a seizure disorder, overactive bladder, and osteoporosis. The patient tells the nurse that she also goes to the natural food store, where she purchases four other supplements. The patient cannot recall the names of the products, but she knows they are to help her mood, her weight, her stiff joints, and her immune system. How should the surgical nurse proceed?

NURSING**TIP**

Herbal Products

Herbal products are consumed by more of the American population than ever before. Whether to improve health or combat illness and pain, this branch of complementary and alternative medicine deserves the nurse's attention. Glucosamine, chondroitin, ephedra, black cohosh, and St. John's wort are just a few of the many herbal products that patients ingest. Since these products are considered dietary supplements in the United States, they are not held to the same level of scrutiny and accountability as medications. Different brands of the same herbal product can have varying levels of potency and purity. Because many people consider these products to be natural, patients rarely consider the possibility of herbal products interacting adversely with one another or with prescription medications. For this reason, patients need to be asked at every encounter which OTC herbal products are being consumed.

about communicable disease at present is human immunodeficiency virus (HIV), the virus responsible for acquired immune deficiency syndrome (AIDS). In recent years, there has also been a major focus on hepatitis C and the growing number of patients diagnosed with it. There is substantial value in asking the patient about possible exposure to communicable diseases, because pathology may not manifest itself until many years after exposure.

"Have you ever been diagnosed with an infectious or communicable disease? Which one(s)?"

"What were your symptoms?"

"How were you treated?"

"Did you have any complications? What were they? Were there any permanent consequences?"

"Have you ever had gonorrhea, syphilis, chlamydia, herpes, or other sexually transmitted diseases?"

"Have you ever had diphtheria, tetanus, pertussis (whooping cough), or tuberculosis?" (If yes, repeat the second, third, and fourth questions from above.)

"Have you ever had hepatitis?" (If yes, repeat the second, third, and fourth questions.)

"Have you ever been told that you are HIV positive?" (If yes, repeat the second, third, and fourth questions.)

"Have you ever been told that you have AIDS?" (If yes, repeat the second, third, and fourth questions.)

"Do you have any tattoos? Where were they done?"

"Do you have any body piercings? Where were they done?"

"Have you ever been exposed to someone who had a communicable disease? Which disease(s)?"

Injuries and Accidents

A patient's injury and accident history can reveal a pattern that is amenable to health promotion. For example, an elderly woman who sustains an injury from slipping on throw rugs in the home would be a candidate for health teaching on maintaining a safe home environment.

"Have you ever been involved in an accident?" **or** "Have you ever been injured in any way?"

"What occurred? Did you lose consciousness?"

"Did you take any precautionary measures? What were they?"
"Were you hospitalized? For how long?"
"Were there any complications? What were they?"
"Were there any long-term effects from this injury/accident?"
"Have you ever sustained an injury in a car accident? Describe."
"Have you ever had a broken bone? Stitches? Burns?"
"Have you ever been assaulted? Raped? Shot? Stabbed?"
"Have you ever been bitten by an animal or insect (e.g., brown recluse spider, tick)?"

Special Needs

The awareness of any cognitive, physical (Figure 3-4), or psychosocial disability is essential to providing individualized health care to a patient. A patient with Down syndrome, a paraplegic, and a sociopathic patient all have unique needs. These patients may receive less than optimal health care if their particular limitations are not identified and considered when planning treatment.

"Do you have any disability or special need? Describe."
"What type of limitations does this disability/special need place on you?"
"What strategies do you use to limit the effect the disability/special need has on your lifestyle?"
"What support systems help you cope with this disability/special need?"
"Does your disability/special need place an extra financial burden on you? How do you handle that?"

Blood Transfusions

The chance of contracting an infectious disease from a blood transfusion is greatest in patients who receive a large number of transfusions, such as hemophiliacs, oncology patients, and trauma victims. The American Red Cross and other organizations are continuously updating their screening tools and history-taking procedures to protect the nation's blood supply. Still, the recipient assumes some risk with every transfusion. Tests are available to screen blood for hepatitis, HIV, and West Nile virus, among others. Unfortunately, no approved diagnostic test is available to screen blood for malaria and other infectious diseases.

"Have you ever received a blood transfusion (whole blood or any of its components)? When?"
"Why did you receive this blood product?"
"What quantity did you receive?"
"Did you experience any reaction to this blood product? What was it?"

Childhood Illnesses

Rarely are adults familiar with a complete history of their childhood illnesses. Ask the patient about specific childhood diseases by name.

"Have you ever had any of the following illnesses: varicella (chickenpox), diphtheria, pertussis (whooping cough), measles, mumps, rubella, polio, rheumatic fever, or scarlet fever?" (This question is eliminated if previously asked during the communicable diseases section.)
"How old were you when the illness occurred?"
"Was an actual diagnosis made? By whom?"
"Were there any complications? What were they?"

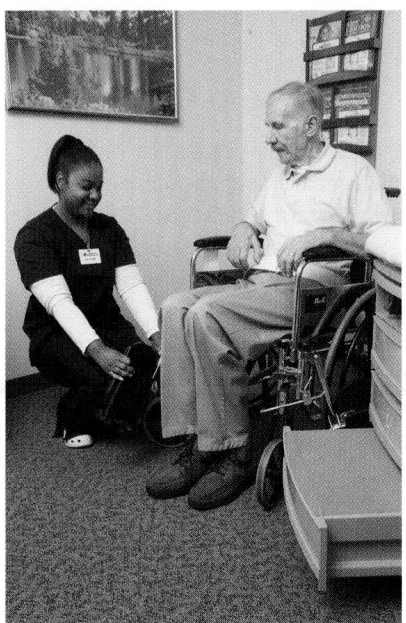

FIGURE 3-4 Patients with physical special needs, such as a wheelchair, need to have this documented in their health history.

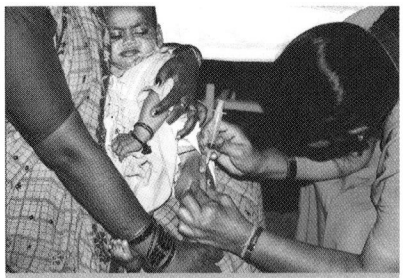

FIGURE 3-5 **Most immunizations are given as injections in childhood.** *Courtesy of WHO/P. Virot.*

Immunizations

The history of immunizations is closely tied to childhood illnesses. Most immunizations are received in childhood (Figure 3-5), though a few may be given in the adult years. The adult patient may not recall the exact dates when the immunizations were given, as with childhood illnesses, but will be aware that "I received everything that I should have." Routine immunizations are also associated with different groups. Health care workers are frequently given the hepatitis B vaccine. Every winter, the adult population, especially those over age 65 and those with chronic diseases, are encouraged to receive the influenza vaccine. In addition, travelers to underdeveloped areas of the world receive numerous vaccines prior to visiting specific regions.

"What immunizations have you received since birth? When?"

"Did you experience any reactions to the immunizations? What were they? Were there any complications?"

"As a child, did you receive the following immunizations: measles-mumps-rubella (MMR), polio, smallpox, diphtheria-pertussis-tetanus (DPT), *Haemophilus influenzae* type b (Hib), hepatitis B?"

"Have you received any immunizations as an adult: varicella, hepatitis A, hepatitis B, influenza, tetanus, pneumococcal, meningococcal, HPV (human papilloma virus [Gardasil]), shingles (Zostavax)?"

"When was your last TB test and what was the result?"

"If born outside the United States, have you received the Bacillus Calmette-Guérin (BCG) vaccine?"

"Have you ever received any other immunizations, perhaps prior to visiting a specific geographical region (malaria, cholera, typhoid fever, yellow fever)?"

FAMILY HEALTH HISTORY

The family health history (FHH) records the health status of the patient, as well as that of immediate blood relatives. At a minimum, the history needs to contain the age and health status of the patient, spouse, children, siblings, and the patient's parents. Ideally, the patient's grandparents, aunts, and uncles should be incorporated into the history as well. Documentation of this information is done in two parts: the genogram, or family tree, and a list of familial diseases. The figure demonstrates the appropriate method for constructing the **genogram**.

The second component of the family health history is the report of occurrences of familial or genetic diseases. Such information is crucial to the patient and may not have been revealed previously because some familial illnesses do not occur in every generation. The pertinent negative findings are documented in the family health history below the genogram. See the genogram below.

You may want to preface the FHH questions with the following statement:

"Different diseases tend to run in families. I would like to ask you about your family and their health to gain a better understanding of your background."

You can then continue with questions about the FHH:

"Tell me about the members of your family: spouse, children, siblings, and parents. How old are they?"

"Do any of these individuals have any medical illnesses or diseases? What are they?"

"Have there been any deaths in your immediate family? What was the cause of death? How old was this person at the time of death?"

"What is the current age of each of the following members of your family: maternal and paternal grandparents, aunts, uncles?"

Repeat questions 2 and 3.

"Has anyone in your family ever had any of the following illnesses: heart disease, sudden cardiac death before age 50, hypertension, stroke, tuberculosis, diabetes mellitus, cancer, kidney disease, blood

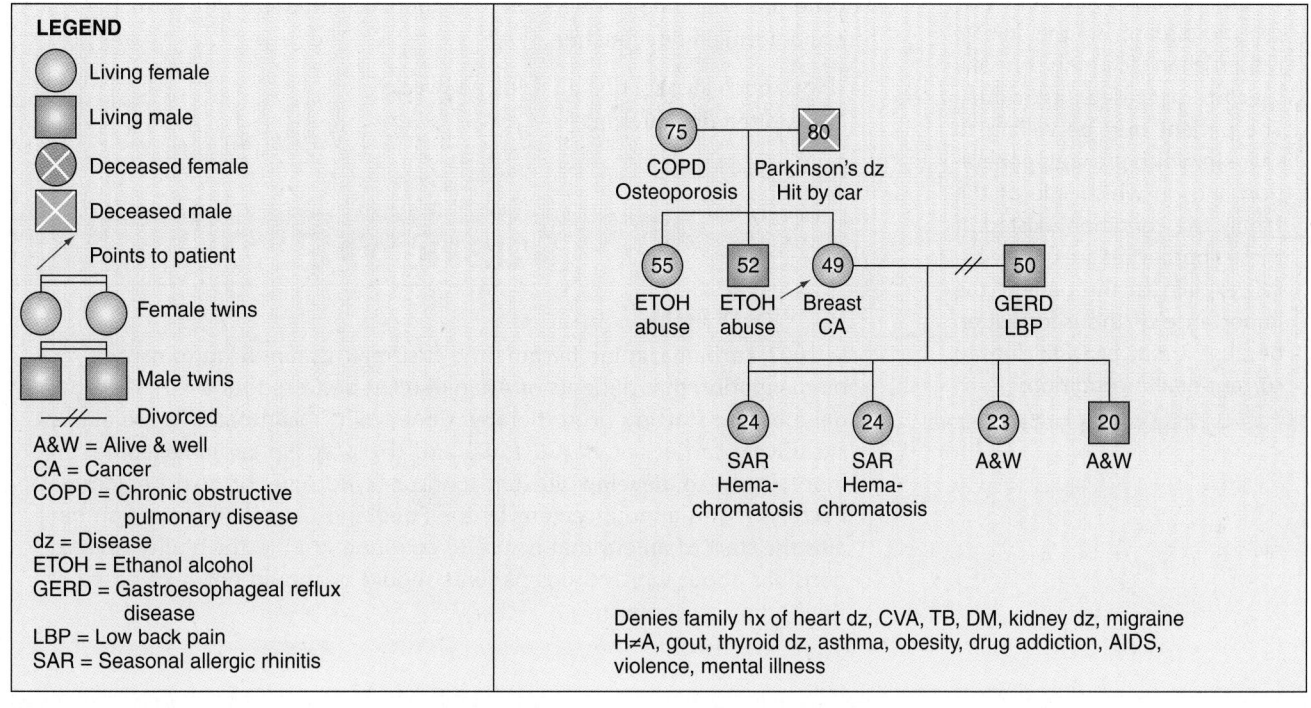

LEGEND
- ○ Living female
- ☐ Living male
- ⊗ Deceased female
- ☒ Deceased male
- / Points to patient
- ○○ Female twins
- ☐☐ Male twins
- —//— Divorced

A&W = Alive & well
CA = Cancer
COPD = Chronic obstructive pulmonary disease
dz = Disease
ETOH = Ethanol alcohol
GERD = Gastroesophageal reflux disease
LBP = Low back pain
SAR = Seasonal allergic rhinitis

75 COPD Osteoporosis — 80 Parkinson's dz Hit by car

55 ETOH abuse | 52 ETOH abuse | 49 Breast CA —//— 50 GERD LBP

24 SAR Hemachromatosis | 24 SAR Hemachromatosis | 23 A&W | 20 A&W

Denies family hx of heart dz, CVA, TB, DM, kidney dz, migraine H≠A, gout, thyroid dz, asthma, obesity, drug addiction, AIDS, violence, mental illness

NURSING**TIP**

Family Health History for a Patient Who Was Adopted

Patients who were adopted have varying degrees of information about their biological parents. Encourage adopted patients to be frank about their FHH. If the FHH of the biological parents is unknown, this is documented.

Likewise, the FHH of adoptive parents can be equally important. Certain environmental factors (such as smoking, drug and alcohol use, and sanitation) may influence the health of the adopted child.

NURSING**TIP**

Family Health History and Cultural Restraints

In some cultures (e.g., Chinese and some American Indian tribes), it is disrespectful to speak of the dead. Thus, the patient may be reluctant to provide detailed information on the family health history of dead relatives. In these cases, you can ask the patient whether there is any history of specific diseases in the family, rather than focusing on any specific deceased individual. The patient may be willing to share in which previous generation and on which side of the family the condition existed. If these approaches are unsuccessful, explain to the patient the importance of this information because it may provide clues to current health conditions.

disorders, sickle cell anemia, arthritis, epilepsy, migraine headaches, gout, thyroid disease, liver disease, asthma, allergic disorders, obesity, alcoholism, mental illness (schizophrenia, depression), mental retardation, drug addiction, AIDS, HIV infection, violent reactions? Who?"

Family Health History and Genomics

Genomics, or the study of the genetic makeup of the human cell, is increasingly becoming an area in which nurses need to be well versed. Over 15 years ago, the U.S. Department of Energy and the National Institutes of Health launched the U.S. Human Genome project. The aim of this project was to identify the approximately 30,000 genes in human DNA and to determine the sequence of the roughly 3 billion chemical pairs that make up human DNA. This information will be used in patient care to prevent disease, provide for early disease detection, develop personalized patient interventions for disease, and, ultimately, provide a cure for disease. All of this is the promise and future of genomics. Though genomics is still in its infancy stages, nurses are involved with fielding questions about genetic screening and testing. One nursing action is the documentation of the patient's genogram. Organizations such as the American Nurses Association (ANA) have Web sites that allow patients to construct their own genogram. This information can help guide genetically based nursing care.

SOCIAL HISTORY

The **social history** (SH) explores information about the patient's lifestyle that can affect health. Introduce this area of questioning with statements similar to the following:

"Now I would like to ask you some questions about your lifestyle. This information is important because of the effects that different practices can have on your health."

Alcohol Use

The intermittent and prolonged use of alcohol can interfere with normal metabolism and normal body function.

"How much alcohol do you drink per week?"
"How often do you drink?"

NURSING**TIP**

Genetic Testing

In 2007, carbamazepine became the first mainstream drug to carry a recommendation that patients of Asian descent be tested for the *HLA-B*1502* gene before starting drug therapy. Genetically, Asian patients are almost exclusively carriers of *HLA-B*1502*, and if placed on carbamazepine, are more likely to develop Stevens-Johnson syndrome or toxic epidermal necrolysis. This announcement by the Food and Drug Administration heralds the start of an era that is sure to continue, that is, the ability to make decisions about which drugs patients should or should not take based on their ethnicity and/or race.

From J. A. Ewing. (1984). "Detecting Alcoholism: The CAGE Questionnaire," in *Journal of the American Medical Association, 252,* 1905–1907.

NURSINGTIP

The CAGE Questionnaire

The CAGE questionnaire is an easily administered alcoholism screening tool that can be used to assess a patient's drinking habits. The four questions in the tool are:

C—Have you ever felt you should **C**ut down on your alcohol intake?

A—Have people **A**nnoyed you by criticizing your alcohol intake?

G—Have you ever felt **G**uilty about your alcohol intake?

E—Have you ever needed alcohol for an **E**ye-opener (morning consumption)?

Positive responses to two or more of these questions necessitate a more thorough history on alcohol consumption.

NURSINGTIP

Dealing with Sensitive Topics

Alcohol, drug use, and sexual practices are some of the most sensitive areas that are addressed in the health history. Some tips for dealing with these sensitive topics are:

- Ask these questions in the later stages of the interview after rapport has been established.
- Use direct eye contact; this demonstrates the importance of the topic to the patient and your lack of embarrassment.
- Pose questions in a matter-of-fact tone.
- Adopt a nonjudgmental demeanor.
- Use the communication technique of normalizing when appropriate (e.g., "Many high school students drink alcohol or use drugs or engage in sexual relationships on a regular basis. Does this happen at your school? With you?").

"What type of alcohol do you prefer (beer, wine, wine coolers, liquor, spirits)?"

"Do you ever consume homemade alcoholic beverages?"

"What quantity do you usually consume at one time?"

"Has your drinking pattern changed? In what way?"

"When did you first start to drink?"

"How long have you been drinking the amount that you are currently consuming?"

"What time of the day do you drink?"

"Where do you obtain your drinks?"

"Do you have a special place to keep your alcohol?"

"Have you ever lost consciousness or blacked out after drinking?"

"Have you ever forgotten what happened when you were drinking?"

"Do you drink alone?"

"Do you drive after drinking?"

"Did you ever drink during pregnancy? How much?" (for women)

"Do you think you have a drinking problem?"

Tobacco Use

Because of the harmful nature of tobacco products, the patient's use of tobacco should be ascertained at each visit. If tobacco is used, it is the role of the nurse to encourage the patient to quit. Many resources are available to the nurse to assist the patient in the smoking cessation process.

The quantity of cigarette smoking is usually described in **pack/year history**. To calculate the patient's pack/year history, multiply the number of packs of cigarettes smoked on a daily basis by the number of years that the patient has smoked. For example, to calculate the pack/year history for a patient who has smoked 2½ packs a day for 30 years:

$$\text{pack/year history} = 2\frac{1}{2} \times 30 = 75$$

Some providers quantify tobacco use in the number of packs per day (PPD) for a specified number of years, for example, 2 PPD × 15 years.

"Do you use or have you ever used tobacco (cigarettes [filtered or nonfiltered], pipe, cigars, chewing tobacco, snuff)?"

"At what age did you start to use tobacco?"

NURSING**TIP**

The Four A's of Smoking Cessation

Ask: At every patient encounter, the nurse *asks* the patient about his or her smoking habits: type, amount, and duration.

Advise: The nurse strongly *advises* the patient that quitting smoking is in his or her best health interest.

Assist: The nurse *assists* the patient in selecting an appropriate nicotine withdrawal method (e.g., "cold turkey," patch, gum, nasal spray, prescription medication, acupuncture, or hypnosis). Advantages and disadvantages of each method can be discussed to empower the patient to make an informed decision.

Arrange: The nurse *arranges* for a close follow-up with the patient once the smoking cessation is started. Studies demonstrate that patients who have a support mechanism (professional or nonprofessional) and encouragement have greater success in quitting smoking. The follow-up can be a scheduled appointment or successive phone calls during which the nurse inquires how the patient is doing in meeting the smoking cessation goals and whether there are any questions about the chosen withdrawal method.

"What quantity do you use on a daily basis?"

"Has this amount changed? In what way?"

"Have you ever tried to kick this habit? How many times? What method(s) did you use? What was the outcome?"

"How long ago did you quit?"

"Do you think you have a smoking (tobacco) problem?"

"Do you live with someone who smokes?"

Drug Use

The questions about use of drugs in the social history section of the complete health history are not to be confused with the medication section under the past health history. The latter includes the use and abuse of OTC and prescription medications, whereas the former refers to the use of illegal substances. You may feel uncomfortable asking the patient whether there has been drug use; remind the patient that the information will be kept confidential and that the withholding of information may delay necessary treatment.

"Do you use or have you ever used marijuana, amphetamines, uppers, downers, cocaine, crack, heroin, PCP, inhalants, or other recreational or street drugs?"

"Do you do club drugs?"

"When did you first start to use drugs?"

"What amount do you use?"

"How often do you use this drug?"

"Has this amount changed? In what way?"

"In what form do you use the drug (pill, needle, snort, other)?"

"Describe how you inject the drug."

"Do you share needles? Do you clean the needles between uses? How?"

"Have you experienced any health problems from the drug use?"

"Have you ever overdosed? What happened?"

"Have you ever been through a drug rehab program? What was the outcome?"

"Do you think you have a drug problem?"

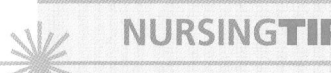

The sexual assault nurse examiner (SANE) is a nurse who has received extensive training in the handling of sexual assault victims. Intensive course work combined with clinical training enables the nurse to sit for the SANE certification exam, which is administered by the International Association of Forensic Nurses (IAFN). The SANE nurse collects evidence with a physical evidence recovery kit (PERK) for legal proceedings and provides much-needed sensitivity during the collection of the physical evidence (e.g., mouth, vaginal, and anal swabs; head and pubic hair; blood samples). The SANE nurse is an expert in providing crisis intervention and support to the patient, as well as guiding the patient to community resources to help with the healing process. Finally, the SANE nurse is responsible for maintaining the chain of custody of the physical evidence so that it is admissible in a court of law. The SANE nurse may be called to testify at these legal proceedings.

REFLECTIVE THINKING

Nursing Care for Drug Users

Twelve-year-old Barbara is brought to the emergency department by her mother, who explains that she heard a loud noise in the bathroom and ran upstairs to find her daughter unconscious on the floor. Barbara was unconscious for approximately 2 minutes. When Barbara awoke, she had no memory of the blackout. Barbara's mother believes that her daughter needs treatment for the multiple cuts to her forehead that she suffered when she fell. Barbara's mother excuses herself to go to the restroom. While she is out of the room, Barbara tells you that she takes LSD occasionally. She then asks, "Do you think that has anything to do with my blackout?"

- How would you respond to Barbara's question?
- Do you exhibit any biases when working with people who take street drugs? Do these biases interfere with your nursing care? If so, what actions do you take to control your bias?
- Explore the legal ramifications of working with patients who take illegal drugs in your city or state. Are there special provisions if the patient is a minor?

Domestic and Intimate Partner Violence

It is estimated that up to 30% of injured women treated in emergency departments (ED) have suffered from domestic or intimate partner violence (IPV) (American College of Obstetricians & Gynecologists, 1995). Violence cuts across both sexes, as well as racial, cultural, geographic, and socioeconomic lines. It is vital to be familiar with your state's statutes regarding reporting actual and suspected violence and abuse.

Domestic and intimate partner violence involves more than physical abuse. It includes psychological, emotional, sexual, and financial abuse or coercion. Just as many health care providers advocate screening for tobacco and alcohol use for both men and women at each health care encounter, some providers recommend routine screening for domestic and intimate partner violence at every health care encounter for women. Though men can be the victims of domestic and intimate partner violence, the majority of victims are women.

Some clues that might alert you to the possibility of domestic and intimate partner violence are as follows:

- Frequent injuries, accidents, or burns
- Previous injuries for which the individual did not seek health care
- Injury is inconsistent with the patient's report of how it occurred
- Refusal of the patient to discuss the injury
- Significant other accompanies the patient to the ED, answers questions for patient, and refuses to leave the patient's side
- Significant other has a history of previous violence or substance abuse
- Vague symptoms such as chronic pain

Using the communication technique of normalizing, the nurse can screen for potential domestic and intimate partner violence. Some appropriate introductory comments might be:

"Almost one-third of injured women who visit the ED have experienced some domestic and intimate partner violence. Is this what happened to you?"

NURSING**TIP**

HITS Screening Tool

Sherin, Sinacore, Li, Zitter, and Shakil (1998) developed the HITS screening tool to assess for domestic and intimate partner violence. This is easily administered in a short period of time. The patient is asked how many times in the past month or year each incident has occurred.

H—Have you been physically **H**urt?

I—Have you been **I**nsulted or did someone talk down to you?

T—Have you been **T**hreatened with physical harm?

S—Has someone **S**creamed at you or cursed you?

From Sherin, K. M., Sinacore, J. M., Li, X. Q., Zitter, R. E., & Shakil, A. (1998)."HITS: A Short Domestic Violence Screening Tool for Use in a Family Practice Setting," in *Family Medicine, 30*(7), 508–512. Reprinted with permission from the Society of Teachers of Family Medicine.

"Domestic and intimate partner violence occur very frequently in our community. Keeping this in mind, I would like to ask you some questions."

A single broad question can also be used to screen for domestic and intimate partner violence:

"In the past year, have you been hit, kicked, punched, or hurt in other ways by someone close to you?"

If the patient answers "yes" to these questions, you need to inquire whether the patient feels safe in his or her current environment or situation. Most EDs have resources available to assist the patient in moving to a climate where he or she can receive help and feel safe.

It is imperative to document physical violence assessment findings concisely and accurately. Incorporate drawings of injury locations or use printed anatomical maps on which injuries can be documented. Many EDs have cameras so that the staff can photograph injuries for the patient's records.

Keep in mind that many victims of IPV experience anxiety, depression, substance abuse, and posttraumatic stress disorder after their attack, and these

REFLECTIVE THINKING

Assessing for Domestic and Intimate Partner Violence

You note that Tasha has come to the ED three times in the past 6 months. Six months ago, she reported falling down the steps and hitting her head. Her old chart documents that she was seen for a mild closed head injury with concussion. Two months ago, Tasha reported falling while ice skating and broke her left arm. Her cast was removed 2 weeks ago. Today, Tasha presents with multiple facial and mouth lacerations. She tells you that she fell off her bike. You note multiple ecchymoses on the exposed areas of her skin.

- What questions would you ask Tasha?
- Describe the physical examination that you would conduct.
- Investigate your agency's policy on reporting actual and suspected violence or abuse.
- Investigate your state's regulations on reporting actual and suspected violence or abuse.

NURSING**TIP**

Eliciting the Sexual History

Be aware that patients may refuse to answer questions pertaining to sexual history; try returning to these questions later. Ask the patient whether a nurse of a different gender would make the patient more comfortable in discussing sexual practice.

The adolescent patient may refuse to answer these questions or may provide false answers if the parent or caregiver is in the room. It may be advisable to ask the caregiver to leave the room at the completion of the health history so that you can ask the patient whether there is anything else that he or she would like to say.

Be alert for cues that demonstrate the patient's desire for sexual education, such as questions or requests for written information. Answer the patient's questions honestly.

conditions can last for years. Specific health care procedures, such as a gynecological examination, may invoke memories of the IPV. The nurse needs to be sensitive to the patient's needs at these times.

Sexual Practice

Sexual practice histories focus on healthy sexual practices as well as the transmission of communicable diseases. Various medications can affect sexual function.

Questioning a patient about sexual practices may be uncomfortable for both patient and nurse. The patient may notice your uneasiness with this topic and may feel embarrassed to answer the questions. Examine your personal feelings on human sexuality and attain a comfort level that will allow ease in questioning. The health histories in Chapters 20 and 21 provide additional information about female and male reproductive health.

"What term would you use to describe your sexual orientation (heterosexual, homosexual, bisexual, transgender)?"

"Does your current sexual orientation represent your past sexual practice? If not, how has it changed?"

"At what age was your first sexual experience?"

"With how many partners are you currently involved? Has this changed?"

"What method of birth control do you use? Do you have any questions about it? Would you like additional information on other methods of birth control?" (for heterosexuals and bisexuals)

"What measures do you use to prevent exchange of body fluids during sexual activity?"

"Do you engage in oral or anal intercourse?"

"Have you ever had a sexual partner who had a sexually transmitted disease?"

"Are there other activities that satisfy your sexual needs?"

"Do you take any prescription or OTC medications to help your sexual performance?"

"Do you use any sexual aid devices?"

"Are you able to be aroused?"

"Are you satisfied with your sexual performance?"

"Do you have any obstacles to achieving sexual satisfaction? (e.g., sexually transmitted disease, children in the house)"

"Do you have any infertility issues? How have you dealt with that?"

"Have you ever been sexually abused? What has transpired since?"

NURSING**ALERT**

Dangerous Sexual Practices

Be alert for individuals who practice potentially lethal sexual practices that involve near strangulation. In adolescents, this practice is often referred to as the "choking game." Individuals literally choke one another with their hands, or they can use noose-like materials such as belts, scarves, and ropes. Adults usually use more sophisticated techniques to have this autoerotic experience. The premise of this "game" is to experience the euphoria that occurs when one is close to unconsciousness or becomes unconscious. In some instances, individuals have died during these activities.

Travel History

Endemic illnesses may be endogenous to specific regions in the world or to a single country. Patients sometimes present with symptoms that cannot or may not be attributed to routine illnesses. For these reasons, a complete travel history is warranted when obtaining a health history.

"Where within the United States have you traveled? Was this a rural or an urban environment? When?"

"Have you ever traveled outside of the United States? Where? When?"

"For what period of time were you within this region?"

"Did you receive any immunizations before you visited that area?"

"Did you need to take any medications prophylactically before or while you were gone?"

"Were you ill when you were there?"

"Was a diagnosis made? By whom? What was it?"

"What treatment did you receive? Were there any complications?"

"Since returning from this area, have you been ill or not feeling normal?"

"If traveling for more than 2 to 4 hours, were you well hydrated? Did you get up and stretch or walk around for a few minutes?"

Work Environment

The work environment can be hazardous. The nature of employment itself may present health hazards, whether or not safety measures are used. Carpentry, for example, is viewed as a relatively safe employment, though over time, carpenters are prone to ischemia of their fingers from repeated exposure to hand-held vibrating tools. Exposure to toxic substances in the work environment, such as asbestos and lead, is an additional factor to consider.

"Describe the work that you do. Is it physically demanding? Is it mentally or emotionally demanding?"

"How many hours a day do you normally work? How long have you held this position?"

"Do you spend the majority of your work day sitting, standing, walking, running, lifting, or biking?"

"Do you work with any chemicals? Raw materials?"

"Are you exposed to radiation? Toxic fumes? Hazardous conditions?"

"What safety measures do you practice at work?"

"Is there pollution near your office?"

"What is the noise level at your place of employment?"

"Have you noticed that you are sick on the weekend or on your days off?"

"Have you had any work-related accidents or injuries?"

"Is there any construction at your work environment?"

"Do you enjoy your work?"

"What other jobs have you held in your lifetime?"

Home Environment

When assessing the patient's home environment, consider both the physical and psychosocial aspects. The physical assessment encompasses a broad spectrum of topics: physical condition of the house, safety from toxic substances, and the presence of modern conveniences such as a refrigerator, furnace, telephones, and electricity. Older houses may have been painted with lead-based paint, which poses a health threat to a young child who eats the paint chips. The presence of radon gas in the home has been a recent health concern.

The psychosocial component of the home environment identifies the relative safety of the neighborhood.

PHYSICAL ENVIRONMENT.

"How old are your living quarters (i.e., house or apartment building)?"

"In what condition are your living quarters?"

"Is your home cleaned regularly?"

"Do you have heat, air conditioning, and electricity? What type of heat do you have? Do you use space heaters?"

"Do you have running water? Do you have a toilet, tub, or shower?"

"What is the temperature on your hot water heater?"

"From what source do you draw your water (e.g., well, reservoir)?"

"Do you have a working telephone?"

"Do you have smoke detectors? Where? Do you inspect the batteries on a regular basis? Do you have a carbon monoxide detector?"

"How many steps separate each floor? Is there a railing?"

"Do you have any throw rugs? Are they taped to the floor?"

"Do you use a nightlight when it is dark?"

"Have you adapted your living quarters to fit any special needs?"

"Do you think your living space is adequate for the number of people who live with you?"

"Have you ever had your living quarters tested for the presence of radon? What was the result?"

"How often do you have your fireplace cleaned?"

"How often do you replace the filter in your ventilation system?"

"What pets do you have? Do they live inside or outside?"

"What type of transportation do you use?"

"Who does your shopping?"

"Do you have easy access to a grocery store? Drug store? Health care facility?"

"Where do you store your medications, cleaning supplies, and other toxic substances? How are they secured?" (if children live in the living quarters)

"Do you have a gun in the house? Where is it stored? How is it stored? Where are the bullets stored? Is the gun loaded?"

"Where do you store gasoline and automotive supplies?"

"Is there a problem with pollution near your home?"

PSYCHOSOCIAL ENVIRONMENT.

"Do you feel safe in your neighborhood?"

"Does your neighborhood have a crime watch prevention program?"

Hobbies and Leisure Activities

Acquiring information on patients' hobbies and leisure activities is necessary because some activities can pose health risks (Figure 3-6). For example, repeated exposure to glue used in constructing model cars and planes can lead to respiratory ailments.

"What hobbies do you have?" **or** "What do you like to do in your spare time?"

"During or after this activity, have you ever felt sick? What happened?"

"Have you ever given up some leisure activity because of the effect it had on your health? What happened?"

"Have you ever had an injury from your hobby?"

"Are the hobbies and leisure activities relaxing?"

Stress

Stress is a physiologically defined response to changes that disrupt the resting equilibrium of an individual. **Distress** is negative stress, or stress that is harmful and unpleasant. **Eustress** is positive stress, stress that challenges the individual, provides motivation, and prevents stagnation.

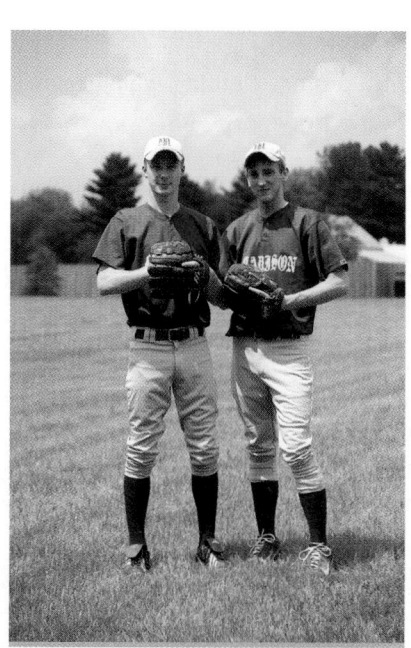

FIGURE 3-6 Many hobbies and leisure activities have some risk of health-related injuries.

NURSING**ALERT**

Internet Addiction

Computers are a vital component of our lives, and they have radically changed how business is conducted. In addition, computers and access to the Internet have altered the way many people now spend their free time. As a consequence, Internet addiction has become a health concern as individuals spend more time in front of computers. Whether the computer user frequents shopping sites, gambling sites, or multiplayer online role-playing games, the outcome can be the same—loss of control, social isolation, difficulties at home and/or work. The issue has become so prevalent that in 2007, the American Psychiatric Association issued a statement on the need for more research on this topic. It is very likely that the next edition of the *Diagnostic and Statistical Manual* will contain criteria for diagnosing this condition.

"What are the current stressors in your life?"

"What do you feel is your greatest stress at the present time?"

"Are there recurring themes with the stress that you experience?"

"Have you ever progressed from the point of being stressed to panic? What were the circumstances? How did you handle it?"

"Are you able to recognize when you become stressed? What happens?"

Education

Elicit information on the patient's ability to read and write, and tailor your questions and information to this level.

"What was the highest grade level that you completed?"

"Describe the type of student that you were."

"Have you completed a GED certification?"

Economic Status

Patients and nurses may be equally uncomfortable discussing financial status. The essence of the information needed is how the patient lives on the income. Patients who lack adequate financial resources may be referred to social services.

"What are the sources of your income?"

"How would you describe your economic status?"

"Are you able to meet food, medication, housing, clothing, and personal expenses for you and your family?"

"Are you able to save any money?"

"Do you hesitate seeking health care because of the cost? What is your insurance coverage?"

"Are you satisfied with your current economic status?"

Military Service

Knowledge of overseas tours of duty may provide a vital link to current health status; a patient may not reveal this information during the travel history because it was work rather than leisure travel. For instance, those military personnel who served in Operation Desert Storm may have been exposed to many chemical agents. Many of them now have a variety of signs and symptoms collectively called Gulf War syndrome. Some of the troops who were in the Middle East for the Iraq conflict have exhibited various illnesses such as malaria and unknown respiratory pathology. The full extent of the impact on these troops may not be known for some time.

"Are you or have you ever been in the military? What branch?"

"How long have you been in the military? Are you on active duty or reserve?"

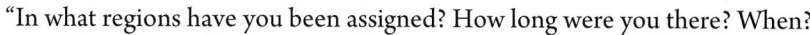

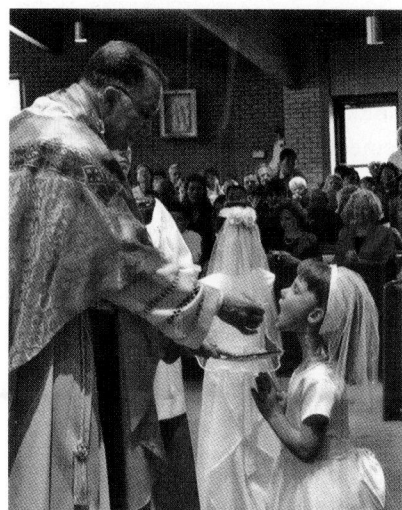

FIGURE 3-7 Assessing a person's religious and spiritual beliefs is an important aspect of nursing care. For example, the young girl in this photo is receiving First Holy Communion in the Roman Catholic Church. She has been required to complete an educational program, fulfill various religious requirements, and fast for a period of time in order to reach this special occasion in her faith.

"In what regions have you been assigned? How long were you there? When?"
"Have you ever been in combat? What were your experiences? Do you have flashbacks?"

Religion

Religion and spirituality can be powerful forces in a patient's life. You need to be aware of and sensitive to implications that spirituality or religious beliefs may have on the patient's health status and health care practices (Figure 3-7). Chapter 6 provides a more detailed assessment on religious and spiritual practices.

"Are you affiliated with a specific religion?"
"Do you currently practice your faith?"
"Do your religious beliefs affect your health status? In what way?"
"Are there any beliefs that you feel are compromised by seeking health care?"
"Are there any religious practices that you may need assistance with?"

Ethnic Background

Closely associated with religious practices is the patient's culture or ethnic background, which can penetrate all facets of a patient's life. Integrate familiarity with various cultures into your knowledge base so you will be sensitive to and more completely understanding of the patient's ethnic heritage. Chapter 5 discusses the cultural assessment in greater detail.

"With what culture or ethnic group do you identify yourself?"

Roles and Relationships

Family roles, work roles, and interpersonal relationships provide clues about possible stressors, areas for health promotion, support systems, and sources of altered psychosocial patterns.

"Who lives with you?"
"What type of relationship do you have with these individuals?"
"What is your role within your family (e.g., caregiver, breadwinner, child, student)?"
"What responsibilities go along with this role?"
"Who do you turn to for support?"
"Describe the relationship that you have with your friends and neighbors."

Characteristic Patterns of Daily Living and Functional Health Assessment

Questions about a patient's usual lifestyle, or **characteristic patterns of daily living**, reveal information about the patient's normal daily timetable: meals, work, and sleep schedules and social interactions (Figure 3-8). If the patient is disabled or impaired physically, anatomically, or psychologically, you need to perform a functional health assessment (see Appendix B). The **functional health assessment** documents a person's ability to perform instrumental activities of daily living (IADL) and physical self-maintenance activities. These data serve as baseline information upon which the effectiveness of nursing interventions can be evaluated.

"Describe a typical day for you, starting from the time you wake up to the time you go to bed."
"Do you need assistance with any activities of daily living? (If yes) Is assistance readily available?"
"Do you socialize, meet, or talk with people outside your house on a daily basis?"
"Does your schedule change on certain days or on the weekend? Describe."

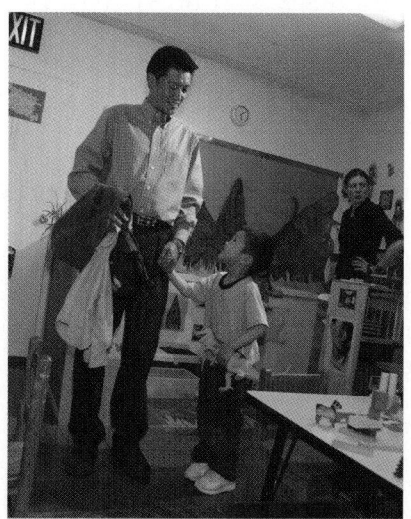

FIGURE 3-8 Part of this child's pattern of daily living is attending child care during the work day.

HEALTH MAINTENANCE ACTIVITIES

Health maintenance activities (HMA) are practices a person incorporates into his or her lifestyle to promote healthy living. You can make the transition from the social history to HMA with the following statements:

"Now I would like to discuss things that you do that promote health."

"There are many things you can do to promote healthy living. I would like us to discuss some of those practices."

Sleep

Many illnesses have sleep pattern disturbances as a characteristic. Increased or decreased sleep patterns can both occur. For this reason, you need to learn about the patient's current and usual sleep habits.

A standardized sleep tool can also be used to assess sleep and wakefulness patterns. One example of this is the Epworth Sleepiness Scale.

"At what time do you usually go to bed? What time do you usually awake?"

"How long does it take you to fall asleep?"

"Is this an adequate amount of sleep for you? How do you feel when you awaken?"

"Is the sleep undisturbed? Do you have difficulty staying asleep? If you awaken, is it easy for you to fall back to sleep?"

"Do you have any discomfort in your legs when you are in bed trying to sleep?"

"Describe the environment in which you sleep (noise level, amount of light, temperature of the room, sleeping arrangement)."

"Are there any bedtime rituals that you practice?"

"What strategies do you use to fall asleep if you are having difficulty (medication, warm milk, other)? How many times per week do you do this?"

"What is your usual emotional state or mental condition when you go to bed? When you awaken?"

"Do you ever have difficulty falling asleep? How often does this occur? Have you ever been told that you have insomnia?"

"Have you ever been told that you snore loudly or excessively?"

"Do you ever have difficulty staying awake? Have you ever been told that you have sleep apnea or narcolepsy?"

"Does the usual time of your sleep-awake cycle change (working rotating shifts)?"

"Do you take a nap during the day? For how long?"

"Do you fall asleep unintentionally at times other than nighttime?"

"Do you have nightmares? How frequent are they?"

"Do you walk in your sleep?"

"Do you experience bedwetting?"

"Do you often wake up with dark circles under your eyes? Puffy eyelids? Blood-shot eyes?"

"Do you ever wake in the night because of pain, dyspnea, or nocturia?"

"Do you have alcohol, nicotine, or caffeine within 2 hours of bedtime?"

"Do you take any prescription medications to help you sleep?"

"Do you have a job that requires rotating shifts or varies the time of work by a number of hours?"

Diet

Refer to Chapter 7 for a more thorough discussion of nutrition and diet history.

"Are you on any special therapeutic diet (soft foods, low salt, low cholesterol, low fat, etc.)?" (Figure 3-9).

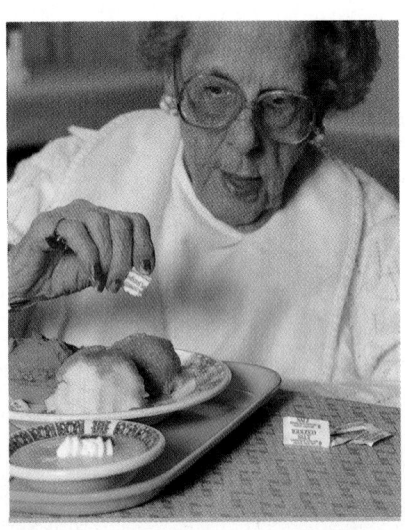

FIGURE 3-9 This woman requires a soft-food-only diet.

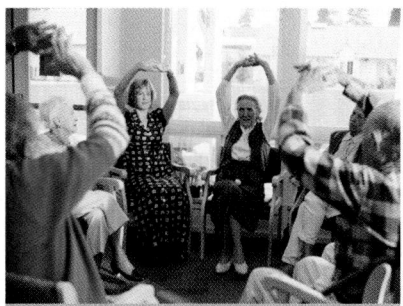

FIGURE 3-10 These older adults are participating in an exercise class at their assisted-living facility.

"Do you follow any particular diet plan (vegetarian, liquid, commercially available diet food, rice diet, Atkins diet, South Beach diet, etc.)?"

"How many meals a day do you eat? At what times do you eat? Do you snack? When?"

"Has your weight fluctuated in the past year? Explain."

Exercise

Aerobic exercise appropriate to the patient's age and physical condition leads to cardiovascular, respiratory, and musculoskeletal fitness as well as mental alertness (Figure 3-10). Combining aerobic exercise with weight lifting (which increases strength) and calisthenics (which enhances flexibility) establishes a complete physical fitness regimen. Nonaerobic activity also has beneficial effects on the body, even though the target heart rate may not be attained.

In 2007, the American College of Sports Medicine and the American Heart Association updated their recommendation on exercise guidelines for healthy adults in the age group 18–65 years. Their guidelines stipulate moderate-intensity aerobic exercise for 30 minutes, 5 days a week, or vigorous-intensity aerobic exercise for 20 minutes, 3 days a week. Combining these exercise levels is also acceptable. In addition, short bouts of exercise that are 10 minutes or more can be combined to meet the new 30-minute goal. Muscle strengthening is also incorporated into the guidelines.

"Do you participate in a formal or informal exercise program?"

"What type of exercise do you do?"

"How many times per week do you exercise?"

"How long do you exercise (in minutes)?"

"What type of warm-up and cool-down exercises do you do?"

"What is your resting heart rate?"

"What is your heart rate at the most intense time of your exercise?"

"For what period of time do you maintain this elevated heart rate?"

"Have you ever experienced any injuries from your exercise regimen? What type?"

"How long have you been involved with this exercise program?"

"Does your health pose any restrictions on your ability to exercise?"

Stress Management

The assessment of stress management practices is vital. Some commonly used stress management techniques are exercise, eating, biofeedback, yoga, progressive

Stress Management Counseling

D.G. is a 42-year-old woman who presents with a gastrointestinal bleed secondary to increased caffeine, alcohol, and aspirin intake. She is transferred from the critical care area to your unit. As soon as D.G. arrives, she asks for a telephone so she can call her office. Suddenly, she bursts into tears and sobs, "I can't handle one more thing! I need to get a handle on life." She asks for your advice.

- How would you respond to D.G.'s statement?
- Is this the appropriate time to conduct a stress management assessment?
- What stress management resources are available in your area or institution?
- What is your bias (if any) with stress management techniques that you do not espouse? How can you become more comfortable in discussing these practices with patients to overcome your bias?

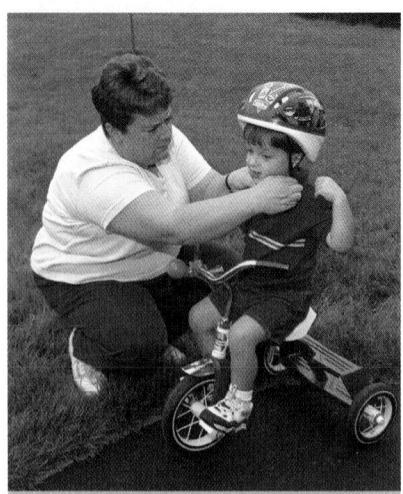

FIGURE 3-11 Wearing safety equipment is essential at all ages.

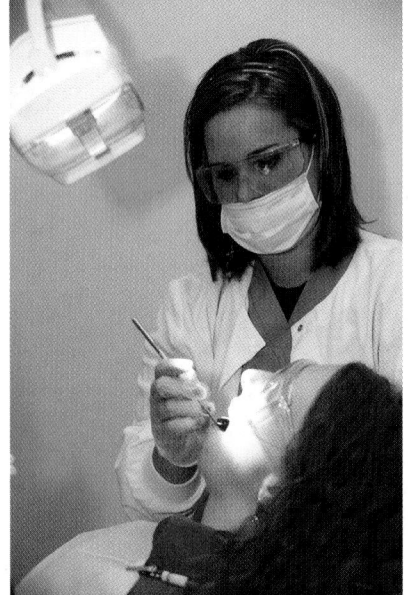

FIGURE 3-12 It is important to ask patients what other health care providers they are seeing, such as the dentist.

muscle relaxation, aromatherapy, imagery, massages, verbalization, praying, humor, pet therapy, music therapy, magnet therapy, reflexology, journaling, storytelling, support groups, and transcendental meditation. For others, stress management techniques include smoking, drinking, drugs, and violence.

"What do you do when you become stressed to help alleviate the stress?"
"When do you use this skill? Is it effective for you?"
"How do you evaluate the effectiveness of this technique?"
"How long do you need to perform this technique before your stress is reduced?"
"How many times per day do you use this technique? Per week?"
"Have you tried other stress management skills? How did they work?"

Use of Safety Devices

The patient's use or lack of use of safety devices on the job, in the home, and in the environment provides a source for teaching health promotion skills (Figure 3-11).

"Do you wear a seat belt when you are in an automobile?"
"Do you wear a helmet when riding a motorcycle?"
"Do your hobbies and leisure activities (e.g., cycling) require the use of safety devices (e.g., helmets)? Do you use them?"
"What precautions do you take when using pesticides or fertilizers?"

Health Check-ups

Health check-up information demonstrates patterns of health care practices by the patient during illness and health, and provides potential sources of health education.

"When was the last time you had the following performed: pulse and blood pressure, complete physical examination, chest X-ray, TB test, EKG, urinalysis, hematocrit, and blood chemistry, including blood sugar and cholesterol? What were the results?"
"How often do you see a dentist (Figure 3-12)? For what reason?"
"How often do you see an eye doctor? For what reason? Have you been checked for glaucoma?"
"How often do you have a gynecological check-up? By whom? What was the date and result of your last Pap smear?" (for women)
"Do you know how to perform a breast self-examination? Who taught you? How often do you perform it? Do you have any questions about it?" (for women)
"What was the date and the result of your last mammogram?" (for women)
"Do you know how to perform a testicular self-examination? Who taught you? How often do you perform it? Do you have any questions about it?" (for men)
"How often do you have a prostate examination? What was the date and result of your last exam?" (for men)

NURSINGTIP

Nontraditional Health Care Sources

As a nurse, you can appreciate the need to base your practice on proven scientific rationale. However, not all patients espouse similar views of health care practices. You need to be sensitive to patients' nontraditional sources of health care, such as curandero, yerbo, espiritualista, voodoo, shaman, or medicine man. It is important to document these caregivers and the usual course of treatment. It may be possible and desired in some instances to allow the nontraditional healer to participate in the patient's care.

"Do you have any other health care providers (psychiatrist, psychologist, podiatrist, occupational or physical therapist, chiropractor, et al.)? For what reason? How often do you see this person?"

REVIEW OF SYSTEMS

The **review of systems** (ROS) is the patient's subjective response to a series of body system–related questions and serves as a double-check that vital information is not overlooked. The ROS covers a broad base of clinical states, but it is by no means exhaustive. The ROS follows a head-to-toe or **cephalocaudal** approach and includes two types of questions: sign or symptom related and disease related. The signs or symptoms and diseases are grouped according to physiological body parts and systems. Some of the diseases may have been discussed earlier in the interview.

Both positive and pertinent negative findings are documented in the ROS. When a response is positive, ask the patient to describe it as completely as possible. Refer to the 10 characteristics of a chief complaint when gathering more information about positive responses. Table 3-1 lists the symptoms and diseases that can be ascertained during the ROS. Many institutions have preprinted ROS sheets. These are convenient to use because positive findings can be circled and noted. Negative responses are not circled. As you become more experienced, you can combine the ROS with the physical examination of the patient. This technique often shortens the interview time with the patient.

Remember to ask the questions in terms that are understood by the patient. An appropriate statement to make the transition from the HMA to the ROS would be:

"Now I would like to ask you if you have experienced a variety of conditions. Most of the questions can be answered with 'yes' or 'no'."

Pose the same question for each item in the ROS:

"Have you ever had . . . ?"

TABLE 3-1 Review of Systems

General	Patient's perception of general state of health at the present, difference from usual state, vitality and energy levels, body odors, fever, chills, night sweats
Skin	Rashes, itching, changes in skin pigmentation, ecchymoses, change in color or size of mole, sores, lumps, dry or moist skin, pruritus, change in skin texture, odors, excessive sweating, acne, warts, eczema, psoriasis, amount of time spent in the sun, use of sunscreen, skin cancer
Hair	Alopecia, excessive growth of hair or growth of hair in unusual locations (hirsutism), use of chemicals on hair, dandruff, pediculosis, scalp lesions
Nails	Change in nails, splitting, breaking, thickened, texture change, onychomycosis, use of chemicals, false nails
Eyes	Blurred vision, visual acuity, glasses, contacts, photophobia, excessive tearing, night blindness, diplopia, drainage, bloodshot eyes, pain, blind spots, flashing lights, halos around objects, floaters, glaucoma, cataracts, use of sunglasses, use of protective eyewear
Ears	Cleaning method, hearing deficits, hearing aid, pain, phonophobia, discharge, lightheadedness (vertigo), ringing in the ears (tinnitus), usual noise level, earaches, infection, piercings, use of ear protection, amount of cerumen

continues

TABLE 3-1 (Continued)

Nose and Sinuses	Number of colds per year, discharge, itching, hay fever, postnasal drip, stuffiness, sinus pain, sinusitis, polyps, obstruction, epistaxis, change in sense of smell, allergies, snoring
Mouth	Dental habits (brushing, flossing, mouth rinses), toothache, tooth abscess, dentures, bleeding or swollen gums, difficulty chewing, sore tongue, change in taste, lesions, change in salivation, bad breath, caries, teeth extractions, orthodontics
Throat and Neck	Hoarseness, change in voice, frequent sore throats, dysphagia, pain or stiffness, enlarged thyroid (goiter), lymphadenopathy, tonsillectomy, adenoidectomy
Breasts and Axilla	Pain, tenderness, discharge, lumps, change in size, dimpling, rash, benign breast disease, breast cancer, results of recent mammogram
Respiratory	Dyspnea on exertion, shortness of breath, sputum, cough, sneezing, wheezing, hemoptysis, frequent upper respiratory tract infections, pneumonia, emphysema, asthma, tuberculosis, tuberculosis exposure, result of last chest X-ray or PPD
Cardiovascular and Peripheral Vasculature	Paroxysmal nocturnal dyspnea, chest pain, cyanosis, heart murmur, palpitations, syncope, orthopnea (state number of pillows used), edema, cold or discolored hands or feet, leg cramps, myocardial infarction, hypertension, valvular disease, intermittent claudication, varicose veins, thrombophlebitis, deep vein thrombosis, use of support hose, result of last EKG
Gastrointestinal	Change in appetite, nausea, vomiting, diarrhea, constipation, usual bowel habits, melena, rectal bleeding, hematemesis, change in stool color, flatulence, belching, regurgitation, heartburn, dysphagia, abdominal pain, jaundice, ascites, hemorrhoids, hepatitis, peptic ulcers, gallstones, gastroesophageal reflux disease, appendicitis, ulcerative colitis, Crohn's disease, diverticulitis, umbilical hernia
Urinary	Change in urine color, voiding habits, dysuria, hesitancy, urgency, frequency, nocturia, polyuria, dribbling, loss in force of stream, bedwetting, change in urine volume, incontinence, urinary retention, suprapubic pain, flank pain, kidney stones, urinary tract infections
Musculoskeletal	Joint stiffness, muscle pain, cramps, back pain, limitation of movement, redness, swelling, weakness, bony deformity, broken bones, dislocations, sprains, crepitus, gout, arthritis, osteoporosis, herniated disc
Neurological	Headache, change in balance, incoordination, loss of movement, change in sensory perception or feeling in an extremity, change in speech, change in smell, syncope, loss of memory, tremors, involuntary movement, loss of consciousness, seizures, weakness, head injury, vertigo, tremor, tic, paralysis, stroke, spasm
Psychological	Irritability, nervousness, tension, increased stress, difficulty concentrating, mood changes, suicidal thoughts, depression, anxiety, sleep disturbances, eating disorders
Female Reproductive	Vaginal discharge, change in libido, infertility, sterility, pelvic pain, pain during intercourse, post-coital bleeding; menses: last menstrual period (LMP), menarche, regularity, duration, amount of bleeding, premenstrual symptoms, intermenstrual bleeding, dysmenorrhea, menorrhagia, fibroids; menopause: age of onset, duration, symptoms, bleeding; obstetrical: number of pregnancies, number of miscarriages or abortions, number of children, type of delivery, complications; type of birth control, hormone replacement therapy
Male Reproductive	Change in libido, infertility, sterility, impotence, pain during intercourse, age at onset of puberty, testicular or penile pain, penile discharge, erections, emissions, hernias, enlarged prostate, type of birth control
Nutrition	Present weight, usual weight, desired weight, food intolerances, food likes and dislikes, where meals are eaten, caffeine intake
Endocrine	Exophthalmos, fatigue, change in size of head, hands, or feet, weight change, heat and cold intolerances, excessive sweating, polydipsia, polyphagia, polyuria, increased hunger, change in body hair distribution, goiter, diabetes mellitus
Lymph Nodes	Enlargement, tenderness
Hematological	Easy bruising or bleeding, anemia, sickle cell anemia, blood type, exposure to radiation

THE SYSTEM-SPECIFIC HEALTH HISTORY

This text uses a system-specific health history in each body system chapter (see Chapters 10–22). The system-specific health history provides detailed information that guides questioning and provides clues of related pathology. Not every item in the complete health history is addressed in every body system history. Only those sections relevant to the body system being assessed are addressed, and this can differ from chapter to chapter due to the nature of the material.

CONCLUDING THE HEALTH HISTORY

After completing the ROS, ask the patient whether there is any additional information to discuss. At the conclusion of the interview, thank the patient for the time spent in gathering the health history. Inform the patient what the next step will be, for example, physical assessment, diagnostic tests, treatment, and when to expect it.

ASSISTIVE DEVICES

Some chapters in this text will contain a section on assistive devices for that body system. These assistive devices are important to assess as they are health care extenders for the patient. Whether the assistive device is supplemental oxygen, a walker, or a feeding tube, they need to be evaluated as you assess the patient. Correct use of these devices will help the patient maintain a current level of health, whereas incorrect use can harm the patient.

ENAP FORMAT

The physical examination chapters in this text use the ENAP format. The "E" represents the examination component, a step-by-step procedure on how to perform each physical examination skill. The "N" states the normal assessment finding for that skill. "A" states many common abnormal findings for the physical examination skill. Finally, the "P" explains the pathophysiology of the abnormal finding. There are reminders at the bottom of each assessment page to remind the reader what these initials mean.

DOCUMENTATION

The documentation of the health assessment and physical examination is the legal record of the patient encounter (Figure 3-13). It also serves as the medium among health professionals for communicating about the patient's condition. The patient record represents a description of the patient's status and the care delivered to the patient. The documentation may be read by a multitude of professionals: nurses; doctors; dieticians; respiratory, physical, speech, and occupational therapists; risk managers; utilization reviewers; quality assurance personnel; accreditation organizations; lawyers; insurance companies; and, ultimately, the patient! Because all of these people have access to the patient's chart, you must document everything in a professional and legally acceptable manner. Table 3-2 outlines general principles to guide your documentation. Table 3-3 provides specific assessment-oriented "do's" and "don'ts" for documentation. Each institution also has its own documentation system. If you perform computerized charting in your workplace, always safeguard your access code to protect yourself.

Many health care facilities have preprinted health history forms that are checklists and require few narrative notes. Other facilities require the nurse to document the health history in its entirety. The health histories that follow illustrate how to document the complete health history of an ill patient and a well patient.

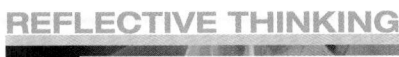

REFLECTIVE THINKING

Assessing Your Documentation

After completing the health history, reflect on the techniques you used to elicit the history. Did you rush the patient? Did you use too many open-ended or closed questions? Was your documentation concise? What could you have done better?

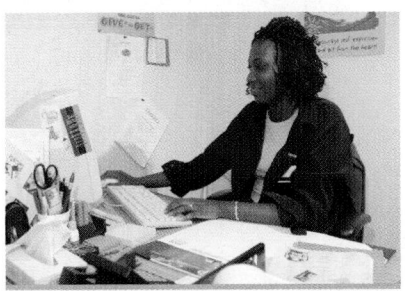

FIGURE 3-13 Documenting the health history is a crucial step in providing patient care.

TABLE 3-2 General Documentation Guidelines

1. Ensure that you have the correct patient record or chart and that the patient's name and identifying information are on every page of the record.

2. Document as soon as the patient encounter is concluded to ensure accurate recall of data (follow institution's guidelines on frequency of charting).

3. Avoid distractions while documenting. This is frequently when errors are made.

4. If interrupted while documenting, reread what you wrote to ensure accuracy.

5. Record date and time of each entry.

6. Sign each entry with your full legal name and with your professional credentials, or per your institution's policy.

7. Do not sign a note that you did not write.

8. Do not leave space between entries.

9. Do not insert information between lines.

10. If an error is made while documenting, use a single line to cross out the error, then date, time, and sign the correction (check institutional policy); avoid erasing, crossing out, or using correction fluid.

11. Never correct another person's entry, even if it is incorrect.

12. Use quotes to indicate direct patient responses (e.g., "I feel lousy").

13. Document in chronological order; if chronological order is not used, state why.

14. Use legible writing.

15. Use a permanent ink pen. (Black is usually preferable because of its ability to photocopy well.)

16. Document in a complete but concise manner by using phrases and abbreviations as appropriate (see the abbreviation list on the inside back cover of this book). Avoid using dangerous abbreviations, acronyms, and symbols as specified by the Joint Commission (formerly the Joint Commission on Accreditation of Health Care Organizations [JCAHO]) and the Institute for Safe Medication Practices (see Appendix C).

17. When writing numbers less than 1, write a zero to the left of the decimal point; this avoids confusion as to the use of a decimal point.

18. Document telephone calls that relate to the patient's case.

19. Always reread your notes for accuracy.

20. Identify the name of an interpreter if one is used.

21. Avoid using words that have more than one meaning.

22. If using electronic medical records, protect your access code and electronic signature.

23. Remember, from a legal standpoint, if you didn't document it, it wasn't done.

TABLE 3-3 Assessment-Specific Documentation Guidelines

1. Record all data that contribute directly to the assessment (i.e., positive assessment findings and pertinent negatives).

2. Document any parts of the assessment that are omitted or refused by the patient.

3. Avoid using judgmental language such as "good," "poor," "bad," "normal," "abnormal," "decreased," "appears to be," and "seems."

4. Avoid evaluative statements (e.g., "Patient is uncooperative," "Patient is lazy"); cite instead specific statements or actions that you observe (e.g., "patient said, 'I hate this place' and kicked trash can").

5. State time intervals precisely (e.g., "every 4 hours," "bid," instead of "seldom," "occasionally").

6. Do not make relative statements about findings (e.g., "mass the size of an egg"); use specific measurements (e.g., "mass 3 cm × 5 cm").

continues

TABLE 3-3 (Continued)

7. Draw pictures when appropriate (e.g., location of scar, masses, skin lesion, decubitus, deep tendon reflex, etc.).

8. Refer to findings using anatomic landmarks (e.g., left upper quadrant [of abdomen], left lower lobe [of lung], midclavicular line, etc.).

9. Use the face of the clock to describe findings that are in a circular pattern (e.g., breast, tympanic membrane, rectum, vagina).

10. Document any change in the patient's condition during a visit or from previous visits.

11. Describe what you observed, not what you did.

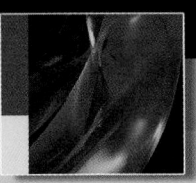

COMPLETE HEALTH HISTORY: WELL PATIENT

Today's Date	January 3, 2010; 9 AM
BIOGRAPHICAL DATA	
Patient Name	Julio Gonzalez, Jr.
Address	4530 176th Place, SE Bellevue, WA 98006
Phone Number H-parents	(206) 603-9122
H-school	(602) 626-6109
Date of Birth	January 27, 1988
Birthplace	Bellevue, WA
Social Security Number	222-56-8765
Occupation	Student
Insurance	Blue Cross/Blue Shield # 987-65-4321, Group No. 108
Usual Source of Health Care	Pediatrician saw pt throughout childhood; he retired and records were lost in a fire last yr
Source of Referral	Parents
Emergency Contact	Julio and Maria Gonzalez (206) 603-9122
SOURCE AND RELIABILITY OF INFORMATION	Self; reliable historian
PATIENT PROFILE	
Age	21
Gender	Male
Race	Hispanic
Marital Status	Single

continues

Complete Health History (continued)

REASON FOR SEEKING HEALTH CARE	"I am home on winter break from college, and I am planning on going to Belize on my spring break c̄ my fraternity brothers and I need to get whatever shots are necessary."
PRESENT HEALTH	Pt describes himself as a healthy college student s̄ any medical problems
PAST HEALTH HISTORY	
Medical History	Seasonal allergies since started college 3 yrs ago; denies any chronic/serious illnesses
Surgical History	Hydrocele repair and Ⓛ inguinal herniorrhaphy age 7 s̄ sequelae
Allergies	NKDA
Medications	
Prescription	Desloratadine 5 mg po daily PRN
OTC	Ibuprofen for H/A PRN
Communicable Diseases	Denies STD, never been tested for HIV
Injuries and Accidents	Scalp sutured age 4 when fell backward off rocking chair, no loss of consciousness, no sequelae
Special Needs	Denies
Blood Transfusions	Denies
Childhood Illnesses	Chickenpox age 6 s̄ sequelae; denies MMR, diphtheria, pertussis, polio, scarlet fever
Immunizations	"My parents say I am up to date; I had a meningitis vaccine before I started college."

FAMILY HEALTH HISTORY

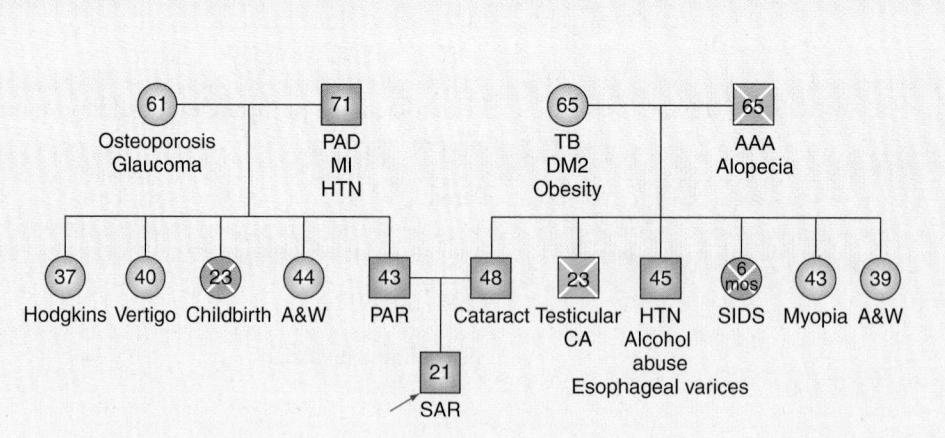

LEGEND

- ◯ Living female
- ▢ Living male
- ⊗ Deceased female
- ⊠ Deceased male
- ↗ Points to patient
- AAA = Abdominal aortic aneurysm
- A&W = Alive & well
- CA = Cancer
- DM = Diabetes mellitus
- dz = disease
- HTN = Hypertension
- MI = Myocardial infarction
- PAD = Peripheral arterial disease
- PAR = Perennial allergic rhinitis
- SAR = Seasonal allergic rhinitis
- SIDS = Sudden infant death syndrome
- sz = Seizure
- TB = Tuberculosis

61 — Osteoporosis, Glaucoma
71 — PAD, MI, HTN
65 — TB, DM2, Obesity
65 — AAA, Alopecia

37 — Hodgkins
40 — Vertigo
23 — Childbirth
44 — A&W
43 — PAR
48 — Cataract
23 — Testicular CA
45 — HTN, Alcohol abuse, Esophageal varices
6 mos — SIDS
43 — Myopia
39 — A&W

21 — SAR

Denies family hx of mental illness, drug addiction, kidney dz, HIV, CVA, liver dz, migraines, sz disorder

continues

Complete Health History (continued)

SOCIAL HISTORY	
Alcohol Use	Beer on the wkends at frat parties, quantity varies; sometimes gets drunk c̄ hangover in AM; denies drinking and driving; denies passing out; believes alcohol use is "typical" for college student
Tobacco Use	Denies
Drug Use	Tried marijuana once at a party freshman yr at college; denies use of anything since then
Domestic and Intimate Partner Violence	Denies
Sexual Practice	Not sexually active nor ever has been; believes he should remain abstinent until marriage
Travel History	Cancun last yr on spring break
Work Environment	N/A
Home Environment	
Physical Environment	Lives in old fraternity house c̄ frat brothers; has kitchen and laundry facilities; has cleaning people for common area; rooms c̄ 2 other brothers; smoke detector is usually disconnected
Psychosocial Environment	Feels safe in house/neighborhood
Hobbies and Leisure Activities	Community service c̄ fraternity, intramural sports program c̄ Interfraternity Council, hanging out c̄ friends
Stress	School, looking for a job p̄ graduation in May
Education	College senior majoring in Environmental Science
Economic Status	Parents pay some tuition and living expenses, has college loans he will need to repay
Military Service	Denies
Religion	Family is Jehovah's Witnesses, pt currently not involved c̄ church while at school
Ethnic Background	Hispanic, grandparents were from Mexico
Roles and Relationships	Only child in a large, extended family; likes to get together c̄ family when he is home on breaks; feels like he can talk to his parents
Characteristic Patterns of Daily Living	"Wow! That varies so much it is hard to say. I can say that I eat at least 2 meals a day, I work out daily, I study, and I play a lot of foosball."
HEALTH MAINTENANCE ACTIVITIES	
Sleep	Tries to get 8 hrs but it can be 4 hrs if there is a party on Thursday night or other social event
Diet	Eats at least 2 meals daily at student dining hall; does not follow any particular diet
Exercise	Basketball, running, racquetball, or lacrosse at least 60 min daily

continues

Complete Health History (continued)	
Stress Management	Exercises, plays foosball
Use of Safety Devices	Wears seat belt
Health Check-ups	Last exam was his pre-college physical; uses student health when sick; dentist q summer
REVIEW OF SYSTEMS	
General	High energy levels, healthy, denies recent illness
Skin	Uses sunscreen when outside more than 1 hr Denies rashes, itching, Δ in skin pigmentation, ecchymoses, pruritus, Δ in moles, sores, lumps, Δ in skin texture, body odors, acne
Hair	Denies alopecia, hirsutism, dandruff, pediculosis, scalp lesions
Nails	Denies Δ in nails, splitting, breaking, onychomycosis
Eyes	Denies use of glasses/contacts; doesn't wear sunglasses on bright days Denies blurry vision, photophobia, ↑ tearing, diplopia, eye drainage, blood-shot eyes, pain, blind spots, floaters, flashing lights, halos around objects, glaucoma, cataracts; can't remember when eyes were last examined
Ears	Denies hearing deficits, hearing aid, pain, discharge, vertigo, tinnitus, ear-aches, infection; Ⓛ ear pierced last yr s̄ sequelae
Nose and Sinuses	SAR per PHH, averages 1–2 colds/yr, denies d/c, itching, postnasal drip, sinus pain, polyps, obstruction, epistaxis, Δ in sense of smell; φ orthodontics
Mouth	Brushes teeth 1–2 ×/d, denies toothache, tooth abscess, caries, bleeding/swollen gums, sore tongue, Δ in taste, lesions, Δ in salivation, halitosis, difficulty chewing
Throat and Neck	Denies hoarseness, Δ in voice, frequent sore throats, dysphagia, pain/stiffness, goiter
Breasts and Axilla	Denies Δ in size, pain, tenderness, d/c, lumps, dimpling, rash
Respiratory	Denies sputum, sneezing, wheezing, hemoptysis, pneumonia, emphysema, EIA, asthma, TB
Cardiovascular and Peripheral Vasculature	Denies paroxysmal nocturnal dyspnea, heart murmur, palpitations, CP, syncope, edema, orthopnea, cold hands/feet, leg cramps, intermittent claudication, varicose veins, thrombophlebitis, anemia, rheumatic heart disease
Gastrointestinal	Regular bowel habit: BM q AM, soft and brown, denies vomiting, diarrhea, constipation, melena, Δ in stool color, hematemesis, ↑ flatulence, belching, heartburn, regurgitation; dysphagia, abdominal pain, jaundice, peptic ulcers, hemorrhoids, hepatitis, gallstones, umbilical hernia
Urinary	Denies Δ in urine color, voiding habits, hesitancy, urgency, frequency, nocturia, polyuria, dribbling, loss in force of stream, bedwetting, suprapubic pain, kidney stones, incontinence, UTIs
Musculoskeletal	Denies bony deformity, weakness, ↓ ROM, swelling, sprains, dislocations, gout, arthritis, herniated disc, back pain

continues

Complete Health History (continued)

Neurological	Denies Δ in balance, incoordination, loss of movement, Δ in sensory perception, Δ in speech, Δ in smell, tremors, syncope, loss of memory, involuntary movement, loss of consciousness, sz, weakness, vertigo, tremors, tics, CVA
Psychological	Anxious about graduating from college in 4 mos Denies nervousness, difficulty concentrating, mood changes, depression, suicidal thoughts
Male Reproductive	Denies impotence, testicular/penile pain, penile d/c, inguinal hernia
Nutrition	Usual and present weight 82 kg (176 lbs) Food preferences: hamburgers and fries Food dislikes: brussel sprouts and peas Denies food intolerances Consumes 2–3 caffeinated drinks daily (sodas)
Endocrine	Denies exophthalmos; Δ in size of head, hands, or feet, cold intolerance, polyuria, polydipsia, polyphagia, Δ in body hair distribution, goiter
Lymph Nodes	Denies enlargement or tenderness
Hematological	Blood type O+ Denies easy bruising/bleeding, anemia

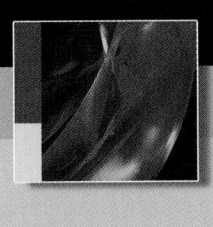

COMPLETE HEALTH HISTORY: ILL PATIENT

Today's Date	December 18, 2009; 11 AM
BIOGRAPHICAL DATA	
Patient Name	Megan Morganstern
Address	2042 Monument Avenue Richmond, VA 23220
Phone Number	(804) 355-2984
Date of Birth	October 21, 1974
Birthplace	El Segundo, CA
Social Security Number	765-09-2348
Occupation	Part-time student, stay-at-home mom
Insurance	Aetna PPO
Usual Source of Health Care	Husband
Source of Referral	Friend

continues

Emergency Contact	Mother: (804) 628-7640
SOURCE AND RELIABILITY OF INFORMATION	Pt cried during most of encounter, deemed reliable historian
PATIENT PROFILE	
Age	35
Gender	Female
Race	Caucasian
Marital Status	Separated
CHIEF COMPLAINT	"My back pain is excruciating. I can't sleep. My husband tried to kill me."
HISTORY OF THE PRESENT ILLNESS	Pt reports that she has had chronic LBP for the past 5 yrs, and that her husband (who is also her doctor) treated her c̄ narcotics. Her legs "go numb" p̄ she has been sitting for 20 min or longer. The pain is a burning sensation that radiates down both legs. Describes daily pain as 6/10 and 10+++/10 when it gets really excruciating. Pt is so debilitated by her LBP that her husband signed for a handicapped parking permit for her. She denies loss of bowel/bladder control, incoordination, falling. She did some physical therapy a yr ago but that did not seem to help. She also tried hypnosis, acupuncture, acupressure, and biofeedback for the pain s̄ success. Her daily pain medication "keeps me sane." In addition, her husband placed her on an antidepressant to help c̄ her mood and restless legs syndrome. Pt states that she usually sleeps about 4 hrs per night and feels tired all the time. This has been very difficult since she is a stay-at-home mom caring for her 2- and 4-yo daughters as well as a PT student pursuing her Master's degree in education. One month ago, pt and her husband got into an argument, and the husband repeatedly threw pt against the wall and started to choke her. Pt's mother came to visit at that time and walked into the house and saw this incident and called the police. Pt's husband currently has a temporary restraining order (TRO) to not be within 100 yards of pt. Pt and her 2 children subsequently moved in c̄ pt's mother.
PAST HEALTH HISTORY	
Medical History	LBP × 5 yrs, started c̄ her 1st pregnancy and has ↑ in severity since then; tx per HPI Restless legs syndrome (RLS) × 3 yrs Depression × 4½ yrs; husband was her therapist Migraine H/A × 4 yrs; triggers—stress and weather Δ Chronic sinusitis × 2 yrs Mitral valve prolapse × 5 yrs, currently observes SBE prophylaxis
Surgical History	C section '05, '07 Tonsillectomy '91
Allergies	Meds: azithromycin—rash Bee stings: respiratory distress (does not have/carry EpiPen) Food: mango—rash Environment: cats—wheezing

continues

Complete Health History (continued)

Medications

Prescription

Bupropion XL 300 mg daily
Ropinirole 4 mg 1 hr ā bedtime
Cyclobenzaprine 5 mg po tid
Oxycodone/acetaminophen 7.5/500 po bid
Zolpidem 10 mg po at bedtime PRN (takes daily)
Naratriptan 2.5 mg po at 1st sign of H/A; may repeat once p̄ 4 hrs; max 5 mg/24 hrs PRN
Amoxicillin 500 mg po, 4 pills po 1 hr ā dental procedures

OTC

MVI po daily
Ca^{++} 500 mg po bid

Communicable Diseases   Denies

Injuries and Accidents   "Too many to count"

Special Needs   Denies

Blood Transfusions   Whole blood—2 units during '05 C section; does not recall details but was hemorrhaging

Childhood Illnesses   Denies, including varicella

Immunizations   Tetanus booster '05, otherwise unknown

FAMILY HEALTH HISTORY

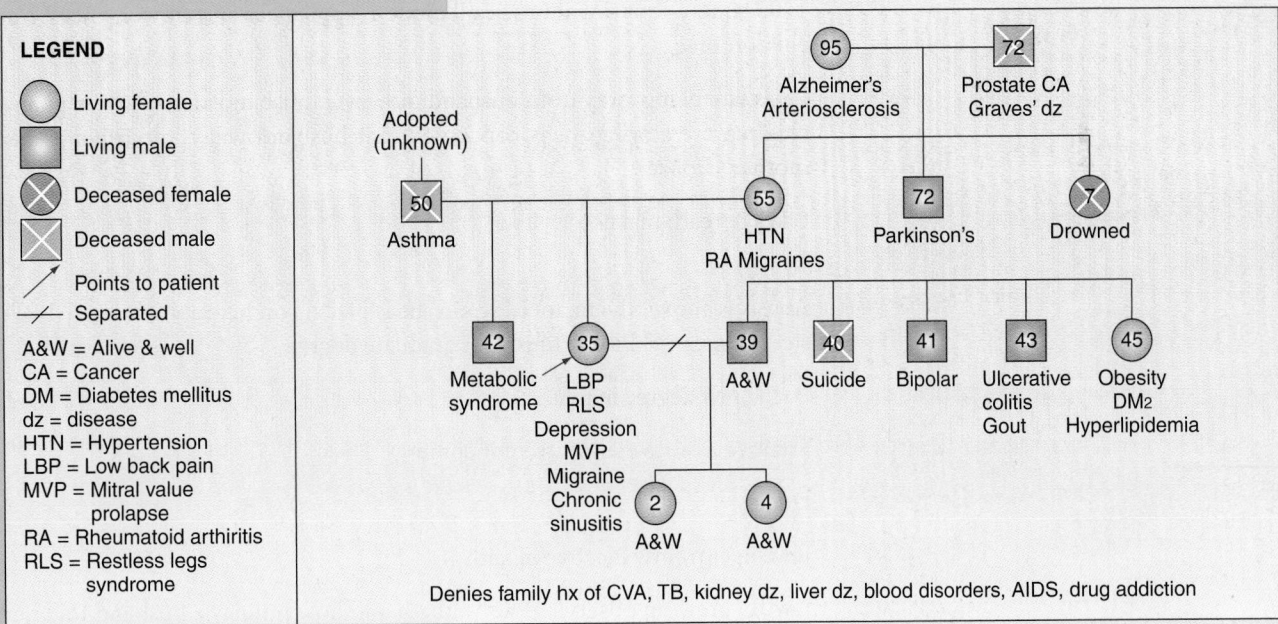

LEGEND

- Living female
- Living male
- Deceased female
- Deceased male
- / Points to patient
- —/ Separated

A&W = Alive & well
CA = Cancer
DM = Diabetes mellitus
dz = disease
HTN = Hypertension
LBP = Low back pain
MVP = Mitral value prolapse
RA = Rheumatoid arthiritis
RLS = Restless legs syndrome

Denies family hx of CVA, TB, kidney dz, liver dz, blood disorders, AIDS, drug addiction

SOCIAL HISTORY

Alcohol Use   Glass of wine on holidays only

Tobacco Use   Denies

Drug Use   Denies

continues

Complete Health History (continued)

Domestic and Intimate Partner Violence	Pt states that she has been verbally abused by her husband for the past 10 yrs. She thought him "hot tempered" but tolerated the verbal abuse and berating "OK." When she became pregnant 5 yrs ago, her husband started pushing her. His rages were unprovoked and took many forms. Most recently, on December 1 of this yr, pt was being choked by husband when her mother arrived for a visit on her way home from work. Pt's mother called police, who responded quickly. Pt refused to press charges. Later she talked to the police, and a TRO was issued to her husband. Pt denied ever losing consciousness, fracturing bones, or having any severe injuries p̄ the physical abuse. She never visited the ER as she was afraid what would happen to her b/c her husband is a physician on staff at the medical center. Her husband told her that she was "unworthy" of love and financial support, and he threatened to leave her. Husband also told her that no one would ever take care of her like he did and she would die s̄ his medical care. With 2 small children at home and not being employed, pt endured these episodes for the welfare of her children and for financial stability. Has phone # for domestic abuse counselor at Women's Center but has not called.
Sexual Practice	Tries to avoid husband as much as possible as he is very rough during sex, sometimes hitting her for arousal
Travel History	Italy for honeymoon 10 yrs ago
Work Environment	N/A
Home Environment	Currently living c̄ mother
Physical Environment	1500-square-foot townhouse c̄ all modern appliances and conveniences; not childproofed
Psychosocial Environment	Feels safe being away from husband; however, husband knows where pt and children are staying; pt is concerned that husband will come p̄ her at her mother's house
Hobbies and Leisure Activities	Likes to read; makes jewelry
Stress	Abuse as above; the financial strain she is placing on her mother; her ↑ LBP; sleeplessness; ability to finish her graduate degree
Education	Bachelor's degree in math
Economic Status	Strained as above; no current income
Military Service	Denies
Religion	Jewish; currently inactive in faith
Ethnic Background	Jewish; grew up observing the Sabbath and holy holidays; husband told her he would not support her in her religious practices
Roles and Relationships	Relationship c̄ husband as previously described; loves and gets along c̄ her mother
Characteristic Patterns of Daily Living	"Right now I am living day to day, and I have no pattern other than caring for my children."

continues

Complete Health History (continued)

HEALTH MAINTENANCE ACTIVITIES

Sleep	4 hrs per night "if I am lucky and that is c̄ my sleeping pill; my restless legs syndrome is getting worse" lies awake at night afraid that her husband may come p̄ her
Diet	Follows no particular diet; due to circumstances of past month, she has lost 10 lbs
Exercise	None
Stress Management	Crying; "I called a therapist, but she can't see me until next wk."
Use of Safety Devices	Wears seat belts; children are placed in car seats
Health Check-ups	Her husband would examine her at home and occasionally send her for blood work; echocardiogram 5 yrs ago; has none of her medical records and can't recall what has been done in the past yr; most recent Pap? Ophth? Dental visit? Does not perform BSE

REVIEW OF SYSTEMS

General	"I'm falling apart. I have no energy for me, my girls, my schoolwork, or my life." Denies recent illness
Skin	Uses sunscreen when outside more than 2 hr, SPF 30 Denies rashes, itching, Δ in skin pigmentation, ecchymoses, warts, eczema, psoriasis, pruritus, Δ in moles, sores, lumps, Δ in skin texture, body odors, acne
Hair	Denies alopecia, hirsutism, dandruff, pediculosis, hair chemicals
Nails	Denies Δ nails, splitting, breaking, onychomycosis
Eyes	Wears Rx sunglasses on bright days. Denies blurry vision, photophobia, tearing, diplopia, eye drainage, bloodshot eyes, pain, blind spots, floaters, flashing lights, halos around objects, glaucoma, cataracts. Can't recall last time she had her eyes examined
Ears	Denies hearing deficits, hearing aid, pain, discharge, vertigo, tinnitus, earaches, infection
Nose and Sinuses	Averages 3–4 sinus infections/yr; never had CT of sinuses; denies discharge, itching, snoring, polyps, obstruction, epistaxis, Δ in sense of smell
Mouth	Brushes teeth 2–3 ×/d; flosses at bedtime; uses OTC rinse c̄ fluoride; denies toothache, tooth abscess, dentures, bleeding/swollen gums, sore tongue, Δ in taste, lesions, Δ in salivation, bad breath, difficulty chewing
Throat and Neck	Denies hoarseness, Δ in voice, frequent sore throats, difficulty swallowing, pain/stiffness, goiter
Breasts and Axilla	Denies Δ in size, pain, tenderness, discharge, lumps, dimpling, rash; no BSE
Respiratory	Denies sputum, sneezing, wheezing, hemoptysis, pneumonia, emphysema, TB exposure, asthma, frequent URIs

continues

Complete Health History (continued)

Cardiovascular and Peripheral Vasculature	MVP dx'd c̄ 1st pregnancy; mod MVP requiring SBE prophylaxis; last echocardiogram was 5 yrs ago; denies paroxysmal nocturnal dyspnea, palpitations, CP, syncope, edema, orthopnea, cold hands/feet, leg cramps, MI, intermittent claudication, varicose veins, thrombophlebitis, anemia, rheumatic heart disease
Gastrointestinal	Regular bowel habit: BM q AM, soft and brown Dyspepsia c̄ stress; ↓ appetite and wt loss per hl hx; denies vomiting, diarrhea, constipation, melena, Δ in stool color, hematemesis; ↑ flatulence, belching, dysphagia, abdominal pain, jaundice, peptic ulcers, hemorrhoids, hepatitis, gallstones
Urinary	Denies Δ in urine color, voiding habits, hesitancy, urgency, frequency, nocturia, polyuria, dribbling, UTIs, suprapubic pain, kidney stones, incontinence
Musculoskeletal	LBP per HPI; states she can walk only 30 yards and the pain becomes unbearable; has not been referred to a pain center; denies bony deformity, weakness, ↓ ROM, swelling, sprains, dislocations, crepitus, gout, arthritis, herniated disc
Neurological	RLS × 3 yrs; on ropinirole for 18 mos, but it does not seem to help, leg mvtment wakes her at night and makes it hard to go to sleep; no lab work done in connection c̄ this; migraine c̄ ↑ stress and precipitated by weather changes, naratriptan usually relieves pain, but the past 3 weeks has had to take it 7 days (5 mg q time); denies Δ in balance, incoordination, loss of movement, Δ in sensory perception, Δ in speech, Δ in smell, tremors, syncope, loss of memory, involuntary movement, loss of consciousness, sz, weakness, vertigo, tremors, spasm, tics
Psychological	Depression for the past 8 yrs, but only started tx 4½ yrs ago; no current thought of suicide or hurting others, feels that she needs more medication now to help her through this experience; has never discussed her abuse c̄ anyone, has never had counseling of any type; ⊕ irritability/difficulty concentrating/anxiety
Female Reproductive	Menarche age 13, menses regular about q 30 days c̄ minimal bleeding and discomfort; no current birth control as husband had vasectomy; ⊕ dyspareunia c̄ occasional postcoital bleeding, admits that sex was difficult the past 2 yrs b/c husband was very rough c̄ no regard for her needs
Nutrition	Present wt: 125 lbs (56.8 kg), usually 135 lbs (61.4 kg); ht: 66″ (167.6 cm) Food likes: sushi and Mexican food when she eats out; prepares balanced meals at home Food dislikes: Thai food, Indian food, and liver Denies food intolerances; no caffeine intake
Endocrine	Denies exophthalmos; Δ in size of head, hands, or feet, cold intolerance; polyuria, polydipsia, polyphagia, Δ in body hair distribution, goiter
Lymph Nodes	Denies enlargement or tenderness
Hematological	Blood type A+ Denies easy bruising/bleeding, anemia

REVIEW QUESTIONS

1. A patient is seen in the clinic 2 days after the initial diagnosis of pneumonia was made. The nurse updates the health history at the second visit. What type of health history is the nurse using?
   a. Complete health history
   b. Episodic health history
   c. Interval health history
   d. Emergency health history
   The correct answer is (c).

2. A patient tells you that he has had a fever and myalgia with the sore throat. What characteristic of a chief complaint do the fever and myalgia represent?
   a. Location
   b. Radiation
   c. Aggravating factors
   d. Associated manifestations
   The correct answer is (d).

3. When drawing a genogram, which symbol is used to represent a living female?
   a. Circle   c. Triangle
   b. Square   d. Rectangle
   The correct answer is (a).

4. A patient reports that he has smoked his entire adult life. Currently, he is smoking one pack of cigarettes per day, and he has done so for the past 10 years. Prior to that, he smoked three packs of cigarettes per day for 25 years. What is his pack/year history?
   a. 10   c. 75
   b. 50   d. 85
   The correct answer is (d).

5. The HITS Screening Tool is used in which of the following situations?
   a. Assessing alcohol use
   b. Assessing domestic abuse
   c. Assessing substance abuse
   d. Assessing tobacco use
   The correct answer is (b).

6. While conducting the Review of Systems (ROS), the nurse asks the patient whether he or she has experienced any fatigue, heat or cold intolerance, polyuria, polyphagia, or increased hunger. In which section of the ROS would this information be documented?
   a. Psychological   c. Gastrointestinal
   b. Endocrine   d. Urinary
   The correct answer is (b).

7. Which of the following chart entries is documented correctly?
   a. The mass is egg-sized.
   b. The mass appears to be smaller than last week.
   c. The mass is located in the left lower quadrant.
   d. The mass does not seem to bother the patient.
   The correct answer is (c).

8. A patient with gout denies that he recently consumed more red meat, beer, or aspirin. What term characterizes the meat, beer, and aspirin?
   a. Chief complaint
   b. Associated manifestations
   c. Aggravating factors
   d. Pertinent negatives
   The correct answer is (d).

9. The patient's social history includes which of the following?
   a. Alcohol use, medications, sleep
   b. Sexual practice, travel history, hobbies, and leisure activities
   c. Communicable diseases, drug use, stress
   d. Work environment, special needs, exercise
   The correct answer is (b).

10. The 4A's of smoking cessation include which of the following?
    a. Asking the patient at the first visit about smoking habits
    b. Advising the patient to quit smoking
    c. Assisting the patient by giving daily medication
    d. Arranging for the patient to return in 6 months for a follow-up visit
    The correct answer is (b).

Visit the Estes online companion resource at
www.delmar.cengage.com
for additional content and study aids.
Click on Online Companions and then select the Nursing discipline.

REFERENCES

American College of Obstetricians & Gynecologists. (1995). *Technical bulletin on domestic violence* (No. 209). Washington, DC: Author.

Ewing, J. A. (1984). Detecting alcoholism: The CAGE questionnaire. *Journal of the American Medical Association, 252,* 1905–1907.

Sherin, K. M., Sinacore, J. M., Li, X. Q., Zitter, R. E., & Shakil, A. (1998). HITS: A short domestic violence screening tool for use in a family practice setting. *Family Medicine, 30*(7), 508–512.

BIBLIOGRAPHY

American Psychiatric Association. *Statement of the American Psychiatric Association on "Video Game Addiction."* Retrieved February 18, 2008, from http://psych.org/news_room/press_releases/07-47videogame addiction_2_pdf

Branson, B. M., Handsfield, H. H., Lampe, M. A., Janssen, R. S., Taylor, A. W., Lyss, S. B., & Clark, J. E. (2006). Revised recommendations for HIV testing of adults, adolescents, and pregnant women in health-care settings. *MMWR. Recommendations and Reports, 55*(RR-14), 1–17.

Correa-de-Araujo, R. (2005). It's your health: Use your medications safely. *Journal of Women's Health, 14*(1), 16–18.

Dowd, T., Kolcaba, K., & Steiner, R. (2006). Development of the healing touch Comfort Questionnaire. *Holistic Nursing Practice, 20*(3), 122–129.

Freeman, C. B. Internet gaming addiction. *The Journal for Nurse Practitioners, 4*(1), 42–47.

Hamilton, N. A., Kitzman, H., & Guyotte, S. (2006). Enhancing health and emotion: Mindfulness as a missing link between cognitive therapy and positive psychology. *Journal of Cognitive Psychotherapy: An International Quarterly, 20,* 123–134.

Haskell, W. L., Lee, I., Pate, R. R., Powell, K. E., Blair, S. N., Franklin, B. A., et al. (2007). Physical activity and public health. Updated recommendation for adults from the American College of Sports Medicine and the American Heart Association. *Circulation, 116,* 1081–1093.

Hill, D. R., Ericsson, C. D., Pearson, R. D., Keystone, J. S., Freedman, D. O., Kozarsky, P. E., et al. (2006). The practice of travel medicine: Guidelines by the Infectious Diseases Society of America. *Clinical Infectious Diseases, 43*(12), 1499–1539.

Hudson, K. L., Holohan, M. K., & Collins, F. S. (2008). Keeping pace with the times—The Genetic Information Nondiscrimination Act of 2008. *New England Journal of Medicine, 358*(25), 2661–2663.

Hung, S. L., Chung, W. H., Jee, S. H., Chen, W. C., Chang, Y. T., Lee, W. R., et al. (2006). Genetic susceptibility to carbamazepine-induced cutaneous adverse drug reactions. *Pharmacogenetics and Genomics, 16*(4), 297–306.

Johns, M. W. (1991). A new method for measuring daytime sleepiness: The Epworth sleepiness scale. *Sleep, 14,* 540–545.

Lugo, N. R. (2007). International traveler health—A national prevention opportunity. *The American Journal for Nurse Practitioners, 11*(3), 51–56.

Lussier-Cushing, M., Repper-DeLisi, J., Mitchell, M. T., Lakatos, B. E., Mahmoud, F., & Lipkis-Orlando, R. (2007). Is your medical/surgical patient withdrawing from alcohol? *Nursing 2007, 37*(10), 50–55.

Mahoney, C. B. (2006). Reducing barriers against routine screening for intimate partner violence. *The American Journal for Nurse Practitioners, 10*(10), 45–58.

Maradiegue, A., & Edwards, Q. T. (2006). An overview of ethnicity and assessment of family health history in primary care settings. *Journal of the American Academy of Nurse Practitioners, 18*(10), 447–456.

Maradiegue, A., Edwards, Q. T., Seibert, D., Macri, C., & Sitzer, L. (2005). Knowledge, perception, and attitudes of advanced practice nursing students regarding medical genetics. *Journal of the American Academy of Nurse Practitioners, 17*(11), 472–479.

Monarch, K. (2007). Documentation, Part 1: Principles for self protection. *American Journal of Nursing, 107*(7), 58–60.

Morgenthaler, T., Kramer, M., Alessi, C., Friedman, L., Boehlecke, B., Brown, T., et al. (2006). Practice parameters for the psychological and behavioral treatment of insomnia: An update. An American Academy of Sleep Medicine report. *Sleep, 29,* 1415–1419.

Mullin, K. A., & Ambrosia, T. (2005). Role of the nurse practitioner in providing health care for the homeless. *The American Journal for Nurse Practitioners, 9*(9), 37–44.

Munoz, C., & Hilgenberg, C. (2005). Ethnopharmacology. *American Journal of Nursing, 105*(8), 40–48.

Nativio, D. G. (2006). Self-inflicted accidental strangulation: The choking game. *The American Journal of Nurse Practitioners, 19*(6), 43–48.

Peterson, J. A. (2007). Get moving! Physical activity counseling in primary care. *Journal of the American Academy of Nurse Practitioners, 19*(7), 349–357.

Reed, D. B., & Claunch, D. T. (2007). Farm safety and family practice: An uncommon partnership for a common goal. *The American Journal for Nurse Practitioners, 11*(11/12), 23–31.

Scholoff, A., Obi-Anyadike, G., Phalak, K., Carrum, G., May, R., & Kamble, R. (2007). Severe systemic reaction to the pneumococcal revaccination. *The Journal for Nurse Practitioners, 3*(3), 178–179.

Schwartz, J. R., & Roth, T. (2006). Shift work sleep disorder: Burden of illness and approaches to management. *Drugs, 66,* 2357–2370.

Smeltzer, S. C. (2007). Improving the health and wellness of persons with disabilities: A call to action too important for nursing to ignore. *Nursing Outlook, 55*(4), 189–195.

Smith, J. P. (2007). Tattoos, body piercing, and nursing: A photo essay. *American Journal of Nursing, 107*(4), 54–57.

Smith, M. C., & Kyle, L. (2008). Holistic foundation of aromatherapy for nursing. *Holistic Nursing Practice, 22*(1), 3–9.

Snyder, M., & Lindquist, R. (Eds.). (2006). *Complementary/alternative therapies in nursing* (5th ed.). New York: Springer.

Summers, M. O., Cristostomo, M. I., & Stepanski, E. J. (2006). Recent developments in the classification, evaluation, and treatment of insomnia. *Chest, 130,* 276–286.

Thompson, R. S., Bonomi, A. E., Anderson, M., Reid, R., Dimer, J., Carrell, D., & Rivara, F. (2006). Intimate partner violence, prevalence, types, and chronicity in adult women. *American Journal of Preventive Medicine, 30*(6), 447–457.

Walker, R., & Buckley, M. (2006). *Probiotic microbes: The scientific basis. A report from the American Academy of Microbiology.* Washington, DC: American Academy of Microbiology.

Wardell, D., Rintala, D., Tan, G., & Duan, Z. (2006). Pilot study of healing touch and progressive relaxation for chronic neuropathic pain in persons with spinal cord injury. *Journal of Holistic Nursing, 24*(4), 231–240.

Woodson, B. T., & Han, J. K. (2005). Relationship of snoring and sleepiness as presenting symptoms in a sleep clinic population. *Annals of Otology, Rhinology, and Laryngology, 114*(10), 762–767.

Zatsick, N. M., & Mayket, P. (2007). Fish oil: Getting to the heart of it. *The Journal for Nurse Practitioners, 3*(2), 104–108.

WEB SITES

American Heart Association Exercise and Fitness:
   http://www.americanheart.org

Centers for Disease Control and Prevention, Traveler's Health:
   http://www.cdc.gov

Evince Clinical Assessments:
   http://www.evinceassessment.com

My Family History Portrait:
   http://familyhistory.hhs.gov

Food and Drug Administration:
   http://www.fda.gov

International Society of Travel Medicine:
   http://www.istm.org

National Coalition Against Domestic Violence:
   http://www.ncadv.org

American Nurses Association:
   http://www.nursingworld.org

National Sexual Violence Resource Center:
   http://www.nsvrc.org

Stop Abuse for Everyone:
   http://www.safe4all.org

National Sleep Foundation:
   http://www.sleepfoundation.org

Transcultural Nursing Society:
   http://www.tcns.org

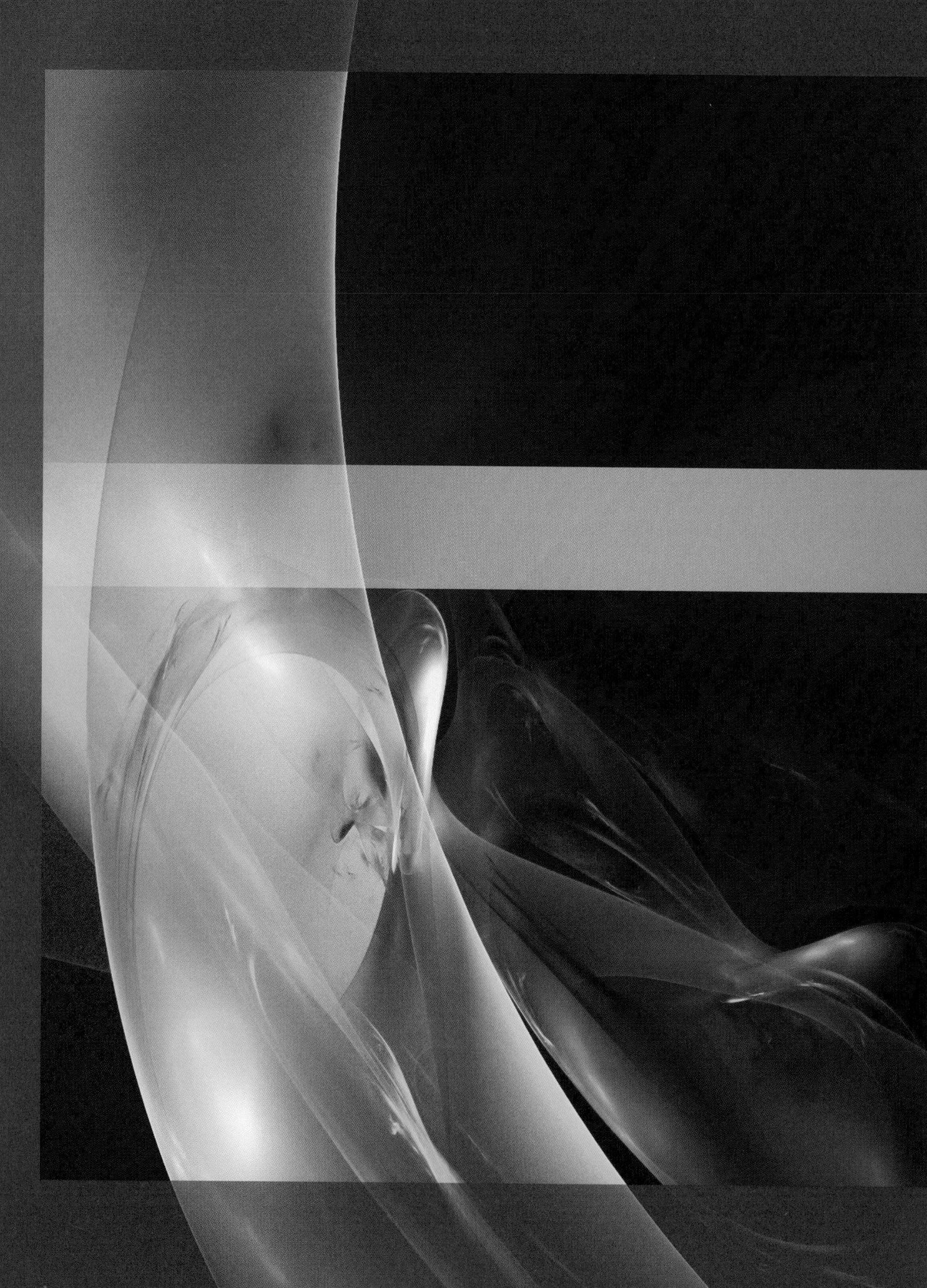

UNIT 2 Special Assessments

People say the effect is only on the mind. It is no such thing. The effect is on the body, too.

—FLORENCE NIGHTINGALE

CHAPTER 4
Developmental Assessment

COMPETENCIES

1. Identify the defining concepts and principles of major developmental theories.

2. Assess patients' developmental levels by applying the major developmental theories.

3. Incorporate appropriate developmental tasks associated with each life stage into a patient's assessment.

4. Select appropriate developmental assessment tools for use in screening a patient for developmental difficulties.

All individuals, from birth to death, pass through identifiable, cyclical stages of growth and development that determine who and what they are and can become. **Growth** refers to an increase in body size and function to the point of optimum maturity. **Development** refers to patterned and predictable increases in the physical, cognitive, socioemotional, and moral capacities of individuals that enable them to successfully adapt to their environments.

Assessing the growth and development status of patients, adults as well as children, is an integral part of patient assessment. It must be noted, however, that although most development is patterned and predictable, you should not impose these expected patterns on a particular patient; assess instead the individual patient's unique development as compared to these general guidelines.

DEVELOPMENTAL THEORIES

A variety of theories have been developed that depict and predict growth and development. The theories most widely used for clinical assessment of patients are the "ages and stages" theories of Piaget (1952), Freud (1946), Erikson (1974), and Kohlberg (1981). The **ages and stages developmental theories** are based on the premise that individuals experience similar sequential physical, cognitive, socioemotional, and moral changes during the same age periods, each of which is termed a **developmental stage**. During each developmental stage, there are specific physical and psychosocial skills known as **developmental tasks** that must be achieved. An individual's readiness for each new developmental task is dependent on success in achieving prior developmental tasks and on the presence of environmental opportunities to develop the new skills. If prior developmental tasks have been insufficiently achieved or appropriate environments in which the tasks can be achieved are not available, mastery of subsequent developmental skills may not occur, may be delayed, or may occur in a defective way, thereby decreasing the individual's capacity to successfully adapt to the environment during his or her lifespan. A key nursing role in assessment is to help identify areas of deficiency and then develop a plan of care designed to address the patient's needs.

A second group of theories include the life events or transitional theories of development. **Life event** or **transitional developmental theories** are based on the premise that development occurs in response to specific events, such as new roles (e.g., parenthood) and life transitions (e.g., career changes). Life events and transitions require adaptive, coping behavior as well as often-significant changes in an individual's life patterns. Each of these events, which can occur singly or together and may be positively or negatively stressful, are not tied to a specific time or stage in the lifespan. Each event, however, does have certain tasks associated with it that must be achieved. For example, getting married is associated with specific developmental tasks that must be achieved regardless of the age of the individual at the time of marriage. The degree of success or failure with these tasks influences the individual's potential for success with concurrent and subsequent developmental tasks that occur in response to any other life events. A variety of factors have been found to affect how an individual responds to life events: biological status, personality, cultural orientation, socioeconomic status, interpersonal support systems, number and intensity of life events, and orientation to life (Aldwin, 2007). Although the stress associated with each life event or transition can serve as an impetus for growth, excessive stress can disrupt the individual's equilibrium and lead to a variety of physical and psychological health problems (Aguilera, 1994; Grey, 1993; Wykle, Kahana, & Kowal, 1992). In identifying life events and stressors, nurses can play a critical role in helping patients maintain health and control stress.

AGES AND STAGES DEVELOPMENTAL THEORIES

The major tenets of Piaget, Freud, Erikson, and Kohlberg are discussed next; these are summarized in Table 4-1.

TABLE 4-1 Summary of Ages and Stages Developmental Theories

STAGE/AGE	PIAGET'S COGNITIVE STAGES	FREUD'S PSYCHOSEXUAL STAGES	ERIKSON'S PSYCHOSOCIAL STAGES	KOHLBERG'S MORAL JUDGMENT STAGES
1. Infancy Birth to 1 year	**Sensorimotor** (birth to 2 years): Begins to acquire language Task: Object permanence	**Oral:** Pleasure from exploration with mouth and through sucking Task: Weaning	**Trust vs. Mistrust** Task: Trust Socializing agent: Mothering person Central process: Mutuality Ego quality: Hope	**Preconventional Level:** 1. **Morality stage:** Avoid punishment by not breaking rules of authority figures
2. Toddler 1 to 3 years	**Sensorimotor** continues **Preoperational** (2 to 7 years) begins: Use of representational thought Task: Use language and mental images to think and communicate	**Anal:** Control of elimination Task: Toilet training	**Autonomy vs. Shame and Doubt** Task: Autonomy Socializing agent: Parents Central process: Imitation Ego quality: Self-control and willpower	2. **Individualism, Instrumental Purpose, and Exchange Stage:** "Right" is relative, follow rules when in own interest
3. Preschool 3 to 6 years	**Preoperational** continues	**Phallic:** Attracted to opposite-sex parent Task: Resolve Oedipus/ Electra complex	**Initiative vs. Guilt** Task: Initiative and moral responsibility Socializing agents: Parents Central process: Identification Ego quality: Direction, purpose, and conscience	
4. School Age 6 to 12 years	**Preoperational** continues **Concrete Operations** (7 to 12 years) begins: Engage in inductive reasoning and concrete problem solving Task: Learn concepts of conservation and reversibility	**Latency:** Identification with same-sex parent Task: Identity with samesex parent and test and compare own capabilities with peer norms	**Industry vs. Inferiority** Task: Industry, self-assurance, self-esteem Socializing agents: Teachers and peers Central process: Education Ego quality: Competence	**Conventional Level** 3. **Mutual Expectations, Relationships, and Conformity to Moral Norms Stage:** Need to be "good" in own and others' eyes, believe in rules and regulations
5. Adolescence 12 to 18 years	**Formal Operations** (12 years to adulthood): Engage in abstract reasoning and analytical problem solving Task: Develop a workable philosophy of life	**Genital:** Develop sexual relationships Task: Establish meaningful relationship for lifelong pairing	**Identity vs. Role Confusion** Task: Self-identity and concept Socializing agents: Society of peers Central process: Role experimentation and peer pressure Ego quality: Fidelity and devotion to others, personal and sociocultural values	4. **Social System and Conscience Stage:** Uphold laws because they are fixed social duties

continues

TABLE 4-1 (Continued)

STAGE/AGE	PIAGET'S COGNITIVE STAGES	FREUD'S PSYCHOSEXUAL STAGES	ERIKSON'S PSYCHOSOCIAL STAGES	KOHLBERG'S MORAL JUDGMENT STAGES
6. **Young Adult** 18 to 30 years	**Formal Operations** continues		**Intimacy vs. Isolation** Task: Intimacy Socializing agent: Close friends, partners, lovers, spouse Central process: Mutuality among peers Ego quality: Intimate affiliation and love	**Postconventional Level:** 5. **Social Contract or Utility and Individual Rights Stage:** Uphold laws in the interest of the greatest good for the greatest number; uphold laws that protect universal rights
7. **Early Middle Age** 30 to 50 years			**Generativity vs. Stagnation** Task: Generativity Socializing agent: Spouse, partner, children, sociocultural norms Central process: Creativity and person-environment fit Ego quality: Productivity, perseverance, charity, and consideration	
8. **Late Middle Age** 50 to 70 years			**Generativity vs. Stagnation** continues	6. **Universal Ethical Principles Stage:** Support universal moral principles regardless of the price for doing so
9. **Late Adult** 70 years to death			**Ego Integrity vs. Despair** (65 years to death) Task: Ego integrity Socializing agent: Significant others Central process: Introspection Ego quality: Wisdom	

Piaget's Theory of Cognitive Development

Jean Piaget's (1952; b. 1896–d. 1980) theory of cognitive development depicts age-related, sequential stages through which all developing children must progress to learn to think, reason, and exercise judgment and to learn the cognitive life skills (e.g., language development, problem solving, decision making, critical thinking, and oral and written communication) needed to successfully adapt to their environments. The individual's cognitive development is influenced by innate intellectual capacity, maturation of the nervous and endocrine systems, and varied environmental interactions during which sensory and motor input is experienced and processed. Piaget divides cognitive development into four periods: sensorimotor stage, preoperational stage, concrete operations stage, and formal operational stage.

SENSORIMOTOR STAGE. During the sensorimotor stage (birth to 2 years), the developing child perceives the world primarily through sensation and action response. The primary cognitive developmental task for this stage is to learn **object permanence**, that is, to form a mental image of an object and to recognize that although the object is removed from view, it still exists. Object permanence is usually achieved by the eight month of life and facilitates the achievement of the second cognitive task, the development of a sense of self separate from one's environment. Beginning to use language and mental representations to think about events before and after they occur is an additional cognitive task that must be achieved during this stage.

PREOPERATIONAL STAGE. The second cognitive development period is the preoperational stage (2 to 7 years), which is characterized by **egocentrism**, that is, viewing the world in terms of self only and interpreting actions and all other events in terms of the consequences they have for self. Learning during this stage usually occurs through imitation of others, physical and cognitive exploration of the environment, and asking numerous questions. Thinking is concrete, and reasoning is intuitive and based on the observable; that is, what is directly seen, heard, or personally experienced. The major cognitive developmental task for this stage is to use language and mental representations to think and communicate about objects and events in the environment.

CONCRETE OPERATIONS STAGE. During the third cognitive development period, the concrete operations stage (7 to 12 years), thinking becomes socialized in that thought becomes less self-oriented and others' points of view are given consideration. Thinking becomes increasingly logical and coherent; facts are organized through sorting, ordering, and classifying; the concept of time evolves; different aspects of situations are dealt with simultaneously; reasoning is inductive; problems are solved concretely and systematically; and communication is enhanced through expanding oral skills and learning to read and write. The major developmental tasks are mastering the concept of **conservation** (understanding that altering the physical state of an object does not change the basic properties of the object) and **reversibility** (understanding that an action does not need to be experienced before one can anticipate the results or consequences of the action).

FORMAL OPERATIONS STAGE. The fourth cognitive development period is the formal operations stage (12 years to adulthood) in which thinking becomes increasingly abstract, logical, analytical, and creative. Ideas are combined to form concepts, and concepts are combined to form constructs and hypotheses. Theories are developed and beginning to be tested, and alternative solutions for problems are generated and examined. The antecedents, moderators, and outcomes of ideas, concepts, situations, and actions are recognized and incorporated into the individual's worldview. The primary cognitive developmental task for this stage is to develop a workable philosophy of life.

Freud's Psychoanalytic Theory of Personality Development

Sigmund Freud (1946; b. 1856–d. 1939) contended that human behavior is motivated by psychodynamic forces within an individual's unconscious mind. Driven to act by these internal forces, individuals repeatedly interact with the external environment. The individual's personality and psychosexual identity are developed through the accumulation of these interactional experiences.

PERSONALITY. Personality, according to Freud, consists of three components with distinctly separate functions: id, ego, and superego. The **id**, evident at birth, is inborn, unconscious, and is driven by biological instincts and urges to seek immediate gratification of needs such as hunger, thirst, and physical comfort. The **ego** is conscious, rational, and emerges during the first year of life as infants begin to test the limits of the world around them. The ego seeks realistic and acceptable ways to meet needs. The **superego**, appearing in early childhood, is the internalization of the moral values formed as children interact with their parents and significant others. The superego acts as a moral arbitrator by blocking unacceptable behavior generated by the id that could threaten the social order, creating feelings of guilt when the internalized moral code is compromised, and generating feelings of pride when the moral code is upheld.

Freud believed individuals experience an ongoing struggle among the id, ego, and superego. Achieving a balance among the three, however, is prerequisite to the development of socially acceptable behavior and an integrated personality. To assist the personality to achieve this balance and to protect itself from excess anxiety created by the ongoing struggle, the ego uses unconscious defense mechanisms such as repression, denial, projection, and rationalization.

PSYCHOSEXUAL STAGES. Freud perceived the desire to satisfy biological needs, primarily sexual, as the major drive governing human behavior. At different psychosexual developmental stages, individuals experience tension associated with a specific body region that prompts them to seek gratification of the needs and conflicts thereby engendered. Each developmental stage is centered on a specific body region and the associated conflicts. If an individual's needs are met during a given stage and conflicts are resolved, development will proceed normally to the next stage, and the developing personality will be integrated in a healthy way. If resolution of the conflict does not occur, however, the individual will become fixated at that stage, and personality and psychosexual identity will be arrested or impaired. Freud identified five psychosexual stages of development: oral, anal, phallic, latency, and genital.

Oral Stage. The oral psychosexual stage (birth to 1 year) is focused on the sensory area of the mouth, lips, and tongue. Sucking, biting, chewing, swallowing, and vocalizing provide pleasure and reduce tension. The major conflict during this stage centers around weaning. Oral personality traits that begin to emerge are optimism versus pessimism, cockiness versus self-belittlement, admiration versus envy, determinism versus submission, and gullibility versus suspiciousness.

Anal Stage. In the anal psychosexual stage (1 to 3 years), the focus is on the anal and urethral sensory areas. Expulsion and retention of body wastes provide pleasure and reduce tension. The major conflict centers around toilet training. Anal personality traits that begin to emerge during this period are orderliness versus messiness, acquiescence versus stubbornness, overgenerosity versus stinginess, rigid punctuality versus tardiness, and expansiveness versus constrictedness.

Phallic Stage. The phallic psychosexual stage (3 to 6 years) is focused on the sensory areas of the genitals. Pleasure is provided and tension is reduced through penile and clitoral exploration and stimulation. The major conflicts center around the controversial **Oedipus** (young boys' sexual attraction toward their mothers and feelings of rivalry toward their fathers) and **Electra** (young girls' sexual attraction toward their fathers and rivalry with their mothers for their fathers' attention) **complexes**, **castration anxiety** (young boys' fear of having their penis cut off or mutilated), and **penis envy** (young girls' desire to have a penis). Phallic personality traits that begin to emerge are gaiety versus sadness, gregariousness versus isolationism, stylishness versus plainness, blind courage versus timidity, and brashness versus bashfulness.

Latency Stage. During the latency psychosexual stage (6 to 12 years), the focus is on the exploration and discovery of the total body's relatedness, coordination, and uses rather than on a specific body region. Channeling generalized psychic and physical activity into knowledge acquisition and vigorous play provides pleasure and reduces tension. The major conflict during this stage centers around identifying with the same-sex parent, learning and testing mental and physical capabilities, and comparing one's capabilities with peer norms.

Genital Stage. The genital psychosexual stage (12 years to adulthood) is focused on full sexual maturity and function. Self and mutual sexual stimulation and the formation of friendships and sexual relationships provide pleasure and reduce tension. The major conflicts during this period center around becoming sexually desirable to others and establishing meaningful relationships in preparation for lifelong pairing.

Erikson's Epigenetic Theory of Personality

The most frequently used theory of personality development is Erikson's (1974; b. 1902–d. 1994) epigenetic theory, which is based on the biological concept that all growing organisms have an inherent plan of growth for all parts of the entity. Each part of a growing entity has a designated time of ascendancy and forms the basis for growth of the next part until the functional whole is fully developed. Erikson's theory was built on Freud's theory of personality but goes beyond it by depicting personality development as a passage through eight sequential stages of ego development from infancy through old age.

According to Erikson, developing individuals must master and resolve, to some extent, a core conflict/crisis during each stage by integrating their personal needs and skills with the social and cultural demands and expectations of their environment. Passage to each developmental stage is dependent on the resolution of the core conflict of the preceding stage. No core conflict is ever completely mastered, however. Rather, in each new life situation, the conflict can be present in a new form that can then be resolved more readily if the conflict was initially resolved favorably. If the conflict was initially resolved unfavorably, subsequent encounters with new forms of the core conflict can provide opportunities to try again to resolve it favorably. Thus, the potential for further development and refinement always exists. For each of the eight core conflicts/crises, there is an associated central process for resolving the conflict, a key socializing agent, and an ego quality that results from the favorable resolution of the core conflict.

TRUST VERSUS MISTRUST STAGE. The core conflict/crisis for the first developmental stage (birth to 1 year) is trust versus mistrust. When developing infants' basic needs are met by prompt, consistent, predictable, loving parent figures, basic, relative trust evolves. If infants' needs are intermittently, inadequately, or perfunctorily met, then mistrust results.

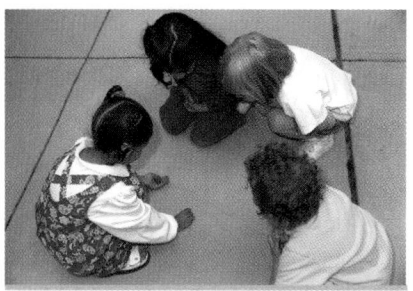

FIGURE 4-1 These young children are taking the initiative to explore their environment as they examine a snail they found on the sidewalk.

REFLECTIVE THINKING

Age-Appropriate Behaviors

While on a home visit, you notice that the mother is spoon feeding her 22-month-old child. You ask the mother why she is spoon feeding her child. The mother tells you that her child is too messy and might dirty her dress and the floor. How would you respond to the mother? What anticipatory guidance would be appropriate?

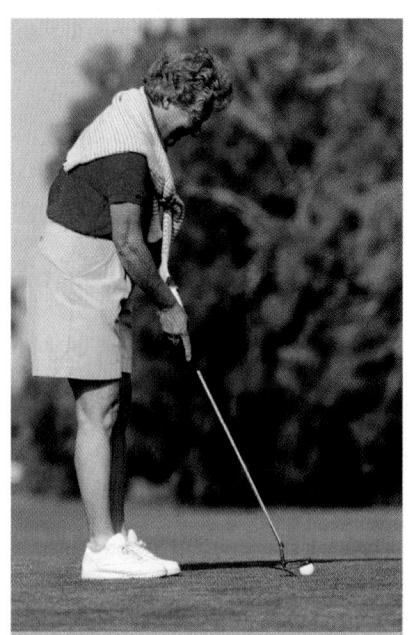

FIGURE 4-2 This older woman is exploring new avenues of enjoyment as she avoids stagnation in her later years.

AUTONOMY VERSUS SHAME AND DOUBT STAGE. The second developmental stage (1 to 3 years) is focused on the autonomy versus shame and doubt core conflict/crisis. If parental figures overprotect their children and overly criticize and punish their attempts to explore and control their environments and body activities, as well as their attempts to make independent decisions, then shame, doubt, and uncertainty about their abilities and themselves will result.

INITIATIVE VERSUS GUILT STAGE. During the third developmental stage (3 to 6 years), the core conflict/crisis is initiative versus guilt. When children are encouraged to explore their environments and to plan and work toward goals that do not infringe on the rights of others, they develop initiative and moral responsibility (Figure 4-1). In contrast, if children are restricted from exploring their environments or are made to feel that their enterprise and active imaginations are bad, they will experience guilt and lose the courage to conceive of and pursue valued goals.

INDUSTRY VERSUS INFERIORITY STAGE. The central conflict/crisis for the fourth developmental stage (6 to 12 years) is industry versus inferiority. Competence is the favorable result of being encouraged to and successfully engaging in achievable tasks and activities, competing and cooperating with others, and learning the rules and norms of a widening social and cultural environment. If children are not given sufficient opportunities or encouragement to develop their abilities or are pushed to achieve beyond their present abilities and thus repeatedly fail, feelings of inadequacy and inferiority result and new learning activities will be increasingly avoided.

IDENTITY VERSUS ROLE CONFUSION STAGE. The fifth stage of development (12 to 18 years) is focused on the identity versus role confusion core conflict/crisis. Adolescents must make the transition from childhood to adulthood, redefine themselves in terms of the roles they hope to play in society, explore life work possibilities, and integrate self-concept and values with those of their peers and society. Supportive, understanding interactions with peers and adult role models help clarify self-identity and lead to the ego quality of fidelity and devotion to others as well as personal and sociocultural values and ideologies. Unfavorable interactions or overidentification with popular teen fads and peer culture heroes can result in role confusion and difficulty clarifying personal identity.

INTIMACY VERSUS ISOLATION STAGE. Intimacy versus isolation is the core conflict/crisis associated with the sixth developmental stage (18 to 30 years). The capacity for intimate affiliation with and the love of significant others is what results from the favorable resolution of this core conflict. Feelings of aloneness and social isolation are the result of unsuccessful resolution.

GENERATIVITY VERSUS STAGNATION STAGE. The seventh developmental stage (30 to 65 years) is focused on the core conflict of generativity versus stagnation. Generativity is when one's focus on meeting the needs of others is of equal concern to that of providing for oneself (Figure 4-2). Qualities of productivity, perseverance, charity, and consideration result from the development of generativity. Generative young and middle-aged adults nourish and nurture the products of their creativity at home, at work, and in their communities. Individuals who are unsuccessful in resolving the core conflict during this stage of development become self-absorbed and feel chronically unfulfilled.

EGO INTEGRITY VERSUS DESPAIR STAGE. During the eighth and last stage of development (65 years to death), the core conflict/crisis is ego integrity versus despair. After reviewing one's life in its entirety, acceptance of what has passed and satisfaction with the present results in a sense of integrity. In contrast, remorse for the past and what might have been results in despair.

Kohlberg's Theory of Moral Development

The basic premise of Kohlberg's (1981; b. 1927–d. 1987) theory of moral development is that when a conflict occurs among any of several universal values (e.g., punishment, affection, authority, truth, law, life, liberty, and justice), the moral choice that must be made and justified requires cognitive capabilities, including systematic problem solving, which constitute moral reasoning. Thus, the development of the individual's moral reasoning and associated behaviors parallels the development of cognitive behavior primarily. According to Kohlberg, moral development is contingent upon children's ability to learn and internalize parental and societal rules and standards, develop the ability to empathize with others' responses, and form their own personal standards of conduct. Moral development progresses through three levels, with two distinct stages per level, for a total of six stages. Keep in mind that Kohlberg's theory of moral development has fallen under heavy criticism because an all-male population was studied.

PRECONVENTIONAL LEVEL. The first level of moral development, the preconventional level, is divided into two stages. In stage 1, the morality stage, individuals have an egocentric point of view and avoid breaking rules and damaging persons and property in order to avoid being punished by authority figures with superior power. In stage 2—the individualism, instrumental purpose, and exchange stage—individuals have a concrete individualistic perspective and follow rules only when doing so is primarily in their own or sometimes in someone else's immediate interest, and because "right" is relative and what is "fair" represents an equal exchange.

CONVENTIONAL LEVEL. The second level of moral development is the conventional level. This level is divided into two stages: stage 3, mutual interpersonal expectations, relationships, and interpersonal conformity, in which individuals can envision the perspective of another and try to live up to the expectations of self and others through conformity to moral norms, have "good" motives, are concerned about others, believe in rules and regulations, and maintain relationships by being trustworthy, loyal, respectful, and appropriately grateful; and stage 4, social system and conscience, in which individuals can differentiate societal points of view from interpersonal agreements and motives, and avoid the breakdown of the social system by recognizing and supporting how the system defines roles and rules, by fulfilling the duties to which they have agreed, and by upholding laws because they are fixed social duties. According to Kohlberg, most adults in the United States have not progressed beyond this stage of moral judgment.

POSTCONVENTIONAL LEVEL. The third level of moral development, the postconventional level, is divided into two stages: stage 5, social contract or utility, and individual rights, in which adult individuals recognize that there are moral and legal points of view that may sometimes be in conflict and that although most rules are relative to the group that makes them, they warrant being upheld in the interest of the greatest good for the greatest number. Individuals in this stage recognize that as people's needs change, laws may need to be changed by working through the system to do so. Nonetheless, laws that protect some universal rights such as life and liberty must be upheld regardless of people's changing opinions or desires. Stage 6, universal ethical principles, occurs when some middle-aged or older adults develop a rational, universal moral perspective and a commitment to laws and social agreements based on universal moral principles of justice, equal rights, and respect for human dignity. When laws violate these moral principles, it

Evaluating Developmental Theories

- Do you agree with the major premises of the developmental theories presented in this chapter?
- Conduct a personal investigation into the research methodologies used by the theorists. Consider the following questions after your research is concluded:
  - What populations did the theorists study when drawing the conclusions upon which their theories are based?
  - Were the appropriate conclusions made on the research data?
  - Would you have approached the study in a different manner? How?
  - Think critically about the research. What conclusions would you draw?

NURSING**TIP**

U.S. Preventive Services Task Force and Lifespan Guidelines

In 1998, the Public Health Service of the Agency for Healthcare Research and Quality convened the U.S. Preventive Services Task Force to function as "an independent panel of experts in primary care and prevention . . . (to) systematically review the evidence of effectiveness and develop recommendations for clinical preventive services" (U.S. Preventive Services Task Force, 2007). After rigorously evaluating all available clinical research and the merits of the preventive measures, screening tests, preventive medications, immunizations, and counseling included, clinical recommendations and guidelines for throughout the lifespan have been developed and periodically updated as more research becomes available. These recommendations and guidelines are made available to health care professionals and the public online, through government publications, and in the medical literature (Sawaya, Guiguis-Blake, LeFevre, Harris, & Petiti, 2007; U.S. Preventive Services Task Force, 2007; Wolff, Guirguis-Blake, Gillespie, & Harris, 2007; Wolff, Gurguis-Blake, Miller, Gillespie, & Harris, 2007).

is the principle, rather than the law, that must be followed regardless of the price that must be paid for doing so. Kohlberg contends that few people attain and even fewer maintain this state of moral development.

DEVELOPMENTAL STAGES, TASKS, AND LIFE EVENTS

As evident from a review of the preceding theories of development, there is no complete agreement about the age associated with each developmental stage. In addition, improved nutrition, medical advances, and healthier lifestyles have contributed to greater longevity in the United States and other Western countries. Indeed, from 1900 when approximately 1 in 25 U.S. citizens were elderly, there are now over 1 in every 8 (Krach & Verkoff, 1999; National Center for Health Statistics, 2007). As a result, what was once considered to be the beginning of late adulthood (55 to 70 years) is now a part of middle adulthood, and what was considered to be the latter part of late adulthood (70+ years) is now recognized as the beginning rather than the end of this period. The developmental assessment process presented in this text, therefore, will be presented using the following stages:

Stage 1: Infancy (birth to 1 year)
Stage 2: Toddler (1 to 3 years)
Stage 3: Preschooler (3 to 6 years)
Stage 4: School-age child (6 to 12 years)
Stage 5: Adolescence (12 to 18 years)
Stage 6: Young adulthood (18 to 30 years)
Stage 7: Early middle adulthood (30 to 50 years)
Stage 8: Late middle adulthood (50 to 70 years)
Stage 9: Late adulthood (70 years to death)

The following section combines the developmental tasks and life events and transitions from each major theory of development, thereby giving a composite of the developmental tasks and possible life events that characterize each developmental stage. The lists of tasks for each stage are not exhaustive, nor do they reflect all the tasks facing the full range of normal human conditions and circumstances. Generally, ask yourself whether the individual's overall development seems consistent with the tasks usually associated with the person's chronological age. In addition, the life events included in each stage are not restricted to that stage but may occur or reoccur during several developmental stages. Failure to meet tasks in one area does not always indicate abnormal development. It is expected that the following will form a general framework on which you can base your assessment of a patient's growth and development. Remember to consider each individual as a whole entity, not just a collection of tasks met or not met.

DEVELOPMENTAL TASKS OF INFANTS (BIRTH TO 1 YEAR)

Infancy is a period of dramatic and rapid physical, motor, cognitive, emotional, and social growth, which marks it as one of the most critical periods of growth and development. During the first year of life, infants change from totally helpless, dependent newborns to unique individuals who actively interact with their environments and form meaningful relationships with significant others. A list of key gross and fine motor, language, and sensory milestones associated with this period can be found in Table 4-2.

One of the major tasks of infancy is weaning, which requires children to give up the breast or bottle, which has been a major source of gratification, and learn to use a cup. Readiness for weaning usually occurs between the ages of 6 months and 12 to 14 months, when the child has learned that good things also come from a spoon, when more motor control has been developed so a cup can be grasped and brought to the mouth, and when the desire for freedom of movement begins to lessen the desire to be held while eating.

Conducting a comprehensive assessment of an infant requires an evaluation of the degree to which the infant has achieved the developmental tasks of infancy. It is important to remember that although individuals experience similar sequential physical, cognitive, socioemotional, and moral changes during the same age periods, there is still a degree of normal variability from one child to another. Developmental tasks that must be achieved during the infancy stage are to:

1. Develop a basic, relative sense of trust.
2. Develop a sense of self as dependent on but separate from others, particularly the mother.
3. Develop and desire affection for and response from others, particularly the mother.
4. Develop a preverbal communication system, including emotional expression, to communicate needs and desires.
5. Begin to develop conceptual abilities and a language system.
6. Begin to learn purposeful fine and gross motor skills, particularly eye-hand coordination and balance (Figure 4-3).

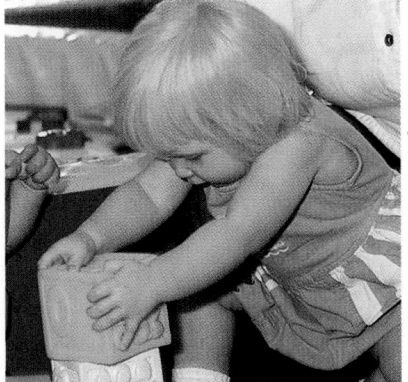

FIGURE 4-3 This 11-month-old girl demonstrates one of the abilities of a child of this age group—creating a tower of two blocks.

REFLECTIVE THINKING

Helping Parents Understand Development

Caregivers are often nervous about their infants and have many questions. Consider how you would respond to each of these questions:

- "My sister's baby was already holding his bottle at 6 months, but my little boy doesn't seem to be able to do that, and he's 2 weeks older than my sister's baby! Is there something wrong with him?"
- "I want to be sure I buy the right toy for my niece. What do you suggest for her? She will be having her third birthday next week."

TABLE 4-2 Growth and Development during Infancy

AGE	GROSS MOTOR	FINE MOTOR	LANGUAGE	SENSORY
Birth to 1 Month	• Assumes tonic neck posture • When prone, lifts and turns head	• Holds hands in fist • Draws arms and legs to body	• Cries	• Comforts with holding and touch • Looks at faces • Follows objects when in line of vision • Alert to high-pitched voices • Smiles
2 to 4 Months	• Can raise head and shoulders when prone to 45°–90°; supports self on forearms • Rolls from back to side	• Hands mostly open • Looks at and plays with fingers • Grasps and tries to reach objects	• Vocalizes when talked to; coos, babbles • Laughs aloud • Squeals	• Smiles • Follows objects 180° • Turns head when hears voices or sounds
4 to 6 Months	• Turns from stomach to back and then back to stomach • When pulled to sitting, almost no head lag • By 6 months, can sit on floor with hands forward for support	• Can hold feet and put in mouth • Can hold bottle • Can grasp rattle and other small objects • Puts objects in mouth	• Squeals	• Watches a falling object • Responds to sounds
6 to 8 Months	• Puts full weight on legs when held in standing position • Can sit without support • Bounces when held in a standing position	• Transfers objects from one hand to the other • Can feed self a cookie • Can bang two objects together	• Babbles vowel-like sounds, "ooh" or "aah" • Imitation of speech sounds ("mama," "dada") beginning • Laughs aloud	• Responds by looking and smiling • Recognizes own name
8 to 10 Months	• Crawls on all fours or uses arms to pull body along floor • Can pull self to sitting • Can pull self to standing	• Beginning to use thumb-finger grasp • Dominant hand use • Has good hand-mouth coordination	• Responds to verbal commands • May say one word in addition to "mama" and "dada"	• Recognizes sounds
10 to 12 Months	• Can sit down from standing • Walks around room holding onto objects • Can stand alone	• Picks up and drops objects • Can put small objects into toys or containers through holes • Turns many pages in a book at one time • Picks up small objects	• Understands "no" and other simple commands • Learns one or two other words • Imitates speech sounds • Speaks gibberish	• Follows fast-moving objects • Indicates wants • Likes to play imitative games such as patty cake and peek-a-boo

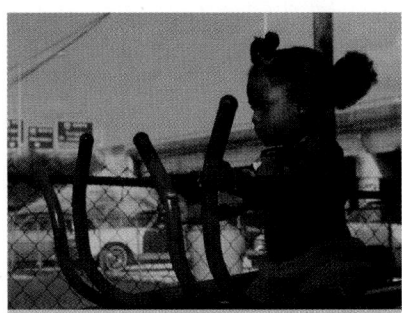

FIGURE 4-4 Refinement of skills and a growing sense of independence are most noted in toddlers.

7. Begin to explore and recognize the immediate environment.
8. Develop object permanence.

DEVELOPMENTAL TASKS OF TODDLERS (1 TO 3 YEARS)

The toddler period is one of steadily increasing motor development and control (Figure 4-4), intense activity and discovery, rapid language development, increasingly independent behaviors, and marked personality development. Key gross and fine motor, language, and sensory milestones associated with the toddler period can be found in Table 4-3.

One of the major developmental tasks for toddlers is toilet training. Readiness for toilet training is usually evident in the infants in the age group of 18 to

TABLE 4-3 Growth and Development during Toddlerhood

AGE	GROSS MOTOR	FINE MOTOR	LANGUAGE	SENSORY
12 to 15 Months	• Can walk alone well • Can crawl up stairs	• Can feed self with cup and spoon • Puts raisins into a bottle • May hold crayon or pencil and scribble • Builds a tower of two cubes	• Says four to six words	• Binocular vision is developed
18 Months	• Runs, falling often • Can jump in place • Can walk up stairs holding on • Plays with push and pull toys	• Can build a tower of three to four cubes • Can use a spoon	• Says 10 or more words • Points to objects or body parts when asked	• Visual acuity 20/40
24 Months	• Can walk up and down stairs • Can kick a ball • Can ride a tricycle	• Can draw a circle • Tries to dress self	• Talks a lot • Approximately 300-word vocabulary • Understands commands • Knows first name, refers to self • Verbalizes toilet needs	
30 Months	• Throws a ball • Jumps with both feet • Can stand on one foot for a few seconds	• Can build a tower of eight blocks • Can use crayons • Learning to use scissors	• Knows first and last name • Knows the name of one color • Can sing • Expresses needs • Uses pronouns appropriately	

Understanding Toilet Training

Parents often have difficulty with "potty training" their child and become frustrated when their first attempts are not successful. What suggestions could you give the caregiver who has been trying unsuccessfully for the past 2 months with her 15-month-old son? She comments that she had absolutely no problems with her first child, a daughter, at this age and cannot understand what the problem is this time.

Preschoolers' Readiness for School

You are performing a physical examination on 5-year-old Jamie for his annual check-up. After the exam, you ask the parents whether they have any questions. Jamie's father expresses concern that the other children in his son's preschool class are printing their names, but Jamie is not. How would you respond to this concern?

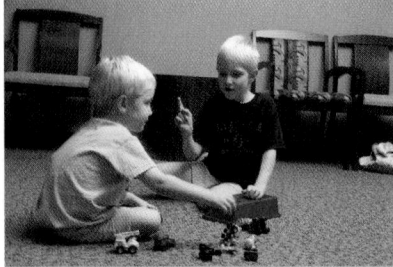

FIGURE 4-5 Play provides these preschoolers with the ability to interact with one another and develop their physical, mental, and social skills.

24 months—girls tend to be ready to toilet train earlier than boys—when the following are present: voluntary control of the anal and urethral sphincters; motor skills of sitting, walking, and squatting; fine motor skills needed to remove clothing; cognitive skills of recognizing the urge to defecate or urinate, and verbalizing the urge to do so; and willingness and ability to please the parents by sitting on the toilet for 5 to 10 minutes. Parental recognition of the child's level of readiness and willingness to invest the necessary time for toilet training are also essential for the toddler's successful mastery of this task.

A variety of life events and transitions may produce stress in the toddler. Among the most stressful are personal injury or illness, death of a parent, or loss through separation or divorce.

Children who have been successful in accomplishing the developmental tasks of infancy enter the toddler period with the basic relative trust needed for the achievement of the next tasks. The principal developmental tasks that must be mastered during the toddler stage are to:

1. Interact with others less egocentrically.
2. Acquire socially acceptable behaviors.
3. Differentiate self from others.
4. Tolerate separation from key socializing agents (mother or parents).
5. Develop increasing verbal communication skills.
6. Tolerate delayed gratification of wants and desires.
7. Control bodily functions (toilet training) and begin self-care (feed and dress self almost completely).

DEVELOPMENTAL TASKS OF PRESCHOOLERS (3 TO 6 YEARS)

During the preschooler period, children are focused on developing initiative and purpose. Play provides the means for physical, mental, and social development and becomes the "work" of children as they use it to understand, adjust to, and work out experiences with their environment (Figure 4-5). Preschoolers demonstrate an active imagination and an ability to invent and imitate. They constantly seek to discover the why, what, and how of objects and events around them; are literal in their thinking; are increasingly sociable with other children and adults other than their parents; and are increasingly aware of their places and roles in their families. Key gross and fine motor, language, and sensory milestones associated with the preschooler period can be found in Table 4-4.

The preschooler stage of development is characterized by the refinement of many of the tasks that were achieved during the toddler stage and the development of the skills and abilities that prepare children for the significant lifestyle change of starting school. Readiness for school is demonstrated by increased attention span and memory, ability to interact cooperatively, ability to tolerate prolonged periods of separation from family, and independence in performing basic self-care activities. Among the principal developmental tasks that must be mastered during the preschooler stage are to:

1. Develop a sense of separateness as an individual.
2. Develop a sense of initiative.
3. Use language for increasing social interaction.
4. Interact in socially acceptable ways with others.
5. Develop a conscience.
6. Identify sex role and function.
7. Develop readiness for school.

TABLE 4-4 Growth and Development during Preschool Years

AGE	GROSS MOTOR	FINE MOTOR	LANGUAGE	SENSORY
3 to 6 Years	• Can ride a bike with training wheels • Can throw a ball over-hand • Skips and hops on one foot • Can climb well • Can jump rope	• Can draw a six-part person • Can use scissors • Can draw circle, square, or cross • Likes art projects, likes to paste and string beads • Can button • Learns to tie and buckle shoes • Can brush teeth	• Language skills are well developed, with the child able to understand and speak clearly • Vocabulary grows to over 2,000 words • Talks endlessly and asks questions	• Visual acuity is well developed • Focused on learning letters and numbers

REFLECTIVE THINKING

Friendship in School-Age Children

Ten-year-old Consuela, who recently immigrated to the United States and speaks broken English, presents with a sore throat. As you are assessing her, she bursts into tears and cries, "Me lonely, me have no friends." What is your response to Consuela?

DEVELOPMENTAL TASKS OF SCHOOL-AGE CHILDREN (6 TO 12 YEARS)

With a well-developed sense of trust, autonomy, and initiative, school-age children increasingly reduce their dependency on the family as their primary socializing agents and move to the broader world of peers (primarily same-sex peers) in their neighborhoods and schools, as well as to teachers and adult leaders of social, sports, and religious groups. They are increasingly exposed to others' views and seek approval from people outside the home. School-age children become industrious workers as they develop the significant physical, social, and intellectual skills needed to operate in the broader and more diverse environment (Figure 4-6). They strive to be a part of a peer group and to achieve a variety of skills that are approved by others; in so doing, they become competent and confident in their own eyes. Key gross and fine motor, language, and sensory milestones associated with this period can be found in Table 4-5.

The principal developmental tasks that must be mastered during the school-age stage are to:

1. Become a more active, cooperative, and responsible family member.
2. Learn the rules and norms of a widening social, religious, and cultural environment.
3. Increase psychomotor and cognitive skills needed for participation in games and working with others.
4. Master concepts of time, conservation, and reversibility as well as oral and written communication skills.
5. Win approval from peers and adults.
6. Obtain a place in a peer group.
7. Build a sense of industry, accomplishment, self-assurance, and self-esteem.
8. Develop a positive self-concept.
9. Exchange affection with family and friends without seeking an immediate payback.
10. Adopt moral standards for behavior.

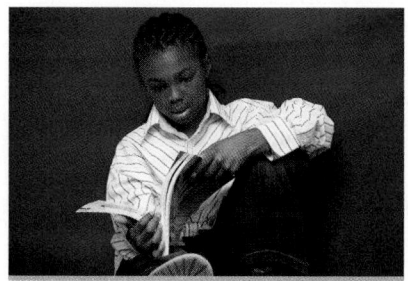

FIGURE 4-6 School-age children are often independent and industrious, with a developing sense of self-confidence.

TABLE 4-5 Growth and Development during School-Age Years

AGE	GROSS MOTOR	FINE MOTOR	LANGUAGE	SENSORY
6 to 12 Years	• Can use in-line skates or ice skates • Able to ride two-wheeler • Plays baseball	• Can put models together • Likes crafts • Enjoys board games, plays cards	• Vocabulary increases • Language abilities continue to develop	• Reading • Able to concentrate on activities for longer periods

REFLECTIVE THINKING

Adolescents' Reactions to Physical Changes

As the school nurse, you are presenting sexual education classes to all students in the junior high school. While you are explaining sexually transmitted diseases, a few of the girls begin to giggle. You overhear one girl saying, "Opal doesn't have to worry about getting that. She's so flat-chested that no guy will even look at her." How would you handle this situation?

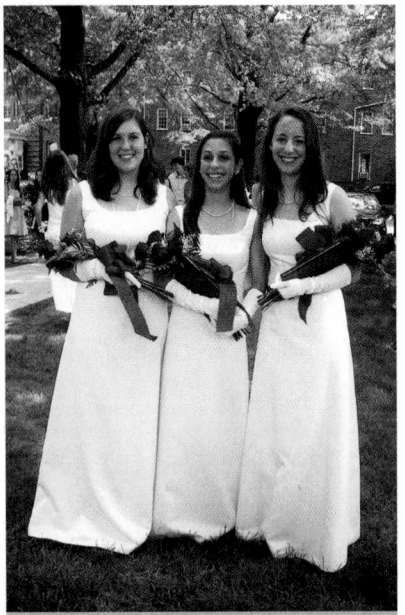

FIGURE 4-7 These adolescents have just graduated and look forward to moving on from high school and adolescence to college and young adulthood.

DEVELOPMENTAL TASKS OF ADOLESCENTS (12 TO 18 YEARS)

The adolescent period is one of struggle and sometimes turmoil as the adolescent strives to develop a personal identity and achieve a successful transition from childhood to adulthood. The biological, social, cognitive, and psychological changes associated with adolescence are the most complex and profound of any developmental period (Neinstein, Gordon, Katzman, Rosen, & Woods, 2007). For example, physical and sexual maturity are reached during adolescence, with girls tending to experience both puberty and a growth spurt earlier than boys. In addition, adolescents develop increasingly sophisticated cognitive and interpersonal skills, test out adult roles and behaviors, and begin to explore educational and occupational opportunities that will significantly influence future adult work life and socioeconomic status (Figure 4-7). Key gross and fine motor, language, and sensory milestones associated with this period can be found in Table 4-6.

Adolescents who have the support and trust of their families as they tackle the developmental tasks of this period are more likely to have a smoother and successful transition from the dependency of childhood to the independence of adulthood. If their parents, however, are too controlling, too permissive, or too confrontational during this period, adolescents will experience difficulty in judging the appropriateness of their behavior and in forming self-identity as competent, worthwhile individuals. If adolescents are able to find sufficient acceptance in a desired peer group or receive more positive than negative responses from the objects of their growing sexual or friendship interests, they will be able to work through feelings of inadequacy and insecurity and become increasingly self-assured and competent in forming and maintaining adult relationships. The principal developmental tasks that must be mastered during the adolescent stage are to:

1. Develop self-identity and appreciate own achievements and worth.
2. Form close relationships with peers.
3. Gradually grow independent from parents.
4. Evolve own value system and integrate self-concept and values with those of peers and society.
5. Develop academic and vocational skills and related social, work, and civic sensitivities.
6. Develop analytic thinking.
7. Adjust to rapid physical and sexual changes.
8. Develop a sexual identity and role.

TABLE 4-6 Growth and Development during Adolescence

AGE	GROSS MOTOR	FINE MOTOR	LANGUAGE	SENSORY
12 to 18 Years	• Muscles continue to develop • At times awkward, with some lack of coordination	• Well-developed skills	• Vocabulary is fully developed	• Development is complete

9. Develop skill in relating to people from different backgrounds.
10. Consider and possibly choose a career.

DEVELOPMENTAL TASKS OF YOUNG ADULTS (18 TO 30 YEARS)

Young adulthood is a time of separation and independence from the family and of new commitments, responsibilities, and accountability in social, work, and home relationships and roles (Figure 4-8). It is also a period when individuals are exposed to more diverse people, situations, and values, and, in recent decades, to a more rapidly changing socioeconomic and technological environment than ever before. For example, the movement, particularly in the Western world, from an industrial to an information era has made extended education and a need to delay complete emancipation from the family, as well as to delay commitment to a lifelong partner, an increasing norm for young adults. Socioeconomic and cultural changes have also legitimized the entry of young adult women into the professional career workforce. Although more young adult women are preparing for and launching lifelong careers outside the home, Leidy and Darling-Fisher's (1995) research indicated that young adult women continue to place a greater focus on intimacy while young men place a greater focus on autonomy.

When parents and young adult offspring are able to resolve normal generational differences in philosophy and lifestyles, mastery of the young adult developmental tasks is greatly facilitated. Among the developmental tasks that the young adult must achieve are to:

1. Establish friendships and a social group.
2. Grow independent of parental care and home.
3. Set up and manage one's own household.
4. Form an intimate affiliation with another and choose a mate.
5. Learn to love, cooperate with, and commit to a life partner.

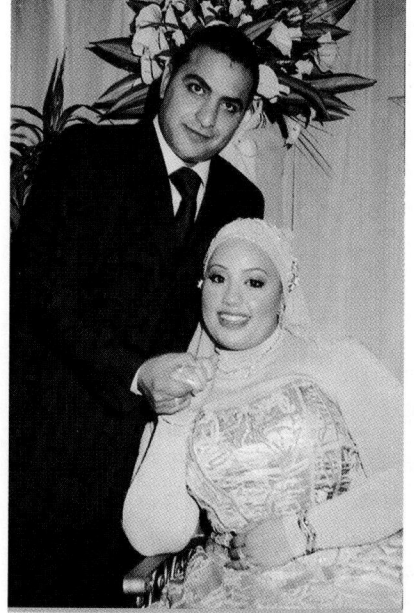

FIGURE 4-8 These young adults look forward to a life together as they celebrate their wedding.

REFLECTIVE THINKING

Young Adult Experiencing Conflict Concerning a Developmental Task

Inger is a 27-year-old astrophysicist. After undergoing her annual gynecological check-up, she tells you that her friends are having babies. Her husband wants children soon. "I'm not ready for kids. I want my career to be first. Maybe I won't ever want kids. My husband is pressuring me, my parents, my in-laws, everybody!" How would you proceed?

6. Develop a personal style of living (e.g., shared or single).
7. Choose and begin to establish a career or vocation.
8. Assume social, work, and civic responsibility and roles in social, professional, political, religious, and civic organizations.
9. Learn to manage life stresses accompanying change.
10. Develop a realistic outlook and acceptance of cultural, religious, social, and political diversity.
11. Form a meaningful philosophy of life and implement it in home, employment, and community settings.
12. Begin a parental role for own or life partner's children or for young people in a broader social framework, for example, teaching, health care, volunteer work.

DEVELOPMENTAL TASKS OF EARLY MIDDLE ADULTHOOD (30 TO 50 YEARS)

Middle age, ranging from 30 to 70 years, is the longest stage of the life cycle and is now often divided into early and late middle adulthood. During early middle adulthood, individuals experience relatively good physical and mental health; settle into their chosen careers, socioeconomic lifestyles, patterns of relationships (married, parental, partnered, single), political, civic, social, professional, and religious affiliations and activities; and achieve maximum productivity in work and in influence over themselves and their environments. It is also a period when individuals experience a need to contribute to the next generation, that is, to raise children or produce something that will be socially useful to others. The generativity that characterizes this period consists of giving, sharing, facilitating the growth of others, and making a contribution that is lasting.

Many who choose to express their generativity through the parental role may, during this period, achieve both the successful launching of their children into responsible adult roles and the associated increase in leisure time and financial resources needed to pursue enjoyable, nonparental goals and activities. Others, following divorce and remarriage, may see a merging of offspring into new family groupings and the return to previous parental cycles. An increasing number of others, during or shortly after launching their young adult children into adult roles, may find themselves having to take on the responsibility of chronically ill, aging parents. Each such life event can generate stress and disruption in individuals' lives with which they must cope. Developing effective coping strategies to manage the stress of life events or role transitions is a developmental task facing individuals in all life stages.

Among the developmental tasks that must be achieved during early middle adulthood are to:

1. Attain a desired level of achievement and status in career (Figure 4-9).
2. Review, evaluate, refine, and redirect career goals consistent with one's personal value system.

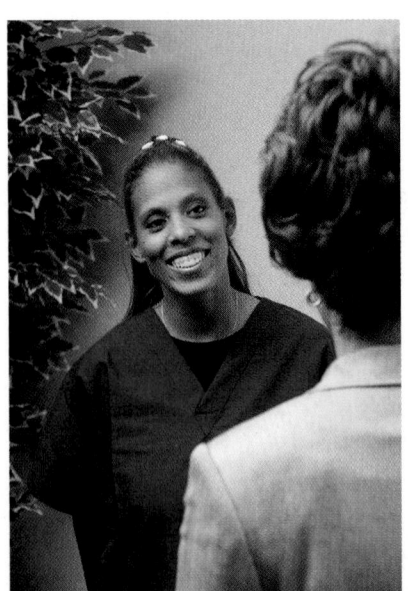

FIGURE 4-9 By middle adulthood, most individuals are established and confident in their careers.

REFLECTIVE THINKING

Early Middle Adult Experiencing an Unexpected Developmental Task

As the hospice nurse for Elly, you visit her daily to assist with her bathing. Elly tells you that she believes she has only a few days left to live. Suddenly, she starts sobbing, saying, "I'm only 35 years old. I have a husband I love and a 7-year-old daughter. I'm too young to die. It's not fair!" What is your response to Elly?

3. Continue to learn and refine competencies in areas of personal and career interests.
4. Manage life stresses accompanying change.
5. Continue developing mature relationships with life partner and significant others.
6. Participate in social, professional, political, religious, and civic activities.
7. Cope with an empty nest and possibly a refilled nest.
8. Adjust to aging parents and help plan for when they will need assistance.
9. Continue currently enjoyable hobbies and leisure activities and begin to develop ones for postretirement.
10. Begin to plan for personal, financial, and social aspects of retirement.

DEVELOPMENTAL TASKS OF LATE MIDDLE ADULTHOOD (50 TO 70 YEARS)

Many individuals during late middle adulthood may be diagnosed for the first time with a chronic health problem, such as arthritis, cardiovascular disease, cancer, diabetes, or asthma. In addition, women generally experience a decrease in estrogen and progesterone production, and undergo menopause during their late 40s or early 50s.

Changes also occur during late middle adulthood in work, family, social, and civic areas. For example, as the nuclear family contracts, parents rediscover being a couple and acquire new roles such as becoming grandparents. In addition, the gender developmental differences related to intimacy and autonomy seen in early adulthood begin to converge during late middle adulthood as men and women tend to take on similar life roles (Leidy & Darling-Fisher, 1995). Women generally become more involved and assume leadership roles in activities outside the home and work, such as politics and other civic activities, while men tend to become more aware and accepting of their nurturing and caring tendencies.

A variety of development tasks must be achieved by individuals during late middle adulthood. Among these tasks are to:

1. Manage life stresses accompanying change.
2. Maintain interest in current political, cultural, and scientific advances, trends, and issues.
3. Maintain affiliation with selected social, religious, professional, civic, and political organizations.
4. Adapt to physical and mental changes and health status accompanying aging.
5. Continue current activities and develop new interests and leisure activities that can be pursued consistent with changing abilities.
6. Adjust to more interaction and time spent with life partner without the presence of children (Figure 4-10).
7. Develop supportive, interdependent relationships with adult children.
8. Help elderly parents and relatives cope with lifestyle changes (may include providing a home for them).
9. Adjust to possible or actual loss of parents, life partner, elder family members, and friends through death or their decreasing abilities to maintain independent living and self-care.
10. Prepare for and adjust to role changes, changing finances, and changing lifestyle resulting from retirement.

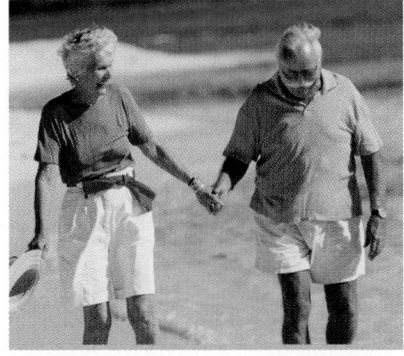

FIGURE 4-10 Adults in late middle adulthood frequently look forward to spending more time with their partner.

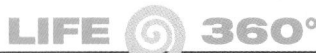

Self-Reflection on Life Events

Reflect on your own personal history and review how you resolved or accomplished each of the developmental tasks and crises according to each major developmental theory presented in this chapter.

- Were there any developmental crises and tasks that you experienced that did not fit the theories presented?
- Are there any tasks and crises for which you think you need additional experiences to master?

When an Elderly Parent Needs Special Care

Jean and Don Allen, 48 and 54 years of age, had finally helped the last of their four children move into his own apartment in another city and had been looking forward to having more time together when Jean's mother, 69 years old and recently widowed, was diagnosed with cancer. Because Jean's mother lives alone, will be receiving chemotherapy on an outpatient basis, and will need a great deal of help during this period, Jean and Don have agreed to have her live with them until the chemotherapy is completed.

- What developmental needs would you anticipate Jean, Don, and Jean's mother to experience?
- What anticipatory counseling would you provide related to these needs?

DEVELOPMENTAL TASKS OF LATE ADULTHOOD (70 YEARS TO DEATH)

How individuals during late adulthood physically and emotionally age and how they confront and adjust to the changes associated with this stage are widely divergent. For those who have achieved the developmental tasks of middle adulthood and are comfortable with the life goals they have achieved, independence from the workplace and time to pursue more leisure activities are welcomed. Although a loss of work-related status and social outlets, reduced income, decline in physical and some cognitive capabilities, decreased resistance to illness, and decreased recuperative powers are inevitable during late adulthood, they are often adjusted to with equanimity. Indeed, a high percentage of individuals will live out their lives managing their activities of daily living independently and in their own homes, enjoying new roles, giving requested advice and moral support to members of younger generations, and sharing leisure activities with new or old friends in their own age group.

One of the most important developmental tasks during late adulthood is conducting a life review (Butler, 2002). A **life review** entails reviewing the experiences, relationships, and events of one's life as a whole, viewing successes and failures from the perspective of age, and accepting one's life and accompanying life choices and outcomes in their entirety. Successful completion of the life-review task provides a sense of having been a meaningful part of human history, provides a sense of integrity, and enables one to face death with equanimity. If, however, one is unsuccessful in achieving the life-review developmental task, a sense of hopelessness, resentment, futility, despair, fear of death, and clinical depression may result.

Among the developmental tasks that must be achieved during late adulthood are to:

1. Maintain and develop new activities that help retain functional capacities.
2. Accept and adjust to changes in mental and physical strength and agility and health status (Figure 4-11).
3. Maintain and develop activities that contribute to a continuing sense of usefulness and self-worth and enhanced self-image.
4. Develop new roles in family as eldest member.
5. Establish affiliation with own age group.
6. Accept and adjust to changing, possibly restricted circumstances—social, financial, and lifestyle.
7. Adapt to loss of life partner, family members, and friends.

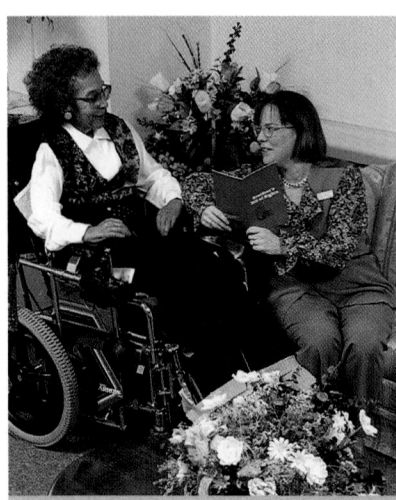

FIGURE 4-11 Adults in late adulthood may need to adapt to a new environment as they age and their health status changes.

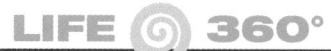

Assessing Family Life Cycle

Today's family can be a heterosexual couple, homosexual or lesbian couple, group home, commune, and so forth. Children are brought into these families by natural birth, artificial insemination, surrogate parent, adoption, and many other routes. Do all these families go through the stages of the family life cycle? Justify your answer.

REFLECTIVE THINKING

Encouraging a Life Review

As the nurse manager of a nursing home, you decide to conduct a weekly class for interested patients who want to share their life experiences.

- How would you prepare for the class?
- What agenda would you establish?
- How would you evaluate the usefulness of the class?

8. Work on life review.
9. Prepare for inevitability of own death.

STAGES OF FAMILY DEVELOPMENT

A review of developmental stages, tasks, and life events is not complete without considering the family context of the child or adult being assessed. Carter and McGoldrick (2005) have described six stages in the life cycle of the average middle-class family and the emotional processes of transition and second-order changes in the family's status required for each developmental stage. Duvall, another family life cycle theorist (Duvall & Miller, 1985), described the family in eight stages, starting with a childless married couple, progressing to a couple with children at various ages, and ending with aging family members and death.

DEVELOPMENTAL ASSESSMENT TOOLS

A variety of developmental assessment tools are available for use by the nurse. Some of the most commonly used tools assess mental, physical, emotional, and social functional status of individuals and families. It should be noted that use of some of these tools requires special training. Table 4-7 summarizes some of the tools that are frequently used.

TABLE 4-7 Developmental Assessment Tools

TOOL	TARGET POPULATION	ASSESSMENT PARAMETERS	SPECIAL CONSIDERATIONS
Brazelton Neonatal Behavioral Assessment Scale (BNBAS)[1]	Newborns	Temperament characteristics: state of arousal, orienting responses to stimuli, ability to deal with disturbing stimuli, social behavior, motor skills	When results are shared with parents, increased and improved newborn-parent interactions have been noted
Denver II[2]	1 month–6 years old	Personal-social, fine motor–adaptive, language, gross motor skills	Standardized for minority populations
Revised Prescreening Developmental Questionnaire (R-PDQ)[3]	1 month–6 years old	Personal-social, fine motor–adaptive, language, gross motor skills	Answered by parents to identify children who need more complete screening

continues

TABLE 4-7 (Continued)

TOOL	TARGET POPULATION	ASSESSMENT PARAMETERS	SPECIAL CONSIDERATIONS
Early Language Milestones Scale (ELM Scale-2)[4]	1 month– 3 years old	Early language development	Tests auditory visual, auditory receptive, expressive language in greater depth than Denver II
Carey Infant and Child Temperament Questionnaires[5]	4 months old– preschoolers	Pattern of temperamental attributes	Influences on child's relationships with parents and other caregivers are assessed
Washington Guide to Promoting Development in the Young Child[6]	Birth–5 years old	Play, motor activities, language, feeding, dressing, toilet training, discipline, sleep	Provides expected tasks for each age group and suggestions about appropriate child-rearing practices
HEADSS (Home, Education, Activities, Drugs, Sex, and Suicide) Adolescent Risk Profile[7]	Adolescents	Home, education, activities, drugs, sex, suicide	Identifies high-risk adolescents, and provides a guide for anticipatory guidance
NGAGED (Now, Growth and Development, Activities of Daily Living, General Health, Environment, and Documentation)[8]	Child with disabilities	Personal, family, social, school	Evaluates degree to which child engages in life activities as function of overall well-being and indicator of areas needing intervention
Stress Scale for Children[9]	Children	Desirable and undesirable life events experienced within last 6 months to 2 years and amount of adjustment that was needed to handle the events	Self-administered; higher scores correlate with increased probability of developing stress-related illness
Recent Life Changes Questionnaire[10]	Adults		
Life Experiences Survey[11]	Young and middle-aged adults	Events that have occurred within the past year and the type and extent of impact the events have had	Self-administered; identifies respondents at high risk for high stress and in need of stress and coping counseling
Everyday Hassles Scale (EHS)[12]	Adults	Everyday irritants that contribute to stress, and behaviors and feelings that promote well-being	Studies have suggested that day-to-day hassles are more strongly correlated with physical and psychosocial problems and outcomes than are life events[13]
Stress Audit[14]	Adults	Experienced and anticipated stressful events, stress symptoms, responses to stress, overall vulnerability to stress	Self-administered; identifies stress profile and provides anticipatory guidance
Sense of Coherence (SOC) Scale[15]	School age–Adults	Sense of coherence (comprehensibility, manageability, meaningfulness)	Gender, culturally, and socioeconomically neutral; results can be used for anticipatory guidance

continues

TABLE 4-7 (Continued)

TOOL	TARGET POPULATION	ASSESSMENT PARAMETERS	SPECIAL CONSIDERATIONS
Functional Activities Questionnaire (FAQ)[16]	Older adults	Level of independence demonstrated in the performance of activities of daily living	Can be completed by significant other or caregiver
Folstein Mini-Mental State Examination (MMSE)[17]	Older adults	Cognitive function	Can be easily administered in any clinical setting. A telephone version is also available.[18] Assists in determining the need for a more definitive neurological examination.
Minimum Data Set (MDS) for Nursing Facility Resident Assessment and Care Screening[19]	Nursing home residents	Cognitive patterns, communication and hearing patterns, vision patterns, physical functioning and structural problems, psychosocial well-being, mood and behavior patterns, activity pursuit patterns, bowel and bladder status, disease diagnoses, health conditions, oral nutritional status, oral and dental status, skin condition, medication use, treatments and procedures, customary activities of daily living routines	Required by federal law for all patients residing in nursing homes
Functional Assessment Screening in the Elderly (FASE)[20]	Older adults	Functional disability	Suggests interventions when abnormal results are present
Beck Depression Inventory (BDI)[21]	Adults	Mood, pessimism, sense of failure, dissatisfaction, guilt, sense of punishment, disappointment in oneself, self-accusations, self-punitive wishes, crying spells, irritability, social withdrawal, indecisiveness, body image, function at work, sleep disturbance, fatigue, appetite disturbance, weight loss, preoccupation with health, loss of libido	Score indicating depression warrants referral to a mental health specialist
Calgary Family Assessment Model (CFAM)[22]	Families	Structural, developmental, and functional	Includes emphasis on diversity issues such as race, culture, ethnicity, gender, and sexual orientation
Friedman Family Assessment Model (FFAM)[23]	Families	Developmental stage and history of a family, environmental data, family structure and functions, family stress and coping	Comprehensive and culturally sensitive

References. [1]Brazelton, 1995; [2]Glascoe, Foster, & Wolraich, 1997; [3]Frankenburg, Dobbs, Archer, Shapiro, & Brisnick, 1996; [4]Caplan & Gleason, 1993; [5]Carey & McDevitt, 1978; Hegvik, McDevitt, & Carey, 1982; Fullard, McDevitt, & Carey, 1984; [6]Powell, 1981; [7]Neinstein, Gordon, Katzman, Rosen, & Woods, 2007; [8]Guillett, 1998; [9]Saunders & Remsberg, 1984; [10]Rahe, 1975; [11]Sarason, Johnson, & Siegal, 1978; [12]Lazarus, 1981; [13]Lazarus & Folkman, 1984; Weinberger, Hiner, & Tierney, 1987; [14]Miller, Smith, & Mehler, 1991; [15]Antonovsky, 1993; [16]McDowell & Newell, 1996; [17]Folstein, Folstein, & McHugh, 1975; [18]Brandt, Spencer, & Folstein, 1988; [19]Carnevali & Patrick, 1993; [20]Resnick, 1994; [21]Gallagher, 1986; [22]Wright & Leahey, 2000; [23]Friedman, Bowden, & Jones, 2002.

CASE STUDY

The Suicidal Adolescent

NOTE: *This case study uses the $H_1E_2A_3D_4S_5$ assessment tool which is discussed in greater detail in Chapter 24.*

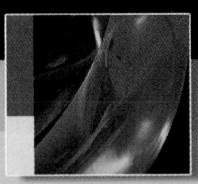

HEALTH HISTORY

Today's Date	January 26, 2009
BIOGRAPHICAL DATA	
Name	James David (JD) Marshall, III
Address	Lynchburg, VA
Phone Number	(434) 685-7703
Date of Birth	September 3, 1993
Birthplace	Arlington, VA
Occupation	Student, 10th grade
Insurance	Blue Cross/Blue Shield (parents' plan)
Usual Source of Health Care	Mandie Rosen, PNP Lynchburg Family Practice
Source of Referral	Mother
Emergency Contact	James and Hillary Marshall, parents, same phone #
SOURCE AND RELIABILITY OF INFORMATION	Mother and pt, reliable historians. Mother in waiting room at pt's request after helping to give health history through family health history
PATIENT PROFILE	
Age	15
Gender	Male
Race	Caucasian
Marital Status	Single
REASON FOR SEEKING HEALTH CARE	Last night mother received call from JD's best friend in Arlington saying she thought JD was in real trouble because although he had e-mailed daily since moving to Lynchburg telling her how awful it was in school and in his new neighborhood, since the holidays ended, he had called every night, sounding more desperate each day and talking about ways to commit suicide. Pt says, "I'm so stressed and so tired. I think I'm going crazy. All I can think about is how I can find some peace . . . like permanently!"

continues

CASE STUDY   (Continued)

The Suicidal Adolescent

PRESENT HEALTH	Describes himself as "physically fit, but emotionally, a misfit."
PAST HEALTH HISTORY	
Medical History	More URIs in the last 7 months than in the last 7 years. "I may be getting some allergies. Who knows?"
Surgical History	Denies
Allergies	None verified
Medications	
OTC	Multivitamin daily; Tylenol, antihistamine and cough syrup for URIs PRN, uses as directed
Communicable Diseases	Denies STD, HIV, TB
Injuries and Accidents	Laceration on chin p̄ diving accident requiring 10 stitches @ age 10 yrs, healed well
Special Needs	Denies
Blood Transfusions	Denies
Childhood Illnesses	Denies
Immunizations	Record indicates up-to-date for age
FAMILY HEALTH HISTORY	

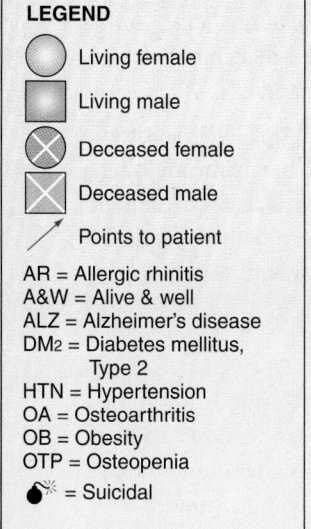

LEGEND

- ⬤ Living female
- ⬛ Living male
- ⊗ Deceased female
- ⊠ Deceased male
- ⬈ Points to patient

AR = Allergic rhinitis
A&W = Alive & well
ALZ = Alzheimer's disease
DM2 = Diabetes mellitus, Type 2
HTN = Hypertension
OA = Osteoarthritis
OB = Obesity
OTP = Osteopenia
💣☀ = Suicidal

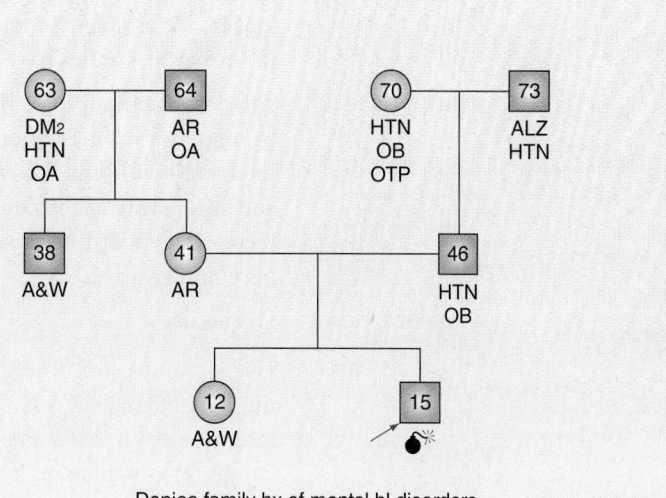

Denies family hx of mental hl disorders

continues

CASE STUDY (Continued)

The Suicidal Adolescent

SOCIAL HISTORY	
H–Home Environment	Just moved from Arlington, VA, where pt lived his entire life. Family moved at beginning of summer break to paternal grandparents' home in Lynchburg, VA, to help care for father's parents, whose health has been deteriorating. Paternal grandfather showing increasing signs of Alzheimer's, and grandmother recently broke her hip while playing tennis and had hip surgery. The grandparents' 6-bedroom, brick colonial home is in a suburb near a well-known religious university. Housekeeper works in home until after dinner 6 days/week. Father left high-level position in the Department of Justice to move back to take care of his parents and take over his father's law firm. Mother left a research position at the National Institute of Nursing Research, NIH, to teach in the BSN program at the nearest state university. Parents thought it would be a good time to move since their daughter would be starting middle school and the pt would be advancing from middle school to high school. Parents thought it would be an easier transition to meet new kids in the summer and early fall.
E–Education	9th grade = 1st year of high school. Was popular member of the drama club and swimming team at middle school. Neither activity available here. Had many long-term friends in Arlington, but has not been accepted by classmates here. "I tried to make friends here, but most everyone just avoided me. I guess I'm too different. Recently some kids have started whispering about me just loud enough for me to hear them call me 'a fag' and a 'queer'." Was an A student taking advanced-placement classes in Arlington. Grades have now fallen to B's and C's.
Exercise	Tried out for and made the track team, but got URIs so often, pt missed a lot of school and practice. Other team members interacted with him "only when absolutely necessary." Patient and sister swim at the country club pool on most weekends. Pt increasingly too tired to swim. Goes now only to watch out for his younger sister.
A–Alcohol	Denies use
Activities	Helps grandfather "find things." Runs some errands for grandmother. Does assigned chores less and less without a lot of reminding by parents. Spends most evenings after dinner on the computer e-mailing his best friend and "messing around."
Attitudes about Life	"Things were great before we moved, life was good. But it's the pits here. I hate it. I know the folks didn't have any choice about coming here to take care of my grandparents, but I feel like the 'me' I used to be has just disappeared here and I can't do anything about it."

continues

CASE STUDY (Continued)

The Suicidal Adolescent

D-Diet	"Not much of an appetite." Five-pound weight loss since moving here 4½ months ago
Drugs	Denies use
Dentist	No cavities. Cleaned every 6 months.
Depression	Decreased interest in activities, admits to being sad, lack of concentration and focus at school; decreased energy level.
S-Sleep	Trouble getting to sleep and staying asleep. Frequently takes a nap after school.
Safety	Denies engaging in any risk-taking behavior.
Sexual Identity and Activity	Always has had girls as buddies but not much interest in them as girlfriends. Started admitting to feelings for same sex last year. Came out to parents, who "have been stressed out about it, especially Dad." Parents planned to find a Parents, Family, and Friends of Lesbians and Gays (PFLAG) group to join, but with the move, have not had time. Briefly dated a boy one grade ahead of him before moving to Lynchburg. Called and e-mailed each other through the summer, less after school started, and stopped around Thanksgiving. "Tried to talk to one guy here who got all upset, wanted to know why I thought he was gay, then told me to get lost. Afraid to approach anyone else, they're so uptight here."
Stressors	See above.
Suicidal Ideation	"I've checked online for ways to do it so it would look like an accident. I wouldn't want my family to feel guilty if I succeed in ending it all."

ASSESSMENT IN BRIEF

Developmental Assessment

- Note the patient's stated chronological age.
- Tailor your questions to the patient's expected level of ability according to developmental parameters until you can accurately assess the actual developmental level.
- When assessing small children, verify information with the caregiver.
- If a third party is assisting in the interview (for an elderly or special needs patient), address all questions to the patient, not the intermediary.

1. The nurse is assessing Anna, a 4-month-old infant, to determine her gross motor development. Which of the following would be age-appropriate development for this infant?
   a. Ability to sit alone without support
   b. Bounces when held in a standing position
   c. Ability to hold head up and use forearms for support
   d. Puts full weight on legs when held in a standing position

   The correct answer is (c).

2. When administering a developmental surveillance exam, the nurse is assessing which of the following?
   a. Parenting behaviors of the child's parents
   b. Task resolution across the developmental years
   c. The child's growth against the norm
   d. Fine and gross motor skills, language, and psychological behavior

   The correct answer is (d).

3. The nurse is teaching the mother of a teenage child what she would note if her child has reached Kohlberg's postconventional stage of development. The teenager would most likely:
   a. Expect to be totally autonomous
   b. Espouse only one moral point of view
   c. Make decisions based on whether they please others or not
   d. Be capable of making decisions after considering different moral approaches

   The correct answer is (d).

4. A first-time mother asks the nurse when she can expect her 2-month-old to start to crawl. The most appropriate response would be:
   a. Four months   c. Eight months
   b. Six months   d. Ten months

   The correct answer is (c).

5. A major development task of early middle age is to:
   a. Evolve one's own value system and integrate it with those of family and society
   b. Form a meaningful philosophy of life and implement it in one's own household
   c. Develop a personal style of living and manage one's own household
   d. Work on a life review consistent with one's philosophy

   The correct answer is (b).

6. While assessing a school-age child's developmental level, the nurse encourages the child to demonstrate

his favorite activity. The nurse is applying the developmental theories of which individuals?
   a. Freud and Erikson   c. Piaget and Erikson
   b. Kohlberg and Freud   d. Piaget and Freud

   The correct answer is (a).

7. What assessment parameter does the Everyday Hassles Scale target?
   a. Desirable and undesirable events in the past 6 months
   b. Events that have occurred within the past year and the type of impact the events had
   c. Anticipated stressful events, stress symptoms, and response to stress
   d. Everyday irritants that contribute to stress, and behaviors that promote well-being

   The correct answer is (d).

8. One of the principal developmental tasks of adolescents is to:
   a. Manage life stress accompanying change
   b. Be independent of parental care and home
   c. Form an intimate affiliation with another
   d. Develop self-identity and appreciate own achievement and worth

   The correct answer is (d).

9. A nurse assessing a toddler would expect to see the child:
   a. Building a tower of four blocks, drawing a circle, and kicking a ball
   b. Pouring liquids, drawing circles, and throwing a ball overhead
   c. Dressing and undressing self, running, jumping, and kicking a ball
   d. Walking up and down stairs, pushing and pulling toys, and jumping rope

   The correct answer is (a).

10. When assessing a preschooler's readiness for school, the nurse would expect to see:
    a. Beginning independence in performing basic self-care activities
    b. Tolerating prolonged periods of separation from family
    c. Differentiating self from others
    d. Knowing his or her first name

    The correct answer is (b).

REFERENCES

Aguilera, D. C. (1994). *Crisis intervention theory and methodology* (7th ed.). Baltimore: Mosby.

Aldwin, C. M. (2007). *Stress, coping and development: An integrative perspective.* New York: Guilford Press.

Antonovsky, A. (1993). The structure and properties of the sense of coherence scale. *Social Science Medicine, 36*(6), 725–733.

Brandt, J., Spencer, M., & Folstein, M. (1988). The Telephone Instrument for Cognitive Status. *Neuropsychiatry, Neuropsychology, and Behavioral Neurology, 1,* 11–17.

Brazelton, T. B., & Nugent, J. K. (1995). *Neonatal behavioral assessment scale* (3rd ed.). London, UK: MacKeith Press.

Butler, R. N. (2002). Age, death, and life review. In K. J. Doka. (Ed.), *Living with grief: Loss in later life.* Hospice Foundation of America. Retrieved January 19, 2008, from www.hospicefoundation.org/teleconference/2002/butler.asp

Caplan, J., & Gleason, J. R. (1993). Test-retest and interobserver reliability of the Early Language Milestone Scale, second edition (Elm Scale-2). *Journal of Pediatric Health Care, 7,* 212–219.

Carey, W. B., & McDevitt, S. (1978). Revision of the infant temperament questionnaire. *Pediatrics, 61,* 735–739.

Carnevali, D. L., & Patrick, M. (1993). *Nursing management for the elderly* (3rd ed.). Philadelphia: J. B. Lippincott.

Carter, B., & McGoldrick, M. (2005). Overview: The expanded family life cycle: Individual, family and social perspectives. In B. Carter & M. McGoldrick (Eds.), *The expanded family life cycle: Individual, family and social perspectives* (3rd ed.). Boston: Allyn & Bacon.

Duvall, E. R. M., & Miller, B. C. (1985). *Marriage and family development* (6th ed.). New York: Harper & Row.

Erikson, E. (1974). *Dimensions of a new identity.* New York: W. W. Norton.

Everall, R. D., Bostick, K. E., & Pauson, B. L. (2005). I'm tired of being me: Developmental themes in a suicidal adolescent. *Adolescence, 40,* 693–708.

Folstein, M. F., Folstein, S. E., & McHugh, P. R. (1975). "Mini-Mental State": A practical method for grading the cognitive state of patients for the clinician. *Journal of Psychiatric Research, 12,* 189–198.

Frankenburg, W. K., Dobbs, J., Archer, P., Shapiro, H., & Brisnick, B. (1996). *The Denver II Technical Manual.* Denver, CO: Denver Developmental Materials, Inc.

Freud, S. (1946). *The ego and the mechanism of defense.* New York: International Universities Press.

Friedman, M. M., Bowden, V. R., & Jones, E. (2002). *Family nursing: Research, theory, and practice* (5th ed.). Upper Saddle River, NJ: Prentice Hall.

Fullard, W., McDevitt, S., & Carey, W. (1984). Assessing temperament in one to three year old children. *Journal of Pediatric Psychology, 9,* 205–217.

Gallagher, D. (1986). The Beck Depression Inventory and older adults: Review of its development and utility. In T. L. Brink (Ed.), *Clinical gerontology: A guide to assessment and intervention* (pp. 149–163). New York: Haworth Press.

Glascoe, F. P., Foster, E. M., & Wolraich, M. L. (1997). An economic analysis of developmental detection methods. *Pediatrics, 99,* 830–837.

Goldston, D. B., Molock, S. D., Whitbeck, L. B., Murakami, J. L., & Hall, G. C. (2008). Cultural considerations in adolescent suicide prevention and psychosocial treatment. *American Psychologist, 63*(1), 14–31.

Grey, M. (1993). Stressors and children's health. *Journal of Pediatric Nursing, 8*(2), 85–91.

Guillett, S. E. (1998). Assessing the child with disabilities. *Home Healthcare Nurse, 16,* 402–409.

Hegvik, R., McDevitt, S., & Carey, W. (1982). The Middle Childhood Temperament Questionnaire. *Journal of Developmental Behavior in Pediatrics, 3,* 197–200.

Kohlberg, L. (1981). *The philosophy of moral development: Moral stages and the idea of justice.* New York: Harper & Row.

Krach, C. A., & Verkoff, V. A. (1999). *Centenarians in the United States* (U.S. Bureau of the Census, Current Population Reports, Series P23-199RV). Washington, DC: U.S. Government Printing Office.

Leidy, N. K., & Darling-Fisher, C. S. (1995). Reliability and validity of the modified Erikson psychosocial stage inventory in diverse samples. *Western Journal of Nursing Research, 17,* 168–187.

Levinson, D. J., Darrow, C. N., & Klein, E. B. (1986). *The seasons of a man's life* (2nd ed.). New York: Ballantine.

McDowell, I., & Newell, C. (1996). *Functional disability and handicap. Measuring health: A guide to rating scales and questionnaires* (2nd ed.). New York: Oxford University Press.

Miller, L. H., Smith, A. D., & Mehler, B. L. (1991). *The stress audit.* Brookline, MA: Biobehavioral Associates.

National Center for Health Statistics. (2007). *Health, United States, 2007: With chartbook on trends in the health of Americans.* CSC, DHHS. Retrieved January 18, 2008, from www.cdc.gov/nchs.hus.htm

Neinstein, L. S., Gordon, C. M., Katzman, D. K., Rosen, D. S., & Woods, E. R. (Eds.). (2007). *Adolescent health care: A practical guide* (5th ed.). New York: Lippincott, Williams and Wilkins.

Piaget, J. (1952). *The origins of intelligence in children.* New York: International Universities Press.

Powell, M. L. (1981). *Assessment and management of developmental changes and problems in children* (2nd ed.). St. Louis: Mosby.

Priwer, S., & Phillips, C. (2006). *Gay parenting: Complete guide to same-sex families.* Far Hills, NJ: New Horizon Press.

Rahe, R. H. (1975). Epidemiological studies in life change and illness. *International Journal of Psychiatry, 6,* 133–146.

Resnick, N. M. (1994). Geriatric medicine & the elderly patient. In L. M. Tierney, Jr., S. J. McPhee, & M. A. Papadakis (Eds.), *Current medical diagnosis & treatment* (33rd ed., pp. 41–60). Norwalk, CT: Appleton & Lange.

Sarason, J. G., Johnson, J. H., & Siegal, J. M. (1978). Assessing the impact of life changes: Development of life experiences survey. *Journal of Consulting Clinical Psychology, 46,* 932–946.

Saunders, A., & Remsberg, B. (1984). *The stress-proof child: A loving parent's guide.* New York: Holt, Rinehart, & Winston.

Sawaya, G. F., Guiguis-Blake, J., LeFevre, M., Harris, R., & Petiti, D. (2007). Update on the methods of the U.S. Preventive Services Task Force: Estimating certainty and magnitude of net benefit. *Annals of Internal Medicine, 147*(12), 871–875.

Schatz, J., McClellan, C. B., Puffer, E. S., Johnson, K., & Roberts, C. W. (2008). Neurodevelopmental screening in toddlers and early preschoolers with sickle cell disease. *Journal of Child Neurology, 23*(1), 44–50.

U.S. Preventive Services Task Force. (2007). *Guide to clinical preventive services: Recommendations of the U.S. Preventive Services Task Force.* Agency for Healthcare Research and Quality, U.S. Department of Health & Human Services. Retrieved January 5, 2008, from http://www.ahrq.gov/clinic/pocketgd.htm

Weinberger, M., Hiner, S. L., & Tierney, W. M. (1987). In support of hassles as a measure of stress in predicting health outcomes. *Journal of Behavioral Medicine, 10,* 19–31.

Wolff, T., Guirguis-Blake, J., Gillespie, M., & Harris, R. (2007). Screening for blockages in the blood vessels to the brain: Recommendations from the U.S. Preventive Services Task Force. *Annals of Internal Medicine, 147*(12), 860–870.

Wolff, T., Guirguis-Blake, J., Miller, T., Gillespie, M., & Harris, R. (2007). Screening for carotid artery stenosis: U.S. Preventive Services Task Force recommendation statement. *Annals of Internal Medicine, 147*(12), 854–859.

Wong, D. L., Hockenberry, J. J., Wilson, D., Winkelstein, M. L., & Kline, N. E. (2003). *Nursing care of infants and children* (7th ed.). Philadelphia: Mosby.

Wright, L. M., & Leahey, M. (2005). *Nurses and families: A guide to family assessment and intervention* (4th ed.). Philadelphia: F. A. Davis.

Wykle, M. L., Kahana, E., & Kowal, J. (Eds.). (1992). *Stress & health among the elderly.* New York: Springer.

BIBLIOGRAPHY

Ash, P. (2008). Suicidal behavior in children and adolescents. *Journal of Psychosocial Nursing and Mental Services, 46*(1), 26–30.

Ashford, J. B., LeCroy, C. W., & Lortie, K. L. (2006). *Human behavior in the social environment* (3rd ed.). Belmont, CA: Thompson Brooks/Cole.

Bonanno, G. A., Galea, S., Bucciarelli, A., & Vlahov, D. (2007). What predicts psychological resilience after disaster? The role of demographics, resources, and life stress. *Journal of Consulting and Clinical Psychology, 75*(5), 671–682.

Carter, A. S., Briggs-Gowan, M. J., & Davis, N. O. (2004). Assessment of young children's social-emotional development and psychopathology: Recent advances and recommendations for practice. *Journal of Clinical Psychology and Psychiatry, 45*(1), 109–134.

Carno, M. A., Hoffman, L. A., Carcillo, J. A., & Sanders, M. H. (2003). Developmental stages of sleep from birth to adolescence, common childhood sleep disorders: Overview and nursing implications. *Journal of Pediatric Nursing, 18*(4), 274–283.

Council on Children with Disabilities. (2006). Identifying infants and young children with developmental disorders in the medical home: An algorithm for developmental surveillance and screening. *Pediatrics, 118*(18), 405–420.

Elbers, J., Macnab, A., McLeod, E., & Gagnon, F. (2008). The Ages and Stages Questionnaires: Feasibility of use as a screening tool for children in Canada. *Canadian Journal of Rural Medicine, 13*(1), 9–14.

Eriksson, M., & Lindstrom, B. (2005). Validity of Antonovsky's Sense of Coherence Scale: A systematic review. *Journal of Epidemiology and Community Health, 59*, 460–466.

Fosarelli, P. D. (2006). *Asap: Ages, stages, and phases: From infancy to adolescence: Integrating physical, social, emotional, intellectual, and spiritual development.* Liguori, MO: Liguori Publications.

Gallo, J. J., Bogner, J. R., Fulmer, T., & Paveza, C. J. (Eds.). (2006). *Handbook of geriatric assessment.* Sudbury, MA: Jones & Bartlett.

Greenfeld, D. A. (2005). Reproduction in same sex couples: Quality of parenting and child development. *Current Opinions in Obstetrics and Gynecology, 17*(3), 309–312.

Hawkins, J. D., Catelano, R. F., Kosterman, R., Abbott, R., & Hill, K. G. (1999). Preventing adolescent health-risk behaviors by strengthening protection during childhood. *Archives of Pediatrics and Adolescent Medicine, 153*, 226–234.

Lester, B. N., & Tronick, E. Z. (2004). History and description of the Neonatal Intensive Care Network Neurobehavioral Scale. *Pediatrics, 111*(3, Pt. 2), 634–640.

Lynch, W. C., Heil, D. P., Wagner, E., & Havens, M. D. (2007). Ethnic differences in BMI, weight concerns, and eating behaviors: Comparisons of Native American, White, and Hispanic adolescents. *Body Image, 4*(2), 179–190.

Murray, R. B., & Zentner, J. P. (2001). *Health promotion strategies through the life span* (7th ed.). Norwalk, CT: Appleton & Lange.

Ostrove, J., & Long, S. M. (2007). Social class and belonging: Implications for college adjustment. *The Review of Higher Education, 30*(4), 363–389.

Ottenbacher, K. J., Msall, M. E., Lyon, N., Duffy, L. C., Ziviani, J., Granger, C. V., et al. (2000). Functional assessment and care of children with neurodevelopmental disabilities. *American Journal of Physical Medicine and Rehabilitation, 79*, 114–123.

Parker, S., Zukerman, B. S., & Augustyn, M. C. (Eds.). (2004). *Developmental and behavioral pediatrics: A handbook of primary care* (2nd ed.). New York: Lippincott Williams & Wilkins.

Penley, J. A., Wiebe, J. S., & Nwosu, A. (2003). Psychometric properties of the Spanish Beck Depression Inventory-II in a medical sample. *Psychological Assessment, 15*(2), 569–577.

Rienzo, B. A., Button, J. W., Sheu, J. J., & Li, Y. (2005). Gay and lesbian perceptions of discrimination in retirement care facilities. *Journal of Homosexuality, 49*(2), 83–102.

Service, K. P., & Hahn, J. E. (2003). Issues in aging: The role of the nurse in the care of older people with intellectual and developmental disabilities. *Nursing Clinics of North America, 38*(2), 291–312.

Sigelman, C. K., & Rider, E. A. (2008). *Lifespan human development* (6th ed.). Belmont, CA: Wadsworth Publishing.

Stewart, J. L. (2003). Children living with chronic illness: An examination of their stressors, coping responses, and health outcomes. *Annual Review of Nursing Research, 21*, 203–243.

Swanson, D. P., Spencer, M. B., Harpalani, V., Dupree, D., Noll, E., Ginzburg, S., et al. (2003). Psychosocial development in racially and ethnically diverse youth: Conceptual and methodological challenges in the 21st century. *Developmental Psychopathology, 15*(3), 743–771.

Swearingen, P. L. (Ed.). (2004). *All-in-one care planning resource: Medical-surgical, pediatric, maternity, and psychiatric nursing care plans.* Philadelphia: Mosby.

Vandwater, E. A., & Stewart, A. J. (2006). Paths to late midlife well-being for women and men: The importance of identity development and social role quality. *Journal of Adult Development, 13*(2), 76–83.

Whitbourne, S. K., & Willis, S. L. (Eds.). (2006). *The baby boomers grow up: Contemporary perspectives on midlife.* Mahwah, NJ: Lawrence Erbaum Associates.

Williams, J., & Holmes, C. A. (2004). Improving the early detection of children with subtle developmental problems. *Journal of Child Health Care, 8*(1), 34–46.

WEB SITES

Agency for Healthcare Research and Quality:
http://ahrq.gov

Centers for Disease Control and Prevention:
http://www.cdc.gov

KidsHealth:
http://kidshealth.org

National Library of Medicine, National Institutes of Health:
http://www.nlm.nih.gov

Gay, Lesbian, Bisexual, and Transgender Health:
http://www.glbthealth.org

CHAPTER 5

Cultural Assessment

COMPETENCIES

1. Assess own cultural values, beliefs, and behaviors.

2. Identify potential areas of cultural conflict between the values and customs of patients and their families and those of health care providers.

3. Identify genetic traits and disorders prevalent in selected ethnic groups.

4. Conduct a comprehensive cultural assessment.

5. Describe the process for providing culturally competent nursing care.

The racial, ethnic, and cultural diversification of American society is accelerating at an unprecedented rate. In 2004, an estimated 69.7% of the U.S. population was Euro-American (predicted to be only 52.8% by the year 2050), and 30.3% were members of ethnic and cultural minority groups: 12.3% African American, 13% Hispanic (the fastest growing minority group in the United States), 4.2% Asian and Pacific Islander, and 0.8% American Indian (U.S. Census Bureau, 2007a). It has been predicted that by the year 2010, nurses in the United States will be interacting with patients from virtually every cultural and ethnic group in the world (Leininger & McFarland, 2002). These changes in the demographic and ethnic composition of the population make it imperative that nurses be able to communicate effectively with a culturally diverse group of patients, make accurate cultural assessments, and plan, provide, and evaluate culturally competent care. Such care must be based on an awareness of, and utilization of, knowledge and theories that explain patients' situations and responses within the context of their cultural, ethnic, gender, and sexual orientations (Campinha-Bacote, 2007; Giger & Davidhizar, 2007; Rundle, Carvalho, & Robinson, 2002; Srivastava, 2006).

CULTURALLY COMPETENT NURSING CARE

The American health care system is now one of **cultural diversity** in that it consists of patients and health care providers from different combinations of ethnic (e.g., Hispanic), racial (e.g., Caucasian), national (e.g., Swiss), religious (e.g., Buddhist), generational (e.g., grandparent), marital status (e.g., single), socioeconomic (e.g., middle class), occupational (e.g., nurse), preference in life partner (e.g., heterosexual), health status (e.g., handicapped), and cultural orientations coexisting in a given location. Kreps and Kunimoto (1994) believe that this cultural diversity should be viewed as an opportunity for health care professionals to experience the benefits of exchange and cooperation across cultures. They note that:

> . . . the exploration of different cultures can help us learn about new ways of interpreting reality and increase our understanding of other people, their experiences, and the world they live in. The demonstration of respect and interest in the cultural perspectives of others can also serve as a foundation for developing supportive and cooperative relationships with people from different cultures. The expression of respect and interest validates the legitimacy and worth of others' cultural backgrounds, encourages their reciprocal interest in our cultural orientation, and provides a basis for communication. (pp. 10–11)

In 2007, the estimate of cultural minorities in the United States reached 100.7 million, or 1 in 4.3 residents (U.S. Census Bureau, 2007b). Recent immigrants from countries such as Mexico, Cuba, the Dominican Republic, El Salvador, the Philippines, China, Vietnam, India, Lebanon, and the former countries of the Union of Soviet Socialist Republics may have very different attitudes toward the health care system, different health behavior patterns, and different types of health problems. Even after these new immigrants undergo **acculturation**—an informal process of adaptation through which the beliefs, values, norms, and practices of a dominant culture are learned by new members born into a different culture—many of their beliefs and attitudes may be an amalgam of their original practices and those of the dominant Euro-American culture. Nurses must develop a perspective of cultural relativity by viewing health beliefs and behaviors within the context of each patient's culture and by working to deliver culturally competent health care.

The ANA Code of Ethics (2001) stipulates that all nurses provide culturally competent care to all patients, being sensitive to the patients' needs while providing nursing care with dignity and respect. **Culturally competent nursing care** is provided by nurses who use **cross-cultural nursing care** models (nursing care provided within the cultural context of patients who are members of a culture or subculture different from that of the nurse) and research to identify health care needs, and to plan and evaluate the care provided within the cultural context of patients. The process of culturally competent nursing care consists of: (1) eliciting statements of cultural values and beliefs so that culturally sensitive approaches to care based on mutual respect can be provided; (2) recognizing and understanding the normal behaviors of different cultural groups and their unique behavioral responses to health and illness; (3) obtaining information on ethnic variations and on normal racial growth patterns to assist in identifying abnormal patterns and designing appropriate interventions; and (4) using an ethic of **cultural relativism** to provide nursing services, that is, the belief that no culture is either inferior or superior to another, that behavior must be evaluated in relation to the cultural context in which it occurs, and that respect, equality, and justice are basic rights for all racial, ethnic, subcultural, and cultural groups.

To provide culturally competent nursing care, the nurse first must be willing and able to confront his or her own cultural biases, or **ethnocentrism** (a condition that occurs when individuals or groups of people perceive their own cultural group and cultural values, beliefs, norms, and customs to be superior to all others and have disdain for the expression and expressor of any way of life but their own) and stereotyping, to whatever extent they exist, and examine the impact these biases will have on the patient. It is also important to understand the dynamics and respond to the challenges inherent in **bilingualism** (the habitual use of two different languages, particularly when speaking), **multiculturalism** (when individuals live and function in two or more cultures simultaneously), and **cultural identity** (the cultural definition or cultural orientation with which an individual self-identifies) of their patients. In addition, consideration should be given to the potential for **culture shock**: the disorientation, uncertainty, and alienation that can occur during the process of adjusting to a new cultural group.

Assessing a patient's cultural beliefs, values, and customs through observation and interview is an essential part of health assessment for culturally competent nursing care. When assessing a patient, a balance is needed between the data related to the specific individual and his or her family who are being assessed and the data related to the cultural group to which they have been **enculturated** (the informal process through which the beliefs, values, norms, and practices of a culture are learned by members born into the culture). The nurse, therefore, needs to have experience with a range of individuals and families from any given cultural group in order to determine where in this range the patient being assessed fits. In addition, knowledge of the patient's racial and ethnic group's physical and biological norm differences, as well as the risks to optimal health that are associated with the patient's racial, ethnic, and cultural group, is also relevant.

During the health assessment interview, the nurse needs to avoid stereotyping the patient by depending too heavily on an "ideal" or normative racial, ethnic, or cultural characteristic or trait list. Summaries of any group are inherently imprecise by virtue of being normative. No one individual or family within a culture or subculture will display all of the characteristics representative of that culture, and normative lists or summaries do not include all of the diversity that may be part of a given culture. An understanding of basic racial, ethnic, and cultural concepts associated with the conduct of culturally competent health assessments, however, can serve as a *guide* for the nurse.

BASIC CONCEPTS ASSOCIATED WITH CULTURALLY COMPETENT ASSESSMENTS

CULTURE

Culture is a learned and socially transmitted orientation and way of life of a group of people. Culture enables members of large groupings of people to find coherence and to survive in the world around them through the development of unique patterns of

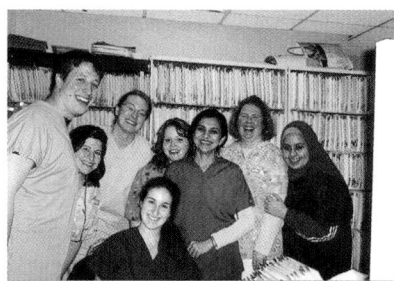

FIGURE 5-1 **This photo shows a subculture of employees who work at a medical practice.**

basic assumptions and shared meanings. The cultural beliefs, values, customs, and norms that result from these assumptions and meanings shape how the group members think, act, and relate to and with others, as well as how they perceive aspects of life such as time, space, health, illness, and family, spousal, parental, work, and community-member roles. The beliefs, values, and norms of a cultural group are passed informally from one generation of group members born into the culture to another, exert a powerful force on all group members, and are very difficult to change.

SUBCULTURE

Subculture refers to membership in a smaller group within a larger culture (Figure 5-1). These smaller groups possess many of the values, beliefs, and customs of the larger culture but have unique characteristics such as age, education, marital status, preference in life partner, generational placement, occupation, socioeconomic level, health status, or religion. Membership in subcultures is generally involuntary. In addition, membership in subcultures is not usually constrained by obvious physical characteristics such as skin color, body build, or mannerisms.

Numerous subcultures exist within each culture. An individual may be simultaneously a member of several subcultures. For example, a 50-year-old (generational), white (race), overweight (health status), Southern (regional), conservative (political value system), heterosexual (sexual orientation), male (special privileges and responsibilities in dominant society), politician (occupation), father of two teenagers (family status), divorced and recently remarried (marital status), Baptist (religious affiliation) of Irish ancestry (genetic) currently living in the Detroit metropolitan area (lifestyle) is a member of at least 13 subcultures. Each subculture influences to some degree the behavior of its members, as does the primary culture.

It is important to recognize that every individual has a combination of cultural influences, derived from membership in the primary culture as well as multiple subcultures, which creates a **multicultural identity.** This unique multicultural identity makes it critical for the nurse to assess each individual patient in context rather than simply as a normative member of a single culture, subculture, race, ethnic, or minority group.

RACIAL GROUPS

Race is defined as the classification of individuals based on shared traits such as skin tone, facial features, and body build that are inherited from biological ancestors and are usually sufficiently obvious to warrant classification as a member of that racial group. Racial characteristics can have an impact on health status and health care; for example, individuals of Asian and American Indian descent have few apocrine glands and therefore perspire little, have mild or no body odor, and have dry ear wax. Also, the incidence of skin cancer in darkly pigmented individuals is much lower than in light-skinned individuals, due to a higher level of melanin in the pigmentation. Nurses need to ask about the patient's self-identified racial group when performing a cultural assessment.

ETHNIC GROUPS

Ethnic group members share a unique national or regional origin and social, cultural, and linguistic heritage. Five ethnic groups are usually recognized in the United States: whites (of European descent such as English, Scottish, Irish, French, Dutch, Polish, Scandinavian, Swiss, Italian, Slavic, and Russian); blacks (of African, Haitian, Jamaican, and Dominican Republic descent); Hispanics (of Spanish-speaking descent such as Cuban, Puerto Rican, Mexican, and Latin and South American); Asian and Pacific Islanders (of Chinese, Japanese, Filipino, Vietnamese, Cambodian, Korean, Hawaiian, Guamanian, East Indian, and Samoan descent);

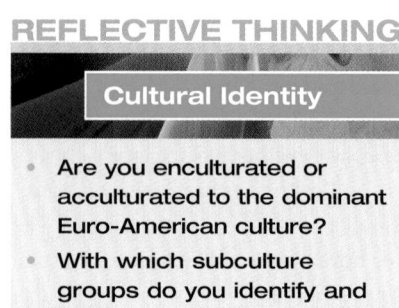

REFLECTIVE THINKING

Cultural Identity

- Are you enculturated or acculturated to the dominant Euro-American culture?
- With which subculture groups do you identify and why?

REFLECTIVE THINKING

HIV-Positive Patient

You are working on an orthopedic unit in a city hospital and have just finished admitting a 26-year-old homosexual male social worker who is HIV positive. The patient sustained multiple lacerations and a compound fracture of his left femur when struck by a speeding car running a red light. As you approach the nurses' station, you overhear the orthopedic intern and a staff nurse making disparaging, homophobic remarks about your new patient.

- What are your thoughts and feelings about working with this patient?
- How would you respond to what you have just overheard?
- How might you help your colleagues increase their cultural sensitivity and ensure the provision of culturally competent care for this patient?
- What research material is available that might support you in your attempt to provide culturally competent care for this patient?

and American Indians (of over 400 American Indian tribes and Eskimo descent) (Leigh, & Huff, 2006). Another ethnic group that is increasingly being recognized in the United States is Middle Easterners (of Egyptian, Persian [Iranian], Armenian, Yemeni, and Arab [Palestinian, Lebanese, Jordanian, Syrian, Saudi Arabian, and Iraqi] descent). Table 5-1 specifies ethnic-specific genetic traits and disorders.

Ethnic identity, or self-identification with an ethnic group, is subjective and not always obvious. For example, Egyptians tend to identify with their country of origin, but Armenians born in a country such as Iran, and Palestinians born in countries such as Lebanon or Israel, identify with their respective cultures of origin rather than their countries of origin (Meleis, Lipson, & Paul, 1992). When conducting a culturally competent assessment, therefore, it is appropriate to determine the patient's self-identified ethnic group as well as place of birth.

MINORITY GROUPS

Minority group members are individuals who are considered by themselves or others to be members of a minority because they have a different racial, cultural, ethnic, gender, or sexual orientation, or different socioeconomic level than do members of the dominant cultural group. Minority group members may receive different or unequal treatment and different degrees of acceptance from members of the dominant group. Although members of a minority may not be a true minority worldwide or even within a given region or nation (e.g., women or nurses), it is their membership in a subculture and the difference in the decisional power they have in influencing the dominant cultural environment that leads to their designation and subsequent treatment as a minority.

VALUES, NORMS, AND VALUE ORIENTATIONS

Cultures and subcultures have a fundamental set of principles known as values that govern the behavior of all members of the group. These values prescribe how each member should think, act, and respond to their internal and external environments. **Cultural values** tend to be acquired subconsciously during the process of enculturation and are a fundamental, often unshakable, unchanging set of principles that serve as the base on which an individual's beliefs, customs, goals, and aspirations are built.

LIFE 360°

Cultural Norms

Assemble a group of colleagues from various cultures and subcultures. Make a composite list of what each believes to be general cultural norms within his or her own culture or subculture, then have each person generate a list of cultural norms from the following topics: breastfeeding in public, law and order, breakfast foods, home remedies for illness, common courtesies, smoking, table manners, and waiting in queues. Compare your lists. What items are similar? What are the differences? Were there any surprises?

TABLE 5-1 Ethnic-Specific Genetic Traits and Disorders

ETHNIC GROUP	GENETIC TRAIT/DISORDER	ETHNIC GROUP	GENETIC TRAIT/DISORDER
Asian Americans		**Middle Eastern**	
Burmese	Hemoglobin E disease	Armenian	Familial Mediterranean fever
Chinese	Adult lactase deficiency		Familial paroxysmal polyserositis
	Alpha thalassemia	Habbanite Jews	Metachromatic leukodystrophy
	Chinese type glucose-6-phosphate dehydrogenase (G-6-PD) deficiency	Iranians	Dubin-Johnson syndrome
	Diabetes mellitus	Iraqian	Ichthyosis vulgaris
	Nasopharyngeal and liver cancer	Karaite Jews	Werdnig-Hoffmann disease
Filipino	Diabetes mellitus	Lebanese	Dyggve-Melchior-Clausen syndrome
	Thalassemia	Libyans (Sephardi Jews)	Cystinuria
	Glucose-6-phosphate dehydrogenase (G-6-PD) deficiency	Saudi Arabian	Metachromatic leukodystrophy
Indian	Cardiovascular disease	Yemenites	Mediterranean type glucose-6-phosphate dehydrogenase (G-6-PD) deficiency
	Lactase deficiency		Phenylketonuria
	Alpha thalassemia	**American Indians**	Chronic liver disease and cirrhosis
	Glucose-6-phosphate dehydrogenase (G-6-PD) deficiency		Diabetes mellitus
Japanese	Acatalasemia		Obesity
	Cleft lip or palate		Tuberculosis
	Oguchi's disease		Hepatitis B
Korean	Lactase deficiency		Asthma—infants
	Osteoporosis		Nasopharyngeal cancer
	Insulin autoimmune syndrome		Trachoma
	Peptic ulcer disease	Eskimos	Congenital adrenal hyperplasia
	Hypertension		Adult lactase deficiency
Papua Melanesian	Burkitt's lymphoma in children		Methemoglobinemia
Polynesians	Clubfoot		Primary narrow-angle glaucoma
Samoan	Diabetes mellitus		Pseudocholinesterase deficiency
Thai	Adult lactase deficiency		Haemophilus influenza type b
	Hemoglobin E disease	Hopi Indians	Tyrosinase-positive albinism
Vietnamese	Lactase deficiency	Navaho Indians	Arthritis
Black Americans			Diabetes mellitus
African	Adult lactase deficiency		Ear anomalies
	African type glucose-6-phosphate dehydrogenase (G-6-PD) deficiency	Yaqui Indians	Diabetes mellitus
	Beta thalassemia	Zuni Indians	Tyrosinase-positive albinism
	Hemoglobin C disease	**White Americans**	
	Hereditary hemoglobin F disease	Amish	
	Hypertension	Adams and Allen Counties, IN	Limb-girdle muscular dystrophy
	Sickle cell anemia	Appalachia	Tuberculosis
	Systemic lupus erythematosus		Coronary heart disease
	Diabetes mellitus		Diabetes mellitus
	Glaucoma	Holmes County, PA	Hemophilia B
Hispanics	Diabetes mellitus	Lancaster County, PA	Ellis-van Creveld syndrome
	Cleft lip or palate		
Mexican American, Latino, Chicano	Hypertension	Mifflin County, OH	Pyruvate kinase deficiency
Costa Rican	Malignant osteoporosis		

continues

TABLE 5-1 (Continued)

ETHNIC GROUP	GENETIC TRAIT/DISORDER	ETHNIC GROUP	GENETIC TRAIT/DISORDER
Bosnia-Herzegovina (Yugoslavia)	Colon cancer Diabetes mellitus	Jews Ashkenazi	Inflammatory bowel disease Gaucher's disease (adult type)
Czechs	Beta thalassemia Familial Mediterranean fever Mediterranean type glucose-6-phosphate dehydrogenase (G-6-PD) deficiency Congenital glaucoma		Niemann-Pick disease (infantile) Tay-Sachs disease (infantile) Hypercholesterolemia Polycythemia vera Stomach cancer Myopia
Danes	Krabbe's disease Phenylketonuria	Sephardi	Ataxia-telangiectasia Cystinuria
English	Cystic fibrosis Hereditary amyloidosis, type III		Familial Mediterranean fever Glycogen storage disease III
Finns	Congenital nephrosis Diastrophic dwarfism Polycystic liver disease Retinoschisis	New Zealanders Norwegians	Asthma Cholestasis-lymphedema Krabbe's disease Phenylketonuria
French Canadians (Quebec)	Hypercholesterolemia Osteoarthritis	Nova Scotia Acadians	Niemann-Pick disease, type D
Greeks	Tay-Sachs disease	Polish	Phenylketonuria
Icelanders	Phenylketonuria	Portuguese	Joseph's disease
Irish	Neural tube defects Phenylketonuria	Scots	Cystic fibrosis Hereditary amyloidosis, type III
Italians	Beta thalassemia Familial Mediterranean fever Mediterranean type glucose-6-phosphate dehydrogenase (G-6-PD) deficiency		Krabbe's disease Phenylketonuria Rett's syndrome Sjögren's syndrome

Based on data reported in *Mosby's Pocket Guide to Cultural Assessment* (4th ed.), by C. E. D'Avanzo, 2007, St. Louis: Mosby; *Transcultural nursing: Assessment & interventions* (5th ed.), by J. N. Giger and R. E. Davidhizar, 2007, Baltimore: Mosby; *Transcultural health care: A culturally competent approach* (3rd ed.), by L. Purnell and F. Paulanka, 2008, Philadelphia: F. A. Davis; *Wong's nursing care of infants and children* (8th ed.), by M. J. Hockenberry, D. Wilson, and C. Jackson, 2006, Philadelphia: Mosby.

Cultural norms are the often unwritten, but generally understood, prescriptions for acceptable behavior in designated situations encountered by group members in the course of their daily lives. Every group member is bound by these norms and may be criticized, punished, or ostracized by other group members when the norms are violated.

All cultures have a fundamental set of values and concurrent **value orientations**, that is, patterned principles that provide order and give direction to individuals' thoughts and behaviors related to the solution of commonly occurring human problems (Giger & Davidhizar, 2007; Kluckhorn & Strodtbeck, 1961; Spector, 2003). Five areas about which cultures have their own unique value orientations have major relevance for culturally competent health assessments and care (Table 5-2). These value orientations are time, human nature, activity, relational, and people to nature.

BELIEFS

Cultural beliefs consist of the explanatory ideas and knowledge that members of a given culture have about various aspects of their world and are based on cultural values and norms, including commonly held opinions, knowledge, and attitudes about

TABLE 5-2 Basic Cross-Cultural Values, Value Orientations, and Beliefs

VALUE	VALUE ORIENTATION AND BELIEFS
Time What is the time orientation of human beings?	*Past* focus: Reverence for long-standing traditions. *Present* focus: Live in the "here and now," perceive time in a linear fashion. *Future* focus: Willing to defer gratification to ensure they can meet a future goal; tend to be disciplined in scheduling and using time.
Human Nature What is the basic nature of human beings?	Human beings are *basically* good. Human beings are *evil* but have a *perfectable* nature. Human beings are a combination of *good* and *evil*, requiring *self-control* to *perfect nature; lapses* occasionally occur and are *accepted*. Human beings are neutral, neither good nor evil.
Activity What is the primary purpose of life?	*Being* orientation: Human beings' value resides in their *inherent existence* and spontaneity. *Becoming-in-being* orientation: Human beings' value is inherent, but they must engage in continuous *self-development* as integrated wholes. *Doing* orientation: Human beings exist to be *active* and to *achieve*.
Relational What is the purpose of human relations?	*Linear* relationships: Welfare and goals of the *hereditary and extended family* are emphasized. Goals of the family take precedence over the individual's. *Collateral* relationships: Welfare and goals of *social and family group* are emphasized. Group goals take precedence. *Individual* relationships: *Individual* goals and accountability for own behavior emphasized.
People to Nature What is the relationship of human beings to nature?	Human beings *dominate nature* and have control over their environment. Human beings *live in harmony with nature* and must maintain that balance. Human beings are *subjugated to nature* and have no control over their environment.

Compiled from information in *Variations in Value Orientations,* by K. Kluckhorn and F. Strodtbeck, 1961, Evanston, IL: Row, Peterson; and *Transcultural Nursing: Assessment and Intervention* (5th ed.), by J. N. Giger and R. E. Davidhizar, 2007, Baltimore: Mosby.

time, relationships, human nature, purpose in life, and nature. Such beliefs influence the meaning individuals attach to health and illness, by whom and how they prefer to treat illness, and the health behaviors in which they are willing to engage. Because health and illness are culturally determined, what may be considered to be health or illness in one culture may not be in another. In addition, many cultures distinguish between a "**folk illness,**" believed to be caused by disharmony or an imbalance or as punishment, and a "**scientific illness,**" in which the presence of pathology is the defining characteristic. In these cultures, a **folk practitioner** (a healer or other individual who is not part of the scientific health care system but is believed to have special knowledge or power to prevent, treat, or provide resources needed to heal folk illnesses) is consulted for a folk illness because health care practitioners are not believed to be knowledgeable in recognizing or treating such illnesses.

Folk Illnesses

Two major types of folk illnesses are usually delineated: naturalistic and personalistic. **Naturalistic illnesses** are believed to be caused by an imbalance or disequilibrium between essentially impersonal factors. For example, the most common imbalance is between "hot" and "cold" (Table 5-3). Illnesses and treatments that are classified as either hot or cold are culturally determined and do not have any

TABLE 5-3 Hot and Cold Conditions, Foods, and Treatments

Hot (*Caliente/Yang*) Conditions	Cold (*Frio/Yin*) Conditions
Constipation	Cancer
Diarrhea	Colds
Fever	Depression
Hypertension	Earache
Infections	Headache
Kidney problems	Infertility
Liver problems	Joint pain
Pregnancy	Lactation
Skin rashes, sores	Malaria
Sore throat	Menstruation
Ulcers	Paralysis
	Pneumonia
	Postpartum psychoses
	Rheumatism
	Stomach cramps
	Teething
	Tuberculosis

Hot (*Caliente/Yang*) foods	Cold (*Frio/Yin*) foods
Aromatic beverages	Avocado
Beans	Barley water
Cereal grains	Bean curds
Cheese	Bland foods
Chili peppers	Bottled whole milk
Chocolate	Cashew nuts
Eggs	Dairy products
Evaporated milk	Fresh vegetables (carrots, turnips, squash, eggplant)
Fried foods	Green vegetables
Goat's milk	Honey
Hard liquor	Meats (chicken, fish, goat)
Meats (beef, lamb, waterfowl)	Raisins
Oils	Tropical fruits (banana, grapefruit, mango, orange, pineapple)
Onions	
Peas	
Spicy, hot foods	
Temperate-zone fruits (apple, grapes, pears, peaches)	
Vinegar	
Wine	

Hot (*Caliente/Yang*) Medicines and herbs	Cold (*Frio/Yin*) Medicines and herbs
Anise	Bicarbonate of soda
Aspirin	Linden
Castor oil	Milk of magnesia
Cinnamon	Orange flower water
Cod-liver oil	Sage
Garlic	
Ginger root	
Iron preparation	
Penicillin	
Tobacco	
Vitamins	

Compiled from data obtained in *Contemporary Psychiatric-Mental Health Nursing* (2nd ed.), by C. R. Kneisl and E. Trigoboff, 2009, Upper Saddle River, NJ: Prentice Hall; and *Transcultural Nursing: Assessment and Intervention* (5th ed.), by J. N. Giger and R. E. Davidhizar, 2007, Baltimore: Mosby.

REFLECTIVE THINKING

Fundamental Cultural Values

- What is your time orientation?
- What do you believe about the basic nature of human beings? What do you believe is your basic nature?
- What do you believe is your primary purpose in life?
- What do you believe about the purpose of human relations?
- What do you believe your relation is to nature and the supernatural?

relationship to the actual temperature of the patient or of the substances used to treat the illness. In general, "hot" illnesses are treated with "cold" substances and vice versa to restore the balance between the two. These beliefs are held by many Hispanic, Arab, and Asian ethnic groups and cultures. Although most cultures who share these beliefs use the hot and cold terminology, among traditional Chinese, these forces are called *yin* (cold) and *yang* (hot).

Understanding the health belief patterns of patients and the meanings attached to symptoms, illnesses, and treatments can be helpful in understanding why patients may refuse to participate in a given treatment regimen or why they insist on a specific treatment. For example, some Hispanic patients may insist on being given penicillin, which is considered to be a *caliente* (hot) treatment, for a viral upper respiratory infection (URI), which is considered to be a *frio* (cold) condition. Explanations about the lack of benefit in treating viral URIs with penicillin and the potential for building a resistance to penicillin when used unnecessarily rarely dissuade those who insist on its use. Substituting another substance such as vitamins, which are also considered to be "hot" treatments, shows an acceptance of their beliefs and "does the least harm."

Personalistic illnesses are believed to occur because an individual has committed some offense and is being punished, or the illness results from acts of aggression (sometimes unintentional) by other individuals. Witchcraft and the "evil eye" are two sources of personalistic illnesses. Witchcraft is believed to be the cause of illness among Haitians, Puerto Ricans, and some black Americans. More often than not, witchcraft is used to punish individuals for an emotional or a physical injury, an illness, or a death they are thought to have caused, or occasionally because they possess something that is coveted by another.

The "evil eye" belief is shared by many Mediterranean (e.g., Italian, Sicilian, and Greek), African, and Spanish-speaking cultures. The "evil eye" is more often than not given unintentionally, for example, by complimenting a child unprotected by an amulet, gold cross, or other protective device or by not touching the child while offering the compliment. It is feared that a child who is complimented for her looks, for example, will lose her good looks (if she was unprotected by a device) or develop symptoms such as severe headache, restlessness, irritability, high fever, diarrhea, weight loss, and sleeplessness if the person complimenting the child was not touching the child at the time.

Self-Care Practices

All cultural groups use a variety of self-care practices that may include the use of "folk medicine" and remedies. Self-care includes practices in which persons engage on their own behalf to aid in health promotion and maintenance, disease or injury prevention or protection, and disease or injury treatment. For example, the Vietnamese American may use *cao gio* (skin rubbing with a coin) to treat diseases he or she believes to be caused by wind entering the body (e.g., upper respiratory infections). After applying oil or an ointment on the skin over the affected body area (chest, shoulders, upper back), the edge of a coin is moved along the skin until ecchymotic stripes appear, demonstrating that the treatment is successful. *Cao gio* is rarely painful or injurious and more often than not is perceived to be helpful by the recipient. Finding these areas of ecchymosis, however, can lead to a misdiagnosis of abuse if knowledge of this folk practice is lacking.

Assessing the Potential for Harm Associated with a Cultural Belief or Behavior

When assessing one's own cultural values and beliefs and the behaviors that result from these values and beliefs, a nurse is often faced with having to decide when it

REFLECTIVE THINKING

Self-Care Practices

- What self-care practices do you use and when do you use them?
- Where or from whom did you learn the self-care practices you use most often?
- Which of these self-care practices are based on medical research and which are not?

- What are the values and beliefs that most characterize each culture and subculture to which you belong, and with which do you agree?
- Do any of your values and beliefs that are derived from membership in one culture or subculture conflict with those from any other?
- If there is any conflict between the values of two or more of the cultures or subcultures with which you identify (e.g., health care professional subculture, religious subculture, socioeconomic subculture, political party subculture), have you resolved these conflicts, and if so, how have you done this and what helped you to reconcile these conflicts?

- Would you assist with a female circumcision?
- Under what conditions would you participate?
- When would you not participate and why?

is appropriate for his or her cultural value orientation to take precedence over that of the patient's. In other words, how culturally competent is a nurse to evaluate and decide when a patient's behavior is adaptive, harmful, or neutral? Sprott (1993) has suggested that nurses might make these judgments using Korbin's (1977) work on assessing whether an ethnic group's child-rearing practices constitute harm.

The conditions cited in Korbin's schema have relevance for evaluating the potential physical or psychological harm that health practices may have on a family member as perceived by health professionals or the agents of the family. Using this schema, a practice would not be considered harmful if:

1. The practice is sanctioned by that culture.
2. The practice is within the limits of deviations that are acceptable in that culture.
3. The practice is important for the acceptance of the patient as a member of the culture.
4. The patient on whom the practice will be carried out perceives that it is an appropriate practice in that situation.
5. The intent of the health care provider or agent of the family is consistent with the cultural "rules" that govern the practice.

For many situations, these five conditions can be quite helpful in clarifying the issues associated with evaluating whether an anticipated health practice is harmful or not. For situations in which the practices of agents of the family, such as folk or traditional practitioners, must be evaluated or when the family requests that the nurse participate in a practice that is in conflict with the nurse's value system, the judgment that must be made is more difficult.

For example, circumcision of young girls (removal of all or part of the clitoris, labia minora, and labia majora) from early childhood through adolescence is widespread in many African countries such as Somalia, Djibouti, Ethiopia, Mali, and northern Sudan; among Muslim groups in the Middle East, the Philippines, Pakistan, Indonesia, and Malaysia; and in some areas of Mexico, Brazil, and Peru (Johnson & Rogers, 1994, World Health Organization, 2000). Although male circumcision is relatively common in the United States, female circumcision is not a part of the dominant Euro-American culture to which most American nurses have been enculturated.

For the health care professional in the United States who is enculturated into the Euro-American value system and bound by the health care professional oath to "do no harm," surgical removal of female genitalia constitutes a physiological and psychological threat to a child from our dominant culture. But does it pose the same threat to a child who is a member of one of the ethnic groups that practice female circumcision and who is now living in the United States? When the female circumcision procedure on a child from one of these ethnic groups is contemplated in the United States, the primary health care provider to the family may be faced with a cultural conflict: to assist with the procedure by ensuring sterile conditions, pain control, and possible anesthesia versus refusing to have anything to do with it and possibly reporting the parents for child abuse if they go through with the circumcision ritual. Each nurse must ultimately resolve this and other such cultural and ethical conflicts on an individual patient basis.

CUSTOMS AND RITUALS

Customs and rituals are culturally learned behaviors that are much easier to observe or learn about through interviewing than are the values and beliefs on which the customs and rituals are based. **Customs** are frequent or common practices carried out by tradition and include communication patterns, family and kinship relations, work patterns, religious and dietary practices (see Chapters 6 and 7), and health behaviors and practices (Table 5-4). **Cultural rituals** are highly

TABLE 5-4 Cultural Characteristics and Health Care Beliefs and Practices

CULTURAL GROUP	COMMUNICATION STYLES	FAMILY, SOCIAL, AND WORK RELATIONSHIPS	HEALTH VALUES AND BELIEFS	HEALTH CUSTOMS AND PRACTICES
Asian-American				
Chinese	Nonverbal and contextual cues important. Silence after a statement is used by a speaker who wishes the listener to consider the importance of what is said. Self-expression repressed. Value silence. Touching limited. May smile when do not understand. Hesitant to ask questions.	Hierarchical, extended family pattern. Deference to authority figures and elders. Both parents make decisions about children. Value self-reliance and self-restraint. Important to preserve family's honor and save face. Value working hard and giving to society.	Health viewed as gift from parents and ancestors and the result of a balance between the energy forces of *yin* (cold) and *yang* (hot). Illness caused by an imbalance. Blood is the source of life and cannot be regenerated. Lack of blood and chi (innate energy) produces debilitation and long illness. Respect for the body and belief in reincarnation dictates that one must die with the body intact. Believe that a good physician can accurately diagnose an illness by simply examining a person using the senses of sight, smell, touch, and listening.	May use medical care system in conjunction with Chinese methods of acupuncture (a *yin* treatment consisting of the insertion of needles to meridians to cure disease or relieve pain) and moxibustion (a *yang* treatment during which heated, pulverized wormwood is applied to appropriate meridians to assist with labor and delivery and other *yin* disorders). Medicinal herbs, e.g., ginseng, are widely used. Fear painful, intrusive diagnostic tests, especially the drawing of blood. May refuse intrusive surgery or autopsy. May be distrustful of physicians who order and use painful or intrusive diagnostic tests. Accept immunizations as valid means of disease prevention. Heavy use of condiments such as monosodium glutamate and soy sauce.
Japanese	Attitude, action, and feeling more important than words. Tend to listen empathically. Touching limited. Direct eye contact considered a lack of respect. Stoic, suppress overt emotion. Value self-control, politeness, and personal restraint.	Close, interdependent, intergenerational relationships. Individual needs subordinate to family's needs. Will endure great hardship to ensure success of next generation. Belonging to right clique or society important to status and success. Obligation to kin and work group. Education highly valued.	Believe illness caused by contact with polluting agents (e.g., blood, skin diseases, corpses), social or family disharmony, or imbalance from poor health habits. Cleanliness highly valued.	Tend to rely on Euro-American medical system for preventive and illness care. Oldest adult child responsible for care of elderly. Care of disabled is a family's responsibility. Take pride in good health of children. Believe in removal of diseased areas. Practice of emotional control may make pain assessment more difficult. When visiting ill, often bring fruit or special Japanese foods.

continues

TABLE 5-4 (Continued)

CULTURAL GROUP	COMMUNICATION STYLES	FAMILY, SOCIAL, AND WORK RELATIONSHIPS	HEALTH VALUES AND BELIEFS	HEALTH CUSTOMS AND PRACTICES
Vietnamese	Respect and harmony most important values. Disrespectful to question authority figures. Avoid direct eye contact. Strong focus on respect through use of titles and terms indicating family and generational relationships. Modesty of speech and action valued. Relaxed concept of time; punctuality less significant than propriety. Use Ya to indicate listening, not understanding. Avoid asking direct questions.	Family close, multigenerational, and primary social network. Filial piety of primary importance. Father is family decision maker. Individual needs are subordinate to family's needs. Training of children shared by extended family. Behavior of individual reflects on total family. Education highly valued.	Believe illness caused by naturalistic (bad food, water), supernaturalistic (punishment for displeasing a deity), metaphysical (imbalance of hot and cold) forces, or from contamination by germs.	Often use both folk medicine and some parts of the scientific health care system such as drugs. Family orally transmits folk medicine information. Health care regarded as family responsibility. Use medicinal herbs, therapeutic diets, hygienic measures to promote health, prevent illness, and treat illness. All means and resources available to family are tried before seeking outside help. Folk care practices include *cao gio* (rubbing skin with coin) for respiratory illnesses; *bat gil* (skin pinching) for headaches; inhalation of aromatic oils and liniments for respiratory and gastrointestinal illnesses. May consult priest, astrologer, shaman, or fortune-teller for prediction or instruction about health, or use hot and cold foods and substances to restore balance.
Filipinos	Personal dignity and preserving self-esteem highly valued. Nonverbal communication important. Eye contact avoided. Avoid direct expressions of disagreement, particularly with authority figures. Sex, socioeconomic status, and tuberculosis too personal to discuss.	Multigenerational matrifocal family with strong family ties. Avoid behavior that shames family. Defer to elderly. Individual interests subordinate to family's interests. Value interpersonal relationships over current events.	Tend to believe illness is related to natural (unhealthy environment), supernatural (God's will and providence), and metaphysical (imbalance between hot and cold) forces. Tend to be fatalistic in outlook on life.	If accessible, may use both folk and scientific medical systems. Folk practices include flushing (stimulating perspiration, vomiting, bowel evacuation), heating (hot and cold substances to maintain internal body temperature), and protection (use of amulets, good luck pieces, religious medals, pictures, statues). Tend to be stoic; believe pain is God's will and He will give one the strength to bear it.

continues

TABLE 5-4 (Continued)

CULTURAL GROUP	COMMUNICATION STYLES	FAMILY, SOCIAL, AND WORK RELATIONSHIPS	HEALTH VALUES AND BELIEFS	HEALTH CUSTOMS AND PRACTICES
Filipinos *continued*	Need to engage in "small talk" before discussing more serious matters.			
Black Americans				
African Americans	Many have high level of caution or distrust of majority group. Expressive use of nonverbal behavior and speech. Many use an English dialect: "black English." Very sensitive to lack of congruence between verbal and nonverbal messages. Value direct eye contact. May "test" health professionals before submitting self to decisions and care of the majority group's health care providers.	Strong kinship bonds in extended family. Families 50% patriarchical, 50% matriarchical. Large social networks of family and unrelated members. Elderly members respected, particularly maternal grandparents. Strong sense of peoplehood; come to aid of others in crisis. Black minister a strong influence in community. Women protect health of family. Worth of education is judged by its "usability in living."	Illness is a collective event that disrupts the total family system. Illness believed to be a natural event resulting from conflict or disharmony in one's life, failure to protect oneself from cold air, pollution, food, and water, or sent by God as punishment. Those more assimilated to dominant culture perceive illness to be due to preventable injury or pathology.	Health is maintained by proper diet, rest, clean environment. Self-care and folk medicine (usually religious in origin) very prevalent. Individuals from more rural backgrounds are more likely to use folk practitioners. Attempt home remedies first; may not seek help from the medical establishment until illness serious; often will elect to retain dignity rather than seek care if values and sensibilities are demeaned. Prayer is common means for prevention and treatment. When ill or hospitalized, visits by family minister are sought, expected, and valued to help cope with illness and suffering.
Haitians	New immigrants and older persons often speak only Haitian Creole. Hand gesturing and tone of voice frequently used to complement speech. Smiling and nodding often do not indicate understanding.	Two-class social system: wealthy and poor. Rural and poor families tend to be matriarchical. Children taught unquestioning obedience to adults. Child-rearing shared by parents and older siblings.	Illness believed to be caused by supernatural forces (angry spirits, enemies, or the dead) or natural forces (irregularities of blood volume, flow, viscosity, purity, color, or temperature [hot and cold]; gas [gaz]; movement and consistency of mother's milk; hot/cold imbalance in the body; bone displacement).	Use medical care and folk medicine simultaneously. Health maintained by good dietary and hygienic habits. Adherence to prescribed treatments directly related to perceived severity of illness; resist dietary and activity restrictions. Hot and cold, and light and heavy properties of food are used to gain harmony with one's life cycle and bodily states.

continues

TABLE 5-4 (Continued)

CULTURAL GROUP	COMMUNICATION STYLES	FAMILY, SOCIAL, AND WORK RELATIONSHIPS	HEALTH VALUES AND BELIEFS	HEALTH CUSTOMS AND PRACTICES
Haitians *continued*	Direct eye contact used in formal and casual conversations. Unassertive—will not ask questions if health care provider appears busy or rushed. Touch is perceived as comforting, sympathetic, and reassuring.	Tend to be status conscious; thus parents often choose children's mate to increase family status.	Believe health is a personal responsibility.	Natural illnesses are first treated by home remedies. Supernatural illnesses treated by healers: herbalist or leaf doctor (*dokte fey*), midwife (*fam saj*), or voodoo priest (*houngan*) or priestess (*mambo*). Use amulets and prayer to protect against supernatural illnesses.
Hispanic Americans **Mexicans**	Most bilingual; may use nonstandard English. Introductory embrace common. Tend to revert to native language in times of stress. Consider prolonged eye contact disrespectful, but value direct eye contact. Appreciate "small talk" before initiating actual conversation topic. Appreciate a nondirect approach with open-ended questions. Hesitant to talk about sex, but may do so more freely with nurse of same sex. Father should be present when speaking with a male child.	Strong kinship bonds among nuclear and extended families including *compadres* (godparents). Strong need for family group togetherness. Respect wisdom of elders. Children highly desired and valued; accompany family everywhere. Entire family contribute to family's financial welfare. Homes frequently decorated with statues, medals, and pictures of saints. Children often reluctant to share communal showers in schools. Relaxed concept of time.	Illness can be prevented by: being good, eating proper foods, and working proper amount of time; also accomplished through prayer, wearing religious medals or amulets, and sleeping with relics at home. Some believe illness is due to: body imbalance between *caliente* (hot) and *frio* (cold) or "wet" and "dry"; dislocation of parts of the body (*empacho*—ball of food stuck to the stomach wall, or *caida de la mollera*—more serious, depression of fontanelle in infant); magic or supernatural (*mal ojo* [evil eye] or punishment from God); strong emotional state (*susto*—soul loss following an extreme fright); or *envidio* (success leads to envy by others resulting in misfortune).	Magico-religious practices common. Usually seek help from older women in family before going to a *Jerbero*, who specializes in the use of herbs and spices to restore balance/health, or *curandero* or *curandera* (holistic healers), with whom they have a uniquely personal relationship and share a common worldview. Prevent and treat illness with "hot" and "cold" food prescriptions and prohibitions. For severe illness, use scientific medical system, but also make promises, visit shrines, use medals and candles, offer prayers—elements of Catholic and Pentecostal rituals and artifacts. Extreme modesty; may avoid seeking medical care and open discussions of sex. Children and adults expected to and do endure pain stoically.

continues

TABLE 5-4 (Continued)

CULTURAL GROUP	COMMUNICATION STYLES	FAMILY, SOCIAL, AND WORK RELATIONSHIPS	HEALTH VALUES AND BELIEFS	HEALTH CUSTOMS AND PRACTICES
Mexicans *continued*			More concerned with present than with future, and therefore may focus on immediate solutions rather than long-term goals. May view hospital as place to go to die.	
Puerto Ricans	Older, newly moved to the mainland often speak only Spanish; others usually bilingual. May use nonstandard English. Personal and family privacy valued. Consider questions regarding family disrespectful and presumptuous. Tend to have a relaxed sense of time.	Paternalistic, hierarchical family; father is family provider and decision maker. Family of central importance. Families usually large. Parents demand absolute obedience and respect from children. Women in family tend to all ill members and dispense all medicines. Children valued—seen as gift from God.	Many believe illness is caused by imbalance of hot and cold, evil spirits, and forces. Many believe in spirits and spiritualism, having visions, and hearing voices. Accept many idiosyncratic behaviors; often perceive behavioral disturbances as symptoms of illness that need to be treated rather than judged. Suspicious and fearful of hospitals.	Use folk practitioners and medical establishment or both. When ill: first seek advice from women in family; if not sufficient, seek help from a *senoria* (woman especially knowledgeable about causes and treatment of common illnesses); if unable to help, consult an *espiritista, curandera, or santeria* (if psychiatric problem), who listens nonjudgmentally; often use herbs, lotions, salves, and massage and *caliente* (hot), *fresco* (cool), and *frio* (cold) treatments; if no relief, may go to a medical physician; if not satisfied, may return to any of the preceding.
Cuban Americans	Most new immigrants are bilingual. Expect some social talk before getting to actual reason for discussion.	Strong family and maternal and paternal kinship ties. Mother tends to explain and reason constantly to obtain child's conformity to family norms. Elderly cared for at home. Mother primary health care provider in home and must be included in all health education programs for family members.	Believe good health results from prevention and good nutrition. Believe plump babies and young children are most healthy and admirable.	Combine use of medical practitioners with religious and nonreligious folk practitioners. Tend to be eclectic in health-seeking practices and, in some instances, may seek assistance of *santeros* (Afro-Cuban healers) and *espiritistas* to complement treatment by medical practitioners. Parents very concerned about eating habits of their children; may spend a considerable part of the family budget on food.

continues

CASE STUDY

An Asian Indian American with Cardiovascular Disease

This case study illustrates the application and objective documentation of the cultural assessment. Patient is accompanied by her husband, Devad Khanna; Mrs. Rajamma Khanna is a 49 yo Asian Indian female presenting for the first time to the Women's Health Center in Fredericksburg, VA, with shortness of breath after mild exercise, easy fatigability, and frequent indigestion of 3 months' duration. Mrs. Khanna's husband reports she did not tell anyone except her mother-in-law about her symptoms until this week. When Mr. Khanna was told by his mother of his wife's symptoms, he immediately made an appointment at this Center because "it has an all-female staff and its cardiovascular physicians and nurse practitioners have excellent reputations!" Mr. Khanna noted that he looked for a center with specialists in cardiovascular medicine because he knows that cardiovascular disease is higher among Asian Indian Americans than in any other immigrant group.

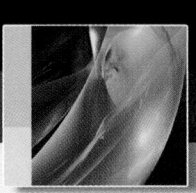

CULTURAL ASSESSMENT

1. **Ethnic Group Affiliation and Racial Background**

   a. **Would you tell me how long you have lived in Fredericksburg, VA?**

   Pt has lived in the Khanna family home in Fredericksburg with her mother- and father-in-law for 25 yrs.

   b. **Where are you from originally?**

   Pt came to the U.S. at the age of 22 after an arranged marriage to her husband, Devad Khanna, a second-generation Asian Indian American and current VP of a regional chain of colonial hotels owned by his family. They have one daughter, 24 yo, in medical school at Georgetown University, and two sons, 21 and 19 yrs, studying at the University of Virginia. Pt received a BA in Musicology before coming to the U.S. and is considered to be an accomplished musician. Pt does not work outside the home.

   c. **With which particular ethnic group would you say you identify? How closely do you identify with this ethnic group?**

   Asian Indian, Hindu. Soft-spoken, speaks English fluently, but with an obvious accent, dressed in a sari. Defers to husband, preferring that he answer most questions. Pt will elaborate on an answer when urged to by husband. Pt admits she has become somewhat Americanized and no longer eats totally vegetarian, but in her heart, she "will always be Indian, Hindu."

   d. **Where have you lived and when? What health problems did you experience or were you exposed to when you lived in each place? What helped you recover from each of the health problems identified?**

   Pt born and raised in an affluent joint family home (grandparents, unmarried sons and daughters, and all married sons and their families) in New Delhi, India. Had no major illnesses, only occasional colds (treated by keeping the body warm, especially the head, throat, chest, and feet, drinking fresh ginger and honey mixed in water for a cough, and eating only boiled or steamed vegetables, hot spice or herbal teas, and vegetable soup); stomachaches (treated with equal parts dry ginger, black pepper, dry mint leaves, and roasted cumin seeds mixed in water, and easily digested foods like rice yogurt, cooked squash, pumpkin, and *mung dal* (green bean dish)—spicy and fried foods with a lot of oil were prohibited; and diarrhea (treated with herbs, i.e., nutmeg, raspberry, and oakbark, a drink made with coriander seeds, and foods "that bind the stool" like bananas, rice, yogurt, pomegranate, and boiled vegetables). "Many Asian Indian Hindus are lactose intolerant, and I have a touch of that."

continues

CASE STUDY (Continued)
An Asian Indian American with
Cardiovascular Disease

2. Major Beliefs and Values

Time orientation: Asian Indian Hindu people are past, present, and future oriented. Past oriented in that they have many traditions and rituals basic to their culture; present oriented in that they perceive time in a linear fashion; and future oriented in that they are focused on performing their duties flaw-lessly to ensure their condition in the next life. Pt notes that their children are more future oriented like most Americans in that they are willing to defer gratification so they can meet a goal in this life and tend to be increasingly disciplined about scheduling as they have matured.

Basic nature of human beings: Pt believes that human beings are a combination of good and evil, which requires self-control, truthfulness, and respect for others to perfect one's self. Pt notes that her entire family, but most especially her mother-in-law and she, have taught this perspective to all of her children and encourage them to engage in daily prayers, *bhajans* (sacred hymns*),* yoga, *pranayama* (breathing exercises), and meditation. She doubts that they are conscientious about doing so daily now that they are all away at school. This worries her.

Purpose of life: Pt and husband believe that humans should have a becoming-in-being orientation in that the value of humans is inherent but that one must engage in continuous, total self-improvement. Thus the raison d'etre for an Asian Indian woman is to become a perfect wife for her husband, to defer to him and never contradict him in public, to speak softly and rarely in public, to be a perfect mother for his children, and to give him sons to follow him. Mr. Khanna says that it is nice to have a "peaceful" home, but that he encourages the pt to say what she wants and to be more open to some of the Ameri-can ways like "letting me know when she first started having symptoms, then I could have gotten her here earlier."

Purpose of human relations: Asian Indian Hindus live in nuclear, joint family homes where mar-ried sons and their families live with or near their parents. The joint family exerts powerful pressures on all family members to uphold their cultural and religious norms and expectations. Individuals are expected to subject their individual desires to the norms of the family. These living arrangements and expectations are not quite as strong among second- and third-generation Asian Indian Americans, although members of the Asian Indian American community maintain very close ties with one another regardless of generation.

Relationship between human beings and nature: Asian Indian Hindus believe humans are subju-gated to nature and must live in harmony with nature inasmuch as they proceed from and will return to *Brahma,* the center of the universe.

3. Health Beliefs and Practices

a. **What does being healthy mean to you?**

Most Asian Indian Hindus believe that the body is made of five elements: earth (bones and muscles), wind (breath), water (phlegm), space (in hollow organs), and fire (gall). A balance among water, wind, and fire is necessary to have good health. Illness is the result of a deficiency or excess of one or more of these elements, which is influenced by one's past and present lifestyle and behaviors and/or the inva-sion of germs. Although pt's beliefs are stronger than her husband's, Mr. Khanna notes that he supports her in her beliefs.

b. **What do you do to help you stay healthy?**

Pt, as do most first-generation Asian Indian Hindus, combines *Ayurvedic* medicine (based on the doctrine that disease has both a germ causation and is the result of an imbalance of the essential body

continues

elements, some of which can be controlled by the individual or a *syanas*, holy man, and some of which cannot) and scientific medicine as practiced in the Western world. Pt believes that personal hygiene, a healthy diet, mostly vegetarian, maintaining self-control of strong emotions, lack of extremism in lifestyle, acquiring accurate knowledge of health and illness cause and effect, and performing one's duties perfectly and without resentment are very important for maintaining health.

c. **What does being ill or sick mean to you?**

Pt stresses that the mother is responsible for the children, her husband, and the home. She must stay well so she can take care of her family.

d. **What do you usually do when you are sick or not feeling well?**
Who do you want to be with when you are sick?
Who in your family is primarily responsible for making health care decisions?

The grandmother is the ultimate source of knowledge about illness and home remedies to treat all family members. Other women of the family may also help care for their own, but the grandmother has the final word on all health matters in the home. Also, it is she who decides whether a sick family member needs to see a *syanas* or a physician and expects both to keep their family's health problems and treatment absolutely confidential. It is important that all family members have total access to the patient when hospitalized. While ill, the patient assumes the sick role without guilt and the family assumes all responsibilities for that time. Family members prefer to protect the patient from knowing the gravity of his or her prognosis or disability because they believe it will make the patient lose hope and hasten his or her death. The husband/father will be the primary spokesman and ultimate decision maker when care is received outside the home.

e. **Are there any cultural or ethnic sanctions or restrictions that you want to or must observe?**

Health care providers should ask permission to perform any examination and explain the rationale for all activities involving disrobing and direct examination of any part, especially with women. Health care providers should avoid exposing the patient's whole body. Daily baths are required and must be taken before breakfast. Asian Indian Hindu Americans are stoic about pain and believe praying for recovery from an illness is the lowest form of prayer.

f. **By whom do you prefer to have your health and medical care provided? Do you prefer that they have the same cultural background or gender as your own?**

Pt prefers female health care providers for all aspects of her care. Pt would like to have an Indian woman assigned to her if possible.

4. **Language Barriers and Communication Styles**

a. **In which language are you most comfortable communicating?**
Do you need an interpreter when discussing health care information and treatments?

Pt is fluent in English and Hindi. Most first-generation Asian Indian Hindu Americans speak English outside their homes and speak Hindi in their homes unless a guest who speaks only English is present.

b. **Are there special ways of showing respect or disrespect in your culture?**
Are there any cultural preferences or restrictions related to touching, social distance, making eye contact, or other verbal or nonverbal behaviors when communicating?

continues

Both men and women tend to be more soft-spoken than the average American. Vitality is generally added to a conversation by head and hand gestures. Men make direct eye contact with one another during greetings and conversations. Women usually look down when speaking with men, thereby showing respect. When introducing oneself to an Asian Indian female, the greeting is first addressed to the father or the oldest female if the father is not present. If it is a married female, the husband is to be greeted first. A man must never make direct eye contact with a woman other than his wife. To do so is considered a seductive gesture and is taboo. Open displays of affection are considered disrespectful. Married Asian Indians display affection only in the privacy of their own home, but not in the presence of their children or elders.

5. **Role of the Family, Spousal Relationship, and Parenting Styles**

a. **What is the composition of your family? Who is considered to be a member of your family?**

In India, one's family lives in the parental home and all are subject to the patriarch's authority. The patriarch controls the family's finances and business ventures, giving each son an allowance from his own earnings. In the pt's family in America, Mr. Khanna's father is the CEO of their family company, and he and his two brothers, as officers in the company, draw their own salaries and manage their own finances. It is expected that if the company expands, all family members will agree to and support such expansion by working faithfully to make it successful. Pt notes that the joint family is much smaller in the U.S. than in India and that her children have already informed their parents that they probably will not be living with the joint family when they finish their education. At this time, only one son plans to join the family company.

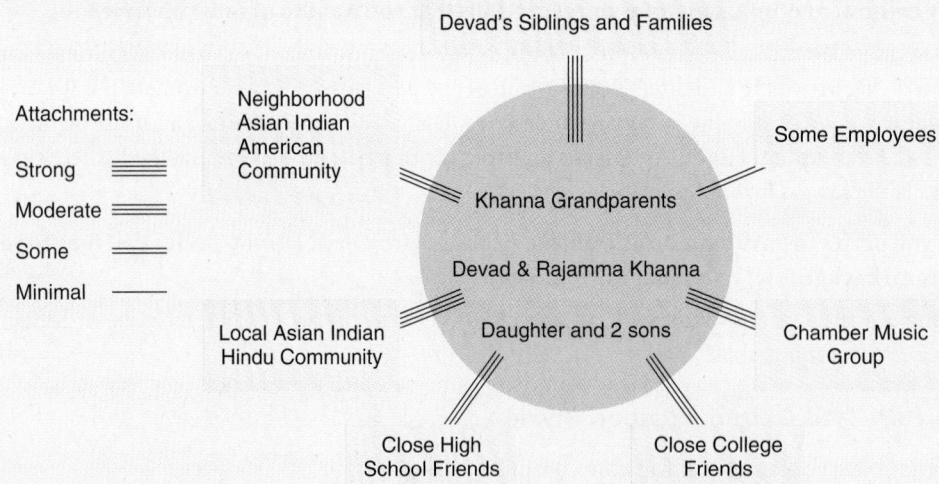

b. **With what ethnic group(s) does your family as a whole identify? How does their ethnic identity and which of their ethnic traditions do you think most affect their health status?**

See above.

c. **Which of your relatives live nearby? With which of your family members and relatives do you interact the most often?**

continues

CASE STUDY (Continued)
An Asian Indian American with
Cardiovascular Disease

A brother and his family live next door to the parent's home, and a sister and her family live across town. All try to get together for major religious events, holidays, birthdays, anniversaries, and the anniversary of the grandparents becoming naturalized citizens of the U.S. Assorted members of each family also enjoy attending activities together at the Kennedy Center, engaging in local Asian Indian American activities, and watching cricket on TV.

d. **In what ways do your family members believe the nurse, physician, and other health care practitioners can help the family members achieve their goals for health and well-being of the family?**

First-generation Asian Indian Hindu Americans believe the *syanas* and physicians are infallible and deserve absolute respect. They value the contributions made by nurses, but see them as working under the direction of the physician. Second- and third-generation family members see less use for *syanas* and trust their health care needs to informed self-care and to scientific medical practitioners. Drugs that must be prescribed by a physician in the U.S. are sold over the counter in India and are used for self-medication. It is important to ask whether such drugs are being or have recently been taken.

e. **With what social (church, community, work, recreation) groups does your family interact, and what is the nature of their social contact and social support?**

Close relations among all Asian Indian American generations are a pivotal part of their culture and religion. First-generation Asian Indian Americans interact primarily with the Asian Indian community. They rarely engage in any strenuous sports or activities. Pt plays in a chamber music group with other family and Asian Indian neighborhood female musicians. The second generation tends to interact with the Asian Indian family plus increasingly more with neighborhood, work, and recreational friends and groups. The third generation typically has close friends in and out of the Asian Indian American communities.

f. **What are the family members' health and social history including health habits, recent major stress events, work patterns, participation in religion, community activities, and recreation patterns?**

As above. Refer to ecogram and family genogram.

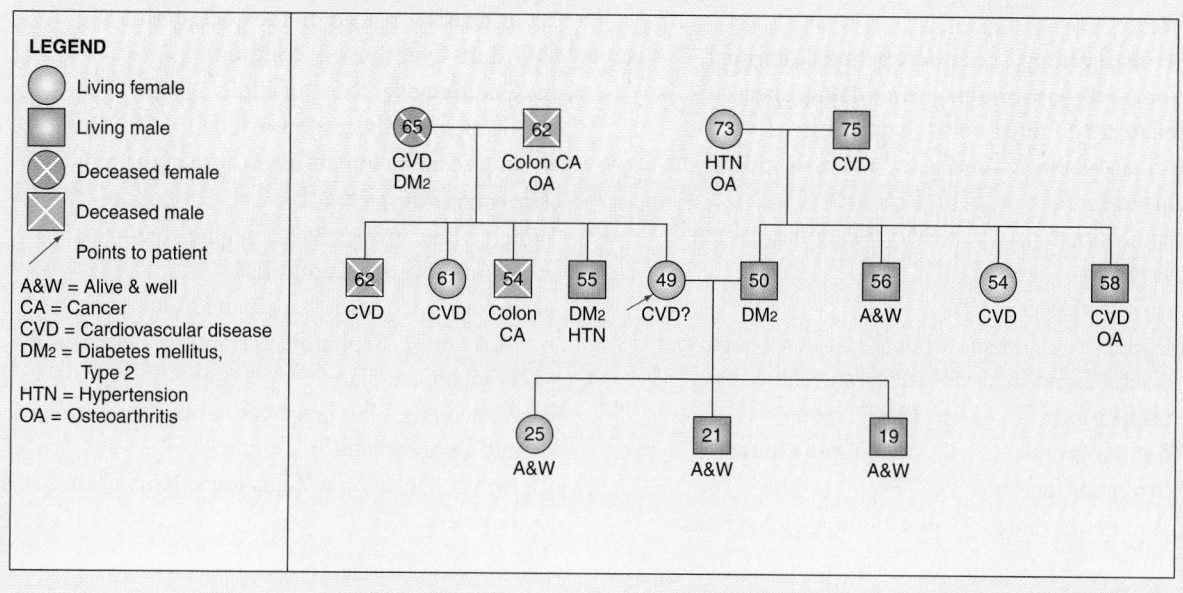

LEGEND

◯ Living female
▢ Living male
⊗ Deceased female
⊠ Deceased male
╱ Points to patient
A&W = Alive & well
CA = Cancer
CVD = Cardiovascular disease
DM2 = Diabetes mellitus, Type 2
HTN = Hypertension
OA = Osteoarthritis

continues

CASE STUDY (Continued)
An Asian Indian American with
Cardiovascular Disease

6. Religious Influences or Special Rituals

Much of the health behaviors among Asian Indians are related to their cultural and Hindu religious beliefs. The Hindu religion is one of the oldest. It consists of disciplined paths of acts and deeds such as self-control, respect for others, *satya* (truthfulness, reality), moral behavior, meditation, yoga, and daily prayer, all of which help Hindus maintain health and spiritual balance. Reincarnation and *karma* (the belief that rebirth is determined by one's moral behavior in previous lives) are central beliefs. The goal is to become more perfect until one achieves *nirvana,* a state of liberation from rebirths and redeaths.

7. Dietary Practices

Mostly vegetables, fruits, grains, yogurt, cheese, and occasional fish or chicken. Breakfast is similar to usual American morning meals. Lunch and dinner are usually Asian Indian dishes. Lunch is usually the largest meal of the day.

REVIEW QUESTIONS

1. The belief that no culture is either inferior or superior to another and that behavior must be assessed from the cultural context in which it occurs is referred to as:
   a. Cultural diversity
   c. Cultural relativism
   b. Ethnocentrism
   d. Multiculturalism
   The correct answer is (c).

2. Cultures have unique value orientations, which provide order and give direction to individuals in which five areas?
   a. Personal, family, social, occupational, spiritual
   b. Good-evil, past-present, being-doing, linear-collateral, domination-subjugation
   c. Human relations, time, place, work, relation to the universe
   d. Time, human nature, activity, relational, people to nature
   The correct answer is (d).

3. People who share a unique national or regional origin and social, cultural, and linguistic heritage are referred to as:
   a. Racial groups
   c. Ethnic groups
   b. Minority groups
   d. Subculture groups
   The correct answer is (c).

4. Mrs. Emma Mason is a 35-year-old Registered Nurse from Maine who attends the Congregational Church, votes Independent, and belongs to a mountain biking club. Health professionals should assess her within the context of the above cultural influences that make up her:
   a. Ethnic identity
   c. Cultural orientation
   b. Value orientation
   d. Multiculturalism
   The correct answer is (d).

5. In collateral families, men are the head of the family, but women play a major role in decision making, and an emphasis is placed on the goals of the:
   a. Adults over those of children
   b. Children over those of adults
   c. Group over those of individuals
   d. Individual members over those of the group
   The correct answer is (c).

6. Which ethnic groups have a higher-than-usual incidence of phenylketonuria?
   a. Poles, Scots, Irish, Danes, and Yemenites
   b. Portuguese, Sephardic, Icelanders, Dutch, and French Canadians
   c. Armenians, Filipinos, Melanesians, East Indians, and Zuni Indians
   d. Amish, Finns, New Zealanders, Norwegians, and Japanese
   The correct answer is (a).

7. Value orientations:
   a. Consist of explanatory ideas and knowledge that members of a given culture have about various aspects of their world
   b. Are culturally learned behaviors associated with a specific culture and include communication patterns, family relations, work patterns, and health practices
   c. Consist of the subjective sense of ethnic definition or social orientation with which an individual self-identifies
   d. Are patterned principles about time, human nature, activity, family relations, and nature, which provide order and give direction to individuals' thoughts and behaviors

   The correct answer is (d).

8. American Indians have an increased incidence of:
   a. Obesity   c. Arthritis
   b. Hemophilia   d. Glaucoma

   The correct answer is (a).

9. Individuals from some cultures believe that certain illnesses are caused by an imbalance or disequilibrium between impersonal factors (hot and cold, *caliente* and *frio, yang* and *yin*). Among the hot (*caliente/yang*) conditions are:
   a. Pneumonia   c. Headache
   b. Cancer   d. Hypertension

   The correct answer is (d).

10. Librada, R.N., is a first-generation Filipino American who travels to the Philippines on a medical mission trip. She is aware that Filipinos have a higher-than-average incidence of which of the following conditions?
    a. Cleft lip and palate and lactase deficiency
    b. Thalassemia and glucose-6-phosphate dehydrogenase deficiency
    c. Tuberculosis and pyruvate kinase deficiency
    d. Hemoglobin E disease and systemic lupus erythematosus

    The correct answer is (b).

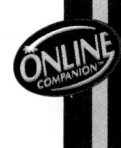

Visit the Estes online companion resource at **www.delmar.cengage.com** for additional content and study aids. Click on Online Companions and then select the Nursing discipline.

REFERENCES

American Nurses Association. (2001). *Code for nurses.* Washington, DC: Author.

Campinha-Bacote, J. (2007). Becoming culturally competent in ethnic psychopharmacology. *Journal of Psychosocial Nursing and Mental Health Services, 45*(6), 27–33.

Coontz, S. (2007). *Modern marriage habits put family structures in catch-up mode.* Retrieved February 10, 2008, from http://www.alternet.org/sex/65402

D'Avanzo, C. E. (2007). *Mosby's pocket guide to cultural health assessment* (4th ed.). St. Louis, MO: Mosby.

De Chesnay, M., & Anderson, B. (2008). *Caring for the vulnerable: Perspectives in nursing theory, practice, and research* (2nd ed.). Sudbury, MA: Jones & Bartlett.

Enas, E. A. (2005). Dyslipidemia among Indo-Asians: Strategies for identification and management. *British Journal of Diabetes and Vascular Disease, 5,* 81–90.

Giger, J. N., & Davidhizar, R. E. (2003). Using role-play to develop cultural competence. *Journal of Nursing Education, 42*(6), 273–276.

Giger, J. N., & Davidhizar, R. E. (2007). *Transcultural nursing: Assessment and intervention* (5th ed.). Philadelphia: Mosby.

Hockenberry, M. J., & Wilson, D. (2006). *Wong's nursing care of infants and children* (8th ed.). Philadelphia: Mosby.

Johnson, K. E., & Rogers, S. (1994). When cultural practices are health risks: The dilemma of female circumcision. *Holistic Nursing Practice, 8*(2), 70–78.

Kemp, C., & Rasbridge, L. A. (Eds.). (2004). *Refugee and immigrant health: A handbook for health professionals.* New York, NY: Cambridge University Press. Retrieved January 16, 2008, from http://www3.baylor.edu/~Charles_Kemp/Indian_health.htm

Kluckhorn, K., & Strodtbeck, F. (1961). *Variations in value orientation.* Evanston, IL: Row, Peterson.

Korbin, J. (1977). Anthropological contributions to the study of child abuse. *Child Abuse and Neglect, 1*(1), 7–24.

Kreps, G. L., & Kunimoto, E. N. (1994). *Effective communication in multicultural health care settings.* Thousand Oaks, CA: Sage.

Leigh, W. A., & Huff, D. (2006). *Women of color health data book: Adolescents to seniors* (3rd ed.). Office of Research on Women's Health, Office of the Director, National Institutes of Health. Retrieved January 8, 2008, from http://orwh.od.nih.gov/pubs/WomenofColor2006.pdf

Leininger, M. M., & McFarland, M. (2002). *Transcultural nursing: Concepts, theory, research, and practice* (3rd ed.). New York: McGraw-Hill Professional.

Markova, T., & Broome, B. (2007). Effective communication and delivery of culturally competent health care. *Urology Nurse, 27*(3): 239–242. Retrieved from http://www3.baylor.edu/~Charles_Kemp/Indian_health.htm

McGoldric, M., Giordano, J., & Garcia-Preto, N. (Eds.). (2005). *Ethnicity and family therapy* (3rd ed.). New York: Guilford Press. Retrieved from http://www3.baylor.edu/~Charles_Kemp/Indian_health.htm

Meleis, A. (2001). Egyptians. In P. Hill, J. G. Lipson, & A. I. Meleis (Eds.), *Caring for women cross-culturally* (pp. 123–141). Philadelphia: F. A. Davis.

Meleis, A., Lipson, J., & Paul, S. (1992). Ethnicity and health among five Middle Eastern immigrant groups. *Nursing Research, 41*(2), 1.

Mohanty, S. A., Woolhandler, S., Himmelstein, D. U., & Bor, D. H. (2005). Diabetes and cardiovascular disease among Asian Indians in the United States. *Journal of General Internal Medicine, 20*(5), 474–478.

Pullen, R. L. (2007). Tips for communicating with a patient from another culture. *Nursing, 37*(10), 48–49.

Purnell, L. D., & Paulanka, B. J. (2008). *Transcultural health care: A culturally competent approach.* Philadelphia: F. A. Davis.

Rundle, A., Carvalho, M., & Robinson, M. R. (2002). *Cultural competence in health care: A practical guide.* San Francisco: Jossey-Bass Publishers.

Simmons, T., & O'Connell, M. (2003). *Married-couple and unmarried-partner households: 2000.* Census 2000 Special Report. Washington, DC: U.S. Department of Commerce, Economics and Statistics Administration, U.S. Census Bureau.

Spector, R. E. (2003). *Cultural diversity in health and illness* (6th ed.). Upper Saddle River, NJ: Prentice Hall Health.

Sprott, J. E. (1993). The black box in family assessment: Cultural diversity. In S. L. Feetham, S. B. Meister, J. M. Bell, & C. L. Gilliss (Eds.), *The nursing of families: Theory, research, education, practice* (pp. 189–199). Norwalk, CT: Sage.

Srivastava, R. (2006). *The healthcare professional's guide to clinical cultural competence.* Baltimore: Mosby.

Swearingen, P. L. (Ed.). (2004). *All-in-one care planning resource: Medical-surgical, pediatric, maternity, and psychiatric nursing care plans.* Philadelphia: Mosby.

U.S. Census Bureau. (2007a). *Minority population tops 100 million.* Retrieved February 2, 2008, from http://www.cencus.gov/Press_Release/www//releases/archives/population/010048.htm

U.S. Census Bureau. (2007b). *Resident population by age and sex: 1980–2006.* Retrieved January 4, 2008, from http://www.census.gov/compendia/statab/tables/08s0007.pdf

Villarruel, A. M., & Konlak-Griffin, D. (2007). Lifestyle behavior interventions with Hispanic children and adults. *Annual Review of Nursing Research, 25,* 51–81.

Wenger, A. F. Z. (1993). Cultural meaning of symptoms. *Holistic Nursing Practice, 7*(2), 22–35.

Wilson, H., & Kneisl, C. (1996). *Psychiatric nursing* (5th ed.). Reading, MA: Addison-Wesley.

World Health Organization. (2000, June). *Female genital mutilation.* Retrieved September 15, 2008, from www.who.int/mediacentre/factsheets/fs241/en/

BIBLIOGRAPHY

Andrews, M. M., & Boyle, J. S. (2007). *Transcultural concepts in nursing care* (5th ed.). Philadelphia: J. B. Lippincott.

Angel, J., & Whitfield, K. E. (2008). *The health of aging Hispanics: The Mexican origin population.* New York: Springer.

Broome, B., & Broome, R. (2007). Native Americans: Traditional healing. *Urology Nurse, 27*(2), 161–163, 173.

Crist, J. D., Woo, S. H., & Choi, M. (2007). A comparison of the use of home care services by Anglo-American and Mexican American elders. *Journal of Transcultural Nursing, 18*(4), 339–348.

Doolen, J., & York, N. L. (2007). Cultural differences with end-of-life care in the critical care units. *Dimensions of Critical Care Nursing, 26*(5), 194–198.

Eggenberger, S. K., Grassley, J., & Restrepo, E. (2006). Culturally competent nursing care: Listening to the voices of Mexican-American women [Online]. *Journal of Issues in Nursing, 19*(11), 7.

Ferdinand, K. C. (2006). Hypertension in minority populations. *Journal of Clinical Hypertension, 8*(5), 365–368.

Fontes, L. A. (2008) *Child abuse and culture: Working with diverse families.* New York: Guilford Press.

Fuligni, A. J., Yip, T., & Tseng, V. (2002). The impact of family obligation on daily activities and psychological well-being of Chinese American adolescents. *Child Development, 73*(1), 302–314.

Geishir-Cantrell, B. (2002). Utilizing traditional storytelling to promote wellness in American Indian communities. *Journal of Transcultural Nursing, 13*(1), 6–11.

Giger, J. N., & Davidhizar, R. E. (2002). Culturally competent care: Emphasis on understanding the people of Afghanistan, Afghanistan Americans, and Islamic culture and religion. *International Nursing Review, 49*(2), 79–86.

Giger, J. N., & Davidhizar, R. E. (2007). Promoting culturally appropriate interventions among vulnerable populations. *Annual Review of Nursing Research, 25,* 293–316.

Goldston, D. B., Molock, S. D., Whitbeck, L. B., Murakami, J. L., & Hall, G. C. (2008). Cultural considerations in adolescent suicide prevention and psychosocial treatment. *American Psychologist, 63*(1), 14–31.

Herek, G. M. (2006). Legal recognition of same-sex relationships in the United States: A social science perspective. *American Psychologist, 61*(6), 607–608.

Hill, P., Lipson, J. G., & Meleis, A. I. (2003). *Caring for women cross-culturally.* Philadelphia: F. A. Davis.

Jaber, L. A., Brown, M. B., Hammad, A., Zhu, Q., & Herman, W. H. (2003). Lack of acculturation is a risk factor for diabetes in Arab immigrants in the U.S. *Diabetes Care, 26*(7), 2010–2014.

Johnson, R. L., Saha, S., Arbelaez, J. J., Beach, M. C., & Cooper, L. A. (2004). Racial and ethnic differences in patient perceptions of bias and cultural competence in health care. *Journal of General Internal Medicine, 19*(2), 101–110.

Jones, E. D., Kennedy-Malone, L., & Wideman, L. (2004). Early detection of type 2 diabetes among older African Americans. *Geriatric Nursing, 25*(1), 24–28.

Katz, R. J. (2004). Addressing the health care needs of American Indians and Alaska Natives. *American Journal of Public Health, 94*(1), 13–14.

Lee, E. E., & Farran, C. J. (2004). Depression among Korean, Korean American, and Caucasian American family caregivers. *Journal of Transcultural Nursing, 15*(1), 18–25.

Leininger, M. M., & McFarland, M. R. (Eds.). (2005). *Culture care diversity & universality: A worldwide nursing theory* (2nd ed.). Sudbury, MA: Jones & Bartlett.

Lipson, J. G., & Dibble, S. L. (Eds.). (2005). *Culture and clinical care.* San Francisco: USCF Nursing Press.

Lovering, S. (2006). Cultural attitudes and beliefs about pain. *Journal of Transcultural Nursing, 17*(4), 389–395.

Luna, E. (2003). Las que curan at the heart of Hispanic culture. *Journal of Holistic Nursing, 21*(4), 326–342.

Meezan, W., & Rauch, J. (2005). Gay marriage, same-sex parenting, and America's children. *Marriage and Child Wellbeing, 15*(2), 97–115.

Munoz, C., & Luckmann, J. (2005). *Transcultural communication in nursing* (2nd ed.). Clifton Park, NY: Thomson Delmar Learning.

Orians, C. E., Erb, J., Kenyou, K. L., Lantz, P. M., Liebow, E. B., Joe, J. R., et al. (2004). Public education strategies for delivering breast and cervical cancer screening in American Indian and Alaska Native populations. *Journal of Public Health Management Practice, 10*(1), 46–53.

Payne, S., Chapman, A., Holloway, M., Seymour, J. D., & Chau, R. (2005). Chinese community views: Promoting cultural competence in palliative care. *Journal of Palliative Care, 21*(2), 111–116.

Rehm, R. S. (2003). Cultural intersections in the care of Mexican American children with chronic conditions. *Pediatric Nursing, 29*(6), 434–439.

Smith, D. M., & Gates, G. J. (2001). *Gay and lesbian families in the United States: Same-sex unmarried partner households.* Washington, DC: Human Rights Campaign.

Tasker, F. (2005). Lesbian mothers, gay fathers, and their children: A review. *Journal of Developmental Behavior in Pediatrics, 26*(3), 224–240.

Vaughn, A. A., & Roesch, S. C. (2003). Psychological and physical health correlates of coping in minority adolescents. *Journal of Health Psychology, 8*(6), 671–683.

Whittemore, R. (2007). Culturally competent interventions for Hispanic adults with type 2 diabetes: A systematic review. *Journal of Transcultural Nursing, 18*(2), 157–166.

Yu, S. M., Huang, Z. J., & Singh, G. K. (2004). Health status and health services utilization among US Chinese, Asian Indian, Filipino, and other Asian/Pacific Islander children. *Pediatrics, 113*(1, Pt. 1), 101–107.

WEB SITES

Culture Grams:
    http://www.culturegrams.com

EthnoMed:
    http://www.ethnomed.org

Gay, Lesbian, Bisexual, and Transgender Health Access Project:
    http://www.glbthealth.org

National Coalition for LGBT Health:
    http://www.lgbthealth.net

Transcultural Nursing Society:
    http://www.tcns.org

United States Census Bureau:
    http://www.census.gov

U.S. Department of State:
    http://travel.state.gov

World Health Organization:
    http://www.who.int

CHAPTER 6

Spiritual Assessment

COMPETENCIES

1. Describe how different spiritual beliefs might influence the patient's view of health, growth and development, illness, and death.

2. Conduct a spiritual assessment on a patient.

3. Identify signs and symptoms that indicate the patient is experiencing spiritual distress.

4. Formulate nursing interventions that promote the patient's spiritual well-being.

5. Identify your personal spiritual beliefs and how they affect your nursing care.

Religion in America

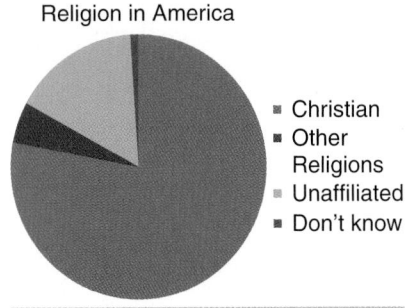

- Christian
- Other Religions
- Unaffiliated
- Don't know

FIGURE 6-1 **Most Americans identify themselves as Christians, but a large percentage are unaffiliated. The unaffiliated category includes secular unaffiliated, religious unaffiliated, atheists, and agnostics. The percentages have been rounded to the nearest whole number.** *Pew Forum, 2008. From: http://religions.pewforum.org/ reports. Retrieved July 21, 2008.*

A patient's spiritual and religious beliefs will influence whether or not he or she will take medication, agree to surgery, follow a special diet, or execute an advanced directive. Those spiritual and religious beliefs may even affect a patient's outcomes and recovery from a major adverse event. Spiritual and religious beliefs may have as weighty an effect on health as does smoking. Studies have shown that religious practices can increase longevity by up to 7 years (14 in African American women), whereas smoking can decrease longevity by up to 7 years (Koenig, 2007b). Just as it would be irresponsible patient care to treat a patient without knowing whether he or she is a smoker, it would be irresponsible patient care to treat a patient without knowing whether he or she has spiritual or religious beliefs.

Most Americans belong to an organized religion. Seventy-eight percent of Americans identify themselves as Christians. Jews, Muslims, Buddhists, New Age, or Hindus; and Native Americans make up an additional 5% of Americans who identify themselves as belonging to a particular religion. A large percentage of Americans identify themselves as "unaffiliated" with any religion. This broad category includes both religious persons who do not identify with a particular religion as well as atheists and agnostics (Pew Forum on Religion and Public Life, 2008). See Figure 6-1.

As an indicator of spirituality, a recent survey showed that most Americans identify religion as being "very important" or "fairly important" to their everyday lives (Newport, 2006). See Figure 6-2. Interestingly, the importance of religion decreased with education level.

When faced with an acute or chronic illness, the dying process, or a major life event, it is clear that many people turn to religious and spiritual practices as powerful coping mechanisms (Chu, 2004; Hampton & Weinart, 2006; Kelly, 2004). In a study of individuals with chronic illnesses, Haynes and Watt wrote:

> The participants were very consistent in relating that family and God were the most important parts of their lives in dealing with a chronic illness. God was considered the constant and unchanging support and source of strength. The support of family and friends was the other key component of helping them get through each day and also served as the focal point in their lives (2008, p. 46).

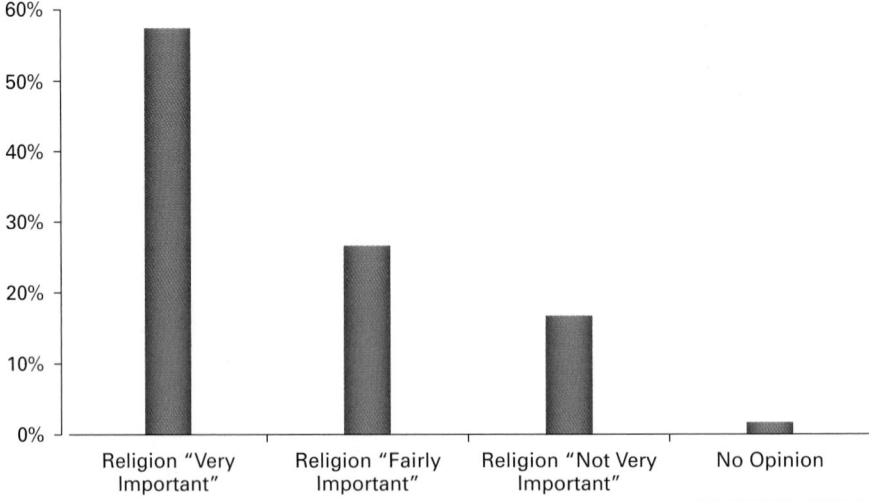

FIGURE 6-2 **An indicator of spirituality is *how important* the religion is to the believer. In this case, most considered their religion important.** *Newport, F. (2006). "Religion most important to Blacks, women and older Americans. Self-reported importance of religion decreases with education." Retrieved July 21, 2008, from http://www.gallup.com/poll/25585/religion-most-important-blacks-women-older-Americans.aspx?version=print.*

For some, spirituality was equivalent to (Hughes et al., 2004) or more important than family support (Astrow & Sulmasy, 2004; Hamilton et al., 2007).

Spiritual beliefs affect decisions about medical care (Astrow & Sulmasy, 2004; Balboni et al., 2007). Religiousness in one study was associated with wanting "all measures" to extend life (Balboni et al., 2007).

Spiritual and religious beliefs are furthermore positively associated with healthy behaviors (Haynes & Watt, 2008), good attitudes (Koenig, George, & Titus, 2004), less pain (Harrison et al., 2005), less depression (Koenig, 2007c), better quality of life (Leak, Hu, & King, 2008), less smoking (Roff et al., 2005), quicker remission after illness (Koenig, 2007c), and reduced morbidity and mortality (Helm et al., 2000; Ostbye et al., 2006). One study reports:

> In a study of 3,851 older adults, *private religious activities (meditation, prayer, or bible study) were a significant predictor of survival among subjects. ... Little or no private religious activity predicted a nearly 50% increase in mortality,* after controlling for demographics, health status, depression, stressful life events, social support and health behaviors (Helm et al., 2000, emphasis added).

One researcher disputes the methodology of most of these studies on religion and health, and denies that religion and spirituality are anything more than helpful coping mechanisms (Sloan, 2000, 2006; Sloan, Bagiella, & Powell, 1999).

Further, not all research shows the benefits of religious and spiritual beliefs. Some studies show no effect on health care outcomes or are ambiguous (Baetz et al., 2004; Koenig, 2004). One study showed a decrease in religiousness as illness became severe (Chen & Koenig, 2006).

In addition, not all spiritual and religious beliefs are helpful influences in health care. Such beliefs can be harmful to the patient and/or family. Spiritual and religious beliefs can lead a patient to make choices against medical advice. Members of Jehovah's Witnesses, for example, refuse even life-saving blood transfusions due to their strict and unique interpretations of the Bible. The Church of Christ, Scientist (Christian Scientists) emphasizes the importance of prayer instead of medical interventions. Devout Christian Scientists may forgo vaccinations, antibiotics, and other life-saving medications. One study identified 172 children who died between 1975 and 1995 due to the religious beliefs of their own parents, beliefs that caused the parents to withhold medical care (Asser & Swan, 1998). In some cases, the parents of these children were prosecuted and served jail time (Margolick, 1990). Dr. Koenig observed that 83% of these cases came from five religious groups, mostly breakaway, dissident Christian, or New Age sects led by a charismatic leader, although the count also includes 28 Christian Science children who died during that period (Koenig, 2007a). The health care team needs to tread carefully in such cases and search for the right balance between respect for the freedom of religious practice and the obligation to treat a patient and protect juveniles who have not reached the age of consent.

Religious and spiritual beliefs can cause conflict in the health care setting when the patient holds different or even conflicting beliefs from those of his or her family. A recent study shows that 24–48% of Americans have changed their religious affiliation during their adult lives (NPR, 2008). Especially in these cases, nurses ought to know what the patient's religious and spiritual beliefs are so that an intelligent understanding of the patient's perspective is attained.

Ignorance of a patient's spiritual and religious beliefs and practices will hamper complete, holistic nursing care of the patient. A complete patient assessment must include a spiritual assessment, which can be done easily and quickly, and yet provides much information crucial to patient care.

Knowing your own spirituality will help you identify and understand your own biases and point of view, which will help you to empathize with patients who make health care decisions based on their spiritual beliefs. Are your own spiritual beliefs more or less important than maintaining your health? If a medical decision forced you to choose between your health and your spiritual or religious beliefs, which would you choose? For instance, imagine that your child is bleeding profusely following an accident and requires a blood transfusion. The transfusion is against your religion. How would you decide what to do?

SPIRITUALITY AND RELIGION

Spirituality is the concern for the meaning and purpose of life. Spirituality integrates values and ultimate concern with oneself, one's relationship with a higher power, and the surrounding environment. Spiritual beliefs help the individual define the self and the self's ultimate purpose in life. For many, health is a concern, but it may not be the primary concern. Factors such as leaving behind a good reputation, passing on morals to the next generation, being in a good relationship with a higher power, and being in harmony with the forces in the universe may be of ultimate concern for the patient and could therefore drive the patient's health care choices.

An example of spirituality is the belief that both animals and human beings can feel pain and joy, and therefore animals must be treated with the same respect shown to humans. A person who has this belief would probably believe the self to be important but only as important as all other beings on the earth. The implication for health care is that this person would likely be a vegetarian and may refuse any treatment (such as a porcine cardiac valve) that resulted from the sacrifice or suffering of an animal.

By contrast, **religion** is an organized system of beliefs usually centered around the worship of a supernatural force or being, which in turn defines the self and the self's purpose in life. Religion exists in group form over time, and is a tradition of shared beliefs. Although many variances may exist among believers within any given religion, there will be common threads uniting the followers. A religious system of beliefs can be highly organized and include **rituals**, which often are solemn, and ceremonial acts that reinforce faith. **Faith** is the assent to the truth of the beliefs and may also refer to the total orientation of the self's entire life to the belief structure. **Dogma** refers to the beliefs of a religion that are so essential to the identity of that religion that to deny them is to deny the religion itself. Religions also include **codes of ethics**, which are codified beliefs and lists of mandatory or prohibited acts that help define the self's relation to the object of worship.

An example of a religion is Judaism. Followers of the Jewish faith worship Yahweh (God) and define humans as the special creations of God who must in turn worship God. Judaism is highly organized. Who God is, why He should be worshipped, and how humans ought to act by virtue of being created by Him are delineated in a system of biblical commentary and teachings by the leaders of the religion. Judaism has different kinds of religious leaders (rabbis, cantors, mohels), codes of ethics (the biblical Ten Commandments is the most well-known example), and rituals (circumcision, bat mitzvah). There are many forms of Judaism, but broadly speaking, implications for health care for a religious Jew could include a special diet (pork-free or kosher) and consultation with a rabbi before any complex bioethical decisions are made.

The relationship between spirituality and religion is illustrated in Figure 6-3. One can be spiritual without being religious. In the example of spirituality given previously, the patient espouses a spiritual belief about the interconnectedness of humans and animals that includes the patient in a harmonious belief system with all living beings on the planet. However, there are not necessarily rituals, involvement of a supernatural force that is being worshipped, or an organized system of beliefs that make this spirituality a religion. Nevertheless, this spirituality can have a profound impact on the person's outlook on life and sense of spiritual well-being.

Likewise, one can be religious without being spiritual. For example, a particular Jew may fulfill religious obligations to attend temple and participate in required rituals without believing in or worshipping Yahweh, which is the central tenet of the religion. The religion may have no impact on the Jew's behavior or outlook on life and may not help define what is important to that person.

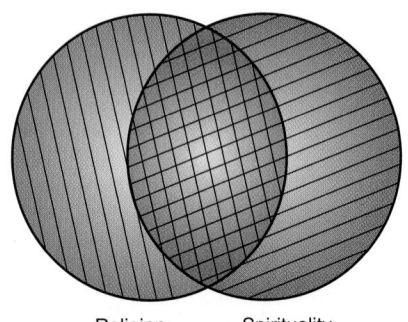

Religion   Spirituality

FIGURE 6-3 **The Relationship between Religion and Spirituality**

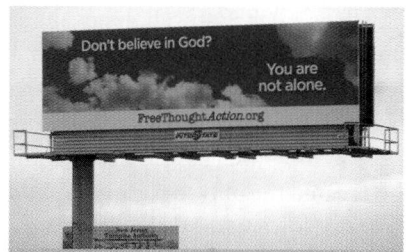

FIGURE 6-4 This billboard reflects the growing prevalence of atheistic views.

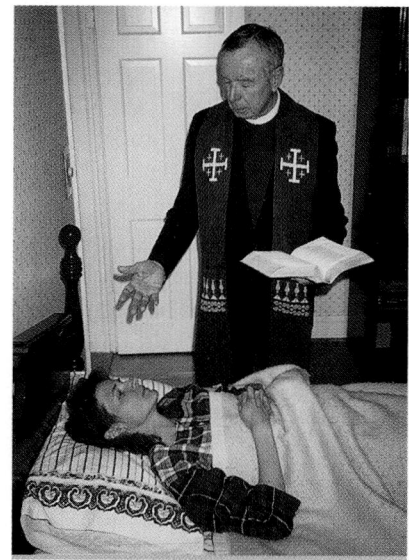

FIGURE 6-5 Rituals such as the sacrament of the Anointing of the Sick are important expressions of religious belief.

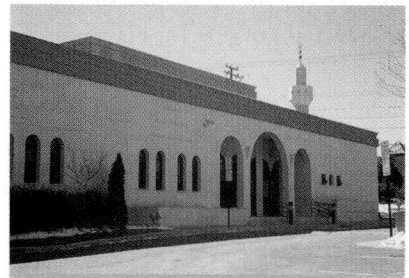

FIGURE 6-6 All Muslims must face Mecca, Saudi Arabia, to pray. Here, the minaret of a mosque is aligned with Mecca.

Finally, one can be both spiritual and religious by participating in a religion and by holding its spiritual core at the center of one's being, actions, and beliefs. For example, a Jew who believes in God and worships God in the manner specified by Judaism, and whose belief in God is manifested in thought, actions, purpose, and identity, exhibits the properties of both religion and spirituality.

Spirituality in health care is not without controversy. At least one researcher, Sloan, has argued that religion is harmful to patient care, raising as it does issues of sin and guilt (Sloan, Bagiella, & Powell, 1999). Introducing spirituality into health care, argues the same researcher, puts health care practitioners in the position of being judges of what are "good" and "bad" religious practices, a judgment that is out of their field of expertise (Sloan, 2006).

Furthermore, a small but growing percentage of Americans identify themselves as being atheists (1.6%) or agnostics (2.4%) (Pew Forum, 2008). See Figure 6-4. Prominent atheists have written best-selling books that are harshly critical, even mocking, of religion (Dawkins, 2006; Hitchens, 2007). The Freedom from Religion Foundation, an atheist advocacy group, sued the Veterans Health Administration (VA) in 2006 because of the VA's integration of spiritual assessment and support into its health care program. The lawsuit alleges that the VA program "unconstitutionally promotes, advances and endorses religion" (Freedom from Religion Foundation, 2008). Such patients may be resentful at being asked about their religious beliefs, may recoil at being prayed over by a nurse or doctor, and may be overtly hostile to any suggestion of seeing a hospital chaplain. Or they may not. Such patients may be very spiritual, and may need nursing assistance or support in a time of illness or major life event to tap into their spiritual support system. "Spirituality" is thus a vague term that has the advantage of being inclusive of most persons with spiritual or religious beliefs. Performing a spiritual assessment will outline the beliefs—spiritual or religious or both—of your patient without offending those who are either very religious or very spiritual. Spirituality is the concern for the meaning and purpose of life. For those patients who are spiritual but not religious, reading a book of poetry or watching a sunset may provide the spiritual support mechanism that will help the patient cope with a difficult treatment. The nurse will know about these important beliefs only by taking a spiritual assessment.

SPIRITUAL THEORY

Almost all religions attempt to explain why human beings suffer from illness and death and how higher powers can affect healing. It is important to realize that religion rarely, if ever, describes disease as resulting from a strictly biological cause that has a scientific solution. Instead, some religious explanations of disease indicate that it was sent directly by the creator or a lesser god, caused by sin or by the poor performance of a ritual act, or resulted from the malevolence of relatives, neighbors, or ancestors. Based on these explanations, the cure for disease is to be found in confessing sin, purification rites, exorcism, or the transmission of power to the patient such as by the sacrament of the Anointing of the Sick (Figure 6-5), plastering, or other rituals. These acts of healing are not performed by physicians and nurses, but by priests, elders, mediums, and other specialists who have access to the higher powers that control disease. It may be more important to the patient to see a neighbor who has had experience with a disease and was successfully able to repel it with certain prayers, for example, than to take a prescribed medication.

Being familiar with various religious and spiritual terms may help you to communicate more effectively with your patients (Figure 6-6). The concept of a **god** may vary from a dispassionate, distant deity to a dynamic, personal, present being. "God" may be called by many names, such as Allah, Yahweh, Jehovah, or Shiva, and one religion, Judaism, considers the name of God to be so sacred that believers are not supposed to pronounce the name at all. **Prayer** is the means by which one communicates with the higher power(s). **Monotheistic religions** such as Judaism, Christianity, and Islam believe in only one all-powerful, omni-present, and omnipotent God (capital **G**), who created the universe. **Polytheistic religions** such as Hinduism recognize many gods (lowercase **g**) that may have different levels of power and status. These gods may even compete with each other, but are all ultimately manifestations of the one true higher power behind existence.

A **sin** exists when someone has gone against the teachings of the belief system. A **heretic** is someone who rejects the official teachings or dogma of a religion or belief system. A **schismatic** is a person who shares the essential beliefs or dogma of a religion but who is separated by political or other disagreements from the group of believers.

A patient may claim to be an **atheist** (a-theist, that is, without God), or one who does not believe in God. An **agnostic** (a-gnosis, that is, without knowledge) is one who is unsure whether God exists. Atheists or agnostics may be very spiritual if they hold certain beliefs to be of utmost importance to their lives, such as attaining great knowledge, living in harmony with humanity, or showing kindnesses to others. **Pagan** is a term with multiple meanings. To members of the three major monotheistic religions (Judaism, Christianity, and Islam), a pagan is someone who is not monotheistic. Another definition of a pagan is someone who believes in an animistic, and usually polytheistic, spirit-filled belief system. Various forms of paganism, as practiced in the Wiccan or Druid faiths, are found throughout the United States. **Animism** is a belief that all components of the universe, including humans, have some form of life force. Many Native American religions contain this concept. **New Age** religion is a popular, heterogeneous, free-flowing spiritual movement that has no holy book, organization, membership, clergy, geographic center, dogma, or creed, but includes a cluster of common beliefs that may be grafted onto an existing religion. Those beliefs include **pantheism**, in which God is believed to be in everything that exists; reincarnation; auras; energy fields; ecology; personal transformation; and evolution toward a new age in which wars and discrimination will not exist, and all will be peace and harmony (Figure 6-7).

A person may belong to a **cult**, which is the religious devotion to a set of beliefs or to a person. Cults are thought to be fanatical and are societally disapproved, but the difference between a religion and a cult may be in the eyes of the person who makes the definition. A patient may be insulted if his or her religion is referred to as a cult, so you must show sensitivity to all expressions of spirituality.

The concept of the **soul** varies from the essential, spiritual part of a person to the part of the person that continues to exist after physical death. This is a concept central to many religions. **Spirit** can encompass the same concept as soul, or may refer to a disembodied being or supernatural force, or may indicate the Christian trinitarian concept of God, as in the Holy Spirit. Many religions and spiritual belief systems contain the belief in life after death, wherein the soul or body of a person continues to live on in some form after physical death. This idea is central to Christianity. **Reincarnation** is the belief that a person is reborn into another life after death. In Hinduism, one seeks, through good deeds, to obtain release from endless reincarnations. Many religions describe a peaceful or joyful place or state one goes to or becomes if the ethics of the religion are followed. Christians, for example, believe in **heaven**, whereas Buddhists believe in **nirvana**, which is the state of perfect blessedness and peace of the soul (Figure 6-8).

FIGURE 6-7 These bumper stickers show an allegiance to New Age religions. The "And We Still Chant" sticker refers to Wiccan and worship.

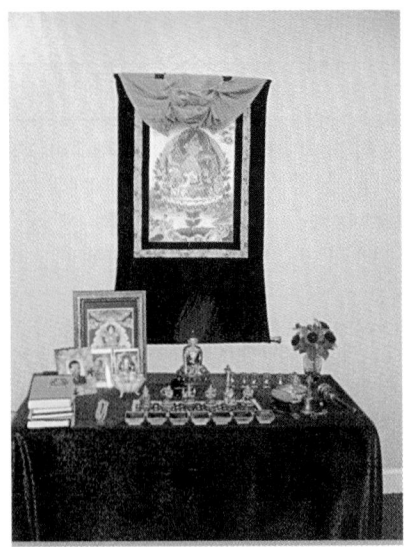

FIGURE 6-8 Some of the fastest growing religions in America are non-Judeo-Christian religions. This photograph shows a Buddhist shrine in a private home. A great deal of attention is paid to the placement of the objects on the shrine.

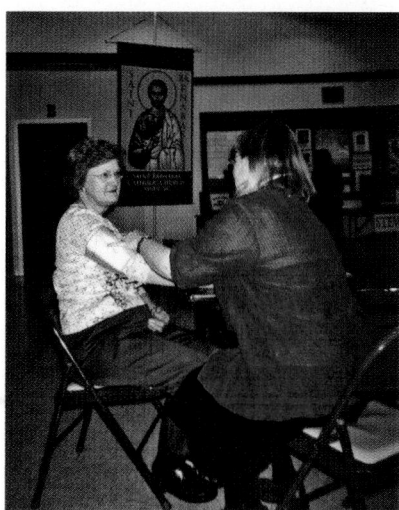

FIGURE 6-9 A parish nurse checks the blood pressure of a church member. Parish nurses perform a variety of functions to promote health care and spiritual well-being.

PARISH NURSING

Parish nursing, also called faith community nursing or congregational nursing, is a relatively new subspecialty in which registered nurses provide and facilitate health care for a religious or spiritual community. Founded by Lutheran minister Reverend Granger Westburg in 1984, parish nursing has grown to about 10,000 nurses in the United States, Canada, Australia, New Zealand, and parts of Africa (VanDover & Pfeiffer, 2007). The Scope and Standards of Practice for Faith Community Nursing were approved by the American Nurses Association in 2005 (ANA, 2005). Parish nursing is defined as "the specialized practice of professional nursing that focuses on the intentional care of the spirit as part of the process of promoting holistic health and preventing or minimizing illness in a faith community" (ANA, 2005, p. 1).

Parish nurses provide health care for individuals already united by their religious and spiritual beliefs, in a setting (the church, or other communal place) to which the individuals are already committed to visit. The parish nurse has many functions, among them, integrator of faith and health, health educator, personal health counselor, referral agent, trainer of volunteers, developer of support groups, and health advocate (Solari-Twadell & McDermott, 2006). The literature provides many examples of the forms parish nursing may take: blood pressure and cholesterol screenings, home visits for shut-ins, CPR classes, lunches for the elderly, walking programs, visits to a hospital or nursing home to support parishioners and their families, arranging for transport, arranging for a priest or minister visit, and the prevention and management of addiction problems (Bard, 2006; Redmond, 2006; VanDover & Pfeiffer, 2007). See Figure 6-9. Congregations with parish nurses provide significant health promotion, disease prevention, and support services for a very low cost or for free (Catanzaro et al., 2007).

In addition to providing health care, parish nurses also provide spiritual care to the patient by means of the health care visit (Shelly, 2002). This aspect of parish nursing is overtly spiritual, and can overlap and support the ministerial project of the church and the role of the minister or priest (Caiger, 2006; Carson & Koenig, 2002; O'Brien, 2003).

REFLECTIVE THINKING

Meeting Patients' Spiritual Needs

What would you do if a patient requested that you participate in a religious practice that conflicted with your own spiritual, religious, or institutional practices? For example, suppose a Hindu family asked a non-Hindu nurse to help move a dying Hindu patient out of his hospital bed and onto the floor, in accordance with their religious beliefs. Or suppose a Muslim family asked a non-Muslim nurse to whisper, "There is no God but Allah, and Mohammed is His Prophet" into the ear of a dying Muslim patient, in accordance with their religious beliefs. What would you do? What would you say? How would you reconcile the institution's policies with the patient's spiritual requests? How would you handle these situations?

REFLECTIVE THINKING

Religious Practices Influencing Care Provided to a Young Child

A 3-year-old child arrives at the emergency department by ambulance after being involved in a head-on collision. All family members with the exception of the father and the patient are dead on arrival. The young child has sustained extensive trauma to the face as a result of being partially thrown through the front windshield. The father accompanied the child in the ambulance and made it known to the paramedics that the family members are Jehovah's Witnesses and, thus, do not permit blood transfusions. This information was relayed to you on the patient's arrival. The child's blood pressure drops from 80/40 to 50/20, and a hematocrit value of 23% comes back from the laboratory. You are asked to call the blood bank for two units of blood.

1. How would you respond to this request?
2. Do your religious beliefs conflict with this family's beliefs?
3. If you feel you cannot assist with the blood resuscitation against the wishes of the father, would you feel comfortable asking a fellow coworker to step in for you?
4. What is your institution's policy?

NURSINGTIP

Gaining Patient Trust

Many people believe that spiritual issues are very private. Patients may fear that they will be ridiculed for their beliefs. It is important, therefore, to build an atmosphere of trust with the patient before you delve into questions about the patient's spiritual beliefs. Begin the health history interview with the expected questions concerning the physical history of the patient. As the patient reveals personal or intimate details about his or her physical being, you will build trust with the patient by remaining nonjudgmental and maintaining an attitude of respect, empathy, and understanding. The trusting patient should gradually feel more comfortable discussing potentially personal issues in the psychological and spiritual portions of the interview.

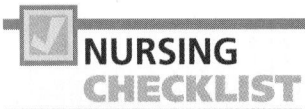

NURSING CHECKLIST

General Approach to Spiritual Assessment

1. If possible, choose a quiet, private room that will be free from interruptions.
2. Ensure that the room's light is sufficiently bright to observe the patient's verbal and nonverbal reactions.
3. Greet the patient, introduce yourself, and explain that you will be taking a health history.
4. Position yourself at eye level with the patient.
5. Portray an interested, non-judgmental manner throughout the interview. Respect silence and diversity.

ROLE OF THE NURSE IN SPIRITUAL CARE

Nurses have a vital role to play in the spiritual care of patients by:

1. Performing a spiritual assessment. (It is impossible to know whether a patient is in a state of spiritual distress or spiritual well-being unless an assessment is done.)
2. Making a nursing diagnosis based on the assessment.
3. Planning, implementing, and evaluating appropriate strategies for spiritual care.

SPIRITUAL ASSESSMENT

The purpose of a spiritual assessment is to collect information in order to understand the patient's religious or spiritual beliefs and practices.

The spiritual assessment is best done as part of the history taking, but can also be performed conversationally during the patient's physical examination or during patient care. It is performed in a supportive and nonjudgmental manner.

Patient History as a Source of Information about Religious and Spiritual Beliefs

Keep in mind that the patient's history may itself raise spiritual and religious issues. For example, the patient may reveal a requirement for a vegetarian diet (Hindu, New Age), or a history of circumcision (Jews), or the fact that his or her hair has never been cut (women: Orthodox Jews; men: Sikhs). Or a patient may reveal that he or she is estranged from family. This may be due to a conversion to a different, even conflicting, religious or spiritual belief, or a rejection of the religious or spiritual belief of the family of origin. The revelation of such facts serves as an invitation to perform the spiritual assessment.

Observe the Patient Closely

Just as you observe the patient for evidence of health and disease, observe the patient for clues to his or her religious and spiritual beliefs. Beyond the obvious Bibles and religious jewelry, look for special clothing (Mormons, Jews, Sikhs), religious objects draped or tied around the body (Catholics, Jews), uncut hair (Orthodox Jews, Sikhs), prayer beads (Buddhists, Catholics), and even knives (Sikhs). Ask about any object with which you are unfamiliar. It may be fashion or it may be sacred. In any case, your observations and questions will open the door to the spiritual assessment.

Non-Christian religions are growing, and it is now common to meet adherents of a much wider variety of religions and spiritualities than even 10 years ago. If the nurse is expecting a patient to pray by folding hands and softly repeating a

REFLECTIVE THINKING

Refusal of Heart Transplant

Your patient has end-stage heart disease and will die unless she receives a heart transplant; however, your patient's religious beliefs forbid her from giving up her own heart. She tells you that she has decided not to pursue a heart transplant and wants to go home once she is medically able to do so. What are your thoughts, knowing that your patient is facing imminent death despite having a surgical therapy available to her that would most likely allow her to live much longer?

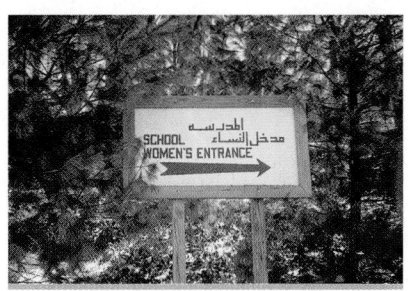

FIGURE 6-10 Awareness of cultural and religious norms and customs will help you deliver appropriate nursing care. Islam separates the sexes in many aspects of public life, as illustrated here.

REFLECTIVE THINKING

Self-Evaluation of Spirituality

Are you spiritual? Are you religious? Are you both? Are you neither? What is most important in your life? What are your beliefs? Have your beliefs changed from when you were younger? How do you feel about people whose beliefs differ markedly from yours?

prayer in the Christian manner, for example, that nurse might overlook expressions of prayer in other traditions. People at prayer may be sitting (Protestant), kneeling (Islam, Catholic), standing (Protestant), rocking (some Jewish), or walking (Buddhist); silent (various religions) or chanting (Muslim, Jewish); with hands folded (Catholic) or arms raised (Protestant); facing a religious object (Orthodox, Catholic, Buddhist) or facing a specific direction (Muslim). An awareness of cultural and religious norms will help you deliver appropriate nursing care (Figure 6-10). It is important to know how different belief systems define acceptable behavior through the life cycle. Table 6-1 illustrates how certain religions view sentinel events, from birth to death.

Beware of stereotyping a patient or jumping to conclusions. Don't assume that a holy book on the table means that the patient is a devout believer. The book may have been left there by a family member or friend, distributed by a missionary group, or donated by a well-meaning volunteer. Additionally, the absence of a holy book does not mean the patient is not spiritual or religious, as some religions (Native American, Unitarian, New Age) do not have holy books. Furthermore, many self-identified members of religious faiths do not follow the teachings of their own religions. A Jew may eat pork, for example, a Jehovah's Witness may accept a blood transfusion, and a Catholic may request birth control. Some atheist patients may want to return to the religion of their youth in a time of crisis. Many patients may blend elements of one religion with those of another religion or spiritual belief. A good understanding of religious and spiritual practices is important, and an understanding of your patient's specific beliefs is crucial.

The Spiritual Assessment Tool

A simple yet complete spiritual assessment tool is one developed by Dr. Christina Puchalski (Pulchalski & Romer, 2000). Its "FICA" formula is short, memorable, and complete. This assessment tool is nonthreatening to everyone from the devout to the atheist, and will glean useful information that will assist in patient care.

F: FAITH AND BELIEF. Ask: "Do you consider yourself spiritual or religious?" "Do you practice a specific Faith?" "Do you have spiritual/religious beliefs that help you cope with stress?" "What gives your life meaning?"

I: IMPORTANCE. Ask: "What Importance does your faith or belief have in your life? Have your beliefs influenced how you take care of yourself?" "What role do your beliefs have in regaining (or maintaining) your health?"

C: COMMUNITY. Ask: "Are you part of a spiritual or religious Community? Does this group support you? How? Is there a group of people you really love or who are important to you?"

Communities such as churches, temples, and mosques, or a group of like-minded friends, can serve as strong support systems for some patients.

A: ADDRESS. Ask: "How would you like the health care team to Address these issues in your health care?"

Record your assessment findings. Communicate them to the health care team as appropriate.

FICA tool used with permission of Christina M. Puchalski, MD, The George Washington Institute for Spirituality and Health (GWish), The George Washington University.

Resistance to the Spiritual Assessment

If your patient is resistant to the spiritual assessment, don't force the conversation. This may be an area more private than the patient's own bowel or sexual habits.

TABLE 6-1 Religions and Health Care

RELIGION	JUDAISM	ISLAM	ROMAN CATHOLIC/ORTHODOX	PROTESTANT
Description	Judaism is an ancient religion dating to about 2000 BCE. It is a monotheistic religion that believes that God (Yahweh) has chosen the Jewish people and made a covenant with them. The covenant is that the Jews will worship God and follow His laws, and in return God will protect and preserve them. Over its long history, Judaism has developed several traditions, among them Orthodox, which believes in a strict interpretation of the Scriptures; Conservative, which allows for some modern interpretation of the Scriptures; and Reform, which is a blending of tradition with modern-day moral demands. Jews are largely concentrated in the Middle East, Europe, and the United States, but can be found worldwide, including Asia, Africa, and South America.	Islam is a monotheistic religion sharing early Judeo-Christian religious roots. It was established when the Prophet Mohammed (d. 632 CE) preached the word of God as revealed to him by an angel. The essence of Mohammed's prophecies is that God (Allah) is the one, true God and is absolutely sovereign. The central tenet of the faith is "There is no God but Allah, and Mohammed is His Prophet." Several versions of Islam have developed, among them Sunni, Sufi, and Shiite. Islam has spread beyond its origins in the Middle East to Europe, Asia, Africa, and the Americas. The five pillars of Islam are regular prayer five times a day facing Mecca, fasting during Ramadan, giving alms to charity, pilgrimage to Mecca if possible, and reciting, at least once in the lifetime, the *shahadaz* (creed): "There is no God but Allah, and Mohammed is His Prophet."	A monotheistic religion and an offshoot of Judaism, Christianity dates from the death and resurrection of Jesus, about 30 AD. Christians believe that Jesus is the son of God, that Jesus died on the cross to serve as a sacrifice for the sins of humanity, that Jesus was resurrected from the dead, and that God exists in three forms: God (Father), Jesus (Son), and the Holy Spirit. Roman Catholicism is the oldest and largest of the Christian denominations, with about 1 billion members worldwide. Rejecting the authority of the Pope (and other political and theological issues), the Eastern Orthodox churches separated from the Roman Catholic Church in 1054 AD and developed into a group of independent churches with separate hierarchies along nationalistic lines (e.g., the Greek Orthodox Church, the Russian Orthodox Church). Roman Catholicism and Orthodoxy are sacramental religions in which sacraments, rituals that impart grace and help from God to the believer, are provided to the believer by bishops, priests, and deacons. There are seven sacraments: Baptism, Holy Eucharist, Confirmation, Holy Matrimony, Confession of Sins, Anointing of the Sick, and Holy Orders. The most important is the Holy Eucharist in which bread and wine are transformed into the true body and blood of Jesus Christ through a miracle of God acting through the priest. These are the distinguishing beliefs of Roman Catholics and Orthodox believers.	The Protestant churches began in the 16th century Reformation, a political and theological break with the Roman Catholic Church. Protestant beliefs are distinguished from Catholic and Orthodox beliefs by: • Rejecting the authority of the Pope and the teaching authority of the Roman Catholic Church. • De-emphasizing the Eucharist and the central role of the priest. • Rejecting the sacramentalism of the Catholic Church. Protestant churches retain two sacraments only: baptism and the Holy Communion, or the Last Supper (in which the bread and wine function as symbols of Jesus only, and not actually as his body and blood). (Lutheran and Episcopal churches retain some sacramentalism and do believe that the bread and wine are more than symbolic of Jesus.) • Emphasizing more the Bible and the individual's interpretation of it. Protestant churches have developed widely along diverse lines, and so vary widely in their theological views.

continues

TABLE 6-1 (Continued)

RELIGION	JUDAISM	ISLAM	ROMAN CATHOLIC/ORTHODOX	PROTESTANT
Religious Leaders	Rabbi: A religious authority of the faith. A rabbi renders decisions interpreting the laws that Jews are required to abide by to preserve their covenant with God. Cantor: A trained person who leads prayer services, performs marriages and funerals, and provides the musical part of prayer services. Mohel: A person trained in the ritual and spiritual aspects of the tradition of circumcision.	Imam: A trained Muslim preacher and teacher.	Bishops: Priests who have been promoted to provide leadership over a certain diocese or area. In the Roman Catholic Church, the bishop of Rome (the Pope) has primary authority over the whole church and appoints all other bishops. Priests: Preside over the Mass and other sacraments, and provide teaching and leadership in the church under the authority of a bishop. Roman Catholic priests must be celibate males, although some married converts have been ordained priests. Orthodox priests may be married but, if married, cannot become bishops. Deacons: Deacons are men, married or unmarried, who function as assistants to priests. They may perform baptisms and preside over funerals, may visit patients in hospitals, and bring already consecrated Eucharist to patients. They cannot preside over a Mass, hear confessions, or anoint the sick. Monks and nuns: Celibate, vowed members of religious orders. Monks may or may not be priests. Monks and nuns function in a wide variety of roles, from cloistered prayer to work as physicians, nurses, hospital chaplains, teachers, and church administrators.	Priests (Episcopal) perform many of the same functions as Roman Catholic priests: anointing the sick, even hearing confessions, and administering the Eucharist. Usually, but not always, wear black or colored clerical shirts and jacket. May be men or women, married, single, or, recently, even noncelibate and homosexual. Ministers (Methodist, Presbyterian, others) and Pastors (Lutherans, Baptists, Pentecostals): Lead worship and prayers, preach the Bible, instruct the faithful, pray over the sick. They may be male or female, married or single, homosexual or heterosexual, depending on the denomination. Likely to wear street clothes, but may wear clerical suits or dress.
Holy Books and Artifacts	Torah: The first five books of the Bible contained in a scroll.	Koran (Qur'an): The collection of the prophecies of Mohammed. The Koran is central to the faith of Muslims.	The Bible, which includes several Old Testament chapters not seen in the Hebrew or Protestant Bible. The Bible is central to the Christian faith.	The Bible, without the Apocrypha (the Old Testament chapters used in the Roman Catholic Bible). Protestants may wear crosses, which emphasize the resurrection of Jesus.

continues

TABLE 6-1 (Continued)

RELIGION	JUDAISM	ISLAM	ROMAN CATHOLIC/ORTHODOX	PROTESTANT
Holy Books and Artifacts *continued*	Bible: A collection of divinely inspired writings concerning God's interaction with and revelations to the Jewish people. Talmud: The tradition of interpretation of holy law. Observant men may wear a small round cap for the top of the head called a *Kipah* (or yarmulke). Men may also wear a prayer shawl called a *Tallith*.	*Shari'a*: The body of Islamic law. *Hadith*: The tradition of Islamic law. Islamic women may wear the Hajib, a cover for their heads, faces, and bodies. Practices vary from no use of the Hajib, to a head scarf only, to a full covering of the face, head, and body. The covering has a Koranic basis, whose purpose is to protect the women from being viewed by men as sexual objects only, and is in part to advertise the women as faithful Muslim women of good character. Dress under the Hajib is to be modest and flowing.	Priests dress distinctively in black with a stiff white collar. Nuns may or may not wear habits, distinctive dress with headgear. Monks may or may not wear distinctive robes. Church members may wear crucifixes, depicting Jesus being crucified on the cross, and may carry rosary beads, a string of beads that aids prayer. Roman Catholics and Orthodox may also use religious medals to remind them of the presence and blessings of God and the saints of God. Devout members may wear scapulars, pieces of cloth embroidered usually with the Virgin Mary or other religious symbol, connected by string, under their clothes. These aid in prayer and also protect the soul after death. It would be important for the devout person to continue to wear these even in the hospital or during surgery.	
Holy Day of the Week	Friday from sundown until Saturday at sundown.	Friday	Sunday	Sunday
Holy Holidays, Festivals, Observances	Rosh Hashana: Jewish new year; it usually occurs in the fall.	Muslims are expected to pray five times a day from before sunup to after sundown. The faithful Muslim prays on a blanket facing Mecca, Saudi Arabia. Prayer should be done in a clean place, and the believer should be clean. A person is considered to be unclean if he or she has	Roman Catholics are required to attend Mass every Sunday, and it is considered a serious sin to miss Mass unless prevented by illness or other circumstances (such as not being able to get to a Mass), or important work (such as providing health care). Other, less important work should not be performed on a Sunday, which is considered a day of rest.	All Protestant churches observe Christmas and Easter, but some denominations eliminate or de-emphasize other observations.

continues

TABLE 6-1 (Continued)

RELIGION	JUDAISM	ISLAM	ROMAN CATHOLIC/ORTHODOX	PROTESTANT
Holy Holidays, Festivals, Observances *continued*	Yom Kippur: Occurs 10 days after Rosh Hashana; a solemn day of atonement and fasting. Sukkot: The feast of tabernacles, a harvest festival; it occurs 5 days after Yom Kippur. Hanukkah: This lesser festival is a 7-day feast of lights. Passover: Usually falls in early spring and recalls the exodus of the Jews from enslavement in Egypt. Shavuot: Festival occurring 50 days after Passover and commemorating the giving of the Torah to Moses on Mt. Sinai.	recently eliminated body wastes, passed flatus, or is asleep. Proper cleansing for prayer includes washing the hands, face, nostrils, ears, arms to the elbows, and feet to the ankles, and moistening the head. After menstruation, childbirth, or sexual intercourse, a complete bath including washing the hair is required before prayer. Muharam 1 Rasal-Sana: The New Year. Ramadan: The ninth month in the Muslim lunar calendar is a time of fasting, meditation, and spiritual purification. Because the Islamic calendar is based on a lunar cycle, the month of Ramadan can fall in any season. Shawwal 1 "Id ad-Fitr": A 3-day celebration following Ramadan. Dhu-al-Hijjah 1–10: This last month of the Muslim calendar is when the journey to Mecca is made. The journey to Mecca is one of the religious pillars of Islam, and Muslims are obligated to go once in their lifetimes if they are able.	In addition, there are six (in the United States, although this varies somewhat by diocese) Holy Days of Obligation in which Mass attendance is also required, and for which it is a serious sin to miss Mass (exceptions the same as above). These days are January 1, the Solemnity of Mary; Ascension Thursday, which occurs 40 days after Easter, although many dioceses have moved this feast to the following Sunday; August 15, the Assumption of the Blessed Virgin Mary; November 1, All Saints Day; December 8, the Immaculate Conception of Mary; and December 25, Christmas. Orthodox Easter is calculated differently and usually falls on a different Sunday than Roman Catholic and Protestant Easter. Other important church observances are: Advent, a 4-week period of penance and preparation before Christmas; Lent, a 40-day period of penance before Easter; Holy Thursday, a day to commemorate the institution of the Eucharist and the priesthood 3 days before Easter; Good Friday, a day of fasting and prayer in commemoration of the Crucifixion of Jesus Christ; Easter, the greatest feast day in the Church, in which the resurrection of Jesus Christ is proclaimed; and Pentecost, a Sunday 6 weeks after Easter in which the coming of the Holy Spirit to the church is remembered.	Attendance at Sunday worship is strongly encouraged, but not required.

continues

TABLE 6-1 (Continued)

RELIGION	JUDAISM	ISLAM	ROMAN CATHOLIC/ORTHODOX	PROTESTANT
Dietary Restrictions	Dietary rules are complex and are not kept by all Jews. Kosher food denotes food prepared according to strict dietary laws, which prohibit pork and any other meat of an animal with a cloven hoof that chews a cud, as well as shellfish. Any meat to be eaten must be ritually slaughtered according to strict laws. Meat and dairy products must not be taken together.	Pork and products made from pork, such as gelatin and lard, are forbidden. Alcohol and street drugs are also forbidden. Strictly speaking, all meat should be ritually slaughtered according to religious laws, but in practice, even religious Muslims are relaxed about this requirement.	Roman Catholics are to refrain from meat on Fridays during Lent. Roman Catholics are supposed to practice some form of penance on all Fridays. This may take the form of refraining from meat, or another form such as extra prayer.	None. Some Protestant denominations (Baptist, Pentecostal) forbid the use of alcohol and tobacco.
Periods of Fasting	Fasting is associated with Yom Kippur and also with some minor holidays. Fasting may be set aside on the advice of a physician.	There is fasting from dawn to sundown during the 28-day month of Ramadan. Pregnant women, menstruating women, and the sick are not required to fast, but they must make up the fast at a later time.	All adult Roman Catholics who are not ill are supposed to fast (that is, eat only one light meal and two smaller meals in one day, and no meat) on Ash Wednesday and Good Friday.	Fasting is de-emphasized in the Protestant tradition.
Medical Treatment	Jews are encouraged to seek medical care and treatment when needed as part of the religious obligation to take care of oneself. Jews hold medicine and physicians in high esteem. Prayers and visitation are proper for the sick.	Healing the sick is considered the highest service to God after religious requirements. Seeking medical treatment for illness is encouraged, and there is no prohibition for doing so. Privacy should be maintained for women and girls during illness and hospitalization. Female bodies should remain covered; gowns should have long sleeves if possible.	Medical treatment is encouraged, even obligated, as part of the obligation to care for oneself. Anointing of the sick with oil and prayers is appropriate at the time of illness. Reception of the Eucharist, if possible, is believed to give special graces to the patient and is considered very important to and for the devout patient.	Same as Roman Catholicism/Orthodoxy, although some Fundamental and Pentecostal offshoots may emphasize prayer and spiritual healing over medical treatment. Mainline Protestants may practice the anointing of the sick. Prayers and visitation are appropriate for the sick.

continues

continues

TABLE 6-1 (Continued)

RELIGION	JUDAISM	ISLAM	ROMAN CATHOLIC/ORTHODOX	PROTESTANT
Birth Control	Sexual relations are permitted only within marriage. Birth control is allowed within marriage.	Sexual relations are permitted only within marriage. Teachings on birth control are contradictory, but in general, the use of birth control within marriage to control family size or to protect the health of the wife is permitted.	Sexual relations are permitted only within marriage. Procreation is one of the celebrated purposes of marriage. Birth control is forbidden by the Roman Catholic Church. Natural family planning, in which intercourse is timed with the menstrual cycle to prevent conception to limit family size or protect the health of the mother, is permitted.	Sexual relations are permitted only within marriage. Birth control is permitted.
Infertility Treatment	A primary purpose of marriage is the procreation of children, and infertility treatments are permitted. Whether to allow the use of gametes from outside the marriage (that is, donor egg or donor sperm) is under discussion.	Procreation is one of the celebrated purposes of marriage, so medical treatment used to treat infertility is acceptable as long as gametes from within the marriage are used and as long as the couple is still married and both husband and wife are alive. Using gametes from outside the marriage (donor egg, donor sperm) would be considered adultery.	Infertility treatment is permitted, with certain important restrictions. Gametes should not leave the body, and only gametes from within the marriage may be used. Thus, medications to stimulate ovulation and surgical treatments to enhance fertility are permitted, but donor egg, donor sperm, in vitro fertilization (IVF), and intracytoplasmic sperm injection (ICSI) are forbidden. The Roman Catholic Church considers all embryos to be human beings and so is against the storage of, destruction of, and research on human embryos.	Infertility treatment is permitted. The use of donor egg or donor sperm is not condemned by most Protestant churches.
Abortion	Judaism has a high respect for life, including prenatal life. However, the fetus is not considered to be fully human until birth. Jewish law does reluctantly permit abortion under some circumstances, such as to preserve the life or welfare of the mother.	Abortion is forbidden after the fetus is "ensouled." There is some controversy as to whether the ensoulment occurs at 40 or 120 days of pregnancy. The father must give permission for the abortion. Abortion after the time of ensoulment is considered murder.	The fetus is considered human from the time of conception. Abortion is therefore prohibited, except when it is done as the effect of another procedure, the purpose of which is not to cause the death of the fetus (for example, a hysterectomy of a pregnant, cancerous uterus is permitted, but the direct abortion of the same fetus is not).	Most Protestant denominations consider fetal life human, but reluctantly allow abortion to preserve the health of the mother. The Southern Baptist Convention recently reversed its pro-choice position and returned to a pro-life position, but it has no authority over its member churches. Many Baptist churches reluctantly allow abortion as a last resort or to save the life of the mother.

TABLE 6-1 (Continued)

RELIGION	JUDAISM	ISLAM	ROMAN CATHOLIC/ORTHODOX	PROTESTANT
Observances at Birth	Circumcision is performed on all males, traditionally at the age of 8 days. Girls may undergo a naming ceremony.	At the time of birth, the baby's father, or nearest male relative, or the mother whispers the central tenet of the Islamic faith into the baby's ear: "There is no God but Allah, and Mohammed is His Prophet." These are the first words the baby should hear. Some Muslim women may refuse to be attended to by male nurses or physicians. A birth is considered legitimate only if it occurs 6 months after marriage.	Baptism is a very important sacrament that should be performed shortly (within a month or so) after birth. Baptism is considered a necessary step for the person to go to heaven. Thus, an ill child of devout Roman Catholic or Orthodox parents should be baptized immediately and can be baptized by any Christian with water and the words, "I baptize you in the name of the Father, and of the Son, and of the Holy Spirit."	Prayers and blessings are customary at the time of birth. If the child is ill at birth, baptism may be performed by most Protestants except Baptists and Pentecostals.
Rites of Initiation	Boys undergo a bar mitzvah at age 13, a celebration of religious adulthood. In the Reform and Conservative traditions, girls may undergo a parallel ceremony called a bat mitzvah.	Males are routinely circumcised at or near birth. Female circumcision is a cultural practice found in parts of Asia and Africa not required by Islam, although it is practiced by some Muslims and justified by them with passages from the Koran.	Baptism is traditionally performed for children as infants. Children are confirmed at about age 12, when they complete instruction about the church.	Protestant churches vary widely over the issue of baptism. Some churches, such as Episcopal, Lutheran, and some Presbyterian churches, baptize infants shortly after birth. Other churches, such as many Baptist and most Pentecostal churches, baptize only older children and adults who confess that Jesus Christ is their Lord and Savior. If a child is ill at birth, some churches will and some will not baptize that infant.
Withdrawal of Life Support	Active euthanasia and assisted suicide are forbidden because of the position of the sanctity of human life and the prohibition of murder. Hastening death is equivalent to murder. The withdrawal of life support is allowed under the right	Active euthanasia and assisted suicide are forbidden because of the position of the sanctity of human life and the prohibition of murder. It is permitted to withdraw life support if the treatment is serving only to prolong the patient's death, or if the patient's condition is medically hopeless.	Suicide and active euthanasia are forbidden because of the principle of the sanctity of life. The withdrawal of life support has been the subject of much controversy in the Church, but is permitted if the condition of the patient is hopeless and as long as the purpose of the withdrawal of support is to reduce pain and suffering, and not to kill the patient.	Suicide is forbidden. Some mainline Protestant denominations have expressed some sympathy for assisted suicide and active euthanasia, but in general, suicide and active euthanasia are forbidden, because of the sanctity of life and the prohibition of murder. The withdrawal of life support is appropriate when the patient's condition is hopeless

continues

TABLE 6-1 (Continued)

RELIGION	JUDAISM	ISLAM	ROMAN CATHOLIC / ORTHODOX	PROTESTANT
Withdrawal of Life Support *continued*				circumstances, as it is simply the removal of impediments to a natural death.		and the treatment is serving only to prolong the patient's death.
Death	Suicide is forbidden. Orthodox Jews may position and wash a dead body. Autopsies are controversial, but are permitted if they will serve to provide information that will save other lives in the future. Burial should be done within 24 hr of death, although this may be extended to 48 hr in special circumstances. Cremation is forbidden. There is a 7-day period of mourning called Shiva that begins the day of the funeral. Some Jews customarily may not shave during this time and may cover mirrors.	Suicide is forbidden. Relatives and friends are normally present when a person dies. There may be an expectation for the patient to say, or for a person to whisper into the ear of the patient, the central tenet of the Islamic faith, "There is no God but Allah, and Mohammed is His Prophet," so that these are the last words the person hears before death. After death the body is washed, usually by a family member. Men wash a man's body, and women wash a woman's body. Autopsies are permitted if they serve to help solve a crime or will provide further medical knowledge. Burial should be commenced without delay, preferably the same day. There are detailed teachings regarding funerals and burials. Attending funerals is a meritorious act. Funerals may be held in absentia for an important person.	Suicide is forbidden. Prayers are appropriate at the time of death. Burial or cremation is permitted. Autopsies are permitted, especially if they will aid medical knowledge.

Devout Roman Catholics and Orthodox at the point of death, or seriously threatened with illness or serious surgery, may request the Last Rites, so called because they involve three sacraments: the Rite of Confession, Anointing of the Sick, and Holy Eucharist. A priest must be called to the bedside to perform these rites. These Last Rites may be performed more than once, if, for example, the patient recovers and then becomes seriously ill again. | Suicide is forbidden, but suicide in the face of suffering at the end of life may be tolerated by some denominations or individual leaders within some denominations. Prayers are appropriate at the time of death. Episcopal priests and Lutheran pastors may administer the Eucharist and anoint the sick. Other pastors and ministers may pray with the family over the sick person, often laying their hands on the sick person as they pray. Bible readings are important to the dying person and the family. |

continues

TABLE 6-1 (Continued)

RELIGION	JUDAISM	ISLAM	ROMAN CATHOLIC/ORTHODOX	PROTESTANT
Organ Donation	Organ donations and receiving transplanted organs are permitted, since the procedure saves lives. One exception is Orthodox Jews, who reject the "brain death" definition of death and agree with the cardiac definition of death only.	Organ donations and receiving transplanted organs are permitted, as are blood transfusions.	Organ donation is permitted.	Organ donation is permitted, though some Baptists or Pentecostals may be against organ donation, believing that they should go to heaven with all their body parts.

RELIGION	CHURCH OF JESUS CHRIST OF LATTER-DAY SAINTS	JEHOVAH'S WITNESSES	CHRISTIAN SCIENCE	UNITARIAN-UNIVERSALIST ASSOCIATION OF CONGREGATIONS (UUA)
Description	The Church of Jesus Christ of Latter-Day Saints (LDS) was founded in 1820. Church members believe that messages and a set of texts were divinely revealed to Joseph Smith, a prophet. The Mormons differ from traditional Christianity in elevating these texts to the level of the Bible, and in believing that the church, as it grew after the resurrection of Christ, was corrupt, and that its authority was replaced by Joseph Smith's followers.	"The Watchtower Bible and Tract Society," commonly known as the Jehovah's Witnesses, was founded in the 1870s. Their beliefs are centered around a unique interpretation of the Bible. They differ from traditional Christianity in their belief that Jesus is God's son but inferior in status to God, and their beliefs concerning the end-time (how and when it will occur and its character) differ as well. Their name for God is Jehovah.	Christian Science is a religious movement founded in the 1860s by American Mary Baker Eddy (1821–1910). Mrs. Eddy experienced a healing after Bible study, and subsequently devoted her life to Bible study and the ministry of healing. Christian Scientists believe that Eddy identified the scientific method and divine laws Jesus used in his healings. The church teaches that Jesus is central to individual salvation, but was not God.	The Unitarians began in Europe in the 1600–1700s. The movement affirms the moral perfection of God but differs from traditional Christianity in that it believes that Jesus was human, and not the son of God (that is, unitarian, not trinitarian). The Universalist movement began in England in the eighteenth century, with the basic belief in a benevolent God and that all humans are inherently good. Unitarians reject the Doctrine of Original Sin held by mainstream Christianity believing instead that humankind does not need redemption by Jesus. The Unitarians and Universalists merged in 1961. UUA is a creedless church that has seven principles that all churches have agreed to, such as respecting

continues

TABLE 6-1 (Continued)

RELIGION	CHURCH OF JESUS CHRIST OF LATTER-DAY SAINTS	JEHOVAH'S WITNESSES	CHRISTIAN SCIENCE	UNITARIAN-UNIVERSALIST ASSOCIATION OF CONGREGATIONS (UUA)
Description *continued*	Church members are properly called "Latter-Day Saints" not "Mormons." "Mormon" refers to one of the four holy books of the Church of LDS.			the worth and dignity of all human beings. Church members live primarily in the United States and Canada, with some churches in Romania and Europe.
Religious Leaders	Bishop: A volunteer lay leader of a local church. Bishops are male and usually serve 5-year terms as church leaders. Home teacher: A male church member assigned to look after a member of the church. The home teacher provides practical as well as spiritual help to his assigned church member. Every member of the church has a home teacher, and that teacher is called in case of an illness. President: The leader of the LDS Church at large. The president is considered a prophet who receives revelation and inspiration directly from God to guide the church.	All baptized persons are considered ordained ministers. Jehovah's Witnesses believe that a clergy class and special titles are improper. Elders or overseers (all male) lead each congregation and lead worship, provide pastoral care, visit the sick, teach, and preach sermons. Ministerial students are young men who assist elders in the functioning of the Kingdom Hall. "Publishers and Pioneers" are active Witnesses who go door to door in an attempt to convert the public.	None. The church is entirely run by laypeople. Christian Science practitioner: A person devoted full time to the ministry of Christian healing. Every practicing Christian Scientist has a practitioner to call in case healing is needed. Christian Science nurse: These nurses are not registered nurses, but undergo 2 to 5 years of training in bedside nursing skills and spirituality. They assist patients with bedside care and prayer while healing is ongoing.	Minister: An ordained male or female church leader who leads worship services.

continues

TABLE 6-1 (Continued)

RELIGION	CHURCH OF JESUS CHRIST OF LATTER-DAY SAINTS	JEHOVAH'S WITNESSES	CHRISTIAN SCIENCE	UNITARIAN-UNIVERSALIST ASSOCIATION OF CONGREGATIONS (UUA)
Holy Books and Artifacts	The "standard works" include: The Bible, *The Book of Mormon*, the *Doctrine and Covenants*, and the *Pearl of Great Price*. Endowed church members, that is, members who have been to a Mormon temple, may also wear special underclothing that is considered sacred.	The *New World Translation* of the Bible, which Jehovah's Witnesses believe to be the most accurate translation of the ancient languages of the Bible. Kingdom Hall is where Jehovah's Witnesses meet and worship. Jehovah's Witnesses reject the Christian symbol of the cross, because they believe that Jesus was crucified on a single upright wooden stake with no cross beam.	The Bible. *Science and Health with Key to the Scriptures* by Mary Baker Eddy. This book is central to the Christian Science theology and is used to interpret the Bible.	The Bible is not a definitive source for the UUA. Many members consider the Bible flawed.
Holy Day of the Week	Sunday	No one day is holier than any other. Most services are held in the evenings during the week or on Sunday.	None Church is attended on Sunday, but this is not a holy day. Short services that include testimonials about healings occur on Wednesdays.	Sunday
Holy Holidays, Festivals, Observances	Church members celebrate Christmas and Easter.	Memorial of Jesus' death: Celebrated annually at the time of the Last Supper of Jesus. Falls in the spring at the time of Passover. Jehovah's Witnesses do not celebrate Christmas or Easter because there is no command by Jesus to do so. Jehovah's Witnesses are forbidden to celebrate "worldly" holidays such as Thanksgiving and Independence Day.	There is a special Thanksgiving service recognized by all Christian Scientists on the American Thanksgiving Day.	UUA members celebrate Christmas and Easter, but the holidays have more cultural than religious significance. Easter is seen as a celebration of spring and new life, rather than a recognition of the resurrection of Jesus.

continues

TABLE 6-1 (Continued)

RELIGION	CHURCH OF JESUS CHRIST OF LATTER-DAY SAINTS	JEHOVAH'S WITNESSES	CHRISTIAN SCIENCE	UNITARIAN-UNIVERSALIST ASSOCIATION OF CONGREGATIONS (UUA)
Dietary Restrictions	Church members abstain from illicit drugs, alcohol, tobacco, tea, and coffee. The church advises all members to practice moderation in all things including diet, and to eat wholesome food, eat meat sparingly, and get rest and exercise.	No food containing blood (such as blood sausages) is allowed, because Jehovah's Witnesses believe it is forbidden to take in blood. Meat should have all blood drained out of it before cooking; meat approved by the American Dietetic Association meets this criterion.	None Most Christian Scientists avoid alcohol, smoking, and caffeine, because these can affect overall well-being.	None
Periods of Fasting	None	None	None	None
Medical Treatment	Church members are encouraged to seek medical care when needed and to exercise their best judgment based on competent medical advice. When sick, church members may call on their home teachers or other church members for the laying on of hands, or a blessing for healing. The blessing is done by two male members of the church at the request of the patient.	Jehovah's Witnesses do seek medical care for all infirmities. The only limitation on their use of health care services is an important religious belief that the Bible forbids the ingestion of blood. This belief prohibits the use of whole blood, packed RBCs, plasma, WBCs, and platelets. Other preparations in which the amount of blood is very minute, such as albumin, immune globulins, and hemophiliac preparations, are up to the conscience of the individual. Autotransfusion is controversial. Jehovah's Witnesses understand the implications (including possible death) of refusing blood. However, full medical treatment is acceptable as long as no blood is used. They appreciate and seek nonblood treatments for bleeding,	There is no prohibition in the Christian Science Church against seeking medical care. However, Christian Scientists believe that illness is caused by a spiritual disruption in the relationship with God. Healing in its most holistic sense is obtained through spiritual guidance. Practicing Christian Scientists avoid hospitals and medical care. There are a few accepted exceptions to this: X-rays and other treatments for broken bones; dental care by a dentist; MD or midwife care during childbirth; and vaccinations and other treatment required by law. In practice, some Christian Science parents avoid vaccinating their children and invoke their religious exemption to vaccinations allowed by most but not all states. In the case of illness, the Christian Scientist would (1) pray and study the Bible and texts, (2) call his or her Christian Science practitioner, (3) seek care from a Christian Science nurse if assistance with activities of daily living is needed, and (4) repeat steps 1 and 2 until the expected healing occurs.	There is no prohibition against seeking medical care and treatment when necessary. The UUA is a socially active organization that has lobbied for the right to health care for all. When UUA members are ill, members of the congregation's caring committee may visit the person and provide practical and spiritual support.

continues

TABLE 6-1 (Continued)

RELIGION	CHURCH OF JESUS CHRIST OF LATTER-DAY SAINTS	JEHOVAH'S WITNESSES	CHRISTIAN SCIENCE	UNITARIAN-UNIVERSALIST ASSOCIATION OF CONGREGATIONS (UUA)
Medical Treatment *continued*		such as Hespan, vasopressors, MAST trousers, intraoperative blood salvage, etc. Bone marrow transplants are a matter of conscience. Jehovah's Witnesses are encouraged to carry cards indicating refusal of blood as well as general advance directives. It is important for the nurse to understand that Jehovah's Witnesses who accept blood or blood products believe that they are committing a serious sin and may thereby forfeit their eternal life.	A few Christian Science parents have been jailed for what has been termed the medical neglect of their children in favor of prayer.	
Birth Control	Sexual relations are permitted only within marriage. Birth control is permitted for family planning but discouraged for family prevention. Surgical sterilization is discouraged unless it is for health reasons. The decision to use birth control is left up to the prayerful decision of the husband and wife, based on competent medical advice.	Sex is permitted only within marriage. Birth control is a matter of personal choice. Birth control that prevents implantation (such as some forms of the pill) are prohibited.	Sex is permitted only within marriage. Birth control is acceptable. Christian Scientists prefer barrier methods over medications such as the pill.	There are no prohibitions against birth control. Sexual relations are permitted between consenting adults in a mutually respectful relationship.

continues

TABLE 6-1 (Continued)

RELIGION	CHURCH OF JESUS CHRIST OF LATTER-DAY SAINTS	JEHOVAH'S WITNESSES	CHRISTIAN SCIENCE	UNITARIAN-UNIVERSALIST ASSOCIATION OF CONGREGATIONS (UUA)
Infertility Treatment	Infertility treatment is a decision left up to the prayerful decision making of husband and wife, based on competent medical advice. Use of surrogate mothers and donor insemination is discouraged.	Infertility treatment is up to the individual conscience. No donor gametes from outside of the marriage are permitted.	Infertility, like other physical problems, is believed to have a spiritual cause; therefore healing should be sought through prayer, not through medical treatment.	There are no prohibitions against seeking treatment for infertility.
Abortion	Abortion is permitted in instances of rape and incest, or when the health of the mother is jeopardized, or is left up to the prayerful consideration between husband and wife, based on competent medical advice.	Abortion is prohibited if it is done solely to prevent the birth of an unwanted child. However, abortion is permitted if needed to save the life of the mother.	There is no official church teaching on abortion. Abortion is very uncommon among Christian Scientists, although it is seen as an individual's choice.	The UUA is in favor of all reproductive rights for women, including the right to an abortion.
Observances at Birth	The child is named and blessed in a church service, usually within 6 weeks of birth.	None.	None. Christian Scientists do not practice baptism.	None.
Rites of Initiation	Baptisms are done at age 8.	Baptism by immersion is done when the child (or adult) can and does give consent to be a Jehovah's Witness, usually at puberty.	None. Christian Scientists do not observe birthdays or anniversaries.	Infants and children can undergo a dedication ceremony in the church.
Withdrawal of Life Support	The decision to withdraw life support is left up to the patient or family, based on competent medical advice.	Life is sacred, and the willful taking of life under any circumstances is wrong. Reasonable and humane effort should be made to sustain and prolong life. However, the Scriptures do not require that extraordinary, complicated, distressing,	Most Christian Scientists have advance directives to avoid medical treatment. Critical illness should be dealt with by prayer, not medical treatment. Withdrawal of medical treatment is in accordance with a practicing Christian Scientist's wishes. A Christian Scientist never prays for death to avoid physical misery. Instead, a Christian	There is no prohibition against withdrawing life support based on competent medical advice.

continues

continues

TABLE 6-1 (Continued)

RELIGION	CHURCH OF JESUS CHRIST OF LATTER-DAY SAINTS	JEHOVAH'S WITNESSES	CHRISTIAN SCIENCE	UNITARIAN-UNIVERSALIST ASSOCIATION OF CONGREGATIONS (UUA)
Withdrawal of Life Support *continued*	or costly measures be taken to sustain a person if such measures would merely prolong the dying process and/or leave the patient with no quality of life. Any advance directives of patients that specifically define what is to be done are to be respected.		Scientist prays for healing, even at an advanced age and in the face of critical illness. No illness is seen as hopeless by Christian Science standards.	UUA members have been in the forefront of the movement to withdraw life support when the quality of life is poor and suffering is great. However, assisted suicide and active euthanasia remain controversial.
Death	Burials are arranged by the church, especially if the person was endowed. Cremation is discouraged. The decision for an autopsy is up to the family.	The soul dies with the body, but resurrection will occur for 144,000 at the end-time, and such will be born again as spiritual sons of God. Euthanasia is forbidden. Suicide is not approved of but understood as the product of mental illness. Autopsies are permitted only if legally necessary, so that the body will not be subjected to unnecessary mutilation. Burial and cremation are permitted.	Death is not a failure. Spiritual life goes on beyond death. When death occurs, the person's Christian Science practitioner should always be notified. Autopsies are permitted. Cremation and memorial service are the usual practices.	Suicide is seen as a tragedy, but not a sin. There are no UUA requirements concerning burial. Autopsies are permitted when necessary.
Organ Donation	The decision for organ donation is left up to the family, based on competent medical advice.	The Jehovah's Witnesses forbade organ transplant in 1967 but reversed this decision in 1980. Organ transplants and organ donations are matters of individual choice. There is no biblical injunction against taking in body tissue or bone as there is against taking in blood.	Christian Scientists do not donate or receive organs, because they believe this is not the way to treat the spiritual cause of organ failure.	There are no UUA restrictions on organ donation.

TABLE 6-1 (Continued)

RELIGION	SHINTO	BUDDHISM	HINDUISM	NATIVE AMERICAN RELIGIONS
Description	Shinto is the ancient, traditional religion of Japan. Although it has been influenced by Buddhism, Shintoism has remained a distinct religion. Shintoism is a polytheistic, animistic religion. Shintoism teaches that the Japanese islands were a special, favored creation by the gods. The religion teaches that the sun goddess Amaterasu sent her grandson down to Earth to rule the world for her. He spawned the long line of emperors that have ruled Japan for hundreds of years. The emperors thus enjoyed a semidivine status until so-called "State Shinto" was outlawed at the end of World War II. "Folk" Shinto still exists. Shintoism centers around shrines, which have a characteristic gate and are built, often at special sites such as the tops of mountains, to house a *kami* (god). Numerous *kamis* exist. There are thousands of shrines in Japan, but fewer than a dozen in the United States.	Buddhism was founded in the 6th century BCE by Siddhartha Gautama, who achieved enlightenment at age 35 by purifying his mind and thus achieved the title of "The Buddha," or "Enlightened One." He spent the remainder of his years preaching the Dharma, or "Way," in an effort to help others reach enlightenment. Buddhism centers around the imagined ideal of the Buddha, the transformation of consciousness, and the transformation of karma (the balance of accumulated sin and merit). The goal in Buddhism is the mind's attainment of Nirvana. The eightfold path to Nirvana includes: right understanding, right thinking, right speech, right conduct, right livelihood, right effort, right mindfulness, and right concentration. There are two forms of Buddhism: Theraveda (found in Burma, Cambodia, Laos, Thailand, Vietnam, and Sri Lanka, and is the most common form of Buddhism in the United States), which emphasizes karma and the worship of Buddha relics; and Mahayana (found in China, Korea, Japan, Tibet, Mongolia, and Russia), which emphasizes ceremony and ritual. Because Buddhism has proved to be so highly adaptable to local culture and religions, it is difficult to	Hinduism is an ancient religion that originated in India around 1500 BCE. It is a complex religion that embraces a variety of gods, practices, and spiritual paths. Hinduism is a polytheistic religion that teaches that ultimately there is only one god, or essence of existence—Brahman. Brahman appears in different forms, most notably in the forms of Krishna, Shiva, and Vishnu. Hinduism teaches that although the universe goes through endless cycles, the divine does not change. Humans are expected to follow the cosmic order (*dharma*) in life and hope to achieve spiritual liberation (*moshka*). This occurs through selfless acts and good thoughts (karma). The cultural caste system of India was early on incorporated into Hinduism. The castes range from brahmins (priest caste) to untouchables (lowest class). Complex social and religious rules govern these castes.	Although there are as many Native American religions as there are Native American tribes, certain common characteristics may serve to illustrate the spirituality of native people. Native beliefs are often not religions per se, but are as much cultural traditions centered around creation and animistic beliefs in the souls and spirits in animals and land surrounding the tribe. In reality, most Native Americans practice some form of Christianity. Some people who claim to follow a Native American religion are really following a New Age religion with Native elements or imitations. True Native American religions are tribe-specific, so a nurse working with someone from a particular tribe should become familiar with that specific tribe's beliefs. The importance of the community is emphasized. Often, the view of humanity is humble and the original or supreme creator god is now withdrawn. There are no temples, holy books, or creeds.

continues

TABLE 6-1 (Continued)

RELIGION	SHINTO	BUDDHISM	HINDUISM	NATIVE AMERICAN RELIGIONS
Description *continued*		isolate one strict Buddhist Dharma, or way. Buddhism has thus become enmeshed with cultures throughout the world.		
Religious Leaders	Priests: Priesthood is a hereditary office limited to males, who are usually married. Only priests are allowed into the holiest part of the shrine, where the *kami* is said to exist. Priests lead worship and conduct ceremonies such as marriages.	Monks and Nuns: Celibate, vowed members of religious orders who wear special robes, have shaved heads, and function as teachers and bearers of Buddhist tradition. A Guru or Spiritual Guide: A highly respected, important teacher who wears special robes and generally travels with attendants. It is not uncommon for devout Buddhists to have a picture or icon of their Guru with them. Kadam: A lay teacher of Buddhism. May have taken some vows, but can be married and wear street clothes. Buddhist tradition also holds that all followers are leaders.	Priests: Offer sacrifices to the gods and idols; control worship. Guru: A teacher of spiritual ways. Sadhu: A "peaceful man," a sort of Hindu holy man, like a monk, but not in a formal order. May wander from village to village. Yogi: A spiritual teacher.	Most often, a specialist in the religion is involved — a medicine man, a teacher, or an elder who is able to communicate with the spirits or the Great Spirit and convey the wishes of the petitioner or people. Such a person may look after sacred objects, organize ceremonies, interpret omens or dreams, know of techniques or remedies for problems, and function as a healer. Some may specialize in one of these functions. Often, such a leader is identified during childhood as having special spiritual gifts and subsequently serves a long apprenticeship. Wisdom is associated with age.
Holy Books and Artifacts	Kojiki: Written 712 CE. Nihongi: Written 720 CE, mostly in Chinese. Both works are important and honored, but are rarely recited or studied by ordinary believers. Believers may have at home a *kami* shelf,	*The Tibetan Book of the Dead*: Intended to be read into the ear of one who is dying or has just died. *The Buddha Dharma*: 100 volumes of the collected words of the Buddha with the commentary of scholars. Statues of the Buddha are common and should be treated with respect,	*The Vedas*: Four ancient (1500 BCE) holy books containing hymns and stories. The hymns are sung to the gods during the presentation of sacrifices. *Upanishads*: A book dating from 500 BCE, including philosophical stories. *Bhagavad Gita*: often called the bible of Hinduism. It details the story of Krishna and explores the themes of destiny and salvation.	Usually, there are no holy books, and the religious tradition is passed on orally and through experience with rituals and festivals. Religious artifacts may include masks, feathers, gourds, drums, shells, a medicine pouch worn around the neck with important

continues

TABLE 6-1 (Continued)

RELIGION	SHINTO	BUDDHISM	HINDUISM	NATIVE AMERICAN RELIGIONS
Holy Books and Artifacts *continued*	where daily prayers are said and offerings made. Daruma dolls, actually representations of the Buddha, are popular. Paper strips, broken arrows, and protective charms may be used by a practicing Shinto.	as should photographs of Buddha statues. Any pictures, statues, or religious books must be treated with respect. Many Buddhists wear mala beads, a string of prayer beads, wrapped around their left wrist. If it becomes necessary to remove them, do so with care and treat them with respect. It is believed to cause bad karma to cut the string of mala beads.	Cows are sacred in Hinduism, symbolizing mother earth, bounty, and Krishna. Feeding a cow is an act of worship. The Ganges River: In India, it is a symbol of life without end, and most Hindus want to bathe in and/or drink its spiritual waters. Other worship artifacts: Statues or dolls depicting various gods are common, as well as sandalwood, flat stones, incense, water, candle or oil lamp, flowers, and food for offerings.	religious symbols inside, and grasses or other sources for incense.
Holy Day of the Week	None.	Buddhist tradition teaches that every day is a holy day. Various cultures and traditions within Buddhism may hold different days as special days (such as the 1st and 15th days of the month).	There is no particular holy day to Hindus. Devotees of particular gods may observe chosen holy days.	None.
Holy Holidays, Festivals, Observances	New Year's Day is popular, with celebrations lasting for 1 to 3 days. The Meiji shrine in Tokyo often is visited on this day. Spring Day, March 20. Children's Day, May 5. Respect for Old Age Persons Day, September 15. Autumn Day, September 23 Thanksgiving for Work Day, November 23.	Wesak: The birth of the Buddha is celebrated for 1 to 15 days. This festival usually falls in April or May. There can be many other holidays, depending on the form of Buddhism.	Divali: New Year, Festival of Lights. Holi: Spring festival dedicated to Krishna. Dasara: 10 days of celebration in honor of Kali. Tarpan: A time of oblation to forefathers. Makar Sankranji/Pongal: A celebration of spring; homage paid to the sun. Shivaratri: A 24-hour celebration and fasting in honor of Lord Siva. Ram Navami: A celebration of Lord Rama's birth. The story of Rama is chanted for 24 hrs.	Festivals are often associated with changes in seasons and with harvests. Often, believers may dress up as well-known spirits or gods.

continues

TABLE 6-1 (Continued)

RELIGION	SHINTO	BUDDHISM	HINDUISM	NATIVE AMERICAN RELIGIONS
Holy Holidays, Festivals, Observances *continued*	Japanese Emperor's Birthday, December 23.		Janmashtami: Lord Krishna's birthday. Ganesh Chaturthi: Day to honor Lord Ganesh. Navaratri: 9-day festival in praise of Lord Rama.	
Dietary Restrictions	None.	Some Buddhists, but not all, are vegetarians. Different schools of thought in Buddhism have different views on diet. Strict Buddhists may refuse strong spices.	Since the cow is sacred, no beef is eaten, although milk and milk products, particularly yogurt, are staples of a Hindu's diet. Some Hindus are vegetarians, others are not. Nonvegetarians do not eat pork. Roasted meat may be eaten after a sacrificial ceremony. If one has dedicated a specific fruit to God, one is forbidden to eat that fruit for the rest of one's life.	Varies.
Periods of Fasting	Priests may fast on a day before a festival by eating no meat or just rice. Fasting is not usually done by lay people.	Some Buddhists may fast as a path to spiritual enlightenment, presenting an opportunity to think and reflect. Other Buddhists may not support fasting.	Fasting is associated with spiritual purposes such as spiritual training and special worship services, some holy festivals, and mourning. At such times, Hindus who eat meat may be vegetarians or may fast altogether.	Fasting may be a special form of prayer, supervised by the elder.
Medical Treatment	Shinto followers with illnesses are encouraged to seek medical treatment. Those with illnesses may go to a shrine to ask for prayers for healing.	Medical treatments that may enhance life and the search for enlightenment are approved of. Buddhism has a high regard for the healing nature of the doctor-patient relationship. Doctors and nurses are respected.	Taking care of the body is seen as a good thing. There is no conflict between religion and seeking medical care, as long as a person is not harmed without purpose. The study of medicine has a long and honored tradition in Hindu culture. Traditional Hindu medicine offers homeopathic, herbal, non-Western care for diseases.	Illness may be related to a sin or an unhappy spirit or god. A specialist in the religion may be consulted to discern the cause of the illness or seek the ritual that will appease the unhappy spirit.
Birth Control	No restrictions.	Birth control is discouraged because it is unnatural.	The traditional Hindu point of view is against birth control because children are seen as a gift, and many children are an even greater blessing.	Usually not practiced. Children are seen as blessings and essential to survival.

continues

TABLE 6-1 (Continued)

RELIGION	SHINTO	BUDDHISM	HINDUISM	NATIVE AMERICAN RELIGIONS
Infertility Treatment	No particular teachings. Medical treatment for infertility is allowed without restrictions.	Infertility may be seen as Buddha's plan. Infertility treatments may be seen as unnatural. This is controversial.	Infertility treatment is permitted, as long as gametes from outside the marriage (donor egg, sperm) are not used. Donor gametes are seen as being against the marriage.	A couple may seek treatment from the tribal elder for infertility, but may be reluctant to seek outside medical assistance.
Abortion	No particular teachings. Abortion is not forbidden but not encouraged.	The morality of abortion would depend on the circumstances. Abortion may be supported if the child is suffering in the womb. Nothing is absolute in Buddhism, however, and in general, any form of killing may be seen as adding to bad karma, and thus abortion would be discouraged. Compassion and wisdom must be emphasized.	The traditional Hindu view prohibits abortion, because it is seen as a form of killing that would lead to the accumulation of bad karma. In modern practice, however, some Hindus practice abortion.	Usually not practiced or tolerated openly.
Observances at Birth	Newborns are commonly taken to a shrine for a blessing and for prayers for good health. Boys are taken on the 31st day of life, girls on the 33rd day of life.	At an early age—from 1 month to 100 days of age—the parents of a new baby give thanks to the Buddha and dedicate the child to Buddha.	On the 10th to 11th day after birth, a priest performs a naming ceremony for the newborn, invoking the blessings of gods and goddesses.	Often a dedication or thanksgiving ceremony.
Rites of Initiation	Children at ages 3, 5, and 7 are blessed with special prayers on Children's Day. At age 20, an adult blessing is received.	It depends on the child. A child may be taken to a temple for a ceremony of further dedication.	Mundan: The first haircut for a boy. Dvija: For boys of the upper three castes, a rite of initiation at age 15. The boy is invested with three strands of the sacred thread, signifying right thought, right speech, right actions.	Often, a boy reaching puberty or adulthood undergoes an initiation rite that includes some shedding of blood, if only a small amount.
Withdrawal of Life Support	No real teachings about withdrawal of life support.	Buddhism values life, but sees death as a natural part of life. Maintenance, comfort care, and withdrawal of life support would be acceptable for those patients who are crossing the threshold of death. But good karma results from saving, prolonging, or .	When the body is beyond repair, Hinduism supports the withdrawal of artificial life support in order to allow for a natural death. The point of life is liberation—moshka—from the endless cycles of life and death through good karma.	Life support is seen as unnatural and therefore not necessary.

continues

TABLE 6-1 (Continued)

RELIGION	SHINTO	BUDDHISM	HINDUISM	NATIVE AMERICAN RELIGIONS
Withdrawal of Life Support *continued*		improving life. The most weighty sin for a Buddhist is to take the life of another living being.		
Death	Upon death, the deceased person becomes a spirit, according to Shinto beliefs. The person's name often is inscribed in wood at the ancestor shrine used by the family. The body is usually, but not always, cremated.	Death is a natural part of life. The state of mind at the time of death is very important: calm and peaceful is preferred as this will cause a happy rebirth. At death, existence for the Buddhist can take a sudden turn for the better or the worse, depending on the good or evil done in life. Suicide is strongly criticized, except for self-sacrifice. Cremation is common. During the entire death process, it is important to keep a calm and serene environment. Touch the patient as little as possible. After death, the body should not be disturbed with movement, talking, or crying.	The atmosphere around the dying person must be peaceful, a spiritual silence, so the last thoughts are of God. Holy water, such as from the Ganges River, is poured into the mouth of the dying person. Hindus prefer to die at home, as close to mother earth as possible, so many prefer to die on the floor or even on the ground. A married woman's nuptial thread (necklace) or amulets are removed just before death to allow the soul's free journey to infinity. The family washes the body, and the eldest son arranges for a funeral and cremation within 24 hrs of death. The body should lie under a white sheet and be disturbed as little as possible. Embalming or beautifying the body are forbidden. Autopsies are discouraged. Children under 2 are buried, and there are no rituals for infants, because the soul from the last life had not yet lived. The names of gods are chanted at the funeral, and the family fasts and wears white for purity. Suicide and active euthanasia are forbidden, because killing accumulates bad karma.	There are complex beliefs about death and the treatment and disposal of the body. Some followers may be forbidden to touch a dead body or be required to undergo a cleansing ritual after touching or being near a dead body. Often, the spirit of the person is believed to live on after death, and ancestor worship is often involved.
Organ Donation	No particular teachings or restrictions. Organ donation is controversial.	This is controversial. Some Buddhists accept the concepts of brain death and organ donation. If the donation of organs would help others, this may bring good karma and be approved of.	Traditional Hindu thought is against receiving organ donations because organ donation is not natural. Donating organs involves disturbing the body after death, which is discouraged.	Organ donation is discouraged because of death and burial practices.

TABLE 6-2 Some "Open Doors" for Discussing Religious and Spiritual Beliefs

- Required queries regarding organ donation and advance directives
- Discussions about difficult treatment options
- When bad news or serious diagnosis is announced
- Ask the patient how his or her spouse or family is "holding up"
- Respond to patient's statement indicating spiritual distress with sympathy and gentle queries about spiritual and religious beliefs
- The patient may ask you about your spiritual or religious beliefs, or those of another health care team member, or make an observation about the hospital chaplain. Turn the conversation around to the patient's beliefs.

REFLECTIVE THINKING

Abortion

What would you say if a patient tells you confidentially that she had an abortion, but that the religion to which she belongs does not approve of abortion?

If the patient is resentful or hostile to questions about religion and spirituality, focus on the patient's support system only. Avoid a debate on the merits of religion and forcing your own views on the patient. Be alert for an opportunity, an "open door," in which it is natural and permissible to ask questions or probe further into the patient's religious and spiritual beliefs and support system. The patient may even "open the door" for you and tacitly invite you to make inquiries in this area (Table 6-2).

The Importance of an Ongoing Assessment

In an ongoing therapeutic relationship with a patient, keep in mind that it is important to reevaluate the patient's spiritual and religious beliefs on a continuous basis. A major life event or health crisis, or the long grind of a chronic illness, can put even long-held spiritual and religious beliefs to the test, and the patient may welcome an intervention previously refused or consider an option previously ruled out.

When caring for a dying patient or end-of-life patient, it may help to inquire of the patient whether he or she is at peace, as a brief means of a spiritual assessment (Steinhauser et al., 2006; Sulmasy, 2006).

NURSING DIAGNOSIS

There are six NANDA-I nursing diagnoses that address the spiritual and religious care of the patient. The first group of nursing diagnoses are *Impaired religiosity, Readiness for enhanced religiosity,* and *Risk for impaired religiosity.* They address "reliance on beliefs and/or participat[ion] in rituals of a particular faith tradition" (NANDA-I, 2009, p. 298). This reliance can be impaired, potentially impaired, or have the potential for increasing religiosity. The second group of nursing diagnoses are *Spiritual distress, Readiness for enhanced spiritual well-being,* and *Risk for spiritual distress.* These NANDA-I diagnoses address an aspect of the ability or inability "to experience and integrate meaning and purpose in life through connectedness with self, others, art, music, literature, nature, and/ or a power greater than oneself" (NANDA-I, 2009, p. 301). The actual diagnoses (*Impaired religiosity* and *Spiritual distress*) are used for patients with an actual disruption in spiritual well-being or their faith. The "Readiness" diagnoses are useful when the nurse perceives that the patient might benefit from spiritual or religious support. The "Risk" diagnoses are useful in the event of a sudden crisis that puts the patient at risk of questioning or needing his or her spiritual or religious supports.

Spiritual distress is the state in which a patient feels that the belief system, or his or her place within it, is threatened. Commonly, the circumstances in which nurses find themselves providing care—birth, accidents, illness, and the dying process— are the same events that provoke spiritual distress. Any threat to one's own life, any reminder of one's own mortality, can serve to evoke both wonderment about

NURSING**TIP**

Clues to a Patient's Spirituality

When you are caring for a patient in the home or in an institution such as a hospital, a hospice, or a nursing home, use your access to the patient to look for clues about the patient's spirituality. Does the patient pray before meals? Do the patient's get-well cards contain religious or spiritual messages? Who visits the patient—family and friends, or also members of the patient's religious or spiritual organization?

the meaning and purpose of life and disquiet about the answers that spirituality or religion provides. Spiritual distress may manifest itself as anxiety, withdrawal, distractedness, hopelessness, or crying behaviors.

NURSING INTERVENTIONS

The following nursing interventions are appropriate for both spiritual nursing diagnoses.

Show Respect for the Patient's Religious and Spiritual Beliefs

A Buddhist in a Christian hospital, for example, may feel awkward displaying an icon of a Guru. Muslims have been singled out for special scrutiny and criticism since 9/11 and may be reluctant to call attention to their religion by praying five times a day in a hospital, where there is little privacy. Even mainstream Christians may find that their religious beliefs are thought of as amusing or quaint to the secular, scientific practitioners of health care.

Allow Patients to Practice Their Religion and Spirituality if They Wish to Do So

Patients may need your permission to practice their religion and spirituality. Without overt permission, some reluctant patients, feeling overwhelmed by unfamiliar institutional surroundings or by their medical treatment regimen, may forgo prayers or rituals that might bring them profound relief at a time of crisis. Giving permission also shows respect for patients' beliefs. There can be real obstacles to religious and spiritual practices in a health care institution, and the nurse will need to use creative interventions to overcome institutional obstacles and make religious and spiritual practice possible for the patient (Table 6-3).

Contact and Mobilize the Patient's Important Spiritual Resources

If the patient so desires, it is important to mobilize the patient's spiritual and religious resources. The patient may be unable to do so, and due to HIPAA privacy laws, the patient's spiritual community may be unable to find out whether one of their own is in a health care institution. This may involve calling the patient's church, contacting the patient's minister, alerting an important group of friends, and so on.

Praying with Patients

Prayer is a means of speaking to God or a higher power. It allows for communication, asks for assistance, and provides reassurance. Certainly, many patients pray for a cure for their disease or help for dealing with a major life event. Studies on the efficacy of prayer in treating ill patients have been decidedly mixed. Some studies showed slight improvements in patients who received intercessory prayer (Harris et al., 1999; Krucoff et al., 2001). Other studies were ambiguous or showed slightly negative results for patients receiving intercessory prayer (Benson et al., 2006; Krucoff et al., 2005). Many have argued that prayer is difficult to study (Churchill, 2007; Dossey, 2005; Krucoff et al, 2006). Sloan (2006) argues that these studies show that prayer is no more useful than other interventions such as music, guided imagery, and touch.

Should nurses pray with patients? It is possible that a strongly religious nurse or doctor might intimidate or even anger a patient by initiating, asking for, or insisting on a shared prayer. In the area of mental health, there is even more danger that such prayer could be coercive. A thorough assessment of the patient's beliefs is important, as is perhaps a mention that the nurse shares (if you do) the patient's beliefs.

TABLE 6-3 Overcoming Obstacles to a Patient's Practice of Religion and Spirituality in the Health Care Setting

OBSTACLES	NURSING INTERVENTIONS
Secular health care practitioners belittle or dismiss the patient's spiritual or religious beliefs.	Show respect for the patient's spiritual and religious beliefs. Educate self and health care team members about the patient's beliefs.
Patient is of a different faith from the mainstream.	Same as above. Encourage the patient to engage in spiritual and religious practices that bring comfort and meaning.
Medical equipment/treatment interferes with patient's practice of religion/spirituality.	Place spiritual/religious objects of importance within view of patient, on patient, or in the patient's hand. For example, holy cards can be taped to an IV pump or ventilator arm. Prayer beads can be placed in the patient's hand. Put the TV on a religious channel of patient's choice. Read or encourage visitors to read religious/spiritual literature to the patient. Mobilize patient's support system to visit. Consult chaplaincy service.
Patient doesn't have proper religious/spiritual equipment (candles, rosary, holy book, prayer blanket, phylacteries, etc.) in the institution.	Contact friends, family, pastor, et al., to bring in necessary equipment. Consult chaplaincy service. An institutional chaplaincy service is likely to have some of the proper equipment available for loan. If proper equipment cannot be used (for example, candles cannot be used if the patient requires oxygen therapy), suggest alternatives (e.g., electric candles).
Lack of privacy to practice religion or spirituality.	Provide privacy as much as possible for spiritual and religious practices.
Religious/spiritual clothing or objects are taken off the patient during the course of treatment.	Religious/spiritual clothing and objects can be draped over the patient or placed on an extremity.

Nevertheless, shared prayer between a patient and a nurse who share beliefs can be comforting and reassuring to the patient. See Table 6-4 for guidelines for praying with patients.

There are no instances when a nurse should be forced to participate in prayer against his or her own religious or spiritual beliefs. An atheist nurse should not have to pray with a devoutly religious patient, although the nurse could stand by politely while the patient prays. A Jewish nurse should not have to say, "There is no God but Allah, and Mohammed is His Prophet," into the ear of a newborn Muslim baby or a dying Muslim patient, but the nurse can allow the baby's parents or Imam into the patient's room to perform this important religious function.

Make Appropriate Referrals to the Hospital Chaplain

Hospital chaplains of any religion generally function as spiritual and religious resource people within a health care institution. Do not fail to take advantage of their expertise just because the patient is Buddhist and the Chaplain is Jewish, for example. The Chaplain should feel comfortable visiting a patient experiencing spiritual distress and discussing the patient's spiritual and religious concerns without judging the patient or trying to convert the patient to the Chaplain's own religion. Occasional problems have been reported in which a hospital chaplaincy

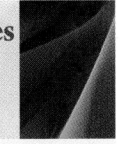

TABLE 6-4 Guidelines for Praying with Patients

Koenig (2007a) suggests these guidelines for praying with patients:

1. In the majority of cases, it is best to allow the *patient* to initiate a prayer with the nurse or other health care providers. If the nurse is uncomfortable praying with a patient, he or she can politely refuse and state a preference for praying alone. Alternatively, the nurse can offer to stand silently with the patient while the patient prays.

2. The nurse or other health care provider may initiate a prayer with a patient when *all* of the following conditions are met:

    a. When a *thorough* spiritual assessment has been performed

    b. When the nurse is *sure* that the patient *shares the beliefs* of the nurse

    c. When the nurse is *sure* that the suggestion of prayer would be welcomed

    d. When there is a *pressing* patient spiritual need

REFLECTIVE THINKING

A Patient Asks for Your Participation

- What would you do if a patient asked you to pray for him?

- What would you do if a patient asked you to pray with him?

- What would you do if a patient asked you to perform a religious ritual (such as a baptism)?

service discriminated against a certain religion (Salmon, 2007) or was proselytizing (Foxnews.com, 2007), so the nurse should make it a practice to become familiar with the chaplain service at a health care institution.

NURSING INTERVENTIONS TO AVOID

There are several nursing interventions to avoid when working with a patient's spirituality, and these are listed in Table 6-5.

When Spiritual and Religious Beliefs May Pose a Risk to Patient Care

When a patient's spiritual and religious beliefs are harmful to patient care, the health care team needs to tread carefully. Showing respect for the patient's rights to his or her own belief system is still appropriate. No one will make headway with a patient by ridiculing—even subtly—the patient's beliefs, or by trying to argue with the patient about them. Patients should not be separated from visitors who support these difficult beliefs, although visitors, even families, may need to be separated and have selected visiting times in order to decrease conflict. Nurses should avoid

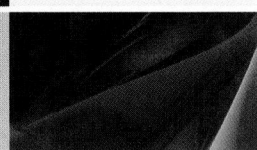

TABLE 6-5 Nursing Actions to Avoid When Intervening in the Patient's Spiritual Condition

It is important to show respect for your patients' religious and spiritual beliefs. These actions are considered disrespectful of such beliefs and should be avoided.

1. Do not proselytize your own spiritual beliefs. You may share your beliefs if the issue comes up, but it is never appropriate to try to convert the patient to another set of beliefs. In a worst-case scenario, you may instill fear in the patient that you will not provide care unless the patient espouses your own beliefs. You may also unwittingly undermine the patient's support system at a time when the patient needs support.

2. Do not instruct the patient in religious or spiritual doctrine. In a time of spiritual distress, a patient needs support, not instruction. Let the religious or spiritual leader take the lead in any instruction that is required, and follow nursing interventions that will enhance spiritual well-being.

3. Do not perform the function of a spiritual advisor for the patient. You and the patient may become confused about your role.

4. Do not respond to the patient with clichés. Well-known and overused clichés such as "no sense crying over spilled milk" or "there's always someone else around who's worse off than you" are inappropriate because they tend to blame or diminish the anguish of the patient. Clichés about religion, such as "God helps those who help themselves" or "it was God's will," are just as inappropriate, because they are patronizing and tend to trivialize both the sufferer's problems and the sufferer's religion. Additionally, most well-known religious clichés are based on Western Judeo-Christian culture and have no bearing on those with other kinds of religions or spiritual beliefs. Respond instead with real, heartfelt words or, in some cases, with silence or with touch, if appropriate.

5. Avoid taking on the role of spiritual advisor, spiritual healer, minister, priest, teacher, guru, and so on. Utilize instead the patient's pastor, imam, priest, or minister or spiritual support systems, family, or the health care institutional chaplain to fill that role.

REFLECTIVE THINKING

Privacy versus Spirituality

In your role as a registered nurse, you recognize a patient who is being admitted to another unit. You have seen her praying at the Shinto shrine where you worship. The patient is asleep after surgery, and her family is not around. She is listed as being in serious condition. Should you notify your priest that the patient has been admitted? How would you decide?

NURSING**TIP**

Answering the "Why Me?" Question

Don't answer. Listen instead.

Nurses care for suffering patients who, in their spiritual distress, may pose the ancient question "Why me?" Different religions and spiritualities answer the question differently. Although you may offer some personal thoughts on the subject, it is a better and more helpful intervention to listen while the patient talks about his or her struggle with the topic. Many times, surprisingly, listening and companionship alone are enough to bring comfort to a suffering patient.

becoming angry with such religiously or spiritually difficult patients, or lecturing or instructing them. A hospital chaplain may be able to help mediate between the patient and the health care team.

If the patient has religious or spiritual beliefs that are or may pose a risk to him or her, it is appropriate to notify the nursing supervisor and possibly obtain an ethics committee consultation to discuss the treatment plan. When a child's health is being harmed by the parents' religious and spiritual beliefs, it is appropriate to invoke your state's statutes on required reporting of possible child abuse. Such reporting will ensure legal representation for the minor patient and move the discussion to the legal realm.

EVALUATION

Evaluate the effect of your nursing interventions by observing the patient. Signs that the patient's spiritual distress has decreased include:

1. Acceptance of spiritual support from the source with which the patient feels most comfortable.

2. Decrease in crying, restlessness, and sleeplessness. There may even be a decrease in complaints of pain or the severity of pain.

3. Decrease in statements of worthlessness and hopelessness.

4. Verbalization of satisfaction with spiritual beliefs and the support and comfort they provide. The patient may talk openly about spiritual beliefs and even offer spiritual insights to other patients, to you, or to other health care professionals. This is a healthy sign that the patient is admitting acceptance of spiritual beliefs.

NURSING**TIP**

Arranging for Pastoral Care

Most institutional chaplains have received special training in **pastoral care**, which is the care and response needed when a person is in a spiritual crisis. Chaplains are employed to visit and support patients in spiritual distress. In their practice of pastoral care, these chaplains can be valuable aids for the patient in spiritual distress. However, some patients, when asked, will refuse a visit with a chaplain based on the incorrect belief that they are present only to visit dying patients, practice their own religious rituals, or preach their own dogmas. If your patient's diagnosis is spiritual distress, initiate a chaplaincy referral. The chaplain will provide a satisfying explanation for the visit, such as "I normally visit with all patients before surgery," and the patient will not miss out on a valuable resource for alleviating spiritual distress.

CASE STUDY

Religious Beliefs Can Lead to Medical Conflict

This case study illustrates the application and objective documentation of the spiritual assessment.
Leaf is an 8-year-old boy admitted to the emergency department with cardiac arrest. He is the son of unmarried parents who live with him. The father reports that the boy had been ill for "a few days." The parents were praying over him when he became unresponsive, at which time the boy's mother called 911. The rescue squad found the boy in cardiac arrest with a blood sugar level of 850 mg/dL. The rescue squad personnel initiated resuscitative measures, administered insulin and a normal saline IV, and transported the patient to the ED. In the ED, a cardiac rhythm was reestablished, and Leaf was intubated and placed on a ventilator. He remains unresponsive with dilated pupils. A loud argument has ensued among the patient's father and mother, and the ED doctor. The father wants to take the boy home immediately. He blames the mother for calling 911. The mother is crying hysterically and accusing the father of killing their son by not allowing her to take him to a doctor earlier. The doctor is loudly threatening to call the police to arrest the parents for child abuse.

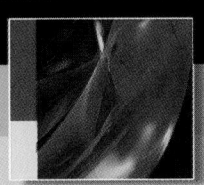

SPIRITUAL HISTORY

PATIENT PROFILE

History of Present Illness

The patient is an 8 yo mixed-race male, currently unconscious

The boy's mother reports that Leaf was in his usual state of health until about 6 months ago, when he began to develop fatigue, thirst, weight loss, and excessive urination.

Leaf's parents took Leaf to see The Bishop, the charismatic leader of their commune. The Bishop prayed over Leaf and then prescribed a special diet of rice, vegetables, and peanut butter. When the boy got worse, the boy's mother took him to the clinic in the next town without the knowledge or permission of The Bishop or the boy's father. Leaf was diagnosed with type I diabetes. The clinic gave the boy insulin for a blood glucose level of 350 mg/dL and instructed the mother on a proper diet and how to administer insulin at home. The mother signed up for classes with the diabetic educator and made an appointment to return the following day. When she returned home, The Bishop and Leaf's mother argued fiercely. The Bishop ordered the mother not to return to the clinic, and he forbade the parents to use "technology" to treat the boy. Leaf's father forbade Leaf and the mother to return to the clinic. The Bishop prayed over the boy and put him on a watermelon-only diet for a week to clean out impurities. By the end of the week, the boy had worsened: The fatigue, thirst, and excessive urination had returned, and he was listless and hot. The Bishop came to the family home at the parents' request and was praying over Leaf when the boy became unresponsive. The mother called 911 over the objections of The Bishop and the boy's father.

continues

CASE STUDY (Continued)

Religious Beliefs Can Lead to Medical Conflict

Spiritual Assessment: FICA Tool

F: Faith and Belief

"Do you consider yourself spiritual or religious?" "Do you practice a specific faith?" "Do you have spiritual/religious beliefs that help you cope with stress?" "What gives your life meaning?"

The parents are devout members of a local religious commune. They believe in organic farming, natural foods, little or no technology, and spiritual prayer. The mother is a lapsed Catholic, and the father was a secular Jew when they met in college. It was there that they met The Bishop, who was in the process of founding a commune. The parents have lived together for 10 years, and Leaf was born in the commune 2 years after they had moved in together. The parents draw strength from the "oneness" of their community.

I: Importance

"What importance does your faith or belief have in your life?" "Have your beliefs influenced how you take care of yourself?" "What role do your beliefs have in regaining (or maintaining) your health?"

The parents dropped out of college and severed their ties to their families of origin in order to join the commune and live there. The father states that they are devout followers of The Bishop. The mother states, "Well, we were until this disaster happened."

C: Community

"Are you part of a spiritual or religious community?" "Does this group support you? How?" "Is there a group of people you really love or who are important to you?"

The parents have lived on the commune for 10 years and have three other children living with them there. The father is a farmer on the commune, and the mother teaches at the small school there. All aspects of life revolve only around their family and those of fellow commune members. They have not left the commune for years, not even for the birth of their children.

A: Address

"How would you like the health care team to address these issues in your son's health care?"

The father is demanding that The Bishop be contacted immediately and be brought into the hospital to pray for the boy. He also wants the boy taken off all life support immediately. The mother wants everything done to save her son. The mother is asking for the nurse to call a Catholic priest. The parents are yelling at each other in the ED.

Nursing Diagnosis

Spiritual distress related to Leaf's medical condition as manifested by parents crying, arguing, and demanding different health care interventions.

ASSESSMENT IN BRIEF

General Approach to Spiritual Assessment

1. If possible, choose a quiet, private room that will be free from interruptions.

2. Ensure that the room's light is sufficiently bright to observe the patient's verbal and nonverbal reactions.

3. Greet the patient, introduce yourself, and explain that you will be taking a health history.

4. Position yourself at eye level with the patient.

5. Portray an interested, nonjudgmental manner throughout the interview. Respect silence and diversity.

6. Use a spiritual assessment tool like FICA to engage the patient:
   Faith and Belief
   Importance
   Community
   Address

REVIEW QUESTIONS

1. Studies on prayer have shown:
   a. That prayer benefits patients
   b. That prayer is helpful only for dying patients
   c. Mixed results
   d. That prayer is measurable
   The correct answer is (c).

2. In the Pew Forum survey of religious identification, what was the largest group after Christian?
   a. Jewish   c. Hindu
   b. New Age   d. Unaffiliated
   The correct answer is (d).

3. Why do Muslim women wear the Hajib?
   a. Their husbands tell them to.
   b. Their tribe tells them to.
   c. Their Koran tells them to.
   d. Their Imam tells them to.
   The correct answer is (c).

4. A negative effect of religious and spiritual beliefs on health care is:
   a. Patients are too busy praying to participate in care.
   b. Patients try to convert their health care workers.
   c. Patients may choose to go against medical advice.
   d. Patients feel guilty for their sins.
   The correct answer is (c).

5. Praying with patients is acceptable if:
   a. The nurse sees a spiritual need.
   b. The patient has a nursing diagnosis of spiritual distress.
   c. The nurse is very religious.
   d. The patient leads the prayer.
   The correct answer is (d).

6. Most Native Americans:
   a. Follow Christianity
   b. Follow their ancient tribal religion
   c. Follow a New Age religion
   d. Follow no religion at all
   The correct answer is (a).

7. If a nurse suspects that parents are neglecting their child due to religious beliefs, the nurse should:
   a. Ask the parents to pray about their actions
   b. Point out the parents' theological errors
   c. Report suspected abuse according to state laws
   d. Not allow the parents or their minister to visit the patient
   The correct answer is (c).

8. A patient wearing a T-shirt with a large atheist slogan on it is admitted to the hospital. The nurse should:
   a. Skip the spiritual assessment, since the patient is an atheist
   b. Cover up the crucifix on the wall, since it's a Catholic hospital
   c. Instruct the hospital chaplain not to visit the patient
   d. Proceed with the spiritual assessment
   The correct answer is (d).

9. A Muslim patient may want to do what activity early in the morning?
   a. Sing hymns
   b. Bathe, obtain a clean blanket, and find out which direction is east
   c. Have a traditional bacon and eggs breakfast
   d. Read the Koran
   The correct answer is (d).

10. Kurt is a 42-year-old male and a home teacher who is assigned to look after a group of teens who are members of his faith community. He meets regularly with the teens, takes them on weekend hiking trips, and is available for spiritual help. What faith does Kurt most likely practice?
   a. Christian Science   c. Buddhism
   b. Jehovah's Witnesses   d. Latter-Day Saints
   The correct answer is (d).

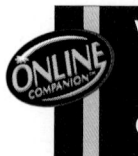
Visit the Estes online companion resource at
www.delmar.cengage.com
for additional content and study aids.
Click on Online Companions and then select
the Nursing discipline.

American Nurses Association and Health Ministries Association (2005). *Faith and community nursing: Scope and standards of parish nursing practice.* Washington, DC: Author.

Asser, S. M., & Swan, R. (1998). Child fatalities from religion-motivated neglect. *Pediatrics, 101*(4), 625–629.

Astrow, A. B., & Sulmasy, D. P. (2004). Spirituality and the patient-physician relationship. *JAMA, 291*(36), 2884.

Baetz, M., Griffen, R., Bowen, R., Koenig, H. G., & Marcoux, G. (2004). The association between spiritual/religious involvement and depressive symptoms in the Canadian populations. *Journal of Nervous and Mental Disorders, 192*(12), 818–822.

Balboni, T. A., Venderwerker, L. C., Block, S. D., Pualk, M. E., Lathan, C. S., Peteet, J. R., & Prigerson, H. G. (2007). Religiousness and spiritual support among advanced cancer patients and association with end-of-life treatment preferences and quality of life. *Journal of Clinical Oncology, 25*(5), 555–560.

Bard, J. (2006). Parish nursing: Faith community nurses and the prevention and management of addiction problems. *Journal of Addictions Nursing, 17*(2), 115–120.

Barnum, B. S. (1996). *Spirituality in nursing: From traditional to new age.* New York: Springer Publishing Co.

Benson, H., Dusek, J. A., Sherwood, J. B., Lam, P., Bethea, C. F., Carpenter, W., et al. (2006). Study of the therapeutic effects of intercessory prayer (STEP) in cardiac bypass patients: A multicenter randomized trial of uncertainty and certainty of receiving intercessory prayer. *American Heart Journal, 151*(4), 934–942.

Bokinskie, J. C., & Kloster, P. K. (2008). Effective parish nursing: Building success and overcoming barriers. *Journal of Christian Nursing, 25*(1), 20–25.

Caiger, B. (2006). *Walking alongside: The essence of parish nursing.* Victoria, BC, Canada: Trafford Publishing.

Carson, V. B., & Koenig, H. G. (2002). *Parish nursing: Stories of service and care.* West Chonshohocken, PA: Templeton Foundation Press.

Catanzaro, A. M., Meador, K. G., Koenig, H. G., Kuchibhatia, M., & Clipp, E. (2007). Congregational health ministries: A national study of pastor's views. *Public Health Nursing, 24*(1), 6–17.

Chen, Y. Y., & Koenig, H. G. (2006). Do people turn to religion in times of stress? An examination of change in religiousness among elderly medically ill patients. *Journal of Nervous and Mental Disease, 194*(2), 114–120.

Chu, J. J. (2004). Critical care extra. *American Journal of Nursing, 104*(2), 72GG–72HH.

Churchill, L. R. (2007). The dangers of looking for the health benefits of religion. *Lancet, 369*(9572), 1509–1510.

Dawkins, R. (2006). *The God delusion.* New York: Houghton Mifflin Co.

Dossey, L. (2005). Are prayer experiments legitimate? Twenty criticisms. *The Journal of Science and Healing, 1*(2), 109–117.

FoxNews.com. (2007, August 30). Florida chaplain says hospital fired him for saying "Jesus" in prayers. Retrieved from www.foxnews.com/story/0.2933.295334.00.html

Freedom from Religion Foundation. (2008). http://ffrf.org/legal/legal12.php#veteran

Gallup Poll. (2006). www.gallup.com/poll/religion

Hamilton, J., Powe, B., Pollard, A., Lee, K., & Felton, A. (2007). Spirituality among cancer survivors: Having a personal relationship with God. *Cancer Nursing, 30*(4), 309–316.

Hampton, J. S., & Weinart, C. (2006). An exploration of spirituality in rural women with chronic illness. *Holistic Nursing Practice, 20*(1), 27–33.

Harris, W. S., Gowda, M., Kolb, J. W., Strychacz, C. P., Vacek, J. L., Jones, P. G., et al. (1999). A randomized controlled trial of the effects of remote intercessory prayer on outcomes in patients admitted to the coronary care unit. *Archives of Internal Medicine, 159*(19), 2273–2278.

Harrison, M. O., Edwards, C. L., Koenig, H. G., Bosworth, H. B., Decastro, L., & Wood, M. (2005). Religiosity/spirituality and pain in patients with sickle cell disease. *Journal of Nervous and Mental Disease, 193*(4), 250–257.

Haynes, D. F., & Watt, P. J. (2008). The lived experience of healthy behaviors in people with debilitating illness. *Holistic Nursing Practice, 22*(1), 44–53.

Helm, H. M., Hays, J. C., Flint, E. P., Koenig, H. G., & Blazer, D. G. (2000). Does private religious activity prolong survival? A six-year follow-up study of 3,851 older adults. *Journal of Gerontology Series A—Biological Sciences and Medical Sciences, 55*(7), M400–M405.

Hitchens, C. (2007). *God is not great: How religion poisons everything.* New York: Hachette Book Group, USA.

Hughes, J. W., Tomlinson, A., Blumenthal, J. A., Davidson, J., Sketch, H. M., & Watkins, L. L. (2004). Social support and religiosity as coping strategies for anxiety in hospitalized cardiac patients. *Annals of Behavioral Medicine, 28*(3), 179–185.

Kelly, J. (2004). Spirituality as a coping mechanism. *Dimensions of Critical Care Nursing, 23*(4), 162–168.

Koenig, H. G. (2007a). *Spirituality in patient care: Why, how, when and what* (2nd ed.). Philadelphia: Templeton Foundation Press.

Koenig, H. G. (2007b). Religion and depression in older medical inpatients. *American Journal of Geriatric Psychiatry, 15*(4), 282–291.

Koenig, H. G. (2007c). Religion and remission of depression in medical inpatients with heart failure/pulmonary disease. *Journal of Nervous and Mental Disease, 195*(5), 389–395.

Koenig, H. G., George, L. K., & Titus, P. (2004). Religion, spirituality and health in medically ill hospitalized older patients. *Journal of the American Geriatrics Association, 52*(4), 554–562.

Krucoff, M. W., Crater, S. W., Gallup, D., Blankenship, J. C., Cuff, M., Guarneri, M., et al. (2005). Music, imagery, touch and prayer as adjuncts to interventional cardiac care: The monitoring and actualization of Noetic training (MANTRA) II randomized study. *Lancet, 366*(9481), 211–217.

Krucoff, M. W., Crater, S. W., Green, C. L., Maas, A. C., Seskevich, J. E., Lane, J. D., et al. (2001). Integrative noetic therapies as adjuncts to percutaneous intervention during unstable coronary syndrome: Monitoring and actualizing of noetic training (MANTRA) feasibility pilot. *American Heart Journal, 142*(5), 760–769.

Krucoff, M. W., Crater, S. W., & Lee, K. L. (2006). From efficacy to safety concerns: A STEP forward or a step back for clinical research and intercessory prayer? The study of therapeutic effects of intercessory prayer (STEP). *American Heart Journal, 151*(4), 762–764.

Leak, A., Hu, J., & King, C. (2008). Symptom distress, spirituality and quality of life in African-American breast cancer survivors. *Cancer Nursing, 31*(1), E15–E21.

Margolick, D. (1990, August 6). In child deaths, a test for Christian Science. *New York Times.*

Matthews, D. A. (2000). Prayer and spirituality. *Rheumatic Disease Clinics of North America, 26*(1), 177–187.

NANDA International. (2009). NANDA-I *Nursing diagnoses: Definitions & classifications 2009–2011.* West Sussex, United Kingdom: John Wiley & Sons, Ltd.

Newport, F. (2006). Religion most important to Blacks, women and older Americans. Self-reported importance of religion decreases with education. Retrieved July 21, 2008, from http://www.gallup.com/poll/25585/religion-most-important-blacks-women-older-Americans.aspx

NPR. (2008, February 26). Religion survey finds many Americans swap faiths. Retrieved from http://www.npr.org/templates/story/story.php?story = 19354039

O'Brien, M. E. (2003). *Parish nursing: Health care ministry within the church.* Sudbury, MA: Jones and Bartlett.

O'Brien, M. E. (2008). *Spirituality in nursing: Standing on holy ground* (3rd ed.). Boston: Jones and Bartlett Publishers.

Ostbye, T., Krause, K. M., Norton, M. C., Tschanz, J., Sanders, L., Hayden, K., et al. (2006). Ten dimensions of health and their relationships with overall self-reported health and survival in a predominantly religiously active elderly populations: The Cache County memory study. *Journal of the American Geriatrics Society, 54*(2), 199–209.

Pew Forum on Religion and Public Life. (2008). Summary of key findings. Retrieved July 7, 2008, from http://religions.pewforum.org/reports

Potter, J. Two controversial religious sects from the 1970s have an impact on Noble County (Indiana). *The News-Sun.* Retrieved from http://kpcnews.net/specialsections/reflections2/reflections36.html

Puchalski, C. M., & Romer, A. L. (2000). Taking a spiritual history allows clinicians to understand patients more fully. *Journal of Palliative Medicine, 3*(1), 129–137.

Redmond, G. M. (2006). Aging matters: Developing programs for older adults in a faith community. *Journal of Psychosocial Nursing, 44*(11), 15–18.

Roff, L. L, Klemmack, D. L., Parker, M., Koenig, H. G., Baker, P., & Allman, R. L. (2005). Religiosity, smoking, exercise and obesity among Southern community-dwelling older adults. *Journal of Applied Gerontology, 24*(4), 337–354.

Salmon, J. L. (2007). Chaplains' complaints of bias rise at NIH. Retrieved September 16, 2008, from www.washingtonpost.com/wp-dyn/content/article/2007/14/13/AR2007041302347_pf.html

Shelly, J. A. (Ed.). (2002). *Nursing in the church.* Madison, WI: NCF Press.

Sloan, R. P. (2000, January–February). Religion, spirituality and medicine. *Freethought Today.* Retrieved from http://ffrf.org/fttoday/2000.jan_feb2000/sloan.html

Sloan, R. P. (2006). *Blind faith: The unholy alliance of religion and medicine.* New York: St. Martin's Press.

Sloan, R. P., Bagiella, E., & Powell, L. (1999). Religion, spirituality and medicine. *Lancet, 353*(9153), 664–667.

Solari-Twadell, P. A., & McDermott, M. A. (Eds.). (2006). *Parish nursing: Development, education and administration.* St. Louis: Mosby.

Steinhauser, K. E., Voils, C. I., Clipp, E. C., Bosworth, B. H., Christakis, N. A., & Tulsky, J. A. (2006). Are you at peace? One item to probe spiritual concerns at the end of life. *Archives of Internal Medicine, 166*(1), 101–105.

Sulmasy, D. P. (2006). Spiritual issues in the care of dying patients. "…it's okay between me and God." *JAMA, 296*(11), 1385–1392.

VanDover, C., & Pfeiffer, J. B. (2007). Spiritual care in Christian parish nursing. *Journal of Advanced Nursing, 57*(2), 213–221.

Watchman Fellowship, Inc. (2000). Faith assembly (Hobart Freeman). Retrieved September 16, 2008, from www.watchman.org/cults/freeman.htm

BIBLIOGRAPHY

Deloria, Y., Jr., Silko, L. M., & Tinker, G. E. (2003). *God is red: A native view of religion.* Golden, CO: Fulcrum Publishing.

Galek, K., Flannelly, K., Vane, A., & Galek, R. (2005). Assessing a patient's spiritual needs: A comprehensive instrument. *Holistic Nursing Practice, 19*(2), 62–69.

Hospice and Palliative Nursing Association. (2007). HPNA Position Paper: Spiritual care. *Journal of Hospice and Palliative Nursing, 9*(1), 15–16.

Mira, L. (2004). Spirituality in Korea: A fog of religion and culture. *Journal of Christian Nursing, 21*(1), 29–31.

Moon, C. (2001). *A medicine woman speaks: An exploration of Native American spirituality.* Franklin Lakes, NJ: The Career Press, Inc.

Newlin, K., Knaff, K., & Melkus, G. D. E. (2002). African-American spirituality: A concept analysis. *Advances in Nursing Science, 25*(2), 57–70.

O'Brien, B. L. (2002). 21st century rural nursing: Navajo traditional and Western medicine. *Nursing Administration Quarterly, 26*(5), 47–51.

O'Rourke, K. D., & Boyle, P. (1999). *Medical ethics: Sources of Catholic teachings* (3rd ed.). Washington DC: Georgetown Press.

Puchalski, C. M. (2006). *A time for listening and caring: Spirituality and the care of the chronically ill and dying.* New York: Oxford University Press.

Solari-Twadell, P. A., & McDermott, M. A. (Eds.). (1999). *Parish nursing: Promoting whole person health within faith communities.* Thousand Oaks, CA: Sage Publications, Inc.

Westburg-McNamara, J. (2006). *Health and wellness: What your faith community can do.* Cleveland, OH: Pilgrim Press.

Winslow, G. R., & Winslow, B. W. (2003). Examining the ethics of praying with patients. *Holistic Nursing Practice, 17*(4), 170–178.

WEB SITES

Adherents: National & World Religion Statistics—Church Statistics—World Religions:
http://www.adherents.com

Beliefnet: Inspiration. Spirituality. Faith:
http://www.beliefnet.com

Duke Center for Spirituality and Health:
http://www.Dukespiritualityandhealth.org

Freedom from Religion Foundation:
http://www.ffrf.org

George Washington University Institute for Spirituality & Health:
http://www.gwish.org

Indiana State University Center for the Study of Health, Religion, and Spirituality:
http://www.indstate.edu/

Religion Facts:
http://www.religionfacts.com

Ontario Consultants on Religious Tolerance:
http://www.religioustolerance.org

International Parish Nurse Resource Center:
http://www.parishnurses.org

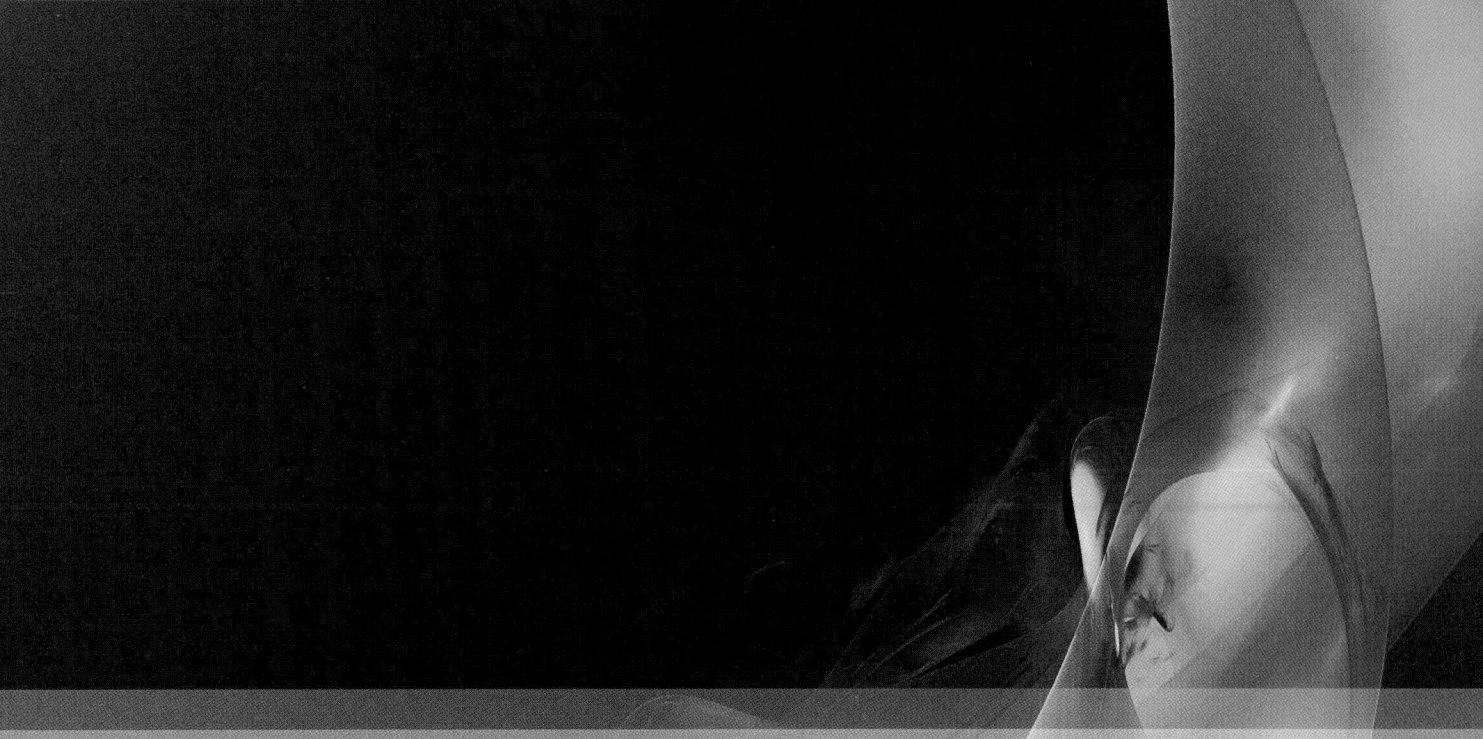

CHAPTER 7

Nutritional Assessment

COMPETENCIES

1. Describe key recommendations of the Dietary Guidelines for Americans 2005.

2. Describe the USDA's food guidance system, MyPyramid. Devise a teaching plan that you can use to educate patients on this nutritional model.

3. Identify nutritional differences for different age groups.

4. Perform a nutritional history and physical assessment.

5. Perform anthropometric measurements.

6. Describe laboratory analyses and their clinical significance to the nutritional assessment.

Nutrition, or the processes by which the body metabolizes and utilizes nutrients, affects every system in the body. We must have food and drink to sustain life, but what type and how much are the questions that must be asked when assessing a person's nutritional health. Health care providers must also understand how the body digests and absorbs nutrients, the importance of meeting daily nutritional requirements, and the causes and results of an imbalance of nutrients and how to assess it. Psychological, social, environmental, financial, and cultural issues must also be considered during a nutritional assessment.

The U.S. Department of Health and Human Services' *Healthy People 2010* public health initiative identified two areas that focus specifically on **nutrition** and food: nutrition and overweight, and food safety. Proper nutrition greatly affects the development and course of many chronic conditions (e.g., coronary artery disease, diabetes mellitus, and hypertension). *Healthy People 2010* strives to increase each American's quality of life and number of years of healthy life, and to eliminate disparities in health by solid dietary practices.

DIETARY GUIDELINES

The Dietary Guidelines Advisory Committee published its 5-year revision of the *Dietary Guidelines for Americans* in 2005. The committee's aim is to reduce the morbidity and mortality of diseases through diet and physical activity. The U.S. Department of Health and Human Services and the U.S. Department of Agriculture (USDA) use this information to formulate programs and policies for the American public. Table 7-1 lists the key recommendations for each subject area.

TABLE 7-1 Dietary Guidelines for Americans 2005

ADEQUATE NUTRIENTS WITHIN CALORIE NEEDS: KEY RECOMMENDATIONS

- Consume a variety of nutrient-dense foods and beverages within and among the basic food groups while choosing foods that limit the intake of saturated and trans fats, cholesterol, added sugars, salt, and alcohol.
- Meet recommended intakes within energy needs by adopting a balanced eating pattern, such as the USDA Food Guide or the DASH Eating Plan.

WEIGHT MANAGEMENT: KEY RECOMMENDATIONS

- To maintain body weight in a healthy range, balance calories from foods and beverages with calories expended.
- To prevent gradual weight gain over time, make small decreases in food and beverage calories and increase physical activity.

PHYSICAL ACTIVITY: KEY RECOMMENDATIONS

- Engage in regular physical activity and reduce sedentary activities to promote health, psychological well-being, and a healthy body weight.
  - To reduce the risk of chronic disease in adulthood: Engage in at least 30 minutes of moderate-intensity physical activity, above usual activity, at work or home on most days of the week.
  - For most people, greater health benefits can be obtained by engaging in physical activity of more vigorous intensity or longer duration.
  - To help manage body weight and prevent gradual, unhealthy body weight gain in adulthood: Engage in approximately 60 minutes of moderate- to vigorous-intensity activity on most days of the week while not exceeding caloric intake requirements.
  - To sustain weight loss in adulthood: Participate in at least 60 to 90 minutes of daily moderate-intensity physical activity while not exceeding caloric intake requirements. Some people may need to consult with a health care provider before participating in this level of activity.
- Achieve physical fitness by including cardiovascular conditioning, stretching exercises for flexibility, and resistance exercises or calisthenics for muscle strength and endurance.

continues

TABLE 7-1 (Continued)

FOOD GROUPS TO ENCOURAGE: KEY RECOMMENDATIONS

- Consume a sufficient amount of fruits and vegetables while staying within energy needs. Two cups of fruit and 2½ cups of vegetables per day are recommended for a reference 2,000-calorie intake, with higher or lower amounts depending on the calorie level.
- Choose a variety of fruits and vegetables each day. In particular, select from all five vegetable subgroups (dark green, orange, legumes, starchy vegetables, and other vegetables) several times a week.
- Consume 3 or more ounce-equivalents of whole grain products per day, with the rest of the recommended grains coming from enriched or whole grain products. In general, at least half the grains should come from whole grains.
- Consume 3 cups per day of fat-free or low-fat milk or equivalent milk products.

FATS: KEY RECOMMENDATIONS

- Consume less than 10% of calories from saturated fatty acids and less than 300 mg/day of cholesterol, and keep trans fatty acid consumption as low as possible.
- Keep total fat intake between 20% and 35% of calories, with most fats coming from sources of polyunsaturated and monounsaturated fatty acids, such as fish, nuts, and vegetable oils.
- When selecting and preparing meat, poultry, dry beans, and milk or milk products, make choices that are lean, low-fat, or fat-free.
- Limit intake of fats and oils high in saturated and/or trans-fatty acids, and choose products low in such fats and oils.

CARBOHYDRATES: KEY RECOMMENDATIONS

- Choose fiber-rich fruits, vegetables, and whole grains often.
- Choose and prepare foods and beverages with little added sugars or caloric sweeteners, such as amounts suggested by the USDA Food Guide and the DASH Eating Plan.
- Reduce the incidence of dental caries by practicing good oral hygiene and consuming sugar- and starch-containing foods and beverages less frequently.

SODIUM AND POTASSIUM: KEY RECOMMENDATIONS

- Consume less than 2,300 mg (approximately 1 tsp) of sodium per day.
- Choose and prepare foods with little salt. At the same time, consume potassium-rich foods, such as fruits and vegetables.

ALCOHOLIC BEVERAGES: KEY RECOMMENDATIONS

- Those who choose to drink alcoholic beverages should do so sensibly and in moderation—defined as the consumption of up to one drink per day for women and up to two drinks per day for men.
- Alcoholic beverages should not be consumed by some individuals, including those who cannot restrict their alcohol intake, women of childbearing age who may become pregnant, pregnant and lactating women, children and adolescents, individuals taking medications that can interact with alcohol, and those with specific medical conditions.
- Alcoholic beverages should be avoided by individuals engaging in activities that require attention, skill, or coordination, such as driving or operating machinery.

From *Dietary Guidelines for Americans, 2005* (6th ed.), by the U.S. Department of Health and Human Services and U.S. Department of Agriculture, 2005, Washington, DC: U.S. Government Printing Office.

Dietary guidelines are published by various government agencies to educate the general population regarding dietary needs. In 1997, the Food and Nutrition Board of the Institute of Medicine developed **Dietary Reference Intakes** (DRIs). DRIs are used to assess an individual's diet and are the basis on which nutritious, balanced diets are devised. DRIs have three components: Adequate Intake (AI), Tolerable Upper Intake Level (UL), and Recommended Dietary Allowances (RDA). AI is the specific intake value that is estimated to provide adequate nutrition for each sex and for various age groups. UL is the maximum level of daily nutrients that is unlikely to pose health risks for most of the general population. **Recommended dietary allowances** (RDA) are the recommended amounts of

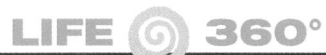

Application of DRIs in Different Settings

Many varieties of multivitamins and supplements are available at drug stores, nutrition centers, natural product stores, and other locations. Visit three different types of businesses and look at their products. Compare the products with the DRIs for individuals (you will first need to access the DRI Web site at www. nap.edu to find the numerical value for each vitamin and mineral). Do you see any similarities? Differences? How can you incorporate this information into your clinical practice?

nutrients that should be eaten daily by healthy individuals. Recommendations differ based on sex, age, and whether the patient is pregnant or lactating. These are recommendations, not requirements. Requirements are the amounts needed to prevent deficiencies. Recommendations exceed the required amounts in order to ensure that the entire population is considered.

Historically, another framework to guide dietary intake was the "Basic Four" food guide. The "Basic Four" food guide, first issued in 1956, divided foods into four groups: milk and dairy, meats, vegetables and fruits, and breads and cereals. The USDA published recommendations in 1992 using the Food Guide Pyramid, which expanded on the original basic four food groups to include guidelines on proportions and moderation. The Food Guide Pyramid was introduced to provide Americans with guidelines to improve their diets. Six different food groups represented specific nutrients. In recent years, the Food Guide Pyramid was criticized because it failed to distinguish among the various fats (e.g., polyunsaturated and Omega-3 fatty acids versus saturated and trans-unsaturated fats), it did not differentiate between high- and low-fat dairy products, and it did not address portion size. Regardless of its shortcomings, the Food Guide Pyramid was the accepted standard until 2005.

In 2005, the USDA published a new food guidance system to replace the original 1992 Food Guide Pyramid. The MyPyramid (see Figure 7-1) plan offers individuals a more personalized approach to nutrition that combines healthy eating with physical activity. MyPyramid is applicable to Americans over age 2. By introducing all Americans to MyPyramid and its slogan, "Steps to a Healthier You," the USDA hopes to help people make informed and healthier food choices. These choices can lead to a decrease in major nutrition-related chronic diseases such as anemia, diabetes mellitus, coronary heart disease, hypertension, and alcoholic cirrhosis.

MyPyramid is the former Food Guide Pyramid tipped on its side. The color bands in MyPyramid represent the types of foods that should be consumed, and the width of the band denotes the approximate relative quantity of each food that should be consumed. In addition, MyPyramid incorporates the concept of physical activity into its design. A person climbing the stairs denotes the importance of physical activity in one's daily life, just as the food groups denote daily food intake. Personalization of one's diet is easy to accomplish by accessing the MyPyramid Web site, where age, gender, and physical activity can be keyed in, and more specific nutrition guidelines are provided. Twelve different pyramids are available on the Web site using these parameters. The 12 pyramids range from daily intake levels of

REFLECTIVE THINKING

Implementing Dietary Guidelines for Americans 2005

- Review the key recommendations of the Dietary Guidelines for Americans 2005 in Table 7-1.
- Perform a personal assessment of how well your diet and physical activity conform to each of the eight focus areas: adequate nutrients within calorie needs, weight management, physical activity, food groups to encourage, fats, carbohydrates, sodium and potassium, and alcoholic beverages.
- Now visit the Dietary Guidelines Web site, www.health.gov/DietaryGuidelines/dga2005/document/, and click on Executive Summary. Explore the key recommendations for specific population groups. Does this information alter the assessment you performed on yourself? How?
- Using the Dietary Guidelines, interview a pregnant woman, a lactating woman, a teenage girl and boy, a man in his 50s, and a woman in her 70s. How do their diet and activity compare with the key recommendations? What chronic diseases do they have? Has their disease led to morbidity? Devise a nursing care plan for each individual.
- What are the strengths of the Dietary Guidelines? Weaknesses? How can you implement the guidelines in your clinical practice?

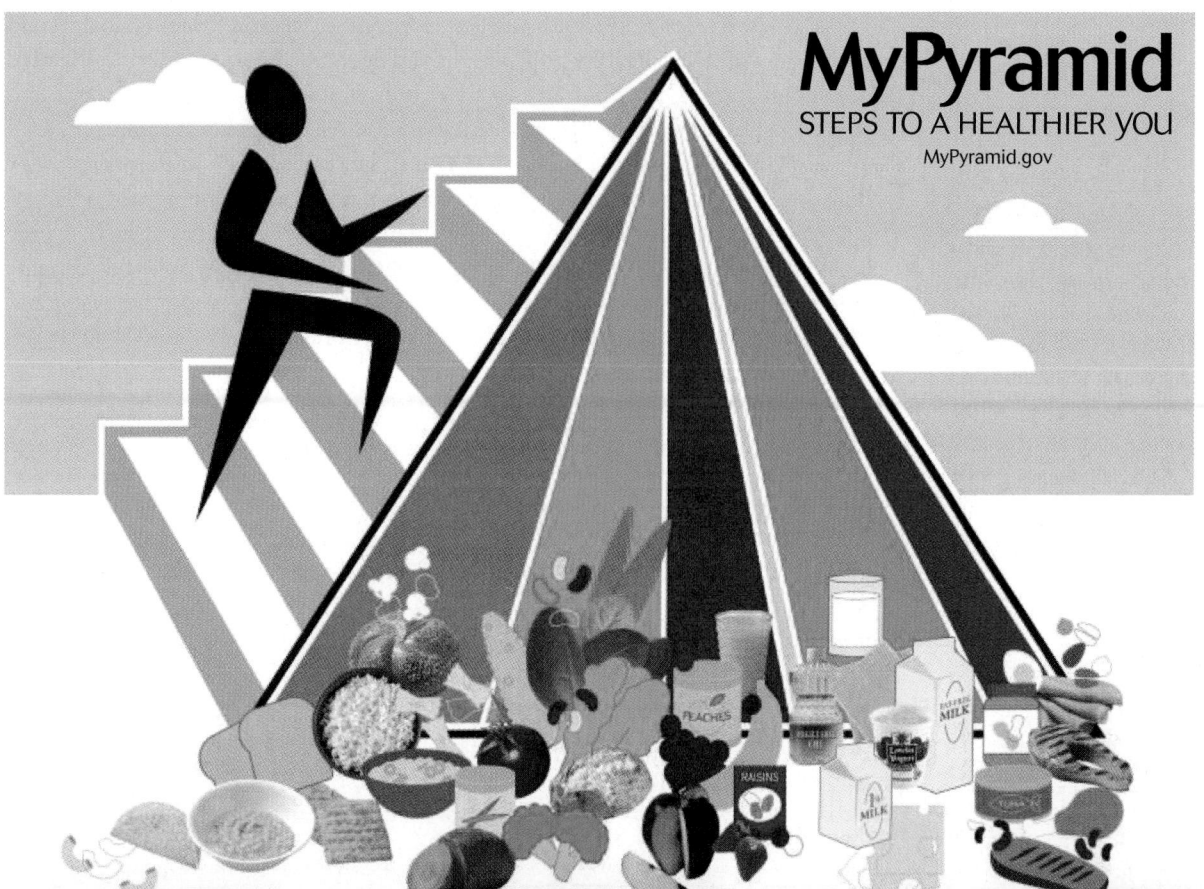

MyPyramid
STEPS TO A HEALTHIER YOU
MyPyramid.gov

GRAINS	VEGETABLES	FRUITS	OILS	MILK	MEAT & BEANS
Make half your grains whole	Vary your veggies	Focus on fruits		Get your calcium-rich foods	Go lean with protein
Eat at least 3 oz. of whole-grain cereals, breads, crackers, rice, or pasta every day 1 oz. is about 1 slice of bread, about 1 cup of breakfast cereal, or ½ cup of cooked rice, cereal, or pasta	Eat more dark-green veggies like broccoli, spinach, and other dark leafy greens Eat more orange vegetables like carrots and sweet potatoes Eat more dry beans and peas like pinto beans, kidney beans, and lentils	Eat a variety of fruit Choose fresh, frozen, canned, or dried fruit Go easy on fruit juices		Go low-fat or fat-free when you choose milk, yogurt, and other milk products If you don't or can't consume milk, choose lactose-free products or other calcium sources such as fortified foods and beverages	Choose low-fat or lean meats and poultry Bake it, broil it, or grill it Vary your protein routine — choose more fish, beans, peas, nuts, and seeds

For a 2,000-calorie diet, you need the amounts below from each food group. To find the amounts that are right for you, go to MyPyramid.gov.

Eat 6 oz. every day	Eat 2½ cups every day	Eat 2 cups every day	Get 3 cups every day; for kids aged 2 to 8, it's 2	Eat 5½ oz. every day

Find your balance between food and physical activity
- Be sure to stay within your daily calorie needs.
- Be physically active for at least 30 minutes most days of the week.
- About 60 minutes a day of physical activity may be needed to prevent weight gain.
- For sustaining weight loss, at least 60 to 90 minutes a day of physical activity may be required.
- Children and teenagers should be physically active for 60 minutes every day, or most days.

Know the limits on fats, sugars, and salt (sodium)
- Make most of your fat sources from fish, nuts, and vegetable oils.
- Limit solid fats like butter, margarine, shortening, and lard, as well as foods that contain these.
- Check the Nutrition Facts label to keep saturated fats, *trans* fats, and sodium low.
- Choose food and beverages low in added sugars. Added sugars contribute calories with few, if any, nutrients.

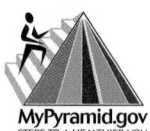

MyPyramid.gov
STEPS TO A HEALTHIER YOU

U.S. Department of Agriculture
Center for Nutrition Policy and Promotion
April 2005
CNPP-15

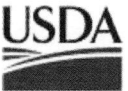

USDA is an equal opportunity provider and employer.

FIGURE 7-1 **MyPyramid Food Guide.** *From the U.S. Department of Agriculture, Center for Nutrition Policy and Promotion, http://www.mypyramid.gov, April 2005.*

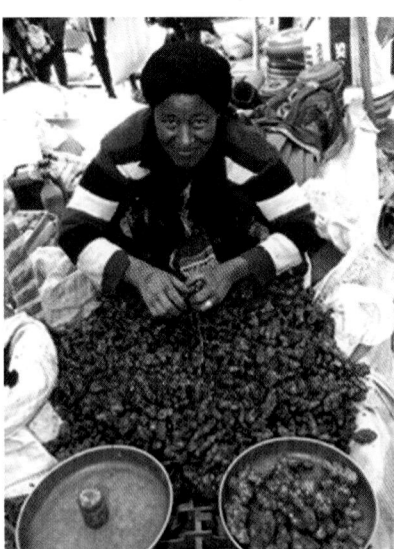

FIGURE 7-2 Accurate nutritional assessment necessitates knowledge of the nutrients within the food. *Courtesy of WHO/P. Virot.*

1,000 to 3,200 calories. By following the appropriate pyramid, an individual should be able to maintain a healthy body weight and decrease the risk of nutrition-related chronic diseases. Quantities are stated in household measures such as cups and ounces instead of the servings that were used in the Food Guide Pyramid.

However, MyPyramid has been criticized by researchers and nutritionists for not addressing the nutritional needs for children under age 2 or pregnant or lactating women. Also, although the interactive nature of MyPyramid is attractive, only highly motivated individuals with access to a computer can reap the full benefits of the system. Last, MyPyramid fails to incorporate the daily amount of water and trans fatty acids that is advisable to consume. Consult the MyPyramid Web site on a regular basis to keep abreast of any changes or additions.

NUTRIENTS

To perform a proper nutritional assessment, you must have a clear understanding of the various nutrients needed to provide an adequate diet, the reason they are needed, and the food sources that provide them (Figure 7-2). **Nutrients** are the substances found in food that are nourishing and useful to the body. Carbohydrates, proteins, fats, vitamins, minerals, and water are the nutrients essential for life.

Carbohydrates, proteins, and fats supply the body with energy, which is measured in units called **kilocalories** (kcal). A kilocalorie (also called calorie) is the amount of heat required to raise 1 gram of water 1 degree centigrade. The USDA guidelines for calculating caloric requirements are based on activity level and the ideal body weight (IBW) multiplied by a specific number of calories per pound.

CALORIES/POUND OF IBW		
Activity	**Females**	**Males**
Sedentary	14	16
Moderate	18	21
Heavy	22	26

A 130-pound female who performs a moderate amount of exercise should have a daily intake of 2,340 calories (18×130), and a 165-pound male who performs a moderate amount of exercise should have an intake of 3,465 calories (21×165). This is compared to a 1,820-calorie intake (14×130) for the 130-pound woman and a 2,640-calorie intake (16×165) for the 165-pound man who lead sedentary lifestyles.

CARBOHYDRATES

The major source of energy for the various functions of the body is **carbohydrates**. Each gram of carbohydrate contains four calories. Adults require 50% to 60% of their daily caloric intake in the form of carbohydrates to prevent ketosis and protein breakdown of muscles.

Carbohydrates help form adenosine triphosphate (ATP), which is needed to transfer energy within the cells. Carbohydrates supply fiber and assist in the utilization of fat. The primary sources of carbohydrates are bread, potatoes, pasta, corn, rice, dried beans, and fruits. Dietary deficiency of carbohydrates can result in electrolyte imbalance, fatigue, and depression. On the other hand, an excess of carbohydrates may produce obesity and tooth decay, and may adversely affect those with diabetes mellitus.

Diets high in fiber have been shown to be beneficial in disease prevention. The possible benefits are decreased weight and decreases in the risks of colon cancer, rectal cancer, heart disease (through decreasing serum cholesterol levels), dental caries, constipation, and diverticulosis.

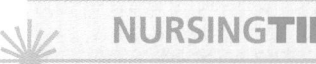

PROTEINS

There are four calories in every gram of protein, but foods usually are a combination of protein and fat (meats, milk) or protein and carbohydrates (legumes). Adults require 0.8 g/kg/day of protein, or approximately 10–20% of their daily caloric intake. **Protein** is required to give the body the nine essential amino acids that the body is unable to synthesize. These are needed to form the basis of all cell structures in the body. Protein is needed to manufacture and repair body tissue; it helps to maintain osmotic pressure within the cells; it is a component of antibodies; and it is ultimately a source of energy. The major sources of protein are meat, poultry, fish, eggs, cheese, and milk. Legumes (dried beans and peas) are a good source of protein when eaten with corn or wheat (e.g., beans and rice provide a good source of protein). This is helpful information for vegetarians and people whose incomes will not cover the purchase of meat and milk products.

FATS

Lipids, or fats, contain nine calories per gram. The recommendation of many health care experts is to use fats in the diet sparingly, and to reduce fat to 20–30% of the total calories consumed. **Fats** supply the essential fatty acids, which form a part of the structure of all cells and must be supplied by the diet. They also help to lower the serum cholesterol. Fats influence the texture and taste of food. The food sources of fat are animal fat (butter, shortening, and lard) and vegetable fat (vegetable oil, margarine, and nuts). The types of fats consumed in the diet should be evaluated. **Saturated fats** come from both animal sources (butter, lard, and fatty meats) and vegetable sources (coconut, palm, and partially hydrogenated oils that occur in some processed foods). Saturated fats have been found to raise the cholesterol level. **Monosaturated fats** (olive and canola oils) lower LDL cholesterol and do not lower HDL cholesterol. **Cholesterol** is a lipid found only in animal products. It is found in muscle, red blood cells, and cell membranes. Cholesterol is transported in the blood by **high-density lipoproteins** (HDL) and **low-density lipoproteins** (LDL). The HDL are useful in carrying cholesterol toward the liver. The LDL carry the cholesterol toward the cells and then tissues, and deposit it there. There is a strong association between high levels of LDL and coronary artery disease (CAD). In contrast, high levels of HDL protect against CAD.

Triglycerides account for most of the lipids stored in the body's tissues. In the bloodstream, triglycerides produce energy for the body. An elevated triglyceride level occurs in hyperlipidemia, a risk factor for CAD.

A deficiency of fat in the diet can cause a decrease in weight, lack of satiety, and skin and hair changes. An excess of fat in the diet contributes to obesity and is linked to CAD. There has also been a correlation between high-fat diets and certain cancers (colon, breast, and prostate, in particular).

VITAMINS

Vitamins are organic substances needed to maintain the function of the body. They are not supplied by the body in sufficient amounts and must be obtained from dietary sources. Vitamins stored in dietary fat and absorbed in the fat portions of the body's cells are **fat-soluble vitamins**. These are vitamins A, D, E, and K. **Water-soluble vitamins** include C, thiamine (B_1), riboflavin (B_2), niacin (B_3), pyridoxine (B_6), folacin (folate), cobalamin (B_{12}), pantothenic acid, and biotin. They are not stored in the body but excreted in the urine. Various disease conditions occur when a vitamin source is lacking. Table 7-2 discusses the signs and symptoms of vitamin deficiencies and excesses.

TABLE 7-2 Fat-Soluble Vitamins and Water-Soluble Vitamins

NAME	FOOD AND OTHER SOURCES	FUNCTIONS	DEFICIENCY/TOXICITY

Vitamin A (retinol)	Animal:
	  Kidney
	  Liver
	  Whole milk
	  Butter
	  Cream
	  Cod liver oil
	Plants:
	  Dark green, leafy vegetables
	  Deep yellow or orange fruit
	  Fortified margarine
		Dim-light vision
		Maintenance of mucous membranes
		Growth and development of bones
			Deficiency:
			  Night blindness
			  Xerophthalmia
			  Respiratory infections
			  Bone growth ceases
			Toxicity:
			  Cessation of menstruation
			  Joint pain
			  Stunted growth
			  Enlargement of liver

Vitamin D (cholecalciferol)	Animal:
	  Eggs
	  Liver
	  Fish liver oils
	  Fortified milk
	Plants:
	  None
	Other:
	  Sunlight
		Bone growth
		Teeth development
			Deficiency:
			  Rickets
			  Osteomalacia
			  Osteoporosis
			  Poorly developed teeth
			  Muscle spasms
			Toxicity:
			  Nephrolithiasis
			  Calcification of soft tissues

Vitamin E (alphatocopherol)	Animal:
	  None
	Plants:
	  Legumes
	  Whole grains
	  Dark green, leafy vegetables
	  Margarines
	  Salad dressing
		Antioxidant	Deficiency:
			  Destruction of RBCs
			Toxicity:
			  Hypertension

Vitamin K	Animal:
	  Egg yolk
	  Liver
	  Milk
	Plants:
	  Green, leafy vegetables
	  Cabbage
		Blood clotting	Deficiency:
			  Prolonged blood clotting
			Toxicity:
			  Hemolytic anemia
			  Jaundice

Thiamin (vitamin B_1)	Animal:
	  Pork
	  Beef
	  Liver
	  Eggs
	  Fish
	Plants:
	  Whole and enriched grains
	  Legumes
		Coenzyme in oxidation of glucose
		Normal appetite
		Healthy nervous system
			Deficiency:
			  Gastrointestinal tract, nervous, and cardiovascular system problems
			Toxicity:
			  None

continues

TABLE 7-2 (Continued)

NAME	FOOD AND OTHER SOURCES	FUNCTIONS	DEFICIENCY/TOXICITY

Riboflavin (vitamin B_2)	Animal:
	  Liver
	  Kidney
	  Milk
	Plants:
	  Green, leafy vegetables
	  Cereals
	  Enriched bread
		Aids release of energy
		  from food
		Healthy skin
		Healthy vision
			Deficiency:
			  Cheilosis
			  Glossitis
			  Photophobia
			Toxicity:
			  None

Pyridoxine (vitamin B_6)	Animal:
	  Fish
	  Poultry
	  Pork
	  Milk
	  Eggs
	Plants:
	  Whole grain cereals
	  Legumes
		Synthesis of nonessential
		  amino acids
		Conversion of tryptophan
		  to niacin
		Antibody production
			Deficiency:
			  Cheilosis
			  Glossitis
			Toxicity:
			  Liver disease

Vitamin B_{12} (cyanocobalamin)	Animal:
	  Seafood
	  Meat
	  Eggs
	  Milk
	Plants:
	  None
		Synthesis of RBCs
		Maintenance of myelin
		  sheaths
			Deficiency:
			  Degeneration of myelin
			    sheaths
			  Pernicious anemia
			Toxicity:
			  None

Niacin (nicotinic acid)	Animal:
	  Milk
	  Eggs
	  Fish
	  Poultry
	Plants:
	  None
		Transfers hydrogen atoms
		  for synthesis of ATP
		Healthy skin
		Healthy nervous system
		Healthy digestion
			Deficiency:
			  Pellagra
			  Dermatitis
			  Dementia
			  Diarrhea
			Toxicity:
			  Vasodilation of blood vessels

Folacin (folic acid)	Animal:
	  Liver
	Plants:
	  Green, leafy vegetables
	  Spinach
	  Asparagus
	  Broccoli
	  Kidney beans
		Synthesis of RBCs	Deficiency:
			  Glossitis
			  Macrocytic anemia
			  Neural tube defects of fetus
			    in pregnant females
			Toxicity:
			  None

Biotin	Animal:
	  Milk
	  Liver
	Plants:
	  Legumes
	  Mushrooms
		Coenzyme in carbohy-
		  drate and amino acid
		  metabolism
		Niacin synthesis from
		  tryptophan
			Deficiency:
			  Dermatitis
			  Loss of hair
			Toxicity:
			  None

continues

TABLE 7-2 (Continued)

NAME	FOOD AND OTHER SOURCES	FUNCTIONS	DEFICIENCY/TOXICITY
Pantothenic acid	Animal: Eggs Liver Salmon Yeast Plants: Mushrooms Cauliflower Peanuts	Metabolism of carbo- hydrates, lipids, and proteins Synthesis of acetylcholine	Deficiency: Burning sensation in feet Toxicity: None
Vitamin C (ascorbic acid)	Animal: None Plants: All citrus Broccoli Tomatoes Brussels sprouts Potatoes	Prevention of scurvy Formation of collagen Healing of wounds Release of stress hormones Absorption of iron	Deficiency: Scurvy Bruises easily Muscle cramps Ulcerated gums Toxicity: Raised uric acid level Hemolytic anemia Kidney stones Rebound scurvy

ATP = adenosine triphosphate; RBC = red blood cell.

MINERALS

Minerals are inorganic elements that regulate body processes and build body tissue. These processes are fluid balance; acid-base balance; nerve cell transmission; vitamin, enzyme, and hormonal activity; and muscle contractions. Minerals are divided into two classifications. **Macrominerals**, or major minerals, are needed by the body in large amounts (>100 mg/day) (Table 7-3). **Microminerals**, or trace minerals, are needed in smaller amounts by the body (<15 mg/day) (Table 7-4).

The most common nutrient deficiency in the world is that of iron. This is particularly prevalent among infants, adolescents, and pregnant and menstruating women. It can result in iron-deficiency anemia.

WATER

Water is essential to life; we cannot survive more than a few days without it. Water accounts for 50% to 60% of the body's weight. The daily amount needed depends on the size of the person, the climate, and the amount of activity. The average adult needs six to eight cups of water a day; athletes and those living in hot, dry climates require more. Thirst may not always be an adequate indicator of water intake needs, especially in infants or very ill individuals who may have a poor thirst mechanism. Those who engage in intense physical activity may have a decreased thirst sensation as well (see Figure 7-3).

In addition, it is important to determine the source of the water intake. Tap water is usually safe in most areas of this country. Since 1971, the CDC has monitored drinking water for contaminants, which include parasites, bacteria, viruses, chemical, and soil deposits. Illnesses from tainted tap water range from gastroenteritis to cancer, hemolytic uremic syndrome, teratogenic effects, and death. However, there is a trend of people consuming more bottled water than tap water (see Nursing Tip, Bottled Water). This may pose potential health problems. Also, people who live in

NURSING**TIP**

Preventing Iron-Deficiency Anemia

- Identify those patients at risk (e.g., children under 2 years of age, adolescents, women with heavy menstrual flow, pregnant women, and individuals with malabsorption syndromes, gastrointestinal bleeding, and gross dietary deficiencies).

- Perform a complete nutritional assessment on these high-risk patients.

- Encourage patients to eat foods high in iron. These include lean meats, poultry, fish, fortified cereals, dark green, leafy vegetables and dried fruits.

TABLE 7-3 Major Minerals

NAME	FOOD SOURCES	FUNCTIONS	DEFICIENCY/TOXICITY

Calcium (Ca++)	Milk
	Cheese
	Sardines
	Salmon
	Green vegetables
		Development of bones and teeth
		Permeability of cell membranes
		Transmission of nerve impulses
		Blood clotting
			Deficiency:
			  Osteoporosis
			  Osteomalacia
			  Rickets
			  Poor tooth formation
			Toxicity:
			  Constipation
			  Increased risk of nephrolithiasis when large amounts are taken in a short period of time

Phosphorus (P)	Milk Cheese Poultry Lean meat Fish Nuts Legumes	Development of bones and teeth Transfer of energy Component of phospholipids Buffer system	Same as calcium

Potassium (K+)	Oranges
	Bananas
	Dried fruits
	Meat
	Cereals
		Contraction of muscles
		Maintaining water balance
		Transmission of nerve impulses
		Carbohydrate and protein metabolism
			Deficiency:
			  Hypokalemia
			  Muscle cramps
			  Irregular heart rhythm
			Toxicity:
			  Hyperkalemia
			  Irregular heart rhythm

Sodium (Na+)	Table salt
	Beef
	Eggs
	Poultry
	Milk
	Cheese
		Maintaining fluid balance in blood
		Transmission of nerve impulses
			Deficiency:
			  Acid-base disturbance
			  Shock (rare)
			Toxicity:
			  Increase in blood pressure
			  Edema

Chloride (Cl-)	Table salt
	Meat
	Eggs
	Seafood
		Gastric acidity
		Regulation of osmotic pressure
		Activation of salivary amylase
			Deficiency:
			  Imbalance in gastric acidity
			  Imbalance in blood pH
			Toxicity:
			  None

Magnesium (Mg++)	Green vegetables
	Milk
	Nuts
	Legumes
	Whole grains
		Synthesis of ATP
		Transmission of nerve impulses
		Activation of metabolic enzymes
		Relaxation of skeletal muscles
			Deficiency:
			  CNS depression
			  Seizures
			Toxicity:
			  Diarrhea
			  Hypersomnolence

Sulfur (S)	Eggs
	Poultry
	Fish
		Maintaining protein structure
		Formation of high-energy compounds
			Deficiency:
			  None
			Toxicity:
			  None

TABLE 7-4 Trace Minerals

NAME	FOOD SOURCES	FUNCTIONS	DEFICIENCY/TOXICITY

Iron (Fe^+)	Meat, organ meats, fish, poultry, dried fruits, beans, fortified cereals, dark green, leafy vegetables	Transports oxygen and carbon dioxide	Deficiency:
			    Iron-deficiency anemia
			Toxicity:
			    Hemochromatosis

Iodine (I^-)	Seafood, iodized salt	Regulates basal metabolic rate	Deficiency:
			    Goiter
			    Cretinism
			    Myxedema
			Toxicity:
			    Rare

Zinc (Zn^+)	Eggs, oysters, liver, legumes, milk	Formation of collagen
		Component of insulin
		Component of many vital enzymes
		Wound healing
			Deficiency:
			    Growth retardation
			Toxicity:
			    Copper and iron absorption are decreased

Selenium (Se^-)	Liver, seafood, grains	Antioxidant	Deficiency:
			    Rare
			Toxicity:
			    Rare

Copper (Cu^+)	Oysters, liver, nuts, legumes, whole grains	Oxidation of glucose	Deficiency:
			    Rare
			Toxicity:
			    Wilson's disease

Manganese (Mn^+)	Nuts, peas, beans, fruits	Component of metabolic enzymes	Deficiency:
			    Rare
			Toxicity:
			    Rare

Fluoride (F^-)	Fluoridated drinking water, seafood	Reduces dental caries	Deficiency:
			    Dental caries
			Toxicity:
			    Mottled-looking teeth

Chromium (Cr)	Eggs, meats, whole grain cereals	Binds insulin to cell membranes	Deficiency:
			    Impaired glucose intolerance (rare)
			Toxicity:
			    Rare

Molybdenum (Mo)	Liver, legumes, whole grains, dark green, leafy vegetables	Metabolism of nucleic acids to uric acid	Deficiency:
			    Headache
			    Tachycardia
			Toxicity:
			    Rare

NURSINGTIP

Bottled Water

Many Americans are now drinking bottled water or a large quantity of bottled water exclusively. The reasons are many: belief that it is purer, safer, and healthier; social status (it is "cool"); transportability; storage; and concerns about the purity of tap water. However, most bottled water does not contain fluoride, so consumers are missing the trace mineral that helps prevent dental caries. Children may need fluoride supplements if they are drinking mostly bottled water.

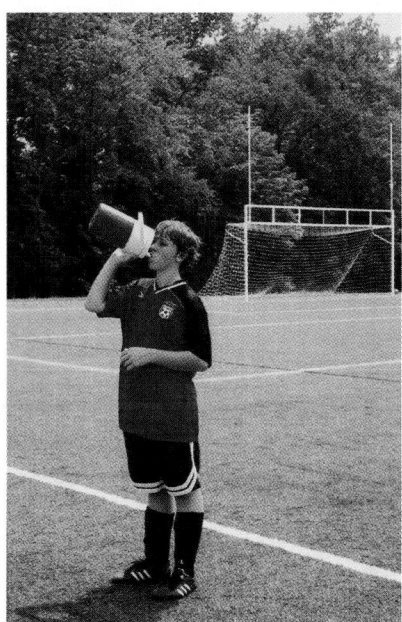

FIGURE 7-3 Hydration is essential to body function, especially when engaged in strenuous activities.

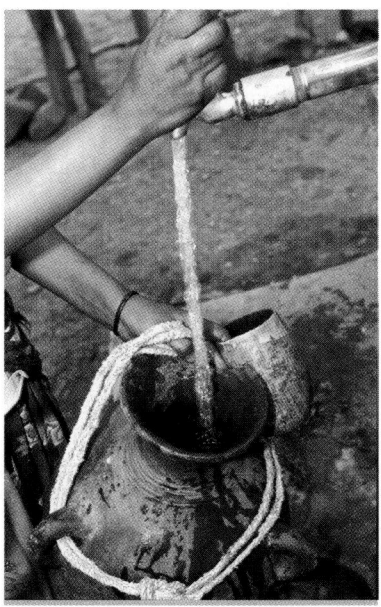

FIGURE 7-4 The source must be considered when evaluating the potability of water. *Courtesy of WHO/P. Virot.*

NURSING**TIP**

Daily Fluid Intake

Approximately 2.3–2.8 liters of fluid are consumed by the average adult on a daily basis. If an adult consumes six 8-oz glasses of fluids per day, the total ingested liquid is 1,440 mL. Added to this total is approximately 700 mL from the water content of food and 200 mL from water produced as the result of oxidation (Roth 2007). All total, this adult's daily intake is 2.3 liters of fluid. If the adult drinks eight 8-oz glasses of fluids in a day, then the total fluid intake increases to 2.8 liters.

NURSING**ALERT**

Signs and Symptoms of Dehydration

- Health history reveals inadequate intake of fluids.
- Decrease in urine output.
- Urine specific gravity >1.035.
- Weight loss (% body weight): 3–5% for mild, 6–9% for moderate, and 10–15% for severe dehydration.
- Eyes appear sunken; tongue has increased furrows and fissures.
- Oral mucous membranes are dry.
- Decreased skin turgor.
- Sunken fontanels in infants.
- Inability to produce tears.
- Changes in neurological status may occur with moderate to severe dehydration.

less populated areas have access only to well water, which must be carefully monitored for health risks. In some rural areas, rusty water pipes with unknown pathogens may be the only source of water (Figure 7-4). In other areas, local streams/rivers may be the only source of water. Unregulated water sources should be monitored by individuals on a regular basis to avoid the risk of illness.

NUTRITION THROUGH THE LIFE CYCLE

Assessment of the patient's developmental needs must always be included with a nutritional assessment. Nutritional needs change throughout the life cycle and are affected by both physical and developmental changes. A clear understanding of those changes, how they affect the patient, and what anticipatory guidance is indicated are needed to conduct a nutritional assessment. **Anticipatory guidance** covers health promotion; informs at-risk individuals of physical, cognitive, psychological, and social changes that may occur; and explains their nutritional needs.

CHILDREN

Recommended daily requirements for children change with each age group. An understanding of development with regard to physical, cognitive, and psychosocial changes is needed to properly assess the nutritional needs of children. This includes educating the caregiver about these changes before they occur. Families can then have more realistic expectations and understand what is within the normal range and what should be cause for concern.

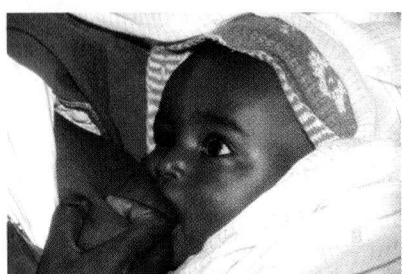

FIGURE 7-5 Breast milk is the preferred source of an infant's nutrition for the first 12 months. *Courtesy of WHO/P. Virot.*

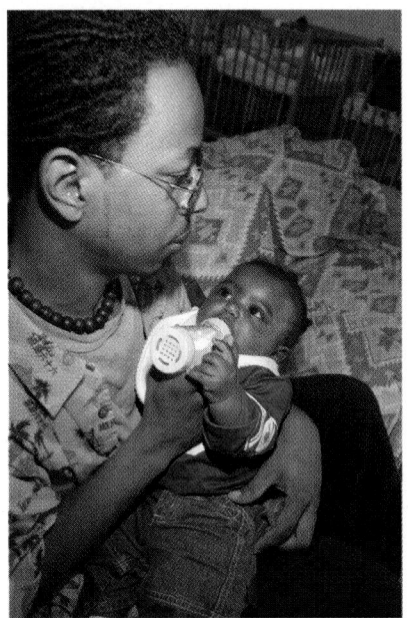

FIGURE 7-6 Many mothers pump their breast milk so that fathers can be involved in infant feedings; fortified infant formulas are also a sound nutritional choice.

Infants

Infants grow more during the first 6 to 12 months of life than at any other time. This is also the time when there is rapid neurological development, which indicates a need for proper nutrients. The American Academy of Pediatrics recommends the use of breast milk for infants instead of formula feeding for the first 12 months (Figure 7-5). If this is not possible, even a few weeks is beneficial, except in cases where the mother is HIV positive, because HIV infection can be transmitted via breast milk. Be prepared to support the caregiver's feeding decision, and discuss schedules, habits, and warning signs of problems or inadequate intake (Figure 7-6).

Infants are born with several reflexes that should be assessed when evaluating their nutritional status—sucking, rooting, and swallowing. Infants are able to feel hunger and express the need to eat by crying. Between 4 and 6 months, infants can feed themselves a cracker. When infants are 8 to 12 months old, they may drink from a cup by themselves. The use of a developmental assessment tool helps you monitor the infant's ability to achieve these milestones (see the DDST II, Chapter 24). Assessing the infant's physical development (such as head control and the ability to sit) is also helpful to determine readiness for solid

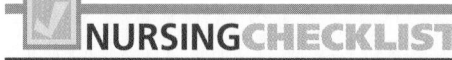

NURSINGALERT

Preventing Choking

Instruct caregivers to:

- Avoid use of foods that may cause choking in infants and small children (up to 3 years old), such as corn, nuts, raw peas and carrots, celery, small candies, hot dogs, popcorn, and any other small, hard food.
- Offer peanut butter only on bread or a cracker.
- Stress the importance of sitting up while eating; prohibit running with food or objects in the mouth.

✓ NURSINGCHECKLIST

Nutritional Assessment of Infants

- If the infant is breastfed, how often and for how long?
- How much formula does the infant take at each feeding, and how often does the infant eat? (Estimate how much is consumed in 24 hours.)
- How is the formula prepared? (It is important to make sure the formula is prepared correctly; this also helps establish how much the infant is eating.) How is the prepared formula stored?
- How does the infant react to eating? Does the infant appear satisfied?
- Does the infant appear to have any respiratory distress or reflux while eating? Are there any problems with constipation or diarrhea, and how is it treated? Have any allergies been discovered?
- Is the infant taking any supplemental food or vitamins?
- Is the infant ever put in bed with a bottle? If the answer is yes, instruct the caregivers about infant bottle caries and the importance of not propping the bottle or placing it in the bed.

NURSINGTIP

Foods to Avoid in Early Infancy

It is advised to not feed infants egg whites or citrus fruits until 12 months of age because of their allergenic potential. Also, infants under 12 months should not have honey because of the possibility of botulism toxicity.

food. Foods should be introduced one at a time to observe for possible allergic reactions. The recommended order of new foods starts with the least allergenic, as outlined in the Nursing Tip, Infant Feeding Guidelines.

Toddlers

Toddlers have their own unique nutritional needs as their physical growth slows. Toddlers' development plays a very important role in their diet (Figure 7-7) and in providing appropriate assessment and anticipatory guidance to the caregivers. As children experience increased independence and control over their bodies, some of this independence is demonstrated in their eating patterns. There is an increased problem with food refusal or the desire for only certain foods. This is a normal response to the developmental stage and should not be a problem unless it is excessive. Toddlers may say "no" even to food they desire to demonstrate that they are in charge.

Instruct parents to offer foods that the toddler can self-feed in small portions and offer only one new food at a time. A serving size should be about 1 to 2 tablespoons of food for each year of age. Toddlers are very good at imitating and often exhibit food dislikes that are shown at home (particularly if there is an older sibling). Encourage routine mealtimes that are enjoyed together to provide the toddler with role models for developing good eating habits.

Preschoolers

Preschoolers continue to have food dislikes and may become picky eaters. They verbalize their likes and dislikes, and show their independence by being in conflict with their caregivers. Giving choices, serving small amounts of foods children can

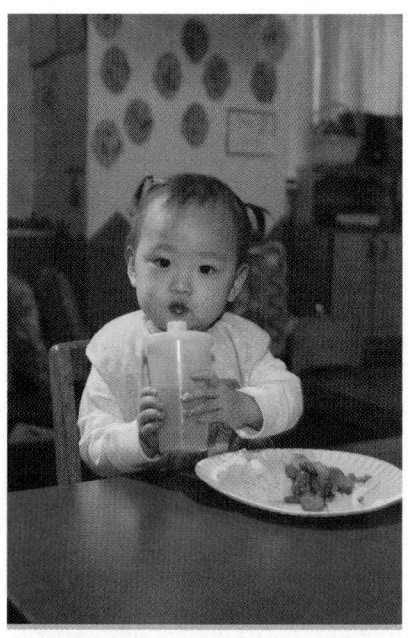

FIGURE 7-7 A toddler's developing motor skills allow the child to exert more independence and control over eating habits.

Lactose Intolerance

Lactose intolerance is the inability of the body, due to an insufficient amount of the enzyme lactase, to digest foods that contain the carbohydrate lactose. Lactose intolerance can affect people of all ages. Typically, people experience abdominal pain and cramping, bloating, flatulence, nausea, and diarrhea. Lactose-digesting enzymes and a lactose-free diet can limit the severity of the symptoms. If these measures are strictly followed by the patient and symptoms persist, then another etiology needs to be explored.

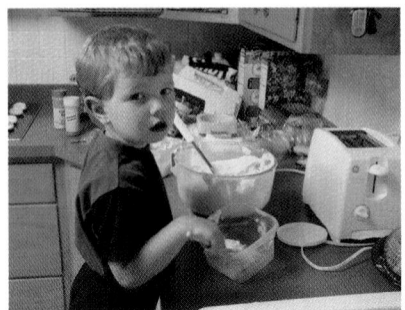

FIGURE 7-8 Preschoolers benefit from helping with meal preparation, especially with foods they like.

eat easily (finger foods), and providing a routine and enjoyable eating environment help to foster good eating habits by decreasing conflicts.

Preschoolers often have smaller appetites compared to toddlers. This may be caused by drinking too many beverages (milk, juice, Kool-Aid), and a slower increase in growth. They often are resistant to new foods and may eat only one food at a time. Encourage the caregivers to offer other foods. Discuss the need to provide healthy snacks and prevent the preschooler from eating foods that are too high in sugar. The preschooler benefits by helping to prepare food (Figure 7-8), setting the table, and making some decisions. Providing preschoolers with acceptable options is an easy way to ensure an appropriate diet.

REFLECTIVE THINKING

Childhood Obesity

The incidence of obesity in childhood is increasing. Many children's favorite activities are sedentary, such as playing computer and video games, and watching television.

- How would you approach a 3-year-old child of average height with a weight of 100 lbs who comes to you for a physical examination? What would you say to the caregiver?
- What health risks does an obese child face? What psychosocial challenges face an obese child?
- How would you present nutrition information to a first grade class? Fourth grade? Seventh grade? Eleventh grade?

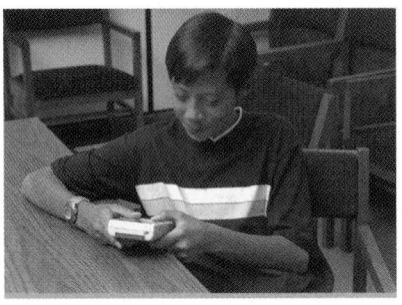

FIGURE 7-9 Playing sedentary games contributes to the childhood obesity epidemic.

Obesity Epidemic in Children

A school-age child comes home from school, grabs a soda, chips, and cookies, and sits in front of the television. After some time, this child may move on to chat with friends on the Internet or play computer games (Figure 7-9). This sedentary lifestyle and the child's dietary practices are some of the reasons for the alarming increase in the rate of childhood obesity. Additional factors include gender, familial history of obesity, ethnic and racial background, socioeconomic status, environment, and concurrent medical conditions. According to the National Heart, Lung, and Blood Institute (NHLBI), more than 12.5 million American children are overweight. With this increase, the number of children diagnosed with diabetes mellitus, hypertension, and hyperlipidemia has also increased. This obesity epidemic demands the attention of all nurses to be involved with identifying those children at risk, and intervening with those children who are already overweight. The NHLBI's We Can! (Ways to Enhance Children's Activity and Nutrition) program, in conjunction with the Association of Children's Museums, strives to reach children ages 8–13 with their educational programs. This science-based program's objectives are to improve food choices, increase physical activity, and decrease sedentary time spent at the computer or playing video games.

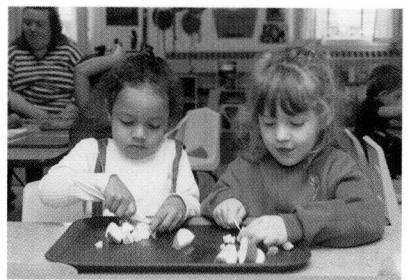

FIGURE 7-10 These school-age children are eating a healthy snack.

School-Age Children

School-age children tend to have erratic growth patterns that are reflected in their equally erratic eating patterns. They also tend to continue having strong likes and dislikes. Encourage families to maintain a balanced diet and to limit highly sweetened snacks and foods (Figure 7-10). Caregivers should be advised to teach children proper nutrition and should be encouraged to show children how to read nutrition and ingredient labels. Advise caregivers and children that pubescent chubbiness is a normal part of growth that often precedes a rapid increase in height.

ADOLESCENTS

Adolescence is a period of rapid growth and change, and adolescents' nutritional needs fluctuate accordingly. Adolescents are concerned with body image and often compare their bodies to those of their peers in an attempt to fit into an identity that is acceptable to them. A poor body image can lead to eating disorders such as anorexia nervosa, bulimia nervosa, and obesity. Although anorexia nervosa and bulimia nervosa can occur at any age, they are frequently seen in adolescents. Anorexia and bulimia are both eating disorders. Anorexia nervosa is characterized by a severely low body weight, defined as being 85% or less of the patient's ideal body weight; a distorted body image in which the individual perceives him-/herself to be fat; a fear of gaining weight; increased exercise patterns; and amenorrhea in women. Bulimia's hallmark is binge eating followed by purging. Purging can take many forms: self-induced vomiting and abuse of laxatives, diuretics, and enemas. These practices can lead to electrolyte imbalances. Bulimic patients frequently complain of a sore throat and heartburn. In addition, the bulimic patient may have an impulsivity and an addictive personality. A third eating disorder, Eating Disorder Not Otherwise Specified, encompasses those individuals who have an eating disorder but do not fit into a specified category. All individuals with eating disorders usually do not present for medical care unless they are hypotensive or have an acute electrolyte imbalance. More commonly, they complain of fatigue, dizziness, and low energy levels.

REFLECTIVE THINKING

Adolescent Issues

- While performing a well-child exam on 14-year-old Beth, she tells you that she is "fat." She is an accomplished ballet dancer who was recently rejected for a lead role in a theater production "because of my weight." You note that she is 64 inches tall and weighs 95 pounds. What would you say to Beth?

- Jamal is the captain of his high school's weight lifting team. During the health history, he informs you that he would like you to write a prescription for a medication to make him stronger. If you don't prescribe a medication, he states he will get it from someone at school. How would you address this situation?

☑ NURSING CHECKLIST

Nutritional Assessment of the Toddler, Preschooler, and School-Age Child

- Do you have any problem or concern with your child's eating?
- Is your child a picky eater, and how is this handled at home?
- Does your family eat together?
- What are your child's food likes or dislikes?
- What does your child eat for snacks?
- Is your child involved in sports or any other physical activity?
- What is your child's meal schedule? Where and when does your child eat?
- How much does your child eat during a meal?
- Does your child eat lunch at school?
- Does your child eat foods from all the groups in MyPyramid?
- Does your child have any food allergies?
- Does your child drink beverages with added sugar (e.g., soda, fruit juices)? How much?

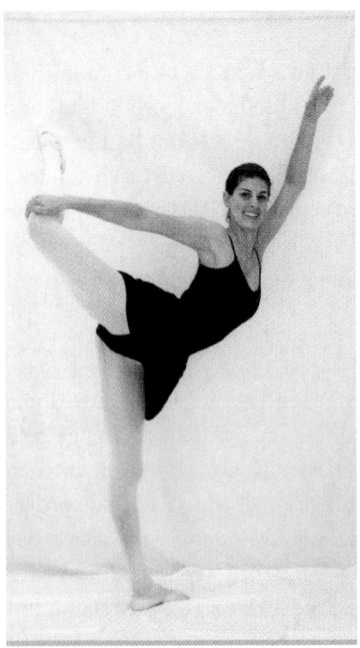

FIGURE 7-11 Adolescent females who participate in activities such as ballet are at risk for eating disorders.

Level of physical activity must also be taken into account for a nutritional evaluation (Figure 7-11). An understanding of the different sports and their requirements may help you screen for potential problems. In some sports (e.g., football), players are encouraged to be large and heavy; this puts them at a risk for possible anabolic steroid use. Toxic effects of steroid use include possible cancer of the liver, short stature, behavioral changes, endocrine problems (acne, impotence, testicular atrophy), and hypertension. In sports where decreased weight is desirable (e.g., wrestling, gymnastics), athletes may try many methods to "make weight." Instruction about proper nutrition to help reduce body fat without compromising health is needed when working with all athletes.

YOUNG AND MIDDLE-AGED ADULTS

Growth and caloric needs usually stabilize in young and middle-aged adults. Eating habits may be altered by changes in activity levels and by the effects of work and life stressors.

Obesity is a weight greater than 120% of the ideal body weight (IBW). Obesity occurs when calories consumed are greater than calories expended. This can occur when there is an increase in food consumption, a decrease in activity level, or both. Obesity can occur at any age but is frequently seen in young and middle-aged adults. The National Center for Health Statistics (2004) estimates from the National Health and Nutrition Examination Study (NHANES, 1999–2002) that 64% of adults in the United States are overweight, with half of them being obese. This represents a doubling in the incidence of obesity among adults 20–74 years of age in the past 20 years. Many factors affect whether a person is prone to obesity: genetic, physiological, psychological, and environmental. Obesity places a person at risk for hyperlipidemia, coronary artery disease (CAD), hypertension, diabetes mellitus, and chronic disorders.

Patients who are overweight or obese frequently experience yo-yo dieting, or weight cycling. In weight cycling, patients diet for some period of time, achieve their goal weights, and cease dieting. The majority of people return to their usual eating habits and regain the lost weight, and may add a few more pounds as well. Because many weight reduction programs neither address behavior modification for eating nor include an exercise regimen, most diets fail. The use of fad diets (i.e., diets that promise results without effectively

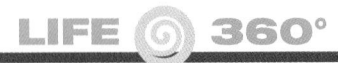

LIFE 360°

Obese Patient

An obese adult woman is concerned about her appearance.

- What are your biases about obesity?
- How would you react to this patient?
- What resources and information would you provide to assist your patient?
- What OTC products are available for weight loss? What are their advantages/disadvantages?
- Compare/contrast commercially available weight loss programs.

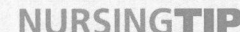

NURSING**TIP**

DASH Diet for Hypertension

The Dietary Approaches to Stop Hypertension (DASH) diet and reduced dietary sodium have been proven to help hypertensive patients eat a nutritionally sound diet while lowering their blood pressure. The DASH diet is low in total fat, cholesterol, saturated fats, red meats, sweets, and sugar-containing beverages, and it is rich in vegetables, fruits, and low-fat dairy products.

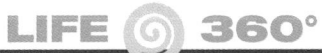

Vitamin D Intake

A postmenopausal woman tells you that she is at low risk for osteoporosis because she does water aerobics three times a week and drinks no milk but takes a multivitamin (MVI) every morning. How would you respond to this woman? What does the current body of literature state is the appropriate vitamin D intake for women of different ages?

NURSING**TIP**

Criteria for Metabolic Syndrome

- Waist circumference > 35" (88 cm) in women
- Waist circumference > 40" (102 cm) in men
- Fasting triglyceride level > 150 mg/dL
- Fasting HDL cholesterol < 50 mg/dL in women
- Fasting HDL cholesterol < 40 mg/dL in men
- Blood pressure of > 130/85 mm Hg
- Fasting serum glucose > 110 mg/dL

From National Cholesterol Education Program (NCEP) Adult Treatment Panel (ATP) III, 2001.

NURSING**TIP**

Alternative Calcium Supplements

Most Americans consume calcium supplements in the form of calcium carbonate and calcium citrate. Calcium carbonate is best absorbed when taken with some food. Calcium citrate can be absorbed well with food or on an empty stomach. Many American men and women combine the food in their daily diet with one of these calcium supplements. Sometimes sufficient quantities of calcium are not consumed with these means to meet the recommended DRI. Additional treatment options are to consume calcium via calcium-fortified beverages (e.g., bottled water, orange juice, milk), calcium-fortified chocolate, calcium-fortified chewables, calcium-fortified aspirin, and calcium-fortified fiber. Corporations are developing new products at an astounding rate to meet the tastes and lifestyles of today's diverse population.

altering lifestyle) and fad exercise regimens (e.g., use of vibrating machines to lose fat, use of saunas to decrease weight) may be deleterious to a person's health. Some fad programs are relatively safe if followed for a short period of time with adequate professional supervision.

Non-insulin-dependent diabetes mellitus, or type 2 diabetes, is a disease usually diagnosed after age 40. It is associated with family history and obesity and is often undiagnosed until there are complications, because until then, the person often has few or mild symptoms.

Coronary artery disease is one of the leading causes of death in the United States. The primary cause is **atherosclerosis**, which is the development of lipid plaques along the coronary arteries. The risk factors for atherosclerosis are discussed in Chapter 16.

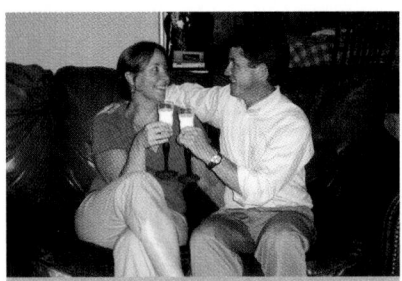

FIGURE 7-12 Calcium consumption is essential for all people. Both men and women can develop osteoporosis.

The metabolic syndrome, previously termed syndrome X, is increasing in prevalence in the United States. In order to be diagnosed with metabolic syndrome, three of these five risk factors need to be present: abdominal obesity, elevated blood pressure, elevated fasting blood glucose, elevated triglycerides, and low HDL. Patients with metabolic syndrome are at an increased risk for diabetes mellitus and CAD, and the majority are already obese. Lifestyle modification is the hallmark of treatment.

Osteoporosis is a disease that reduces bone mass. It is more common in women (Figure 7-12), and it is often not detected until a person falls and fractures a bone. Suspect anorexia nervosa in a young, thin female with osteoporosis. See Chapter 18 for additional information.

PREGNANT AND LACTATING WOMEN

It is important to assess and counsel a pregnant woman regarding nutrition to promote a healthy pregnancy. Proper nutrition for the mother from the time of conception is required for the development of a healthy infant. The infant is at risk of being small for gestational age if the woman does not gain adequate weight, and the woman is at risk for gestational diabetes and hypertension if the weight gain is excessive. Target weight gain is dependent on the woman's weight at conception. The woman at IBW should gain 24 to 28 pounds. If she is more than 20% above IBW, she should gain 15 to 20 pounds, and 30 to 35 pounds if she is 10% under IBW. Assessment includes a general knowledge of physical changes and their relationships to nutrition. Some of the common complaints experienced during pregnancy (e.g., heartburn, constipation, nausea, and vomiting) can be alleviated by dietary changes such as small, frequent meals; increased fluid intake; and a well-balanced diet.

Iron supplements are given routinely during pregnancy because diet alone is not adequate in meeting the body's requirements. Prenatal vitamins are usually prescribed for all pregnant women. There is evidence that folic acid helps to reduce the risk of neural tube defects, especially when the folic acid supplement is instituted 3 months prior to pregnancy. The U.S. Public Health Service recommends that all women of childbearing age consume 0.4 mg of folic acid per day. An additional 300 calories per day is recommended during pregnancy and an additional 500 calories per day during lactation; also recommended is an increase in milk consumption, which increases both protein and caloric intake. Fluid intake is important, and pregnant women are encouraged to drink

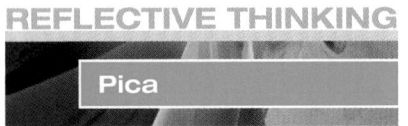

REFLECTIVE THINKING

Pica

You suspect a pregnant patient in the hospital practices pica. She keeps a box of starch by the bed and is diagnosed with anemia.

- How would you approach the patient?
- What are your own feelings toward those who practice pica?
- What would be your plan of care?
- How could you rule out pica as the cause of her anemia?

✓ NURSINGCHECKLIST

Nutritional Assessment of Pregnant Women

- What was your prepregnancy weight? (Take ideal body weight from Table 7-8 to determine targeted pregnancy weight gain.)
- What is your activity level and are there any changes since you became pregnant?
- Do you take any supplemental vitamins?
- Do you have a history of problems during previous pregnancies? What were they? How were they resolved?
- How often do you use caffeine, artificial sweeteners, and alcohol?
- Do you experience constipation, nausea, vomiting, or heartburn?
- Do you have any food cravings?
- Do you have cravings for substances other than food?

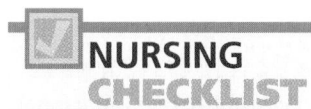

NURSING CHECKLIST

Nutritional Assessment of Older Adults

- Do you have any physical limitations that affect your eating?

- Do you have any difficulty swallowing? (history of cerebrovascular accident, neuromuscular disorders)

- Do you have any dental problems that interfere with eating?

- Who buys and prepares the food?

- Do you eat alone or with someone?

- How are your eating habits different from 10 years ago? 30 years ago?

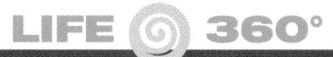

LIFE 360°

Investigate what resources are available in your community for older adults who need help with meals or food acquisition.

six to eight glasses of fluid daily (in the form of water, fruit juices, and milk). Lactating women need additional fluid intake and may need 2 to 3 quarts of fluid daily.

Pica, or cravings for substances other than food, is a phenomenon documented primarily in pregnant women. It is the practice of eating dirt, clay, starch, or even ice cubes, and may lead to nutritional difficulties, including an increased risk of anemia.

OLDER ADULTS

Good eating habits and nutrition established early in life will benefit adults as they age, whereas poor eating habits may contribute to disease processes (e.g., hypertension, diabetes mellitus, CAD, and obesity). Caloric needs decrease as a person ages, due to the reduction in basal metabolic rate, so health teaching should focus on modifications in portion size to coincide with reduced activity and decreased caloric requirements. Planning with the patient to include modifications that are acceptable and providing education and support help to ensure compliance.

Possible problems that may be noted when assessing the elderly are difficulty chewing (oral problems), difficulty swallowing (possible stroke or Parkinson's disease), decreased appetite, decreased ability to feed self (musculoskeletal diseases, such as osteoarthritis, and neurological diseases, such as stroke), and decreased taste and smell. There is also a decreased emptying time of the esophagus, making the older adult more susceptible to aspiration. The older adult should eat in a sitting position to avoid aspiration. Constipation, due to a decrease in gastrointestinal motility, is a common problem that can be alleviated through adequate fluid intake and foods high in fiber. It is significant to note that one-third of hospitalized older adults as well as those in long-term care facilities experience protein calorie malnutrition (Jensen, 1996).

There are numerous socioeconomic conditions that can affect the nutrition of older adults: income, transportation, and social support. First, many older adults do not work and therefore have no regular source of income, or they are on a fixed income. Their limited financial resources can adversely affect their food choices. Without adequate public or personal transportation, elders may not have the means to obtain their food. Lastly, in the United States, eating is a social as well as nutritional ritual (Figure 7-13). Cooking responsibilities are often shared in a family, and eating is a bonding, congenial event. Many older adults live alone and may not "feel" like eating because of their solitary nature, depression, or both.

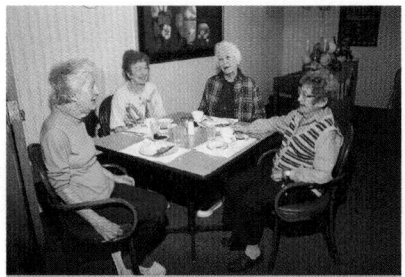

FIGURE 7-13 Eating is a nutritional as well as a social time. These women are enjoying camaraderie as well as a nutritional meal at their local senior center.

NURSING**TIP**

Psychosocial Implications of Food

The psychosocial implications of food and eating cannot be stressed enough. Food elicits certain memories and feelings of when we were younger (e.g., the smell of our mom's pie baking or the taste of Aunt Edna's cookies). It is also important to take into account other aspects of the nutritional history. If an older adult lives alone, there may be a problem obtaining food or preparing it; loneliness at mealtimes may also be a factor.

CULTURAL DIFFERENCES

It is not possible to have knowledge of all cultural differences, but an open and understanding attitude and acceptance of various religious and cultural beliefs is imperative. Certain foods may have special meanings and memories for individual patients or may be traditional among many with the same cultural backgrounds (e.g., turkey for Thanksgiving). There may also be regional considerations, food preferences, and religious beliefs that restrict certain foods and their consumption. An understanding of the food practices for various cultural groups is needed to provide appropriate nutritional assessment and education. This understanding is also helpful to establish rapport and individualize the nutritional plan. Be sure to inquire about various cultural and religious influences on dietary practices during the nutritional assessment; refer to Chapters 5 and 6 for a more in-depth discussion.

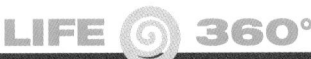

Culturally Based Nutritional Practices

- Your Islamic patient has been fasting during Ramadan. He is diabetic and continues to become hypoglycemic. What would be your plan of care? How would you help him balance his religious and nutritional needs?
- LoAn is a pregnant Vietnamese female who is HIV positive. She incorporates the observance of *yin* and *yang* into her daily rituals. LoAn confides that she is looking forward to breastfeeding her child. You realize that pregnancy is a *yang* condition and lactation is a *yin* condition, which is in line with LoAn's beliefs. What information would you discuss with LoAn, knowing that a female who is HIV positive is advised against breastfeeding?

HEALTH HISTORY

The nutritional history or subjective information gathered is one of the most significant aspects of the nutritional assessment. It gives an understanding of the patient's dietary habits and practices. Information about nutrition is gathered throughout the entire health history.

The nutritional health history provides insight into the link between a patient's lifestyle and nutritional information and pathology.

PATIENT PROFILE	*Diseases that are age- and gender-specific for nutrition are listed.*
Age	Anorexia nervosa (adolescents)
	Bulimia (adolescents)
Gender	
Female	Over 90% of patients with anorexia nervosa are female.
CHIEF COMPLAINT	*Common chief complaints for nutrition are defined, and information on the characteristics of each sign and symptom is provided.*
1. Anorexia	Lost or decreased interest and desire for food
Quantity	Amount of food consumed in relation to patient's normal intake
Associated Manifestations	Physical weakness, fatigue, nausea, cramps, dietary intolerances, weight loss, abdominal distension, abdominal fullness, anxiety, depression

continues

Health History (continued)

Aggravating Factors	Smoking, sleeplessness, odors, pain, emotional status, cardiorespiratory distress
Timing	Early morning, afternoon, bedtime, continuous, days, weeks, months, during pregnancy
2. Dysphagia	Difficulty swallowing; associated with damage to the 9th or 10th cranial nerve, causing paralysis of the swallowing mechanism or disorders of the throat, neck, or esophagus
Associated Manifestations	Weight loss, choking, or difficulty breathing when swallowing
Aggravating Factors	Solid or liquid foods
Alleviating Factors	Position, throat lozenges
Timing	Associated with specific times and meals during the day
3. Weight Gain	Number of pounds gained above usual weight
Associated Manifestations	Use of medications (corticosteroids, insulin, OCP, antidepressants), pregnancy, sedentary lifestyle, high-calorie diet, high-fat diet, increased appetite
Setting	Stress, depression, and negative body image
Timing	Over what period of time
4. Weight Loss	Number of pounds lost below usual weight
Associated Manifestations	Nausea, vomiting, diarrhea, use of laxatives or diuretics, medication side effects, decreased appetite, increase in exercise, malabsorption diseases, diseases increasing demand of nutrients
Setting	Stress, depression, and negative body image, following a particular diet, participating in a structured weight-loss program (e.g., Weight Watchers)
Timing	Over what period of time
PAST HEALTH HISTORY	*The various components of the past health history are linked with nutrition pathology and nutrition-related information.*
Medical History	
Nutrition Specific	Obesity, malnutrition, malabsorption diseases, anorexia nervosa, bulimia nervosa, dysphagia, weight cycling, metabolic syndrome
Non–Nutrition Specific	Diabetes mellitus, coronary artery disease, increased cholesterol level, burns, cerebrovascular accident, hypertension, cancer, diverticulosis, muscular dystrophy, multiple sclerosis, Parkinson's disease, Crohn's disease, ulcerative colitis, gout, pancreatitis, cholelithiasis, dental disease, dialysis, cystic fibrosis, Wilson's disease, phenylketonuria
Surgical History	Gastric reduction (bypass, lap band, or stapling), jaw wiring to reduce intake of food in morbid obesity, any surgical procedure that would alter food intake from postsurgical complications, nausea, or normal recovery
Allergies	Gastrointestinal disturbances may occur with medication, food, and environmental allergies; infants may manifest allergies as dietary disturbances (lactose intolerance)
Medications	Review all medications for actual or potential side effects that may affect appetite or growth (antibiotics may cause gastrointestinal disturbances, methylphenidate may cause anorexia, and long-term steroid use may affect linear growth), vitamins, supplements, orlistat, sibutramine
Communicable Diseases	Children with AIDS: failure to thrive; adults with AIDS: wasting syndrome

continues

Health History (continued)

Injuries and Accidents	Affect eating or the ability to self-feed, such as facial or mouth trauma; need for nasogastric tube feeding, gastrostomy
Special Needs	Affect ability to cut, handle, chew, or swallow food
FAMILY HEALTH HISTORY	*Nutritional diseases that are familial are listed.*
	Food allergies and intolerances, eating disorders, obesity, as well as any medical conditions that may contribute to nutritional problems (e.g., diabetes mellitus, hyperlipidemia, hypertension, CAD, celiac disease, cancer, gout, osteoporosis, alcoholism)
SOCIAL HISTORY	*The components of the social history are linked to nutritional factors and pathologies.*
Alcohol Use	Alcohol has very little nutrient value, and abuse may lead to nutritional deficiencies. These include an inadequate intake of food, decreased sense of taste and smell, altered metabolism of nutrients (by decreasing storage and increasing excretion of nutrients), and decreased absorption through intestinal mucosa. There is also an increased excretion of calcium with alcohol consumption, which increases the risk of osteoporosis. In a pregnant woman, chronic alcohol consumption can lead to a low-birth-weight baby and fetal alcohol syndrome in a newborn.
Tobacco Use	Smoking is associated with decreased estrogen levels in women, which increases their risk of osteoporosis. Tobacco is also an appetite suppressant that may stimulate weight gain when the person quits smoking. Tobacco may also alter the senses of taste and smell.
Drug Use	Drug abuse alters nutrition due to the patient's increased dependence on the substance and decreased intake of proper nutrients. Many drugs alter food intake by causing anorexia (e.g., amphetamines) and decreasing sense of smell and taste (e.g., cocaine).
Travel History	Recent travel may cause gastrointestinal disturbances. It may also temporarily change the normal dietary habits of the patient.
Hobbies and Leisure Activities	Food-related hobbies or food activities (gourmet cooking), or the amount of physical activity
Education	Education level may not necessarily translate into an adequate knowledge of nutritional needs.
Economic Status	Resources for purchase of adequate food and transportation to grocery store
Religion	See Chapter 6 for religious restrictions on diet.
Ethnic Background	See Chapter 5 for ethnic considerations regarding diet.
HEALTH MAINTENANCE ACTIVITIES	*This information provides a bridge between health maintenance activities and nutritional function.*
Sleep	Stress increases when a patient is sleep deprived, which may contribute to nutritional problems.
Diet	See Table 7-6 for questions to be asked during the diet history.
Exercise	Patients with anorexia nervosa may exercise to excess.
Stress Management	Increasing or decreasing food consumption
Health Check-ups	Lipid panel results, fasting serum glucose, weight, height, waist circumference, anthropometric measurements, blood pressure, and any other laboratory or diagnostic results

EQUIPMENT

- Wall-mounted unit (stadiometer), rod attached to the scale that has a right-angle headboard
- Tape measure
- Scale (preferably a balance-beam scale or electronic scale)
- Skinfold calipers (ideally one with a spring-loaded lever)

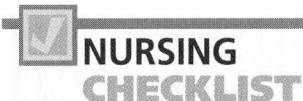

NURSING CHECKLIST

General Approach to Nutritional Assessment

1. Explain all procedures to patients and family members.
2. Ask patient to remove shoes prior to height measurement.
3. Have older children or adults remove heavy clothing (an adult may wear a hospital gown).
4. Explain and review results with patient and family.

NUTRITIONAL ASSESSMENT

Table 7-5 illustrates a comprehensive nutritional assessment. It includes the nutritional history, physical assessment, anthropometric measurements, laboratory data, and diagnostic data.

THE NUTRITIONAL HISTORY

The first step in the nutritional assessment is the nutritional history. A comprehensive history is always warranted when the patient has a chronic medical condition or an unexplained weight loss or gain. Specific diet information is obtained via the Diet History (Table 7-6). The food intake history may be obtained in a variety of ways. The first is the 24-hour recall. In this approach, the patient relates what has been consumed in the past day. Patients may also keep a food diary recording what foods and drinks were consumed over a specific 72-hour period. These histories can provide essential information; however, they may not truly represent a typical diet for the patient. It is possible for the patient to change the usual dietary habits, omit foods that were eaten, or record incorrect entries, knowing that the information will be evaluated by the nurse. Such instances can lead to invalid information and incorrect diagnoses and treatment plans.

Direct observation of the food and drink consumed by the patient and recorded by the nurse constitutes another method to record food intake patterns. Caloric intake can then be calculated. This is most easily done with the hospitalized patient.

Once the food intake history is recorded, the nurse evaluates the diet. Many frameworks can be used to evaluate food consumption. The Dietary Guidelines for Americans, the MyPyramid, the American Heart Association diets, and the American Dietetic Association diets are just a few standards against which a patient's diet can be evaluated.

PHYSICAL ASSESSMENT

Certain physical signs may indicate poor nutrition. See Table 7-7 for a list of signs and symptoms of poor nutritional status.

ANTHROPOMETRIC MEASUREMENTS

Anthropometric measurements are the various measurements of the human body, including height, weight, and body proportions. They measure growth patterns in children and changes in nutritional status in adults.

Measurements are easily obtained and can assist in an objective assessment that can be compared over time. Standardized charts should be used to compare the specific measurements with expected norms.

Height

A standing height is obtained for patients 3 years and older (see Figure 7-14).

E 1. Have the patient stand erect with back and heels against the wall or measuring device.

2. Place the headboard at a right angle to the wall and along the crown of the patient's head.

3. Record height to the nearest 1/8 inch or 1 mm.

N Compare to standardized charts (see Table 7-8). Bear in mind that patients will reflect familial growth patterns. Also compare to the patient's height and weight at the last visit.

 Examination   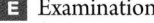 Normal Findings   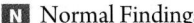 Abnormal Findings   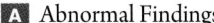 Pathophysiology

TABLE 7-5 Comprehensive Nutritional Assessment

NUTRITIONAL HISTORY (refer to Health History)

PHYSICAL ASSESSMENT

1. General appearance
2. Skin
3. Hair
4. Nails
5. Eyes
6. Mouth
7. Head and neck
8. Heart and peripheral vasculature
9. Abdomen
10. Musculoskeletal system
11. Neurological system
12. Female genitalia

ANTHROPOMETRIC MEASUREMENTS

Height: _____ in or cm
Weight: _____ lbs or kg

% Ideal Body Weight: _____
% Usual Body Weight: _____
% Weight Change: _____
Body Mass Index: _____

Waist Circumference: _____ in or cm
Waist/Hip Ratio: _____
Triceps Skinfold: _____ mm
Mid-Arm Circumference: _____ cm
Mid-Arm Muscle Circumference: _____ cm

LABORATORY DATA

Hematocrit (Hct): _____ %
Cholesterol: _____ mg/dL
Triglycerides: _____ mg/dL
Transferrin: _____ mg/dL
TIBC: _____ µg/dL
Iron: _____ µg/dL
Total Lymphocyte Count: _____ cells/mm³
Antigen Skin Testing:
Prealbumin: _____ mg/dL
Glucose: _____ mg/dL
HbA1c: _____ %
CHI: _____ %
Nitrogen Balance: _____ g
Vitamin D: _____ ng/mL

Hemoglobin (Hgb): _____ g/dL
HDL: _____ mg/dL
LDL: _____ mg/dL

Albumin: _____ g/dL

DIAGNOSTIC DATA

X-rays _____   DEXA Scan _____

TABLE 7-6 Diet History

PART 1: GENERAL DIET INFORMATION

Do you follow a particular diet?

What are your food likes and dislikes?

Do you have any especially strong cravings?

How often do you eat fast food?

How often do you eat at restaurants?

Do you have adequate financial resources to purchase your food?

How do you obtain, store, and prepare your food?

Do you eat alone or with a family member or other person?

Do you consume any food supplements (e.g., high-caloric beverages)?

In the last 12 months have you:

• Experienced any change in weight?
• Had a change in your appetite?
• Had a change in your diet?
• Experienced nausea, vomiting, or diarrhea from your diet?
• Changed your diet because of difficulty in feeding yourself, eating, chewing, or swallowing?

PART 2: FOOD INTAKE HISTORY (24-HOUR RECALL, 3-DAY DIARY, DIRECT OBSERVATION)

Time	Food/Drink	Amount	Method of Preparation	Eating Location

TABLE 7-7 Physical Signs and Symptoms of Poor Nutritional Status

	SUBJECTIVE	OBJECTIVE
1. General appearance	Fatigue, poor sleep, change in weight, frequent infections	Dull affect, apathetic, increased weight, decreased weight
2. Skin	Pruritus, swelling, delayed wound healing	Dry, rough, scaling, flaky, edema, lesions, decreased turgor, changes in color (pallor, jaundice), petechiae, ecchymoses, xanthomas (slightly elevated yellow nodules)
3. Hair	Easily falls out, brittle	Less shiny, dry, changes in color pigment
4. Nails	Brittle	Dry, splinter hemorrhages, spoon-shaped, pale
5. Eyes	Vision changes, night blindness, eye discharge	Hardening and scaling of cornea, conjunctiva pale or red
6. Mouth	Mouth sores	Lips: cracked, dry, swollen, fissures around corners Gums: recessed, swollen, bleeding, spongy Tongue: smooth, beefy red, magenta, pale, fissures, sores, increased or decreased in size, increased or decreased papillae Teeth: missing, caries
7. Head and neck	Headaches, decreased hearing	Xanthelasma, irritation and crusting of nares, swollen cheeks (parotid gland enlargement), goiter
8. Heart and peripheral vasculature	Palpitations, swelling	Cardiac enlargement, changes in blood pressure, tachycardia, heart murmur, edema
9. Abdomen	Tender, changes in appetite, nausea, changes in bowel habits	Edema, hepatosplenomegaly, vomiting, diarrhea
10. Musculoskeletal system	Weakness, pain, cramping, frequent fractures	Muscle tone is decreased, flabby muscles, muscle wasting, bowing of lower extremities
11. Neurological system	Irritable, changes in mood, numbness, paresthesia	Slurred speech, unsteady gait, tremors, decreased deep tendon reflexes, loss of position and vibratory sense, paresthesia, decreased coordination
12. Female genitalia	Changes in menstrual pattern	None

A Insufficient growth is abnormal.

P Chronic malnutrition may result in a decrease in height because the body does not have the nutrients necessary for proper growth.

P A patient with osteoporosis may demonstrate a decrease in height due to thinning of the bones and possible vertebral compression fractures. A patient with degenerative disc disease may also lose stature due to the nature of the musculoskeletal changes.

A Excessive growth is abnormal.

P Hormone abnormalities may cause excessive growth, as in acromegaly, giantism, and precocious puberty.

P Genetic and metabolic syndromes that affect growth are Marfan's syndrome and Klinefelter's syndrome.

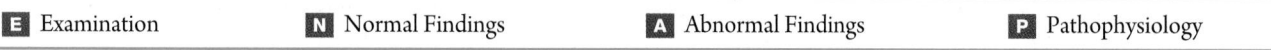

E Examination   **N** Normal Findings   **A** Abnormal Findings   **P** Pathophysiology

TABLE 7-8 Suggested Weights for Adults

HEIGHT (without shoes)	WEIGHT IN POUNDS WITHOUT CLOTHES	
	19 to 34 years	35 years and over
5'0"	97–128	108–138
5'1"	101–132	111–143
5'2"	104–137	115–148
5'3"	107–141	119–152
5'4"	111–146	122–157
5'5"	114–150	126–162
5'6"	118–155	130–167
5'7"	121–160	134–172
5'8"	125–164	138–178
5'9"	129–169	142–183
5'10"	132–174	146–188
5'11"	136–179	151–194
6'0"	140–184	155–199
6'1"	144–189	159–205
6'2"	148–195	164–210
6'3"	152–200	168–216
6'4"	156–205	173–222
6'5"	160–211	177–228
6'6"	164–216	182–234

The higher weights in the ranges generally apply to men, who tend to have more muscle and bone; the lower weights more often apply to women, who have less muscle and bone.

From *Dietary Guidelines for Americans*, 3rd ed., by U.S. Departments of Agriculture and Health and Human Services, 1990. Retrieved January 22, 2008, from http://www.nal.usda.gov/fnic/dga/weight.htm.

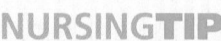

NURSINGTIP

Measuring Height of the Bedridden Patient

When a patient is bedridden or immobile, measure recumbent length with a rod or yardstick.

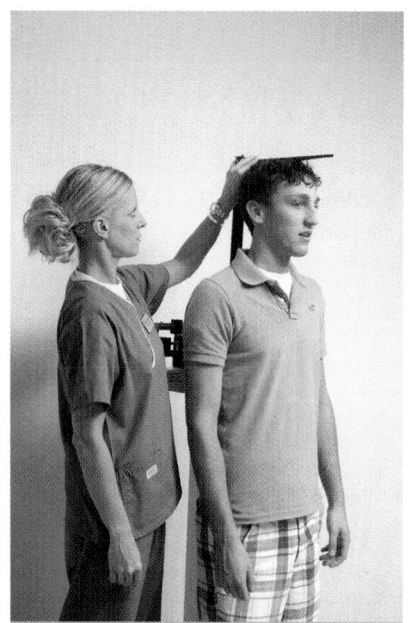

FIGURE 7-14 Measuring Patient Height

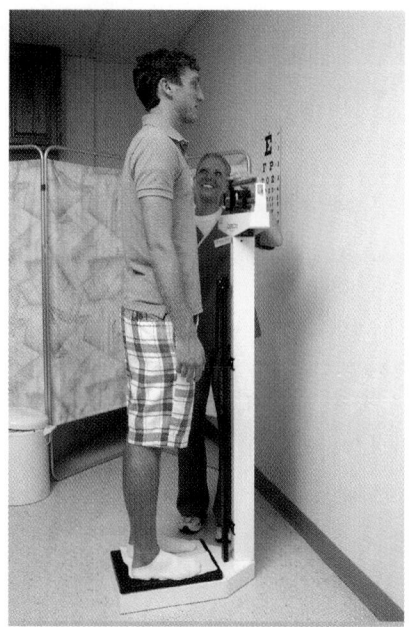

FIGURE 7-15 Measuring Patient Weight

Weight

E 1. Have the patient stand on scale, facing the weights (Figure 7-15).

2. Slide the weight until balanced.

3. Read and record to the nearest 100 g or ¼ lb (10 g or ½ oz for infants).

4. Calculate percentage of ideal body weight (IBW) using the formula:

$$\% \text{ Ideal Body Weight} = \frac{\text{Current Weight}}{\text{Ideal Body Weight (IBW)}^*} \times 100$$

*IBW can be obtained from Table 7-8.

5. Calculate the percentage of usual body weight using the formula:

$$\% \text{ Usual Body Weight} = \frac{\text{Current Weight}}{\text{Usual Body Weight}} \times 100$$

6. Calculate the percentage of weight change using the formula:

$$\% \text{ Weight Change} = \frac{\text{Usual Weight} - \text{Current Weight}}{\text{Usual Weight}} \times 100$$

N Compare weight to standardized charts (see Table 7-8).

A Obesity is abnormal. Mild obesity occurs when the patient is 20–40% above the IBW; moderate obesity occurs when the patient is 40–100% above the IBW; and morbid obesity occurs when a patient is more than 100% above the IBW.

P Obesity occurs when there is excess body fat because of increased food intake, decreased activity level, or both.

P Some medications may contribute to weight gain (e.g., steroids).

P Some disease processes, such as hypothyroidism, may contribute to weight gain because of decreased metabolic rate.

P Genetics may influence weight gain.

A A weight under 90% of IBW is termed undernutrition. A weight between 80% and 90% of the IBW is mild undernutrition, between 70% and 80% is moderate undernutrition, and below 70% is severe undernutrition.

P Decreased food intake may occur with dental problems, depression, medications, alcoholism, anorexia nervosa, and poverty.

P Inadequate nutrition may occur with impaired absorption, as present in malabsorption diseases (e.g., celiac disease), AIDS, and small bowel disease.

P There may be a loss of nutrients with diarrhea, vomiting, and diabetes mellitus.

P Increased demand for nutrients may be present in malignancies, fever, burns, and hyperthyroidism. This increased demand may account for the weight loss that occurs early in cancer even when calories are not decreased. If this continues, the patient exhibits signs of extreme malnutrition and wasting, which is called **cachexia**.

Body Mass Index

Body Mass Index (BMI) is a measurement that indicates body composition. The degree of overweight or obesity, as well as the degree of underweight, can be determined. The BMI can be associated with increased mortality at specific levels with patients with known chronic diseases and those without.

The BMI takes into account a person's height as well as weight. The formula to determine BMI is:

$$\text{BMI} = \frac{\text{Weight (in kg)}}{\text{m}^2}$$

The BMI can be difficult to calculate because few people know their height in meters squared. In this case, the BMI can be determined by two different methods:

E 1. Determine the BMI measurement by using the patient's height and weight in Table 7-9. OR

2. Multiply the weight in lbs by 703.

3. Multiply the height in inches by the height in inches.

4. Divide the first number in step 2 by the second number in step 3.

5. The answer is the BMI.

For example: weight = 107 lbs, height = 60 inches

$107 \times 703 = 75221$

$60 \times 60 = 3600$

$75221 \div 3600 = 20.9 \text{ or } 21$

N A BMI of 20 to 25 is considered within normal limits.

A A BMI of 25 to 29.9 is considered overweight. A BMI of 30 to 34.9 is considered obese (Obesity Class I), 35 to 39.9 is moderately obese (Obesity Class II), and greater than 40 is extremely obese (Obesity Class III).

P A BMI greater than 25 is associated with an increased morbidity and mortality from cardiovascular disease, cancer, and other diseases.

A A BMI less than 20 is abnormal.

P A BMI less than 20 is underweight and can be associated with possible malnutrition. A BMI less than 18 is associated with definite malnutrition. The malnutrition can be self-induced (e.g., anorexia nervosa, bulimia), caused by illness (e.g., cancer, AIDS), or it can be from a lack of available adequate nutrition.

| **E** Examination | **N** Normal Findings | **A** Abnormal Findings | **P** Pathophysiology |

TABLE 7-9 Body Mass Index (BMI)

HEIGHT (inches)	19	20	21	22	23	24	25	26	27	28	29	30	31	32	33	34	35
							BODY WEIGHT (pounds)										
58	91	96	100	105	110	115	119	124	129	134	138	143	148	153	158	162	167
59	94	99	104	109	114	119	124	128	133	138	143	148	153	158	163	168	173
60	97	102	107	112	118	123	128	133	138	143	148	153	158	163	168	174	179
61	100	105	111	116	122	127	132	137	143	148	153	158	164	169	174	180	185
62	104	109	115	120	126	131	136	142	147	153	158	164	169	175	180	185	191
63	107	113	118	124	130	135	141	145	152	158	163	169	174	180	185	191	197
64	110	116	122	128	134	140	145	151	157	163	169	174	180	185	192	197	204
65	114	120	126	132	138	144	150	156	162	168	174	180	186	192	198	204	210
66	118	124	130	136	142	148	155	161	167	173	179	186	192	198	204	210	216
67	121	127	134	140	146	153	159	166	172	178	185	191	198	204	211	217	223
68	125	131	138	144	151	158	164	171	177	184	190	197	203	210	216	223	230
69	128	135	142	149	155	162	169	176	182	189	196	203	209	216	223	230	236
70	132	139	146	153	160	167	174	181	188	189	196	203	209	216	223	230	236
71	136	143	150	157	165	172	179	186	193	200	208	215	222	229	236	243	250
72	140	147	154	162	169	177	184	191	199	206	213	221	228	235	242	250	258
73	144	151	159	166	174	182	189	197	204	212	219	227	235	242	250	257	265
74	148	155	163	171	179	186	194	202	210	218	225	233	241	249	256	264	272
75	152	160	168	176	184	192	200	208	216	224	232	240	248	256	264	272	279
76	156	164	172	180	189	197	205	213	221	230	238	246	254	263	271	279	287

From *Clinical Guidelines on the Identification, Evaluation, and Treatment of Overweight and Obesity in Adults,* by the National Institutes of Health and National Heart, Lung, and Blood Institute, June 1998, Bethesda, MD: Authors. Reprinted with permission.

Waist Circumference and Waist to Hip Ratio

Body fat distribution is linked to morbidity and mortality. This is frequently referred to as the "pears" and "apples" distribution. Women tend to deposit fat more in their hips and buttocks, giving them a pear-shaped appearance. Men, on the other hand, tend to deposit fat around the abdominal midline, thus giving them an apple-shaped appearance. The latter is usually connected more with the adverse effects associated with obesity. The waist circumference and waist to hip ratio is a simple method to determine one's body fat distribution.

E 1. Measure the waist in inches around the narrowest point of the waist between the 12th rib and the iliac crest. This is the waist circumference.

2. Measure the hips at the widest point.

3. Divide the waist measurement by the hip measurement. This is the waist to hip ratio. For example:

waist = 25 inches, hips = 35 inches

$25 \div 35 = 0.71$

N A waist circumference ≤ 35″ (88 cm) in women and ≤ 40″ (102 cm) in men is considered within normal limits. A waist to hip ratio less than 0.8 is normal in women. A waist to hip ratio less than 1.0 is normal in men.

A A waist to hip ratio greater than 0.8 in women and 1.0 in men is abnormal.

A A waist circumference >35" (88 cm) in women and >40" (102 cm) in men is abnormal.

P These measurements are associated with the adverse morbidity and mortality of obesity, cardiovascular disease, and diabetes.

Skinfold Thickness

Skinfold thickness is used to determine body fat stores and nutritional status. It is a more reliable indicator of body fat than is weight, because more than half of the body's total fat is located in the subcutaneous tissue. The most common measurement site is the **triceps skinfold** (TSF). Measurements can also be performed in subscapular and suprailiac skinfolds.

E
1. Place the patient in a sitting or standing position.
2. Take the measurements on the nondominant arm, with the patient in a relaxed position.
3. Make a mark on the posterior portion of the upper arm midway between the acromion process and the olecranon process.
4. Using your nondominant hand, grasp the skin and pull it free from the muscle.
5. Apply the caliper with your dominant hand and align the markers (Figure 7-16).
6. Note the measurement to the nearest 0.5 mm.
7. Release the skin and repeat two or three times.
8. Average the findings to determine the TSF.

N See Table 7-10. Normal measurements fall between the 5th and 95th percentiles.

A See abnormal findings and pathophysiology under Mid-Arm and Mid-Arm Muscle Circumferences.

Mid-Arm and Mid-Arm Muscle Circumferences

The **mid-arm circumference** (MAC) provides information on skeletal muscle mass. This measurement alone is not of great significance, but it is used to calculate the **mid-arm muscle circumference** (MAMC).

E
1. Instruct patient to flex the arm at the elbow.
2. Measure the circumference of the upper arm (MAC) midway between the acromion process and the olecranon process.
3. Calculate MAMC using the formula:

$$\text{MAMC (cm)} = \text{MAC (cm)} - [3.14 \times \text{TSF* (cm)}]$$

*The TSF is measured in mm. You need to convert the TSF from mm to cm in order to calculate the MAMC.

N See Table 7-11. Normal measurements fall between the 5th and 95th percentiles.

A Results less than the 5th percentile on the standard charts are abnormal.

P **Kwashiorkor**, or protein malnutrition, is a severe deficiency in good-quality protein. This can develop even if the patient is consuming an adequate number of calories. Because of the decrease in visceral proteins (especially albumin), edema may develop, particularly in the abdomen. This can also lead to a decreased immune function. The TSF, MAC, and weight can be within

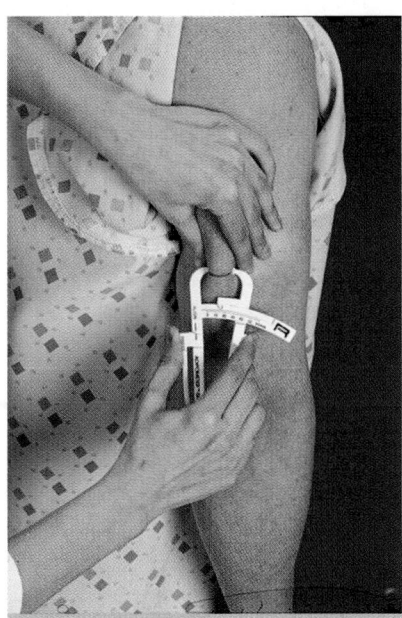

FIGURE 7-16 **Measuring Triceps Skinfold**

E Examination **N** Normal Findings **A** Abnormal Findings **P** Pathophysiology

TABLE 7-10 Triceps Skinfold Percentiles[†]

				TRICEPS SKINFOLD PERCENTILES (mm²)											
AGE (yr)				MALES								FEMALES			
	n	5	10	25	50	75	90	95	n	5	10	25	50	75	90	95

AGE (yr)	n	5	10	25	50	75	90	95	n	5	10	25	50	75	90	95
1–1.9	228	6	7	8	10	12	14	16	204	6	7	8	10	12	14	16
2–2.9	223	6	7	8	10	12	14	15	208	6	8	9	10	12	15	16
3–3.9	220	6	7	8	10	11	14	15	208	7	8	9	11	12	14	15
4–4.9	230	6	6	8	9	11	12	14	208	7	8	8	10	12	14	16
5–5.9	214	6	6	8	9	11	14	15	219	6	7	8	10	12	15	18
6–6.9	117	5	6	7	8	10	13	16	118	6	6	8	10	12	14	16
7–7.9	122	5	6	7	9	12	15	17	126	6	7	9	11	13	16	18
8–8.9	117	5	6	7	8	10	13	16	118	6	8	9	12	15	18	24
9–9.9	121	6	6	7	10	13	17	18	125	8	8	10	13	16	20	22
10–10.9	146	6	6	8	10	14	18	21	152	7	8	10	12	17	23	27
11–11.9	122	6	6	8	11	16	20	24	117	7	8	10	13	18	24	28
12–12.9	153	6	6	8	11	14	22	28	129	8	9	11	14	18	23	27
13–13.9	134	5	5	7	10	14	22	26	151	8	8	12	15	21	26	30
14–14.9	131	4	5	7	9	14	21	24	141	9	10	13	16	21	26	28
15–15.9	128	4	5	6	8	11	18	24	117	8	10	12	17	21	25	32
16–16.9	131	4	5	6	8	12	16	22	142	10	12	15	18	22	26	31
17–17.9	133	5	5	6	8	12	16	19	114	10	12	13	19	24	30	37
18–18.9	91	4	5	6	9	13	20	24	109	10	12	15	18	22	26	30
19–24.9	531	4	5	7	10	15	20	22	1,060	10	11	14	18	24	30	34
25–34.9	971	5	6	8	12	16	20	24	1,987	10	12	16	21	27	34	37
35–44.9	806	5	6	8	12	16	20	23	1,614	12	14	18	23	29	35	38
45–54.9	898	6	6	8	12	15	20	25	1,047	12	16	20	25	30	36	40
55–64.9	734	5	6	8	11	14	19	22	809	12	16	20	25	31	36	38
65–74.9	1,503	4	6	8	11	15	19	22	1,670	12	14	18	24	29	34	36

[†]The Lange caliper was used in these studies.

Reprinted with permission from "New Norms of Upper Limb Fat and Muscle Areas for Assessment of Nutrition Status," by A. R. Frisancho, 1981, *American Journal of Clinical Nutrition*, 34, p. 2540, American Society for Clinical Nutrition.

TABLE 7-11 MAC and MAMC Percentiles

	ARM CIRCUMFERENCE (mm)							ARM MUSCLE CIRCUMFERENCE (mm)						
Age Group	5	10	25	50	75	90	95	5	10	25	50	75	90	95
							Males							
1–1.9	142	146	150	159	170	176	183	110	113	119	127	135	144	147
2–2.9	141	145	153	162	170	178	185	111	114	122	130	140	146	150
3–3.9	150	153	160	167	175	184	190	117	123	131	137	145	148	153
4–4.9	149	154	262	171	180	186	192	123	126	133	141	148	156	159
5–5.9	153	160	167	175	185	195	204	128	133	140	147	154	161	169
6–6.9	155	159	167	179	188	209	228	131	135	142	151	161	170	177
7–7.9	162	167	177	187	201	223	230	137	139	151	160	168	177	190

continues

TABLE 7-11 (Continued)

Age Group	ARM CIRCUMFERENCE (mm)							ARM MUSCLE CIRCUMFERENCE (mm)						
	5	10	25	50	75	90	95	5	10	25	50	75	90	95
8–8.9	162	170	177	190	202	220	245	140	145	154	162	170	182	187
9–9.9	175	178	187	200	217	249	257	151	154	161	170	183	196	202
10–10.9	181	184	196	210	231	262	274	156	160	166	180	191	209	221
11–11.9	186	190	202	223	244	261	280	159	165	173	183	195	205	230
12–12.9	193	200	214	232	254	282	303	167	171	182	195	210	223	241
13–13.9	194	211	228	247	263	286	301	172	179	196	211	226	238	245
14–14.9	220	226	237	253	283	303	322	189	199	212	223	240	260	264
15–15.9	222	229	244	264	284	311	320	199	204	218	237	254	266	272
16–16.9	244	248	262	278	303	324	343	213	225	234	249	269	287	296
17–17.9	246	253	267	285	308	336	347	224	231	245	258	273	294	312
18–18.9	245	260	276	297	321	353	379	226	237	252	264	283	298	324
19–24.9	262	272	288	308	331	355	372	238	245	257	273	289	309	321
25–34.9	271	282	300	319	342	362	375	243	250	264	279	298	314	326
35–44.9	278	287	305	326	345	363	374	247	255	269	286	302	318	327
45–54.9	267	281	301	322	342	362	376	239	249	265	281	300	315	326
55–64.9	258	273	296	317	336	355	369	236	245	260	278	295	310	320
65–74.9	248	263	285	307	325	344	355	223	235	251	268	284	298	306
Females														
1–1.9	138	142	148	156	164	172	177	105	111	117	124	132	139	143
2–2.9	142	145	152	160	167	176	184	111	114	119	126	133	142	147
3–3.9	143	150	158	167	175	183	189	113	119	124	132	140	146	152
4–4.9	149	154	160	169	177	184	191	115	121	128	136	144	152	157
5–5.9	153	157	165	175	185	203	211	125	128	134	142	151	159	165
6–6.9	156	162	170	176	187	204	211	130	133	138	145	154	166	171
7–7.9	164	167	174	183	199	216	231	129	135	142	151	160	171	176
8–8.9	168	172	183	195	214	247	261	138	140	151	160	171	183	194
9–9.9	178	182	194	211	224	251	260	147	150	158	167	180	194	198
10–10.9	174	182	193	210	228	251	263	148	150	159	170	180	190	197
11–11.9	185	194	208	224	248	276	303	150	158	171	181	196	217	223
12–12.9	194	203	216	237	256	282	294	162	166	180	191	201	214	220
13–13.9	202	211	223	243	271	301	328	169	175	183	198	211	226	240
14–14.9	214	223	237	252	272	304	322	174	179	190	201	216	232	247
15–15.9	208	221	239	254	279	300	322	175	178	189	202	215	228	244
16–16.9	218	224	241	258	283	318	334	170	180	190	202	216	234	249
17–17.9	220	227	241	264	295	324	350	175	183	194	205	221	239	257
18–18.9	222	227	241	258	281	312	325	174	179	191	202	215	237	245
19–24.9	221	230	247	265	290	339	345	179	185	195	207	221	236	249
25–34.9	233	240	256	277	304	342	368	183	188	199	212	228	246	264
35–44.9	241	251	267	290	317	356	378	186	192	205	218	236	257	272
45–54.9	242	256	274	299	328	362	384	187	193	206	220	238	260	274
55–64.9	243	257	280	303	335	367	385	187	196	109	225	244	266	280
65–74.9	240	252	274	299	326	356	373	185	195	208	225	244	264	279

Reprinted with permission from "New Norms of Upper Limb Fat and Muscle Areas for Assessment of Nutrition Status," by A. R. Frisancho, 1981, *American Journal of Clinical Nutrition*, 34, p. 2540, American Society for Clinical Nutrition.

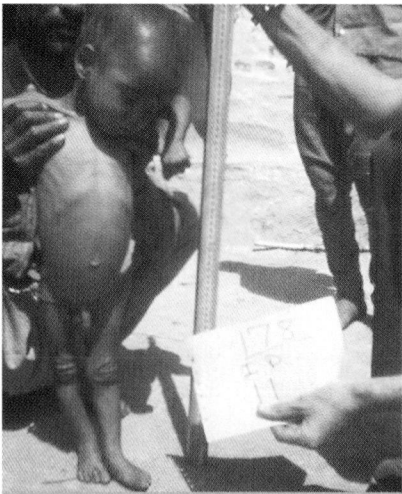

FIGURE 7-17 Patients with kwashiorkor can have a normal weight as well as TSF and MAC. Edema is common. *Courtesy of the Centers for Disease Control and Prevention.*

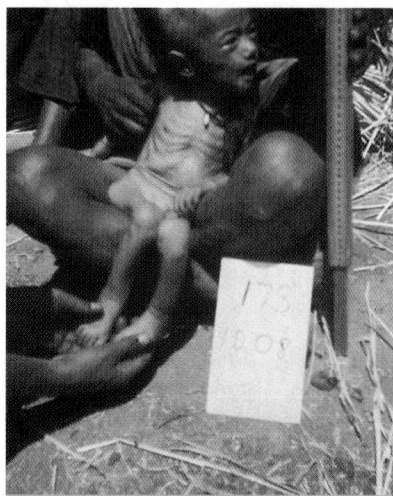

FIGURE 7-18 Marasmus is characterized by decreased weight, TSF, MAC, and muscle wasting. *Courtesy of the Centers for Disease Control and Prevention.*

normal limits. Additional physical signs are scaly, flaky skin, depigmentation of the hair, enlarged liver, and mental apathy (Figure 7-17). It can occur with the ingestion of liquid diets that are low in protein, malabsorption diseases, hypermetabolic states, cancer, and AIDS.

P **Marasmus,** or protein-calorie malnutrition, is a severe nutritional disorder in which there is an inadequate intake of protein and calories. As a result, there is a wasting of skeletal muscle and subcutaneous fat. This disorder can also occur from poor absorption of proteins, such as with burns, anorexia nervosa, tuberculosis, cancer, AIDS, and malabsorption diseases. Patients with marasmus have symptoms similar to kwashiorkor except that they appear more emaciated and do not have edema (Figure 7-18). If severe enough, these patients can have impaired cell-mediated immunity.

P Mixed marasmus and kwashiorkor is a severe form of protein-calorie malnutrition. It is typically seen in patients who are in a severe hypermetabolic state (such as trauma or burns), as well as a near starvation state. There is a reduction in subcutaneous tissue, visceral proteins, and somatic proteins.

A Results greater than the 95th percentile on the standard charts are abnormal.

P Obesity is suggested.

P If edema is present on the assessed body parts, the measurement may not be a reliable indicator of nutritional status.

LABORATORY DATA

Laboratory analysis is used for screening for potential nutritional problems and to assist with diagnosis when problems are suspected after a thorough history and a physical are conducted. Caution must be exercised when interpreting these laboratory values because many pathophysiological processes can affect the values. The lab data need to be considered in context with the patient's history, physical examination, and anthropometric measurements.

Hematocrit and Hemoglobin

Hematocrit determines the percentage of red cells to volume of whole blood. It reflects the body's iron supply. **Hemoglobin** is the iron component of the

---

E Examination   **N** Normal Findings   **A** Abnormal Findings   **P** Pathophysiology

TABLE 7-12 Normal Values for Hematocrit and Hemoglobin		
	NORMAL VALUES	
Age	Hematocrit (%)	Hemoglobin g/dL
1 mo	33–55	10.7–17.1
12 mo	33–41	11.3–14.1
1–2 yr	32–40	11.0–14.0
12–14 yr		
Female	34–44	11.5–15.0
Male	35–45	12.0–16.0
18–44 yr		
Female	35–45	12.0–15.0
Male	39–49	13.0–17.0
45–64 yr		
Female	35–47	12.0–16.0
Male	39–50	13.0–17.0
65–74 yr		
Female	35–47	12.0–16.0
Male	37–51	13.0–17.0

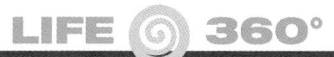

Nutritional Assessment of Cardiac Status

You are scheduled to perform a history and physical on a 52-year-old man. He does not drink alcohol, use tobacco, or salt his food. He runs 4 miles, 5 days a week. His BMI and body weight are appropriate for his age and height. However, the patient's father and grandfather both died of massive heart attacks in their 40s. You inform the patient that you would like to have him obtain blood work for his lipid profile since it has not been checked in more than 10 years. The patient tells you that this is unnecessary because he observes a heart-healthy lifestyle. What would you say to the patient? How would you proceed with the rest of the history and physical examination?

blood that transports oxygen. Both values are obtained from a venous blood sample.

N Hemoglobin and hematocrit results should fall within expected values, as shown in Table 7-12. Increased hematocrit and hemoglobin may normally occur in people living in high altitudes, due to the decrease in partial pressure of oxygen in those areas.

A Decreased hematocrit and hemoglobin are abnormal.

P Moderate to severe anemia may indicate decreased iron intake, leukemia, cirrhosis, hyperthyroidism, hemorrhage, hemodilution, or hemolytic reactions.

P Increased hematocrit and hemoglobin are abnormal.

P Chronic hypoxia, such as in cyanotic heart defects, can result in polycythemia. Severe dehydration may also result from hemoconcentration.

Lipids

In 2001, the Third Report of the National Cholesterol Education Program (NCEP) Expert Panel on Detection, Evaluation, and Treatment of High Blood Cholesterol in Adults (ATP III) published guidelines to assist health care providers in assessing and managing hyperlipidemia. Keep in mind that the laboratory values are obtained from a fasting patient. The following values are drawn from ATP III:

N *Total Cholesterol* (in mg/dL)

< 200	Desirable
200–239	Borderline high
> 240	High

HDL Cholesterol (in mg/dL)

< 40	Low
> 60	High

LDL Cholesterol (in mg/dL)

< 100	Optimal
100–129	Near optimal/above optimal
130–159	Borderline high
160–189	High
> 190	Very high

Triglycerides (in mg/dL)

< 150	Normal
150–199	Borderline high
200–499	High
> 500	Very high

A Elevated cholesterol, LDL, and triglycerides above desirable range are abnormal. HDL less than 40 mg/dL is abnormal in adults.

P Elevated cholesterol and/or triglycerides can be due to increased fat intake, genetics, and some medications (e.g., steroids, estrogens, cyclosporin). These elevations can lead to an increased risk of cardiac disease.

Transferrin, Total Iron-Binding Capacity (TIBC), and Iron

Transferrin is a protein that regulates iron absorption. Transferrin can be measured by the **total iron-binding capacity** (TIBC) (the amount of iron with which it can bind).

Serum iron is the amount of transferrin-bound iron. These data are obtained from a venous blood sample. Serum transferrin can be calculated using the following formula:

$$\text{Transferrin} = (0.8 \times \text{TIBC}) - 43$$

N Normal adult levels are:
Transferrin: 170–250 mg/dL
TIBC: 240–450 mcg/dL
Serum iron (women): 65–165 mcg/dL
Serum iron (men): 75–175 mcg/dL

A An increase in transferrin is abnormal.

P Increased levels of transferrin are found in inadequate dietary iron, iron-deficiency anemia, hepatitis, and oral contraceptive use.

A Decreased levels of transferrin are abnormal.

P Decreased levels of transferrin are found in pernicious anemia, sickle cell anemia, anemia associated with infection or chronic diseases, cancer, and malnutrition.

A Increases in serum iron levels are abnormal.

P Increases in serum iron levels are found in hemolytic anemias and lead poisoning.

A Decreases in serum iron levels are abnormal.

P Decreases in serum iron levels are found in iron deficiency, chronic diseases, third-trimester pregnancy, and severe physiological stress.

Total Lymphocyte Count

Total lymphocyte count (TLC) is measured in the complete blood count with differential and measures immune function and visceral protein status. When the white blood cell count is abnormally elevated or decreased, such as in bacterial infections or AIDS, respectively, the TLC is not always a reliable indicator of nutritional status.

N Normal adult levels are 1,500–1,800 cells/mm^3.

A A decrease in the total lymphocyte count of less than 1,500 indicates moderate protein deficiency, whereas less than 900 indicates severe protein deficiency.

P Protein deficiency occurs when the body is malnourished, such as when a patient is immunocompromised.

Antigen Skin Testing

Antigen skin testing is another test of immune function. Intradermal injections of various antigens can be used. Antigens commonly used are PPD tuberculin skin tests, mumps virus, *Candida albicans*, streptokinase, *Streptococcus*, *coccidioidin*, and *Trichophyton*. Results are read at 24 and 48 hours postinjection.

N A negative skin reaction (no induration or erythema) after being tested with various antigens is normal. These are antigens to which most people have been exposed and have developed an antibody response.

A A positive reaction to antigens placed intradermally is abnormal, which is indicated by a red area or induration 5 mm or more around the test site 24 hours or more after the injection. A negative reaction to only one of the antigens tested or a delayed positive reaction may occur with malnutrition.

P Poor antibody response occurs in patients who are immunocompromised. They have a decreased ability to fight infection and build antibodies. Protein malnutrition has been shown to decrease immune function. This diminished reaction to antigens is called **anergy**. Antigen skin testing is often called anergy panels.

Prealbumin

Prealbumin (also called thyroxine-binding prealbumin) is the transport protein for thyroxine and retinol-binding protein. The half-life is 24 to 48 hours, so it is an excellent value to monitor the effects of recent nutritional support and changes in nutritional status.

N The normal range for prealbumin is 10–40 mg/dL.

A Liver disease, such as cirrhosis and hepatitis, as well as severe stress from infection, burn injury, sepsis, prolonged surgery, hyperthyroidism, and cystic fibrosis can all lead to decreased prealbumin levels.

P Severe acute conditions in which severe catabolism occurs tend to lower the prealbumin level. In the case of liver disease, the levels are lower because of decreased hepatic synthesis of proteins.

Albumin

Albumin is formed in the liver. It transports nutrients, blood, and hormones, and helps maintain osmotic pressure. Albumin must have functioning liver cells and an adequate amount of amino acids to be synthesized. It is an indicator of visceral protein status. Because albumin has a long half-life (about 20 days), it is not an indicator of subtle or early changes in nutritional status. It is measured from a venous blood sample.

N The normal range for serum albumin is 3.5 to 5.0 g/dL.

A Less than 3.5 g/dL is abnormal.

P Decreased levels of albumin may indicate malnutrition because of a decrease in visceral protein stores, or a decrease in the amount of protein stored in organs. The decrease may not be seen until the protein deficiency reaches a chronic stage.

P Decreased levels of albumin are also found in massive hemorrhage, burns, and kidney disease.

Glucose

Serum glucose tests the body's ability to metabolize glucose. It is best assessed after a fasting period and from a venous blood sample.

N The normal glucose levels are:

Adult:	Fasting serum:	70–110 mg/dL
	Nonfasting:	85–125 mg/dL
Child:		60–100 mg/dL

A An increase in glucose level is abnormal.

P **Hyperglycemia** occurs in diabetes mellitus, impaired glucose tolerance, vitamin B_1 deficiency, and convulsive states. This indicates that glucose is not being transported into the cells by insulin.

A A decrease in serum glucose level is abnormal.

P **Hypoglycemia** occurs in pancreatic disorders, liver disease, decreased food intake, and insulin overdose. This occurs when there is too much insulin and not enough glucose in the blood.

Glycosylated Hemoglobin (HbA1c)

Glycosylated hemoglobin represents the amount of glucose that is permanently bound to hemoglobin. It is a long-term measure of blood sugar control, as it reflects the average serum glucose over a 2- to 3-month period. For this reason, it is usually not checked more than once every 3 months.

E Examination	**N** Normal Findings	**A** Abnormal Findings	**P** Pathophysiology

The normal HbA1c is 4.0–6.0%.

A value over 6.0% is abnormal.

A HbA1c greater than 6.0% is found in diabetic patients. The higher the value, the more uncontrolled the diabetes. The HbA1c treatment goal is stated as 6.5% by the American Association of Clinical Endocrinologists and 7.0% by the American Diabetes Association.

Creatinine Height Index (CHI)

Creatinine is a substance normally excreted in the urine; it is dependent on the amount of skeletal muscle mass, and it measures the amount of protein reserves. Urine creatinine is tested after collecting a 24-hour urine sample. An ideal urine creatinine level by height table is used to establish the denominator in the equation used to calculate CHI. Use the following equation to calculate creatinine height index:

$$CHI = \frac{\text{actual 24-hour creatinine excretion}}{\text{ideal 24-hour creatinine excretion}} \times 100$$

The CHI is not an accurate indicator of skeletal muscle mass in dehydrated patients or in patients with renal dysfunction.

Normal CHI values are greater than 90%.

CHI between 80% and 90% indicates mild protein deficiency.

CHI between 70% and 80% indicates moderate protein deficiency.

CHI of less than 70% indicates severe protein deficiency.

Protein malnutrition may be indicated by the loss of lean body mass, which can occur in severe trauma, prolonged fever, and stress.

Nitrogen Balance

Nitrogen is usually taken into the body in the form of food protein sources. It is one of the compounds of amino acids. Nitrogen is incorporated into protein and excreted in urine and feces. This balance of nitrogen intake to nitrogen output is compared, usually with a 24-hour urine sample. The nitrogen balance can be calculated using this formula:

$$\text{Nitrogen Balance} = \frac{\text{grams of protein eaten}}{6.25} - (\text{UUN}^* + 4)$$

*UUN = 24-hour urine urea nitrogen (in grams)

A zero balance is normal. A positive balance indicates tissue formation, found in growing children and in pregnant women.

A negative nitrogen balance is abnormal and indicates a catabolic state (i.e., the body excretes more nitrogen than is consumed).

More nitrogen is excreted than taken in, which means there is destruction or wasting of tissue. This can occur in malnutrition and in catabolic states (e.g., burns, severe stress, trauma, surgery).

Vitamin D

Table 7-2 shows that vitamin D is essential for proper bone growth and teeth development. Vitamin D is unique because dietary consumption can help meet nutritional needs, but the body, with sufficient ultraviolet light radiation exposure, can also produce vitamin D. Thus, vitamin D is actually a hormone and not a vitamin. A dietary deficiency of vitamin D levels can lead to vitamin D

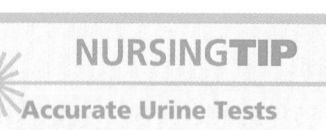

NURSING**TIP**

Accurate Urine Tests

Urine samples for CHI and nitrogen balance require the observance of strict collection procedures. Check your institution's procedure manual to ensure accuracy of the 24-hour samples.

E Examination   **N** Normal Findings   **A** Abnormal Findings   **P** Pathophysiology

insufficiency, as can the lack of adequate sun exposure and/or the use of sunscreen agents. Extensive research is being conducted worldwide on the larger role that vitamin D may have in osteoporosis, decreased muscle strength, myopathy, and cancer. The laboratory marker that is used to evaluate vitamin D is the total 25-hydroxyvitamin, or vitamin D 25-OH, which is a combination of 25-hydroxyvitamin D_2 and D_3.

N The normal vitamin D 25-OH is 25–80 ng/mL.

A A serum vitamin D 25-OH less than 25 ng/mL is suboptimal.

P Hypovitaminosis D, or vitamin D deficiency, in adults can result in osteoporosis, osteomalacia, hepatobiliary disease, and calcium malabsorption and in children can result in rickets.

DIAGNOSTIC DATA

Radiographic studies are used to determine bone formation and to assess development. Rickets and scurvy are both examples of long-term nutritional deficiencies that have radiographic manifestations. Rickets is a deficiency of vitamin D, and scurvy is a deficiency of vitamin C; both are characterized by softening and deformities of the bones. A bone density, or dual-energy X-ray absorptiometry (DEXA), scan is a low-radiation, noninvasive test that assesses the hip, lumbar spine, femoral neck, and wrist for osteoporosis. Though osteoporosis can result from many variables, nutrition is one of the leading etiologies in various age groups.

CASE STUDY

The Patient with Metabolic Syndrome

This case study illustrates the application and objective documentation of the nutritional assessment.
Diane visits the health clinic for a physical examination. She wants to enter a weight-loss program and needs medical clearance.

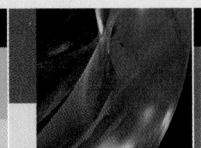

HEALTH HISTORY

PATIENT PROFILE	52 yo SWF
REASON FOR SEEKING HEALTH CARE	"I want to lose this weight once and for all. I have tried many programs, and this one seems the best suited for me, but I need medical clearance to enroll in the program."
PRESENT HEALTH	Pt has been overwt since her early 30s. She reports that she eats when she gets bored. Her job is sedentary, and she consumes a lg lunch daily. She has tried many diets in the past and has been successful c̄ a wt loss of a few lbs in 2–3 mos but then gets tired of the diet and puts the wt back on. Pt does not want to be on so much medication and expresses the desire to get off some of her meds. Her PCP has been stressing the need for her to lose wt in the hopes that she can come off some medication. Pt sees her PCP q 3 mos. Pt has researched different wt loss programs and is committed to "finally doing it."

continues

CASE STUDY (Continued)

The Patient with Metabolic Syndrome

PAST HEALTH HISTORY	
Medical History	Gyn told her this yr that she is menopausal
	OAB: age 49
	DM 2: age 48
	HTN: age 37
	Hyperlipidemia: age 37
	GERD: age 31
	AR: age 29
	Sees PCP q 3 mos
Surgical History	Appendectomy: age 32 (general anesthesia); no sequelae
	SCC excision Ⓛ face: age 50 (local anesthesia); no sequelae
Allergies	Niacin: tachycardia, palpitations
	Nickel: contact dermatitis
Medications	Solifenacin 5 mg po daily
	Metformin 500 mg 2 po BID
	Exenatide 10 mg subcutaneous BID
	Metoprolol XL 25 mg po daily
	Ezetimibe/simvastatin 10/20 mg po daily
	Esomeprazole 40 mg po daily
	Fluticasone aqueous nasal spray 1–2 sprays q nostril q AM PRN
	MVI po q AM
	Calcium 500 mg po BID
	Vitamin C 1,000 mg po daily
Communicable Diseases	Denies STDs/hepatitis/⊕ HIV
Injuries and Accidents	Fx Ⓛ wrist when fell on ice age 44; healed c̄ cast and s̄ sequelae
Special Needs	Denies
Blood Transfusions	Denies
Childhood Illnesses	Varicella 45 yrs ago, some facial scarring
Immunizations	Usual childhood immunizations per recollection; last dT 5 yrs ago; receives annual influenza vaccine

continues

CASE STUDY (Continued)

The Patient with Metabolic Syndrome

FAMILY HEATH HISTORY

LEGEND

 Living female

 Living male

Deceased female

Deceased male

Points to patient

Divorced

AR = Allergic rhinitis
COPD = Chronic obstructive
      pulmonary disease
DM2 = Diabetes mellitus type 2
GERD = Gastroesophageal
      reflux disease
HTN = Hypertension
MS = Multiple sclerosis
OAB = Overactive bladder

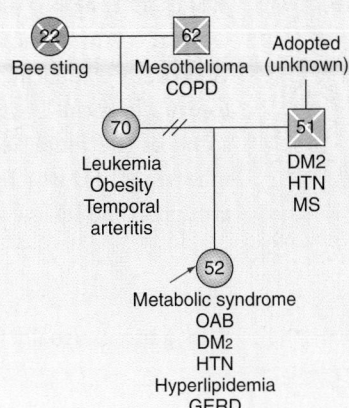

Denies FHH of food allergies/intolerances, eating disorders, celiac dz, malabsorption syndromes

SOCIAL HISTORY

Alcohol Use	Wine c̄ dinner on wkends
Tobacco Use	Smoked 1PPD × 25 yrs; quit 7 yrs ago
Drug Use	Denies
Domestic and Intimate Partner Violence	Denies
Sexual Practice	Heterosexual; presently not involved in any re/ship
Travel History	Visits family in Adirondacks every summer
Work Environment	Receptionist at surgeon's office in a new office park complex 25 min from home; access restricted to tenants p̄ nl business hrs; bldg has security staff
Home Environment	Lives alone in apt; has CO and smoke detectors, but forgets to check them
Hobbies and Leisure Activities	Gourmet cooking; participates in monthly gourmet cooking group for singles
Stress	Job; health status due to lg # of meds that she is taking
Education	HS diploma
Economic Status	Lives modestly c̄ little money left over
Military Status	Denies
Religion	Jewish; goes to temple on special occasions
Ethnic Background	Raised in strict Jewish family; bat mitzvah at age 13; drifted from faith when she left home at age 21; lost some relatives in the WWII Holocaust

continues

CASE STUDY (Continued)

The Patient with Metabolic Syndrome

Roles and Relationships	Talks c̄ parents and siblings in NY q wk; adopted "aunt" to a friend's child in PA
Characteristic Patterns of Daily Living	Wakes at 6:30, has breakfast and gets ready for work. Arrives at work at 8 AM. Lunch hour is from 1 to 2 PM; lunches are provided daily by pharmaceutical reps or other companies, and tends to eat a lg meal. Leaves work at 5 PM, and usually takes home some of the lunch leftovers for dinner. Likes to read cooking magazines and watch the cooking channel on TV. Goes to bed around 10:30 PM.

HEALTH MAINTENANCE ACTIVITIES

Sleep	8 hrs q night; usually feels rested in AM
Diet	
Diet History	• Does not follow any particular diet • Likes all foods, especially sweets • Has strong cravings at night to cook gourmet food from the recipes she read earlier that evening • Fast foods occasionally on wkends • At home eats alone; once a month she has dinner c̄ her gourmet group • Occasional heartburn even on esomeprazole, especially p̄ lg, fatty meals • Gained 10 lbs in past yr; no change in appetite; denies N/V/D • No dentures, no dysphagia

Food Intake History (24-hour recall)

TIME	FOOD/ DRINK	AMOUNT	METHOD OF PREPARATION	EATING LOCATION
7 AM	Breakfast burrito	2	Microwave	Home
	Orange juice	8 oz	Fresh	"
	Coffee	12 oz	Brewed	"
10 AM	Banana	1	Fresh	Office
	Donut	1	In office	"
1 PM	Chinese food	2 helpings	Brought to office	Office
	Cake or cookies	"big dessert"	"	"
	Soft drink (not diet)	16 oz	Bottled	"
4 PM	Cookies/candy	4	Store-bought	"
7 PM	Usually same as lunch			Home

continues

CASE STUDY (Continued)

The Patient with Metabolic Syndrome

Exercise	Walks ⅛ mile from car to office and back
Stress Management	Eats whatever she can find
Use of Safety Devices	Wears seat belt
Health Check-ups	Last visit c̄ PCP was 2 mos ago Dentist q few yrs Gyn checks q 1–2 yrs

NUTRITIONAL ASSESSMENT

Physical Assessment

	SUBJECTIVE	OBJECTIVE
1. General appearance	"I am too big."	Obese
2. Skin	c/o frequent rashes beneath breasts	Intact; Ø rashes
3. Hair	None	WNL
4. Nails	None	Fingernails—WNL
5. Eyes	Hard to drive at night	Conjunctiva pink
6. Mouth	None	Lips/gums/tongue/teeth WNL
7. Head and neck	None	Gross hearing WNL, nares patent, no discharge
8. Heart and peripheral vasculature	Palpitations c̄ stairs	BP: 148/95 HR: 96 and reg
9. Abdomen	Some constipation	Lg rounded abd, ⊠ BS, Ø mass, Ø HSM
10. Musculoskeletal system	None	Flabby muscles, FROM all joints
11. Nervous System	None	Mental status, DTR, and cerebellar fx all WNL

Height: 66"
Weight: 252 lbs (Nl for ht: 130–167 lbs)
% IBW: $252/167 \times 100 = 151\%$
BMI: $252 \times 703 = 177{,}156$

$\qquad 66 \times 66 = 4{,}356$

$\qquad 177{,}156/4{,}356 = 40.6$ (Obesity Class III)
Waist circumference: 52 inches (132 cm) (Nl: less than 35 inches)

continues

CASE STUDY (Continued)

The Patient with Metabolic Syndrome

Waist to hip ratio: 52/63 = 0.825 (Nl: less than 0.8)

TSF: 40 mm (95th percentile)

MAC: 384 mm (95th percentile)

MAMC: 38.4 − (3.14 × 4.0) = 25.8 cm (approximately 90th percentile)

LABORATORY DATA

Hct: 40% (Nl: 35–47%)

Hgb: 13.5 g/dL (Nl: 12–16 g/dL)

Lipids:

      Total cholesterol: 233 mg/dL (Nl: less than 200 mg/dL)

      HDL: 38 mg/dL (Nl: greater than 50 mg/dL in women)

      LDL: 175 mg/dL (Nl: less than 100 mg/dL)

      Triglycerides: 222 mg/dL (Nl: less than 150 mg/dL)

Transferrin/TIBC/Iron: Not performed

Total Lymphocyte Count: Not performed

Antigen Skin Testing: Not performed

Prealbumin: Not performed

Albumin: 4.9 g/dL (Nl: 3.5–5.0 g/dL)

Glucose: 132 mg/dL (fasting) (Nl: 70–110 mg/dL)

HbA1c: 7.7% (Nl: 4.0–6.0%)

Creatinine Height Index: Not performed

Nitrogen Balance: Not performed

Vitamin D: 40 ng/mL (Nl: 25–80 ng/mL)

DIAGNOSTIC DATA

X-rays: Not performed

DEXA Scan: Discussed need to get baseline in near future

ASSESSMENT IN BRIEF

Nutritional Assessment

Nutritional History

Physical Assessment

Anthropometric Measurements

- Height
- Weight
- Body mass index
- Waist circumference and waist to hip ratio
- Skinfold thickness
- Mid-arm and mid-arm muscle circumferences

Laboratory Data

- Hematocrit and hemoglobin
- Lipids
- Transferrin, total iron-binding capacity, and iron

- Total lymphocyte count
- Antigen skin testing
- Prealbumin
- Albumin
- Glucose
- HbA1c
- Creatinine height index
- Nitrogen balance
- Vitamin D

Diagnostic Data

- X-rays
- DEXA scan

REVIEW QUESTIONS

1. Which of the following statements reflects the recommendation of the Dietary Guidelines for Americans 2005?
   a. Consume less than 2,300 mg of sodium per day
   b. Consume less than 20% of calories from saturated fatty acids per day
   c. Consume one cup of fat-free or low-fat milk or equivalent milk products per day
   d. Consume up to two alcoholic beverages for women per day and up to three drinks per day for men
   The correct answer is (a).

2. The MyPyramid schematic representation can be an effective motivating tool for patients for which of the following reasons?
   a. It addresses the nutritional needs of patients of all ages to ensure a healthy body.
   b. Patients can track their progress on a Web site that is tailored to their specifications.
   c. It tells patients the amount of water that should be consumed daily to avoid dehydration.
   d. The length of the color band instructs patients on the quantity of food and the amount of physical activity that should be maintained on a daily basis to be fit.
   The correct answer is (b).

3. A deficiency of vitamin B_{12} results in which of the following conditions?
   a. Xerophthalmia
   b. Osteomalacia
   c. Cheilosis
   d. Pernicious anemia
   The correct answer is (d).

4. Phosphorus is a major mineral with which of the following functions?
   a. Maintaining protein structure
   b. Transmission of nerve impulses
   c. Regulation of osmotic pressure
   d. Development of bones and teeth
   The correct answer is (d).

5. Which of the following patients meets the criteria for the metabolic syndrome?
   a. A 32-year-old male with high HDL, high triglycerides, high fasting serum glucose
   b. A 75-year-old woman with high blood pressure, high LDL, abdominal obesity

   c. A 21-year-old male with high cholesterol, high HbA1c, high blood pressure
   d. A 44-year-old woman with abdominal obesity, high blood pressure, high triglycerides
   The correct answer is (d).

6. A 39-year-old woman is 5′2″ tall and weighs 149 lbs. What conclusion do you make about her BMI?
   a. Normal BMI   c. Obese
   b. Overweight   d. Moderately obese
   The correct answer is (b).

7. A patient presents for his annual physical examination. He currently weighs 285 lbs. One year ago, he weighed 235 lbs. What is this patient's percentage of weight change?
   a. 21.3%   c. 82.4%
   b. 28.5%   d. 121.0%
   The correct answer is (a).

8. A female patient has a waist of 32″ and hips that are 46″. What conclusion do you make about her waist to hip ratio?
   a. It is normal.
   b. It is associated with anorexia.
   c. It is associated with an increase in morbidity.
   d. It is associated with an "apple" appearance.
   The correct answer is (a).

9. The nurse is evaluating laboratory data on a 44-year-old female patient. Which of the following values is cause for concern and follow-up?
   a. HDL = 75 mg/dL
   b. Total lymphocyte count = 1,500 cells/mm^3
   c. Hemoglobin = 9.2 g/dL
   d. Nonfasting serum glucose = 110 mg/dL
   The correct answer is (c).

10. A patient has a TSF of 18 mm and a MAC of 27.4 cm. What is the MAMC?
    a. 2.68 cm   c. 268 mm
    b. 26.8 mm   d. 268 cm
    The correct answer is (c).

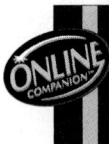

Visit the Estes online companion resource at
www.delmar.cengage.com
for additional content and study aids.
Click on Online Companions and then select
the Nursing discipline.

REFERENCES

Frisancho, A. R. (1981). New norms of upper limb fat and muscle areas for assessment of nutrition status. *American Journal of Clinical Nutrition, 34,* 2540.

Krauss, R. M., Eckel, R. H., Howard, B., Appel, L. J., Daniels, S. R., Deckelbaum, R. J., et al. (2000). AHA Dietary Guidelines. Revision 2000: A statement for healthcare professionals from the Nutrition Committee of the American Heart Association. *Circulation, 102*(18), 2296.

National Academy of Sciences, Food and Nutrition Board. (1997). *Dietary reference intakes: Recommended intakes for individuals.* Retrieved September 19, 2008, from http://www.nap.edu

National Center for Health Statistics. (2004). *Prevalence of overweight and obesity among adults: United States, 1999–2002.* Retrieved September, 19, 2008, from http://www.cdc.gov/nchs/products/pubs/pubd/hestats/obese/obse99.htm

National Heart, Lung, and Blood Institute, National Institutes of Health. (2001). *Third report of the National Cholesterol Education Program (NCEP) expert panel on detection, evaluation, and treatment of high blood cholesterol in adults (Adult Treatment Panel III), Executive summary* (NIH Publication No. 01-3670). Bethesda, MD: Authors.

National Institutes of Health and National Heart, Lung, and Blood Institute. (1998, June). *Clinical guidelines on the identification, evaluation, and treatment of overweight and obesity in adults.* Bethesda, MD: Authors.

Roth, R. A., & Townsend, C. E (2007). *Nutrition and diet therapy* (9th ed.). Clifton Park, NY: Delmar Cengage Learning.

U.S. Department of Agriculture. (2005). *MyPyramid food intake pattern calorie levels.* Retrieved January 22, 2008, from http://www.mypyramid.gov/professionals/pdf_calorie_levels.html

U.S. Department of Health and Human Services and U.S. Department of Agriculture. (2005). *Dietary guidelines for Americans, 2005* (6th ed.). Washington, DC: U.S. Government Printing Office.

BIBLIOGRAPHY

American Psychiatric Association. (2000). *Diagnostic and statistical manual of mental disorders* (4th ed.), *Text Revision.* Washington, DC: Author.

Barlow, S., & Dietz, W. (1998). Obesity evaluation and treatment: Expert committee recommendations. *Pediatrics, 102*(3), e29.

Bischoff-Ferrari, H. A. (2007). How to select the doses of vitamin D in the management of osteoporsis. *Osteoporosis International, 18*(4), 401–407.

Chalupka, S. (2005). Tainted water on tap. *American Journal of Nursing, 105*(11), 40–52.

Dansinger, M. L., Tatsioni, A., Wong, J. B., Chung, M., & Balk, E. M. (2007). Meta-analysis: The effect of dietary counseling for weight loss. *Annals of Internal Medicine, 47*(1), 41–50.

Doolen, J. L., & Miller, S. K. (2005). Primary care management of patients following bariatric surgery. *Journal of the American Academy of Nurse Practitioners, 17*(11), 446–450.

Fischbach, F. (2008). *A manual of laboratory and diagnostic tests* (8th ed.). Philadelphia: Lippincott.

Hudson, J., & Rapee, R. (Eds.). (2005). *Psychopathology and the family.* Amsterdam, The Netherlands: Elsevier.

Janssen, I., Katzmarzyk, P. T., & Ross, R. (2004). Waist circumference and not body mass index explains obesity-related health risk. *American Journal of Clinical Nutrition, 79*(3), 347–349.

Jockers, B. S. (2007). Vitamin D sufficiency: An approach to disease prevention. *The American Journal for Nurse Practitioners, 11*(1), 43–50.

Killip, S., Bennett, J. M., & Chambers, M. D. (2007). Iron deficiency anemia. *American Family Physician, 75*(5), 671–678.

Mahan, K., & Escott-Stump, S. (2007). *Krause's food and nutrition therapy.* Philadelphia: Saunders.

Mitrou, P. N., Kipnis, V., Thiebaut, A. C. M., Reedy, J., Subar, A. F., Wirfalt, E., et al. (2007). Mediterranean dietary pattern and prediction of all-cause mortality in a US population. *Archives of Internal Medicine, 167*(22), 2461–2468.

Moore, N. L., & Kiebzak, G. M. (2007). Suboptimal vitamin D status is a highly prevalent but treatable condition in both hospitalized patients and the general population. *Journal of the American Academy of Nurse Practitioners, 19*(12), 642–651.

Ogden, C. L., Carroll, M. D., Curtin, L. R., McDowell, M. A., Tabak, C. J., & Flegal, K. M. (2006). Prevalence of overweight and obesity in the United States, 1999–2004. *JAMA, 295*(13), 1549–1555.

Prussian, K. H., Barksdale-Brown, D. J., & Dieckmann, J. (2007). Racial and ethnic differences in the presentation of metabolic syndrome. *The Journal for Nurse Practitioners, 3*(4), 229–239.

Reavis, C. (2005). Rural health alert: *Helicobacter pylori* in well water. *Journal of the American Academy of Nurse Practitioners, 17*(7), 283–289.

Shils, M. E., Shike, M., Ross, A. C., Caballero, B., & Cousins, R. J. (Eds.). (2006). *Modern nutrition in health and disease* (10th ed.). Philadelphia: Lippincott Williams & Wilkins.

U.S. Department of Health and Human Services, Public Health Services, Office of Disease Prevention and Health Promotion. (1994). *Clinician's handbook of preventive services: Put prevention into practice.* Washington, DC: U.S. Government Printing Office.

Walker, K. J., & Beckstrand, R. L. (2006). Omega-3 fatty acid consumption in the reduction of sudden cardiac death: A critical appraisal. *The American Journal for Nurse Practitioners, 10*(11/12), 11–24.

Williams, P. M., Goodie, J., & Motsinger, C. D. (2008). Primary care management of eating disorders reviewed. *American Family Physician, 77*(2), 187–195.

WEB SITES

American Association of Clinical Endocrinologists:
   http://www.aace.com

American Diabetes Association:
   http://www.diabetes.org

American Dietetic Association:
   http://www.eatright.org

American Dietetic Association Home Food Safety:
   http://www.homefoodsafety.org

American Heart Association:
   http://www.americanheart.org

The DASH Diet Eating Plan:
   http://www.dashdiet.org

USDA MyPyramid For Kids:
   http://www.mypyramid.gov

USDA MyPyramid Tracker:
   http://www.mypyramidtracker.gov

WeightWatchers:
   http://www.weightwatchers.com

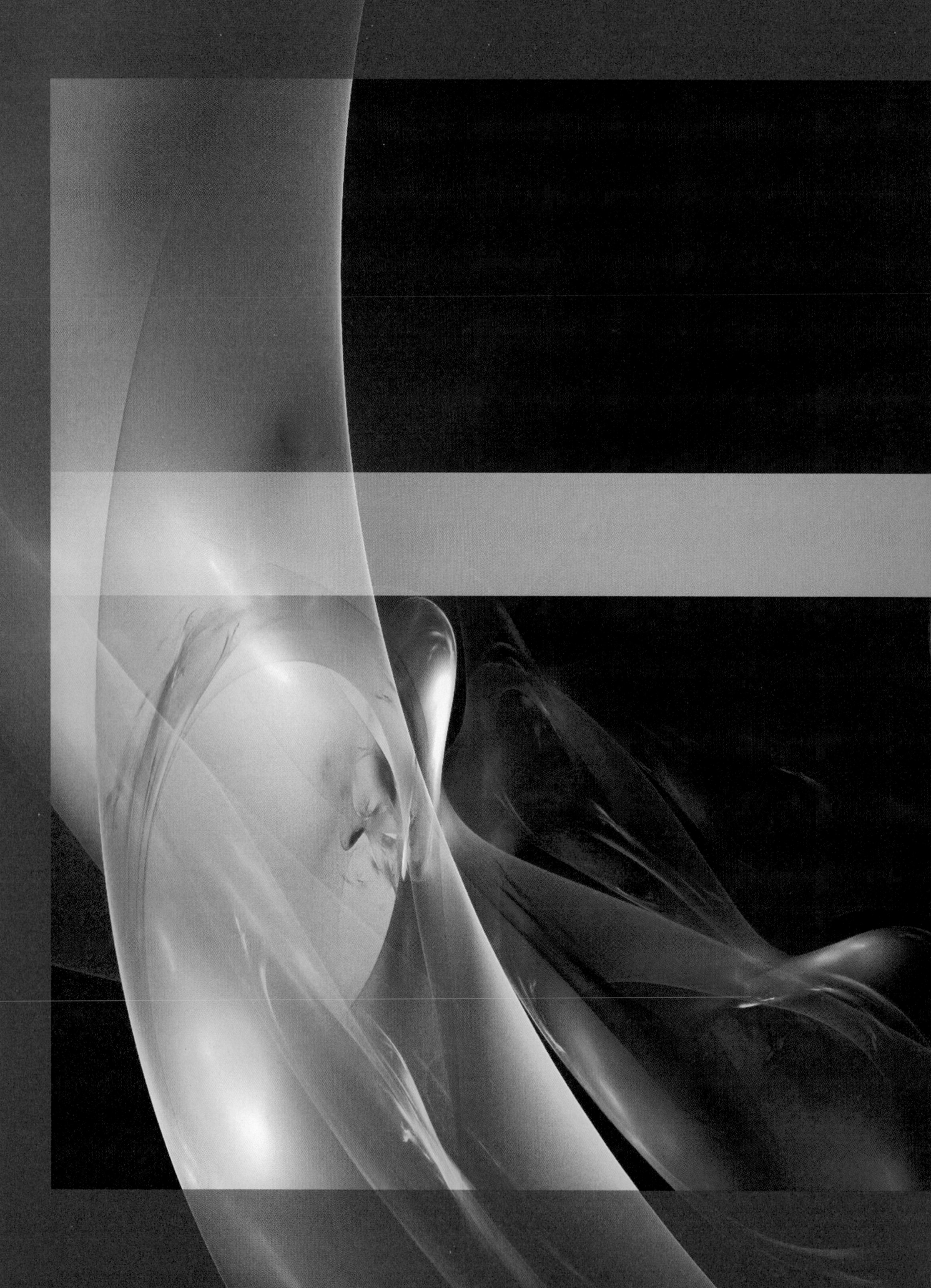

UNIT 3 | Physical Examination

What is a nurse there for if she cannot observe these things
for herself?

—FLORENCE NIGHTINGALE

CHAPTER 8

Physical Assessment Techniques

COMPETENCIES

1. Describe how to maintain Standard Precautions and Transmission-Based Precautions during the physical assessment.

2. Establish an environment suitable for conducting a physical assessment.

3. Describe how to perform inspection, palpation, percussion, and auscultation, and identify which areas of the body are assessed with each technique.

4. Demonstrate inspection, palpation, percussion, and auscultation in the clinical setting.

Inspection, palpation, percussion, and auscultation are the techniques used by the nurse to assess the patient during a physical examination. This chapter introduces the assessment techniques and equipment used to conduct physical examinations.

ASPECTS OF PHYSICAL ASSESSMENT

Physical assessment of a patient serves many purposes:

1. Screening of general well-being. The findings will serve as baseline information for future assessments.
2. Validation of the complaints that brought the patient to seek health care.
3. Monitoring of current health problems.
4. Formulation of diagnoses and treatments.

The need for physical assessment depends on, among other factors, the patient's health status, concept of health care, and accessibility to health care. For example, a person with brittle diabetes with arthritis and glaucoma who has access to health care is likely to enter the health care delivery system more often than a healthy college student.

ROLE OF THE NURSE

The professional nurse plays a vital role in the assessment of patient problems. Educational preparation and the clinical setting in part determine the extent to which the nurse participates in the assessment process. For example, a nurse in primary care may perform a comprehensive physical assessment of patients, while a critical care nurse may conduct selected patient assessments to monitor and evaluate current health problems. In either case, nurses are expected to be familiar with and comfortable using physical assessment skills. Today's nurses are sophisticated professionals who require information in order to make clinical decisions. The physical assessment findings provide this information.

STANDARD PRECAUTIONS AND TRANSMISSION-BASED PRECAUTIONS

The transmission of hepatitis, human immunodeficiency virus (HIV), and other infectious diseases is a primary concern for the nurse and for the patient. **Standard Precautions**, formerly known as "universal precautions," were developed by the Centers for Disease Control and Prevention (CDC) to protect health care professionals and patients. The primary goal of Standard Precautions is to prevent the exchange of blood and body fluids (Figure 8-1). Standard Precautions should be practiced with every patient throughout the entire encounter, whether or not the patient has a known or suspected infectious process.

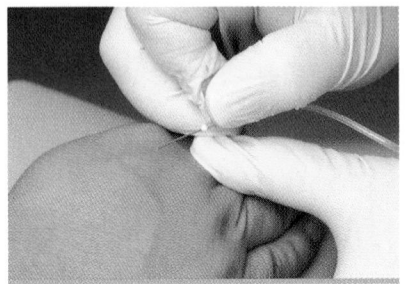

FIGURE 8-1 The nurse is using Standard Precautions to draw blood.

- You are preparing to perform a genital exam when the patient says, "I've changed my mind. I don't want to do this." What is your best course of action?

- While performing a breast exam on a patient, the patient shrieks, "What do you think you are doing?" How would you respond to this patient?

- During deep palpation of the abdomen, your patient responds, "Ouch, you hurt me!" How would you respond?

- You are auscultating the lungs of a 42-year-old man. He tells you that he is thinking of suing his previous health care provider. The patient tells you, "The real problem these days is that no one bothers to listen to the patient anymore." What would be an appropriate response?

- What strategies can you incorporate into your practice to decrease your legal liability?

In 2007, the CDC added three elements to the list of Standard Precautions:

1. Respiratory Hygiene/Cough Etiquette
2. Safe injection practices
3. Use of masks for any invasive procedure involving the spinal or epidural spaces

The Respiratory Hygiene/Cough Etiquette recommendation is based on the recent experience with the severe acute respiratory syndrome coronavirus (SARS-CoV) and avian influenza in humans. Simple infection control practices were not used in some instances and may have aided the pathogen's transmission. Safe injection practices are reinforced in the new guidelines because of the continued incidence of hepatitis B and hepatitis C in outpatient settings.

Lastly, the use of masks in invasive procedures involving the spinal area was advised because of research that demonstrated an increased risk of contracting *Neisseria meningitidis* from respiratory secretions during invasive spinal procedures. Figure 8-2 illustrates the Standard Precautions recommended by the CDC.

The CDC has developed another level of precautions called **Transmission-Based Precautions**. These precautions are to be used in conjunction with Standard Precautions. Contact, droplet, and airborne transmissions of microorganisms that are known to exist in a patient or are suspected in a patient are targeted. Contact transmission pathogens, such as in impetigo, scabies, varicella zoster virus, and multidrug-resistant organisms (e.g. MRSA), can be spread directly from person to person. Contact precautions must also be implemented when the patient has fecal incontinence, excessive wound drainage, or other body secretions, because of the risk for environmental contamination and subsequent transmission. Microorganisms can also be spread indirectly from a contaminated inanimate object to a person. Droplet transmission occurs when microorganisms are deposited on susceptible body parts via respiratory secretions (sneezing and coughing). Typically, the pathogens in the droplet remain infectious for only a short period of time. Suctioning a patient can also transmit droplets. *Bacillus pertussis*, *Haemophilus influenzae*, rhinovirus, adenovirus, group A *Streptococcus*, and *N. meningitidis* are examples of pathogens contracted through this mode of transmission. Airborne transmission spreads microorganisms by air currents and inhalation. These pathogens are infectious over long distances when they are airborne. They can also be passed through ventilation systems. Measles, the varicella virus, and *Mycobacterium tuberculosis* can spread in this mode. Transmission-Based Precautions are used in every encounter in every health care setting in addition to Standard Precautions, as some diseases can have more than one mode of transmission (e.g., SARS-CoV). Additional information can be viewed on the CDC Web site.

Hand Washing

The most important infection control practice is hand washing. You must begin every physical assessment with a thorough hand wash (see Figure 8-3). Some nurses perform this in the assessment area with the patient present. It is a nonthreatening way to start the physical assessment and allows the patient time to ask questions concerning the process.

The CDC's *Guideline for Hand Hygiene in Healthcare Settings* recommends the use of an alcohol-based hand rub (see Figure 8-4), an antimicrobial soap and water, or a nonantimicrobial soap and water when the hands are visibly contaminated with body fluids. Your institution may provide some or all of these methods of hand washing; regardless, the most important factor is that you use them with every patient interaction.

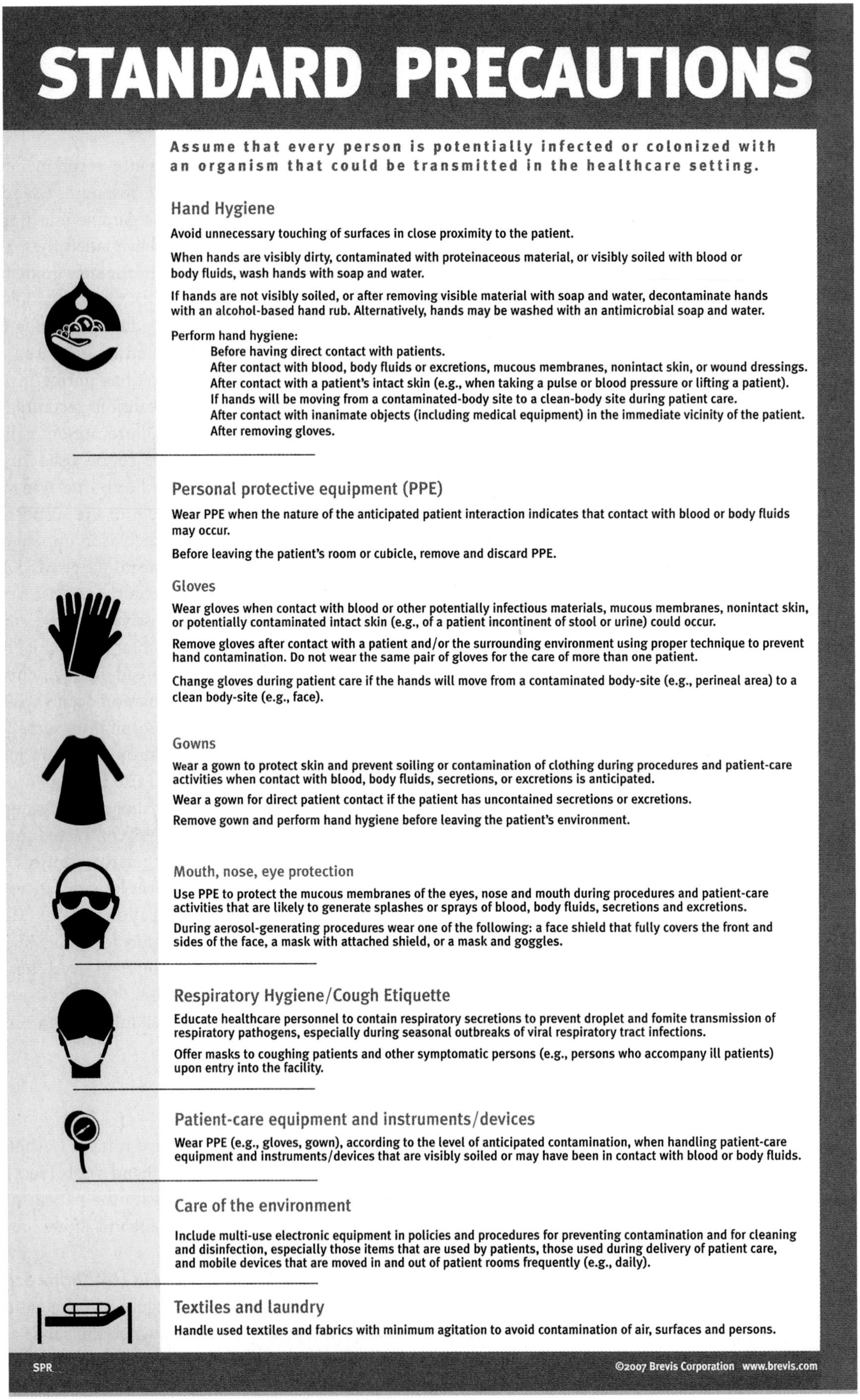

STANDARD PRECAUTIONS

Assume that every person is potentially infected or colonized with an organism that could be transmitted in the healthcare setting.

Hand Hygiene

Avoid unnecessary touching of surfaces in close proximity to the patient.

When hands are visibly dirty, contaminated with proteinaceous material, or visibly soiled with blood or body fluids, wash hands with soap and water.

If hands are not visibly soiled, or after removing visible material with soap and water, decontaminate hands with an alcohol-based hand rub. Alternatively, hands may be washed with an antimicrobial soap and water.

Perform hand hygiene:
    Before having direct contact with patients.
    After contact with blood, body fluids or excretions, mucous membranes, nonintact skin, or wound dressings.
    After contact with a patient's intact skin (e.g., when taking a pulse or blood pressure or lifting a patient).
    If hands will be moving from a contaminated-body site to a clean-body site during patient care.
    After contact with inanimate objects (including medical equipment) in the immediate vicinity of the patient.
    After removing gloves.

Personal protective equipment (PPE)

Wear PPE when the nature of the anticipated patient interaction indicates that contact with blood or body fluids may occur.

Before leaving the patient's room or cubicle, remove and discard PPE.

Gloves

Wear gloves when contact with blood or other potentially infectious materials, mucous membranes, nonintact skin, or potentially contaminated intact skin (e.g., of a patient incontinent of stool or urine) could occur.

Remove gloves after contact with a patient and/or the surrounding environment using proper technique to prevent hand contamination. Do not wear the same pair of gloves for the care of more than one patient.

Change gloves during patient care if the hands will move from a contaminated body-site (e.g., perineal area) to a clean body-site (e.g., face).

Gowns

Wear a gown to protect skin and prevent soiling or contamination of clothing during procedures and patient-care activities when contact with blood, body fluids, secretions, or excretions is anticipated.

Wear a gown for direct patient contact if the patient has uncontained secretions or excretions.

Remove gown and perform hand hygiene before leaving the patient's environment.

Mouth, nose, eye protection

Use PPE to protect the mucous membranes of the eyes, nose and mouth during procedures and patient-care activities that are likely to generate splashes or sprays of blood, body fluids, secretions and excretions.

During aerosol-generating procedures wear one of the following: a face shield that fully covers the front and sides of the face, a mask with attached shield, or a mask and goggles.

Respiratory Hygiene/Cough Etiquette

Educate healthcare personnel to contain respiratory secretions to prevent droplet and fomite transmission of respiratory pathogens, especially during seasonal outbreaks of viral respiratory tract infections.

Offer masks to coughing patients and other symptomatic persons (e.g., persons who accompany ill patients) upon entry into the facility.

Patient-care equipment and instruments/devices

Wear PPE (e.g., gloves, gown), according to the level of anticipated contamination, when handling patient-care equipment and instruments/devices that are visibly soiled or may have been in contact with blood or body fluids.

Care of the environment

Include multi-use electronic equipment in policies and procedures for preventing contamination and for cleaning and disinfection, especially those items that are used by patients, those used during delivery of patient care, and mobile devices that are moved in and out of patient rooms frequently (e.g., daily).

Textiles and laundry

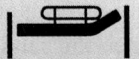

Handle used textiles and fabrics with minimum agitation to avoid contamination of air, surfaces and persons.

SPR   ©2007 Brevis Corporation   www.brevis.com

FIGURE 8-2 **Standard Precautions.** *Courtesy of Brevis Corporation.*

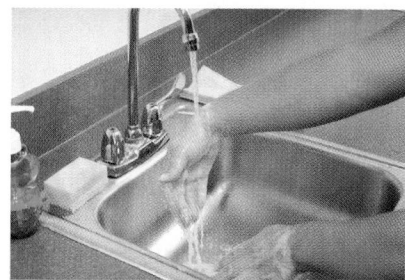

FIGURE 8-3 Hand Washing Using Soap and Water

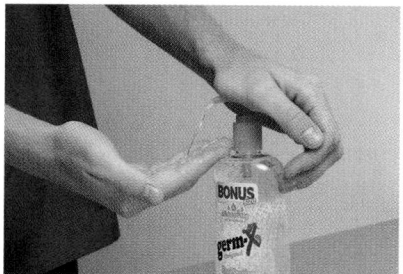

FIGURE 8-4 Hand Washing Using an Alcohol-Based Hand Rub

LEGAL ISSUES

In today's litigious society, you must be ever vigilant when engaging in nursing practice. Documentation issues have previously been addressed. Equally important is how you execute the nursing assessment. Establishing a trusting and caring relationship is the primary element in avoiding malpractice claims. While performing each step in the physical assessment process, you need to inform the patient of what to expect, where to expect it, and how it will feel. Protests by the patient need to be addressed prior to continuing the examination. Otherwise, the patient may claim insufficient informed consent, sexual abuse, or physical harassment.

All assessments and procedures, including any injury that was caused during the physical assessment, must be completely documented. The institutional policy regarding patient injury in the workplace must be followed.

ASSESSMENT TECHNIQUES

Physical assessment findings, or objective data, are obtained through the use of four specific diagnostic techniques: inspection, palpation, percussion, and auscultation. Usually, these assessment techniques are performed in this order when body systems are assessed. An exception is in the assessment of the abdomen, when auscultation is performed after inspection. Percussion and palpation can alter bowel motility, so they are performed after auscultation. These four techniques validate information provided by a patient in the health history, or they can verify a suspected physical diagnosis.

Usually, the easiest assessment skills to master are inspection and basic auscultation. Percussion and palpation may take more time and practice to perfect. With time and practice, the physical assessment techniques become second nature, and you will develop your own rhythm and style. You may not perform all assessment skills in the same order as they are presented in this text. This practice is acceptable as long as basic guidelines are observed.

INSPECTION

"A conscientious nurse is not necessarily an observing nurse; and life or death may lie with the good observer." This statement by Florence Nightingale provides inspiration and direction for inspection, which is usually the first assessment technique used during the assessment process. **Inspection** is an ongoing process that you use throughout the entire physical assessment and patient encounter. Inspection is the use of one's senses of vision and smell to consciously observe the patient.

Vision

Use of sight can reveal many facts about a patient. Visual inspection of a patient's respiratory status, for example, might reveal a rate of 38 breaths per minute and cyanotic nailbeds. In this case, the patient is tachypneic and possibly hypoxic, and would need a more thorough respiratory assessment. The process of visual inspection necessitates full exposure of the body part being inspected, adequate overhead lighting, and when necessary, **tangential lighting** (light that is shone at an angle on the patient to accentuate shadows and highlight subtle findings).

Smell

The nurse's olfactory sense provides vital information about a patient's health status. The patient may have a fruity breath odor characteristic of diabetic ketoacidosis. The classic odor emitted by a *Pseudomonas* infection is another well-recognized smell to the experienced nurse.

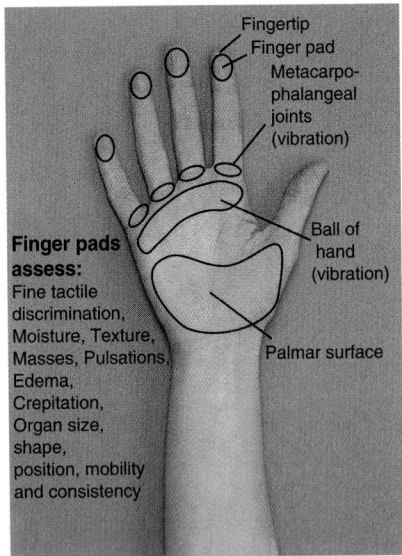

Finger pads assess:
Fine tactile discrimination, Moisture, Texture, Masses, Pulsations, Edema, Crepitation, Organ size, shape, position, mobility and consistency

A. Palmar Surface

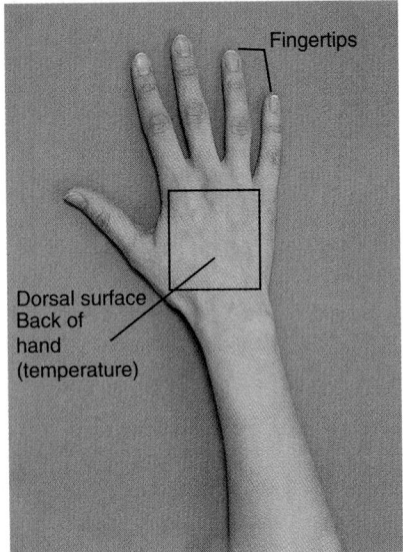

B. Dorsal Surface

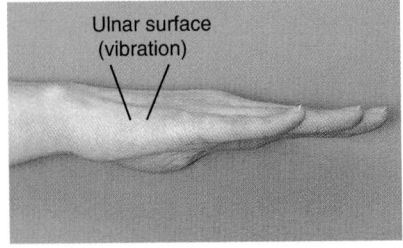

C. Ulnar Surface

FIGURE 8-5 **Parts of the Hand Used in Palpation**

PALPATION

The second assessment technique is **palpation**, which is the act of touching a patient in a therapeutic manner to elicit specific information. Prior to palpating a patient, some basic principles need to be observed. You should have short fingernails to avoid hurting the patient as well as yourself. Also, you should warm your hands prior to placing them on the patient; cold hands can make a patient's muscles tense, which can distort assessment findings. Encourage the patient to continue to breathe normally throughout the palpation. If pain is experienced during the palpation, discontinue the palpation immediately. Most significantly, inform the patient where, when, and how the touch will occur, especially when the patient cannot see what you are doing. In this way, the patient is aware of what to expect in the assessment process.

Your hands are the tools used to perform the palpation process. Different sections of the hands are best used for assessing certain areas of the body. The dorsum of the hand is most sensitive to temperature changes in the body. Thus, it is more accurate to place the dorsum of the hand on a patient's forehead to assess the body temperature than it is to use the palmar surface of the hand. The palmar surface of the fingers at the metacarpophalangeal joints, the ball of the hand, and the ulnar surface of the hand best discriminate vibrations, such as a cardiac thrill and fremitus. The finger pads are the portion of the hand used most frequently in palpation. The finger pads are useful in assessing fine tactile discrimination, skin moisture, and texture; the presence of masses, pulsations, edema, and crepitation; and the shape, size, position, mobility, and consistency of organs (Figure 8-5).

Remember to observe Standard Precautions when you are performing palpation. Gloves must be worn when examining any open wounds, skin lesions, or a body part with discharge, as well as internal body parts such as the mouth and rectum.

There are two distinct types of palpation: light and deep palpation. Each of these techniques is briefly described here and covered in greater detail in chapters describing body systems in which palpation is specifically used.

Light Palpation

Light palpation is done more frequently than deep palpation and is always performed before deep palpation. As the name implies, **light palpation** is superficial, delicate, and gentle. In light palpation, the finger pads are used to gain information on the patient's skin surface to a depth of approximately 1 cm below the surface. Light palpation reveals information on skin texture and moisture; overt, large, or superficial masses; and fluid, muscle guarding, and superficial tenderness. To perform light palpation:

1. Keeping the fingers of your dominant hand together, place the finger pads lightly on the skin over the area that is to be palpated. The hand and forearm will be on a plane parallel to the area being assessed.

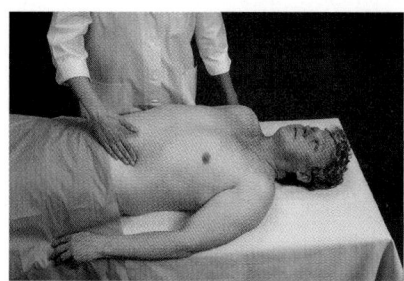

FIGURE 8-6 Technique of Light Palpation

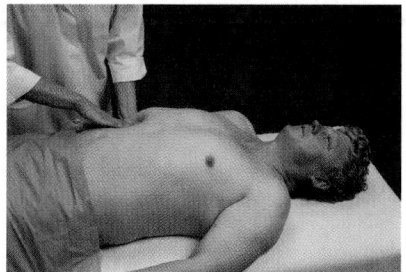

FIGURE 8-7 Technique of Deep Palpation

2. Depress the skin 1 cm in light, gentle, circular motions.
3. Keeping the finger pads on the skin, let the depressed body surface rebound to its natural position.
4. If the patient is ticklish, lift the hand off the skin before moving it to another area.
5. Using a systematic approach, move the fingers to an adjacent area and repeat the process.
6. Continue to move the finger pads until the entire area being examined has been palpated.
7. If the patient has complained of tenderness in any area, palpate this area last. Figure 8-6 shows how light palpation is performed.

Deep Palpation

Deep palpation can reveal information about the position of organs and masses, as well as their size, shape, mobility, and consistency, and areas of discomfort. Deep palpation uses the hands to explore the body's internal structures to a depth of 4–5 cm or more (Figure 8-7). This technique is most often used for the abdominal and the male and female reproductive assessments. Variations in this technique are single-handed and bimanual palpation, and are discussed in Chapter 17.

PERCUSSION

Percussion is the technique of striking one object against another to cause vibrations that produce sound. The density of underlying structures produces characteristic sounds. These sounds are diagnostic of normal and abnormal findings. The presence of air, fluid, and solids can be confirmed, as can organ size, shape, and position. Any part of the body can be percussed, but only limited information can be obtained in specific areas such as the heart. The thorax and abdomen are the most frequently percussed locations.

Percussion sound can be analyzed according to its intensity, duration, pitch (frequency), quality, and location. **Intensity** refers to the relative loudness or softness of the sound. It is also called the amplitude. **Duration** of percussed sound describes the time period over which a sound is heard when elicited. Frequency describes the concept of **pitch**. Frequency is caused by the sound's vibrations, or the highness or lowness of a sound. Frequency is measured in cycles per second (cps) or hertz (Hz). More rapidly occurring vibrations have a pitch that is higher than that of slower vibrations. Figure 8-8 illustrates this concept. The **quality** of a

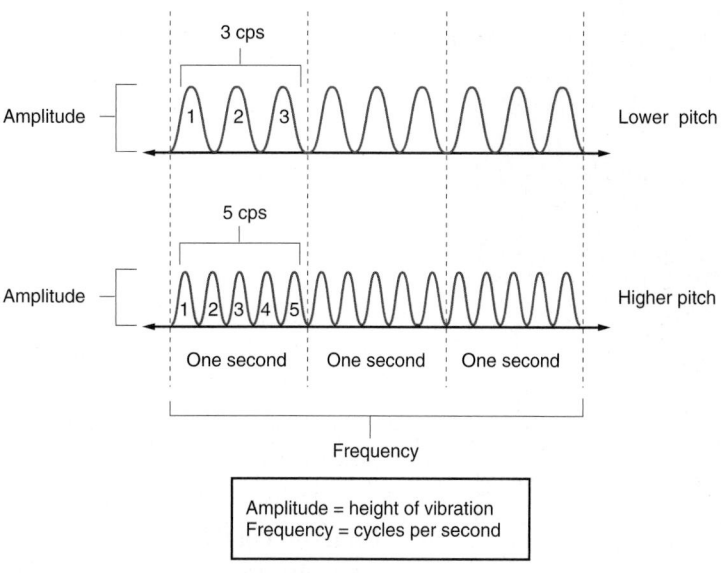

FIGURE 8-8 Percussion Pitch

TABLE 8-1 Characteristics of Percussion Sounds

SOUND	INTENSITY	DURATION	PITCH	QUALITY	NORMAL LOCATION	ABNORMAL LOCATION	DENSITY
Flatness	Soft	Short	High	Flat	Muscle (thigh) or bone	Lungs (severe pneumonia)	Most dense
Dullness	Moderate	Moderate	High	Thud	Organs (liver)	Lungs (atelectasis)	
Resonance	Loud	Moderate-long	Low	Hollow	Normal lungs	No abnormal location	
Hyperresonance	Very loud	Long	Very low	Boom	No normal location in adults; normal lungs in children	Lungs (emphysema)	
Tympany	Loud	Long	High	Drum	Gastric air bubble	Lungs (large pneumothorax)	Least dense

sound is its timbre, or how one perceives it musically. Location of sound refers to the area where the sound is produced and heard.

The process of percussion can produce five distinct sounds in the body: **flatness, dullness, resonance, hyperresonance,** and **tympany.** Specific parts of the body elicit distinct percussible sounds. Therefore, when an unexpected sound is heard in a particular part of the body, the cause must be further investigated.

Table 8-1 illustrates each of the five percussion sounds in relation to its respective intensity, duration, pitch, quality, location, and relative density. In addition, examples are provided of normal and abnormal locations of percussed sounds.

Sound waves are better conducted through a solid medium than through an air-filled medium because of the increased concentration of molecules. The basic premises underlying the sounds that are percussed are:

1. The more solid a structure, the higher its pitch, the softer its intensity, and the shorter its duration.
2. The more air filled a structure, the lower its pitch, the louder its intensity, and the longer its duration.

There are four types of percussion techniques: direct (immediate), indirect (mediate), direct fist percussion, and indirect fist percussion. It is important to keep in mind that the sounds produced from percussion are generated from body tissue up to 5 cm below the surface of the skin. If the abdomen is to be percussed, the patient should have the opportunity to void before the assessment.

Direct Percussion

Direct percussion or **immediate percussion** is the striking of an area of the body directly. To perform direct percussion:

1. Spread the index or middle finger of the dominant hand slightly apart from the rest of the fingers.
2. Make a light tapping motion with the finger pad of the index finger against the body part being percussed.
3. Note what sound is produced.

Percussion of the sinuses (Figure 8-9) illustrates the use of direct percussion in the physical assessment.

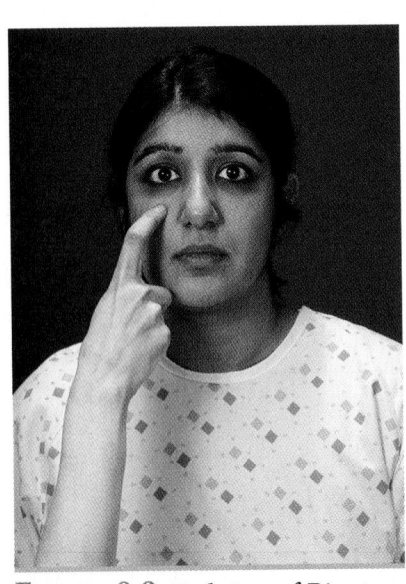

FIGURE 8-9 Technique of Direct Percussion

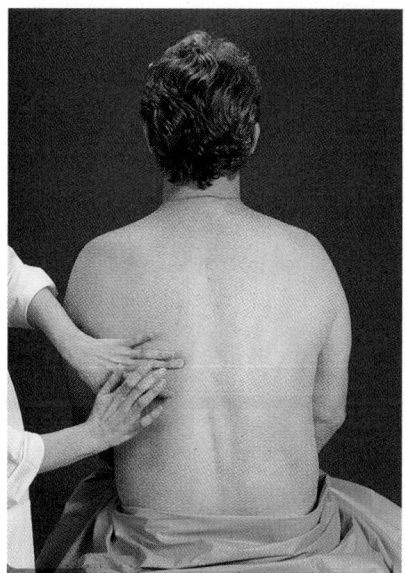

A. Position of Hands for Posterior Thorax Percussion

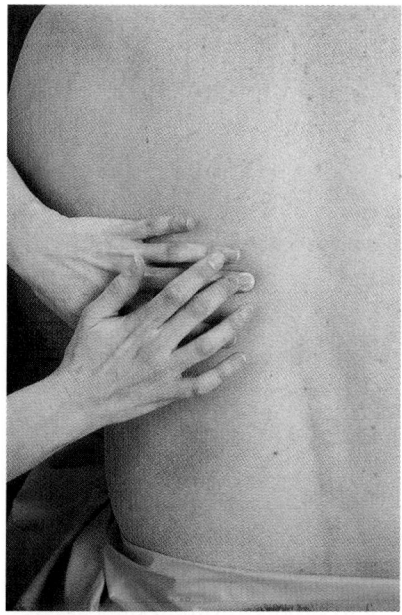

B. Percussion Strike

FIGURE 8-10 Technique of Indirect Percussion

Indirect Percussion

Indirect percussion is also referred to as **mediate percussion**. This is a skill that takes time and practice to develop and use effectively. Most sounds are produced using indirect percussion. Follow these steps to perform indirect percussion (Figure 8-10):

1. Place the nondominant hand lightly on the surface to be percussed.
2. Extend the middle finger of this hand, known as the **pleximeter**, and press its distal phalanx and distal interphalangeal joint firmly on the location where percussion is to begin. The pleximeter will remain stationary while percussion is performed in this location.
3. Spread the other fingers of the nondominant hand apart and raise them slightly off the surface. This prevents interference, and thus dampening, of vibrations during the actual percussion.
4. Flex the middle finger of the dominant hand, called the **plexor**. The fingernail of the plexor finger should be very short to prevent undue discomfort and injury to the nurse. The other fingers on this hand should be fanned.
5. Flex the wrist of the dominant hand and place the hand directly over the pleximeter finger of the nondominant hand.
6. With a sharp, crisp, rapid movement from the wrist of the dominant hand, strike the pleximeter with the plexor. At this point, the plexor should be perpendicular to the pleximeter. The blow to the pleximeter should be between the distal interphalangeal joint and the fingernail. Use the finger pad rather than the fingertip of the plexor to deliver the blow. Concentrate on the movement to create the striking action from the dominant wrist only.
7. As soon as the plexor strikes the pleximeter, withdraw the plexor to avoid dampening the resulting vibrations. Do not move the pleximeter finger.
8. Note the sound produced from the percussion.
9. Repeat the percussion process one or two times in this location to confirm the sound.
10. Move the pleximeter to a second location, preferably the contralateral location from where the previous percussion was performed. Repeat the percussion process in this manner until the entire body surface area being assessed has been percussed.

Recognizing Percussion Sound

When using direct and indirect percussion, the change from resonance to dullness is more easily recognized by the human ear than is the change from dullness to resonance. It is often helpful to close your eyes and concentrate on the sound in order to distinguish whether a change in sounds occurs. This concept has implications

NURSING TIP

At-Home Practice of Percussion

- Percuss two glasses—one filled with water, the other empty. Compare the sounds.
- Percuss the wall of a room and listen for the change in tones when a stud is reached.
- Percuss your thigh. Puff your cheeks and percuss them. Compare the sounds.

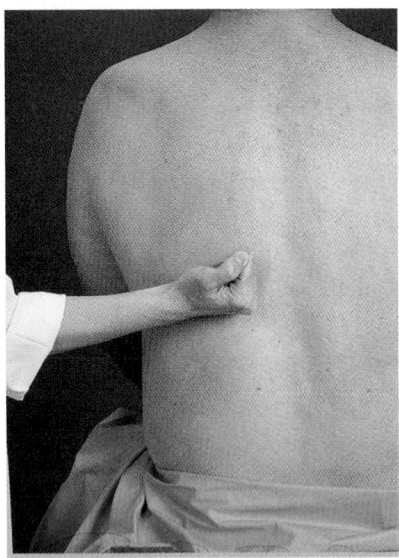

FIGURE 8-11 Technique of Direct Fist Percussion: Left Kidney

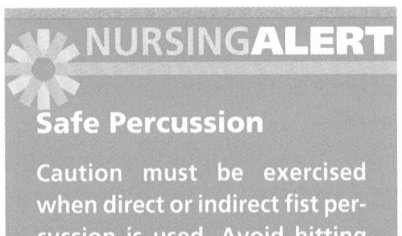

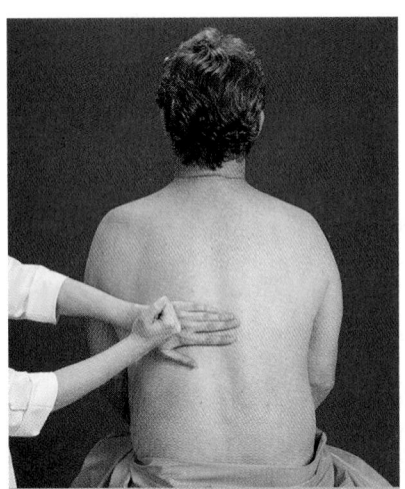

FIGURE 8-12 Technique of Indirect Fist Percussion: Left Kidney

for patterns of percussion in areas of the body where known locations have distinct percussible sounds. For example, the techniques of diaphragmatic excursion and liver border percussion can proceed in a more defined pattern because percussion can be performed from an area of resonance to an area of dullness. Another helpful hint is to validate the change in sounds by percussing back and forth between the two areas where a change is noted to confirm this change.

As stated earlier, the percussion technique can take considerable time to develop and perfect. Practicing the technique in the home environment can be a helpful learning experience; see the Nursing Tip, At-Home Practice of Percussion.

Direct Fist Percussion

Direct fist percussion is used to assess the presence of tenderness and pain in internal organs such as the liver or the kidneys. To perform direct fist percussion (Figure 8-11):

1. Explain this technique thoroughly so the patient does not think you are hitting him or her.
2. Draw the dominant hand up into a fist.
3. With the ulnar aspect of the closed fist, directly hit the area where the organ is located. The strike should be of moderate force, and it may take some practice to achieve the right intensity.

The presence of pain in conjunction with direct fist percussion indicates inflammation of that organ or a strike of too high an intensity.

Indirect Fist Percussion

The purpose of **indirect fist percussion** is the same as that of direct fist percussion. In fact, the indirect method is preferred over the direct method. It is performed in the following manner (Figure 8-12):

1. Place the palmar side of the nondominant hand on the skin's surface over the organ to be examined. Place the fingers adjacent to one another and in straight alignment with the palm.
2. Draw up the dominant hand into a closed fist.
3. With the ulnar aspect of the closed fist, use moderate intensity to hit the outstretched nondominant hand on the dorsum.

The nondominant hand absorbs some of the force of the striking hand. The resulting intensity should be of sufficient force to produce pain in the patient if organ inflammation is present.

AUSCULTATION

Auscultation is the act of active listening to body organs to gather information on a patient's clinical status. Auscultation includes listening to sounds that are voluntarily and involuntarily produced by the body. A deep inspiration a patient takes with the lung assessment illustrates a voluntary sound, and heart sounds illustrate involuntary sounds. A quiet environment is necessary for auscultation. Auscultated sounds should be analyzed in relation to their relative intensity, pitch, duration, quality, and location. There are two types of auscultation: direct and indirect.

Direct Auscultation

Direct or **immediate auscultation** is the process of listening with the unaided ear. This can include listening to the patient from some distance away or placing the ear directly on the patient's skin surface. An example of direct auscultation is

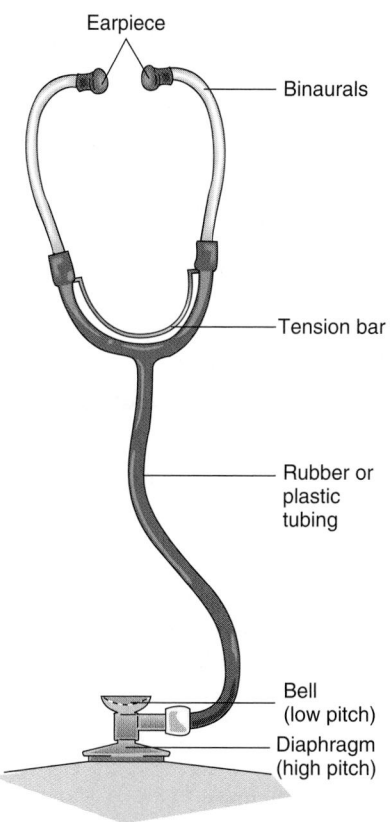

Earpiece

Binaurals

Tension bar

Rubber or
plastic
tubing

Bell
(low pitch)

Diaphragm
(high pitch)

FIGURE 8-13 Acoustic Stethoscope

NURSING**TIP**

Headpiece Mnemonic

The word "bellow" can be used
to remember which frequency
is transmitted by the headpiece
of the stethoscope. The "bell"
transmits "low" sounds.

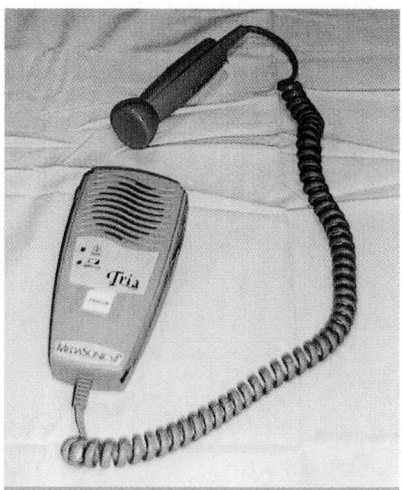

**FIGURE 8-14 Doppler Ultrasonic
Stethoscope**

listening to the wheezing that is audible to the unassisted ear in a person having a severe asthmatic attack.

Indirect Auscultation

Indirect or **mediate auscultation** describes the process of listening with some amplification or mechanical device. The nurse most often performs indirect auscultation with an acoustic stethoscope, which does not amplify the body sounds, but instead blocks out environmental sounds. Amplification of body sounds can be achieved with the use of a Doppler ultrasonic stethoscope. This text describes the use of an acoustic stethoscope.

Figure 8-13 illustrates the acoustic stethoscope. The earpieces come in various sizes. Choose an earpiece that fits snugly in the ear canal without causing pain. The earpieces block out noises in the environment. The earpieces and binaurals should be angled toward the nose. This angle permits the natural direction of the ear canal to be accessed. In this manner, sounds will be directed toward the adult tympanic membrane. The rubber or plastic tubing should be between 30.5 and 40 cm (12–18 in.). Stethoscopes with longer tubing will diminish the body sounds that are auscultated.

The acoustic stethoscope has two listening heads: the bell and the diaphragm. The diaphragm is flat, and the bell is a concave cup. The diaphragm transmits high-pitched sounds, and the bell transmits low-pitched sounds. Breath sounds and normal heart sounds are examples of high-pitched sounds. Bruits and some heart murmurs are examples of low-pitched sounds. Another commonly used stethoscope has a single-sided, dual-frequency listening head. This stethoscope has a single chestpiece. The nurse applies different pressures on the chestpiece to auscultate high- and low-pitched sounds. In addition, some practitioners are using digital stethoscopes to enhance sound clarity. These stethoscopes can amplify natural sounds up to 30 times, and they can also function as a traditional acoustic stethoscope with the bell and the diaphragm. The volume can be adjusted on the digital stethoscope, and a mute feature to block the sound of crying children is available.

Prior to auscultating, remove dangling necklaces or bracelets that can move during the examination and cause false noises. Warm the headpieces of the stethoscope in your hands prior to use, because shivering and movement can obscure assessment findings. To use the diaphragm, place it firmly against the skin surface to be auscultated. If the patient has a large quantity of hair in this area, it may be necessary to wet the hair to prevent it from interfering with the sound that is being auscultated. Otherwise, a grating sound may be heard. To use the bell, place it lightly on the skin surface that is to be auscultated. The bell will stretch the skin and act like a diaphragm and transmit high-pitched sounds if it is pressed too firmly on the skin. In both instances, auscultation requires a great deal of concentration. It may be helpful to close your eyes during the auscultation process to help you isolate the sound. Sometimes you can hear more than one sound in a given location. Try to listen to each sound and concentrate on each separately. It is important to clean your stethoscope after each patient to prevent the transfer of pathogens. Remember, auscultation is a skill that requires practice and patience. Do not expect to become an expert overnight!

Amplification of body sounds can also be achieved with the use of a Doppler ultrasonic stethoscope (Figure 8-14). Water-soluble gel is placed on the body part being assessed, and the Doppler ultrasonic stethoscope is placed directly on the patient. The device amplifies the sounds in that region. Fetal heart tones and unpalpable peripheral pulses are frequently assessed via a Doppler ultrasonic stethoscope.

EQUIPMENT

The physical assessment will proceed in an efficient manner if you have gathered all of the necessary equipment beforehand. The equipment needed to perform a complete physical examination of the adult patient includes:

- Pen and paper
- Marking pen
- Tape measure
- Ruler
- Clean gloves
- Penlight or flashlight
- Scale (You may need to walk the patient to a central location if a scale cannot be brought to the patient's room.)
- Thermometer
- Sphygmomanometer
- Gooseneck lamp
- Tongue depressor
- Stethoscope
- Otoscope
- Nasal speculum
- Ophthalmoscope
- Transilluminator
- Visual acuity charts
- Visual occluder
- Tuning fork
- Reflex hammer
- Sterile needle
- Cotton balls
- Odors for cranial nerve assessment (coffee, lemon, flowers, etc.)
- Small objects for neurological assessment (paper clip, key, cotton ball, pen, etc.)
- Lubricant
- Various sizes of vaginal speculums
- Cervical brush
- Cotton-tip applicator
- Cervical spatula
- Slide and fixative
- Guaiac material
- Specimen cup
- Goniometer

The use of these items is discussed in the chapters describing the assessments for which they are used. Figure 8-15 illustrates some of the equipment used in the physical assessment.

FIGURE 8-15 Equipment Used in Physical Assessment

1. Tuning Fork
2. Visual Occluder
3. Ruler
4. Visual Acuity Chart
5. Reflex Hammer (brush at bottom)
6. Reflex Hammer
7. Pen and Marking Pen
8. Penlight
9. Thermometer
10. Sphygmomanometer
11. Slide and Fixative
12. Specimen Cup
13. Vaginal Speculum
14. Lubricant
15. Goniometer
16. Clean Gloves
17. Cervical Spatula (Ayre Spatula)
18. Cervical Brush (Cytobrush)
19. Cotton-Tip Applicator
20. Tongue Depressor
21. Guaiac Material
22. Tape Measure
23. Stethoscope
24. Ophthalmoscope
25. Otoscope with Speculum
26. Objects for Neurological Examination (key and cotton ball)
27. Sterile Needle

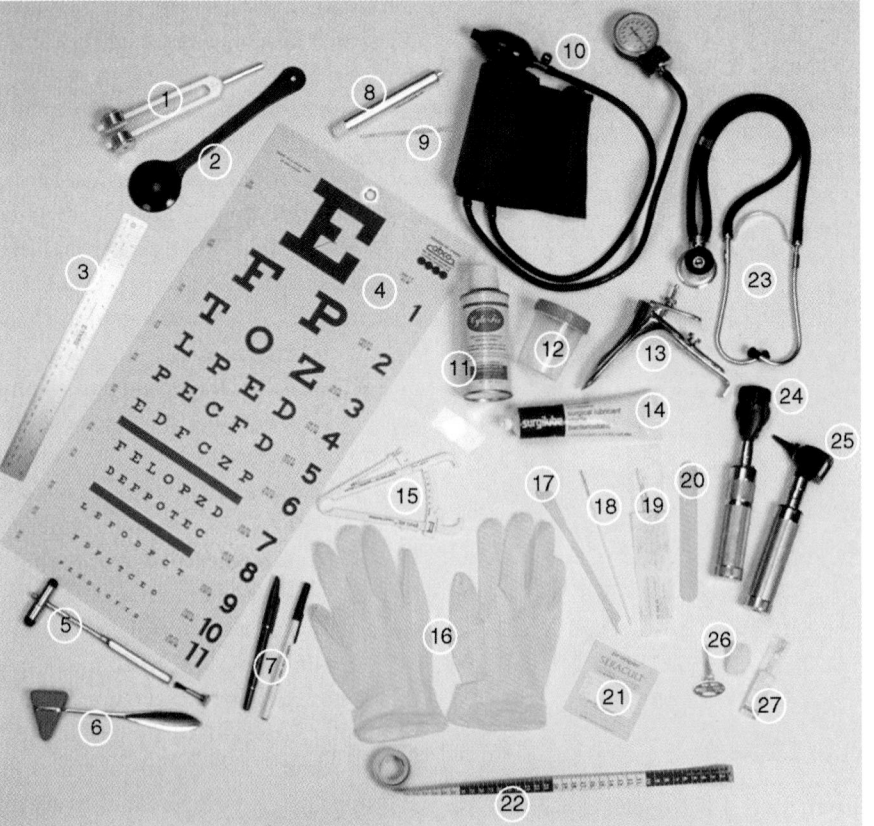

✓ NURSINGCHECKLIST

Preparing for a Physical Assessment

- Always dress in a clean, professional manner; make sure your name pin or workplace identification is visible.
- Remove all bracelets, necklaces, or earrings that can interfere with the physical assessment.
- Be sure that your fingernails are short and your hands are warm for maximum patient comfort.
- Be sure your hair will not fall forward and obstruct your vision or touch the patient.
- Arrange for a well-lit, warm, and private room.
- Ensure that all the necessary equipment is ready for use and within reach.
- Introduce yourself to the patient: "My name is Veronica Rojas. I am the nurse who is caring for you today. I need to assess how your lungs are today."
- Clarify with the patient how he or she wishes to be addressed: Miss Jones, José, Dr. Casy, Rev. Grimes, etc.
- Explain what you plan to do and how long it will take; allow the patient to ask questions.
- Instruct the patient to undress; the underpants can be left on until the end of the assessment; provide a gown and drape for the patient and explain how to use them.
- Allow the patient to undress privately; inform the patient when you will return to start the assessment.
- Have the patient void prior to the assessment.
- Wash your hands in front of the patient to show your concern for cleanliness.
- Observe Standard Precautions and Transmission-Based Precautions, as indicated.
- Ensure that the patient is accessible from both sides of the examining bed or table.
- If a bed is used, raise the height so that you do not have to bend over to perform the assessment.
- Position the patient as dictated by the body system being assessed; see Figure 8-16 for positioning and draping techniques.
- Enlist the patient's cooperation by explaining what you are about to do, where it will be done, and how it may feel.
- Warm all instruments prior to their use (use your hands or warm water).
- Examine the unaffected body part or side first if a patient's complaint is unilateral.
- Explain to the patient why you may be spending a long time performing one particular skill: "Listening to the heart requires concentration and time."
- If the patient complains of fatigue, continue the assessment later (if possible).
- Avoid making crude or negative remarks; be cognizant of your facial expression when dealing with malodorous and dirty patients or with disturbing findings (infected wounds, disfigurement, etc.).
- Conduct the assessment in a systematic fashion every time. (This decreases the likelihood of forgetting to perform a particular assessment.)
- Thank the patient when the physical assessment is concluded; inform the patient what will happen next.
- Document assessment findings in the appropriate section of the patient record.

NURSINGTIP

Golden Rules for Physical Assessment

- Stand on the right side of the patient; establishing a dominant side for assessment will decrease your movement around the patient.
- Perform the assessment in a head-to-toe approach.
- Always compare the right- and left-hand sides of the body for symmetry.
- Proceed from the least invasive to the most invasive procedures for each body system.
- Always perform the physical assessment using a systematic approach; if it is performed the same way each time, you are less likely to forget some part of the assessment.

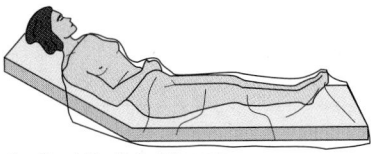

A. Semi-Fowler's 45° angle

Skin, head, and neck; eyes, ears, nose, mouth, and throat; thorax and lungs; heart and peripheral vasculature; musculoskeletal; neurological; patients who cannot tolerate sitting up at a 90° angle

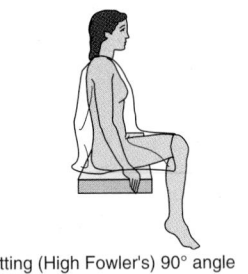

B. Sitting (High Fowler's) 90° angle

Skin, head, and neck; eyes, ears, nose, mouth, and throat; back; posterior thorax and lungs; anterior thorax and lungs; breasts; axillae; heart and peripheral vasculature; musculoskeletal; neurological

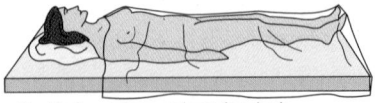

C. Horizontal recumbent (supine)

Breasts; heart and peripheral vasculature; abdomen; musculoskeletal

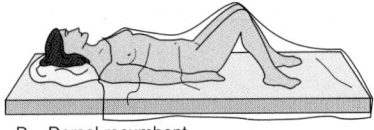

D. Dorsal recumbent

Female genitalia; anterior thorax and lungs; breasts; axillae; heart and peripheral vasculature; abdomen; musculoskeletal

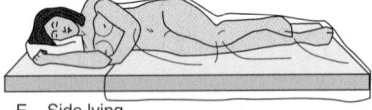

E. Side lying

Skin; thorax and lungs; bedridden patients who cannot sit up

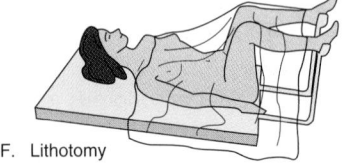

F. Lithotomy

Female genitalia and rectum

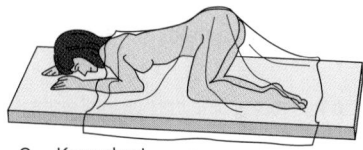

G. Knee-chest

Rectum and prostate

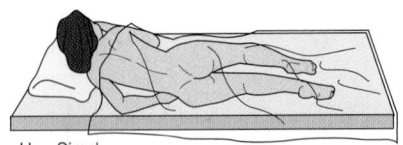

H. Sims'

Rectum and female genitalia

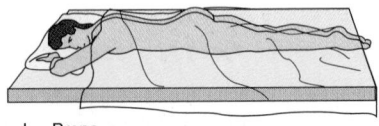

I. Prone

Skin; posterior thorax and lungs; hips

FIGURE 8-16 Positioning and Draping Techniques

ASSESSMENT IN BRIEF

Physical Assessment Techniques

Inspection

- Vision
- Smell

Palpation

- Light palpation
- Deep palpation

Percussion

- Direct, or immediate percussion
- Indirect, or mediate percussion
- Direct fist percussion
- Indirect fist percussion

Auscultation

- Direct, or immediate auscultation
- Indirect, or mediate auscultation

REVIEW QUESTIONS

1. The newest component of the CDC's infection control practices is called:
   a. Transmission Precautions
   b. Respiratory Hygiene/Cough Etiquette
   c. Contact Precautions
   d. Universal Hygiene
   The correct answer is (b).

2. The nurse palpates the patient's abdomen, assessing skin texture, moisture, and muscle guarding. Which assessment skill is most likely being used?
   a. Light palpation   c. Deep palpation
   b. Direct percussion   d. Indirect percussion
   The correct answer is (a).
   Questions 3 and 4 refer to the following situation:

   > A 62-year-old man is admitted to your unit with a bowel obstruction.

3. In what order would you conduct the physical assessment of the abdomen?
   a. Percussion, inspection, palpation, auscultation
   b. Inspection, auscultation, percussion, palpation
   c. Auscultation, palpation, percussion, inspection
   d. Palpation, percussion, inspection, auscultation
   The correct answer is (b).

4. What position best facilitates the abdominal assessment?
   a. Sims'   c. Horizontal recumbent
   b. Lithotomy   d. High Fowler's
   The correct answer is (c).

5. Temperature is best palpated with which section of the hand?
   a. Fingertips   c. Ulnar surface
   b. Finger pads   d. Dorsal surface
   The correct answer is (d).

6. Which percussion sound is soft in intensity, short in duration, high in pitch, and has a flat quality?
   a. Flatness   c. Resonance
   b. Dullness   d. Tympany
   The correct answer is (a).

7. Which percussion technique is usually used to assess costovertebral tenderness of a kidney?
   a. Direct percussion   c. Direct fist percussion
   b. Indirect percussion   d. Indirect fist percussion
   The correct answer is (d).

8. Which characteristics best describe hyperresonance?
   a. Soft intensity, short duration, high pitch
   b. Moderate intensity, moderate duration, high pitch
   c. Loud intensity, long duration, high pitch
   d. Very loud intensity, long duration, very low pitch
   The correct answer is (d).

9. The bell of the stethoscope is used to assess which of the following sounds?
   a. Breath sounds   c. Carotid bruit
   b. Bowel sounds   d. Apical heart rate
   The correct answer is (c).

10. Which of the following positions is the best to assess the female genitalia and conduct a Pap smear when a woman cannot tolerate the lithotomy position?
    a. Semi-Fowler's   c. Sims'
    b. Horizontal recumbent d. Prone
    The correct answer is (c).

Visit the Estes online companion resource at
www.delmar.cengage.com
for additional content and study aids.
Click on Online Companions and then select the Nursing discipline.

BIBLIOGRAPHY

Brashers, V. L. (2006). *Clinical application of pathophysiology: Assessment, diagnostic reasoning and management* (3rd ed.). St. Louis: Mosby.

Daniels, R., Nosek, L., & Nicoll, L. H. (2007). *Contemporary medical-surgical nursing*. Clifton Park, NY: Delmar Cengage Learning.

Fauci, A. S., Braunwald, E., Kasper, D. L., Hauser, S. L., Longo, D. L., Jameson, J. L., et al. (2008). *Harrison's principles of internal medicine* (17th ed.). New York: McGraw-Hill.

Lashley, F. R., & Durham, J. D. (2007). *Emerging infectious diseases: Trends and issues* (2nd ed.). New York: Springer.

Markel, H. (2006). The stethoscope and the art of listening. (2006). *The New England Journal of Medicine, 354*(6), 551–553.

Martin, R. (2007). HIPAA privacy complaints. *Advance for Nurse Practitioners, 15*(6), 23.

Paskawicz, J. (2005). Latex allergy revisited. *Clinician Reviews, 15*(11), 66–75.

Peters, W. (2007). *Atlas of tropical medicine and parasitology* (6th ed.). St. Louis: Mosby.

Severe Acute Respiratory Syndrome (SARS). *Guidelines and recommendation: Clinical guidance on the identification and evaluation of possible SARS-CoV disease among persons presenting with community-acquired illness*. Retrieved November 26, 2007, from http://www.cdc.gov/ncidod/sars/clinicalguidance.htm.

Shaw, K. (2006). The 2003 SARS outbreak and its impact on infection control practices. *Public Health, 120*, 8–14.

Siegel, J. D., Rhinehart, E., Jackson, M., Chiarello, L., & the Healthcare Infection Control Practices Advisory Committee. (2007, June). *Guideline for isolation precautions: Preventing transmission of infectious agents in healthcare settings*. Retrieved September 21, 2008, from http://www.cdc.gov/ncidod/dhqp/gl_isolation.html.

U.S. Preventive Services Task Force. (2007). *The guide to clinical preventive services, 2007*. Rockville, MD: U.S. Department of Health and Human Services.

Wenzel, R. P. (2003). *Prevention and control of nosocomial infections* (4th ed.). Philadelphia: Lippincott Williams & Wilkins.

WEB SITES

American Academy of Allergy, Asthma & Immunology: http://www.aaaai.org

American Association of Legal Nurse Consultants: http://www.aalnc.org

American Latex Allergy Association: http://www.latexallergyresources.org

Centers for Disease Control and Prevention: Morbidity and Mortality Weekly Report: http://www.cdc.gov.mmwr

My Stethoscope: The Leading Provider of Stethoscopes: http://www.mystethoscope.com

CHAPTER 9

General Survey, Vital Signs, and Pain

COMPETENCIES

1. Describe general assessment observations.

2. Discuss factors affecting respiratory rate and heart rate.

3. Describe the characteristics that are included in an assessment of pulse.

4. Discuss factors influencing body temperature.

5. Describe factors influencing blood pressure and blood pressure measurement.

6. Obtain a patient's vital signs.

7. Conduct an assessment on a patient experiencing pain.

A complete physical examination is initiated by performing general observations of a patient, obtaining the patient's **vital signs**, and assessing the patient for pain. These initial observations can provide data about the patient's general state of health. Vital signs include the patient's respirations, pulse, temperature, and blood pressure (BP). These measurements provide information about the patient's basic physiological status. The presence of pain can affect a patient's physical, emotional, and mental health; pain is thus often referred to as the fifth vital sign.

EQUIPMENT

- Stethoscope
- Watch with a second hand
- Thermometer (gloves and lubricant if using a rectal thermometer)
- Sphygmomanometer

NURSING**TIP**

Environmental Cues

In addition to observing the patient, look around the room for clues about the patient's health status. For example, an inhaler, nasal spray, a hearing aid, or used tissues may all provide information about the patient's health.

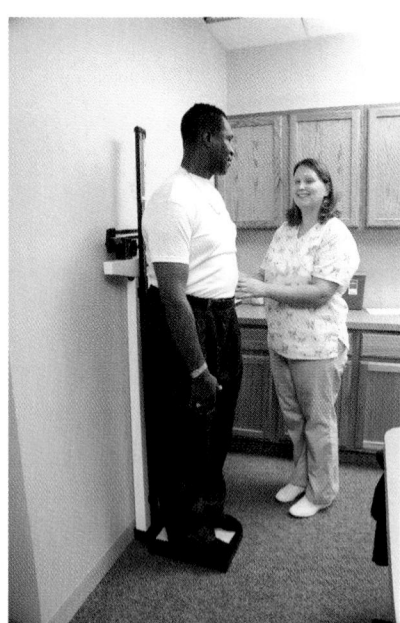

FIGURE 9-1 The nurse can make observations about the patient's general appearance while talking with the patient and preparing for the physical examination.

GENERAL SURVEY

Initial observations include collecting information about the patient's physical presence, psychological presence, and signs and symptoms of distress.

PHYSICAL PRESENCE

Observe the patient's:

E 1. Stated age versus apparent age

2. General appearance

3. Body fat

4. Stature

5. Motor activity

6. Body and breath odors

Stated Age versus Apparent Age

N The patient's stated chronological age should be congruent with the apparent age.

A It is significant for a patient to appear older or younger than the stated chronological age.

P Endocrine deficiencies of growth hormone associated with dwarfism can manifest in a younger-than-chronological-age appearance in younger life and premature aging later in life.

P Genetic syndromes (e.g., Turner's) manifest in an "old-person" facial appearance.

P Chronic disease, severe illness (such as cancer and AIDS), and prolonged sun exposure that causes facial wrinkling can all lead to a patient looking older than his or her chronological age.

General Appearance

E Observe body symmetry, any obvious anomaly, and the patient's apparent level of wellness (Figure 9-1). In addition, note any gross observation, such as use of a walker, assistance from a caregiver, or distinctive markings (e.g., multiple piercings, tattoos).

N The patient should exhibit body symmetry, no obvious deformity, and a well appearance. The level of gross normal observations is varied.

A Asymmetry is seen when a paired body part does not look the same on the contralateral side.

P The unilateral facial drooping of Bell's palsy, a limb appearing at an abnormal angle, and unilateral paralysis are examples of body asymmetry.

A A missing limb, cleft lip, and burned facial skin are examples of obvious anomalies.

P The pathophysiology of each of these is varied and needs to be investigated further via history and physical assessments.

A The patient who appears ill is abnormal.

P A patient who appears ill usually is ill and needs to be carefully assessed via the history and physical examination.

Body Fat

N Body fat should be evenly distributed. Body fat composition is difficult to estimate accurately without the use of immersion tanks or calipers. Research has indicated, however, that it is body fat content, not body weight, that is most closely linked to pathology. For example, a person can be within normal limits on height and weight charts but have a high proportion of body fat to lean body mass.

A Obesity occurs when there are large amounts of body fat. This poses a serious health risk to the patient and warrants a comprehensive nutritional assessment (see Chapter 7).

P Excess caloric intake and decreased energy expenditure are the most common causes of obesity.

P Some disease processes, such as hypothyroidism, which slows the basic metabolic rate, may result in obesity.

A Cushing's syndrome manifests in a rounded, moonlike face, truncal obesity, fat pads on the neck, and relatively thin limbs.

P Excessive production of cortisol resulting from an anterior pituitary tumor or large doses of prolonged steroid therapy produces Cushing's syndrome.

A A thin or frail appearance occurs when there are limited body fat stores. Severely limited fat stores can be a life-threatening condition.

P Energy expenditures that exceed caloric intake will result in decreased fat stores. This may be caused by several conditions, including:

- Anorexia nervosa, which results in inadequate intake of calories from food and overexpenditure of energy by means of exercise.
- Hyperkinetic states, in which the body's metabolic needs are greater than the ability to ingest calories. Adolescent growth spurts result in tall, thin teens because the increased metabolic demands for growing tissue exceed the calories teens can consume.
- Many chronic disease processes may be due to hyperkinetic states or a result of malabsorption diseases.

Stature

N Limbs and trunk should appear proportional to body height; posture should be erect. A person's arm span (fingertip to fingertip) should be approximately equal to a person's height, and body length (crown to pubis) should be about equal to the length from the pubis to the feet.

A A slumped or humpbacked appearance is abnormal.

P Osteoporosis, especially in postmenopausal women, may cause a slumped or humpbacked appearance.

E Examination **N** Normal Findings **A** Abnormal Findings **P** Pathophysiology

P   Patients experiencing depression may also present with a slumped posture.

A   Long limbs relative to trunk length are abnormal.

P   Marfan's syndrome, an inherited disease, can result in the development of long limbs; long, thin fingers; a tall, thin appearance; and poorly developed muscles due to a defect in the elastic fibers of connective tissues. The patient's arm span is greater than the patient's height.

Motor Activity

N   Gait as well as other body movements should be smooth and effortless. All body parts should have controlled, purposeful movement.

A   An unsteady gait or movements that are slow, absent, or require great effort are abnormal. Tremors or movements that seem uncontrollable by the patient are also abnormal.

P   Arthritis can result in slow and difficult movement because joint movement is painful. See Chapter 18 for additional information.

P   Neurological disturbances can result in tics, paralysis, or ataxia, and can cause difficulty with the smoothness of movement. See Chapter 19 for additional information.

Body and Breath Odors

N   Normally, there is no apparent odor from patients. It is normal for some people to have bad breath related to the types of foods ingested or due to individual digestive processes and reflux.

A   Severe body or breath odor is abnormal.

P   Poor hygiene can cause body odors due to perspiration and bacteria left on the skin.

P   An alcohol smell on the breath can result from alcohol ingestion or from ketoacidosis in a diabetic patient.

P   Bad breath can result from poor oral hygiene, allergic rhinitis, or from infections such as tonsillitis, rhinosinusitis, or pneumonia.

P   Severe vaginal infections can result in an offensive body odor.

PSYCHOLOGICAL PRESENCE

Observe the patient's:

E   1. Dress, grooming, and personal hygiene

2. Mood and manner

3. Speech

4. Facial expressions

REFLECTIVE THINKING

Assessing the Patient with Severe Odors

A patient has severe halitosis and you need to conduct a physical exam. Describe your approach and list the questions you would pose to discover the cause of the odor, while maintaining respect for the patient's dignity.

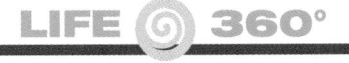

LIFE 360°

Assessing Facial Expressions

You are eliciting a health history from a female patient who presents for an illness. During the history taking, the patient looks away from you, then at her feet while playing with her hair. Her replies are quiet and mumbled. The patient's husband jumps up from his chair, shakes his wife, and says, "You answer the questions NOW! I am tired of you in every way. You quit your job because you couldn't handle the stress, you aren't taking care of the kids, and you sleep all day!" What is your assessment of this situation? How would you proceed?

Dress, Grooming, and Personal Hygiene

N Normally, patients should appear clean and neatly dressed. Clothing choice should be appropriate for the weather. Norms and standards for dress and cleanliness may vary among cultures.

A A disheveled, unkempt appearance or clothing that is inappropriate for the weather (such as a wool coat in hot weather) is abnormal.

P Psychological or psychiatric disorders such as depression (characterized in part by lethargy, mood swings, anhedonia [or lack of pleasure in activities], fatigue, etc.), psychotic disorders (characterized by a distortion in thinking), and dementia (processes that alter perceptions of reality) may be reflected in inappropriate appearance (hair, makeup) or through inappropriate clothing selection.

P Poor self-esteem or a homeless lifestyle may be reflected by general neglect of personal hygiene, grooming, and dress.

P An unshaven, unclean appearance may reflect abuse or neglect of the patient by the patient's caregiver.

Mood and Manner

N Generally, a patient should be cooperative and pleasant.

A An uncooperative, hostile, or tearful adult or an adult who seems unusually elated or who has a flat affect needs further assessment.

P Psychiatric conditions such as depression, manic disorders, paranoid disorders, and psychotic disorders produce a distortion in reality (distorted thinking and perceptions), resulting in abnormal behaviors. Dementia or confusion in the elderly can also result in disturbances of mood and manner. See Chapter 19 for a more complete discussion.

Speech

N The patient should respond to questions and commands easily. Speech should be clear and understandable. Pitch, rate, and volume should be appropriate to the circumstances.

A Speech that is slow, slurred, mumbled, very loud, or rapid needs to be assessed further.

P Hyperthyroidism can cause rapid speech because of hormones that are stimulatory in nature and result in hypermetabolism and hyperactivity.

P Alcohol ingestion can cause slow, mumbled, or slurred speech because alcohol affects the central nervous system, causing transient brain dysfunction.

P Hearing difficulties may be associated with loud speech because individuals with decreased ability to hear may not be able to hear themselves at normal conversational decibels.

P Strokes can result in aphasia if the speech center in the brain is affected.

Facial Expressions

N The patient should appear awake and alert. Facial expressions should be appropriate for what is happening in the environment and should change naturally.

E Examination   **N** Normal Findings   **A** Abnormal Findings   **P** Pathophysiology

A Unchanging or flat facial expression, inappropriate facial expression, tremors, or tics are abnormal.

P Apathy or depression may cause lack of facial expression due to feelings of lethargy or sadness.

P Dementia may cause inappropriate facial expressions because the patient's perception of reality is distorted.

P Bell's palsy, a condition resulting in paralysis of the muscles in the face, may cause the mouth to droop and the affected side of the face to appear flaccid, with the inability to completely close the eye on the affected side.

DISTRESS

Observe for:

E 1. Labored breathing, wheezing or cough, or labored speech.

2. Painful facial expression, sweating, or physical protection of painful area.

3. Serious or life-threatening occurrences such as seizure activity, active and severe bleeding, gaping wounds, and open fractures.

4. Signs of emotional distress or anxiety that may include, but are not limited to, tearfulness; nervous tics or laughter; avoidance of eye contact; cold, clammy hands; excessive nail biting; inability to pay attention; autonomic responses such as diaphoresis; or changes in breathing patterns.

N Breathing should be effortless, without cough or wheezing. Speech should not leave a patient breathless. The face should be relaxed, and the patient should be willing to move all body parts freely. There should be no serious or life-threatening conditions. The patient should not perspire excessively or show signs of emotional distress such as nail biting or avoidance of eye contact (Figure 9-2).

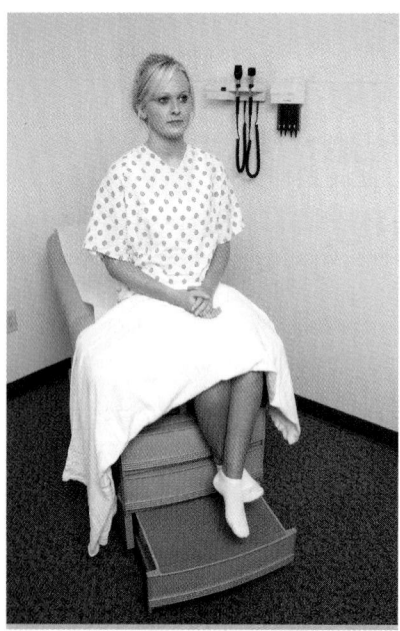

FIGURE 9-2 The general survey includes assessing every patient for signs of distress.

A The presence of shortness of breath with labored speech, wheezing, or cough is abnormal.

P Pulmonary disease may be present. See Chapter 15 for additional information.

A Pain as evidenced by facial grimacing, crying, moaning, sweating, or protection of a body part is an abnormal finding.

P Tissue damage results in pain and needs further investigation into the character, location, intensity, and occurrence of the pain, as well as factors associated with increased and decreased pain.

A Excessive nail biting, avoidance of eye contact, nervous laughter, tearfulness, or lack of interest may be indicators of emotional distress or emotional pain.

P Nervous habits are often displayed when a person is in an uncomfortable or new situation. A tearful or sad affect can result from emotional pain related to situations the patient may be experiencing or has experienced. Often, there is an attempt made to disguise emotional distress.

VITAL SIGNS

Vital sign measurements include respiration, pulse, temperature, and blood pressure.

NURSING**TIP**

Assessing Vital Signs

Vital signs should be assessed at the beginning of each visit. If the patient is hospitalized, vital signs should be assessed as often as prescribed or as often as the patient's condition requires.

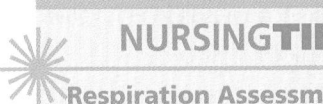

NURSINGTIP

Respiration Assessment

Most frequently, respirations can be measured while measuring radial or apical pulse. If respirations are shallow and the patient is supine, put the patient's arm across the chest while taking a radial pulse and feel the chest rise while observing for respirations.

☑ NURSINGCHECKLIST

General Approach to Vital Sign Assessment

1. Gather equipment.
2. Explain the procedure to the patient.
3. Select equipment according to the patient's age, size, and developmental level and the site selected for assessment. Specific decision-making criteria are discussed under each section.
4. Warm the stethoscope headpiece before touching the patient with it.
5. Assess vital signs and record findings.

RESPIRATION

Respiration is the act of breathing. Breathing supplies oxygen to the body and occurs in response to changes in the concentration of oxygen (O_2), carbon dioxide (CO_2), and hydrogen (H^+) in the arterial blood. Inhalation, or inspiration, occurs when air is taken into the lungs. Exhalation, or expiration, refers to the airflow out of the lungs.

Inspiration occurs when the diaphragm and the intercostal muscles contract. This can be observed by the movement of the abdomen outward and the movement of the chest upward and outward, resulting in the lungs filling with air. Expiration occurs when the external intercostal muscles and the diaphragm relax. The abdomen and the chest return to a resting position.

Respiratory rate is measured in breaths per minute. One respiratory cycle consists of one inhalation and one expiration. A complete discussion of respiratory assessment is found in Chapter 15.

To assess respiratory rate:

E 1. Stand in front of or to the side of the patient.

2. Discreetly observe the patient's breathing (rise and fall of the chest). These observations are best done with the patient unaware of what you are doing. If the patient is aware that you are counting respirations, the breathing pattern may be altered.

3. Count the number of respiratory cycles that occur in 1 minute.

N Table 9-1 lists the normal respiratory rates for different ages. Respiratory rates decrease with age and may vary with excitement, anxiety, fever, exercise, medications, and altitude.

A Tachypnea is a respiratory rate greater than 20 breaths per minute in an adult.

P Hypoxia and metabolic acidosis are common causes of tachypnea. The increased respiratory rate is a compensatory mechanism to provide the body with more oxygen and eliminate excess hydrogen ions when the body's metabolism is increased.

P Stress and anxiety cause the release of catecholamines, which can elevate the respiratory rate.

A Bradypnea is a respiratory rate less than 12 breaths per minute in an adult at rest.

P Head injury resulting in increased intracranial pressure in the respiratory center of the brain can cause bradypnea.

P Medications or chemicals such as narcotics, barbiturates, or alcohol depress the respiratory center of the brain and can cause bradypnea.

TABLE 9-1
Respiratory Rate

AGE	RESTING RESPIRATORY RATE (BREATHS/ MINUTE)	AVERAGE
Newborn	30–50	40
1 Year	20–40	30
3 Years	20–30	25
6 Years	16–22	19
10 Years	16–20	18
14 Years	14–20	17
Adult	12–20	18

E Examination	**N** Normal Findings	**A** Abnormal Findings	**P** Pathophysiology

P A lower metabolic rate that occurs during normal sleep can result in bradypnea.

A **Apnea** is the absence of spontaneous breathing for 10 or more seconds.

P Many causes of apnea are unknown.

P Traumatic brain injury may lead to apnea from injury of the brain stem. Death ensues in the absence of respirations and pulse.

PULSE

As the heart contracts, blood is ejected from the left ventricle (stroke volume) into the aorta. A pressure wave is created as the blood is carried to the peripheral vasculature. This palpable pressure is the **pulse**. Pulse assessment can determine heart rate, rhythm, and the estimated volume of blood being pumped by the heart.

Rate

Pulse rate is the number of pulse beats counted in 1 minute. Several factors influence heart rate or pulse rate. These include:

- The SA node, which fires automatically at a rate of 60 to 100 times per minute and is the primary controller of pulse rate and heart rate.
- Parasympathetic or vagal stimulation of the autonomic nervous system, which can result in decreased heart rate.
- Sympathetic stimulation of the autonomic nervous system, which results in increased heart rate.
- Baroreceptor sensors, which can detect changes in blood pressure and influence heart rate. Elevated blood pressure can decrease heart rate, whereas decreased blood pressure can increase heart rate.

Other factors influencing heart rate include:

- Age: The heart rate generally decreases with age.
- Gender: The average female's heart rate is higher than a male's heart rate.
- Activity: The heart rate increases with activity. Athletes will have a lower resting heart rate than the average person because of their increased cardiac strength and efficiency.
- Emotional status: Heart rate increases with anxiety.
- Pain: Heart rate increases with pain.
- Environmental factors: Temperature and noise level can alter the heart rate.
- Stimulants: Caffeinated beverages and tobacco elevate the heart rate.
- Medications: Drugs such as digoxin decrease the heart rate, and drugs such as amphetamines increase the heart rate.
- Disease state: Abnormal clinical conditions can affect the heart rate (e.g., increased heart rate in hyperthyroidism, fever, and hemorrhage).

Rhythm

Pulse rhythm refers to the pattern of pulses and the intervals between pulses. Pulses can be regular or irregular. A regular pulse occurs at regular intervals with even intervals between each beat. Normal sinus rhythm is an example of a regular pulse.

An irregular pulse can be regularly irregular or irregularly irregular. A regular irregular rhythm is one in which an abnormal conduction occurs in the heart, but at regular intervals. Ventricular bigeminy is an example of a regularly irregular rhythm. In ventricular bigeminy, the irregular conduction, called a premature ventricular complex (PVC), occurs prior to the expected QRS complex. This PVC occurs at a regular rhythm (every other beat).

An irregularly irregular rhythm has no predictable pattern. Atrial fibrillation is an example of an irregularly irregular rhythm. Refer to the Bibliography for additional information on heart rhythms.

Volume

Pulse volume (also called pulse strength or amplitude) reflects the stroke volume and the **peripheral vasculature resistance** (afterload). It can range from absent to bounding. Table 9-2 displays the two most commonly used scales: a 3-point and a 4-point scale. When reporting pulse volume, 2+/4+ indicates a normal pulse (2+) on a 4-point scale, whereas 2+/3+ indicates a normal pulse (2+) on a 3-point scale. Refer to the Nursing Tip, Documenting Pulses, for schematic representations. If a pulse is not palpable, then attempt to ascertain its presence with a Doppler ultrasonic stethoscope. The letter "D" in a pulse chart or stick figure represents the pulse that was detected by using this mechanical device.

Site

Peripheral pulses can be palpated where the large arteries are close to the skin surface. There are nine common sites for assessment of pulse, as indicated in Figure 9-3. When routine vital signs are assessed, the pulse is generally measured at one of two sites: radial or apical.

Measuring the apical pulse is indicated for patients with irregular pulses or known cardiac or pulmonary disease. The assessment of apical pulse can be accomplished through palpation but is most commonly accomplished through auscultation.

RADIAL PULSE.

To palpate the radial pulse:

 1. Place the pad of your first, second, and/or third finger on the site of the radial pulse, along the radial bone on the thumb side of the inner wrist (see Figure 9-4).

2. Press your fingers gently against the artery with enough pressure so that you can feel the pulse. Pressing too hard will obliterate the pulse.

3. Count the pulse rate using the secondhand of your watch. If the pulse is regular, count for 30 seconds and multiply by 2 to obtain the pulse rate per minute. If the pulse is irregular, count for 60 seconds.

4. Identify the pulse rhythm as you palpate (regular or irregular).

5. Identify the pulse volume as you palpate (using scales from Table 9-2).

N/A/P   Refer to section on Rate.

APICAL PULSE.

To assess the apical pulse:

 1. Place the diaphragm of the stethoscope on the apical pulse site.

2. Count the pulse rate for 30 seconds if regular, 60 seconds if irregular.

3. Identify the pulse rhythm.

4. Identify a **pulse deficit** (apical pulse rate greater than the radial pulse rate) by listening to the apical pulse and palpating the radial pulse simultaneously.

N/A/P   Refer to section on Rate.

Rate

N   Normal pulse rates vary with age. Table 9-3 depicts ranges for normal pulse rates by age. The heart rate normally increases during periods of exertion. Athletes commonly have resting heart rates below 60 beats per minute because of the increased strength and efficiency of the cardiac muscle.

A   **Tachycardia** refers to a pulse rate faster than 100 beats per minute in an adult.

TABLE 9-2
Scales for Measuring Pulse Volume

3-POINT SCALE	
SCALE	**DESCRIPTION OF PULSE**
0	Absent
1+	Thready/weak
2+	Normal
3+	Bounding

4-POINT SCALE	
SCALE	**DESCRIPTION OF PULSE**
0	Absent
1+	Thready/weak
2+	Normal
3+	Increased
4+	Bounding

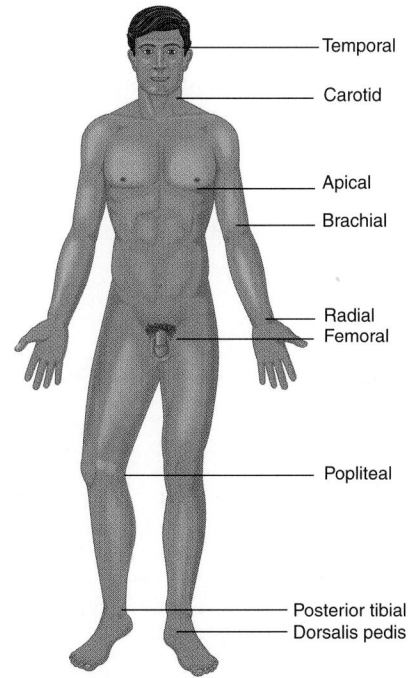

- Temporal
- Carotid
- Apical
- Brachial
- Radial
- Femoral
- Popliteal
- Posterior tibial
- Dorsalis pedis

FIGURE 9-3 **Peripheral Pulse Sites**

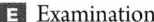 Examination	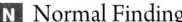 Normal Findings	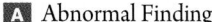 Abnormal Findings	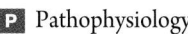 Pathophysiology

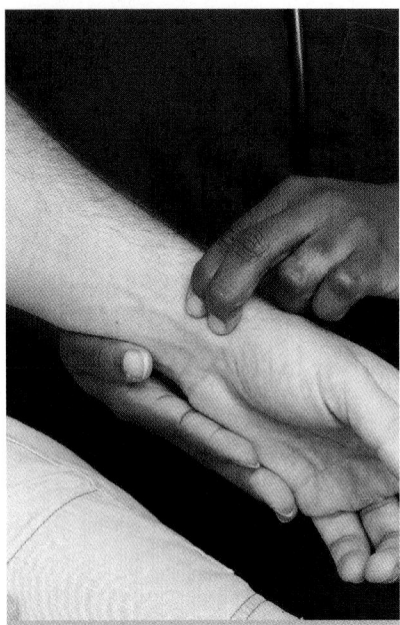

FIGURE 9-4 Palpation of the Radial Pulse

P Psychophysiological stressors such as trauma, blood volume losses, anemias, infection, fear, fever, pain, hyperthyroidism, shock, and anxiety can increase pulse rate because of increased metabolic demands placed on the body.

P Some tachycardia may not have clinical significance; however, in patients with myocardial disease, tachycardia can be a sign of decreased cardiac output, congestive heart failure, myocardial ischemia, or dysrhythmias.

A **Bradycardia** refers to slow pulse rates. Pulse rates that fall below 60 in adults are considered to be bradycardic.

P Medications such as cardiotonics (digoxin) and beta blockers decrease the heart rate.

P Bradycardia usually occurs with excessive vagal stimulation or decreased sympathetic tone. Conditions that may cause bradycardia are eye surgery, increased intracranial pressure, myocardial infarction, hypothyroidism, and prolonged vomiting.

A **Asystole** refers to the absence of a pulse. Palpate or auscultate for a pulse for 10 to 15 seconds to establish asystole.

P Cardiac arrest resulting from biological or clinical death can result in asystole.

P Pulseless electrical activity (electromechanical dissociation) caused by, for example, hypovolemia, pneumothorax, cardiac tamponade, or acidosis results in the absence of a pulse despite the presence of electrical activity in the heart muscle.

A A pulse deficit occurs when the apical pulse rate is greater than the radial pulse rate.

P Dysrhythmias (such as atrial fibrillation, premature ventricular contractions, second-degree heart block, and third-degree heart block) and heart failure can cause pulse deficits because some heart contractions are too weak to produce a pulse pressure to the peripheral site. Severe vascular disease can also cause pulse deficits.

Rhythm

N Normal pulse rhythm is regular, with equal intervals between each beat.

A **Dysrhythmias,** or **arrhythmias,** refer to pulse rhythms that are not regular. They may consist of irregular beats that are random, or irregular beats that present in a regular pattern.

P Cardiac dysrhythmias that are atrial and ventricular in origin cause abnormal rhythms, such as atrial flutter and ventricular fibrillation.

Volume

N The pulse volume is normally the same with each beat. A normal pulse volume can be felt with a moderate amount of pressure of the fingers and obliterated with greater pressure.

A Small, weak pulses are referred to as weak or thready pulses or as pulses easily obliterated with light pressure.

P Decreased cardiac stroke volume caused by heart failure, hypovolemic shock, and cardiogenic shock can result in weak pulses.

P A low pulse amplitude occurs in states of increased peripheral vascular resistance, such as in aortic stenosis and constrictive pericarditis.

P Weak pulses occur in conditions when ventricular filling time is decreased, such as in dysrhythmias.

A Bounding pulses are full, forceful pulses that are difficult to obliterate with pressure.

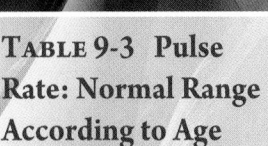

TABLE 9-3 Pulse Rate: Normal Range According to Age

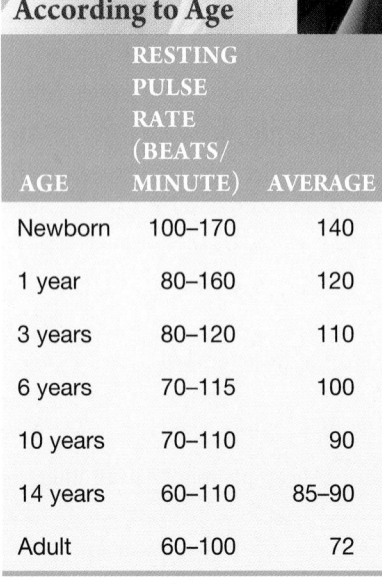

AGE	RESTING PULSE RATE (BEATS/ MINUTE)	AVERAGE
Newborn	100–170	140
1 year	80–160	120
3 years	80–120	110
6 years	70–115	100
10 years	70–110	90
14 years	60–110	85–90
Adult	60–100	72

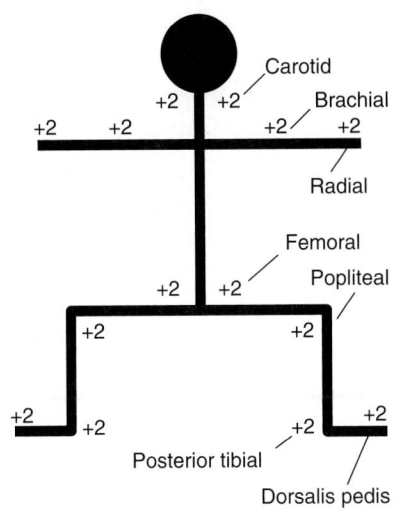

Scale = 3+

A. Stick Figure Peripheral Pulse Documentation

	Carotid	Brachial	Radial	Femoral	Popliteal	PT	DP
R	2+	2+	2+	1+	1+	D	D
L	2+	2+	2+	2+	1+	1+	1+
Scale = 4+							
D = Doppler Ultrasonic Stethoscope							

B. Tabular Peripheral Pulse Documentation

FIGURE 9-5 **Methods to Chart Peripheral Pulses**

P Hyperkinetic states such as exercise, fever, anemia, anxiety, and hyperthyroidism can cause bounding pulses.

P Early stages of septic shock are characterized by bounding pulses because of decreased peripheral vascular resistance.

TEMPERATURE

Scales, variables, routes, and measurement methods for assessing temperature are outlined.

Temperature Scales

Both the Celsius and the Fahrenheit scales are commonly used to measure **temperature**, which is the degree of core body heat. Patients are most often familiar with the Fahrenheit scale, whereas institutions often use the Celsius scale. Therefore, it is important that you know temperature scale correlations. Figure 9-6 summarizes these correlations and gives the conversion formulas.

Variables Affecting Body Temperature

Core body temperature is established by the temperature of blood perfusing the area of the hypothalamus (the body's temperature control center), which triggers the body's physiological response to temperature. An ideal thermometer would accurately measure central brain stem temperature at the hypothalamus. Invasive procedures that provide temperatures of the arterial blood, esophagus, or bladder are reliable indicators of core temperature, but are impractical. More practical methods for measurement of body temperature are less reliable and can result in variations in body temperature readings. In addition, there are physiological variables that affect body temperature. These include:

- **Circadian rhythm** patterns: Normal body temperature (as well as pulse and blood pressure) fluctuates with a patient's activity level and the time of day. Core body temperature is lower during sleep than during waking activities, being the lowest in the early morning just before awakening from sleep, and the highest in the afternoon or early evening. A 0.5°C to 1.0°C, or a 1°F to 2°F, fluctuation in body temperature throughout the day is considered within the normal range.

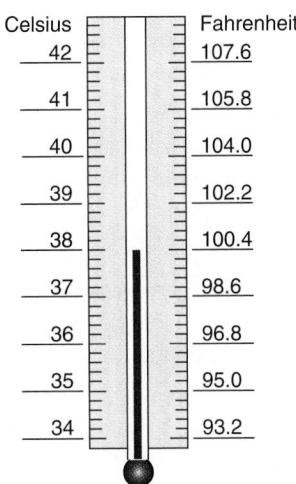

To convert:
(9/5 x temperature in Celsius) + 32° = temperature in Fahrenheit

5/9 x (temperature in Fahrenheit − 32°) = temperature in Celsius

FIGURE 9-6 **Correlation between Celsius and Fahrenheit Scales**

E Examination	**N** Normal Findings	**A** Abnormal Findings	**P** Pathophysiology

- Hormones: In women, increased production of progesterone at the time of ovulation raises the basal body temperature about 0.35°C, or 0.5°F.
- Age: Infants and young children are affected by the environmental temperature to a much greater extent than adults because their thermoregulation mechanisms are not fully developed. The elderly are more sensitive to extremes of environmental temperature due to a decrease in thermoregulatory controls.
- Exercise: Body temperature rises due to increased metabolic activity.
- Stress: Stimulation of the sympathetic nervous system increases the production of epinephrine, resulting in increased metabolic activity and higher body temperature.
- Environmental extremes of hot or cold.
- Health status: Temperature deviations can occur in illnesses such as infections as well as hypothalamus dysfunction.

Measurement Routes

There are four basic routes by which temperature can be measured: oral, rectal, axillary, and tympanic. Each method has advantages and disadvantages. The advantages and disadvantages of each route are summarized in Table 9-4.

TABLE 9-4 Advantages and Disadvantages of Four Routes for Body Temperature Measurement

ROUTE	NORMAL RANGE	ADVANTAGES	DISADVANTAGES
Oral Average 37.0°C or 98.6°F	36.0°–38.0°C 96.8°–100.4°F	Convenient; accessible	**Safety:** Glass thermometers with mercury can be bitten and broken, causing patient injury. Glass thermometers are no longer used in health care institutions. Patients need to be alert and cooperative and cognitively capable of following instructions for safe use. **Physical abilities:** Patients need to be able to breathe through the nose and be without oral pathology or recent oral surgery; route not applicable for comatose or confused patients. **Accuracy:** Oxygen therapy by mask, as well as ingestion of hot or cold drinks immediately before oral temperature measurement, affects accuracy of the reading.
Rectal Average 0.4°C or 0.7°F higher than oral	36.7°–38.0°C 98.0°–100.4°F	Considered most accurate	**Safety:** Contraindicated following rectal surgery. Risk of rectal perforation in children less than 2 years of age. Risk of stimulating Valsalva maneuver in cardiac patients. **Physical aspects:** Invasive, uncomfortable, and possibly embarrassing
Axillary Average 0.6°C or 1°F lower than oral	35.4°–37.4°C 95.8°–99.4°F	Safe; noninvasive	**Time frame:** Glass thermometer must be left in place for 5 minutes to obtain accurate measurement. Glass and mercury thermometers are no longer used in health care facilities. Placement and position of thermometer tip affect reading.
Tympanic Calibrated to oral or rectal scales	See oral or rectal	Convenient; fast; safe; noninvasive. Does not require contact with any mucous membrane.	**Accuracy:** Research is inconclusive as to accuracy of readings and correlations with other body temperature measurements. Technique affects reading. Tympanic membrane is thought to reflect the core body temperature.

Measurement

ORAL METHOD.

E
1. Place the thermometer (Figure 9-7) at the base of the tongue and to the right or left of the frenulum, and instruct the patient to close the lips and to avoid biting the thermometer. Ensure that it has been at least 15 minutes since the patient has consumed a hot or cold beverage or food.
2. Leave the thermometer in the mouth until the device has signaled that the maximum body temperature has been reached.
3. Remove the thermometer from the patient's mouth.

RECTAL METHOD.

E
1. Position patient with the buttocks exposed. Adults may be more comfortable lying on the side (with the knees slightly flexed), facing away from you, or prone.
2. Put on clean gloves.
3. Lubricate the tip of the thermometer with a water-soluble lubricant.
4. Ask the patient to take a deep breath; insert the thermometer into the anus 0.5 to 1.5 inches, depending on the patient's age.
5. Do not force the insertion of the thermometer or insert into feces.
6. Leave the thermometer in the rectum until the device has signaled that the maximum body temperature has been reached.
7. Remove the thermometer from the patient's rectum.

AXILLARY METHOD.

E
1. Place the thermometer into the middle of the axilla (Figure 9-8) and fold the patient's arm across the chest to keep the thermometer in place.
2. Leave the thermometer in the axilla until the device has signaled that the maximum body temperature has been reached.
3. Remove the thermometer from the patient's axilla.

ELECTRONIC THERMOMETER.

E
1. Remove the electronic thermometer from the charging unit (Figure 9-9).
2. Attach a disposable cover to the probe.
3. Using a method described (oral, rectal, or axillary), measure the temperature.

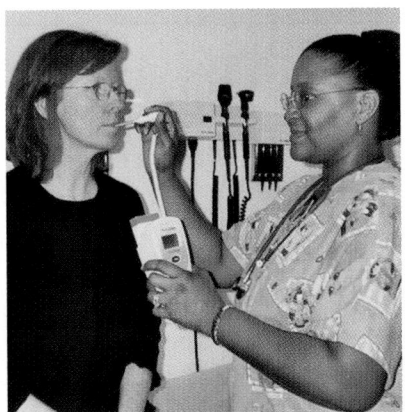

FIGURE 9-7 Taking a Patient's Oral Temperature with an Electronic Thermometer

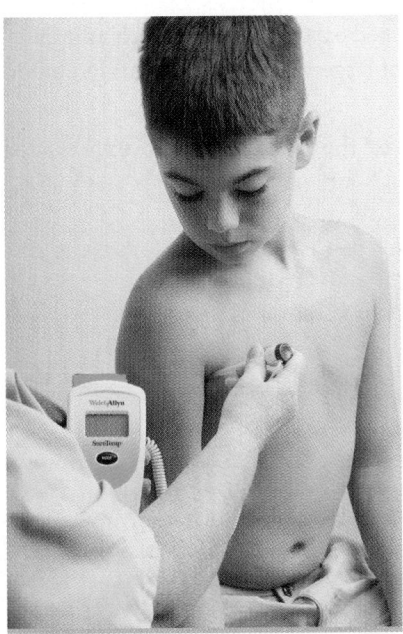

FIGURE 9-8 Taking a Patient's Axillary Temperature

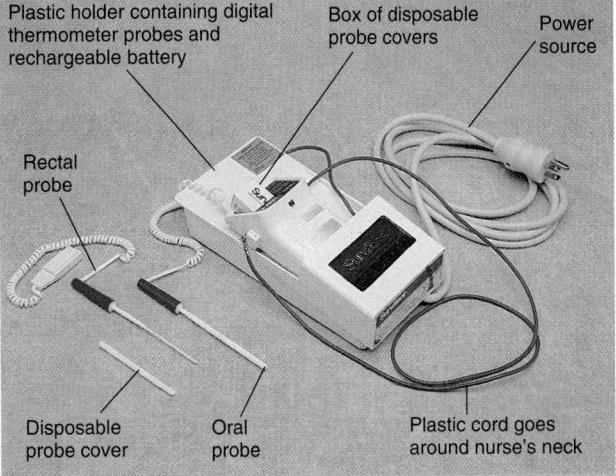

Plastic holder containing digital thermometer probes and rechargeable battery

Box of disposable probe covers

Power source

Rectal probe

Disposable probe cover

Oral probe

Plastic cord goes around nurse's neck

FIGURE 9-9 An Oral, Battery-Operated Thermometer

| **E** Examination | **N** Normal Findings | **A** Abnormal Findings | **P** Pathophysiology |

4. Listen for the sound or look for the symbol that indicates maximum body temperature has been reached.

5. Observe and record the reading.

6. Remove and discard the probe cover.

7. Return the electronic thermometer to the charging unit.

TYMPANIC THERMOMETER.

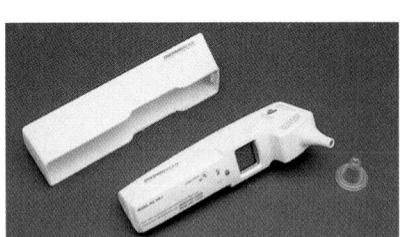

FIGURE 9-10 A Tympanic Thermometer

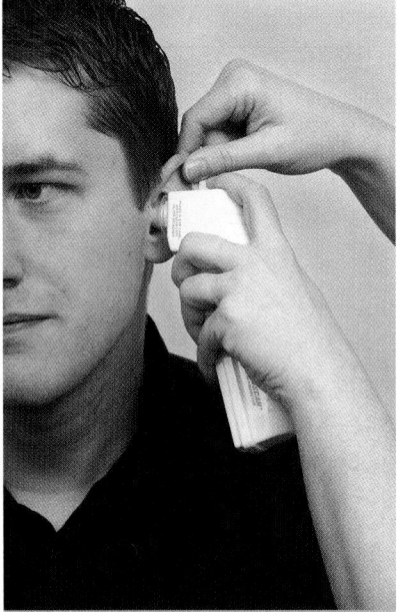

FIGURE 9-11 Taking a Patient's Temperature with a Tympanic Thermometer

E 1. Attach the probe cover to the nose of the thermometer (Figure 9-10).

2. Gently place the probe of the thermometer over the entrance to the ear canal. If the patient is under 3 years old, pull the pinna down, aiming the probe toward the opposite eye. If the patient is over 3 years old, grasp the pinna and pull gently up and back, aiming the probe toward the opposite ear (Figure 9-11). Make sure there is a tight seal.

3. Press the start button on the thermometer handle.

4. Wait for the beep, remove the probe from the ear, and read the temperature.

5. Discard the probe cover.

6. Return the tympanic thermometer to the charger unit.

N Normal body temperatures are described in Table 9-4.

A **Hyperthermia**, pyrexia, or fever are conditions in which body temperatures exceed 38.5°C, or 101.5°F. Clinical signs of hyperthermia include increased respiratory rate and pulse, shivering, pallor, and thirst.

P There can be many causes of hyperthermia (including infection), which results from an increased basal metabolic rate.

A **Hypothermia** occurs when the body temperature is below 34°C, or 93.2°F. Clinical signs of hypothermia include decreased body temperature and initial shivering that ceases as drowsiness and coma ensue. Hypotension, decreased urinary output, lack of muscle coordination, and disorientation also occur as hypothermia progresses.

P Hypothermia can be caused by prolonged exposure to cold such as immersion in cold water or administration of large volumes of unwarmed blood products.

P Hypothermia can be induced to decrease the tissues' need for oxygen, such as during cardiac surgery.

REFLECTIVE THINKING

Assessing Temperature in a Reluctant Patient

You are the rural health nurse substituting for a sick colleague. Today, you are visiting 3-year-old Amalia, who has been followed for many months since her congenital heart repair. Her mother tells you that Amalia feels hot and that she has been unable to find a thermometer to take Amalia's temperature. You prepare to assess Amalia's rectal temperature when she tells you that she doesn't want you to touch her. She will let only Nurse McElroy take care of her. What is your best course of action?

E Examination   **N** Normal Findings   **A** Abnormal Findings   **P** Pathophysiology

BLOOD PRESSURE

Blood pressure measures (in millimeters of mercury [mm Hg]) the force exerted by the flow of blood pumped into the large arteries. Arterial blood pressure is determined by blood flow and the resistance to blood flow as indicated in the following formula:

$$MAP = CO \times TPR$$

mean arterial pressure (MAP) = cardiac output (CO) × total peripheral resistance (TPR)

Changes in blood pressure can be used to monitor changes in cardiac output. Ineffective pumping, decreased circulating volume, as well as changes in the characteristics of the blood vessels, can affect blood pressure. There is a diurnal variation in blood pressure as characterized by a high point in the early evening and a low point during the early deep stage of sleep.

Korotkoff Sounds

Korotkoff sounds are generated when the flow of blood through the artery is altered by inflating the blood pressure cuff that is wrapped around the extremity. Korotkoff sounds may be heard by listening over a pulse site that is distal to the blood pressure cuff. As the air is released from the bladder of the cuff, the pressure on the artery changes from that which completely occludes blood flow to that which allows free flow. As the pressure against the artery wall decreases, five distinct sounds occur. These are:

Phase I: The first audible sound heard as the cuff pressure is released. Sounds like clear tapping and correlates to systolic pressure (the force needed to pump the blood out of the heart).

Phase II: Sounds like swishing or a murmur. Created as the blood flows through blood vessels narrowed by the inflation of the blood pressure cuff.

Phase III: Sounds like clear, intense tapping. Created as blood flows through the artery, but cuff pressure is still great enough to occlude flow during diastole.

Phase IV: Sounds are muffled and are heard when cuff pressure is low enough to allow some blood flow during diastole. The change from the tap of Phase III to the muffled sound of Phase IV is referred to as the first diastolic reading.

Phase V: No sounds are heard. Occurs when cuff pressure is released enough to allow normal blood flow. This is referred to as the second diastolic reading.

Measuring Blood Pressure

Systolic pressure represents the pressure exerted on the arterial wall during **systole**, when the ventricles are contracting. Diastolic pressure represents the pressure in the arteries when the ventricles are relaxed and filling. Blood pressure is recorded as a fraction, with the top number representing the systole and the bottom number(s) representing the **diastole**. If first and second diastolic sounds are recorded, the first diastolic sound is written over the second. For example, 120/90/80 indicates that 120 mm Hg is the systolic pressure, 90 mm Hg is the first diastolic sound, and 80 mm Hg is the second diastolic sound. **Pulse pressure** is the difference between the diastolic and systolic blood pressures.

Measurement Sites

There are several potential sites for blood pressure measurement. The preferred site is the brachial pulse site, where the brachial artery runs across the antecubital fossa. The posterior thigh, where the popliteal artery runs behind the knee joint, can also be used. A site should not be used if there is pain or injury around or near the site; for instance, a postmastectomy patient should have blood pressure assessed on the unaffected side. Surgical incisions; intravenous, central venous, or

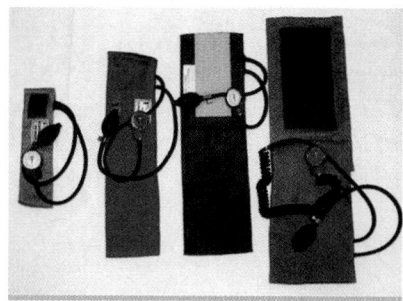

FIGURE 9-12 **Blood pressure cuffs come in various sizes.**

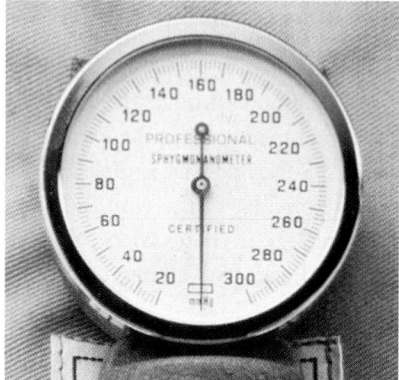

FIGURE 9-13 **An Aneroid Sphygmomanometer Dial**

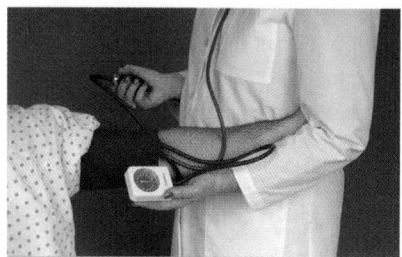

FIGURE 9-14 **Taking a Patient's Blood Pressure**

arterial lines; or areas with poor perfusion should be avoided for blood pressure measurement. Patients with arteriovenous (AV) fistulas or AV shunts should not have blood pressure measured in those extremities.

Equipment

Blood pressure is measured indirectly with a stethoscope or Doppler and a **sphygmomanometer**, which consists of the blood pressure cuff, connecting tubes and air pump, and manometer. Blood pressure cuffs come in several sizes (Figure 9-12). The size of the cuff bladder should be 80% of the circumference of the limb being assessed (JNC 7, 2003). The cuff should completely encircle the limb.

A manometer is attached to the cuff via a second tube. The **aneroid manometer** is a calibrated dial with a needle that points to numbers representing the air pressure within the cuff (Figure 9-13).

A Doppler ultrasonic stethoscope can also be used to obtain blood pressure. It is especially useful when blood pressure sounds are difficult to hear, such as with infants or very obese patients.

E 1. Ensure that the patient has not had any caffeine or tobacco products in the past 30 minutes. Allow the patient to rest for 5 minutes before you take the blood pressure.

2. Select an appropriate size cuff.

3. Position the patient. The patient may be sitting, standing, or supine. At the first encounter, all three positions are recommended.

4. Position the arm or leg to be used so that the extremity is at a level equal to the heart to prevent a false reading (Figure 9-14). At subsequent encounters, the sitting position is usually the position of choice. Ensure that the patient's feet are firmly on the floor in this position.

5. Apply the deflated blood pressure (BP) cuff:

   a. Upper arm: Wrap the BP cuff snugly around the bare upper arm. The bottom of the BP cuff should be 1–2 in. above the antecubital fossa. The center of the bladder should be directly above the brachial artery.

   b. Leg: Wrap the BP cuff around the bare thigh, with the bottom of the BP cuff slightly above the knee. The popliteal artery below the cuff is used for BP measurement. This is usually easier if the patient is in the prone position.

6. Establish a baseline systolic blood pressure (palpating the blood pressure), if needed:

   a. Palpate the brachial or radial artery with the finger pads of your nondominant hand distal to the BP cuff.

   b. Inflate the BP cuff, and note when the artery pulsation is no longer palpable.

   c. Release the air from the BP cuff, and wait 1 to 2 minutes.

7. Palpate the pulse distal to the BP cuff.

8. Place the bell of the stethoscope over the blood pressure site (the diaphragm may be used if sounds are hard to hear):

   a. If a Doppler ultrasonic stethoscope is to be used, apply conducting gel to the site where the pulse was palpated.

   b. Place the Doppler transducer over the site.

9. Inflate the BP cuff to approximately 20 mm Hg above the established baseline blood pressure or 20 mm Hg above where the Korotkoff sounds disappear.

NURSINGTIP

Home Blood Pressure Monitoring Devices

Many patients monitor their blood pressure at home to document their body's response to antihypertensive medications. Brachial artery-based monitors are the most accurate of home monitoring devices. Periodically, patients should be instructed to bring their home devices to their appointments. You can observe how patients take their blood pressure and assess the process for accuracy. Reinforcing correct technique can positively influence patient compliance with the medical regimen.

It is also appropriate to compare the blood pressure reading on the home device with that obtained in the office. The measurements should correlate within 5 mm Hg of each other. This allows you to determine if the readings from home accurately reflect the patient's actual blood pressure.

NURSINGALERT

Palpating the Blood Pressure

If you are unable to hear a patient's blood pressure and there is no electronic monitor or amplification device available, you can use the palpation method. Conduct the blood pressure as described in steps 1–6 using the brachial artery. When releasing air from the cuff, note when the brachial artery is palpable. This correlates with the systolic pressure. This blood pressure is then documented as a number over palpated (e.g., 115/P)

10. Slowly open the valve and release the pressure at a rate of 2 to 3 mm Hg per second.

11. Listen for the Korotkoff sounds:

   a. Onset of Korotkoff sounds correlates to systolic pressure.

   b. Muffling or disappearance of sounds correlates to diastolic pressures.

12. Deflate the BP cuff completely.

13. Record the blood pressure reading(s). The extremity used and position of the patient are important data to record along with the blood pressure reading. Refer to the Nursing Tip, Documenting Blood Pressure.

N Normal blood pressure varies with age. As a person ages, blood pressure generally increases. Table 9-5 presents general ranges for normal blood pressure at different ages. Normally, baroreceptors (receptors located in the walls of most of the great arteries that sense hypotension and initiate reflex vasoconstriction and tachycardia to bring the blood pressure back to normal) help a patient to maintain normal blood pressure when changing from a supine to a sitting or a standing position. Processes increasing cardiac output, such as exercise, will normally increase blood pressure. Pulse pressure is normally 30 to 40 mm Hg. Table 9-6 lists errors in blood pressure measurement.

A **Hypertension**, or high blood pressure, is usually confirmed when an adult patient has blood pressure readings remaining consistently above 120 mm Hg systolic and 80 mm Hg diastolic on two consecutive visits after an initial screening. See Table 9-7 for the classification and management of hypertension.

P The cause of hypertension in 90% of patients who have it is unknown. It is thought that the mechanisms that maintain the therapeutic fluid volume in the body (e.g., the heart, kidneys, nervous system, renin-angiotensin-aldosterone system) may be abnormal. The other 10% of the population who have high blood pressure have secondary hypertension. All of the following pathophysiologies of hypertension are secondary in nature.

P Arteriosclerosis reduces arterial compliance. Elastic and muscular tissues of arteries are replaced with fibrous tissue as part of the normal aging process,

NURSINGTIP

Documenting Blood Pressure

The position of the patient during the blood pressure measurement should be recorded. Use the following symbols to depict patient position:

O— supine   Q sitting   Q standing

Also, record where the blood pressure was taken. Use the following abbreviations:

RA = right arm   LA = left arm
RL = right leg   LL = left leg

Examples of blood pressure readings are:

O— 160/122 LL (left leg, supine)

Q 98/52 RA (right arm, sitting)

Q 118/85 LA (left arm, standing)

| **E** Examination | **N** Normal Findings | **A** Abnormal Findings | **P** Pathophysiology |

(Figure 9-15)

NURSING**ALERT**

Automatic Blood Pressure Cuffs

Your patient may be receiving a drug such as heparin, aspirin, or other thrombolytic therapy that makes him or her susceptible to bleeding complications (Figure 9-15). If you are using an automatic blood pressure cuff on your patient, take these precautions to prevent any bleeding complications that may occur in the arm that is being used for noninvasive blood pressure monitoring:

1. Adjust the maximal inflation pressure on the automatic blood pressure machine to your patient's last systolic blood pressure. Otherwise, the blood pressure cuff could inflate as high as a systolic blood pressure of 200 mm Hg.
2. Once your patient's blood pressure is stable, increase the intervals between measurements. If you do not, the blood pressure cuff could inflate as often as every minute. Also, you can switch the mode to manual from automatic so that you avoid unnecessary inflations of the blood pressure cuff.
3. Place the blood pressure cuff on the arm opposite any intravenous infusions. If this is not possible, then try the thigh as a site for blood pressure measurement.
4. Whenever permissible, rotate the cuff site and remember to remove it at least every shift to assess the patient's skin.

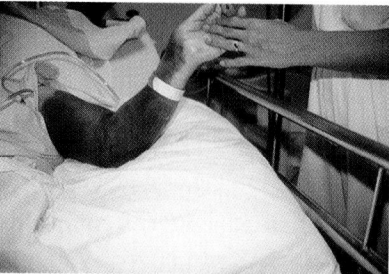

FIGURE 9-15 Proper placement and monitoring of an automatic blood pressure cuff will reduce the risk of injury or trauma to the patient. This Caucasian patient had an automatic blood pressure cuff placed on the left arm while also receiving a heparin infusion in that arm.

making the vessels less able to contract and relax in response to systolic and diastolic pressures. When the systolic pressure alone is elevated in the elderly, it is called isolated systolic hypertension.

P Processes decreasing the size of arterial lumen cause hypertension. Hypercholesterolemia results in deposits of plaque along the inner walls of the vessels, reducing the size of the arterial lumen and increasing blood pressure.

P Processes that increase the viscosity of the blood, such as sickle cell crisis, cause greater friction between molecules of the blood and, thus, higher blood pressure.

P Chronic steroid use, Cushing's syndrome, thyroid disease, and parathyroid dysfunction can all cause hypertension.

P High blood pressure may result from diseases affecting other regulatory blood pressure processes. For example, kidney disease, which affects the production of antidiuretic hormone, a hormone that helps control

TABLE 9-5 Blood Pressure: Normal Range According to Age and Gender*

AGE (FEMALE)	SYSTOLIC (mm Hg)	DIASTOLIC (mm Hg)
1	97–103	52–56
5	103–109	66–70
10	112–118	73–76
15	120–127	78–81
≥ 18	< 120	< 80
AGE (MALE)	**SYSTOLIC (mm Hg)**	**DIASTOLIC (mm Hg)**
1	94–103	49–54
5	104–112	65–70
10	111–119	73–78
15	122–131	76–81
≥ 18	< 120	< 80

*The National Heart, Lung, and Blood Institute of the National Institutes of Health developed pediatric blood pressure guidelines based on gender, age, and height percentiles. The measurements listed for pediatric patients are consolidated for ease in reporting. Normal blood pressure is defined as the systolic (SBP) and diastolic (DBP) blood pressures that are below the 90th percentile for age and gender. High-normal blood pressure is defined as the SBP or DBP being at the 90th percentile and above, but not including, the 95th percentile. Hypertension is defined as the SBP or DBP being greater than or equal to the 95th percentile on three different occasions.

E Examination   **N** Normal Findings   **A** Abnormal Findings   **P** Pathophysiology

TABLE 9-6 Errors in Blood Pressure Measurement

IF READING SHOWS:	SUSPECT:
Inaccurately high blood pressure	Blood pressure cuff is too short or too narrow (e.g., using a regular blood pressure cuff on an obese arm), or the brachial artery may be positioned below the heart. The patient may also be stressed, be in an emotional state, or have just completed physical activity.
High diastolic blood pressure	Unrecognized **auscultatory gap** (a silent interval between systolic and diastolic pressures that may occur in hypertensive patients or because you deflated the blood pressure cuff too rapidly); immediate reinflation of the blood pressure cuff for multiple blood pressure readings (resultant venous congestion makes the Korotkoff sounds less audible); if the patient supports his or her own arm, then sustained muscular contraction can raise the diastolic blood pressure by 10%.
Inaccurately low blood pressure	Blood pressure cuff is too long or too wide; the brachial artery is above the heart.
Low systolic blood pressure	Unrecognized auscultatory gap (a rapid deflation of the cuff or immediate reinflation of the cuff for multiple readings can result in venous congestion, thus making the Korotkoff sounds less audible and the pressure appear lower).

TABLE 9-7 Classification and Management of Blood Pressure for Adults 18 Years or Older

BP CLASSIFICATION	SBP* (mm Hg)	DBP* (mm Hg)	LIFESTYLE MODIFICATION	MANAGEMENT — INITIAL DRUG THERAPY** WITHOUT COMPELLING INDICATIONS	MANAGEMENT — INITIAL DRUG THERAPY** WITH COMPELLING INDICATIONS
Normal	<120	and <80	Encourage	N/A	N/A
Prehypertension	120–139	or 80–89	Yes	No antihypertensive drug indicated	Drug(s) for compelling indications**
Stage 1 hypertension	140–159	or 90–99	Yes	Thiazide-type diuretics for most. May consider ACEI, ARB, BB, CCB, or a combination	Drug(s) for the compelling indications** Other antihypertensive drugs (diuretics, ACEI, ARB, BB, CCB) as needed
Stage 2 hypertension	≥160	or ≥100	Yes	Two-drug combination for most*** (usually thiazide-type diuretic and ACEI, ARB, BB, or CCB)	Drug(s) for the compelling indications** Other antihypertensive drugs (diuretics, ACEI, ARB, BB, CCB) as needed

BP = blood pressure; SBP = systolic BP; DBP = diastolic BP; ACEI = angiotensin-converting enzyme inhibitor; ARB = angiotensin receptor blocker; BB = ß-blocker; CCB = calcium channel blocker

*Treatment determined by highest BP category.

**Treat patients with chronic kidney disease or diabetes to BP goal of less than 130/80 mm Hg.

***Initial combined therapy should be used cautiously in those at risk for orthostatic hypotension.

From "The Seventh Report of the Joint National Committee on Prevention, Detection, Evaluation, and Treatment of High Blood Pressure," by A. V. Chobanian, G. L. Bakris, H. R. Black, W. C. Cushman, L. A. Green, J. L. Izzo, Jr., et al., 2003. Retrieved May 28, 2008, from http://www.nhlbi.nih.gov/guidelines/hypertension/jnc7full.pdf.

body fluid balance, can cause hypertension. An adrenal gland tumor, or pheochromocytoma, can increase blood pressure because of epinephrine and norepinephrine secretion.

P Overload of fluids from poor renal function or indiscriminant intravenous fluid administration (particularly in children) can result in hypertension.

P Stress can increase blood pressure. Stimulation of the sympathetic nervous system increases cardiac output and vasoconstriction, thus increasing blood pressure.

P A patient's stress level can increase when in the presence of a health care provider. Patients who have elevated blood pressure in an office or hospital environment only are said to have "white coat syndrome." When these patients have their blood pressure taken in the community, it is frequently within an acceptable range.

A Blood pressure falling below normal range is considered to be **hypotension**, or low blood pressure, which results in inadequate tissue perfusion and oxygenation. If the standing systolic blood pressure is more than 30 mm Hg below the supine systolic pressure, it may indicate that the person has orthostatic hypotension. See Chapter 16. Slow response by baroreceptors when an individual transitions from a lying to a standing position can result in transitory orthostatic hypotension. When this occurs, the individual may feel dizzy and is at risk for falls.

P Processes drastically reducing circulatory blood volume, such as hypovolemic shock, cause hypotension.

P Medications such as nitroglycerin or antihypertensives lower blood pressure.

P Anaphylactic shock, resulting from massive histamine release, and circulatory collapse cause severe hypotension.

A A difference of greater than 10 to 15 mm Hg between the blood pressure in both arms is abnormal.

P This difference in blood pressure between arms can be caused by coarctation of the aorta, aortic aneurysm, atherosclerotic obstruction, and subclavian steal syndrome. These conditions all result in an increased pressure proximal to the narrowing and a decreased pressure distal to the narrowing of the aorta or whatever is causing the obstruction.

A A systolic blood pressure that is greater in the arms than in the legs is abnormal.

P This blood pressure difference between the arms and the legs is caused by constriction or obstruction of the aorta, which can result from an increase in stroke volume ejection velocity, increased cardiac output, peripheral vasodilation, and decreased distensibility of the aorta or major arteries.

A A decreased pulse pressure is abnormal.

P A decreased pulse pressure can result from a decreased stroke volume (cardiac tamponade, shock, and tachycardia) or increased peripheral resistance (aortic stenosis, coarctation of the aorta, mitral stenosis or mitral regurgitation, and cardiac tamponade).

A An increased pulse pressure is abnormal.

P An increased pulse pressure can result from increased stroke volume (aortic regurgitation) or increased peripheral vasodilatation (fever, anemia, heat, exercise, hyperthyroidism, and arteriovenous fistula).

LIFE 360°

The Accuracy of Vital Signs

A first-semester nursing student shows you the vital signs of her 23-year-old male patient who is scheduled for an inguinal herniorrhaphy this morning. The vital signs are:

Temperature: 95.8°F (tympanic)
Pulse: 56
Respirations: 6
Blood Pressure: 69/55 LA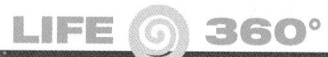

Are these vital signs accurate? Describe why some of the vital signs may be inaccurate and what errors the nursing student may have committed when obtaining them.

| **E** Examination | **N** Normal Findings | **A** Abnormal Findings | **P** Pathophysiology |

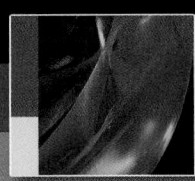

PAIN

Pain is "an unpleasant sensory or emotional experience associated with actual or potential tissue damage, or described in terms of such damage" (IASP, 1979). It is a complex sensory experience that has been receiving more clinical attention in the last 40 years. Pain has become the focus of many clinical research projects as a single clinical phenomenon, not just as a symptom of clinical pathology.

NOCICEPTIVE PAIN

Nociceptive pain arises from somatic or visceral stimulation. **Nociception**, or pain perception, is a multistep process that involves the nervous system as well as other body systems (Figure 9-16). A noxious stimulus occurs, which stimulates the **nociceptors** (receptive neurons of pain sensation that are located in the skin and various viscera). The noxious stimulus can be many things (e.g., trauma, burn, chemical exposure, internal body inflammation, or internal body growth of tissue). Transduction of the noxious stimulus travels to the spinal cord via the nociceptors. This transduction causes the conversion of one energy (traveling stimulus) from another (noxious stimulus). Cell damage from the noxious stimulus causes the release of certain chemicals or sensitizing nociceptors. Prostaglandins (PG), bradykinins (BK), serotonin (5 HT), substance P (SP), hydrogen (H^+), potassium (K^+), histamine (H), and leukotrienes are all sensitizing substances. Substance P is unique because it is released only when pain fibers are stimulated.

Activating the sensitizing substances leads to an action potential in which the pain sensation is moved via afferent nerves to the spinal cord. Two types of nerve fibers participate in the action potential: A-delta fibers are myelinated neurons that transmit acute, sharp, shooting, and localized pain; C fibers are nonmyelinated neurons that transmit dull, throbbing, and poorly localized pain. These nerve fibers carry the pain impulse from the spinal cord via the spinothalamic tract to the brain stem and thalamus. The thalamus relays information to the cortex (which is capable of identifying past pain memories) and to the limbic system (where the emotional component of pain is formed). It is in these areas of the brain that pain is consciously perceived.

The last step of nociception is modulation. Modulation is the inhibition of nociceptor impulses. Neurons from the brain stem release neurotransmitters (e.g., serotonin, norepinephrine [NE], gamma-aminobutyric acid [GABA], 5 HT, and endogenous opioids [e.g., enkephalins, dynorphins, and β-endorphins]) as the pain message descends from the brain stem to the spinal cord. Collectively, these substances block the transmission of pain and produce analgesia.

NEUROPATHIC PAIN

Neuropathic pain can result from lesions in the central nervous system (CNS) or the peripheral nervous system (PNS). It is often characterized as a severe burning or tingling, such as that experienced with herpes zoster. Neuropathic pain may be difficult to treat clinically.

TYPES OF PAIN

Pain can be grouped by its origin as well as its duration. Cutaneous, somatic, visceral, and referred pain are the types of pain grouped by origin. Cutaneous pain arises from the stimulation of cutaneous nerves. This pain usually has a burning quality. Somatic pain originates from bone, tendons, ligaments, muscles, and nerves and is frequently caused by musculoskeletal injury. Visceral pain arises from the organs. Diseased organs can change size, usually resulting in stretching of the organ, leading to pain. Acute appendicitis is an example of visceral pain. Referred pain is perceived in a location other than where the pathology is occurring. The location of the referred pain is in the dermatome of the spinal cord that is innervating the affected viscera and where the organ was located in its embryonic stage. An example of referred pain is the pain of pancreatitis felt on the left shoulder.

continues

Pain (continued)

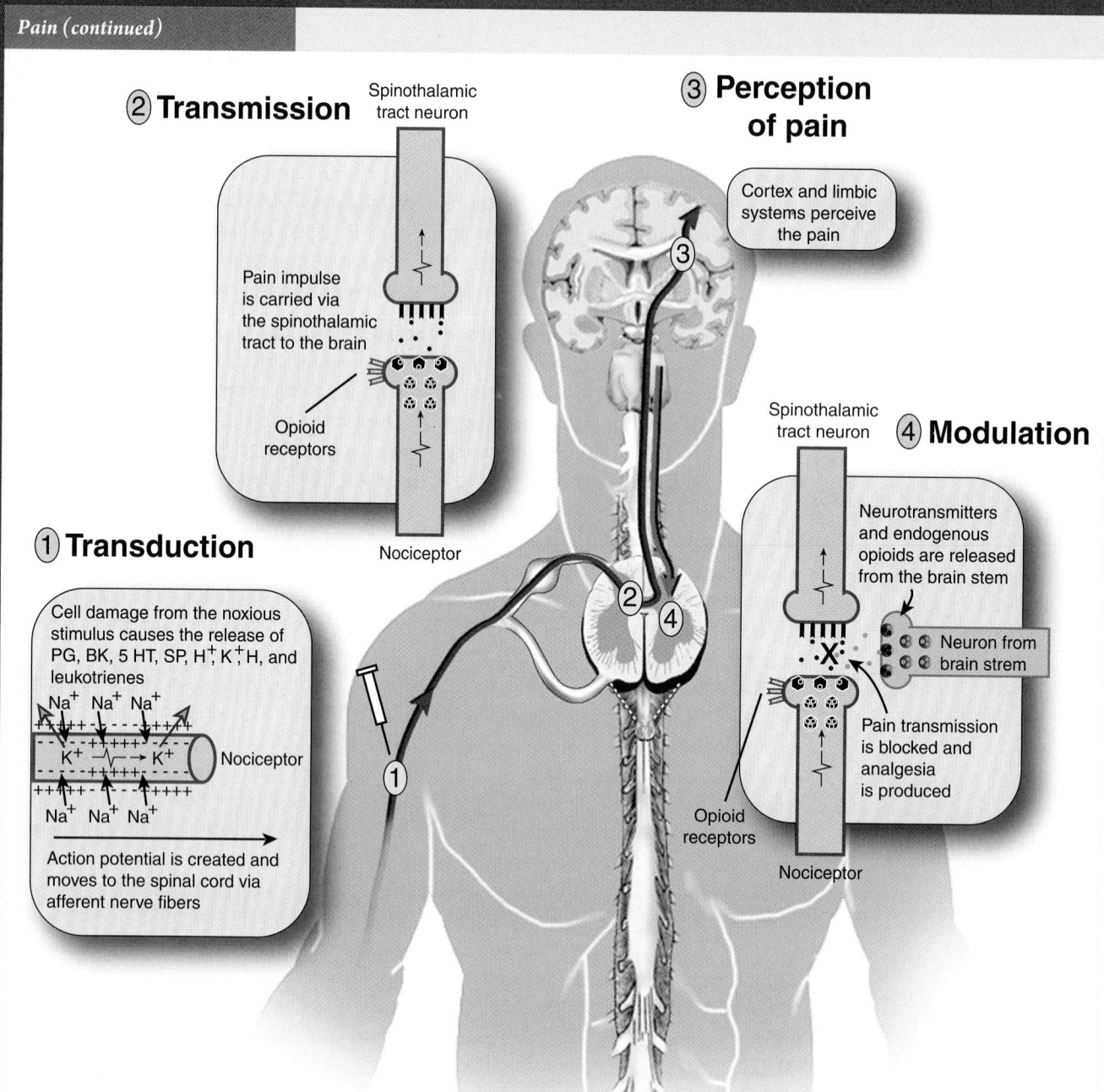

② **Transmission**
Spinothalamic tract neuron

Pain impulse is carried via the spinothalamic tract to the brain

Opioid receptors

Nociceptor

③ **Perception of pain**

Cortex and limbic systems perceive the pain

③

④ **Modulation**
Spinothalamic tract neuron

Neurotransmitters and endogenous opioids are released from the brain stem

Neuron from brain strem

Pain transmission is blocked and analgesia is produced

Opioid receptors

Nociceptor

① **Transduction**

Cell damage from the noxious stimulus causes the release of PG, BK, 5 HT, SP, H^+, K^+H, and leukotrienes

Na^+ Na^+ Na^+

K^+ → K^+ Nociceptor

Na^+ Na^+ Na^+

Action potential is created and moves to the spinal cord via afferent nerve fibers

②
④
①

FIGURE 9-16 Nociception

Acute, chronic malignant, and chronic nonmalignant pain are examples of pain grouped by their duration. Acute pain has a sudden onset, is of short duration, and is self-limiting. It ranges in intensity from mild to severe. It usually has an identifiable cause, such as surgery or trauma. Chronic malignant pain is pain of more than 6 months' duration, for example, in a patient with cancer. This persistent pain can be due to a tumor, inflammation, blocked ducts, pressure on other body parts, and necrosis. Chronic nonmalignant pain also lasts more than 6 months. It can occur with and without an identifiable cause. The pain can remain even after an initial injury is healed. Back pain and fibromyalgia are examples of chronic nonmalignant pain.

VARIABLES AFFECTING PAIN

A patient's sex, age, previous experience with pain, and cultural expectations can affect an individual's response to pain. Studies have shown that females have a lower pain tolerance or threshold than males and report pain more frequently. Females tend to

continues

Pain *(continued)*

dwell on the psychological aspects of pain, whereas males emphasize its physiological aspects (Berkeley & Holdcroft, 1999; Fillingim & Maixner, 1995).

Regarding the effect of age on pain, typically, young children become sensitized to pain and may be greatly affected by the pain experience. As they reach adolescence, children may become more stoic about pain. Older adults, especially those who have chronic pain, may also not complain about their pain until it becomes debilitating. This failure to seek treatment for pain is frequently due to the perception that the pain means something is seriously wrong, or the patient may not have the resources to seek treatment. Older adults also have a lifetime of experiences with different types of pain, and that greatly influences how they choose to deal with new pain. Lastly, cultural norms can help determine what the patient's pain experience will be. Refer to Chapter 5.

EFFECTS OF PAIN ON THE BODY

Pain affects everyone in different ways. Acute pain usually manifests itself differently from chronic pain, although there are some common elements. Physiological responses to pain include tachycardia, tachypnea, hypertension, diaphoresis, dilated pupils, and an altered immune response. Additional responses to pain include complaints of pain, crying, moaning, frowning, anger, fear, anxiety, depression, suicidal ideation, decreased appetite, sleep deprivation, altered concentration, pacing, rubbing the affected body part, and protecting or splinting the affected body part. These responses to pain are by no means all-inclusive. Pain can affect every system in the human body, and unrelieved pain can take its toll on the health of the patient over time. Just as pain is a unique experience for the person in pain, so is the patient's response to pain.

ASSESSING PAIN

The Joint Commission mandates that a comprehensive pain assessment be conducted on each patient in a health care setting, or that a patient be referred for a pain assessment as determined by the patient's health status and the availability of care. Pain assessment is to be measured in terms of intensity and quality appropriate to the patient's age and then documented in the patient's record. Subsequently, assessment of pain is not optional in health care. Pain is a critical vital sign of a patient's well-being.

However, many patients present to the health care system with a chief complaint of pain. The 10 characteristics used to gain information about a chief complaint are likewise used to elicit information on a patient's pain.

- Location: Where is the pain located?
- Radiation: Does the pain move to another part of the body?
- Quality: How does the pain feel?
- Quantity: How severe is the pain?
- Associated manifestations: What other signs and symptoms are occurring with the pain?
- Aggravating factors: What makes the pain worse?
- Alleviating factors: What makes the pain better?
- Setting: Where were you (physically or emotionally or both) when the pain started?
- Timing: When did the pain start? How long does it last? How frequently does it occur?
- Meaning and impact: Does this pain have any special significance to you? How has it affected your life?

Many pain assessment tools are available to guide accurate pain assessment and pain control. McCaffery and Pasero (1999) and Schechter, Berde, and Yaster (2003) have developed tools that can be used in the clinical setting. Many institutions have also developed their own pain assessment flow sheet.

Pain intensity rating scales are available to assess the severity of a patient's pain experience. The Visual Analog Scale, described in Chapter 3, is perhaps the easiest to use in any setting because it requires no additional resources. The nurse uses scale imagery to

continues

Pain (continued)

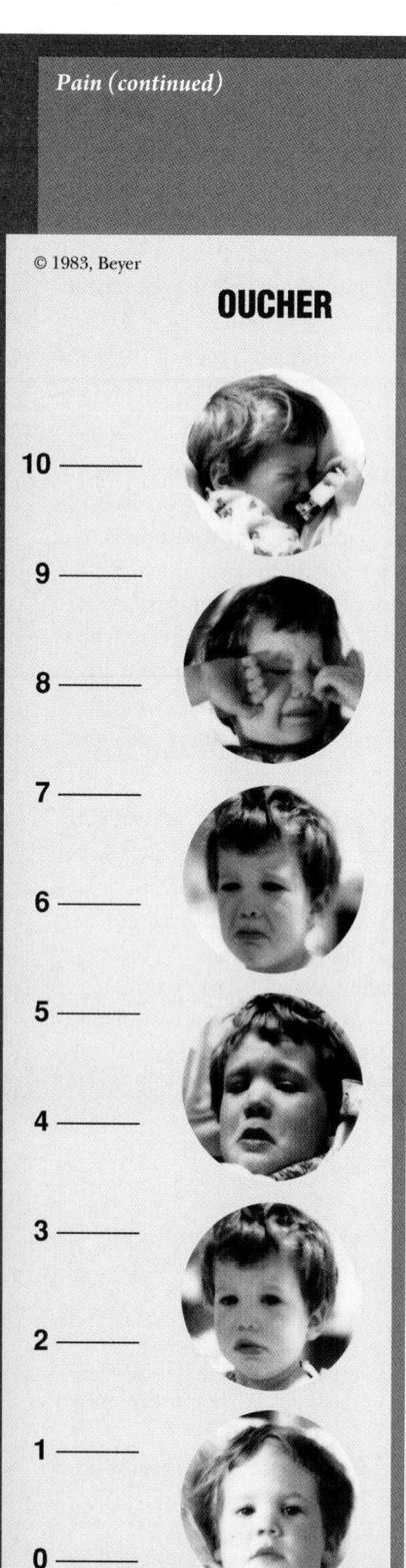

© 1983, Beyer

OUCHER

10
9
8
7
6
5
4
3
2
1
0

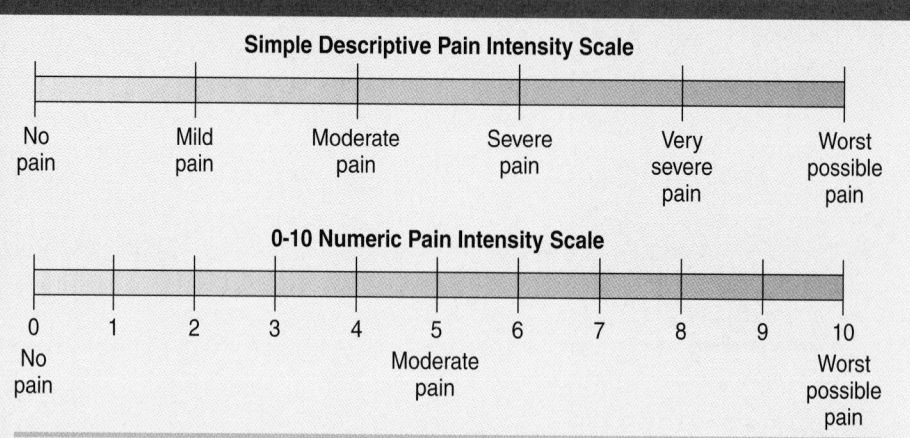

Simple Descriptive Pain Intensity Scale

No pain | Mild pain | Moderate pain | Severe pain | Very severe pain | Worst possible pain

0-10 Numeric Pain Intensity Scale

0 1 2 3 4 5 6 7 8 9 10

No pain | Moderate pain | Worst possible pain

FIGURE 9-17 **Pain Intensity Scale.** *From Acute Pain Management: Operative or Medical Procedures and Trauma. Clinical Practice Guideline (AHCPR Publication No. 92-0032), by the Acute Pain Management Guideline Panel, 1992, Rockville, MD: Agency for Health Care Policy and Research.*

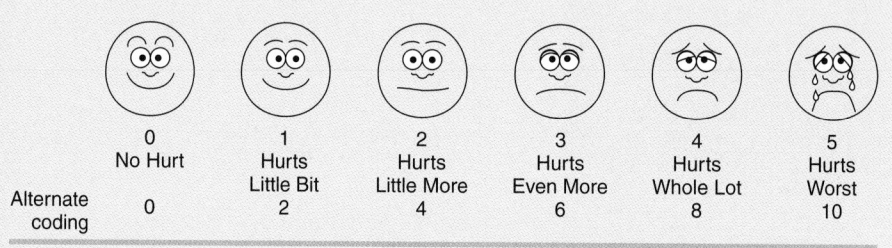

0 No Hurt	1 Hurts Little Bit	2 Hurts Little More	3 Hurts Even More	4 Hurts Whole Lot	5 Hurts Worst

Alternate coding: 0 | 2 | 4 | 6 | 8 | 10

FIGURE 9-18 **Wong-Baker FACES Pain Rating Scale.** *From Hockenberry, M. J., Wilson, D., & Winkelstein, M. L., Wong's Essentials of Pediatric Nursing, 7th ed., St. Louis, 2005, p. 1259. Used with permission. Copyright, Mosby.*

assess the intensity of a patient's pain. Flow sheets are often used to trend the patient's verbal reports of pain.

Three additional pain intensity scales are the Pain Intensity Scale (Acute Pain Management Guideline Panel, 1992), the Wong-Baker FACES Pain Rating Scale (Hockenberry et al., 2003), and the Oucher Pain Assessment Tool (Beyer, 1983). With each scale, the patient has control over each of his or her own pain assessment encounters. Trending these reports provides information on whether the patient's pain is alleviating or worsening. This information allows the nurse to evaluate the effectiveness of the patient's pain regimen.

The Pain Intensity Scale (Figure 9-17) is a quick assessment tool that is easily understood. The Wong-Baker FACES Pain Rating Scale (Figure 9-18) is recommended for children over the age of 3 years. The nurse needs to explain this scale to the child with each assessment encounter. The Oucher Pain Assessment Tool (Figure 9-19) is used with children 3–12 years old. The scale should be explained to the child at each assessment. Caucasian, Hispanic, and African American versions of this tool are available.

FIGURE 9-19 **Oucher Pain Assessment Tool.** *From The Caucasian version of the Oucher, developed and copyrighted by Judith E. Beyer, RN, PhD, 1983.*

Using Clinical Judgment When Taking Vital Signs

Mr. Goldstein is a 75-year-old man hospitalized for pneumonia. He is wearing a 40% oxygen face mask. Mr. Goldstein has a history of confusion and combative behavior, particularly at night. His IV had to be replaced last night because, in his confusion and agitation, he pulled it out. You are working the night shift, and it is 2:00 AM. Mr. Goldstein is sleeping comfortably. He has vital signs ordered every 4 hours. His signs were last taken at 10:00 PM and were as follows:

Respirations: 14

Pulse: 90

Blood pressure: 132/88 (LA)

Temperature: 37.1°C (rectal)

- What are the major issues related to taking Mr. Goldstein's vital signs right now?
- What are the possible actions you could take, and what are the potential consequences of each?

ASSESSMENT IN BRIEF

General Survey, Vital Signs, and Pain

General Survey

- Physical presence
  - Stated age versus apparent age
  - General appearance
  - Body fat
  - Stature
  - Motor activity
  - Body and breath odors
- Psychological presence
  - Dress, grooming, and personal hygiene
  - Mood and manner

  – Speech
  – Facial expression
- Distress

Vital Signs

- Respiration
- Pulse
- Temperature
- Blood pressure

Pain

REVIEW QUESTIONS

1. You are assessing a patient's physical presence and note that the patient looks thin and frail. What condition might this patient have?
   a. Cushing's syndrome
   b. Hypokinetic state
   c. Malabsorption disease
   d. Hypothyroidism
   The correct answer is (c).

2. Smelling an alcohol odor on a patient may indicate which of the following conditions?
   a. Vaginal infection   c. Tonsillitis
   b. Allergic rhinitis   d. Ketoacidosis
   The correct answer is (d).

Questions 3 to 8 refer to the following situation:

A patient is brought to the emergency room after being hit by a car while riding a bicycle. His vital signs are: T 97.1°F (tympanic); P 142; R 32; BP 78/45/38.

3. What conclusion do you make about the patient's temperature?
   a. The patient's temperature is within normal limits.
   b. The rectal route is the best method to use in a trauma patient to determine temperature.
   c. Tympanic thermometers are inaccurate if the patient has lost a lot of blood.
   d. The Celsius scale is the most accurate scale to use when documenting temperature.
   The correct answer is (a).

4. The patient's respiratory rate is called:

  a. Hyperpnea   c. Bradypnea

  b. Dyspnea   d. Tachypnea

The correct answer is (d).

5. The patient is connected to a heart monitor. You recognize the patient's electrical rhythm as atrial fibrillation. You also palpate the patient's carotid pulse. Which of the following describes the rhythm of the heart rate and pulse?

  a. Regular   c. Regularly irregular

  b. Regularly regular   d. Irregularly irregular

The correct answer is (d).

6. The patient's pulse volume is documented as 1+/4+. This means the patient's pulse is:

  a. Absent   c. Normal

  b. Thready   d. Bounding

The correct answer is (b).

7. The patient's blood pressure is 78/45/38. The second diastolic reading corresponds to which Korotkoff sound?

  a. Phase II   c. Phase IV

  b. Phase III   d. Phase V

The correct answer is (d).

8. A blood pressure of 78/45/38 in this patient indicates which of the following conditions?

  a. Anaphylactic shock

  b. Hypovolemic shock

  c. Septic shock

  d. Cardiogenic shock

The correct answer is (b).

9. A patient's blood pressure in the right arm is 138/92 and 145/89 in the left arm. According to JNC 7, into which category does the place the patient?

  a. Normal

  b. Prehypertension

  c. Stage 1 hypertension

  d. Stage 2 hypertension

The correct answer is (c).

10. A 4-year-old patient is hospitalized after the repair of an inguinal hernia. Which pain scale would be the most appropriate to use with this patient?

  a. Visual analog scale

  b. Pain intensity scale

  c. The McCaffery and Pasero scale

  d. Wong-Baker FACES scale

The correct answer is (d).

Visit the Estes online companion resource at
www.delmar.cengage.com
for additional content and study aids.
Click on Online Companions, then select the Nursing discipline.

REFERENCES

Acute Pain Management Guideline Panel. (1992). *Acute pain management: Operative or medical procedures and trauma. Clinical practice guideline* (AHCPR Publication No. 92-0032). Rockville, MD: Agency for Health Care Policy and Research. (Telephone: 800-358-9295 or 301-495-3453; or write Acute Pain Management Guideline, AHCPR Publications Clearinghouse, P.O. Box 8547, Silver Spring, MD 20907).

Berkeley, K. J., & Holdcroft, A. (1999). Sex and gender differences in pain. In P. D. Wall & R. Melzack (Eds.), *Textbook of pain* (4th ed.). Edinburgh: Churchill Livingstone.

Beyer, J. (1983). *The Caucasian version of the Oucher.* Developed and copyrighted by Judith E. Beyer, RN, PhD, 1983.

Classification and Management of Blood Pressure for Adults 18 Years or Older. *Note. From "The Seventh Report of the Joint National Committee on Prevention, Detection, Evaluation, and Treatment of High Blood Pressure,"* by A. V. Chobanian, G. L. Bakris, H. R. Black, W. C. Cushman, L. A. Green, J. L. Izzo, Jr., et al., 2003. Retrieved May 28, 2008, from http://www.nhlbi.nih.gov/guidelines/hypertension/jnc7full.pdf

Fillingim, R. B., & Maixner, W. (1995). Gender differences in response to noxious stimuli. *Pain Forum, 4*, 209–211.

Hockenberry, M., Wilson, D., Winkelstein, M., & Kline, N. (2003). *Wong's nursing care of infants and children* (7th ed.). St. Louis: Mosby.

International Association for the Study of Pain. (1979). *IASP pain terminology.* Retrieved December 23, 2004, from http://www.iasp-pain.org/terms-p.html

Joint National Committee on Prevention, Detection, Evaluation, and Treatment of High Blood Pressure and the National High Blood Pressure Education Program Coordinating Committee. (2003). The seventh report of the Joint National Committee on Prevention, Detection, Evaluation, and Treatment of High Blood Pressure (NIH Publication No. 03-5233). *Archives of Internal Medicine, 157.*

McCaffery, M., & Pasero, F. (1999). *Pain: Clinical manual for nursing practice.* St. Louis: Mosby.

Schecter, N. L., Berde, C. B., & Yaster, M. (Eds.). (2003). *Pain in infants, children, and adolescents* (2nd ed.). Baltimore: Williams & Wilkins.

BIBLIOGRAPHY

Allcock, N., Elkan, R., & Williams, J. (2007). Patients referred to a pain management clinic: Beliefs, expectations and priorities. *Journal of Advanced Nursing, 60*(3), 248–256.

Altman, G. (2004). *Delmar's fundamental advanced nursing skills handbook.* Clifton Park, NY: Delmar Cengage Learning.

Behrman, R., Kliegman, R., & Jenson, H. (Eds.). (2008). *Nelson textbook of pediatrics* (18th ed.). Philadelphia: Saunders.

Chevlen, E. (2005). Unraveling the pathophysiology of neuropathic pain. *Journal of the American Academy of Nurse Practitioners [Supplement], 17*(6), 4–7.

Elkin, M. K., Perry, A. G., & Potter, P. A. (2008). *Nursing interventions & clinical skills* (4th ed.). St. Louis: Mosby.

Guyton, A. C., & Hall, J. (2006). *Textbook of medical physiology* (11th ed.). Philadelphia: Saunders.

Hockenberry, M., Wilson, D., & Winkelstein, M. (2005). *Wong's essentials of pediatric nursing* (7th ed.). St Louis: Mosby.

Old, J. L., & Swagerty, D. L., Jr. (2007). *A practical guide to palliative care.* Philadelphia: Lippincott Williams & Wilkins.

Quatrara, B., Coffman, J., Jenkins, T., Mann, K., McGough, K., Conway, M., et al. (2007). The effect of respiratory rate and ingestion of hot and cold beverages on the accuracy of oral temperatures measured by electronic thermometers. *MEDSURG Nursing, 16*(2), 105–108.

Richards, T., Johnson, J., Sparks, A., & Emerson, H. (2007). The effect of music therapy in patients' perceptions and manifestation of pain, anxiety, and patient satisfaction. *MEDSURG Nursing, 16*(1), 7–14.

Smeltzer, S. C., & Bare, B. G. (Eds.). (2006). *Brunner and Suddarth's textbook of medical-surgical nursing* (11th ed.). Philadelphia: Lippincott.

Teenier, P., & Sender, S. (2007). Assessing pain in the home care environment. *Home Healthcare Nurse, 25*(7), 471–476.

Waldman, S. D. (2007). *Pain management.* Philadelphia: Saunders.

Waldman, S. D. (2008). *Atlas of common pain syndromes* (2nd ed.). Philadelphia: Saunders.

WEB SITES

American Heart Association:
http://www.americanheart.org

American Heart Association Go Red for Women:
http://www.goredforwomen.org

American Pain Society:
http://www.ampainsoc.org

International Association for the Study of Pain:
http://www.iasp-pain.org

The Joint Commission:
http://www.jointcommission.org

National Heart, Lung, and Blood Institute:
http://www.nhlbi.nih.gov

CHAPTER 10

Skin, Hair, and Nails

COMPETENCIES

1. Describe the anatomy and physiology of the integumentary system.

2. Explain the process of describing and classifying skin lesions.

3. Identify common skin lesions and discuss possible etiologies.

4. Identify pathophysiological changes to hair and nails and discuss possible etiologies.

5. State the warning signs of carcinoma in pigmented lesions.

6. Describe methods used to assess integumentary changes in both light- and dark-skinned patients.

The skin, also known as the **integumentary system,** or cutaneous tissue, is the largest organ system of the body. It shelters most of the other organ systems, and if assessed carefully, it can provide a noninvasive window to observe the body's level of functioning.

This chapter provides a review of the skin and its appendages: hair and nails. Techniques for examination of the integumentary system are addressed, as is an approach to evaluating skin lesions.

ANATOMY AND PHYSIOLOGY

The skin, hair, and nails, along with their functions, are discussed.

SKIN

The surface area of the skin covers approximately 20 square feet in the average adult, with a thickness varying from 0.2 to 1.5 mm, depending on the region of the body and the patient's age. Morphologically speaking, the skin is composed of three main layers: the epidermis, the dermis, and the subcutaneous tissue, or hypodermis (Figure 10-1).

Epidermis

The **epidermis** is a multilayered outer covering consisting of four layers throughout the body, except for the palms of the hands and soles of the feet, where there are five layers (see Figure 10-2). The deepest layer of the epidermis is the **stratum germinativum,** or basal cell layer. It is composed of columnar-shaped cells that rest on a basement membrane. These columnar cells undergo continuous mitosis to produce new cells that replace the cells that are lost from the top layer of the epidermis. This layer provides the skin with tone and also creates pigment-producing melanocytes, which filter ultraviolet light. The **stratum spinosum** overlays the stratum germinativum. The stratum spinosum consists of layers of polyhedral-shaped cells.

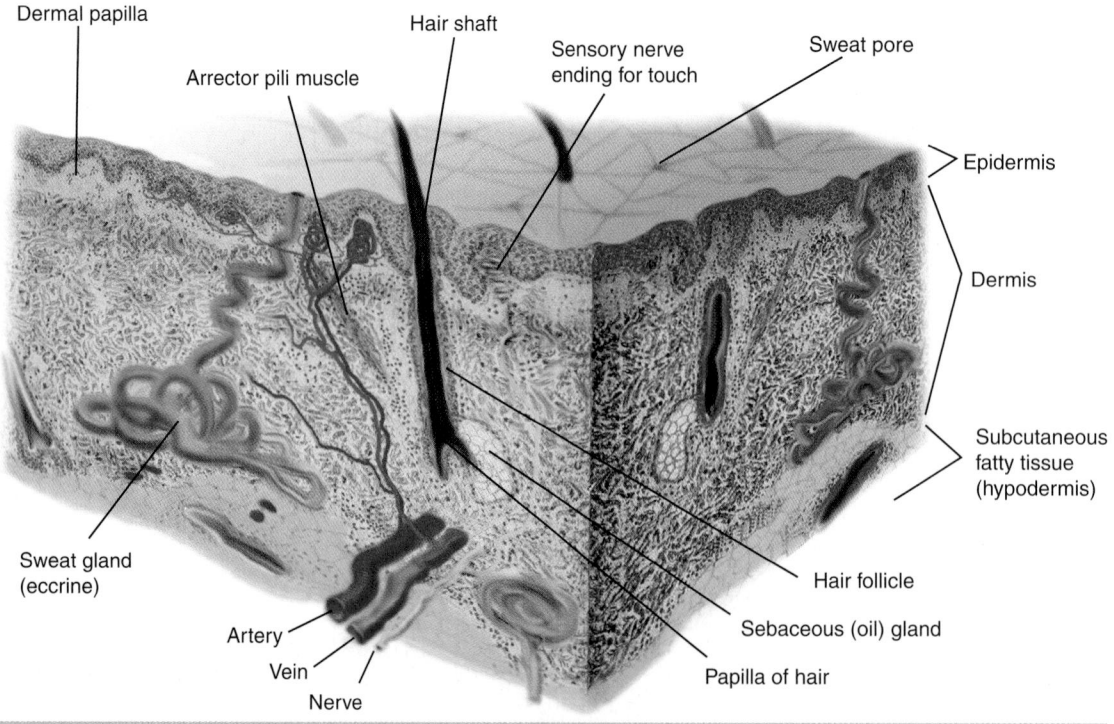

Dermal papilla

Hair shaft

Arrector pili muscle

Sensory nerve ending for touch

Sweat pore

Epidermis

Dermis

Subcutaneous fatty tissue (hypodermis)

Sweat gland (eccrine)

Artery

Vein

Nerve

Hair follicle

Sebaceous (oil) gland

Papilla of hair

FIGURE 10-1 **Structures of the Skin**

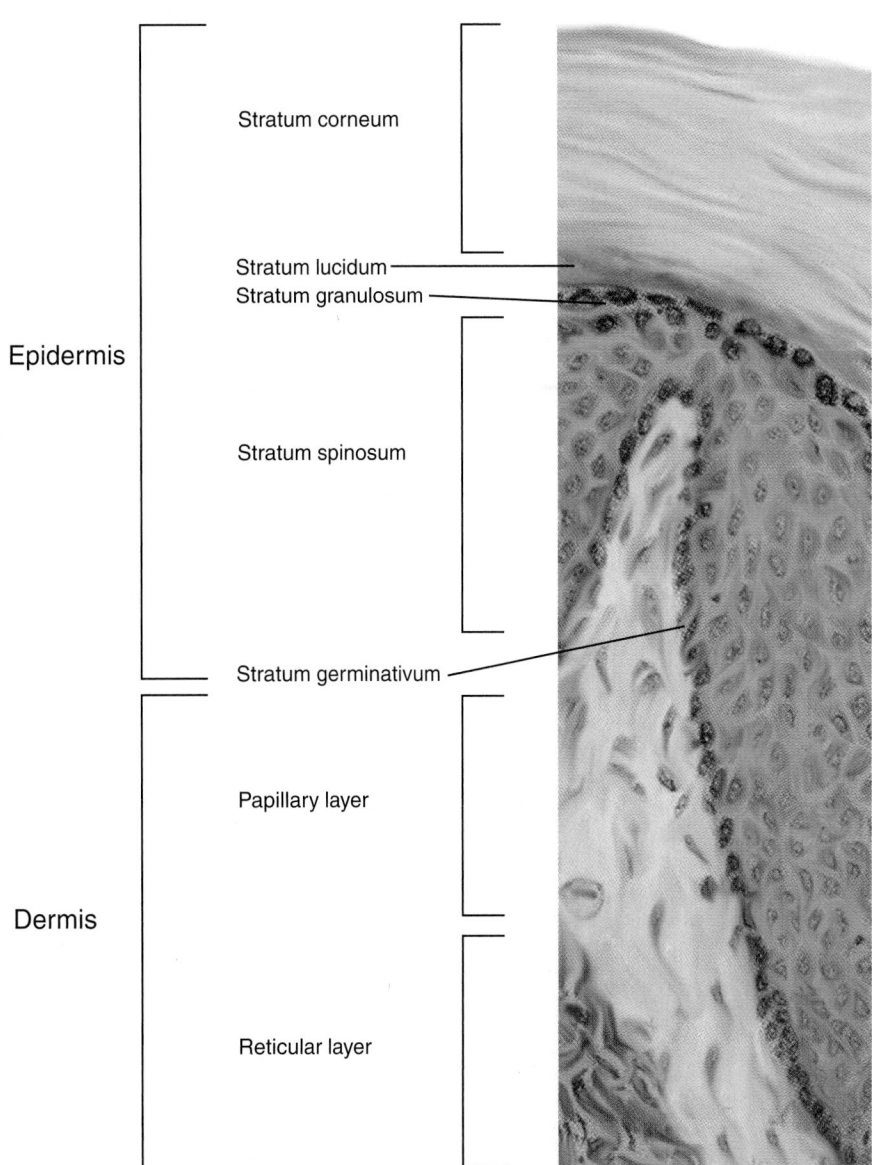

Epidermis

Stratum corneum

Stratum lucidum
Stratum granulosum

Stratum spinosum

Stratum germinativum

Dermis

Papillary layer

Reticular layer

FIGURE 10-2 Epidermal and Dermal Layers of the Skin

Intercellular bridges provide for the irregular shape. Skin cell death occurs in the **stratum granulosum**, which overlays the stratum spinosum. The stratum granulosum is composed of cells with shriveled nuclei and strands of keratin.

The additional layer, which is found exclusively on the palmar and plantar surfaces, is the **stratum lucidum**. It contains a thin layer of translucent eleidin that aids in the formation of keratin. Finally, the **stratum corneum**, also known as the horny layer, completes the epidermis. The stratum corneum is composed of enucleated dead epithelial cells. These cells contain keratin, which provides a waterproof barrier. This layer is in a continual state of **desquamation** (shedding), as new skin cells are pushed up from the lower layers; a complete turnover of cells occurs every 3 to 4 weeks.

The epidermis, with the exception of the palmar and plantar surfaces, is normally smooth. All epidermal surfaces are devoid of blood vessels. Despite the absence of vessels, blood pigments, such as oxyhemoglobin and reduced hemoglobin in the corium or dermis, are responsible for the vascular color transmitted to the skin's surface. Other factors that affect the skin's color are various pigments such as melanin and carotene. Epidermal thickness and the ability of the skin to reflect light, known as the Tyndall effect, also influence integumentary color.

Dermis

The **dermis**, or corium, is the second layer of the skin. It is approximately 20 times thicker than the epidermis in certain areas of the body and can be divided into two layers: the papillary layer and the reticular layer (see Figure 10-2). The **papillary layer**, or upper layer, is composed primarily of loose connective tissue, small elastic fibers, and an extensive network of capillaries that serve to nourish the epidermis. The **reticular layer**, the lower layer of the dermis, is formed by a dense bed of vascular connective tissue that also includes nerves and lymphatic tissue. This layer also provides structural support for the skin. In the deeper portions of the reticular layer, collagen fibers in combination with elastic fibers are surrounded in a gelatinous matrix. Intermeshed with the connective tissue are hair follicles, sweat glands, sebaceous glands, and adipose tissue.

The fibrous connective tissue in the dermis gives the skin its strength and elasticity. The fibrous tissues provide structural support for the epidermis and form dermal "ridges" to which the epidermis conforms and anchors, creating "epidermal ridges" known as fingerprints. These ridges develop during the first trimester of fetal development and although they enlarge with growth, their pattern remains the same throughout life and enhances with age.

In general, the dermis is thicker over the dorsal and lateral surfaces such as the palmar and plantar surfaces. It is much thinner over the ventral and medial surfaces, and is especially thin in areas such as the eyelids, scrotum, and penis.

Subcutaneous Tissue

Beneath the dermis is the **subcutaneous tissue**, or superficial fascia. It is composed of either loose areolar connective tissue or adipose tissue, depending on its location in the body. The subcutaneous layers attach the skin to the underlying bones. These layers act as a temperature insulator and help regulate body heat; they also encompass fat stores for energy use and contain an extensive venous plexus layer, which acts as a reservoir for the blood that warms the surface of the skin.

Distributed around the dermal blood vessels and the subcutaneous tissue are the skin's mast cells. These cells number from 7,000 to 20,000 per cubic centimeter of skin. **Mast cells** are the body's major source of tissue histamine and trigger the body's reaction to allergens.

Glands of the Skin

There are two main groups of glands in the skin: the sebaceous glands and the sweat glands.

SEBACEOUS GLANDS. The **sebaceous glands** are sebum-producing glands that are found almost everywhere in the dermis except for the palmar and plantar surfaces. They are also part of the apparatus that contains the hair follicle and the **arrector pili muscle**, which causes contraction of the skin and hair, resulting in "goose bumps." The ducts of the sebaceous glands open into the upper part of the hair follicle and are responsible for producing **sebum**, an oily secretion that is thought to retard evaporation and water loss from the epidermal cells. Sebaceous glands are most prevalent in the scalp, forehead, nose, and chin.

SWEAT GLANDS. The two main types of **sweat glands** are **apocrine glands**, which are associated with hair follicles, and **eccrine glands**, which are not associated with hair follicles. The secretory apparatus of both types of sweat glands is located in the subcutaneous tissue. Eccrine glands open directly onto the skin's surface and are widely distributed throughout the body. Apocrine glands are found primarily in the axillae, genital and rectal areas, nipples, and navel. These glands become functional during puberty, and secretion occurs during emotional stress or sexual stimulation. After puberty, apocrine glands are responsible for the characteristic body odor when sweat mixes with the natural bacterial flora normally present on the skin surface.

HAIR

With few exceptions (the palmar and plantar surfaces, lips, nipples, and the glans penis), hair is distributed over the entire body surface. Its abundance and texture are dependent on an individual's age, gender, race, and heredity. **Vellus hair**, or fine, faint hair, covers most of the body. In general, **terminal hair** is the coarser, darker hair of the scalp, eyebrows, and eyelashes. In the axillary and pubic areas, terminal hair becomes increasingly evident in both males and females with the onset of puberty. Males will also tend to develop coarser, thicker chest and facial hair.

Specialized epidermal cells are located in depressions at the base of each hair follicle and are responsible for the formation of each individual hair shaft. The cells are nourished by blood vessels in the dermis so that they grow and divide, pushing the older cells toward the surface of the skin.

Most hair shafts are composed of three layers: the cuticle, or outer layer; the cortex, or middle layer; and the medulla, or innermost layer. Hair color is determined by the **melanocytes** produced in the cells at the base of each follicle; an abundance of pigment produces darker hair color, and smaller amounts produce a lighter color.

NAILS

Nails are composed of keratinized, or horny, layers of cells that arise from undifferentiated epithelial tissue called the **matrix**. The **nail plate**, tissue that covers the distal portion of the digits and provides protection, is approximately 0.5- to 0.75-mm thick. The nails consists of the **nail root**, which lies posteriorly to the cuticle and is attached to the matrix; the **nailbed**, which is the vascular bed located beneath the nail plate; and the **periungal tissues**, which surround the nail plate and the free edge of the nail (Figure 10-3). At the proximal end of each nail is a white, crescent-shaped area known as the **lunula**. This structure is obscured by the cuticle in some individuals.

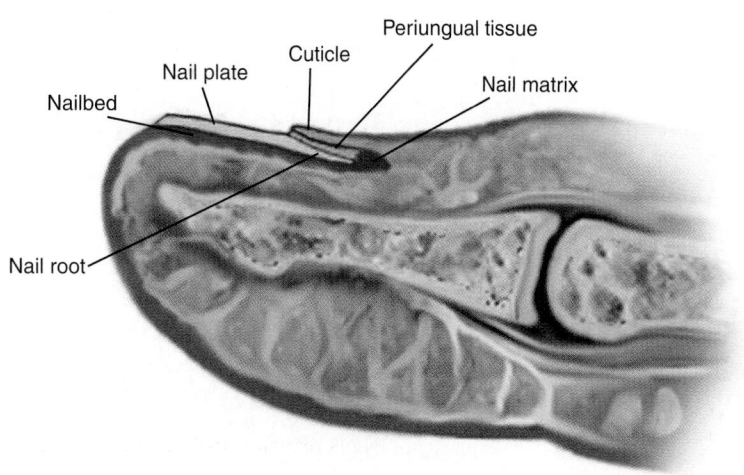

FIGURE 10-3 **Structures of the Nail**

The normally translucent nail plate is given a pinkish cast by the underlying vascular bed in light-skinned individuals and a brownish cast in dark-skinned individuals. In many disease processes, the color of the nailbed may vary. For instance, a decrease in oxygen content of the blood will cause the nailbeds to appear **cyanotic**, or blue.

The nail plate is formed continuously as the plate is pushed forward by new growth from the germinative layer of the matrix. Normal growth for an adult is 0.1 to 1.0 mm per day, but growth varies with age, season, nutrition, climate, health status, and activity.

FUNCTION OF SKIN

The skin has many functions, but perhaps the most important one is its ability to serve as a protective barrier against invasion from environmental hazards and pathogens. It provides boundaries against materials that might enter the body, such as toxic chemicals, and provides boundaries for fluids and mobile tissues, such as blood, within the body. An intact integument is also responsible for the protection of underlying organs, which would otherwise be vulnerable to injury because of exposure.

Temperature regulation is carried out by the skin through the production of perspiration. During states of increased body temperature, large quantities of sweat are produced by the eccrine glands. As perspiration reaches the skin's surface, rapid evaporation takes place, and the body's temperature begins to decrease. The skin's vascular system also plays a role in heat control. When vasodilation occurs, much of the heat can be lost through radiation and conduction. Conversely, vasoconstriction helps to maintain body heat.

The skin contains receptors for pain, touch, pressure, and temperature. These receptors originate in the dermis and terminate as either free nerve endings throughout the skin's surface or as special touch receptors that are encapsulated and found predominantly in the fingertips and lips. Each hair found on the body also contains a basal nerve fiber that acts as a tactile receptor. Sensory signals that help determine precise locations on the skin are transmitted along rapid sensory pathways, and less distinct signals such as pressure or poorly localized touch are sent via slower sensory pathways.

The skin acts as an organ of excretion for substances such as water, salts, and nitrogenous wastes. The skin produces cells for wound repair and is the site for the production of vitamin D. The skin is also an indicator of nonverbal language and emotions via blushing and facial expressions. The skin may further be used for the purpose of identification via fingerprints and birthmarks.

FUNCTION OF HAIR

Hair provides warmth, protection, and sensation to the underlying systems. Terminal hair of the scalp and face provides warmth, shields against ultraviolet light, and filters dust and particulate matter. Vellus hair enhances tactile sensation and sensory perception. In many cultures, hair is a status symbol of beauty and wealth.

FUNCTION OF NAILS

Nails provide protection to the distal surface of the digits and can be used for self-protection. In many cultures, nail length in both men and women is a qualifier of social and economic status.

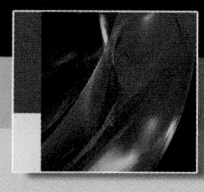

HEALTH HISTORY

The skin, hair, and nails health history provides insight into the link between a patient's life/lifestyle and skin, hair, and nails information and pathology.

PATIENT PROFILE

Diseases that are age-, gender-, and race-specific for the skin, hair, and nails are listed.

Age

Skin

Fungal infections, diseases of sebaceous glands, such as acne vulgaris (13–26 years)

Lupus erythematosus, psoriasis, hyperpigmented macular lesions, skin tags (acrochordon), dermatophyte infections (25–60 years)

Basal cell carcinoma (older adults)

Hair

Male pattern alopecia (adolescence to young adulthood)

Thinning, graying, loss of hair in axillary and pubic areas, excessive facial hair (middle to old age)

Gender

Skin

Male: Skin pathology is consistently more prevalent among males than females; dermatophyte infections, skin tumors, fungal infections, and increased incidence of tumors related to occupational hazards and hygiene; Kaposi's sarcoma associated with immunodeficiency conditions

Hair

Female: Female pattern alopecia, increased facial hair with aging

Male: Alopecia, increased coarse nose and ear hair with aging

Race

Dark Skinned

Keloid formation, dermatosis papulosa nigra, hyper- and hypopigmentation, traumatic marginal alopecia, seborrheic dermatitis, pseudofolliculitis barbae, acne keloidalis, granuloma inguinale, Mongolian spots, albinism, hypopigmented sarcoidosis, granulomatosis skin lesions

Light Skinned

Squamous and basal cell carcinoma, actinic keratosis, psoriasis

CHIEF COMPLAINT

Common chief complaints for the skin, hair, and nails are defined, and information on the characteristics of each sign and symptom is provided.

1. Pruritus

Cutaneous itching that may have a multitude of etiologies

Location

Generalized or localized

Quality

Superficial or deep sensation of itching, intensity of itching, interference with sleep habits

Associated Manifestations

Rashes, lesions, edema, angioedema, anaphylaxis, excoriation or ulcers as the result of scratching, **lichenification** (thickening of the skin), systemic disease

Aggravating Factors

Exposure to chemicals, sunlight, plants, food, animals, stress, climate, parasites, xerosis, drug reaction, systemic disease processes, contact dermatitis, types of clothing (frequently wool)

continues

Alleviating Factors	Dietary changes, medications, antihistamines, biofeedback, cool baths, types of clothing (frequently cotton), increased skin hydration, ultraviolet-band light therapy
Setting	Work, home, school, or recreational environment
Timing	Pre- or postprandial, nocturnal, seasonal, during periods of stress, associated with menstrual cycle
2. Rash	A cutaneous eruption that may be localized or generalized
3. Lesion	A circumscribed pathological change in the tissues
Location	Location of where it started and spread, distribution over the body, percent of body involved, following dermatomes
Quantity	"Grouping or arrangement": discrete, grouped, confluent, linear, annular, polycyclic, generalized, zosteriform
Quality	"Morphology": macule, patch, papule, plaque, nodule, cyst, wheal, vesicle, pustule, bullae, tumor, lichenification, crust, erosion, fissure, ulcer, or atrophy
Associated Manifestations	Edema, angioedema, anaphylaxis, excoriation or ulcers as the result of scratching, lichenification, systemic disease, allergies, fever, induration
Aggravating Factors	Exposure to chemicals, sunlight, plants, food, animals, stress, climate, parasites, xerosis, drug reaction, systemic disease processes, contact dermatitis, radiation, types of clothing (frequently wool)
Alleviating Factors	Dietary changes, medications, antihistamines, biofeedback, cool baths, types of clothing (frequently cotton), increased skin hydration, ultraviolet-band light therapy, surgery
Setting	Work, home, school, or recreational environment
Timing	When it started, pre- or postprandial, nocturnal, seasonal, during periods of stress, associated with menstrual cycle
PAST HEALTH HISTORY	*The various components of the past health history are linked to skin, hair, and nails pathology and skin-, hair-, and nails-related information.*
Medical History	
Skin Specific	Allergies, eczema, atopic dermatitis, melanoma, albinism, vitiligo, psoriasis, skin cancer, athlete's foot, birthmarks, body piercing, tattoos, urticaria
Non–Skin Specific	Renal disease, diabetes mellitus, lupus erythematosus, peripheral vascular disease, idiopathic thrombocytopenia purpura (ITP), Rocky Mountain spotted fever, liver disease, hepatitis, collagen diseases, cardiac dysfunction, sexually transmitted diseases, Lyme disease, arthritis, lymphoma, thyroid disease, pregnancy, Addison's disease, pernicious anemia, HIV, cytomegalovirus, Epstein-Barr virus, measles, mumps, rubella, coxsackievirus, adenovirus, drug hypersensitivities, varicella, herpes zoster, herpes simplex, Kawasaki disease, toxic shock syndrome, carcinoma, tuberculosis, viral syndromes
Hair Specific	Allergies, alopecia, lice, bacterial or fungal infections of the scalp, brittle hair, rapid hair loss, trichotillomania, trauma, congenital anomalies

continues

Health History (continued)

Non–Hair Specific	Renal disease, diabetes mellitus, cardiac dysfunction, peripheral vascular disease, thyroid disease, pregnancy, Addison's disease, HIV, anemia, malnutrition, stress, chemotherapy, radiation therapy
Nail Specific	Allergies, psoriasis, bacterial or fungal infections, trauma, brittle nails, nail biting, congenital anomalies
Non–Nail Specific	Iron deficiency anemia, chronic infection, malnutrition, Raynaud's disease, hypoxia, acute infections, syphilis
Surgical History	Keloid and scar formation, plastic surgery for birthmarks, skin grafts, reconstructive surgery, excision biopsy
Allergies	Medication, insect stings, foods, soaps, laundry detergent, chemicals, fibers (wool), metals (nickel), animal dander, pollens, grasses, cosmetics, signs/symptoms of first manifestation of allergic reaction
Medications	Reaction manifested in skin changes after use of prescription or OTC drugs
Communicable Diseases	Varicella, roseola, measles, scabies, bacterial or fungal infections, HIV Sexually transmitted diseases: syphilis, gonorrhea, chancroid, genital warts (See Chapters 20, 21, and 22 for further information.)
Injuries and Accidents	Chemical inhalation, trauma, burns, toxin contamination
Special Needs	Poor eyesight can lead to poor hygiene; frequent skin trauma prevents early detection and treatment of skin diseases; bedridden or wheelchair bound with possibility of pressure trauma and compromise of skin integrity
Blood Transfusions	Skin eruptions, pruritus
Childhood Illnesses	Refer to section on communicable diseases.
FAMILY HEALTH HISTORY	*Skin, hair, and nail diseases that are familial in nature are listed.*
Skin Specific	Allergies, eczema, melanoma, albinism, vitiligo, psoriasis, nonmelonanomatous skin cancer
Hair Specific	Allergies, alopecia, brittle hair, hair loss
Nail Specific	Brittle nails
SOCIAL HISTORY	*The components of the social history are linked to skin, hair, and nail factors/pathology.*
Alcohol Use	Hepatotoxicity and subsequent skin manifestations that accompany liver failure, such as jaundice and pruritus; skin bruising and trauma from falls and ataxia; telangiectasia of the nose, neck, and upper chest
Tobacco Use	Yellow discoloration of fingertips on smoking hand, leathery facial appearance
Drug Use	Skin manifestations from intravenous drug use, such as injection sites or tracks; these are especially prevalent in the forearms, behind the knees, toe webs, finger webs, and under the nails
Sexual Practice	Various sexually transmitted diseases may manifest in the genital region; these are discussed in Chapters 20, 21, and 22.

continues

Travel History	Tropical regions: fungal infections, contact dermatitis, tropical eczema, leishmaniasis
	Insect bites: insects indigenous to certain climates, such as the tsetse fly in Africa and the deer tick in wooded areas of the northern and southeastern United States
	High-altitude areas: light-sensitive eruptions and winter eczema
	Southeastern United States, Mississippi and Ohio River valleys, and South America: blastomycosis most likely caused by infected soil
Work Environment	Chemical: contact dermatitis and burns
	Sunlight: skin eruptions, increased incidence of basal or squamous cell carcinoma, burns, wrinkles, senile freckles, lightened hair, excessive exposure to ultraviolet radiation
	Excessive exposure to water: drying and cracking of skin, pruritus, soft nails, damaged hair shafts
	Insect bites: rashes, urticaria, edema, angioedema, pruritus
	Operating heavy or sharp equipment: trauma, laceration
	Excessive exposure to wind and cold temperatures: aging, drying, and cracking of skin
	Pollution: contact dermatitis
	Tar and pitch: act as both photosensitizers and carcinogens
Home Environment	Chemicals used in cleaning can cause contact dermatitis; excessive exposure to water can cause dry, cracked skin, soft nails, and damaged hair shafts; excessive heat in the home can dry skin and cause pruritus; infected kittens and puppies may lead to tinea capitis.
Hobbies and Leisure Activities	Gardening with exposure to chemicals, sunlight, contact dermatitis (e.g., poison ivy, poison oak), and insect bites; outdoor summer sports or activities increase sun and insect-bite exposure; outdoor winter activities increase frostbite and exposure; excessive exposure to chlorine and salt water damages hair; excessive use of tanning salons may lead to skin carcinoma.
Stress	Skin eruptions such as eczema, urticaria, acne, and psoriasis may have a psychological component in some cases; body image disorder as a result of skin disease and hair loss.
Economic Status	People of lower socioeconomic status may develop skin eruptions associated with poor hygiene because of insufficient resources, infestations associated with overcrowding, and infections associated with malnutrition.
Ethnic Background	
Scandinavian and Northern European	Psoriasis
Mexican American	Lupus erythematosus
Central and South American	Fungal infections, contact dermatitis, tropical ulcers, and eczema related to increased heat and humidity; light-sensitivity eruptions and winter eczema related to high altitude
HEALTH MAINTENANCE ACTIVITIES	*This information provides a bridge between the health maintenance activities and the skin, hair, and nails function.*

continues

Health History (continued)

Sleep	Sleep disturbances caused by symptoms such as itching or burning
Diet	Allergies to food can cause skin eruptions such as urticaria; diets high in fat and cholesterol may be connected to the development of xanthelasmatous lesions; vitamin deficiencies result in skin, hair, and nail changes; see Chapter 7 for further information.
Exercise	Increased risk for cutaneous trauma associated with contact sports and sun exposure with outdoor sports and activities
Use of Safety Devices	Sunblock with appropriate sun protection factor (SPF) to prevent ultraviolet exposure; lotions and creams to prevent drying and cracking of skin; protective gloves when handling harsh, irritating chemicals
Health Check-ups	Moles and birthmarks assessed for changes in size, shape, or color; skin lesions from sun exposure assessed

NURSING**ALERT**

Skin Cancer Risk Factors

- Ultraviolet radiation exposure that is repeated and unprotected
- Family history of skin cancer
- Second-degree burns before age 18
- Acute sun burns
- Outdoor employment
- Melanocytic precursor lesion
- Fair skin
- Smoking
- Male gender
- Chemical exposure
- Radiation exposure
- Long-term or severe skin inflammation or injury
- Psoralens and ultraviolet light treatment (PUVA) treatment for psoriasis
- Xeroderma pigmentosum
- Basal cell nevus syndrome
- Reduced immunity
- Human papillomavirus

✓ NURSING**CHECKLIST**

Specific Health History Questions Regarding the Skin, Hair, and Nails

Skin Care Habits
- Do you use lotions, perfumes, cologne, cosmetics, soaps, oils, shaving cream, after-shave lotion, electric or standard razor?
- What type of home remedies do you use for skin lesions and rashes?
- How often do you bathe or shower?
- Do you use a tanning bed or salon?
- What type of sun protection do you use?
- Have you ever had a reaction to jewelry that you wore?
- Do you wear hats, visors, gloves, long sleeves or pants, sunscreen when in the sun?
- How much time do you spend in the sun?

Hair Care Habits
- Do you use shampoo, conditioner, hair spray, setting products?
- Do you color, dye, bleach, frost, or use relaxants on your hair?
- What products do you use?
- Do you wear a wig or hairpiece?
- Do you have graying hair or hair loss?
- Do you use a hair dryer, heated curlers, hair straightener, or curling iron?
- Do you tightly braid your hair?

Nail Care Habits
- Do you get manicures or pedicures?
- What type of nail care do you practice (trimming, clipping, use of polish, nail tips, acrylics)?
- Do you bite your nails?
- Do you suffer from nail splitting or discoloration?

NURSINGALERT

Manicures and Pedicures

There is a risk of contracting hepatitis B and C in commercial salons from manicures and pedicures if strict sterilization protocols are not followed. Advise your patients to verify that the facilities in which they obtain these types of cosmetic treatments sterilize the equipment between clients. Also advise patients to bring their own equipment to be used during the manicures or pedicures.

NURSINGTIP

Reducing Exposure to Integumentary Irritants

- In the workplace, always follow Occupational Safety and Health Administration (OSHA) and employer's safety guidelines.
- Follow the directions on the labels of all products; pay special attention to warning labels.
- If using a personal care product for the first time, perform a patch test to evaluate for sensitivity.
- Use rubber gloves when handling toxins or caustic substances.
- Contact a poison control center for treatment guidelines if exposed to toxic or caustic substances.
- Notify HAZMAT officials if a dangerous chemical or toxin exposure occurs.

NURSINGCHECKLIST

General Approach to Skin, Hair, and Nails Assessment

1. Ensure that the room is well lit. Daylight is the best source of light, especially when determining skin color. However, if daylight is unavailable, overhead fluorescent lights should be added.
2. Use a hand-held magnifying glass to aid in inspection when simple visual inspection is not adequate.
3. Explain to the patient each step of the assessment process prior to initiating the assessment.
4. Ensure patient privacy by providing drapes.
5. Ensure the comfort of the patient by keeping the room at an appropriate temperature.
6. Warm hands by washing them in warm water prior to the assessment.
7. Gather equipment on a table prior to initiating the assessment.
8. Ask the patient to undress completely and put on a patient gown, leaving the back untied.
9. Perform the assessment in a cephalocaudal fashion.
10. For episodic illness, the skin examination is incorporated into the regional physical exam.

EQUIPMENT

- Magnifying glass
- Good source of natural light
- Penlight
- Clean gloves
- Microscope slide
- Small centimeter ruler

For Special Techniques

- Wood's lamp
- #15 scalpel blade
- Microscope slide with cover slips
- Mineral oil
- Microscope

ASSESSMENT OF THE SKIN, HAIR, AND NAILS

INSPECTION OF THE SKIN

In each area, observe for: color, bleeding, ecchymosis, vascularity, lesions, moisture, temperature, texture, turgor, and edema.

E 1. Facing the patient, inspect the color of the skin of the face, eyelids, ears, nose, lips, and mucous membranes.

2. Inspect the anterior and lateral aspects of the neck, then behind the ears.

3. Inspect arms and dorsal and palmar surfaces of the hands. Pay special attention to the webs between the fingers.

4. Have the patient move to a supine position with arms placed over the head.

5. Lower gown to uncover chest and breasts.

6. Inspect intramammary folds and ridges. Pendulous breasts may need to be raised to complete this inspection.

7. Assess axillae, and then cover chest and breasts with gown.

8. Raise gown to uncover abdomen and anterior aspect of the lower extremities; place a sheet over the genital area.

9. Inspect abdomen, anterior aspect of the lower extremities, dorsal and plantar surfaces of the feet, and toe webs.

10. Don gloves and uncover genital area.

11. Inspect inguinal folds and genitalia.

12. Remove and discard gloves.

13. Have the patient turn to a side-lying position on the examination table so the patient's back is facing you.

14. Inspect back and posterior neck and scalp. Specifically look for nevi or other lesions.

15. Inspect posterior aspect of the lower extremities.

16. Don clean gloves and raise the gluteal cleft and inspect the gluteal folds and perianal area; then remove and discard the gloves.

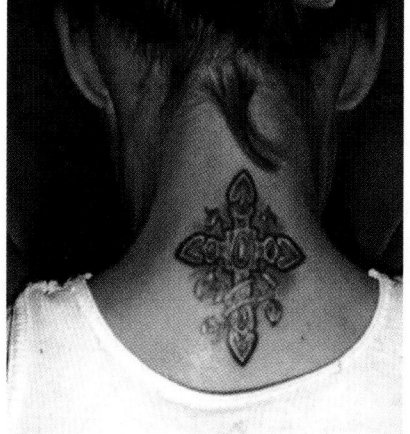

A. This patient developed cellulitis from the tattoo ink. Note the erythematous areas in the upper half of the tattoo.

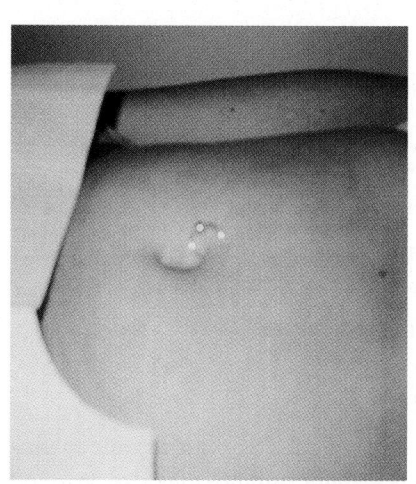

B. Note the presence of all body piercings. Assess the skin at the pierced site.

FIGURE 10-4 Tattoos and Body Piercings

NURSING**TIP**

Tattoos and Body Piercings

It is important to inspect the skin and note the presence and location of tattoos and body piercings (Figure 10-4). Some patients react to the ink in the tattoo and develop various skin disorders. Body piercing sites should be assessed for signs of infection (e.g., erythema, purulent discharge, increased skin temperature). Remember to assess all body areas. The ears, umbilicus, eyebrows, lips, nares, tongue, vagina, and scrotum are often pierced. Document the location of all tattoos and body piercings.

A recent study by Carroll, Riffenburg, Roberts, & Myhre (2002) suggests that adolescents with tattoos and body piercings may be more likely to engage in high-risk behaviors (e.g., drug use, violence). For this reason, you should consider screening patients with tattoos and body piercings for diseases such as hepatitis and HIV, among others.

E Examination	**N** Normal Findings	**A** Abnormal Findings	**P** Pathophysiology

17. Cover the patient and assist him or her back to a sitting position.

18. Wash hands.

Color

E Assess for coloration.

N Normally, the skin is a uniform whitish-pink or brown color, depending on the patient's race. Exposure to sunlight results in increased pigmentation of sun-exposed areas. Dark-skinned persons may normally have a freckling of the gums, tongue borders, and lining of the cheeks; the gingiva may appear blue or variegated in color.

A The appearance of cyanotic (dusky blue) fingers, lips, or mucous membranes is abnormal in both light- and dark-skinned individuals. In light-skinned individuals, the skin has a bluish tint. The earlobes, lower eyelids, lips, oral mucosa, nailbeds, and palmar and plantar surfaces may be especially cyanotic. Dark-skinned individuals have an ashen-gray to pale tint, and the lips and tongue are good indicators of cyanosis.

P Cyanosis occurs when there is greater than 5 g/dL of deoxygenated hemoglobin in the blood. In order for cyanosis to be an accurate indicator of arterial oxygen (PaO_2), two conditions must be met. The patient must have normal hemoglobin and hematocrit as well as normal perfusion. For example, a patient with **polycythemia** (elevated number of red blood cells) can be cyanotic but have adequate oxygenation. The problem lies in the fact that the patient has too many red blood cells rather than too little oxygen. Conversely, a patient with **anemia** (reduced number of red blood cells) can be hypoxemic but not cyanotic. In this case, the patient has too little hemoglobin. Central cyanosis is secondary to marked heart and lung disease; peripheral cyanosis can be secondary to systemic disease, or vasoconstriction stimulated by cold temperatures or anxiety.

A The appearance of **jaundice** (yellow-green to orange cast or coloration) of skin, sclera, mucous membranes, fingernails, and palmar or plantar surfaces in the light-skinned individual is abnormal (Figure 10-5A). Jaundice in dark-skinned individuals may appear as yellow staining in the sclera, hard palate, and palmar or plantar surfaces.

P Jaundice is caused by an increased serum bilirubin level of greater than 2 mg/dL associated with liver disease or hemolytic disease. Severe burns and sepsis also can produce jaundice.

A A yellow discoloration of the palmar and digital creases is abnormal.

P Xanthoma striata palmaris is caused by hyperlipidemia.

A Orange-yellow coloration of palmar and plantar surfaces and forehead, but no involvement of the mucous membranes, is abnormal.

P **Carotenemia**, elevated levels of serum carotene, results from the excessive ingestion of carotene-rich foods such as carrots.

A A grayish cast to the skin is abnormal.

P A grayish cast is seen in renal patients and is associated with chronic anemia along with retained urochrome pigments. Slight jaundice may also be found in the renal patient.

A A combination of pallor and ecchymosis with a jaundiced appearance is abnormal.

E Examination   **N** Normal Findings   **A** Abnormal Findings   **P** Pathophysiology

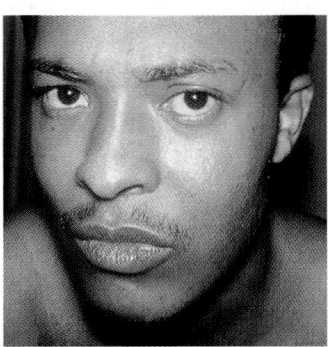

A. Jaundice. Note the yellowing of the skin as well as the eyes. *Courtesy of the Centers for Disease Control and Prevention.*

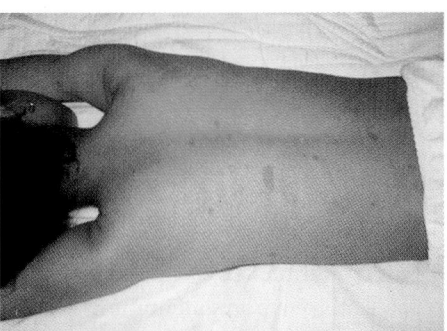

B. Café au Lait Spots

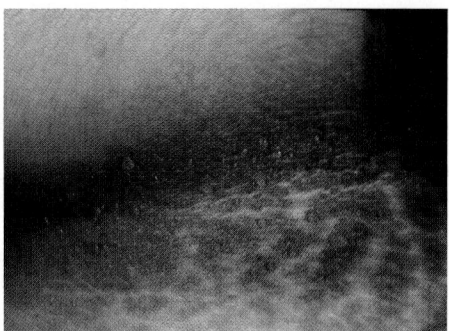

C. Acanthosis Nigricans. *Courtesy of Robert A. Silverman, M.D., Clinical Associate Professor, Department of Pediatrics, Georgetown University.*

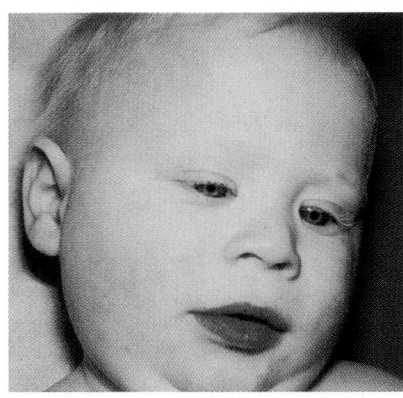

D. Note the lack of coloration in this child with albinism. *Courtesy of Robert A. Silverman, M.D., Clinical Associate Professor, Department of Pediatrics, Georgetown University.*

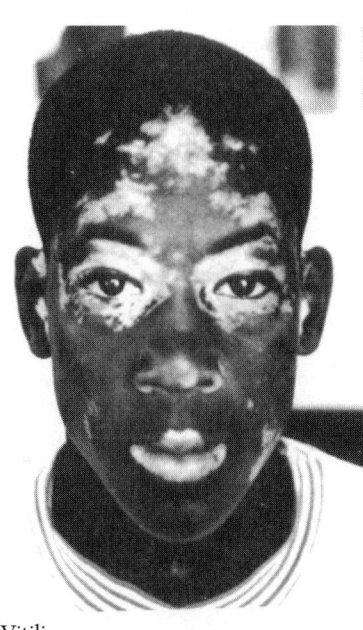

E. Vitiligo

FIGURE 10-5 **Skin Color Abnormalities**

P Uremia secondary to renal failure results in serum urochrome pigment retention.

A Sustained bright red or pink coloration in light-skinned individuals is abnormal. Dark-skinned individuals may have no underlying change in coloration. Palpation may be used to ascertain signs of warmth, swelling, or induration.

P Hyperemia occurs because of dilated superficial blood vessels, increased blood flow, febrile states, local inflammatory condition, or excessive alcohol intake.

A A bright red to ruddy, sustained appearance that is evident on the integument, mucous membranes, and palmar or plantar surfaces is abnormal in both light- and dark-skinned individuals.

P Polycythemia, as noted earlier, is an increased number of red blood cells and results in this ruddy appearance.

A A dusky rubor of the extremities when in a dependent position, which can be associated with tissue necrosis, is abnormal.

P Venous stasis results from venule engorgement and diminished blood flow, which occurs in congestive heart failure and atherosclerosis.

A A pale cast to the skin that may be most evident in the face, mucous membranes, lips, and nailbeds is abnormal in light-skinned individuals. A yellow-brown to ashen-gray cast to the skin along with pale or gray lips, mucous membranes, and nailbeds is abnormal in dark-skinned individuals.

P Pallor is due to decreased visibility of the normal oxyhemoglobin. This can occur when the patient has decreased blood flow in the superficial vessels, as in shock or syncope, or when there is a decreased amount of serum oxyhemoglobin, as in anemia. Localized pallor may be secondary to arterial insufficiency.

A A brown cast to the skin can be generalized or discrete.

P A brown coloration occurs when there is a deposition of melanin, which can be caused by genetic predisposition, pregnancy, Addison's disease (deficiency in cortisol leads to enhanced melanin production), café au lait spots (Figure 10-5B), and sunlight.

P Acanthosis nigricans is a condition in which the skin becomes brownish and thicker, almost leathery in appearance (Figure 10-5C). This usually occurs in the axillae, on the flexoral surfaces of the groin and neck, and around the umbilicus. Acanthosis nigricans occurs in obesity, diabetes mellitus, and with medications such as steroids.

A A white cast to the skin as evidenced by generalized whiteness, including of the hair and eyebrows, is abnormal (see Figure 10-5D).

P This lack of coloration is caused by **albinism**, a congenital inability to form melanin.

A **Vitiligo** is a condition marked by patchy, symmetrical areas of white on the skin and is abnormal (see Figure 10-5E).

P This condition can be caused by an acquired loss of melanin. Trauma can also lead to hypopigmentation, especially in dark-skinned individuals.

A An erythematous, confluent eruption in a butterfly-like distribution over the face is abnormal.

P Systemic lupus erythematosus, a connective tissue disorder, is the most likely etiology.

Bleeding, Ecchymosis, and Vascularity

E Inspect the skin for evidence of bleeding, ecchymosis, or increased vascularity.

N Normally, there are no areas of increased vascularity, ecchymosis, or bleeding.

A Bleeding from the mucous membranes, previous venipuncture sites, or lesions should be considered abnormal.

P Spontaneous bleeding can be indicative of clotting disorders, trauma, or use of antithrombolytic agents such as coumadin or heparin.

A **Petechiae** are violaceous (red-purple) discolorations of less than 0.5 cm in diameter (see Figure 10-6A). Petechiae do not blanch. In dark-skinned individuals, evaluate for petechiae in the mucous membranes and axillae.

P Petechiae can indicate an increased bleeding tendency or embolism; causes include intravascular defects or infections.

A **Purpura** is a condition characterized by the presence of confluent petechiae or confluent ecchymosis over any part of the body (see Figure 10-6B).

P Purpura or peliosis is characterized by hemorrhage into the skin and can be caused by decreased platelet formation. Lesions vary based on the type of purpura; pigmentation changes may become permanent.

A **Ecchymosis** is a violaceous discoloration of varying size, also called a black-and-blue mark (see Figure 10-6C). In dark-skinned patients, these discolorations are deeper in color.

P Ecchymosis is caused by extravasation of blood into the skin as a result of trauma and can also occur with heparin or coumadin use or liver dysfunction.

A An erythematous dilation of small blood vessels is abnormal (see Figure 10-6D).

P This erythematous dilation describes a telangiectasia. They tend to appear on the face and thighs, and occur more frequently in women.

A **Spider angiomas** are bright red and star-shaped (see Figure 10-6E). There is often a central pulsation noted with pressure, and this pressure results in blanching in the extensions. Most often, these lesions are noted on the face, neck, and chest. They are a type of telangiectasia.

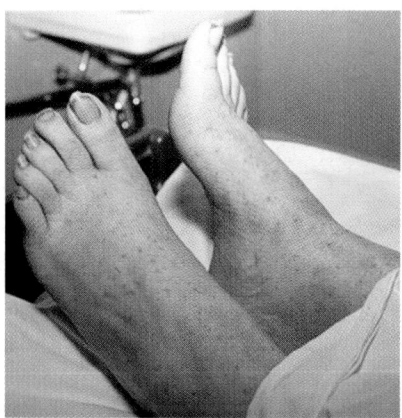

A. Petechiae. *Courtesy of Dr. Mark Dougherty, Lexington, KY.*

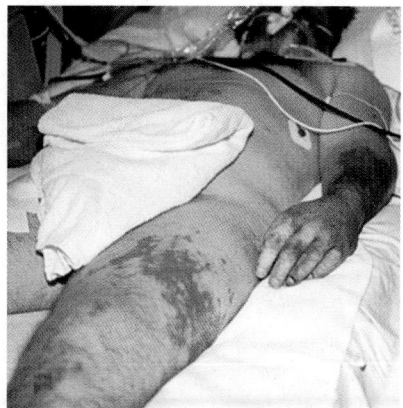

B. Purpura. *Courtesy of Dr. Mark Dougherty, Lexington, KY.*

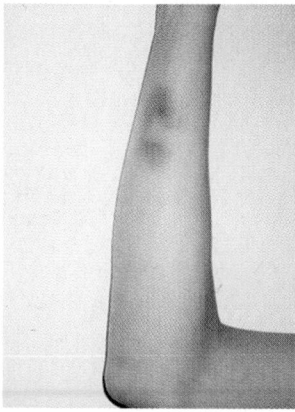

C. Ecchymosis

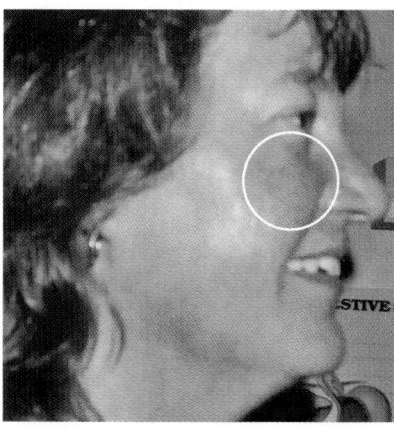

D. Telangiectasia usually occurs in women and on the face.

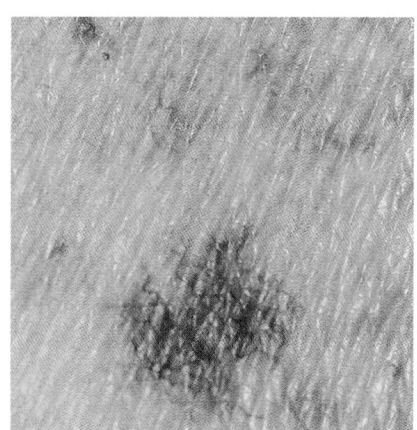

E. Spider Angioma

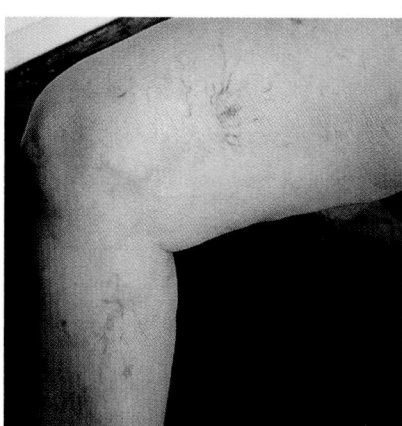

F. Venous Star

FIGURE 10-6   Bleeding, Ecchymosis, and Vascular Abnormalities of the Skin *continues*

P Causes of spider angiomas include pregnancy, liver disease, and hormone therapy. They are normal in a small percentage of the population and are more prevalent in women.

A **Venous stars** are linear or irregularly shaped, blue vascular patterns that do not blanch with pressure (Figure 10-6F). These are often noted on the legs near veins or on the anterior chest.

P Venous stars are caused by increased venous pressure in the superficial veins.

A **Cherry angiomas** are bright red, circumscribed areas that may darken with age (see Figure 10-6G). They can be flat or raised and may show partial blanching with pressure. Most often, they are found on the trunk.

P These vascularities are of unknown etiology and are pathologically insignificant except for cosmetic appearance.

A A bright red, raised area that has well-defined borders and does not blanch with pressure is abnormal (see Figure 10-6H).

E Examination   **N** Normal Findings   **A** Abnormal Findings   **P** Pathophysiology

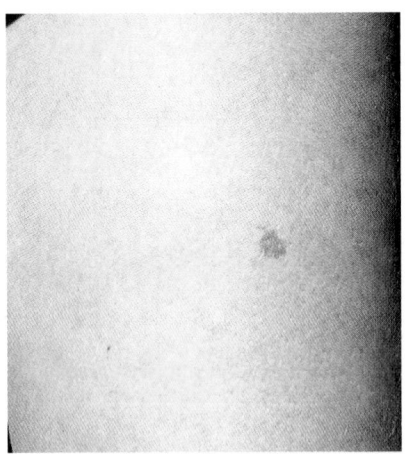

G. Cherry Angioma

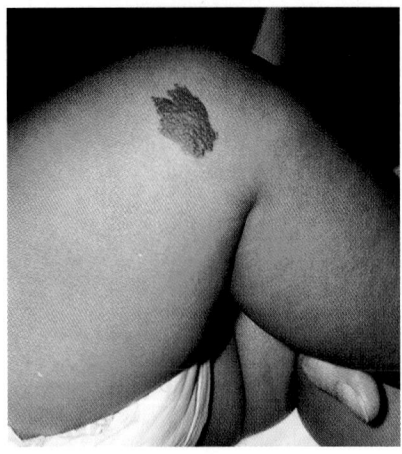

H. Strawberry Hemangioma

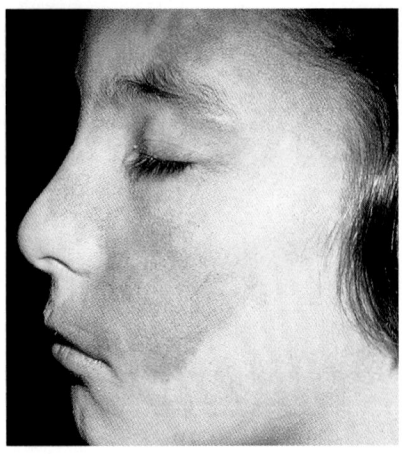

I. Nevus Flammeus. *Courtesy of Robert A. Silverman, M.D., Clinical Associate Professor, Department of Pediatrics, Georgetown University.*

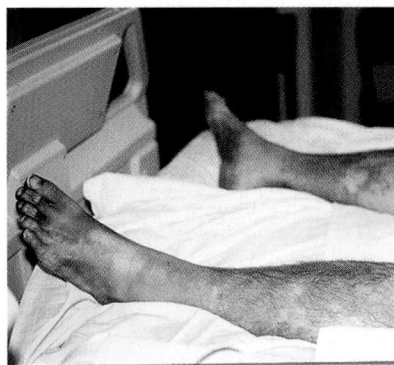

J. Necrosis. *Courtesy of Dr. Mark Dougherty, Lexington, KY.*

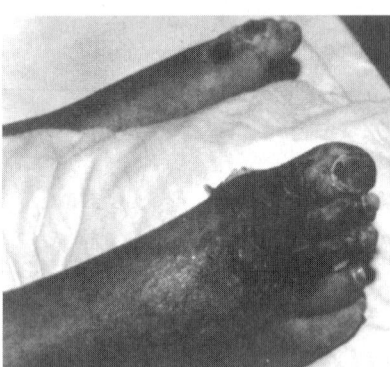

K. Gas Gangrene

FIGURE 10-6 **Bleeding, Ecchymosis, and Vascular Abnormalities of the Skin** *continued*

P Strawberry hemangiomas, or strawberry marks, are congenital malformations of closely packed, immature capillaries. This condition is also known as nevus vascularis. They regress as the child grows and are usually gone in a few years.

A A burgundy, red, or violaceous macular/vascular patch that is located along the course of a peripheral nerve is abnormal (Figure 10-6I).

P This macular/vascular patch is a port-wine stain, or nevus flammeus. The port-wine stain is composed of mature, but thin-walled, capillaries. The lesion is usually present at birth and is frequently located on the face. A port-wine stain can be indicative of underlying disorders, such as Sturge-Weber syndrome.

A In light-skinned individuals, a purple to black discoloration is abnormal (Figure 10-6J). In dark-skinned individuals, very dark to black discoloration is abnormal.

P These findings can indicate different stages of necrosis, or tissue death. Conditions that starve the affected body part of oxygen, whether in acute

E Examination   **N** Normal Findings   **A** Abnormal Findings   **P** Pathophysiology

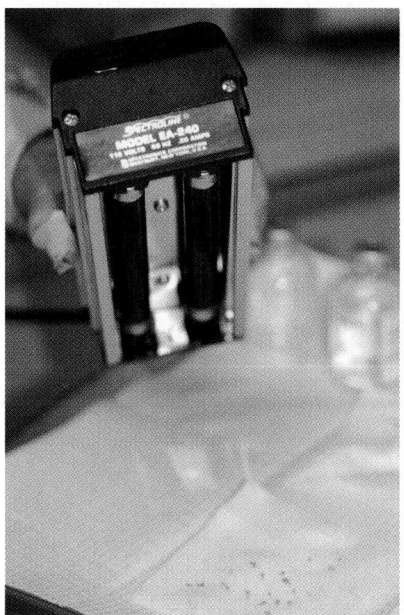

FIGURE 10-7 **Wood's Lamp.** *Courtesy of Robert A. Silverman, M.D., Clinical Associate Professor, Department of Pediatrics, Georgetown University.*

NURSINGTIP

Enhancement Techniques

Magnification: Use of a magnifying glass may be beneficial in the evaluation of lesions and discolorations for morphology.

Wood's Lamp: Also known as an ultraviolet light, it is valuable in the diagnosis of certain skin and hair diseases (Figure 10-7). Dermatophytosis and erythrasma are easily diagnosed by the fluorescent changes that occur under ultraviolet exposure. Dermatophytosis in the hair shaft will appear green to yellow, and erythrasma will appear coral red.

Diascopy: Consists of pressing a microscope slide over a skin lesion. Diascopy is useful in determining whether a red lesion's coloration is due to erythema, which will blanch, or extravasation of blood, which will not blanch. Diascopy can also be useful in the detection of the glassy, yellow-brown appearance of papules found in tuberculosis of the skin, lymphoma, and sarcoidosis.

or chronic situations, can cause necrosis. Diabetes mellitus, disseminated intravascular coagulation, acute hypovolemia, and severe electric charge are some of the conditions that can cause necrosis.

A Dark brown or blackened areas of skin that are edematous and painful are abnormal (see Figure 10-6K). These areas may drain a thin liquid that has a sweet, foul odor. Crepitus may be palpated in the affected areas.

P Gas gangrene, or clostridial myonecrosis, is a gram-positive infection that affects skeletal muscles that have decreased oxygenation. The clostridia organisms are endogenous to the gastrointestinal tract and are also found in the soil. Patients who experience circulatory compromise, such as in diabetes mellitus, arterial insufficiency, trauma, and constricting casts, are at risk for developing gas gangrene. Patients who have contaminated wounds and decreased vascularity to the affected area are also at risk for developing gas gangrene.

Lesions

E 1. Inspect the skin for lesions, noting the anatomic location. Lesions can be localized, regionalized, or generalized. They can involve exposed areas or skin folds (see Table 10-1).

2. Note the grouping or arrangement of the lesions: discrete, grouped, confluent, linear, annular, polycyclic, generalized, or zosteriform (see Figure 10-8).

3. Inspect the lesions for elevation (flat or raised).

4. Using a ruler, measure the lesions.

5. Describe the color of the lesions.

6. Note any exudate for color or odor.

7. Note the morphology of the skin lesions. Skin lesions can be primary, originating from previously normal skin, or secondary, originating from primary lesions. For specific descriptions of primary lesion morphology, see Figure 10-9. For specific descriptions of secondary lesion morphology, refer to Figure 10-10.

NURSINGTIP

ABCDE Mnemonic for Evaluating Skin Lesions

A (Asymmetrical): Is the lesion asymmetrical?

B (Borders): Are the borders of the lesion irregular?

C (Color): Is the color of the lesion uneven, irregular, or multicolored?

D (Diameter): Has the lesion's diameter changed recently?

E (Elevation): Has the lesion become elevated?

TABLE 10-1 Anatomic Locations of Various Skin Lesions

LESION	LOCATION
Basal cell carcinoma	Medial and lateral canthi and nasolabial fold
Rosacea	Face
Acne vulgaris	Face, back, shoulders, chest
Furuncle	Nose, neck, face, axillae, and buttocks
Lesions resulting from light exposure (squamous cell carcinoma, solar lentigo, solar keratosis)	Forehead, cheeks, tops of the ears, neck, dorsal surface of hands and forearms, and lateral arms
Seborrheic keratosis, spider angioma	Face, trunk, and upper extremities
Impetigo, verruca vulgaris (warts)	Arms, legs, buttocks, face, hands, fingers, and knees
Herpes zoster	Along the cutaneous spinal nerve tracks, almost always unilateral
Kaposi's sarcoma	Widespread: trunk, head, tip of nose, periorbital, penis, legs, palms, and soles
Erythema nodosum	Lower legs
Stasis dermatitis	Sock area
Cutaneous moniliasis	Moist folds behind the ears, under the breasts, in the axilla, umbilicus, along the inguinal and pudendal regions, and in the gluteal and perineal areas
Adult atopic eczema	Mainly flexor surfaces of the body
Psoriasis	Mainly scalp, elbows, and extensor surfaces of the body (rarely on the face and skin folds)
Contact dermatitis	Affects surfaces in contact with irritating agents
Pediculosis pubis	Pubic and axillary areas

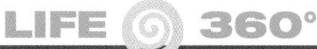

LIFE 360°

Curious Skin Findings

A 65-year-old Vietnamese woman comes to the clinic because of the increasing frequency and intensity of her headaches. Her English-speaking and -comprehension abilities are limited. After conducting the health history, you start your physical examination. You note that 75% of her back is covered with ecchymoses in various stages. You know that the woman believes in *bat gil*, or skin pinching, as a remedy for headaches. You have also read in the patient's chart that this woman has been the victim of domestic violence in recent years. How would you proceed with this patient?

LESIONS	EXAMPLES	LESIONS	EXAMPLES

A.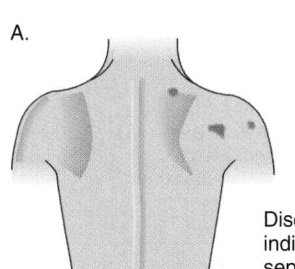

Discrete: individual, separate, and distinct

Insect bites

B.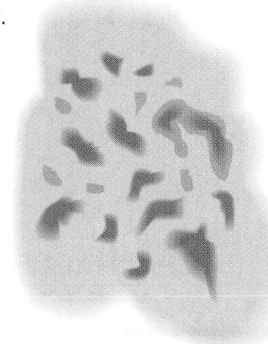

Grouped: lesions are clustered

Herpes simplex

C.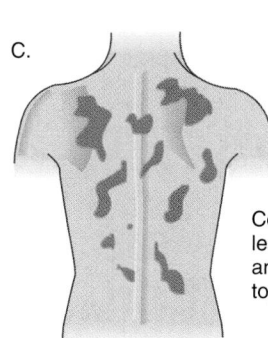

Confluent: lesions merge and run together

Childhood exanthema

D.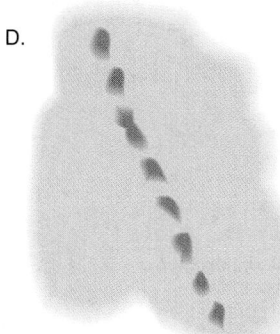

Linear or serpiginous: lesions that form a line or snakelike shape

Poison ivy, dermatitis, hookworm

E.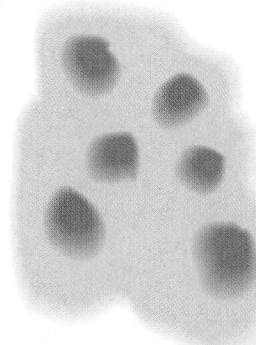

Annular: lesions arranged in a circular pattern

Ringworm

F.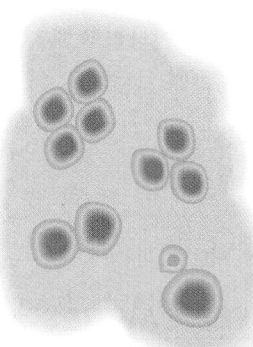

Polycyclic or targetoid: lesions arranged in concentric circles resembling a bull's-eye

Eruptions from drug reactions such as urticaria, erythema multiforme

G.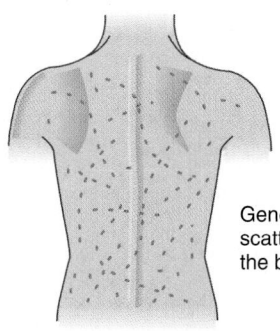

Generalized: scattered over the body

Measles

H.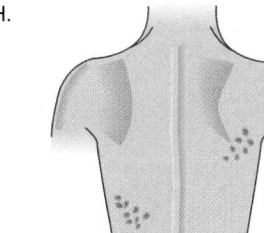

Zosteriform: linear arrangement along a nerve root

Herpes zoster

FIGURE 10-8 Arrangement of Lesions

NONPALPABLE

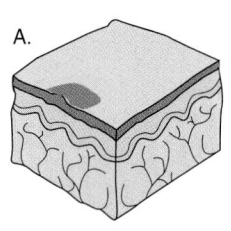

A.

Macule:
Localized changes in skin color of less than 1 cm in diameter
Example:
Freckle

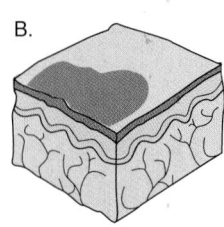

B.

Patch:
Localized changes in skin color of greater than 1 cm in diameter
Example:
Vitiligo, stage 1 of pressure ulcer

PALPABLE

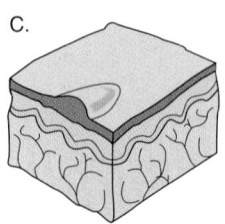

C.

Papule:
Solid, elevated lesion less than 0.5 cm in diameter
Example:
Warts, elevated nevi, seborrheic keratosis

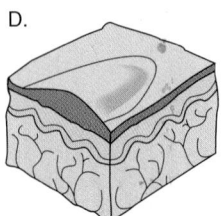

D.

Plaque:
Solid, elevated lesion greater than 0.5 cm in diameter
Example:
Psoriasis, eczema, pityriasis rosea

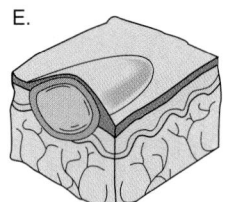

E.

Nodules:
Solid and elevated; however, they extend deeper than papules into the dermis or subcutaneous tissues, 0.5-2.0 cm
Example:
Lipoma, erythema nodosum, cyst, melanoma, hemangioma

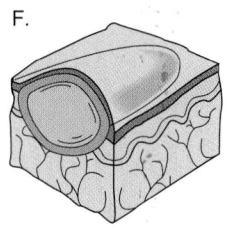

F.

Tumor:
The same as a nodule only greater than 2 cm

Example:
Carcinoma (such as advanced breast carcinoma); **not** basal cell or squamous cell of the skin

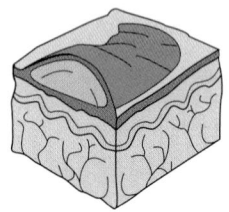

G.

Wheal:
Localized edema in the epidermis causing irregular elevation that may be red or pale
Example:
Insect bite, hive, angioedema

FLUID-FILLED CAVITIES WITHIN THE SKIN

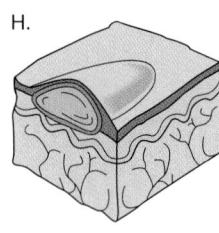

H.

Vesicle:
Accumulation of fluid between the upper layers of the skin; elevated mass containing serous fluid; less than 0.5 cm
Example:
Herpes simplex, herpes zoster, chickenpox, scabies

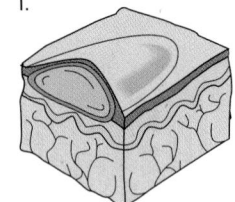

I.

Bullae:
Same as a vesicle only greater than 0.5 cm
Example:
Contact dermatitis, large second-degree burns, bullous impetigo, pemphigus

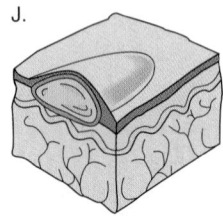

J.

Pustule:
Vesicles or bullae that become filled with pus, usually described as less than 0.5 cm in diameter
Example:
Acne, impetigo, furuncles, carbuncles, folliculitis

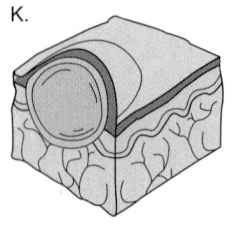

K.

Cyst:
Encapsulated fluid-filled or a semi-solid mass in the subcutaneous tissue or dermis
Example:
Sebaceous cyst, epidermoid cyst

FIGURE 10-9 Morphology of Primary Lesions

ABOVE THE SKIN SURFACE

A.
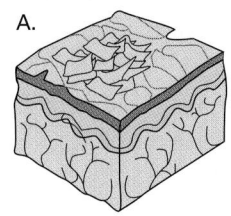

Scales:
   Flaking of the skin's surface
Example:
   Dandruff, psoriasis, xerosis

B.
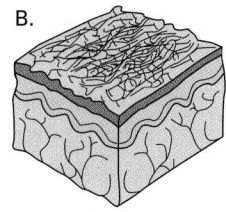

Lichenification:
   Layers of skin become
   thickened and rough as a
   result of rubbing over a
   prolonged period of time
Example:
   Chronic contact dermatitis

C.
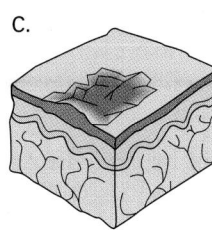

Crust:
   Dried serum, blood, or pus
   on the surface of the skin
Example:
   Impetigo, acute eczematous
   inflammation

D.
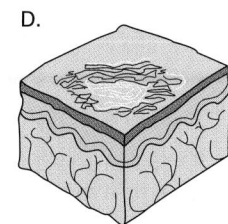

Atrophy:
   Thinning of the skin surface
   and loss of markings
Example:
   Striae, aged skin

BELOW THE SKIN SURFACE

E.
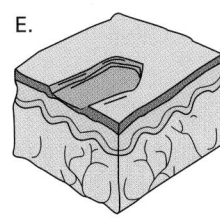

Erosion:
   Loss of epidermis
Example:
   Ruptured chickenpox vesicle

F.
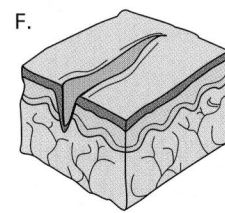

Fissure:
   Linear crack in the epidermis
   that can extend into the dermis
Example:
   Chapped hands or lips,
   athlete's foot

G.
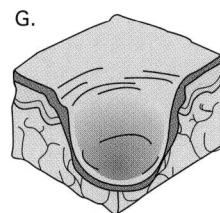

Ulcer:
   A depressed lesion of
   the epidermis and upper
   papillary layer of the dermis
Example:
   Stage 2 pressure ulcer

H.
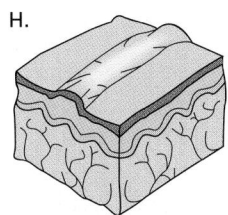

Scar:
   Fibrous tissue that replaces
   dermal tissue after injury
Example:
    Surgical incision

I.
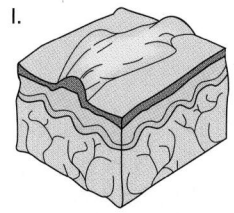

Keloid:
   Enlarging of a scar past
   wound edges due to excess
   collagen formation (more
   prevalent in dark-skinned
   persons)
Example:
   Burn scar

J.

Excoriation:
   Loss of epidermal layers
   exposing the dermis
Example:
   Abrasion

FIGURE 10-10 Morphology of Secondary Lesions

NURSING**TIP**

Wound Evaluation

If a wound is present, remove the dressing and assess the wound for location, color, drainage, odor, size, and depth. Measure the borders of the wound with a centimeter ruler and draw a picture in your notes, if necessary, to depict necrotic areas, drains, and so on.

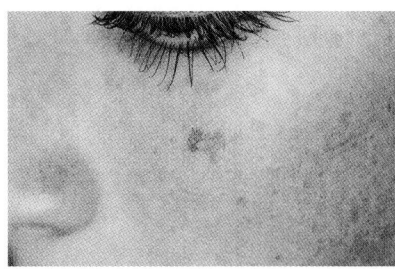

A. A lentigo occurs in sun-exposed areas of the body. *Courtesy of Robert A. Silverman, M.D., Clinical Associate Professor, Department of Pediatrics, Georgetown University.*

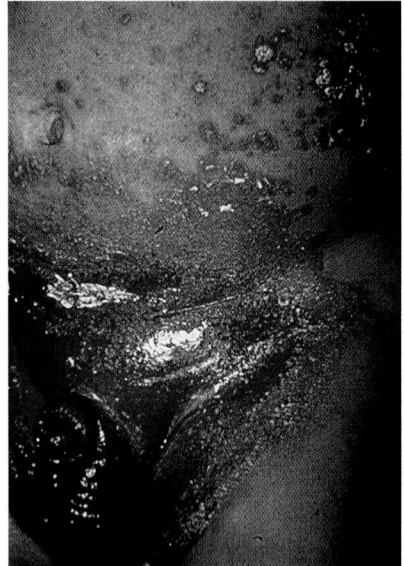

B. Moniliasis. *Courtesy of the Centers for Disease Control and Prevention.*

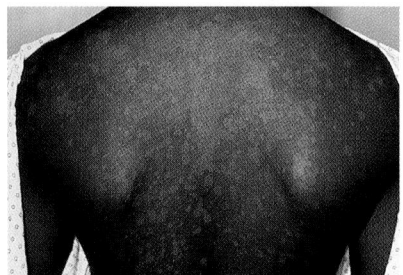

C. Tinea Versicolor. *Courtesy of Robert A. Silverman, M.D., Clinical Associate Professor, Department of Pediatrics, Georgetown University.*

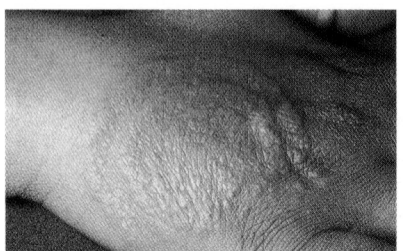

D. Tinea Corporis. *Courtesy of Robert A. Silverman, M.D., Clinical Associate Professor, Department of Pediatrics, Georgetown University.*

N No skin lesions should be present except for freckles, birthmarks, or moles (**nevi**), which may be flat or elevated.

A A nonpalpable lesion that is less than 2 cm in size, light brown in color, and appearing on the face, arms, and hands is abnormal (Figure 10-11A).

P This nonpalpable lesion describes a lentigo. It is a hyperpigmented disorder that occurs in body areas that are exposed to the sun. They can increase in size as the person ages.

A Intertriginous exudative patches that are beefy red in color, well demarcated, pruritic, and erythematous are abnormal.

P Moniliasis, also known as candidiasis, is a yeast infection that may invade numerous areas of the body but normally occurs in the axillae, inframammary areas, groin, and gluteal regions (Figure 10-11B).

A Scaly macular patches of white, reddish brown, or tan hyperpigmentation, or hypopigmentation, of the skin are abnormal (Figure 10-11C).

P These occur in tinea versicolor, which is caused by superficial fungal infections. The lesions usually occur on the trunk and proximal extremities.

A A pink to red papulosquamous annular lesion with raised borders that expands peripherally and has a clearing center is abnormal.

P Tinea corporis is caused by *Trichophyton*, a dermatophyte (fungal) infection (Figure 10-11D).

A Toe web lesions that are macerated and have scaling borders are abnormal.

P Tinea pedis (athlete's foot) is very common and often erupts in the third and fourth interdigital spaces; with time, the lesions will spread over the plantar surface. Tinea pedis is caused by *Trichophyton mentagrophytes* (Figure 10-11E).

A A slightly erythematous, rose- or fawn-colored, round or oval patch that may have slightly raised borders is abnormal (Figure 10-11F).

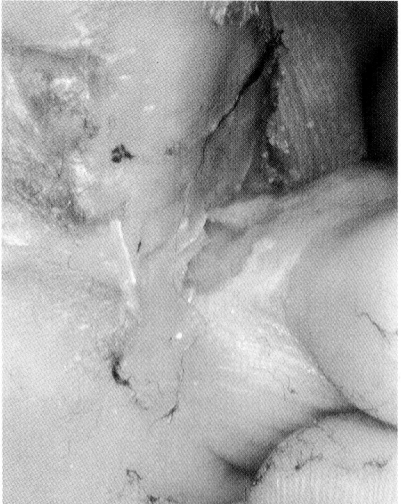

E. Tinea Pedis. *Courtesy of Robert A. Silverman, M.D., Clinical Associate Professor, Department of Pediatrics, Georgetown University.*

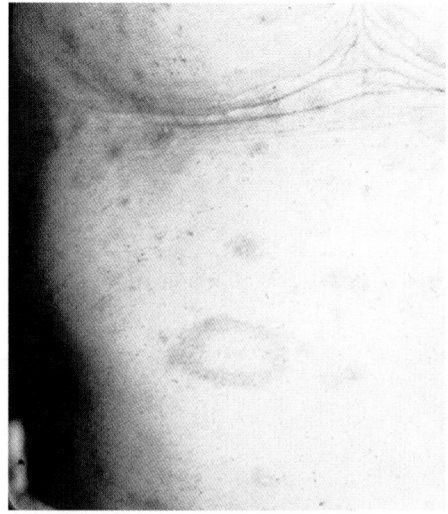

F. Pityriasis Rosea. *Courtesy of the Centers for Disease Control and Prevention.*

FIGURE 10-11 **Common Skin Lesions** *continues*

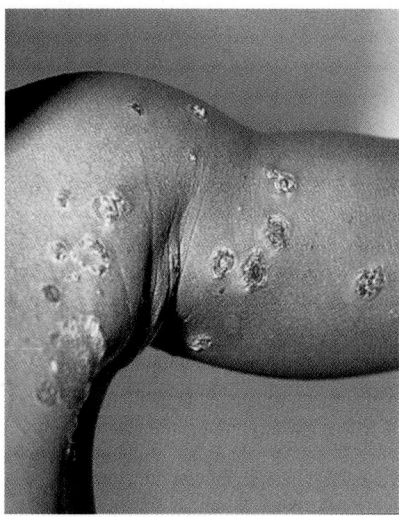

G. Impetigo. *Courtesy of Robert A. Silverman, M.D., Clinical Associate Professor, Department of Pediatrics, Georgetown University.*

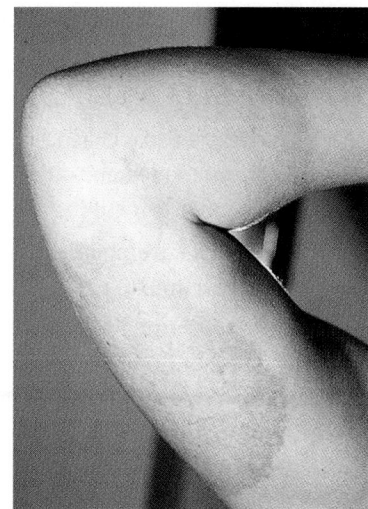

H. Erysipelas. *Courtesy of Robert A. Silverman, M.D., Clinical Associate Professor, Department of Pediatrics, Georgetown University.*

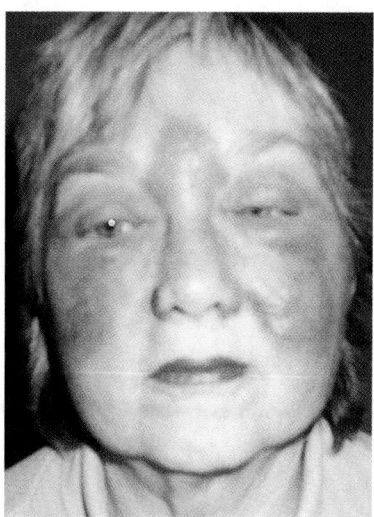

I. Cellulitis

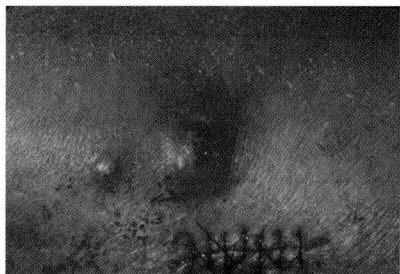

J. Furuncle. *Courtesy of Robert A. Silverman, M.D., Clinical Associate Professor, Department of Pediatrics, Georgetown University.*

FIGURE 10-11 **Common Skin Lesions** *continues*

P A herald patch is normally found on the trunk and is indicative of pityriasis rosea. This benign, self-limiting condition is often seen in young adults and may resemble ringworm. The herald patch is normally followed in 5 to 10 days by a generalized eruption of similar lesions. The etiology is thought to be viral.

A Vesicles or bullae that measure 1 to 2 cm and become pustular and rupture easily, discharging straw-colored fluid, are abnormal. The purulent drainage becomes thick as it dries, producing light brown or golden-honey–colored crusts (Figure 10-11G).

P Impetigo is usually caused by group A streptococcus or *Staphylococcus aureus* and is highly contagious. It is typically found in preschoolers in the late summer and can be associated with poor hygiene, crowding, contact sports, and minor skin trauma that is untreated.

A Red, shiny, indurated (with a peau d'orange appearance), and warm edematous lesions are abnormal. These lesions may be elevated, have defined margins, and may be painful. Vesicles and bullae may also be present (Figure 10-11H).

P Erysipelas is a type of superficial cellulitis that is usually found in older adults and in young children. Erysipelas can originate in cuts or incisions infected by group A streptococcus either from the patient's respiratory tract or the respiratory tract of someone who was in close contact with the patient.

A A diffuse red area that is warm, edematous, painful, and indurated is abnormal (Figure 10-11I).

P These findings suggest cellulitis, an acute bacterial infection (usually staphylococcal or streptococcal) of the skin and subcutaneous tissues. Cellulitis can result from trauma to the skin, foreign bodies in the skin, and underlying infection.

P A lesion that starts as a tender, deep red papule and develops into a well-defined, erythematous, and painful mass with purulent material (Figure 10-11J) is abnormal. This describes a furuncle, commonly called a boil. It can be a firm or fluctuant lesion. Furuncles are usually caused by staphylococci.

A A flat or raised lesion with a black interior is abnormal.

P A comedo, or blackhead, is usually seen on the face, chest, shoulders, or back. Comedones are due to increased keratinization in the hair follicle from an unknown etiology. They are associated with acne.

A Comedones accompanied by pustules (with yellow or white centers), red papules (Figure 10-11K), nodules, and cysts are abnormal.

P Acne vulgaris usually occurs in the middle to late teen years and is caused by an inflammation of the sebaceous follicles. Acne vulgaris is associated with hormonal changes. It can be located on the face, chest, shoulders, and back. Lesions that appear punched out may be present from scarring of previously active acne lesions (Figure 10-11L).

A Redness, with dilatation of the blood vessels on the cheeks and forehead, and acne are abnormal.

P Acne rosacea is a chronic inflammation seen primarily in middle-aged and older adults. The cause is unknown, although it is aggravated by alcohol, spicy food, hot liquids, sunlight, extremes in temperature, exercise, and stress (Figure 10-11M).

A Rosacea that is red or purple on the lower nose and is accompanied by thickening of the affected skin and enlargement of the follicular orifices is abnormal (Figure 10-11N).

P This condition is rosacea rhinophyma. The pathophysiology is the same as for rosacea.

A Reddish-salmon–colored macular lesions are abnormal.

A Elevated purple to brown lesions (in light-skinned patients) and bluish lesions (in dark-skinned patients) that are spongy, painful, and pruritic are abnormal (Figure 10-11O).

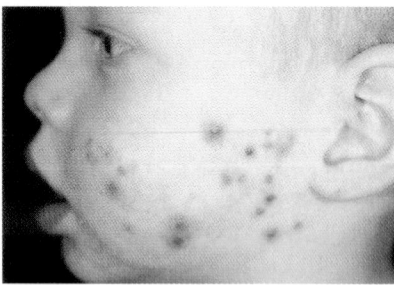

K. Acne papules and nodules are visible on this child's face. *Courtesy of Robert A. Silverman, M.D., Clinical Associate Professor, Department of Pediatrics, Georgetown University.*

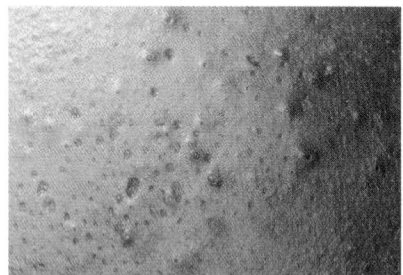

L. Acne Scarring. *Courtesy of Robert A. Silverman, M.D., Clinical Associate Professor, Department of Pediatrics, Georgetown University.*

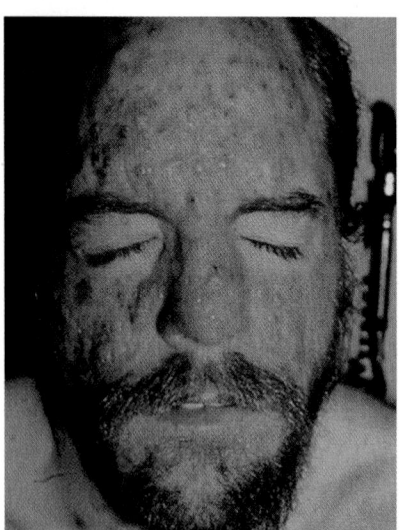

M. Acne Rosacea. *Courtesy of Timothy Berger, M.D., San Francisco, CA.*

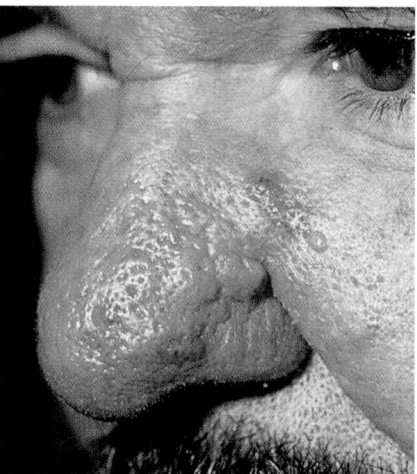

N. Rosacea Rhinophyma. *Courtesy of Robert A. Silverman, M.D., Clinical Associate Professor, Department of Pediatrics, Georgetown University.*

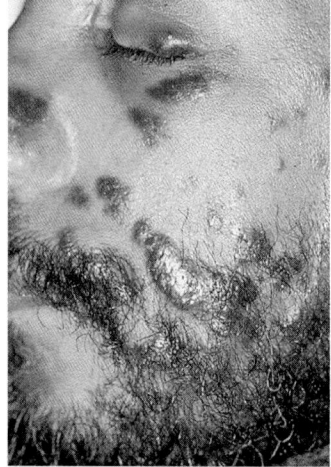

O. Kaposi's Sarcoma. *Courtesy of Robert A. Silverman, M.D., Clinical Associate Professor, Department of Pediatrics, Georgetown University.*

FIGURE 10-11 **Common Skin Lesions** *continues*

NURSING**ALERT**

MRSA Infections

Within the past few years, the incidence of skin and soft tissue infections caused by methicillin-resistant *Staphylococcus aureus* (MRSA) has significantly increased in the outpatient population. What is of concern is that many of these infections occur in an otherwise healthy individual and are more severe than infections of past years. Deaths due to MRSA infections have occurred in young and old alike. Risk factors are close living quarters (e.g., military barracks, dormitories, prisons) and poor hygiene (e.g., sharing towels and other personal items, and skin contact with unclean athletic equipment). All suspect lesions need to be cultured.

LIFE 360°

Limiting MRSA Infections

Consider the following sports: wrestling, football, gymnastics, and bodybuilding. What are possible modes of transmission of MRSA infections in each sport? How can transmission be minimized? Devise a teaching plan for athletes in these sports.

LIFE 360°

Teenage Acne

Rachana is an 18-year-old female who is scheduled to have her annual physical examination today. At the conclusion of the exam, the pediatric nurse practitioner tells Rachana that she is a healthy teenager. Rachana begins to cry and states that she hates herself because she is so ugly because of her acne and it is ruining her life. What could the nurse say to Rachana? What treatment options could be discussed?

P Both of these abnormal findings are typical lesions of Kaposi's sarcoma. The reddish-salmon lesions are early findings, and the purplish or bluish lesions are more advanced lesions. Kaposi's sarcoma is a neoplastic disorder that is thought to have a genetic, hormonal, and viral etiology. It is frequently found in patients infected with the AIDS virus, immunocompromised patients, and older adults.

A Pruritic, silvery scales of the epidermis that have clearly demarcated borders and underlying erythema are abnormal. These lesions are circular and are found primarily on the elbows, knees, and behind the ears (see Figure 10-11P).

P The etiology of psoriasis is unknown, but it has a genetic component and may be aggravated by cold weather, trauma, and infection.

P On rare occasions, psoriasis can progress to pustular psoriasis (see Figure 10-11Q). Erythema develops throughout the body, especially in flexural areas. Pustules develop over the erythema and can easily rupture. The patient is often febrile. Death can ensue from sepsis.

A A chronic superficial inflammation of the face, scalp, buttocks, or extremities that evolves into pruritic, red, weeping, crusted lesions is abnormal (see Figure 10-11R).

P Eczema, also known as atopic dermatitis, is a multifaceted disease process that is often associated with asthma and allergic rhinitis. The etiology is unknown, and a family history of related disorders is usually noted.

A It is abnormal to have edema and erythema along with red, pruritic vesicles that may discharge an exudate that leads to crusting (see Figure 10-11S).

P This describes allergic contact dermatitis. In Figure 10-11S, the allergen is poison oak. The patient must come in direct contact with the irritant to develop the dermatitis. Contact dermatitis is also caused by metals such as nickel, detergents, cosmetics, rubber, topical medications, food, shampoo, hair dye, and clothing.

REFLECTIVE THINKING

Adult Patient with Chickenpox

Kara is a monogamous 35-year-old married woman who develops painful, red, maculopapular, itchy lesions on her vulva. She shows them to her husband, who insists that she has had an extramarital affair. She presents to the county clinic for evaluation of her lesions. When you enter the room, you see a distressed woman who is crying. What questions would you ask this woman? How would you proceed with the examination?

| **E** Examination | **N** Normal Findings | **A** Abnormal Findings | **P** Pathophysiology |

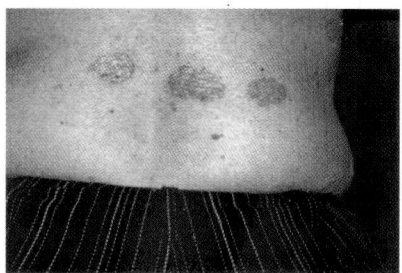

P. Psoriasis

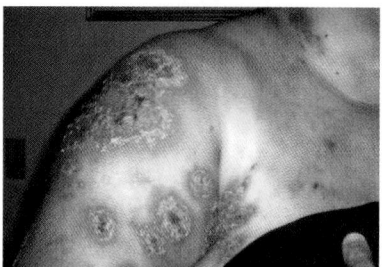

Q. Pustular Psoriasis

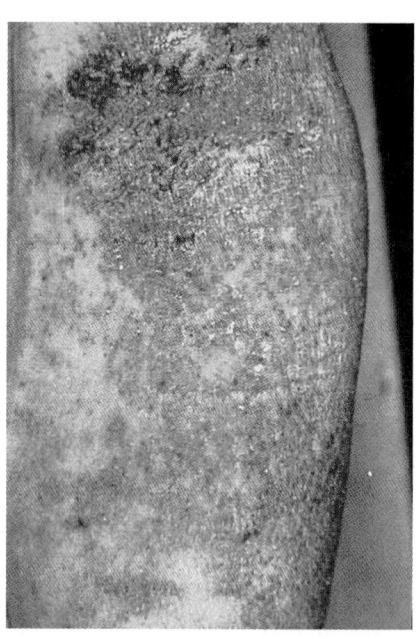

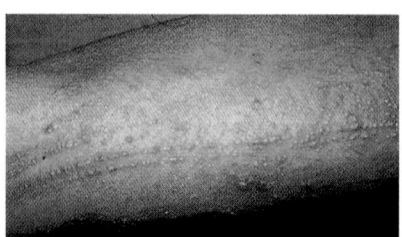

S. Allergic Contact Dermatitis. *Courtesy of the Centers for Disease Control and Prevention.*

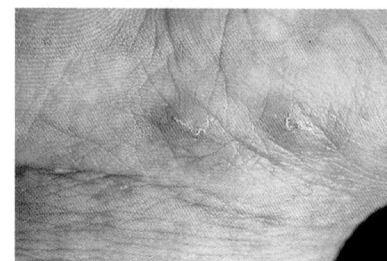

T. Scabies. *Courtesy of Robert A. Silverman, M.D., Clinical Associate Professor, Department of Pediatrics, Georgetown University.*

R. Eczema. *Courtesy of the Centers for Disease Control and Prevention.*

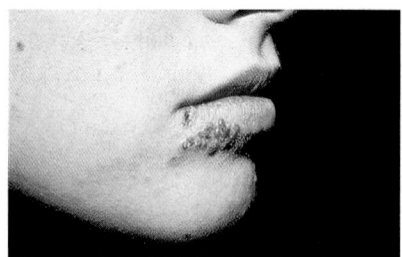

U. Herpes Simplex Virus I. *Courtesy of Robert A. Silverman, M.D., Clinical Associate Professor, Department of Pediatrics, Georgetown University.*

FIGURE 10-11 **Common Skin Lesions** *continues*

A Red, pruritic papules or vesicles with S-shaped or straight-line burrows are abnormal (Figure 10-11T). These lesions can be intensely pruritic.

P Scabies is caused by the *Sarcoptes scabiei* mite, and may be visible as a small, dark area within the vesicle. It is highly contagious and can sometimes be spread through infected clothing or bedding.

A Red papules, vesicles, open sores, and crusting on the face, in the mouth, or on the genitalia are abnormal (Figure 10-11U).

P Herpes simplex virus I is usually responsible for these lesions, which are more common on the face and in the mouth. After the initial exposure, the patient can often predict an outbreak because of the presence of numbness, burning, itching, or soreness at the eruption site.

A Red macular and papular lesions that are intensely pruritic are abnormal (see Figure 10-11V).

P Varicella, or chickenpox, usually starts on the trunk and proceeds to the extremities. Papules progress to thin-walled vesicles, pustules, and crusts. The patient may exhibit all of the different lesions simultaneously. Varicella is caused by the varicella-zoster virus, which is highly contagious, especially in children.

A Red, extremely painful vesicles with paresthesia that are closely grouped in a dermatomal pattern are abnormal (see Figure 10-11W).

P Herpes zoster, or shingles, is caused by a reactivation of the varicella-zoster virus. The virus remains dormant after the initial varicella inoculation. It frequently occurs in elderly individuals. The lesions are similar to those of varicella, but they tend to develop more slowly.

P Herpes zoster that involves the ophthalmic branch of the fifth cranial nerve is called herpes zoster ophthalmicus (see Figure 10-11X).

| **E** Examination | **N** Normal Findings | **A** Abnormal Findings | **P** Pathophysiology |

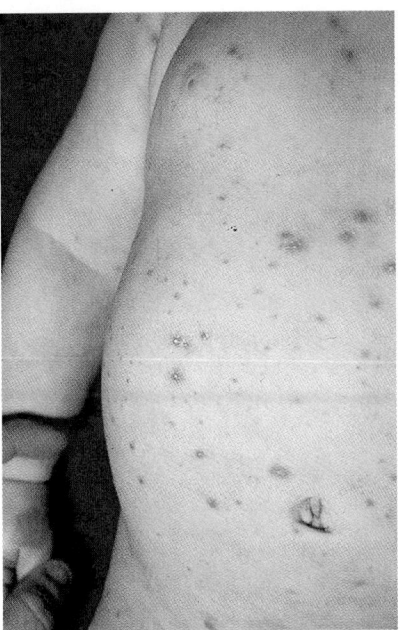

V. Varicella. *Courtesy of Robert A. Silverman, M.D., Clinical Associate Professor, Department of Pediatrics, Georgetown University.*

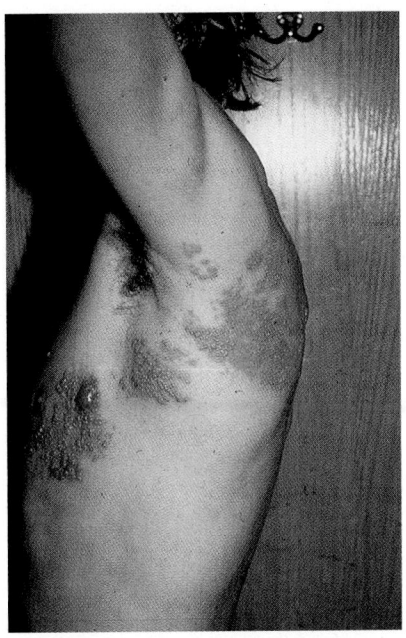

W. Herpes Zoster. *Courtesy of Robert A. Silverman, M.D., Clinical Associate Professor, Department of Pediatrics, Georgetown University.*

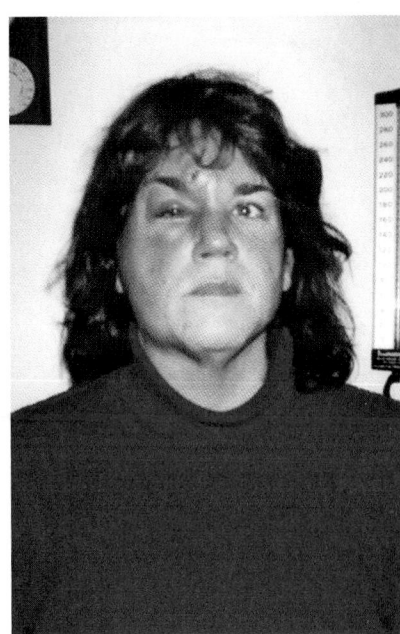

X. Herpes Zoster Ophthalmicus

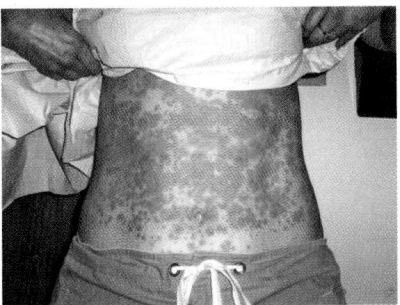

Y. Stevens-Johnson Syndrome

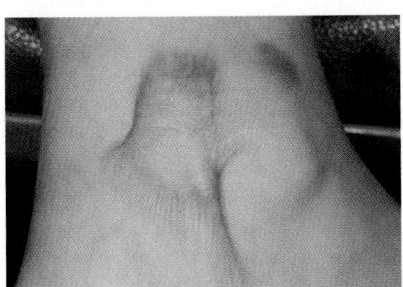

Z. Keloid. *Courtesy of Robert A. Silverman, M.D., Clinical Associate Professor, Department of Pediatrics, Georgetown University.*

FIGURE 10-11 **Common Skin Lesions** *continues*

Anterior uveitis, keratitis, optic neuritis, and retinal necrosis are possible complications of this condition. These patients need to be evaluated by an ophthalmologist within 24 hours.

A Flat, purpuric macules or atypical target lesions that are widespread and/or located on the thorax and progress to blistering are abnormal (Figure 10-11Y).

P These lesions are characteristic of Stevens-Johnson syndrome. Medications such as phenytoin, sulfonamides, and penicillin are frequently the causative agent. Serious complications can occur with this condition if not diagnosed and treated early.

A An excessive enlarging of a scar past wound edges is abnormal (Figure 10-11Z).

P Keloids are formed from excess collagen formation.

A Discrete pink macules or papular lesions with clear halos are abnormal. These lesions usually start on the trunk and progress to the face, neck, and extremities a few days after the patient has had a high fever (see Figure 10-11AA).

P Roseola, or exanthem subitum, is most likely viral in origin.

A A maculopapular rash that is brownish pink and starts around the ears, face, and neck and then progresses over the truck and limbs is abnormal (see Figure 10-11BB).

P Rubeola (measles) is a viral infection that is highly contagious, and is characterized by high fever, cough, rash, and Koplik's spots (whitish-blue spots with a red halo) on the buccal or labial mucosa (see Figure 10-11CC).

A Rubella (German measles) displays a fine, pinkish, macular rash that becomes confluent and pinpoint after the second day (see Figure 10-11DD).

P Rubella is an RNA virus in nature and spreads from the face and neck to the trunk.

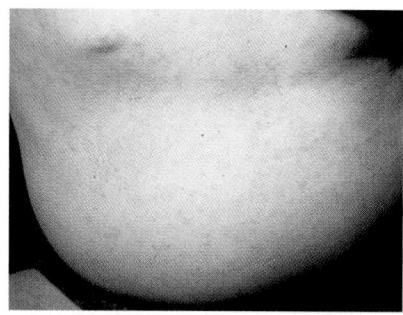

AA. Roseola. *Courtesy of Robert A. Silverman, M.D., Clinical Associate Professor, Department of Pediatrics, Georgetown University.*

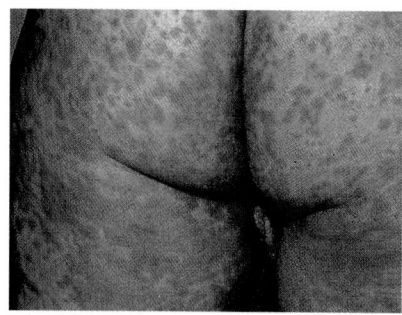

BB. Rubeola. *Courtesy of the Centers for Disease Control and Prevention.*

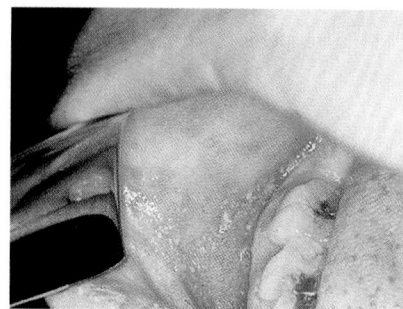

CC. Koplik's Spots in Rubeola. *Courtesy of the Centers for Disease Control and Prevention.*

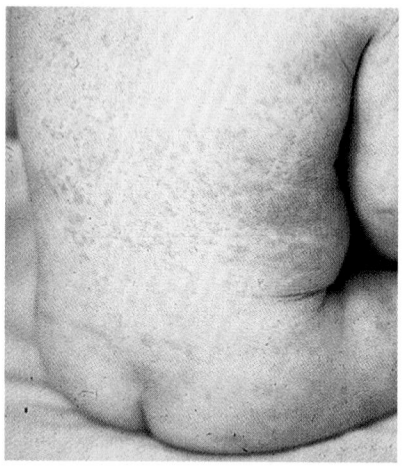

DD. Rubella. *Courtesy of the Centers for Disease Control and Prevention.*

EE. Scarlet Fever. *Courtesy of the Centers for Disease Control and Prevention.*

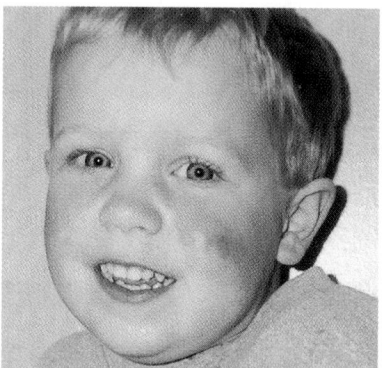

FF. Erythema Infectiosum

FIGURE 10-11 **Common Skin Lesions** *continues*

A A diffuse, pinkish-red flush of the skin that is confluent over the entire body surface is abnormal (Figure 10-11EE).

P Scarlet fever (scarlatina) is caused by streptococcal bacteria (usually group A) and is associated with a strawberry tongue, circumoral pallor, fever, and chills. Linear petechiae (Pastia's sign) may be found in skin folds such as the antecubital fossa.

A A blotchy, maculopapular rash that may be reticular is abnormal (Figure 10-11FF).

P Erythema infectiosum (fifth disease) usually starts on the cheeks and spreads to the arms and trunk. It gives a "slapped cheek" appearance. Its cause is human parvovirus B19. Erythema infectiosum is usually a benign condition, but it can cause severe complications in pregnant women.

A A maculopapular rash with erythemic borders that appears first on the wrists, ankles, palms, soles, and forearms and is associated with a high fever is abnormal (see Figure 10-11GG).

P Rocky Mountain spotted fever is associated with a history of tick bites. This febrile disease is caused by *Rickettsia rickettsii* and is transmitted by several types of ticks. Severe headaches, myalgia, and vomiting can occur.

| **E** Examination | **N** Normal Findings | **A** Abnormal Findings | **P** Pathophysiology |

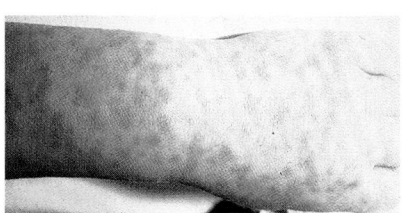

GG. Rocky Mountain Spotted Fever. *Courtesy of the Centers for Disease Control and Prevention.*

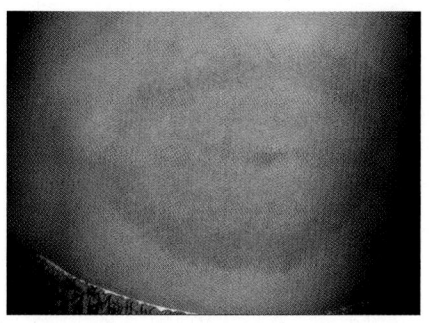

HH. Erythema Migrans of Lyme Disease. *Courtesy of Robert A. Silverman, M.D., Clinical Associate Professor, Department of Pediatrics, Georgetown University.*

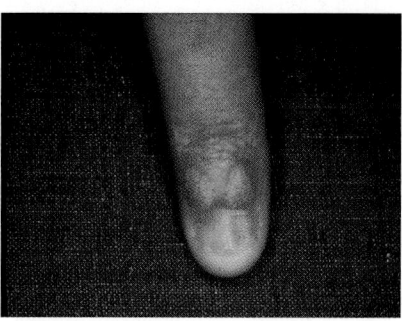

II. Verruca Vulgaris (Wart). *Courtesy of Robert A. Silverman, M.D., Clinical Associate Professor, Department of Pediatrics, Georgetown University.*

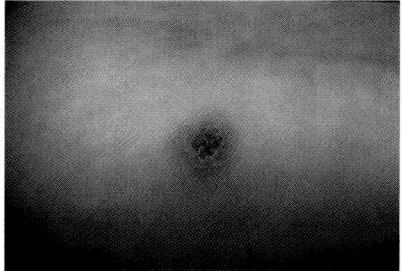

JJ. Plantar Wart. *Courtesy of Robert A. Silverman, M.D., Clinical Associate Professor, Department of Pediatrics, Georgetown University.*

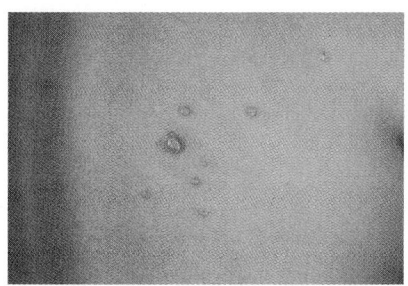

KK. Molluscum Contagiosum. *Courtesy of Robert A. Silverman, M.D., Clinical Associate Professor, Department of Pediatrics, Georgetown University.*

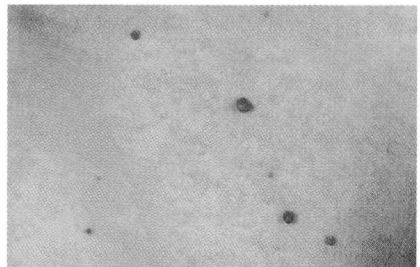

LL. Skin Tags. *Courtesy of Robert A. Silverman, M.D., Clinical Associate Professor, Department of Pediatrics, Georgetown University.*

FIGURE 10-11 **Common Skin Lesions** *continues*

A A red papule that progresses to an erythematous circular lesion with central clearing (Figure 10-11HH) is abnormal.

P This lesion is erythema migrans, the characteristic skin lesion of Lyme disease. Lyme disease is caused by the spirochete *Borrelia burgdorferi*. It is transmitted by infected ticks, especially in the northern and mid-Atlantic states. The area of the skin lesion is the site of the tick bite.

A Flesh-colored, hyperkeratotic papules (Figure 10-11II) that have black dots on them are abnormal.

P Common warts, or verruca vulgaris, are viral in origin. The black dots represent thrombosed blood vessels. Warts that occur on the feet are called plantar warts (Figure 10-11JJ).

A Discrete, flesh-colored, dome-shaped papules that are slightly umbilicated in the center (Figure 10-11KK) are abnormal.

P This describes molluscum contagiosum, a self-limiting viral infection. The papules may be found anywhere on the body except the palmar and plantar surfaces. When found on the genitalia of children, sexual abuse must be considered.

A A flesh-colored or brown pedunculated nodule is abnormal.

P Skin tags, or achrochordon, are benign nodules (Figure 10-11LL). They are frequently removed if they are in an area that receives repeated movement such as a bra line, or if they are annoying to the patient.

A Small, pinkish-brown papules that are slightly raised and retract beneath the skin when compressed are abnormal.

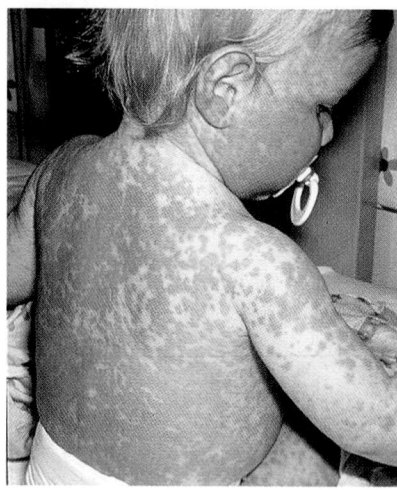

MM. Exanthematous Drug Eruption. *Courtesy of Robert A. Silverman, M.D., Clinical Associate Professor, Department of Pediatrics, Georgetown University.*

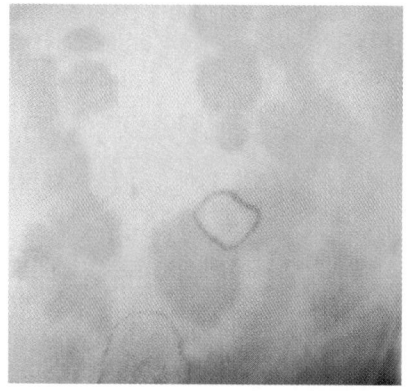

NN. Urticaria. *Courtesy of Robert A. Silverman, M.D., Clinical Associate Professor, Department of Pediatrics, Georgetown University.*

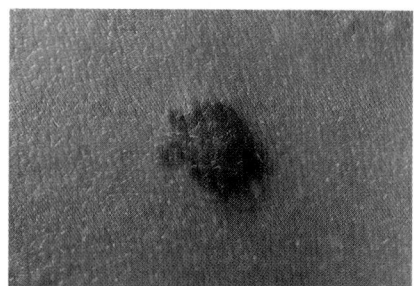

OO. Malignant Melanoma. *Courtesy of Robert A. Silverman, M.D., Clinical Associate Professor, Department of Pediatrics, Georgetown University.*

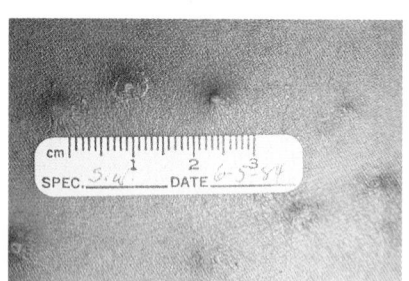

PP. Folliculitis. *Courtesy of Robert A. Silverman, M.D., Clinical Associate Professor, Department of Pediatrics, Georgetown University.*

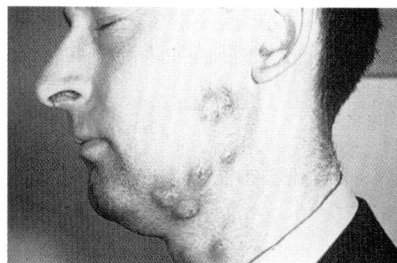

QQ. Tinea Barbae. *Courtesy of the Centers for Disease Control and Prevention.*

FIGURE 10-11 **Common Skin Lesions** *continues*

P These are dermatofibromas, or benign papules. Occasionally, they may also be scaly in appearance.

A Pruritic, red wheals (urticarial rash) that vary in size from very small to large and are sometimes accompanied by maculopapular eruptions, vesicles, and bullae are abnormal (Figure 10-11MM).

P Urticaria can be acute or chronic in nature. This itchy skin lesion is linked to histamine release within the body (Figure 10-11NN). Exposure to food, drugs, infections, chemicals, physical stimuli (pressure, sun, cold weather or water, exercise) are among the causes of urticaria.

A Lesions that are brownish-tan, red, white, blue, pink, purple, or gray and that have irregular borders and notching are abnormal. These lesions can be flat or elevated.

P Malignant melanoma (Figure 10-11OO) is a cancerous lesion that is associated with repeated sun exposure. Those individuals with light skin and blue eyes are particularly at risk for malignant melanoma. These neoplastic lesions can also be related to precancerous lesions such as nevi.

A Perifollicular papules are abnormal.

P Pseudofolliculitis barbae, or ingrown hair, is caused by hair tips that penetrate into the skin rather than exiting through the follicular orifice. It usually occurs in the beard area, particularly in African American men, because their hair may be curly and leave the skin at a sharp angle.

A Pustules at the opening of the hair follicle are abnormal (Figure 10-11PP).

P Folliculitis is an inflammation of the hair follicle. Figure 10-11PP depicts a staphylococcal folliculitis; however, the causative agent may be fungal and the inflammation therefore called tinea barbae (Figure 10-11QQ).

A Multiple pedunculated papules, nodules, or tumors, which are violaceous and soft (see Figure 10-11RR), are abnormal.

P This describes neurofibromas, one of the hallmark findings of neurofibromatosis, type I (or von Recklinghausen's disease). Six or more café au lait spots are concurrently found on the patient's skin in neurofibromatosis, type I.

E Examination   **N** Normal Findings   **A** Abnormal Findings   **P** Pathophysiology

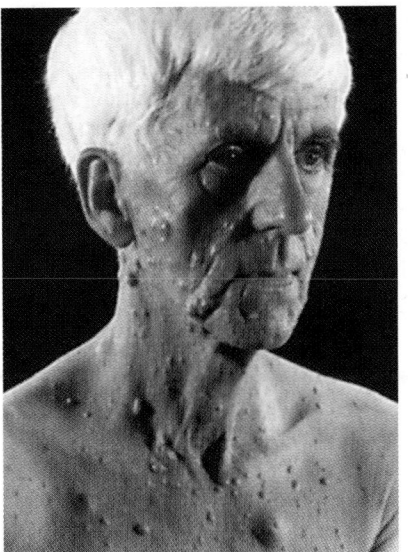

RR. Type I Neurofibromatosis (von Recklinghausen's Disease)

FIGURE 10-11 Common Skin Lesions *continued*

NURSING**ALERT**

Danger Signs in Potentially Cancerous Lesions

1. Rapid change in size
2. Change in coloration
3. Irregular border or butterfly-shaped border
4. Elevation in a previously flat mole
5. Multiple colorations in a lesion
6. Change in surface characteristics, such as oozing
7. Change in sensation, such as pain, itching, or tenderness
8. Change in surrounding skin, such as inflammation or induration
9. Bleeding or ulcerative appearance in a mole

Patient referral is required for any of the above-mentioned abnormal findings because of the risk of carcinoma.

NURSING**TIP**

Wound Healing

Wound healing includes reepithelialization, which is the migration of epithelial cells inward from the wound edges and from any surrounding hair follicles or eccrine glands. Scab formation may prohibit reepithelialization because of diminished moisture. Granulation tissue is a combination of inflammatory cells, new vessels, and white blood cells that forms a matrix at the base of the wound. The granulation tissue provides a foundation on which reepithelialization occurs. Scar formation may take several months. New scars are thick, darkened, and vascular in appearance. Over time, the scar tissue flattens and becomes less vascular; however, old scars remain slightly darker or discolored compared to the surrounding tissue.

NURSING**ALERT**

Stages of Pressure Ulcers

Uniform standards for staging pressure ulcers are used for patients with pressure sores on any portion of the body.

Stage 1 In light-skinned patients, the area is reddened, but the skin is not broken; in dark-skinned patients, the pigmentation is enhanced (Figure 10-12A).

Stage 2 Epidermal and dermal layers have sustained injury (Figure 10-12B).

Stage 3 Subcutaneous tissues have sustained injury (Figure 10-12C).

Stage 4 Muscle tissue and perhaps bone have sustained injury (Figure 10-12D).

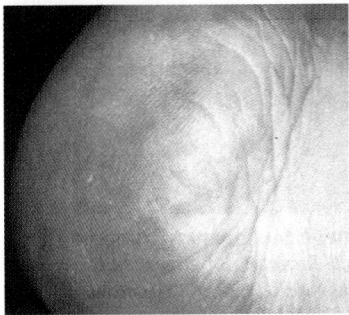

A. Stage 1

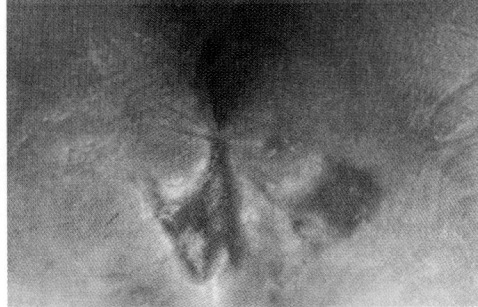

B. Stage 2

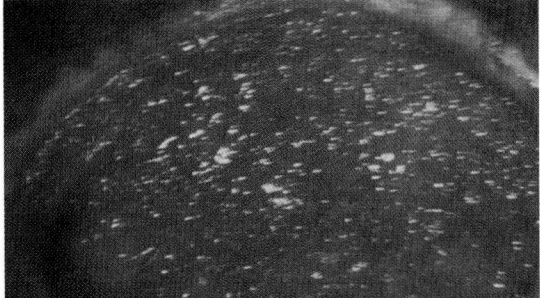

C. Stage 3

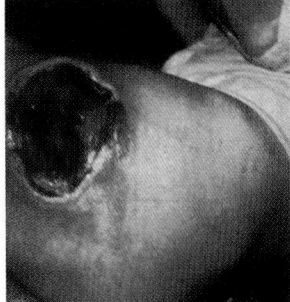

D. Stage 4

FIGURE 10-12 **Pressure Ulcers.** *Courtesy of Emory University Hospital, Atlanta, Georgia.*

A burn patient frequently has varying degrees of injury on the body. Parts of the body may have first-degree burns, and other parts may have second-, third-, or fourth-degree burns. The following descriptions and photographs will assist you in identifying burn injuries:

First-Degree Burn (superficial thickness) (Figure 10-13A): the epidermis is injured or destroyed; there may be some damage to the dermis; hair follicles and sweat glands are intact; the skin is red and dry; painful, no blisters.

Second-Degree Burn (partial thickness, superficial or deep) (Figure 10-13B): the epidermis and upper layers of the dermis are destroyed; the deeper dermis is injured; hair follicles, sweat glands, and nerve endings are intact; the skin is red and blistery with exudate; painful. Blisters are present.

Third-Degree Burn (full thickness) (Figure 10-13C): the epidermis and dermis are destroyed; subcutaneous tissue may be injured; hair follicles, sweat glands, and nerve endings are destroyed; the skin is white, red, black, tan, or brown with a leathery-looking appearance; painless because nerve endings are destroyed.

Fourth-Degree Burn (full thickness) (Figure 10-13D): the epidermis and dermis are destroyed; subcutaneous tissue, muscle, and bone may be injured; hair follicles, sweat glands, and nerve endings are destroyed; the skin is white, red, black, tan, or brown with exposed and damaged subcutaneous tissue, muscle, or bone; painless.

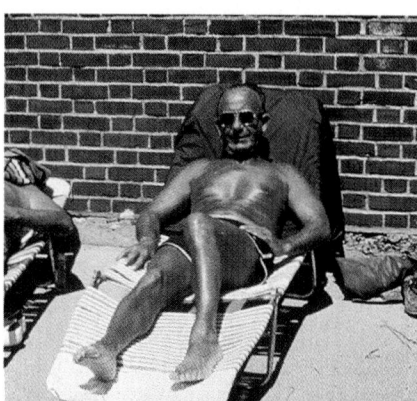

A. First-Degree Burn

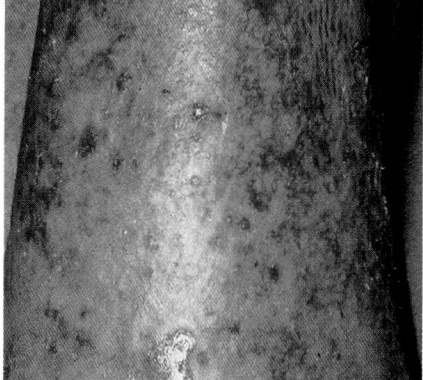

B. Second-Degree Burn

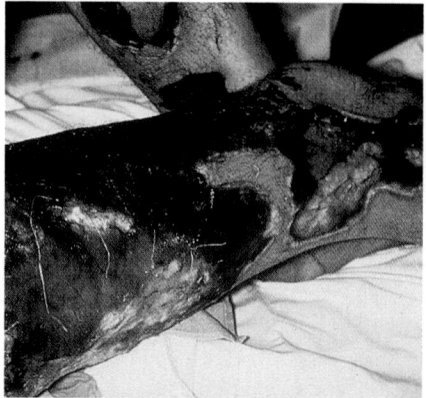

C. Third-Degree Burn

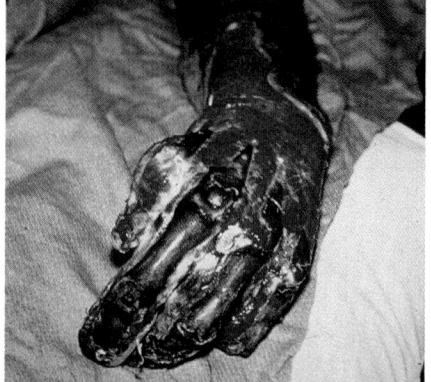

D. Fourth-Degree Burn

FIGURE 10-13 **Types of Burns.** *Courtesy of the Phoenix Society for Burn Survivors, Inc.*

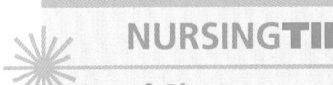

NURSING**TIP**

Use of Gloves

Use gloves for palpation of the skin only if there is any probability of contact with body fluids or if the patient is in isolation.

FIGURE 10-14 **Ichthyosis Vulgaris.**
Courtesy of Robert A. Silverman, M.D., Clinical Associate Professor, Department of Pediatrics, Georgetown University.

PALPATION OF THE SKIN

Moisture

E Palpate all nonmucous membrane skin surfaces for moisture using the dorsal surfaces of the hands and fingers.

N Normally, the skin is dry with a minimum of perspiration. Moisture on the skin will vary from one body area to another, with perspiration normally present on the hands, axilla, face, and in between the skin folds. Moisture also varies with changes in environment, muscular activity, body temperature, stress, and activity levels. Body temperature is regulated by the skin's production of perspiration, which evaporates to cool the body.

A Excessive dryness of the skin, **xerosis**, as evidenced by flaking of the stratum corneum and associated pruritus, is abnormal.

P Hypothyroidism and exposure to extreme cold and dry climates can lead to xerosis.

A Very dry, large scales that are light colored or brown are abnormal (Figure 10-14).

P Ichthyosis vulgaris is a skin abnormality originating from a keratin disorder. It can be associated with atopic dermatitis.

A Diaphoresis is the profuse production of perspiration.

P Causes include hyperthyroidism, increased metabolic rate, sepsis, anxiety, or pain.

Temperature

E Palpate all nonmucosal skin surfaces for temperature using the dorsal surfaces of the hands and fingers.

N Skin surface temperature should be warm and equal bilaterally. Hands and feet may be slightly cooler than the rest of the body.

A **Hypothermia** is a cooling of the skin and may be generalized or localized.

P Generalized hypothermia is indicative of shock or some other type of central circulatory dysfunction. Localized hypothermia is indicative of arterial insufficiency in the affected area.

A Generalized **hyperthermia** is the excessive warming of the skin and may be generalized or localized.

P Generalized hyperthermia may be indicative of a febrile state, hyperthyroidism, or increased metabolic function caused by exercise. Localized hyperthermia may be caused by infection, trauma, sunburn, or windburn.

Tenderness

E Palpate skin surfaces for tenderness using the dorsal surfaces of the hands and fingers.

N Skin surfaces should be nontender.

A Tenderness over the skin structures can be discrete and localized or generalized.

P Discrete tenderness may indicate a localized infection such as cellulitis, and generalized tenderness can indicate systemic illness such as lymphoma or allergic reaction.

E Examination   **N** Normal Findings   **A** Abnormal Findings   **P** Pathophysiology

Texture

E 1. Evaluate the texture of the skin using the finger pads.

2. Evaluate surfaces such as the abdomen and medial surfaces of the arms first.

3. Compare these areas to areas that are covered with hair.

N Skin should normally feel smooth, even, and firm except where there is significant hair growth. A certain amount of roughness can be normal.

A Roughness can occur on exposed areas such as the elbows, the soles of the feet, and the palms of the hands.

P Roughness can be due to wool clothing, cold weather, occupational exposures, or the use of soap. In addition, generalized roughness can be associated with systemic diseases such as scleroderma, hypothyroidism, and amyloidosis. Localized thickening and roughness can be a result of chronic pruritus (lichenification) due to scratching, which causes a thickening of the epidermis.

A Areas of hyperkeratosis and increased roughness that are found in the lower extremities are abnormal.

P This type of texture change may be indicative of peripheral vascular disease, which causes abated circulation and diminished nourishment of cutaneous layers.

A The skin can feel very soft and silk-like.

P Generalized softness can result from hyperthyroidism secondary to elevated metabolism.

Turgor

Palpate the skin **turgor**, or elasticity, which reflects the skin's state of hydration.

E 1. Pinch a small section of the patient's skin between your thumb and forefinger. The anterior chest, under the clavicle, and the abdomen are optimal areas to assess.

2. Slowly release the skin.

3. Observe the speed with which the skin returns to its original contour when released (Figure 10-15).

N When the skin is released, it should return to its original contour rapidly.

A Decreased skin turgor is present when the skin is released and it remains pinched, and slowly returns to its original contour.

P **Dehydration**, or lack of fluid in the tissues, is the main cause of decreased skin turgor. The aging process and scleroderma can also decrease the turgor of the skin.

A Increased turgor or tension causes the skin to return to its original contour too quickly.

P Increased turgor can be indicative of connective tissue disease caused by an increase of granulation tissue.

Edema

Palpate the skin for **edema**, or accumulation of fluid in the intercellular spaces.

E 1. Firmly imprint your thumb against a dependent portion of the body, such as the arms, hands, legs, feet, ankle, or sacrum.

2. Release pressure.

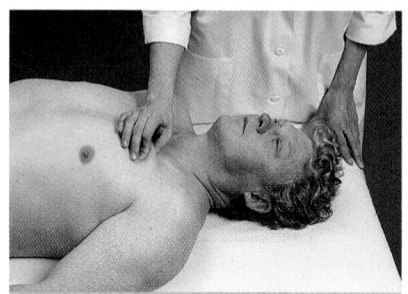

FIGURE 10-15 Assessment of Skin Turgor

NURSING ALERT

Evaluation of Edema

If the edema is severe enough, it can prohibit the evaluation of pathological conditions that are manifested by coloration changes. Two plus (2+) edema warrants referral if it is newly onset. Significant, severe edema (3+–4+) warrants immediate evaluation.

| **E** Examination | **N** Normal Findings | **A** Abnormal Findings | **P** Pathophysiology |

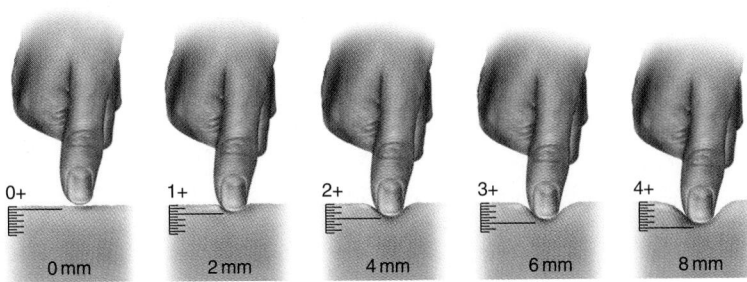

0+ No pitting edema
1+ Mild pitting edema. 2 mm depression that disappears rapidly.
2+ Moderate pitting edema. 4 mm depression that disappears in 10–15 seconds.
3+ Moderately severe pitting edema. 6 mm depression that may last more than 1 minute.
4+ Severe pitting edema. 8 mm depression that can last more than 2 minutes.

FIGURE 10-16 Pitting Edema Grading Scale

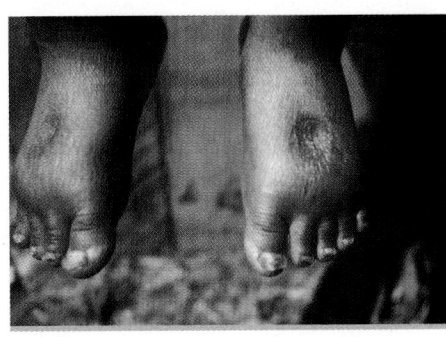

FIGURE 10-17 **Assessment of Pitting Edema.** *Courtesy of the Centers for Disease Control and Prevention.*

3. Observe for an indentation on the skin.

4. Rate the degree of edema. Pitting edema is rated on a 4-point scale (Figure 10-16).

5. Check for symmetry and measure circumference of affected extremities.

N Edema is not normally present.

A Edema is present if the skin feels puffy and tight. It can be localized in one area (Figure 10-17) or generalized throughout the body. There are many different types of edema (Table 10-2).

TABLE 10-2 Types of Edema	
TYPE	**DESCRIPTION**
Pitting	Edema that is present when an indentation remains on the skin after applying pressure
Nonpitting	Edema that is firm with discoloration or thickening of the skin; results when serum proteins coagulate in tissue spaces
Angioedema	Recurring episodes of noninflammatory swelling of skin, brain, viscera, and mucous membranes (Figure 10-18); onset may be rapid, with resolution requiring hours to days
Dependent	Localized increase of extracellular fluid volume in a dependent limb or area
Inflammatory	Swelling due to an extracellular fluid effusion into the tissue surrounding an area of inflammation
Noninflammatory	Swelling or effusion due to mechanical or other causes not related to congestion or inflammation
Lymphedema	Edema due to the obstruction of a lymphatic vessel

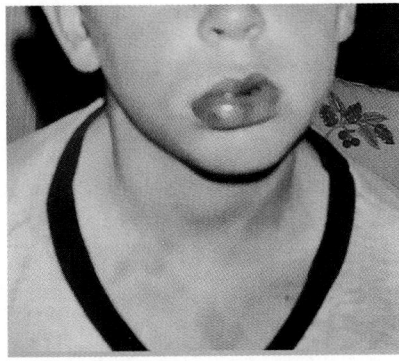

FIGURE 10-18 **Angioedema of the Lips**

P Localized edema may be due to dependency; however, generalized or bilateral edema is caused by increased hydrostatic pressure, decreased capillary osmotic pressure, increased capillary permeability, or obstruction to lymph flow. This occurs in congestive heart failure or kidney failure.

INSPECTION OF THE HAIR

Color

E Inspect scalp hair, eyebrows, eyelashes, and body hair for color.

N Hair varies from dark black to pale blonde based on the amount of melanin present. As melanin production diminishes, hair turns gray. Hair color may also be chemically changed.

A Patches of gray hair that are isolated or occur in conjunction with a scar are abnormal.

P Patches of gray hair not associated with aging can be indicative of nerve damage.

Distribution

E Evaluate the distribution of hair on the body, eyebrows, face, and scalp.

N The body is covered in vellus hair. Terminal hair is found in the eyebrows, eyelashes, and scalp, and in the axilla and pubic areas after puberty. Males may experience a certain degree of normal balding and may also develop terminal facial and chest hair. Native Americans, Asians, and those from the Pacific Rim may have a light distribution of hair.

A The absence of pubic hair, unless purposefully removed, is abnormal in the adult.

P Diminished or absent pubic hair may be indicative of endocrine disorders, such as anterior pituitary adenomas, or chemotherapy.

A Male or female pattern baldness (**alopecia**) may be abnormal in some individuals if associated with pathology. Alopecia areata is a circumscribed bald area (see Figure 10-19A).

P Androgenetic alopecia is a common, progressive hair loss that is caused by a combination of genetic predisposition and androgenetic effects on the hair follicle; however, alopecia may be secondary to chemotherapy and radiation, infection, stress, drug reactions, lupus, and traction. A pathological etiology of alopecia should be ruled out.

A Total scalp baldness, or alopecia totalis, is abnormal.

P Autoimmune diseases, emotional crisis, stress, or heredity can cause alopecia totalis.

A Hair loss in linear formations is abnormal (see Figure 10-19B).

P Linear alopecia can be caused by frequent pressure on hair follicles leading to their inability to produce new hair. In addition, traction alopecia can be caused by the use of curlers and wearing the hair in a tightly pulled ponytail, whereby traction is continually applied. This is common among individuals who wear cornrows.

E Examination   **N** Normal Findings   **A** Abnormal Findings   **P** Pathophysiology

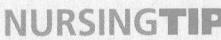
A Excess facial and body hair is abnormal (see Figure 10-19C).

P **Hirsutism** is manifested by excessive body hair. It is indicative of endocrine disorders such as hypersecretion of adrenocortical androgens and polycystic ovary syndrome. In women, this disorder is manifested as excess facial and chest hair.

P Hirsutism can also result as a side effect of medications such as cyclosporin.

A Areas of broken-off hairs in irregular patterns with scaliness, but no infection, are abnormal (see Figure 10-19D).

P Trichotillomania is the manipulation of the hair by twisting and pulling, leading to reduced hair mass. This can be an unconscious action or a sign of psychiatric illness.

A Broken-off hairs with scaliness and follicular inflammation are abnormal (see Figure 10-19E). The area may be painful and purulent with boggy nodules.

P Tinea capitis (ringworm) is a fungal infection, frequently caused by dermatophytic trichomycosis.

A The scalp is covered with yellow-brown scales and crusts. The scalp may be oily. Edema may be present (see Figure 10-19F).

P Seborrheic dermatitis is caused by increased production of sebum by the scalp.

Lesions

E 1. Don gloves and lift the scalp hair by segments.

2. Evaluate the scalp for lesions or signs of infestation.

N The scalp should be pale white to pink in light-skinned individuals and light brown in dark-skinned individuals. There should be no signs of infestation or lesions. **Seborrhea**, commonly known as dandruff, may be present.

A Abnormal manifestations include head lice.

P Head lice (pediculosis capitis) may be distinguished from dandruff in that dandruff can be easily removed from the scalp or hair, whereas nits (see Figure 10-19G), which are the lice larvae, are attached to the hair shaft and are difficult to remove. Both seborrhea and head lice may cause itching.

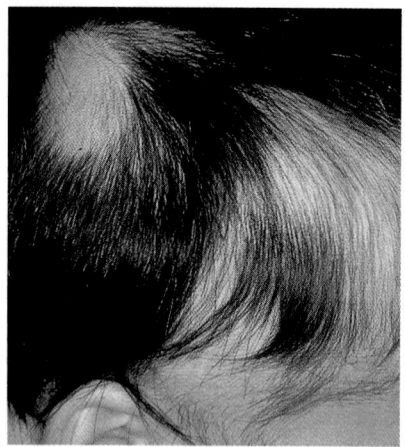

A. Alopecia Areata. *Courtesy of Robert A. Silverman, M.D., Clinical Associate Professor, Department of Pediatrics, Georgetown University.*

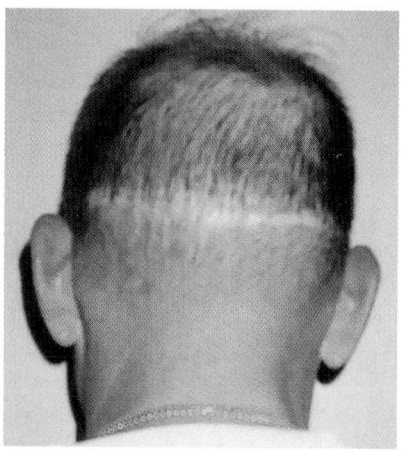

B. Linear alopecia developed in this man from daily wearing of his military uniform cap.

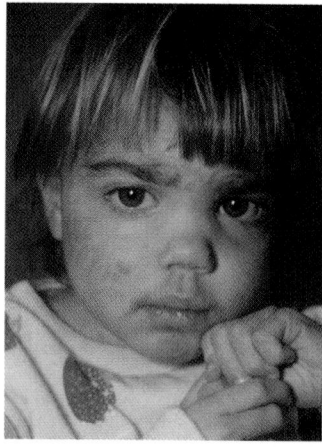

C. Hirsutism Caused by the Drug Cyclosporin. *Courtesy of Robert A. Silverman, M.D., Clinical Associate Professor, Department of Pediatrics, Georgetown University.*

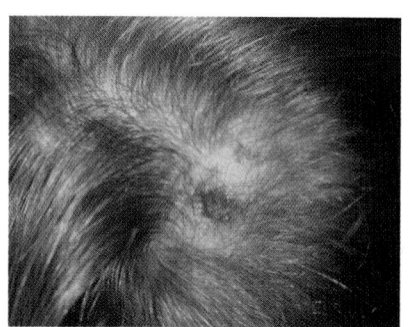

D. Trichotillomania. *Courtesy of Robert A. Silverman, M.D., Clinical Associate Professor, Department of Pediatrics, Georgetown University.*

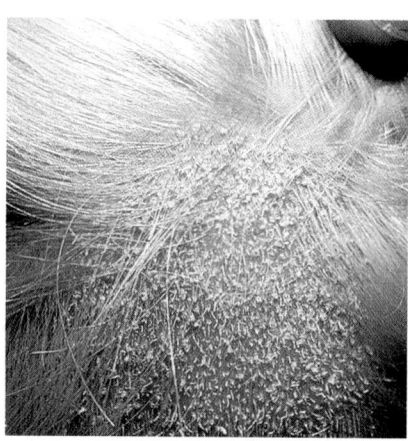

E. Tinea Capitis. *Courtesy of Robert A. Silverman, M.D., Clinical Associate Professor, Department of Pediatrics, Georgetown University.*

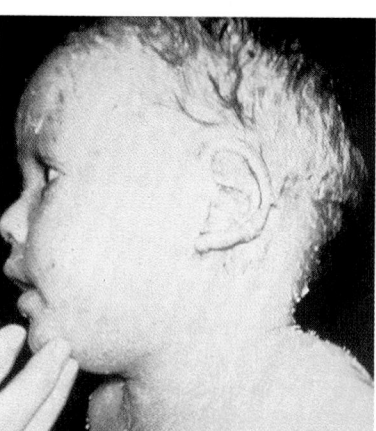

F. Seborrheic Dermatitis. *Courtesy of the Centers for Disease Control and Prevention.*

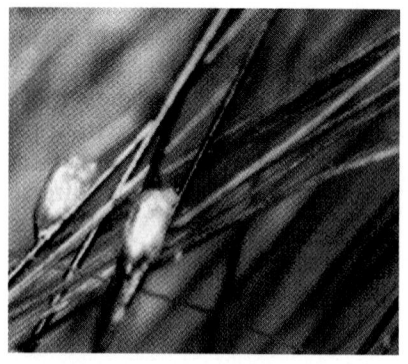

G. Head Lice. *Courtesy of Hogil Pharmaceutical Corporation.*

FIGURE 10-19 **Abnormalities of the Head and Scalp**

PALPATION OF THE HAIR

Texture

E 1. Palpate the hair between your fingertips.

2. Note the condition of the hair from the scalp to the end of the hair.

N Hair may feel thin, straight, coarse, thick, or curly. It should be shiny and resilient when traction is applied and should not come out in clumps in your hands.

A Brittle hair that easily breaks off when pulled or hair that is listless and dull is abnormal.

P Brittle, dull hair or hair that is broken off can be indicative of malnutrition, hyperthyroidism, use of chemicals such as permanents, or infections secondary to damage of the hair follicle.

| **E** Examination | **N** Normal Findings | **A** Abnormal Findings | **P** Pathophysiology |

INSPECTION OF THE NAILS

Color

E 1. Inspect the fingernails and toenails, noting the color of the nails.

2. Check capillary refill by depressing the nail until blanching occurs.

3. Release the nail and evaluate the time required for the nail to return to its previous color.

4. Perform a capillary refill check on all four extremities.

N Normally, the nails have a pink cast in light-skinned individuals and are brown in dark-skinned individuals. Capillary refill is an indicator of peripheral circulation. Normal capillary refill may vary with age, but color should return to normal within 2 to 3 seconds.

A White striations or dots in the nailbed are abnormal (Figure 10-20A).

P Leukonychia (Mees bands) may result from trauma, infections, vascular diseases, psoriasis, and arsenic poisoning.

A An entire nail plate that is white is abnormal (Figure 10-20B).

P Leukonychia totalis may result from hypercalcemia, hypochromic anemia, leprosy, hepatic cirrhosis, and arsenic poisoning.

A A brown color in the nail plate is abnormal (Figure 10-20C).

P Melanonychia may result from Addison's disease and malaria.

A Bluish nails are abnormal.

P Bluish nails may result from cyanosis, venous stasis, and sulfuric acid poisoning.

A Red or brown linear streaks in the nailbed are abnormal (Figure 10-20D).

P Splinter hemorrhages can result from subacute bacterial endocarditis, mitral stenosis, trichinosis, cirrhosis, and nonspecific causes.

A It is abnormal for the proximal end of the nailbed to be white and the distal portion to be pink.

P Lindsey's nails (half-and-half nails) can result from chronic renal failure and hypoalbuminemia.

A A yellow or white hue in a hyperkeratotic nailbed is abnormal (Figure 10-20E).

P Onychomycosis is a fungal infection of the nail.

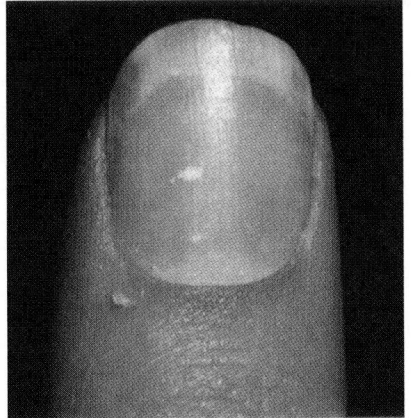

A. Leukonychia

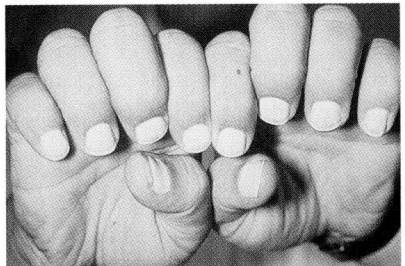

B. Leukonychia Totalis. *Courtesy of Robert A. Silverman, M.D., Clinical Associate Professor, Department of Pediatrics, Georgetown University.*

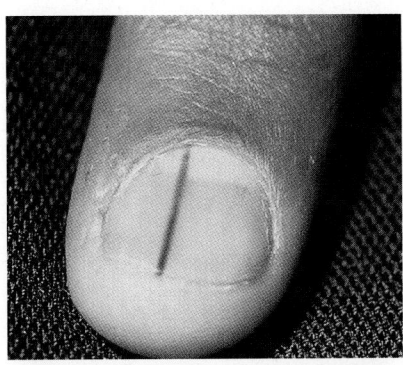

C. Longitudinal Melanonychia. *Courtesy of Robert A. Silverman, M.D., Clinical Associate Professor, Department of Pediatrics, Georgetown University.*

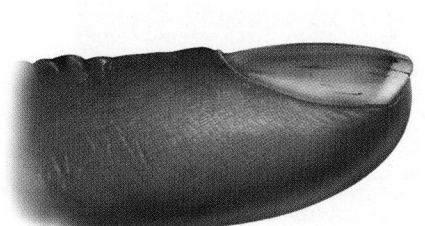

D. Splinter Hemorrhages

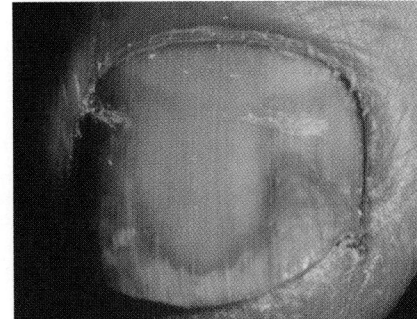

E. Onychomycosis. *Courtesy of Robert A. Silverman, M.D., Clinical Associate Professor, Department of Pediatrics, Georgetown University.*

FIGURE 10-20 Abnormal Color Changes of the Nailbed

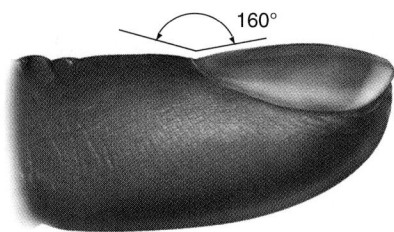

A. Normal Nail Angle

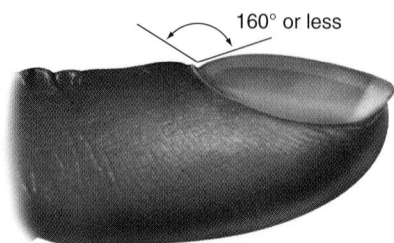

B. Curved Nail Variant of Normal

FIGURE 10-21 **Evaluate the angle of the nail base.**

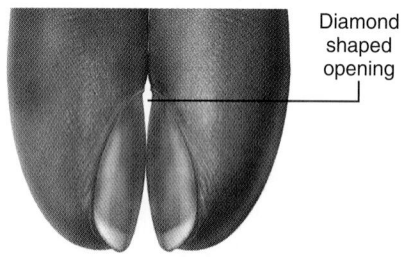

Diamond shaped opening

FIGURE 10-22 **Assess the nailbeds' configuration.**

Shape and Configuration

E 1. Assess the fingernails and toenails for shape, configuration, and consistency.

2. View the profile of the middle finger and evaluate the angle of the nail base (Figure 10-21).

3. Have the patient bring the distal phalanxes together, as illustrated in Figure 10-22. Note the position of the nailbeds in relation to each other.

N The nail surface should be smooth and slightly rounded or flat. Curved nails are a normal variant. Nail thickness should be uniform throughout, with no splintering or brittle edges. The angle of the nail base should be approximately 160°. Longitudinal ridging is a normal variant. There is a diamond-shaped opening at the base of the nailbeds in nails that are normal when assessed, as in Figure 10-22.

A An angle of the nail base greater than 160°, along with sponginess of the nailbed, is abnormal.

A Nailbeds that do not meet medially and do not have a diamond-shaped opening at their base are abnormal (Figure 10-23).

P Clubbing can result from long-standing hypoxia and lung cancer.

A Thin nail plates with cuplike depressions and concave, or spoon-shaped, nails are abnormal (see Figure 10-24A).

P Koilonychia can result from iron deficiency anemia, chronic infections, malnutrition, or Raynaud's disease.

A A transverse furrow in the nail plate is abnormal (see Figure 10-24B).

P Beau's line is caused by an arrest of nail growth at the matrix. It can be associated with an acute phase of an infectious disease, malnutrition, and anemia.

A Separation of the nail from the nailbed is abnormal (see Figure 10-24C).

P Onycholysis can result from hypo- and hyperthyroidism, repeated trauma, Raynaud's disease, syphilis, eczema, and acrocyanosis.

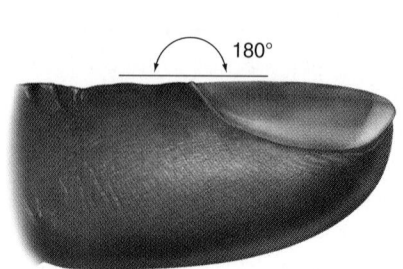

A. Early Clubbing

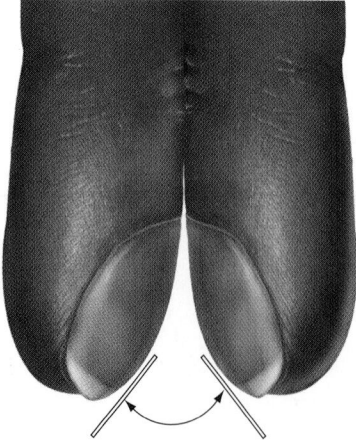

B. Clubbing Seen From a Lateral View

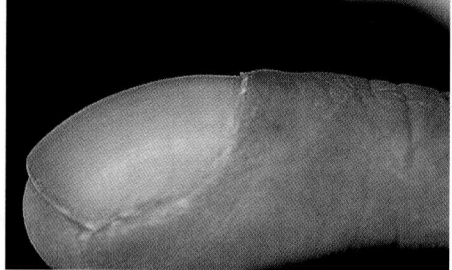

C. Established Clubbing. *Courtesy of Robert A. Silverman, M.D., Clinical Associate Professor, Department of Pediatrics, Georgetown University.*

FIGURE 10-23 **Clubbing**

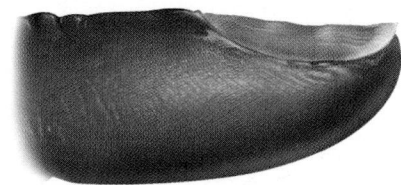

A. Koilonychia

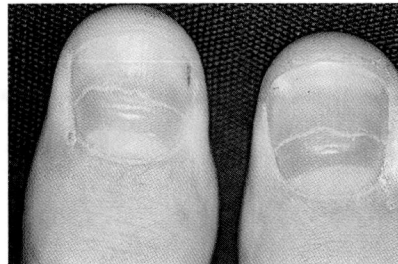

B. Beau's Lines. *Courtesy of Robert A. Silverman, M.D., Clinical Associate Professor, Department of Pediatrics, Georgetown University.*

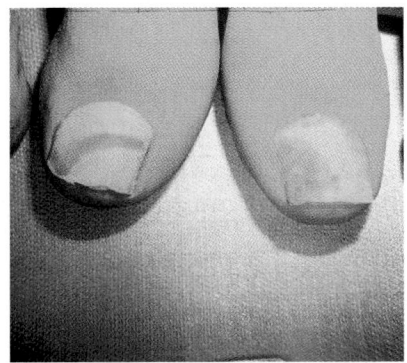

C. Onycholysis with Hyperkeratosis.
Courtesy of Judith A. Mysliborski, M.D., Albany, NY.

A Painful, red swelling of the nail fold is abnormal (Figure 10-24D).

P Paronychia can be caused by *Candida albicans*, bacteria, and repeated exposure of the nails to moisture.

A Numerous horizontal depression ridges or a depression down the middle of the nail is abnormal.

P Habit tic deformity is caused by continuous picking of the cuticle and nail by a finger of the same hand. Trauma ensues to the nail base and nail matrix.

A Purpura or ecchymosis under the nail plate is abnormal (Figure 10-24E).

P Subungual hematoma is caused by trauma to the digit and nail, leading to hemorrhage into the matrix and nailbed.

A The distal portion of the nail plate is embedded in periungual tissues (Figure 10-24F). The periungual tissues may become inflamed and have purulent discharge.

P Onychocryptosis (ingrown nail) is caused by growth of the distal nail plate into periungual tissues, secondary to increased lateral nail pressure, resulting in trauma to the tissues.

A Nails that become white, thin, and curved under the free edge are abnormal (Figure 10-24G).

P Eggshell nails may be caused by systemic diseases, medications, dietary deficiencies, nervous disorders, or sleeping with the hand fisted.

A Nails that atrophy, shrink, and fall off are abnormal (Figure 10-24H).

P Onychatrophia may result from injury to the nail matrix and from systemic diseases.

A Nails that hypertrophy (become abnormally thick and overgrown) are abnormal (Figure 10-24I).

P Onychauxis is caused by systemic infection, electrolyte imbalance, and hereditary predisposition.

A Nails deformed in shape are abnormal (Figure 10-24J).

P Onychophagy results from excessive biting of the nails.

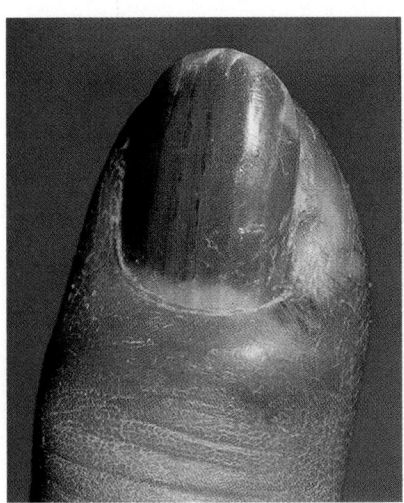

D. Paronychia

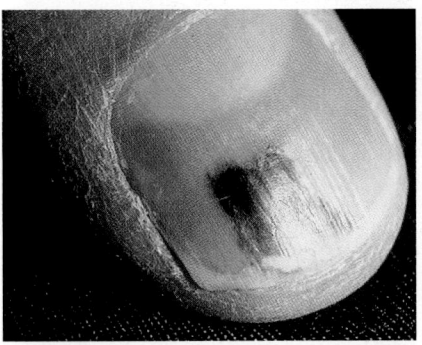

E. Subungual Hematoma. *Courtesy of Robert A. Silverman, M.D., Clinical Associate Professor, Department of Pediatrics, Georgetown University.*

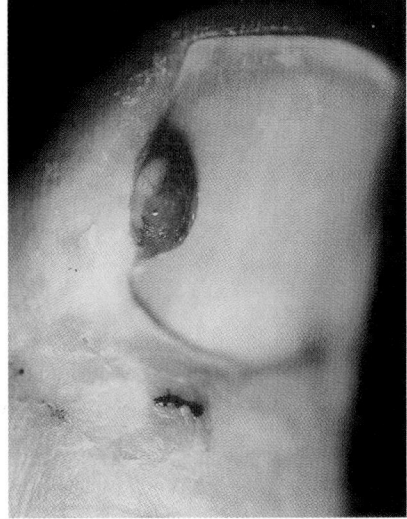

F. Ingrown Nail

FIGURE 10-24 **Abnormalities of the Shape and Configuration of the Nail** *continues*

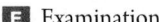

E Examination   **N** Normal Findings   **A** Abnormal Findings   **P** Pathophysiology

1. Place a drop of mineral oil on a sterile #15 scalpel blade.

2. Scrape the suspected papule or known scabies burrow vigorously in order to excavate the top of the papule or burrow. Flecks of blood will mix with the oil.

3. Place some of the oil and skin scrapings onto a microscope slide and cover with a cover slip.

4. Examine the slide for mites, ova, or feces.

A A nail that is split or brittle with lengthwise ridges is abnormal (Figure 10-24K).

P Onychorrhexis may result from trauma to the nail, toxic exposure to solvents, or harsh nail filing.

A It is abnormal for the cuticle to overgrow the nail and become attached to the nail (Figure 10-24L). The cuticle growth may persist to the free edge.

P Pterygium can occur in Raynaud's disease.

PALPATION OF THE NAILS

Texture

E 1. Palpate the nail base between your thumb and index finger.

2. Note the consistency.

N The nail base should be firm on palpation.

A A spongy nail base is an early indication of clubbing.

P Clubbing is the result of impaired tissue oxygenation over a prolonged period of time, as in chronic bronchitis, emphysema, and heart disease. See Chapters 15 and 16 for further information.

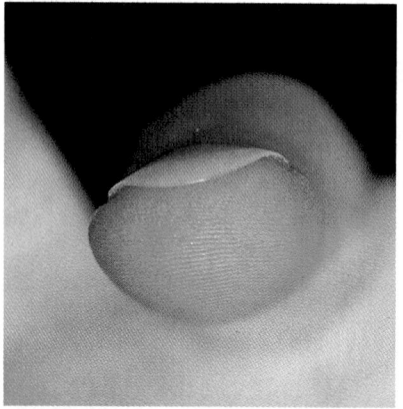

G. Eggshell Nail

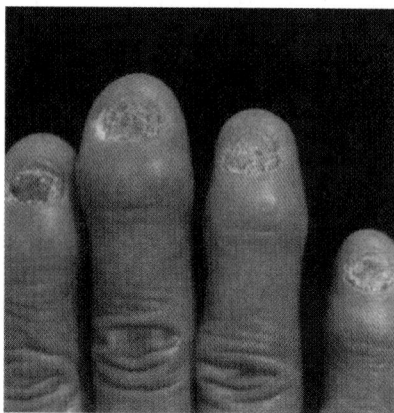

H. Onychatrophia

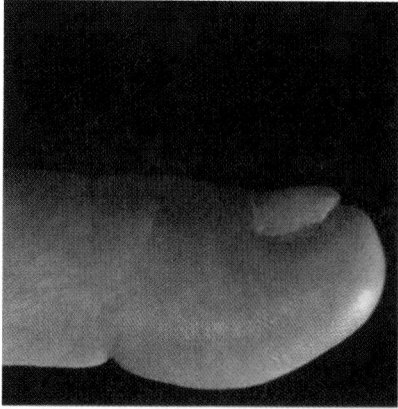

I. Onychauxis

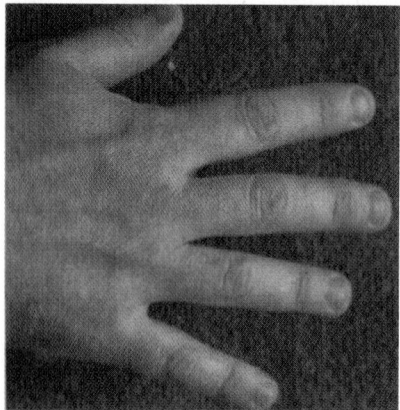

J. Onychophagy

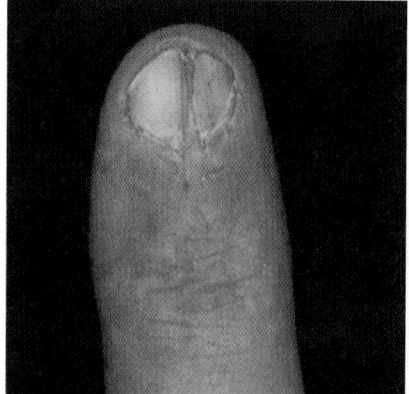

K. Onychorrhexis

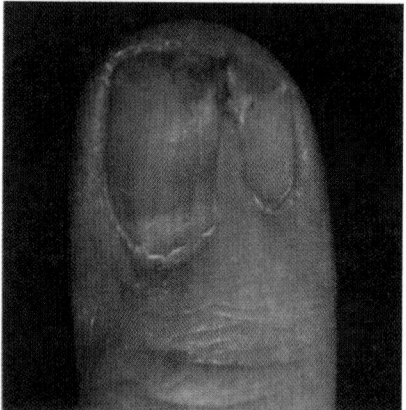

L. Pterygium

FIGURE 10-24 **Abnormalities of the Shape and Configuration of the Nail** *continued*

| 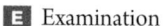 Examination | 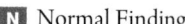 Normal Findings | 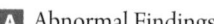 Abnormal Findings | 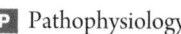 Pathophysiology |

The Patient with Herpes Zoster

This case study illustrates the application and objective documentation of the skin, hair, and nails assessment.
Arjetta presents with an abdominal rash.

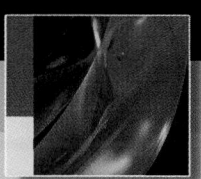

HEALTH HISTORY

PATIENT PROFILE   62 yo MHF

CHIEF COMPLAINT   "I have this painful rash on my lower tummy."

HISTORY OF PRESENT ILLNESS   4 days ago, pt reported burning RLQ pain, malaise, and a 99.5°F temperature. The pain started as a 1–2/10 and progressed over the next 24 hrs to 8/10. Pt denied radiation of pain, or N/V/D, constipation. Denies h/o Crohn's dz, ulcerative colitis, and diverticulitis; pt still has appendix. Ibuprofen did not help the pain. Nothing made the pain worse. Pt was concerned and went to the local ED, fearful of appendicitis. Pt had blood work and an abd CT, which were neg. Pt was sent home c̄ instructions to follow up c̄ her PCP. Last night, pt noted a rash on her lower abd and presents today for evaluation.

PAST HEALTH HISTORY

Medical History   Hypothyroidism age 52
Malaria age 35 and multiple times since
Eczema since age 12

Surgical History   Wisdom teeth extraction age 19 s̄ sequelae

Allergies   Denies medication, bee sting/insect, food, and environmental

Medications   Levothyroxine 100 mcg po q AM
Hydrocortisone valerate 0.2% cream bid prn to affected areas
MVI prn
Ca⁺⁺ 500 mg po bid prn
Ibuprofen 200–600 mg po prn q 6 hrs

Communicable Diseases   Denies

Injuries and Accidents   Wrist fx age 12 when she fell jumping over a fence; mother "rigged" up a splint for her; never had medical care for the fx
Husband has sutured her in various places over the course of their married life when she has had deep cuts.

Special Needs   Denies

Blood Transfusions   Denies

Childhood Diseases   Not sure—had a few illnesses c̄ rashes and fever

continues

CASE STUDY (Continued)

The Patient with Herpes Zoster

Immunizations	No immunizations as a child due to economic status; also, mother did not believe in vaccinations; believes she was fully immunized at age 23 ā she went overseas; since age 23, has received whatever she was told to get for her job (location dependent)

FAMILY HEALTH HISTORY

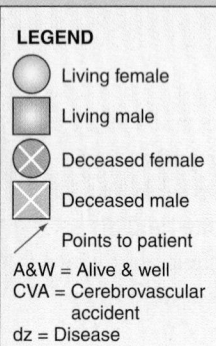

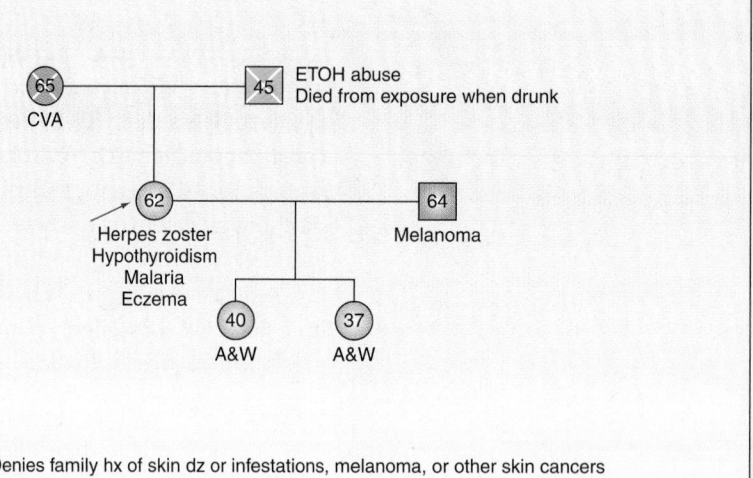

LEGEND
- Living female
- Living male
- Deceased female
- Deceased male
- Points to patient

A&W = Alive & well
CVA = Cerebrovascular accident
dz = Disease
ETOH = Ethanol alcohol

65 CVA — 45 ETOH abuse / Died from exposure when drunk

62 Herpes zoster / Hypothyroidism / Malaria / Eczema — 64 Melanoma

40 A&W   37 A&W

Denies family hx of skin dz or infestations, melanoma, or other skin cancers

SOCIAL HISTORY

Alcohol Use	Denies; has aversion to those who drink even in moderation
Tobacco Use	Denies
Drug Use	Denies
Domestic and Intimate Partner Violence	States she was physically abused by her father growing up; he frequently came home drunk and would "beat up" her and her mother; denies sexual abuse
Sexual Practice	Husband of 40 yrs only partner
Travel History	Pt has lived and worked in 3rd-world countries most of her adult life; refer to work environment
Work Environment	Pt lived in the US until her mid-20s. She and her husband were missionaries and lived in Bolivia, the Philippines, Kenya, and Papua New Guinea. Usually, she was miles from public transportation and medical care. In severe instances, the missionary headquarters would evacuate via helicopter if available. She has lived and worked in the most rural and primitive environments. Pt and husband returned to the U.S. 2 yrs ago. She works PT for the mission at her home and travels around the region speaking to various churches.

continues

CASE STUDY (Continued)

The Patient with Herpes Zoster

Home Environment	Currently resides in 1-level house c̄ all modern appliances; has lived in various houses throughout her life, ranging from mud-hut houses, to wood houses with no running water or any appliances
Hobbies and Leisure Activities	Enjoys sewing clothes for grandchildren and reading
Stress	Current pain; would like to repair re/ship c̄ older daughter
Education	HS grad
Economic Status	"We don't need much. We are fine." Has retirement pension
Military Service	Denies
Religion	Evangelical Christian; "God is the most important focus in my life. God is the reason for my being."
Ethnic Background	Hispanic; parents are from Peru
Roles and Relationships	Happily married for 40 yrs to husband. "He is my soul mate. The Lord put us together, and together we have grown closer to Him." Enjoys re/ship c̄ younger daughter and her 3 grandchildren, who live 30 miles away. "I pray that the Lord will repair my re/ship c̄ my older daughter. Her faith in the Lord is strong, but we have never seemed able to communicate." Older daughter lives in Bolivia. Pt sees her for 3 mos every other yr when she is home on furlough.
Characteristic Patterns of Daily Living	States her schedule changes daily. The most important times of her day are her prayer time and the time spent c̄ her husband. Her commitment to these never waivers.
HEALTH MAINTENANCE ACTIVITIES	
Sleep	Has difficulty falling asleep and staying asleep; never tried any sleep aid
Diet	Predominantly vegetarian; does not oppose the consumption of meat, but got used to going s̄ for so many yrs in the past that she forgets to buy meat for meals
Exercise	Walks 30–60 minutes daily, weather permitting
Stress Management	"I pray."
Use of Safety Devices	Wears seat belt
Health Check-ups	"In the past, I always had medical checks ā we went overseas, now I just seek medical care when I am sick . . . really sick."

continues

CASE STUDY (Continued)

The Patient with Herpes Zoster

PHYSICAL ASSESSMENT

Inspection of Skin

Color
Uniformly brown

Bleeding, Ecchymosis, and Vascularity
No bleeding, ecchymosis, or ↑ vascularity

Lesions
20–30 vesicles of varying sizes over lower abd, dermatomal level T 9–10 with extended base of erythema; mild edema of area, no crusting of vesicles

Palpation of the Skin

Moisture
Mild xerosis

Temperature
Hands/feet/trunk all warm and =

Tenderness
Nontender $\bar{x}$ for hyperesthesia in regions inferior and superior to abd lesions

Texture
Smooth

Turgor
Skin returns to original contour immediately.

Edema
No edema $\bar{x}$ as noted above

Inspection of the Hair

Color
Black $\bar{c}$ gray roots, shiny

Distribution
Ø hirsutism or alopecia

Lesions
Ø infestations

Palpation of Hair

Texture
Mildly coarse, Ø brittle

Inspection of Nails

Color
Light brown $\bar{c}$ brisk cap refill

Shape and Configuration
Smooth and flat; no splintering or brittle edges; nail edge less than 160°

Palpation of Nails

Texture
Firm

ASSESSMENT IN BRIEF

Skin, Hair, and Nails Assessment

Inspection of the Skin

- Color
- Bleeding, ecchymosis, and vascularity
- Lesions

Palpation of the Skin

- Moisture
- Temperature
- Tenderness
- Texture
- Turgor
- Edema

Inspection of the Hair

- Color
- Distribution
- Lesions

Palpation of the Hair

- Texture

Inspection of the Nails

- Color
- Shape and configuration

Palpation of the Nails

- Texture

Advanced Technique

- Skin scraping for scabies

REVIEW QUESTIONS

1. Which layer of the skin is found exclusively on the palmar and plantar surfaces and aids in the formation of keratin?

   a. Stratum corneum   c. Stratum spinosum
   b. Stratum lucidum   d. Stratum germinativum
   The correct answer is (b).

2. Which integumentary structure is responsible for sweat gland secretion in the axillary, genital, and rectal areas?

   a. Apocrine glands   c. Eccrine glands
   b. Arrector pili muscles d. Periungal tissues
   The correct answer is (a).

3. While inspecting the skin of a patient, you note thick, leathery-looking skin in the back of the neck and on the abdomen. What medical condition might you suspect this patient has?

   a. Psoriasis   c. Ichthyosis vulgaris
   b. Second-degree burns d. Diabetes mellitus
   The correct answer is (d).

4. A patient complains of pruritus all over the body. You note polycyclic lesions arranged in concentric circles resembling a bull's-eye. What is a possible etiology of these lesions?

   a. Ringworm   c. Drug reaction
   b. Herpes zoster   d. Dermatitis
   The correct answer is (c).

5. While conducting the health history interview, you note that the patient repeatedly scratches her left forearm. You ask the patient about her scratching, and she tells you that she is constantly itchy and the scratching helps relieve the itch temporarily. What skin change would you expect to see in this area?

   a. Crusting   c. Atrophy
   b. Lichenification   d. Scaling
   The correct answer is (b).

6. Macular patches of white, reddish-brown, or tan hyperpigmentation that occur in the posterior thorax are most likely caused by which of the following?

   a. Fungal infection   c. *Streptococcus* infection
   b. *Staphylococcus* infection d. Syphilis infection
   The correct answer is (a).

7. A chronic superficial inflammation of the face and extremities that evolves into pruritic, red, weeping, crusted lesions is usually associated with which of the following conditions?

a. Contaminated clothing and bedding

b. Poison oak contact

c. Cold weather and trauma

d. Asthma and allergic rhinitis

The correct answer is (d).

8. The classic skin lesion that may be seen in Lyme disease is best described by which of the following findings?

a. A maculopapular rash with erythemic borders that appears first on the wrists

b. A blotchy maculopapular rash that appears first on the cheeks

c. A red papule that progresses to an erythematous circular lesion with central clearing

d. Flesh-colored, hyperkeratotic papules that are slightly umbilicated

The correct answer is (c).

9. A patient in congestive heart failure is noted to have 3^+ pitting edema. This means that the nurse was able to indent a finger to what depth into the patient's foot?

a. 2 mm   c. 6 mm

b. 4 mm   d. 8 mm

The correct answer is (c).

10. A 43-year-old male bites his nails during the health history interview. You inquire about this practice, and the patient tells you that he has been doing this since his teen years. What condition would you expect to find on inspection of the nails?

a. Onychatrophia   c. Onychorrhexis

b. Onychauxis   d. Onychophagy

The correct answer is (d).

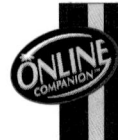

Visit the Estes online companion resource at **www.delmar.cengage.com** for additional content and study aids. Click on Online Companions and then select the Nursing discipline.

REFERENCE

Carroll, S. T., Riffenburgh, R. H., Roberts, T. A., & Myhre, E. B. (2002). Tattoos and body piercings as indicators of adolescent risk-taking behaviors. *Pediatrics, 109*, 1021–1027.

BIBLIOGRAPHY

Babic, M. J. (2007). Eczema vaccinatum: A reaction to the smallpox vaccine. *The American Journal of Nursing, 107*(8), 30–31.

Barber, S. (2008). A clinically relevant wound assessment method to monitor healing progression. *Ostomy Wound Management, 54*(3), 42–49.

Depietropaolo, D. L., Powers, J. H., Gill, J. M., & Foy, A. J. (2005). Diagnosis of Lyme disease. *American Family Physician, 72*(2), 297–304, 309.

Ersser, S. J., Getliffe, K., Voegeli, D., & Regan, S. (2005). A critical review of the interrelationship between skin vulnerability and urinary incontinence and related nursing interventions. *International Journal of Nursing Studies, 42*(7), 823–835.

Flinders, D. C., & de Schweinitz, P. (2004). Pediculosis and scabies. *American Family Physician, 69*(2), 341–350.

Frankel, D. H. (2006). *Field guide to clinical dermatology* (2nd ed.). Philadelphia: Lippincott Willams & Wilkins.

Guillen, S., & Khachemoune, A. (2006). Psoriasis: Disease management with a brief review of new biologies. *Dermatology Nursing, 18*(1), 40–43.

Habif, T. P. (2004). *Clinical dermatology: A color guide to diagnosis and treatment* (4th ed.). St. Louis: Mosby.

Klevins, R. M., Morrison, M. A., Nadle, J., Petit, S., Gershman, K., Ray, S., et al. (2007). Invasive Methicillin-resistant *Staphylococcus aureus* infections in the United States. *JAMA, 298*(15), 1763–1771.

Mendyk, M. K. (2008). Community-associated MRSA: Coming to a patient near you? *The Nurse Practitioner: The American Journal of Primary Health Care, 33*(3), 32–33.

Moore, J., & Miller, C. B. (2007). Skin, hair, and other infections associated with visits to barber's shops and hairdressing salons. *American Journal of Infection Control, 35*(3), 203–204.

Oxman, M. N., Levin, M. J., Johnson, G. R., et al., for the Shingles Prevention Study Group. (2005). A vaccine to prevent herpes zoster and postherpetic neuralgia in older adults. *NEJM, 352*(22), 2271–2284.

Rhoads, J. (2007). Epidemiology of the brown recluse spider bite. *The Journal of the American Academy of Nurse Practitioners, 19*(2), 79–87.

Scudder, L., & Edmunds, M. W. (2006). Addressing the physical and mental symptoms of shingles. *The Journal for Nurse Practitioners, 2*(4), 229–235.

Singer, A., Lee, C., & Thode, H. Jr. (2006). Epidemiology of burns in the ED, 1996–2004. *Annals of Emergency Medicine, 50*(3), S63–S65.

Wolff, K., Johnson, R. A., & Suurmond, R. (2005). *Fitzpatrick's color atlas & synopsis of clinical dermatology* (5th ed.). New York: McGraw Hill.

Xu, F., Sternberg, M. R., Kotteri, B. J., McQuillan, G. M., Lee, F. K., Nahmias, A. J., et al. (2006). Trends in herpes simplex virus type 1 and type 2 seroprevalence in the United States. *JAMA, 296*(8), 964–973.

WEB SITES

American Burn Association:
   http://www.ameriburn.org

American Cancer Society:
   http://www.cancer.org

Dermatology Nurses' Association:
   http://www.dnanurse.org

Dermatology Nursing Institute:
   http://www.dermatologynursing.net

International Society for Burn Injuries:
   http://www.worldburn.org

National Pressure Ulcer Advisory Panel:
   http://www.npuap.org

Skin Cancer Foundation:
   http://www.skincancer.org

CHAPTER 11

Head, Neck, and Regional Lymphatics

COMPETENCIES

1. Identify the anatomic structures of the head and neck.

2. Identify the lymph nodes of the head and neck.

3. Describe the system-specific health history for the head and neck.

4. Demonstrate the physical examination of the head and neck.

5. Describe normal findings in the physical assessment of the head and neck.

6. List common abnormalities found in physical assessment of the head and neck.

7. Explain the pathophysiology of common abnormalities found in physical assessment of the head and neck.

Assessment of the head and neck is the gateway to a wide range of critical clues about the functions of various body systems. As you assess the head and neck, you will learn about the skin, endocrine function, musculoskeletal integrity, and neurological function.

ANATOMY AND PHYSIOLOGY

The skull, face, neck, thyroid, lymphatics, and blood supply are discussed in the following sections.

SKULL

The skull is a complex bony structure that rests on the superior end of the vertebral column (Figure 11-1). The skull protects the brain from direct injury and provides a surface for the attachment of the muscles that assist with mastication and produce facial expressions.

Cranial bones of the skull are connected by immovable joints called **sutures**. The most prominent sutures are the coronal suture, the sagittal suture, and the lambdoidal suture. The junction of the coronal and sagittal sutures is called the **bregma**.

FACE

The face of every individual has its own unique characteristics influenced by factors such as race, state of health, emotions, and environment. Facial structures are symmetrical so that the eyes, eyebrows, nose, mouth, nasolabial folds, and palpebral fissures look the same on both sides.

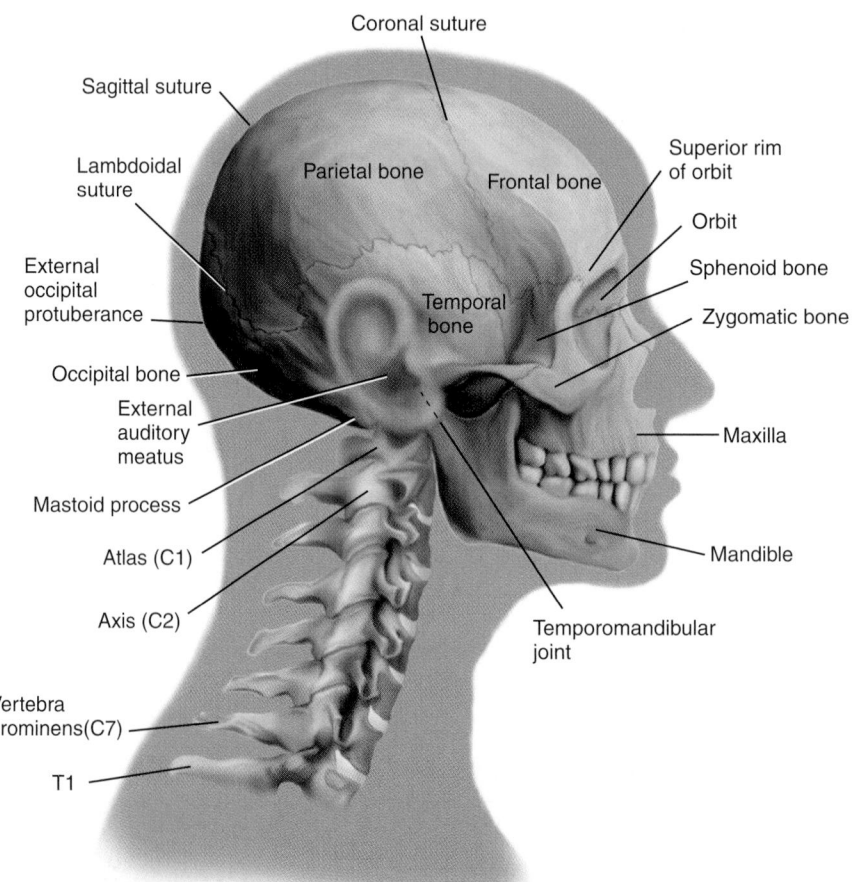

FIGURE 11-1 **Bones of the Face and Skull (Lateral View)**

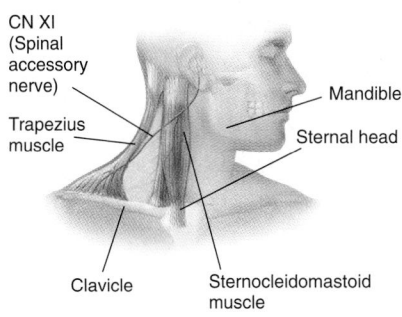

FIGURE 11-2 **Major Cervical Muscles**

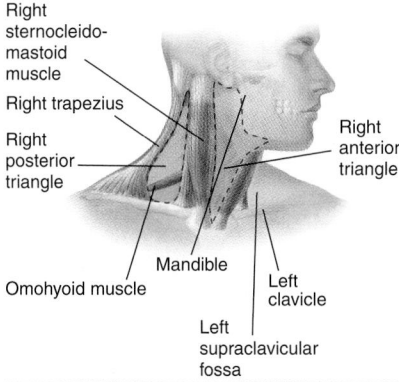

FIGURE 11-3 **Anterior and Posterior Cervical Triangles**

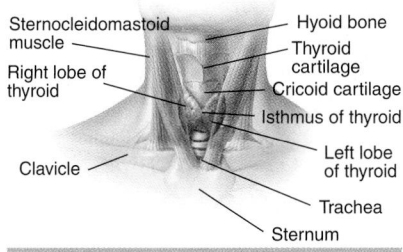

FIGURE 11-4 **Structures of the Thyroid Gland**

NECK

The neck is made up of seven flexible cervical vertebrae that support the head while allowing it maximum mobility. The first cervical vertebra, the **atlas**, articulates with the occipital condyles to support and balance the head. The second vertebra, the **axis**, has an odontoid process that extends into the ring of the atlas, allowing it to pivot as the head is turned from side to side. The seventh cervical vertebra has a long spinous process called the **vertebra prominens**, which serves as a useful landmark during physical assessment of the neck, back, and thorax.

The major muscles of the neck are the sternocleidomastoids and the trapezii (Figure 11-2). The sternocleidomastoid muscles extend from the upper portion of the sternum and the clavicle to the mastoid process and allow the head to bend laterally, rotate, flex, and extend. They also divide each side of the neck into two triangles: the anterior cervical and the posterior cervical, which serve as assessment landmarks. The **anterior triangle** is formed by the mandible, the trachea, and the sternocleidomastoid muscle and contains the anterior cervical lymph nodes, the trachea, and the thyroid gland. The **posterior triangle**, the area between the sternocleidomastoid and the trapezius muscles with the clavicle at the base, contains the posterior cervical lymph nodes (Figure 11-3).

The trapezii extend from the occipital bone down the neck to insert at the outer third of the clavicles, at the acromion process of the scapula, and along the spinal column to the level of T12. They allow the shoulders and scapula to move up and down, and rotate the scapula medially.

THYROID

The thyroid gland, the largest endocrine gland in the body, secretes thyroxine (T_4) and triiodothyronine (T_3), which regulate the rate of cellular metabolism. The gland, a flattened, butterfly-shaped structure with two lateral lobes connected by the **isthmus**, weighs about 25 to 30 grams and is slightly larger in females (Figure 11-4). The isthmus rests on top of the trachea, inferior to the cricoid cartilage.

LYMPHATICS

An extensive system of lymphatic vessels drains the head and neck and is an important part of the immune system (Figure 11-5). Lymphatic tissue in the nodes is responsible for the filtering and sequestration of pathogens and other harmful substances. Lymph nodes are usually less than 1 cm, round or ovoid in shape, and smooth in

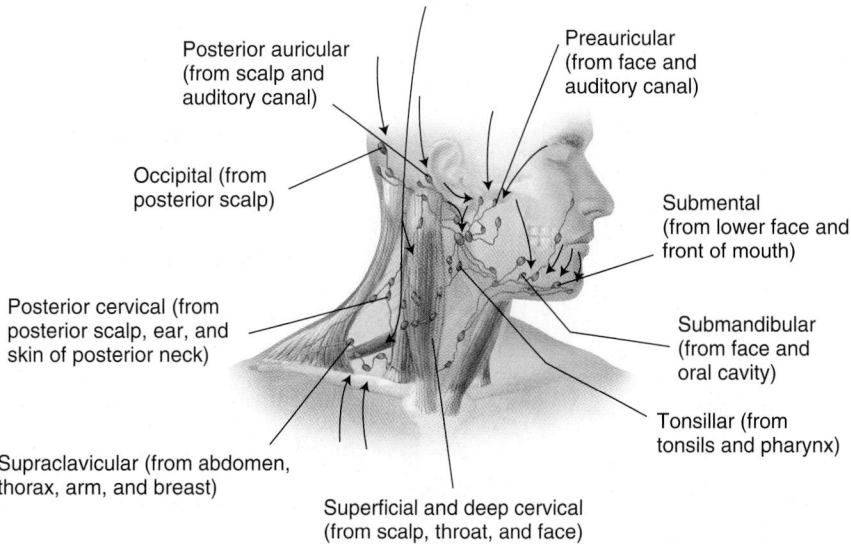

FIGURE 11-5 **Lymph Nodes of the Head and Neck and Drainage Patterns**

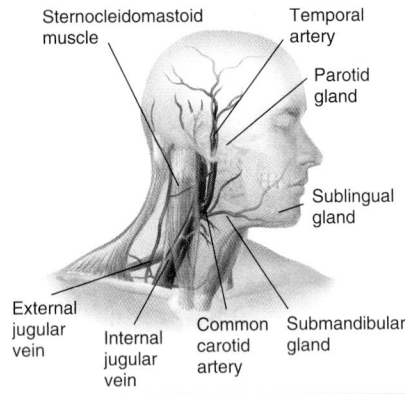

Sternocleidomastoid muscle
Temporal artery
Parotid gland
Sublingual gland
External jugular vein
Internal jugular vein
Common carotid artery
Submandibular gland

FIGURE 11-6 Major Veins and Arteries of the Neck

consistency. When nodes are enlarged or tender, it is important to assess for infection or malignancy. Note the direction in which each node drains (Figure 11-5). If a tender or enlarged lymph node is found on the clinical examination, assess the entire lymph node area, as well as the area that the involved node drains. For example, if a patient's posterior cervical node is enlarged, examine the posterior scalp, the ear (both externally and internally), and the skin of the posterior neck for pathology.

BLOOD SUPPLY

The blood supply to the head and neck is quite extensive, with arterial and venous patterns. Major arteries that carry blood to the head and neck include the common carotids (which bifurcate into the internal and external carotid arteries), the brachiocephalic artery (the right common carotid artery branches from this), the subclavian arteries, and the temporal arteries. Deoxygenated blood from the head and neck is returned to the heart via the internal and external jugular veins, the brachiocephalic vein, and the subclavian veins (Figure 11-6).

NURSING**TIP**

Cranial Nerve Assessment

The 12 cranial nerves that innervate the head and neck are integrated into this portion of the examination; see also Chapters 12 and 19.

HEALTH HISTORY

The head and neck health history provides insight into the link between a patient's life/lifestyle, and head and neck information and pathology.

PATIENT PROFILE

Diseases that are age- and gender-specific for the head and neck are listed.

Age

Lymphadenopathies related to Hodgkin's disease (11–29 years)
Cervical spine trauma (young adults)
Hyperthyroidism (reproductive years in young women)
Temporal arteritis (elderly)
Decreased mobility of the cervical spine related to an inflammatory or degenerative process (elderly)

Gender

Female

Hypo- or hyperthyroidism, thyroid cancer
Degenerative cervical bone disease

Male

Lymphadenopathy related to Hodgkin's disease
Trauma-related cervical spine injury

CHIEF COMPLAINT

Common chief complaints for the head and neck are defined, and information on the characteristics of each sign or symptom is provided.

1. Stiff Neck

Painful movement of the neck that restricts range of motion

Quality

Limited range of motion, either passive or active

Associated Manifestations

Headache, neck tenderness, swelling, fever, numbness and tingling in arms or hands

continues

Aggravating Factors	Position (sitting, standing, lying down), immobilization of position for a prolonged period, mobility, stress, weather
Alleviating Factors	Immobility or rest, certain position, analgesics, heat
Setting	Work, driving, stress
Timing	With all movements, with rotating movements only, with flexion and extension only, with weather changes; after falls, motor vehicle or other accidents
2. Hoarseness	Husky or harsh quality of the voice
Quality	Audible, inaudible
Associated Manifestations	Fever, sore throat, malaise, reflux, vocal cord mass
Aggravating Factors	Inhalation of chemicals or noxious fumes, smoking, overuse of voice, alcohol use, recent upper respiratory infections, recent head and neck surgery, intubation, neck trauma
Alleviating Factors	Medications, adequate hydration, voice rest
Setting	Public speaking, singing, yelling, normal speech
Timing	Continuous, intermittent
3. Neck Mass	Discrete area of swelling found in the neck
Quality	Mobile, nonmobile, smooth, irregular, tender, nontender
Associated Manifestations	Shortness of breath, hoarseness, weight loss, fever and chills, dysphagia, ear pain
Aggravating Factors	Eating, talking, movement, tight clothing around the neck, swallowing
Alleviating Factors	Avoidance of tight clothing, analgesic medications, decreased dietary intake
Timing	Long-standing, recent
4. Headache	Pain felt within the head, behind the eyes, or at the nape of the neck (Table 11-1)
Location	Temporal, frontal, occipital, orbital, hemicranial, neck, and upper shoulders
Quality	Neck pain: aching, sore, dull, sharp; head pain: throbbing, sharp, dull, aching
Associated Manifestations	Neck pain: fever, headache, swelling, tenderness; head pain: nausea and vomiting, aura, diplopia, blurred vision, irritability, sneezing, rhinorrhea, weakness, dizziness, photophobia, phonophobia
Aggravating Factors	Neck pain: stress, trauma, aging, position, mobility, weather changes; head pain: stress, fatigue, foods, noxious odors, caffeine intake, coughing, alcohol intake, smoke, hunger, season, menstruation, chemicals, toxins
Alleviating Factors	Medications such as analgesics, anti-inflammatory agents, ergotamine, caffeinated drugs, antidepressants, or triptan medications; position change; rest; sleep; shaking head; food intake
Setting	Work, outdoors, relationship to biologic events, stressful environment, change in weather
Timing	Neck pain: with movement, at rest, weather changes; head pain: constant, intermittent, in the morning, at the end of the day, premenstrual, seasonal
5. Head Injury	
Quality	Open, closed

continues

Health History (continued)

Associated Manifestations	Lightheadedness, photophobia, phonophobia, poor attention and concentration, sleep disturbances, depression, neck pain, nausea, vomiting, projectile vomiting, dizziness or vertigo, associated laceration, headache, seizure activity, loss of consciousness, amnesia, visual disturbances, gait disturbances, speech disturbances, confusion, drowsiness, abnormal behavior, abnormal movement of extremities, change in respiratory pattern, discharge from nose or ear, head or neck lacerations/abrasions/ecchymoses
Alleviating Factors	Ice, analgesics, rest, surgical intervention
Setting	Mechanism of injury, use of helmet or protective headgear, use of seat belt, violent activity, fall, sports injury, motor vehicle accident (MVA), alcohol or drug use, concurrent history of seizure disorder, heart disease, or diabetes mellitus
PAST HEALTH HISTORY	*The various components of the past health history are linked to head and neck pathology and head- and neck-related information.*
Medical History	
Head and Neck Specific	Hypo- or hyperthyroidism, hypo- or hyperparathyroidism, sinus infections, migraine headache, cancer, closed head injury, skull fracture, Bell's palsy, Cushing's syndrome
Non-Head and Neck Specific	Pheochromocytoma
Surgical History	Thyroidectomy, parathyroidectomy, facial reconstruction, cosmetic surgery, neurosurgery, other surgery related to the head or neck
Medications	Antibiotics, steroids, anticonvulsants, chemotherapy, thyroxine, propranolol, analgesics, oral contraceptives, radioiodine (^{131}I), propylthiouracil, methimazole
Communicable Diseases	Meningitis, encephalitis
Injuries and Accidents	Obstruction caused by foreign bodies, trauma to the head or neck, chemical splashes to the face, noxious fumes, sports injuries, motor vehicle accidents
Special Needs	Tracheostomy, paralysis
FAMILY HEALTH HISTORY	*Head and neck diseases that are familial are listed.*
	Thyroid disease, migraines
SOCIAL HISTORY	*The components of the social history are linked to head and neck factors or pathology.*
Alcohol Use	Predisposes to accidents and head injury
Work Environment	Risk of head injury, exposure to toxins or chemicals, carbon monoxide
Home Environment	Risk of falls and head injury due to loose throw rugs or absence of handrails, carbon monoxide
Stress	Demands of employment, home, school
HEALTH MAINTENANCE ACTIVITIES	*This information provides a bridge between the health maintenance activities and head and neck function.*
Sleep	May be increased due to head injury
Diet	Recent weight gain or loss
Use of Safety Devices	Protective headgear for sports and work

TABLE 11-1 Classification of Headaches

VASCULAR ETIOLOGIES

Migraine headaches

Cluster headaches

Subarachnoid hemorrhage

Subdural hematoma

Infarction

Cerebral aneurysm

Temporal arteritis

Vasculitis

MUSCLE CONTRACTION

Tension headache

INTRACRANIAL ETIOLOGIES

Brain tumors

Increased intracranial pressure from hydrocephalus, pseudotumor cerebri

Intracranial infection (e.g., meningitis, encephalitis, abscess)

Ischemic cerebrovascular disease

SYSTEMIC ETIOLOGIES

Infection

Post-lumbar puncture

Hypertension

Exertion from coitus, cough, exercise

Postictal

Pheochromocytoma

Premenstrual syndrome

FOOD-RELATED ETIOLOGIES

Nitrites (e.g., hot dogs, bacon)

Tyramine (e.g., red wine, cheese, chocolate)

Monosodium glutamate (e.g., Chinese food)

Food allergy

FACIAL OR CERVICAL ETIOLOGIES

Sinusitis

Temporomandibular joint dysfunction

Dental lesions

Trigeminal neuralgia

Cervical spine radiculopathy

OCULAR-RELATED ETIOLOGIES

Narrow angle glaucoma

Uveitis

Extraocular muscle paralysis

Eye strain

METABOLIC ETIOLOGIES

Hypoxia

Hypercapnia

Hypoglycemia

DRUG ETIOLOGIES

Alcohol and alcohol withdrawal

Caffeine withdrawal

Nitrates

Oral contraceptives

Estrogen

ENVIRONMENTAL ETIOLOGIES

Change in barometric pressure (from weather or altitude)

Carbon monoxide poisoning

Tobacco smoke

Glaring or flickering lights

Odors

MISCELLANEOUS ETIOLOGIES

Fever

Influenza

Head trauma

Otitis media

Parotitis

Pregnancy

Fatigue and decreased sleep

Psychogenic disorders

NURSING ALERT

Risk Factors for Migraine Headache

- Ages 5–50
- Female
- Family history of migraines
- Allergies
- Raynaud's phenomenon
- History of motion sickness in childhood
- Increased stress
- Estrogen supplementation
- Caffeine intake
- Tyramine, MSG, sulfites, or nitrite consumption
- Sleep disorders
- Oral contraceptive use

NURSING TIP

Nonpharmaceutical Headache Remedies

The patient may benefit from instructions on methods to reduce or alleviate headaches by nonchemical means. Some suggestions include: relaxation techniques, a quiet environment, a dark room, lying down, walking, music, muscle stretching, warm or cool compresses to the head, herbal tea, and a neck or temple massage. Encourage the patient to experiment with these techniques to determine what is effective, and to use the effective method when headaches occur.

REFLECTIVE THINKING

The Patient with Migraines

You are a home health nurse visiting a 54-year-old female who had surgery 4 days ago. As you are performing the dressing change, the woman tells you that she has had migraine headaches all her life and she "can't take them anymore." She confides to you that all her past health care providers dismissed her headaches as "nothing." How would you respond to this patient? What questions would you ask her?

Preventing Head and Neck Injury

Ivan is a 20-year-old bicycle courier for a large business in the downtown area. He presents to the clinic with a swollen ankle that he sustained after running a red light and colliding with a car. You note that Ivan has extensive bruises on his face. You inquire about his use of a helmet. He replies, "I'm careful. I don't need it." How would you respond to this comment? What teaching strategies might you use?

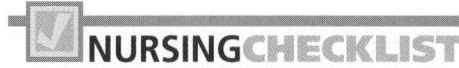

NURSINGCHECKLIST

General Approach to Head and Neck Assessment

1. Greet the patient and explain the assessment techniques that you will be using.
2. Ensure that the environment is at a warm, comfortable room temperature to provide the patient comfort.
3. Use a quiet room that will be free from interruptions.
4. Ensure that the light in the room provides sufficient brightness to allow adequate observation of the patient.
5. Place the patient in an upright sitting position on the examination table, or gain access to the head of the supine, bedridden patient by removing nonessential equipment or bedding (for patients who cannot tolerate the sitting position).
6. If the patient is wearing a wig or headpiece, ask the patient to remove it.
7. Visualize the underlying anatomic structures during the assessment process to permit an accurate description of the location of any pathology.
8. Always compare the right and left sides of the head, neck, and face to one another.
9. Use the same systematic approach every time the assessment is performed.

EQUIPMENT

- Stethoscope
- Cup of water

ASSESSMENT OF THE HEAD AND NECK

INSPECTION OF THE SHAPE OF THE HEAD

E 1. Have the patient sit in a comfortable position.

2. Face the patient, with your head at the same level as the patient's head.

3. Inspect the head for shape and symmetry.

N The head should be normocephalic and symmetrical.

A **Hydrocephalus** is an enlargement of the head without enlargement of the facial structures (see Figure 11-7A).

P Hydrocephalus is caused by an abnormal accumulation of cerebrospinal fluid within the skull.

A **Acromegaly** is an abnormal enlargement of the skull and bony facial structures.

P Acromegaly is caused by excessive secretion of growth hormone from the pituitary gland (see Figure 11-7B).

A Craniosynostosis is characterized by abnormal shape of the skull or bone growth at right angles to suture lines, exophthalmos, and drooping eyelids (see Figure 11-7C).

P Craniosynostosis is caused by the premature closure of one or more sutures of the skull before brain growth is complete.

| **E** Examination | **N** Normal Findings | **A** Abnormal Findings | **P** Pathophysiology |

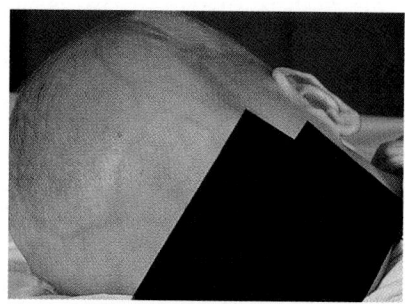

A. Hydrocephalus. *Courtesy of Armed Forces Institute of Pathology.*

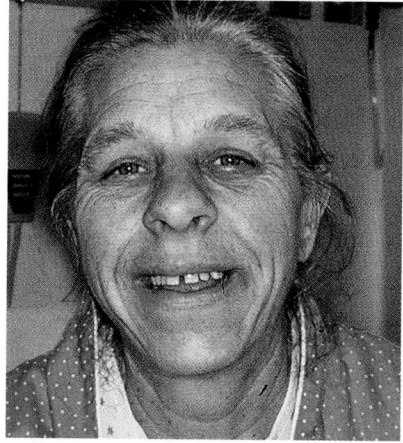

B. Acromegaly. Note wide nose, spaced-teeth, and large lips. *Courtesy of Matthew C. Leinung, M.D., Acting Head, Division of Endocrinology, Albany Medical College, Albany, NY.*

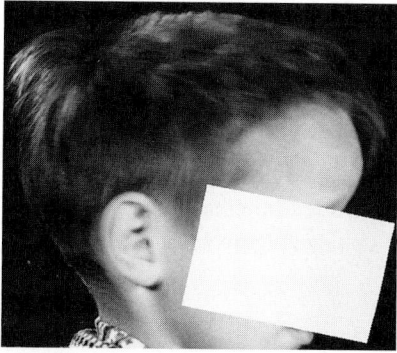

C. Craniosynostosis. *Courtesy of Armed Forces Institute of Pathology.*

FIGURE 11-7 **Abnormal Head Shapes**

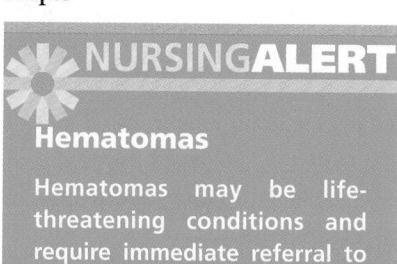

NURSING**ALERT**

Hematomas

Hematomas may be life-threatening conditions and require immediate referral to a physician.

PALPATION OF THE HEAD

E 1. Place the finger pads on the scalp and palpate all of its surface, beginning in the frontal area and continuing over the parietal, temporal, and occipital areas.

2. Assess for contour, masses, depressions, and tenderness.

3. Palpate the temporal artery, which is located anterior to the tragus of the ear.

N The normal skull is smooth, nontender, and without masses or depressions. The temporal artery is usually a weaker peripheral pulse (1+/4+ or 1+/3+) than the other peripheral pulses of the body. The artery is nontender, smooth, and readily compressible.

A Masses in the cranial bones that feel hard or soft are abnormal.

P These types of masses may be carcinomatous metastasis from other regions of the body or may result from lymphomas, multiple myeloma, or leukemia.

A Palpation elicits localized edema over the bony frontal portion of the skull.

P Osteomyelitis of the skull may develop following acute or chronic sinusitis if the infection extends out from the sinuses into the surrounding bone.

A Firm palpation reveals a softening of the outer bone layer.

P **Craniotabes** is a softening of the skull caused by hydrocephalus or demineralization of the bone due to rickets, osteogenesis imperfecta or syphilis.

A A temporal artery that is hard in consistency and tender is abnormal.

P This can indicate temporal arteritis. In temporal arteritis, the temporal arteries may also be more tortuous.

INSPECTION AND PALPATION OF THE SCALP

E 1. Part the hair repeatedly all over the scalp and inspect the scalp for lesions or masses.

2. Place the finger pads on the scalp and palpate for lesions or masses.

N The scalp should be shiny, intact, and without lesions or masses.

A A laceration or a laceration with bleeding is abnormal.

P Direct trauma can cause lacerations to the scalp.

A A gaping laceration with profuse bleeding is abnormal.

P If the laceration on the scalp is gaping, it indicates a deep wound that may further indicate a compound skull fracture as a result of some type of trauma.

A Palpation reveals a localized, easily movable accumulation of blood in the subcutaneous tissue.

P Hematomas can result from direct trauma to the skull.

A Palpation may reveal either single or multiple masses that are easily movable. They are round, firm, nontender, and arise from either the skin or the subcutaneous tissue.

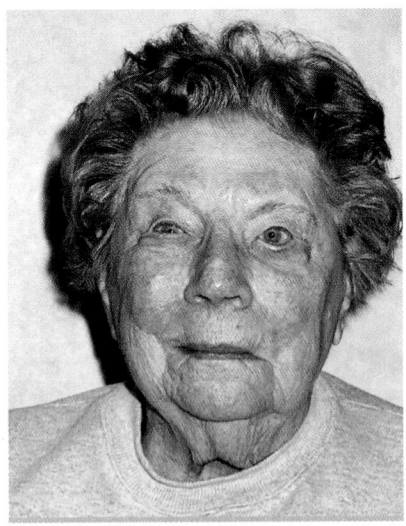

FIGURE 11-8 Bell's Palsy. Note the drooping left lower eyelid and left side of the mouth. *Courtesy of Mary A. Hitcho.*

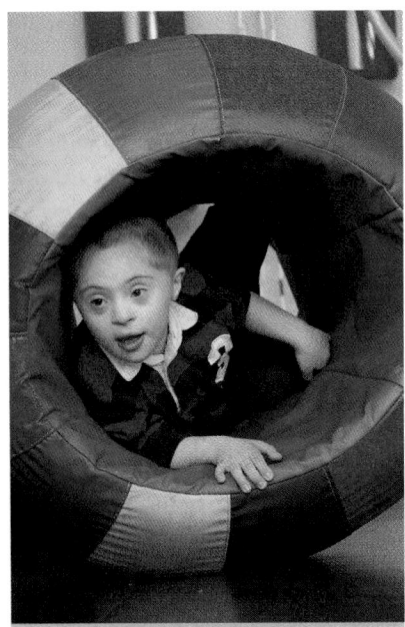

FIGURE 11-9 Down Syndrome

P These are sebaceous cysts that form as a result of retention of secretions from sebaceous glands.

A Nonmobile, fatty masses with smooth, circular edges may be palpated deeper in the scalp.

P These masses are benign fatty tumors known as **lipomas**.

INSPECTION OF THE FACE

Symmetry

E 1. Have the patient sit in a comfortable position facing you.

2. Observe the patient's face for expression, shape, and symmetry of the following structures: eyebrows, eyes, nose, mouth, ears.

N The facial features should be symmetrical. Both palpebral fissures should be equal and the nasolabial fold should present bilaterally. It is important to remember that slight variations in symmetry are common. Slanted eyes with inner epicanthal folds are normal findings in patients of Asian descent.

A Structures are absent or deformed. There is a definite asymmetry of expression, the palpebral fissures, the nasolabial folds, and the corners of the mouth.

P Asymmetry of the palpebral fissures, nasolabial folds, the mouth, and facial expression may indicate damage to the nerves innervating facial muscles (cranial nerve VII), as in stroke or **Bell's palsy** (Figure 11-8).

Shape and Features

E 1. Face the patient.

2. Observe the shape of the patient's face.

3. Note any swelling, abnormal features, or unusual movement.

N The shape of the face can be oval, round, or slightly square. There should be no edema, disproportionate structures, or involuntary movements.

A Inspection of the face may reveal slanted eyes with inner epicanthal folds; a short, flat nose; and a thick, protruding tongue.

P These findings are likely to indicate the presence of **Down syndrome**, or Trisomy 21, a chromosomal aberration (Figure 11-9).

A An abnormally wide distance between the eyes is **hypertelorism**.

P Hypertelorism is a congenital anomaly.

E Examination   **N** Normal Findings   **A** Abnormal Findings   **P** Pathophysiology

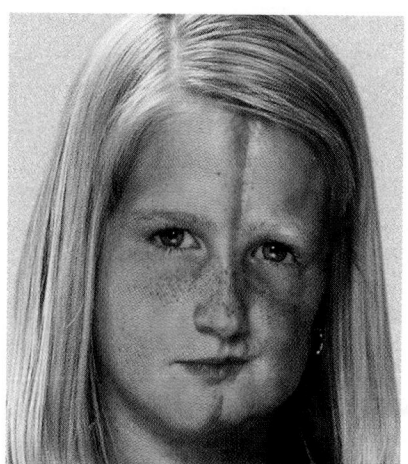

FIGURE 11-10 Scleroderma. *Courtesy of the Scleroderma Foundation (www.scleroderma.org).*

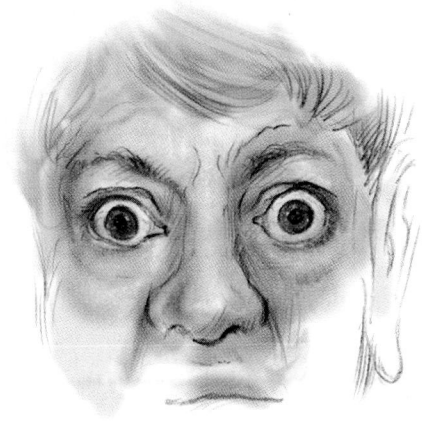

FIGURE 11-11 Exophthalmos of Graves' Disease

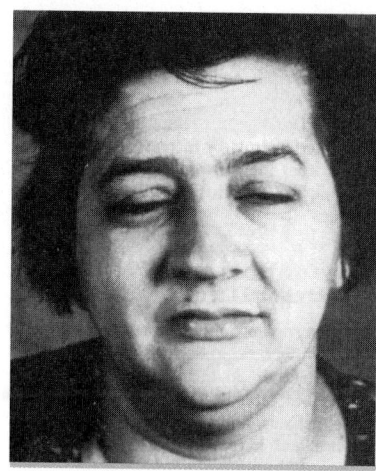

FIGURE 11-12 Myxedema

REFLECTIVE THINKING

Facial Piercing

Your patient has a history of acne, chronic sinusitis, and allergies. She informs you that she plans to get her eyebrows and nares pierced. How would you respond to her? How would you counsel this patient to have her body piercing done safely?

REFLECTIVE THINKING

Sensitivity to Patients with Severe Facial Burns

During your first day working in the burn unit, you are assigned to care for a patient who has multiple second-degree burns to his face and upper extremities. As you meet him for the first time, he says, "I look horrible; you won't be able to stand to look at me." How would you respond verbally and nonverbally to his comment and his disfigurement?

A Facial skin is shiny, contracted, and hard. The face appears to have furrows around the mouth (Figure 11-10).

P Scleroderma is a collagen disease of unknown cause. Sclerosis of the skin, as well as visceral organs (esophagus, lungs, heart, muscles, and kidneys) occurs.

A The face is thin with sharply defined features and prominent eyes (exophthalmos) in Graves' disease (Figure 11-11).

P Graves' disease is an autoimmune disorder associated with increased circulating levels of T_3 and T_4.

A The patient's face is round and swollen with characteristic periorbital edema and dry, dull skin (Figure 11-12).

P This condition is known as myxedema and is associated with hypothyroidism.

A The eyes are sunken and the cheeks are hollow in cachexia (see Figure 11-13).

P Cachexia is a profound state of wasting of the vital tissues that is associated with cancer, malnutrition, and severe chronic illnesses.

A The patient's face is immobile and expressionless with a staring gaze and raised eyebrows in Parkinson's disease (see Figure 11-14).

P Parkinson's disease is the degeneration of basal ganglia, resulting from a deficiency of the neurotransmitter dopamine.

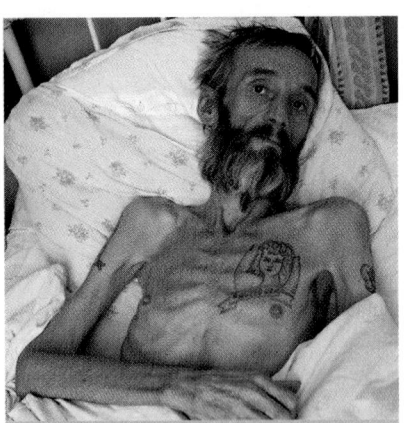

FIGURE 11-13 This is cachectic face in a 40-year-old man with tuberculosis. Also note his cachectic torso. *Courtesy of WHO/STB/Colors Magazine/J. Mollison.*

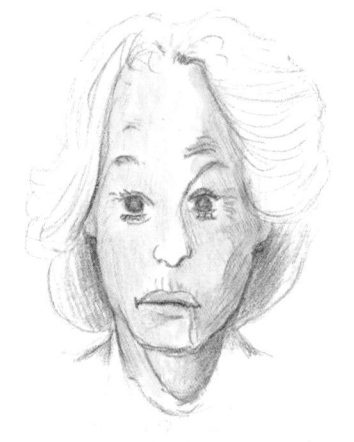

FIGURE 11-14 Parkinson's Disease

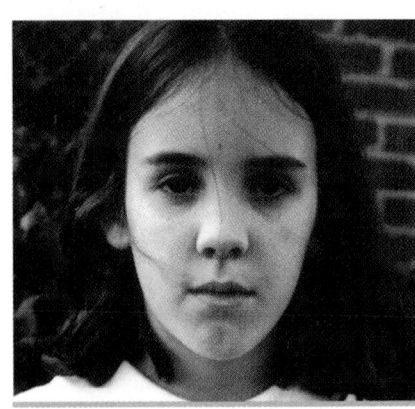

FIGURE 11-15 Allergic Facies

A The faces of some Caucasians show a dusky blue discoloration beneath the eyes ("allergic shiners") along with creases below the lower eyelids (Dennie's lines) and open mouth due to mouth breathing (Figure 11-15).

P The patient with chronic allergies or allergic rhinitis develops this characteristic allergic facies or allergic gape. This can occur in seasonal or perennial allergic rhinitis.

A A transverse crease is noted across the nose.

P This is a characteristic finding in patients with allergies and allergic rhinitis who frequently are observed to do the "nasal salute" or upward wiping of the nose (Figure 11-16).

A The patient has a rounded "moon face" along with red cheeks and excess hair on the jaw and upper lip (Figure 11-17).

P This is the facies of Cushing's syndrome, which is caused by increased production of adrenocorticotropic hormone (ACTH) or prolonged steroid ingestion.

PALPATION AND AUSCULTATION OF THE MANDIBLE

E 1. Use the fingertips of both index and middle fingers to locate the temporomandibular joint anterior to the tragus of the ear on both sides.

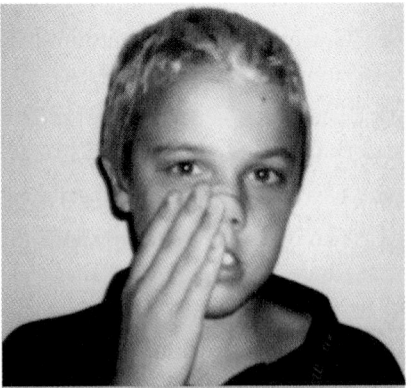

FIGURE 11-16 This young boy has a characteristic nasal crease from the repeated action of the "nasal salute" caused by allergies.

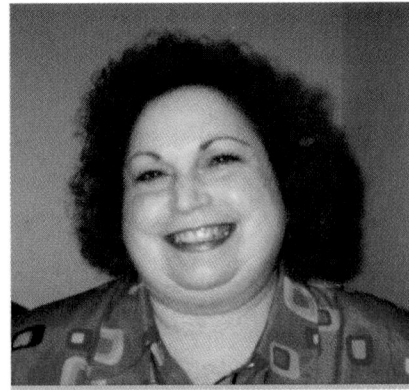

FIGURE 11-17 Cushing's Syndrome

2. Hold the fingertips firmly in place over the joints and ask the patient to open and close the mouth.

3. As the patient opens and closes the mouth, observe the relative smoothness of the movement and whether or not the patient notices any discomfort.

4. Remove the hands.

5. Hold the bell of the stethoscope over the joint.

6. Listen for any sound while the patient opens and closes the mouth.

N The patient should experience no discomfort with movement. The temporomandibular joint should articulate smoothly and without clicking or crepitus.

A The patient complains of tenderness when the mouth is opened and closed. Palpation or auscultation reveals clicking or crepitus.

P Tenderness in the joint may be from the inflammation of migratory arthritis.

A Crepitus is present from the articulation of irregular bone surfaces found in osteoarthritis.

P Clicking may follow a "snapping" sound if there is displaced cartilage.

A The mouth remains in an open and fixed position.

P Following a wide yawn or trauma to the chin, the temporomandibular joint is dislocated and will not function. This condition requires reduction.

INSPECTION AND PALPATION OF THE NECK
Inspection of the Neck

E 1. Have the patient sit facing you, with the head held in a central position.

2. Inspect for symmetry of the sternocleidomastoid muscles anteriorly, and the trapezii posteriorly.

3. Have the patient touch the chin to the chest, to each side, and to each shoulder.

4. Assess for limitation of motion.

5. Note the presence of a stoma or tracheostomy.

N The muscles of the neck are symmetrical with the head in a central position. The patient is able to move the head through a full range of motion without complaint of discomfort or noticeable limitation. The patient may be breathing through a stoma or tracheostomy.

A Asymmetry of the neck is abnormal (see Figure 11-18).

P Asymmetrical masses can be benign or malignant, but they all must be evaluated further.

A The patient complains of pain with flexion or rotation of the head.

P Pain with flexion can be associated with the pain and muscle spasm caused by meningeal irritation of meningitis (see Chapter 19). Generalized discomfort may be related to trauma, spasm, inflammation of muscles, or diseases of the vertebrae.

NURSINGALERT

Neck Injury

If a neck injury is suspected, stabilize the neck and do not proceed with the assessment. Refer the patient immediately to a qualified specialist for further evaluation.

| **E** Examination | **N** Normal Findings | **A** Abnormal Findings | **P** Pathophysiology |

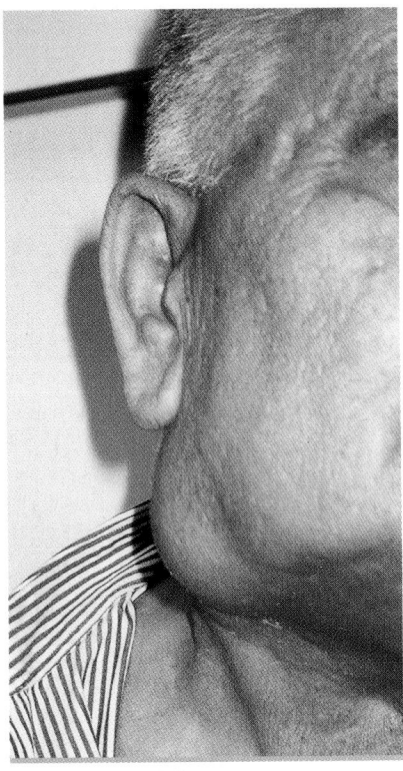

FIGURE 11-18 **This right neck mass was identified as squamous cell carcinoma.** *Courtesy of Dr. Daniel D. Rooney.*

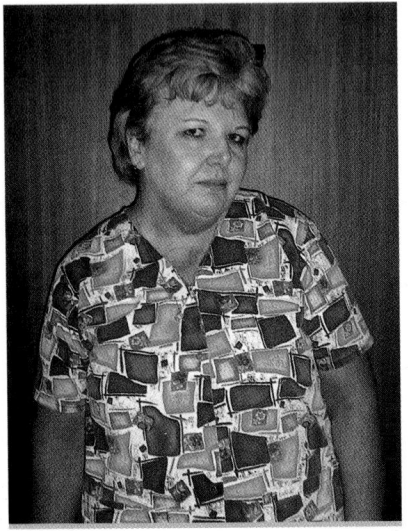

FIGURE 11-19 **Torticollis**

NURSINGTIP

Assessment of the Trachea

It is appropriate to assess the trachea at this point in the examination; refer to Chapter 15 for a description of the technique.

A There is a slight or prominent lateral deviation of the patient's neck. The sternocleidomastoid muscles, and to a lesser extent the trapezius and scalene muscles, may also be prominent on the affected side. The muscles frequently hypertrophy as the result of powerful contractions.

P This condition is called **torticollis** (Figure 11-19). Causes can be:

1. Congenital: resulting from a hematoma or partial rupture at birth of the sternocleidomastoid, causing a shortening of the muscle.

2. Ocular: a head posture assumed to correct for ocular muscle palsy and resulting diplopia.

3. Acute spasm: commonly associated with the inflammation of viral myositis or trauma such as sleeping with the head in an unusual position.

4. Other: hysteria, phenothiazine therapy, and Parkinson's disease as the result of increased cholinergic activity in the brain.

A Range of motion of the neck is reduced.

P Degenerative changes of osteoarthritis may result in decreased ability for full range of motion. This condition is usually painless unless nerve root irritation has occurred. Crepitus, or a crunching sound on hyperextension of the neck, may also be observed.

Palpation of the Neck

E
1. Stand in front of the patient.
2. With the finger pads, palpate the sternocleidomastoid muscles.
3. Note the presence of masses or tenderness.
4. Stand behind the patient.
5. With the finger pads, palpate the trapezius.
6. Note the presence of masses or tenderness.

N The muscles should be symmetrical without palpable masses or spasm.

A A mass is palpated in the musculature.

P A mass may be a tumor, either primary or metastatic.

A A spasm may be felt in the muscles.

P Muscle spasm may be due to varied causes such as infections, trauma, chronic inflammatory processes, or neoplasms.

INSPECTION OF THE THYROID GLAND

E
1. Secure tangential lighting, and shine it at an oblique angle on the patient's anterior neck.
2. Face the patient.
3. Ask the patient to look straight ahead with the head slightly extended.
4. Have the patient drink a sip of water and swallow twice.
5. As the patient swallows, observe the front of the neck in the area of the thyroid and the isthmus for masses and symmetrical movement.

N Thyroid tissue moves up with swallowing, but often the movement is so small that it is not visible on inspection. In males, the thyroid cartilage, or Adam's apple, is more prominent than in females.

| **E** Examination | **N** Normal Findings | **A** Abnormal Findings | **P** Pathophysiology |

A A mass or enlargement of the thyroid that moves upward with swallowing is not normal.

P Many **goiters** (enlarged thyroid glands) or thyroid nodules are visible and may indicate a variety of thyroid diseases (Figure 11-20).

PALPATION OF THE THYROID GLAND

Palpation of the thyroid gland may be done using both anterior and posterior approaches (Figure 11-21).

Posterior Approach

E 1. Have the patient sit comfortably. Stand behind the patient.

2. Have the patient lower the chin slightly in order to relax the neck muscles.

3. Place the thumbs on the back of the patient's neck and bring the other fingers around the neck anteriorly with their tips resting on the lower portion of the neck over the trachea.

4. Move the finger pads over the tracheal rings.

5. Instruct the patient to swallow. Palpate the isthmus for nodules or enlargement.

6. Have the patient incline the head slightly forward.

7. Press the fingers of the left hand against the left side of the thyroid cartilage to stabilize it while placing the fingers of the right hand gently against the right side.

8. Instruct the patient to swallow sips of water.

9. Note consistency, nodularity, and tenderness as the gland moves upward.

10. Repeat on the other side.

N/A/P Refer to Anterior Approach.

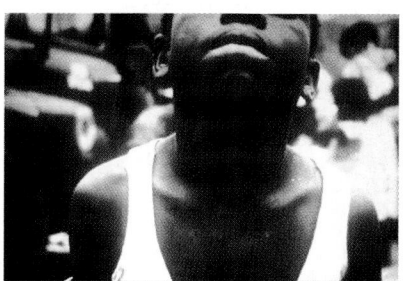

FIGURE 11-20 Goiter. *Courtesy of the Centers for Disease Control and Prevention (CDC).*

NURSINGTIP
Assessment of the Neck's Vasculature

It is important to assess the carotid arteries and the jugular veins at this point in the examination; refer to Chapter 16 for a description of the technique.

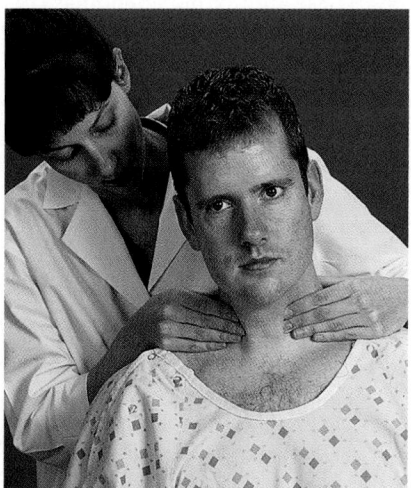
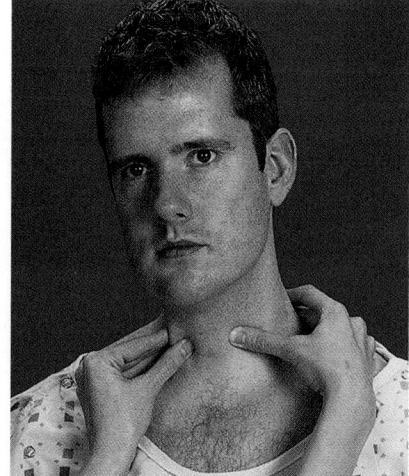

A. Posterior Approach   B. Anterior Approach

FIGURE 11-21 Examination of the Thyroid Gland

Anterior Approach

P 1. Stand in front of the patient.

2. Ask the patient to flex the head slightly forward.

3. Place the right thumb on the thyroid cartilage and displace the cartilage to the patient's right.

4. Grasp the elevated and displaced right lobe of the thyroid gland with the thumb and index and middle fingers of the left hand.

5. Palpate the surface of the gland for consistency, nodularity, and tenderness.

6. Have the patient swallow, and then palpate the surface again.

7. Repeat the procedure on the opposite side.

N No enlargement, masses, or tenderness should be noted on palpation.

A Palpation reveals the gland to be smooth, soft, and slightly enlarged but less than twice the size of a normal thyroid gland.

P This is referred to as physiological hyperplasia and can be seen premenstrually, during pregnancy, or from puberty to young adulthood in females. Symmetrical enlargement may also be noted in patients who live in areas of iodine deficiency. These are referred to as nontoxic diffuse goiters or endemic goiters.

A Palpation reveals the gland to be two to three times larger than normal size.

P This is diffuse toxic hyperplasia of the thyroid, or Graves' disease, an autoimmune disorder that is the most common type of hyperthyroidism. Table 11-2 distinguishes between the signs and symptoms of thyroid disorders. In addition, Table 11-3 identifies signs and symptoms of parathyroid disease. Since the parathyroid glands can be affected with thyroid manipulation, it is imperative that clinical knowledge of pathology of the parathyroid glands is known.

A Asymmetrical enlargement of the thyroid and the presence of two or more nodules are found.

P These are thyroid adenomas (benign epithelial tumors) that usually occur after the age of 30. A nontoxic, diffuse goiter may become nodular as the patient ages.

A Palpation reveals a solitary nodule in the thyroid tissue.

P A solitary nodule is suggestive of carcinoma (Figure 11-22).

A Lateral deviation of the trachea is noted on palpation, but you are unable to identify a specific goiter.

P This may be a retrosternal goiter. This type of goiter sometimes occurs in a patient with a short neck or may be a goiter with many adenomatous nodules.

A Tenderness of the thyroid is found on palpation.

P Tenderness of an enlarged, firm thyroid suggests thyroiditis.

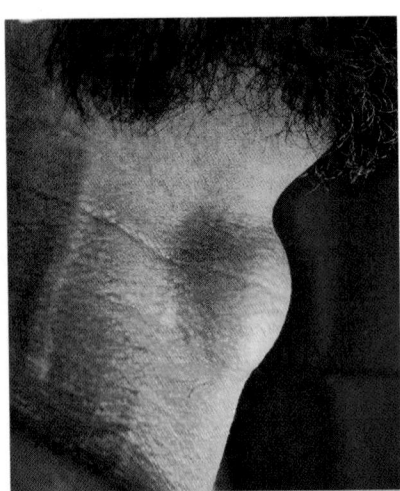

FIGURE 11-22 Solitary Thyroid Nodule. *Courtesy of Dr. Andrew B. Silva, Pediatric Otolaryngology.*

E Examination   **N** Normal Findings   **A** Abnormal Findings   **P** Pathophysiology

TABLE 11-2 Signs and Symptoms of Thyroid Disease

Hypothyroidism and hyperthyroidism are diseases that can occur from birth until later years of life. They can be congenital or acquired. The primary laboratory tests that are used to screen for these conditions are the thyroid stimulating hormone (TSH), T_3 and T_4.

SYSTEM	HYPOTHYROIDISM	HYPERTHYROIDISM
General	Tired, weak	Fatigue, weak
Skin	Dry, cold, coarse	Sweaty, warm
Hair	Alopecia	Thin hair
Head and Neck	Hoarseness, puffy face	Lid lag, exophthalmos, goiter
Ears and Mouth	Impaired hearing, macroglossia	None
Respiratory	Dyspnea	Tachypnea
Cardiovascular	Bradycardia, cool extremities, peripheral edema	Tachycardia, palpitations
Gastrointestinal	Constipation	Diarrhea
Musculoskeletal	Carpal tunnel syndrome	Muscle weakness
Neurological	Difficulty concentrating, decreased memory, paresthesia, decreased deep tendon reflexes (DTRs)	Hyperactivity, irritability, tremor, insomnia
Reproductive	Amenorrhea	Oligomenorrhea, gynecomastia, decreased libido
Endocrine	Cold intolerance	Heat intolerance
Weight	Weight gain with decreased appetite	Weight loss with increased appetite

TABLE 11-3 Signs and Symptoms of Parathyroid Disease

Hypoparathyroidism and hyperparathyroidism are diseases that can occur congenitally or be acquired in life. Both are primarily conditions of calcium imbalance. In hypoparathyroidism, the patient is in a state of hypocalcemia, and in hyperparathyroidism, the patient is hypercalcemic. The body has four parathyroid glands, located posterior to the thyroid. Occasionally, they are accidentally removed when a patient undergoes thyroid surgery. The parathyroid glands are not accessible to direct physical examination, but parathyroid conditions can be detected by astute history taking and physical assessment data synthesis.

HYPOPARATHYROIDISM	HYPERPARATHYROIDISM
Muscle spasms	Recurrent nephrolithiasis
Facial grimacing	Peptic/duodenal ulcers
Laryngeal spasm	Mental status changes
Seizures	Proximal muscle weakness
Mental status changes	Fatigue
Tetany	Muscle atrophy
⊕ Chvostek's sign (see Chapter 18)	Osteitis fibrosa cystica
⊕ Trousseau's sign (see Chapter 18)	
Respiratory arrest	

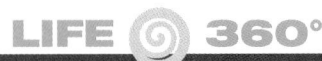

AUSCULTATION OF THE THYROID GLAND

If the thyroid is enlarged, auscultation should be performed.

E 1. Stand in front of the patient.

2. Place the bell of the stethoscope over the right thyroid lobe.

3. Auscultate for bruits.

4. Repeat on the left thyroid lobe.

N Auscultation should not reveal bruits.

A Auscultation reveals the presence of a bruit over an enlarged thyroid gland.

P Bruits occur with increased turbulence in blood vessels and are due to the increased vascularization of a thyroid gland that is enlarged due to diffuse toxic goiter.

INSPECTION OF THE LYMPH NODES

E 1. Stand in front of the patient.

2. Expose the area of the head and neck to be assessed.

3. Inspect the nodal areas of the head and neck for any enlargement or inflammation.

N Lymph nodes should not be visible or inflamed.

A Enlargement and inflammation is present in specific nodes.

P Lymph nodes can be enlarged and inflamed when there is a localized or generalized infection in the body. This attempt to prevent the spread of infection occurs as a part of the body's immune response to infection.

PALPATION OF THE LYMPH NODES

E 1. Have the patient sit comfortably.

2. Face the patient and conduct the assessment of both sides of the neck simultaneously.

3. Move the pads and tips of the middle three fingers in small circles of palpation using gentle pressure.

4. Follow a systematic, routine sequence beginning with the preauricular, postauricular, occipital, submental, submandibular, and tonsillar nodes. Moving down to the neck, evaluate the anterior cervical chain, the posterior cervical chain, and the supraclavicular nodes (see Figure 11-23).

5. Note size, shape, delimitation (discrete or matted together), mobility, consistency, and tenderness.

N Lymph nodes should not be palpable in the healthy adult patient; however, small, discrete, movable nodes are sometimes present but are of no significance.

A Palpable lymph nodes are abnormal.

P Palpable lymph nodes are frequently seen in acute bacterial infections such as streptococcal pharyngitis. The anterior cervical nodes are usually affected and may be warm, firm, tender, and mobile.

P An enlarged postauricular node is sometimes found in patients with ear infections.

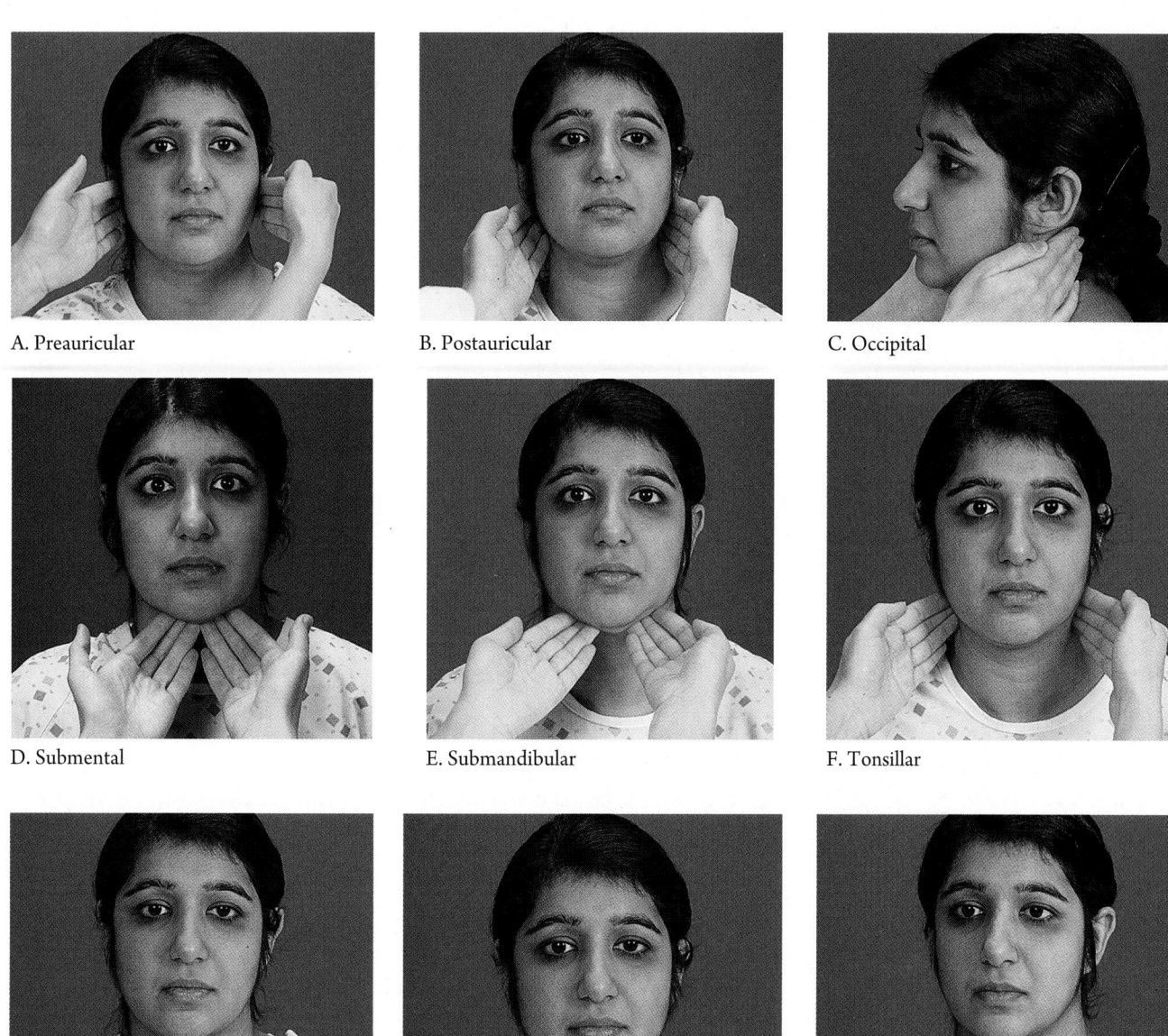

A. Preauricular

B. Postauricular

C. Occipital

D. Submental

E. Submandibular

F. Tonsillar

G. Anterior Cervical Chain

H. Posterior Cervical Chain

I. Supraclavicular

FIGURE 11-23 **Palpation of Lymph Nodes**

> **P** Enlarged, hard, tender nodes are seen in lymphadenitis (inflammation of the lymph nodes). The affected node is the site of the inflammation.

> **P** Enlarged nodes, particularly of the anterior and posterior cervical chains, may be found in infectious mononucleosis. These nodes are usually tender.

> **P** An enlarged node in the left supraclavicular area (Virchow's node) may point to malignancy in the abdominal or thoracic regions.

> **P** Nontender, firm, or hard nodes that are nonmobile may indicate a malignancy in the head and neck area, or metastasis from the region that the lymph node drains.

| **E** Examination | **N** Normal Findings | **A** Abnormal Findings | **P** Pathophysiology |

P Patients with malignant lymphomas may also present with nodes that are firm, hard, or rubbery; nontender; and fixed. In Hodgkin's disease, the cervical nodes are frequently the first to be palpable.

P Palpable lymph nodes can result from a variety of other pathological processes, including blood dyscrasias, AIDS, tuberculosis, surgical procedures that traumatize the nodes, blood transfusions, or chronic illness.

CASE STUDY

The Patient with Thyrotoxicosis

This case study illustrates the application and objective documentation of the head, neck, and regional lymphatics assessment. James Calhoun is a 54-year-old man who has not been feeling well the past few months.

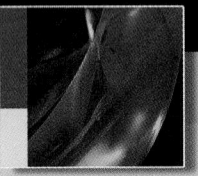

HEALTH HISTORY

PATIENT PROFILE	59 yo MWM
CHIEF COMPLAINT	"I just haven't felt right for the past 2 mos."
HISTORY OF PRESENT ILLNESS	Pt reports that he was doing well until 9 mos ago, when he saw his hl care provider for his 6-mos check for HTN and hyperlipidemia. At that time, he was noted to have Ⓡ tonsillar enlargement and was referred to an ENT. Pt was dx'd c̄ SCC of the tonsils. His tonsils were removed and pt received a 6-wk course of external beam radiation to the Ⓡ tonsillar region. Pt did well postop and resumed work. About 2 mos ago, pt developed sx of myalgias and general weakness. Denies dysphagia, hoarseness, fever, SOB, palpitations, diarrhea, tremor, heat intolerance. He has lost 10 lbs since his sgy. Pt is concerned about the effects of his current hl status b/c he has no more sick time this yr due to his earlier sgy and radiation therapy treatments.

PAST HEALTH HISTORY

Medical History	HTN × 14 yrs, controlled c̄ meds; takes BP at home every other day and records Hyperlipidemia × 10 yrs, takes med and watches diet
Surgical History	Appendectomy 1973 s̄ sequelae Ⓡ ACL repair 2004 s̄ sequelae Tonsillectomy 2009 (per HPI)
Allergies	PCN (hives), sulfa (hives, angioedema)
Medications	Metoprolol XL 50 mg po daily Ezetimibe 10 mg po daily ASA 81 mg po daily

continues

E Examination	**N** Normal Findings	**A** Abnormal Findings	**P** Pathophysiology

CASE STUDY (Continued)

The Patient with Thyrotoxicosis

Communicable Diseases	Chickenpox age 3; believes he had gonorrhea or syphilis while in the military in the early 1970s, tx by military MD
Injuries and Accidents	2003 playing basketball and tore Ⓡ ACL, repaired early 2004; superficial GSW to leg in Vietnam in 1970; denies recent injury/trauma
Special Needs	Denies
Blood Transfusions	Denies
Childhood Illnesses	Mumps age 5
Immunizations	Believes he was UTD when in the military; doesn't recall last tetanus

FAMILY HEALTH HISTORY

LEGEND

 Living female

 Living male

Ⓧ Deceased female

☒ Deceased male

A&W = Alive & well
BPH = Benign prostatic hypertrophy
CA = Cancer
COPD = Chronic obstructive pulmonary disease
dz = disease
MVA = Motor vehicle accident
OA = Osteoarthritis
SCC = Squamous cell carcinoma

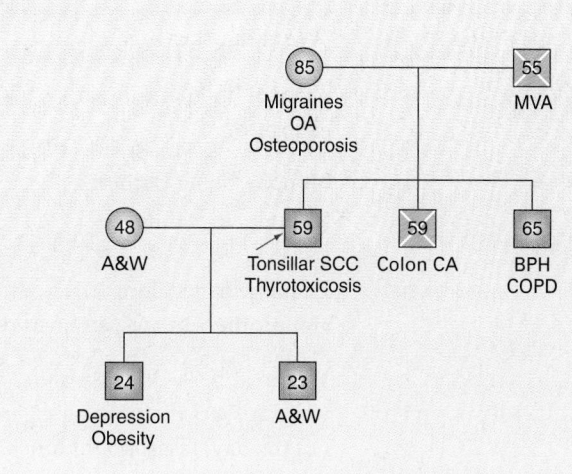

Denies family hx of thyroid dz

SOCIAL HISTORY

Alcohol Use	2–3 beers Q PM p̄ work; sometimes goes out to drink c̄ friends from work
Tobacco Use	½ PPD for 9 mos; prior to this he smoked 2 PPD × 35 yrs; cigars on the weekend
Drug Use	Marijuana in high school; continued use on irregular basis until age 30; denies injectable/snortable drugs
Domestic and Intimate Partner Violence	Denies

continues

CASE STUDY (Continued)

The Patient with Thyrotoxicosis

Sexual Practice	Monogamous c̄ wife of 30 yrs; many partners while in Vietnam
Travel History	Travels to NC frequently to watch NASCAR races; has not been outside the US in 20 years
Work Environment	Manager of postal service vehicles maintenance staff × 25 yrs; crowded, dirty office c̄ exhaust from cars all day long
Home Environment	Lives c̄ wife and mother-in-law in townhouse; requires little maintenance; 3 levels, 2½ baths, uses wood-burning fireplace q wkend in winter; has smoke detectors but never checks them; no carbon monoxide detectors
Hobbies and Leisure Activities	Poker once a month, watching NASCAR on TV
Stress	"My health and bills, bills, bills and work, work, work"
Education	Finished high school
Economic Status	"We aren't starving."
Military Service	Tour of Vietnam in early 1970s for 18 mos; ⊕ Agent Orange exposure
Religion	Nonpracticing Lutheran
Ethnic Background	No association c̄ any group
Roles and Relationships	Pt and wife get along "OK"; estranged from oldest child; "tolerates mother-in-law"; strained re/ship c̄ his work superior
Characteristic Patterns of Daily Living	Wakes at 5:30 AM, showers, has coffee and cereal; arrives at work at 7 AM; smokes a cigarette q hr; black coffee throughout the day; fast food for lunch, but lately has been trying to cut down on fried food; leaves work at 4 PM, may go to bar c̄ friends for 1–2 beers; arrives home 7 PM; eats dinner wife prepared and then watches TV; in bed by 11 PM
HEALTH MAINTENANCE ACTIVITIES	
Sleep	6½ hrs per night; usually feels rested
Diet	"It should be low-fat, low-cholesterol c̄ lots of fish; I am trying to be better about my diet."
Exercise	None
Stress Management	"A good beer cures all."
Use of Safety Devices	"I can't say that we all follow OSHA guidelines all the time."

continues

CASE STUDY   (Continued)

The Patient with Thyrotoxicosis

Health Check-ups	Had been q 6 mos since HTN dx'd, increased visits c̄ dx of tonsillar SCC
PHYSICAL ASSESSMENT	
Inspection of the Shape of the Head	Normocephalic and symmetrical
Palpation of the Head	Skull smooth, s̄ tenderness, masses, or depressions; temporal artery 1+/4+ c̄ mild tenderness, mildly stiff vessel
Inspection and Palpation of the Scalp	Scalp smooth and intact s̄ lesions or masses
Inspection of the Face	
Symmetry	Symmetrical s̄ involuntary movements or swelling
Shape and Features	Round, s̄ edema or involuntary movements; no exophthalmos
Palpation and Auscultation of the Mandible	TMJ articulates smoothly s̄ clicking or crepitus
Inspection of the Neck	Muscles symmetrical c̄ FROM
Palpation of the Neck	Muscles s̄ palpable masses/spasms
Inspection of the Thyroid Gland	Moves c̄ swallowing
Palpation of the Thyroid Gland	No enlargement, no discrete nodules, nontender
Auscultation of the Thyroid Gland	Ø bruits
Inspection of the Lymph Nodes	Ø enlargement
Palpation of the Lymph Nodes	Ø adenopathy
LABORATORY VALUES	CBC—WNL
	Complete Metabolic Panel—WNL

	PT'S VALUES	NORMAL RANGE
TSH	< 0.003 mU/L/mL	0.465–4.680 mU/L/mL
Free T$_4$	> 6.5 ng/dL	0.78–1.85 ng/dL
Free T$_3$	> 22.8 pg/mL	2.77–5.27 pg/mL
Thyroperoxidase Ab, S	8.8 IU/mL	< 9.0 IU/mL
ESR	82 mm/hr	0–20 mm/hr (Westergren method)

continues

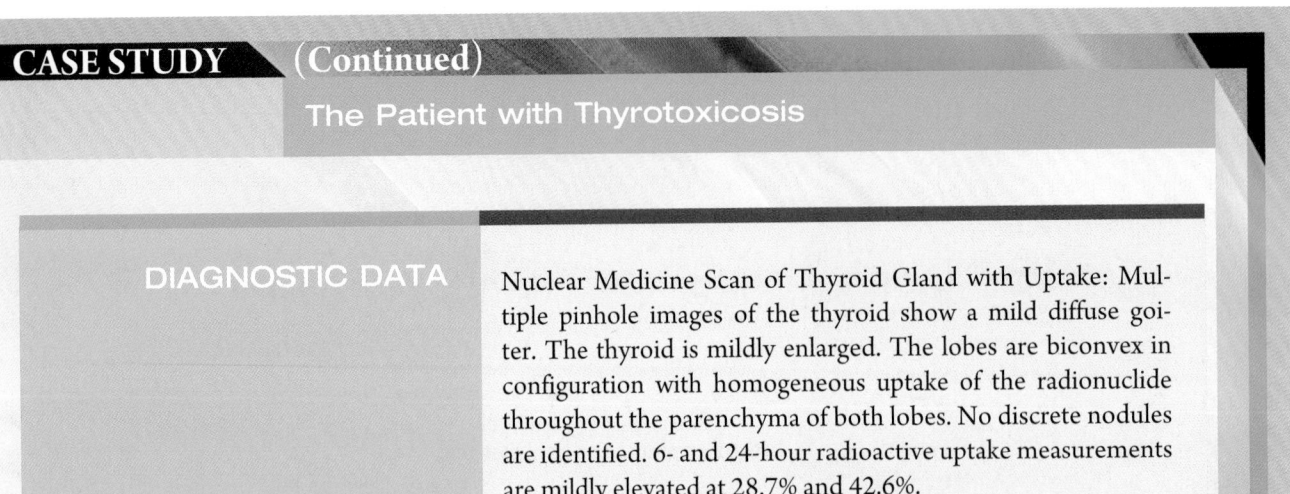

CASE STUDY (Continued)

The Patient with Thyrotoxicosis

DIAGNOSTIC DATA	Nuclear Medicine Scan of Thyroid Gland with Uptake: Multiple pinhole images of the thyroid show a mild diffuse goiter. The thyroid is mildly enlarged. The lobes are biconvex in configuration with homogeneous uptake of the radionuclide throughout the parenchyma of both lobes. No discrete nodules are identified. 6- and 24-hour radioactive uptake measurements are mildly elevated at 28.7% and 42.6%. Impression: Mild diffuse toxic goiter.

ASSESSMENT IN BRIEF

Head, Neck, and Regional Lymphatics Assessment

Inspection

- Shape of the head
- Scalp
- Face
  - Symmetry
  - Shape and features
- Neck
- Thyroid gland
- Lymph nodes

Palpation

- Head
- Scalp
- Mandible
- Neck
- Thyroid gland
  - Posterior approach
  - Anterior approach
- Lymph nodes

Auscultation

- Mandible
- Thyroid gland

REVIEW QUESTIONS

1. Which skull suture connects the frontal and parietal bones?
   a. Coronal
   b. Lambdoidal
   c. Sagittal
   d. Zygomatic
   The correct answer is (a).

2. The posterior triangle of the neck is formed by the:
   a. Mandible, trachea, and sternocleidomastoid muscle
   b. Omohyoid muscle, trachea, and trapezius muscle
   c. Sternum, sternocleidomastoid muscle, and mandible
   d. Sternocleidomastoid muscle, trapezius muscle, and the base of the clavicle
   The correct answer is (d).

3. The preauricular node drains which areas of the head and neck?
   a. Tonsils and pharynx
   b. Face and auditory canal
   c. Scalp, throat, and face
   d. Posterior scalp, ear, and skin of the posterior neck
   The correct answer is (b).

4. While inspecting a patient's face, you note the patient's slanted eyes with inner epicanthal folds; a short, flat nose; and a thick, protruding tongue. What condition do these findings suggest?
   a. Hydrocephalus   c. Bell's palsy
   b. Craniosynostosis   d. Down syndrome
   The correct answer is (d).

5. A patient with sharply defined facial features and exophthalmus is most likely experiencing:
   a. Hypothyroidism   c. Hypoparathyroidism
   b. Hyperthyroidism   d. Hyperparathyroidism
   The correct answer is (b).

6. Which of the following assessment findings describe the patient with Cushing's syndrome?
   a. Red cheeks, increase in hair on the upper lip, large cheeks
   b. An abnormally wide distance between the eyes
   c. Facial skin that is shiny, contracted, and hard
   d. Sunken eyes and hollow cheeks
   The correct answer is (a).

7. Risk factors for thyroid cancer include:
   a. Thyroid adenoma, male gender, diet high in sodium
   b. Exposure to nuclear fallout, female gender, diet high in phosphates
   c. History of thyroid radiation, male gender, diet low in potassium
   d. Genetics, female gender, diet low in iodine
   The correct answer is (d).

8. Upon inspecting a patient, you note that the patient's neck deviates sharply to the left. The patient also has a prominent left sternocleidomastoid muscle. What may be causing this patient's condition?
   a. Osteoarthritis   c. Trigeminal neuralgia
   b. Acute spasm   d. Thyroid cancer
   The correct answer is (b).

9. Which of the following is a normal finding of lymph node assessment?
   a. Small, discreet, movable nodes
   b. Enlarged node in the left supraclavicular area
   c. Nontender, fixed, hard node
   d. Nonmobile, rubbery, erythematous node
   The correct answer is (a).

10. When palpating a patient's thyroid, the examiner places his or her right thumb on the thyroid cartilage and displaces the cartilage to the right. Why is this technique used?
    a. To decrease the discomfort of the assessment
    b. To better assess whether the thyroid cartilage moves with swallowing
    c. To stabilize the thyroid for palpation
    d. To best auscultate for thyroid bruits
    The correct answer is (c).

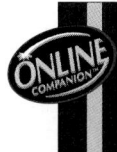

Visit the Estes online companion resource at
www.delmar.cengage.com
for additional content and study aids.
Click on online companions, and then select
the Nursing discipline.

BIBLIOGRAPHY

Benatar, M., & Edlow, J. (2004). The spectrum of cranial neuropathy in patients with Bell's palsy. *Archives of Internal Medicine, 164*(21), 2383–2385.

Bindra, A., & Braunstein, G. D. (2007). Thyroiditis. *American Family Physician, 73*(10), 1769–1776.

Burman, K. (2007). *Thyroid disorders: An issue of endocrinology and metabolism clinics.* Philadelphia: Saunders.

Camacho, P. M., Gharib, H., & Sizemore, G. W. (2006). *Evidence-based endocrinology* (2nd ed.). Philadelphia: Lippincott Williams & Wilkins.

Chen, A. Y., & Halpern, M. (2007). Factors predictive of survival in advanced laryngeal cancer. *Archives of Otolaryngology, 133*(12), 1270–1276.

Colosimo, C., Bologna, M., Lamberti, S., Avanzino, L., Marinelli, L., Fabbrini, G., et al. (2006). A comparative study of primary and secondary hemifacial spasm. *Archives of Neurology, 63*(3), 441–444.

Davies, L., & Welch, G. (2006). Increasing incidence of thyroid cancer in the United States, 1973–2002. *JAMA, 295*(18), 2164–2167.

Diamond, S., Bigal, M. E., Silberstein, S., Loder, E., Reed, M., & Lipton, R. B. (2007). Patterns of diagnosis and acute and preventive treatment for migraine in the United States: Results from the American Migraine Prevalence and Prevention study. *Headache, 47*(3), 355–363.

Dunphy, L. M., Winland-Brown, J. E., Porter, B. O., & Thomas, D. J. (2007). *Primary care: Art & science of advanced practiced nursing* (2nd ed.). Philadelphia: F. A. Davis.

Jones, R. (2007). Primary hyperparathyroidism. *Clinician Reviews, 17*(7), 27–33.

Kronenberg, H. M., Melmed, S., Polonsky, K. S., & Larsen, P. R. (2008). *Williams textbook of endocrinology* (11th ed.). Philadelphia: Saunders.

Kurth, T., Gaziano, M., Cook, N. R., Bubes, V., Logroscino, G., Diener, H., & Buring, J. E. (2007). Migraine and risk of cardiovascular disease in men. *Archives of Internal Medicine, 167*(8), 795–801.

Merati, A. L., & Bielamowicz, S. A. (Eds.). (2006). *Textbook of laryngology.* San Diego: Plural Publishing.

Moore, A. (2007). Migraine prevention overview. *The American Journal for Nurse Practitioners, 11*(7, Editorial Supplement), 10–29.

Pereira, K., & Brown, A. J. (2008). Postpartum thyroiditis. *The Journal for Nurse Practitioners, 4*(3), 175–182.

Tiemstra, J. D., & Khatkhate, N. (2007). Bell's palsy: Diagnosis and management. *American Family Physician, 76*(7), 997–1002.

Uphold C. K., & Graham, M. V. (2003). *Clinical guidelines in family practice* (4th ed.). Gainesville, FL: Barmarrae Books.

Utiger, R. D. (2005). The multiplicity of thyroid nodules and carcinomas. *The New England Journal of Medicine, 352*(23), 2376–2378.

Vujevich, K. (2007, September). What makes women's migraines different. *The Clinical Advisor*, 33–38.

WEB SITES

American Academy of Allergy, Asthma & Immunology:
http://www.aaaai.org

American Academy of Otolaryngology—Head and Neck Surgery:
http://www.entnet.org

American Association of Clinical Endocrinologists:
http://www.aace.com

American Board of Otolaryngology:
http://www.aboto.org

American Society of Preventive Oncology:
http://www.aspo.org

The Endocrine Society:
http://www.endo-society.org

ENT Nursing:
http://www.entnursing.com

The Mayo Clinic:
http://www.mayoclinic.com

Scleroderma Foundation:
http://www.scleroderma.org

CHAPTER 12

Eyes

COMPETENCIES

1. Identify the structures of the eyes.

2. Discuss the system-specific history for the eyes.

3. Describe normal findings in the physical assessment of the eyes.

4. Describe common abnormalities found in the physical assessment of the eyes.

5. Explain the pathophysiology of common abnormalities of the eyes.

6. Perform the physical assessment of the eyes.

Physical examination of the eyes provides information about the patient's nutritional, endocrine, cardiovascular, gastrointestinal, and neurological systems. This chapter provides a comprehensive guide to examining the eye and the factors that affect it.

ANATOMY AND PHYSIOLOGY

EXTERNAL STRUCTURES

The external structures of the eyes comprise the eyelids or palpebra, the conjunctiva, the lacrimal glands, and the extraocular muscles. The eyelids consist of smooth muscle covered with a very thin layer of skin; they admit light to the eye while protecting and maintaining lubrication of the eye. The interior surface of the lid muscle is covered with a pink mucous membrane called the **palpebral conjunctiva**. Contiguous with the palpebral conjunctiva is the **bulbar conjunctiva**. The bulbar conjunctiva folds back over the anterior surface of the eyeball and merges with the cornea at the **limbus**, the junction of the sclera and the cornea (Figure 12-1). The conjunctiva contains blood vessels and pain receptors that respond quickly to outside insult. Eyelashes are evenly spaced along lid margins and curve outward to protect the eye by filtering particles of dirt and dust from the external environment. Eyebrows are symmetrical and evenly distributed above the eyelids.

The opening between the eyelids is called the **palpebral fissure**. Upper and lower eyelids meet at the inner **canthus** on the nasal side and at the outer canthus on the temporal side. Embedded just beneath the lid margins are the meibomian glands, which secrete a lubricating substance onto the surface of the eye. The **tarsal plates** are connective tissue that gives shape to the upper lids.

Lacrimal Apparatus

The **lacrimal apparatus** is made up of the lacrimal gland and ducts. The lacrimal glands, located above and on the temporal side of each eye, are responsible for the production of tears, which lubricate the eye. Tears drain through the inferior and superior **puncta** at the inner canthus through the nasolacrimal duct and the lacrimal sac to the inferior turbinate in the nose. The **caruncle**, which contains sebaceous glands, is the round, red structure in the inner canthus.

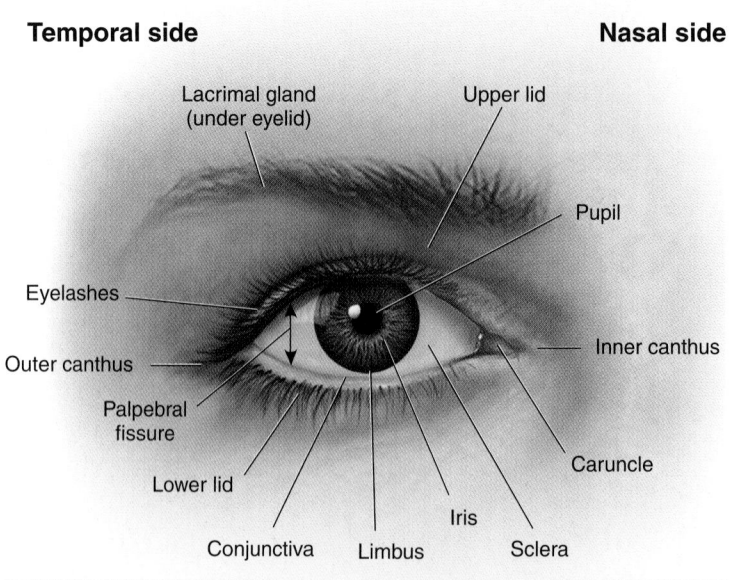

FIGURE 12-1 External View of the Right Eye

Extraocular Muscles

Six extraocular muscles extend from the scleral surface of each eye and attach to the bony orbit. These voluntary muscles work in concert to move the eyes with great precision in several directions to provide a single image to the brain. These muscles are the superior, inferior, medial, and lateral recti, and the superior and inferior obliques.

INTERNAL STRUCTURES

The globes of the eyes are spherical structures that are encased in the protective bony orbits of the face along with the lacrimal gland and extrinsic muscles of the eye. Only a small portion of the anterior surface of the eye is exposed. The eye itself is approximately 1 inch in diameter and has three layers: a tough, outer, fibrous tunic (sclera); a middle, vascular tunic; and the innermost layer, which contains the retina (Figure 12-2).

Outer Layer

The outer tunic consists of the transparent cornea on the outer portion, which is continuous with the **sclera**, an opaque material that appears white and covers the structures inside the eye. The **cornea** is a nonvascular, transparent surface that covers the iris and is continuous with the conjunctival epithelium. The sclera protects the eye and is a surface for the attachment of the extraocular muscles. The posterior portion of the sclera contains an opening for the entrance of the optic nerve and various blood vessels.

Middle Layer

The pigmented, middle, vascular tunic, or uveal layer, is composed of the **choroid**, the ciliary body, and the iris. The choroid is a vascular tissue that lines the inner surface of the eye just beneath the retina. It provides nutrition to the retinal pigment epithelium and helps absorb excess light.

The **ciliary body** is an anterior extension of the uveal tract; it siphons serum from the systemic blood flow to produce the aqueous humor needed to nourish the corneal endothelium. Zonules are small strands of tissue extending from the ciliary body to the crystalline **lens**. Zonules hold the lens in place and allow it to change shape in order to refract light from various focusing distances. The **iris**, the most anterior portion of the uveal tract, provides a distinctive color for the eye. It is comprised of

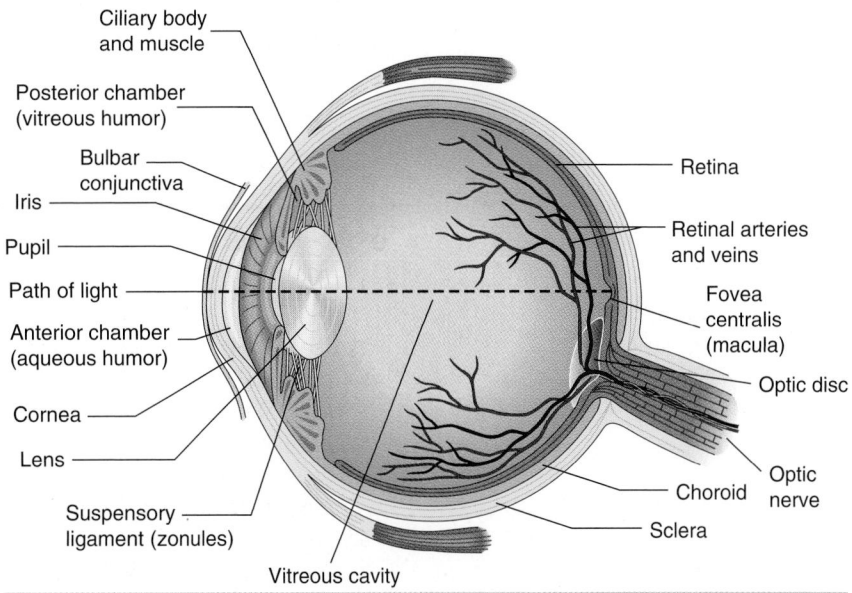

FIGURE 12-2 Lateral Cross Section of the Interior Eye

smooth muscle that regulates the entrance of light. The **pupil**, an opening in the center of the iris, regulates the amount of light entering the eye. The pupil reacts to light and the closeness of objects by stimulation of the sympathetic nervous system, which dilates it, and the parasympathetic nervous system, which constricts it.

The central cavity of the eye posterior to the lens is filled with a clear, gelatinous material called **vitreous humor**, which helps maintain the shape of the eye and the position of the internal structures.

Visual images pass through the structures and aqueous humor of the **anterior chamber**, the space anterior to the pupil and iris, and the vitreous humor of the **posterior chamber**, the space immediately posterior to the iris, to the fundus of the eye, where the retina is located.

Inner Layer

The innermost layer of the eyeball, or the **retina**, is an extension of the optic nerve, which lines the inside of the globe and receives light impulses to be transmitted to the occipital lobe of the brain. Paired retinal arteries and veins branch from the optic disc toward the periphery, growing smaller as they extend outward. Generally, retinal arteries are smaller and a lighter red than veins and often have a silver-looking "arterial light reflex." Normal arterial-to-venous width is a ratio of 2:3 or 4:5.

The **optic disc** is a round or oval area with distinct margins located on the nasal side of the retina. Retinal fibers join at the optic disc to form the optic nerve. Nerve fibers from the temporal visual fields cross at the optic chiasm.

The **physiologic cup** is a pale, central area in the optic disc occupying one-third to one-fourth of the disc. In the temporal area of the retina, the tiny, darker **macula**, with the **fovea centralis** at its center, contains a high concentration of **cones** necessary for color vision, reading ability, and other tasks requiring fine visual discrimination. The fovea is the area of sharpest vision. Other portions of the retina contain a high concentration of **rods**, which provide dark and light discrimination and peripheral vision.

VISUAL PATHWAY

Objects in the field of vision reflect light, which is received by sensory neurons in the retina; these images are received upside down and reversed. From there they pass along nerve fibers through the optic disc and the optic nerve. Fibers from the left half of each eye pass through the optic chiasm to the right side of the brain, and fibers from the right side of each eye pass to the left side of the visual cortex of the occipital lobe of the brain (see Figure 12-3).

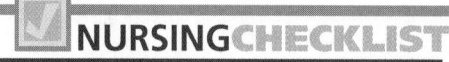

NURSINGCHECKLIST

General Approach to Eye Assessment

1. Greet the patient and explain the assessment techniques that you will be using.
2. Use a quiet room that will be free from interruptions.
3. Ensure that the light in the room provides sufficient brightness to allow adequate observation of the patient.
4. Place the patient in an upright sitting position on the examination table.
5. Visualize the underlying structures during the assessment process to allow adequate description of findings.
6. Always compare right and left eyes.
7. Use a systematic approach that is followed consistently each time the assessment is performed.

LEFT VISUAL FIELD   **RIGHT VISUAL FIELD**

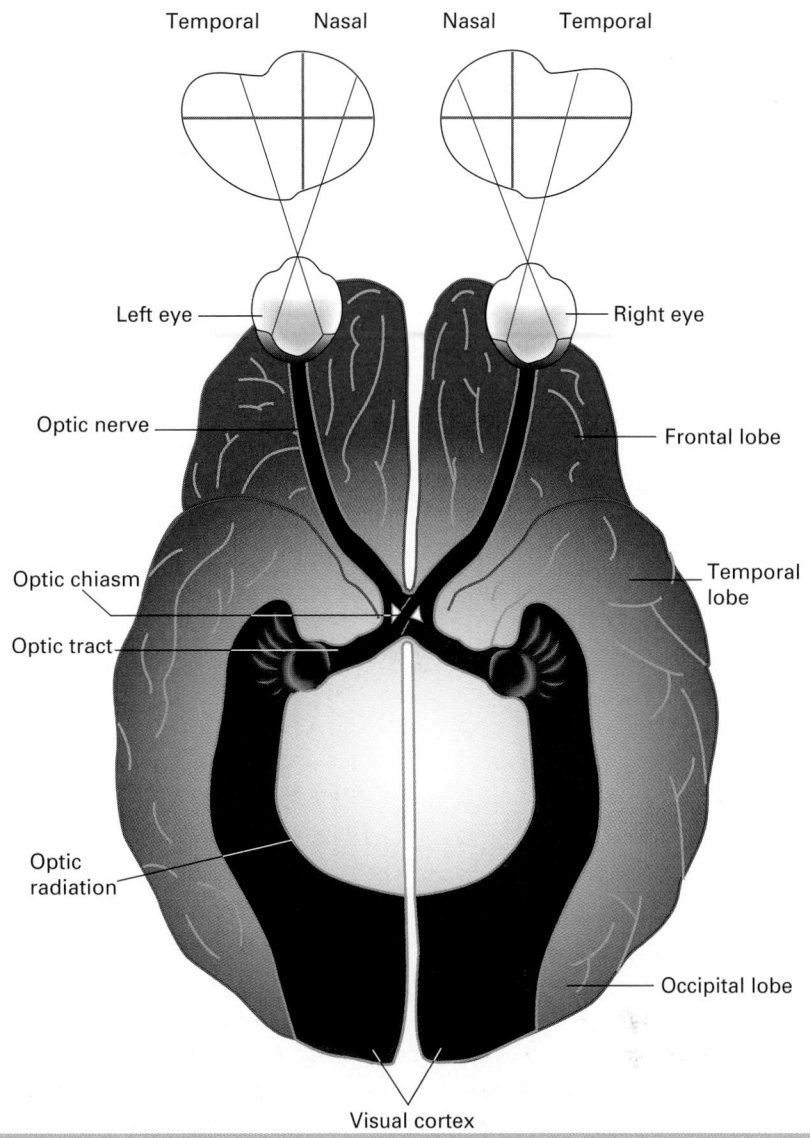

FIGURE 12-3   Visual Pathway

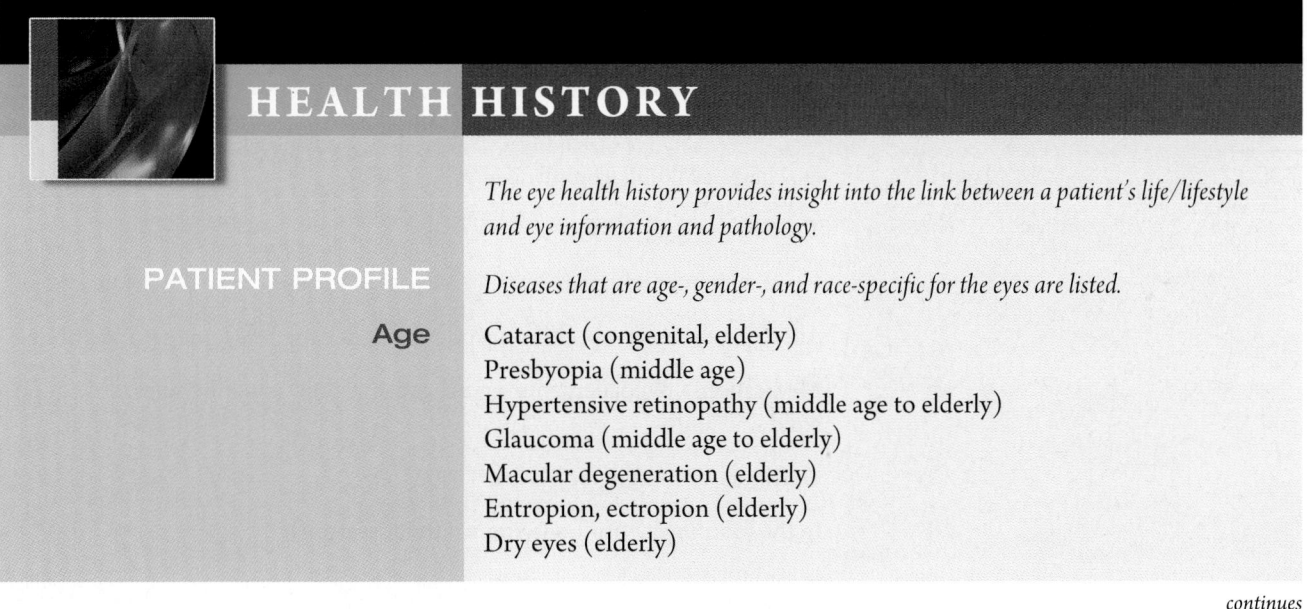

HEALTH HISTORY

The eye health history provides insight into the link between a patient's life/lifestyle and eye information and pathology.

PATIENT PROFILE

Diseases that are age-, gender-, and race-specific for the eyes are listed.

Age   Cataract (congenital, elderly)
Presbyopia (middle age)
Hypertensive retinopathy (middle age to elderly)
Glaucoma (middle age to elderly)
Macular degeneration (elderly)
Entropion, ectropion (elderly)
Dry eyes (elderly)

continues

Gender	Female: dry eyes, thyroid-related ophthalmopathy
Race	Glaucoma (African Americans), melanoma of the eye (Caucasians)
CHIEF COMPLAINT	*Common chief complaints for the eyes are defined, and information on the characteristics of each sign or symptom is provided.*
1. Changes in Visual Acuity	Change in ability to see clearly
Location	One eye or both eyes
Quality	Dimming of vision, blurred vision, diplopia, visual field loss, legal blindness
Associated Manifestations	Headache, rhinorrhea, sneezing, vertigo, "floaters" (spots of different sizes that float across the visual field and are caused by changes in the vitreous humor), flashes of light, aura, nausea and vomiting, generalized muscle weakness, eye pain or pressure, infection (herpes simplex/herpes zoster or cytomegalovirus)
Aggravating Factors	Allergens, stress, lack of sleep, decreased lighting, darkness (night), refractive changes, systemic diseases
Alleviating Factors	Improved lighting, medication, corrective glasses, rest or sleep, adequate hydration
Setting	Work environment, increased reading, computer work, night driving
Timing	With aging, at night, after trauma, with or after a headache, seasonal, sudden onset, gradual onset
2. Pain	Discomfort in the eye
Quality	Aching, sharp, throbbing, burning
Associated Manifestations	Drainage, conjunctival injection, decreased vision, herpes simplex/herpes zoster, increased tearing, headache
Aggravating Factors	Foreign body in the eye, sunlight or very bright light, contact lenses, trauma, allergens
Alleviating Factors	Closing of eye or eyes, removal of contacts, medications, sunglasses, avoiding allergens
Setting	Work environment (increased reading or computer work), recreational area, outdoors
Timing	Sudden onset, gradual onset, with reading
3. Drainage	Discharge of liquid from the eye
Quality	Type, color
Associated Manifestations	Crusting on the lids, pain, itching, redness of the eye or the lids, headache
Aggravating Factors	Allergens, eye makeup, chlorine, poor hygiene, upper respiratory infection
Alleviating Factors	Medications, hypoallergenic or no eye makeup, avoiding allergens, good hand washing
Setting	Outdoors, swimming pool
Timing	In the morning, continuous, intermittent, seasonal

continues

Health History (continued)

4. Itching	Irritation that causes the patient to scratch or rub
Quality	Mild, severe
Associated Manifestations	Rhinitis, sneezing, drainage, burning sensation in the eye, gritty sensation in the eye, conjunctivitis, headache
Aggravating Factors	Allergens, contact lenses, eye makeup
Alleviating Factors	Medications, cold compresses to the eyes, removal of contacts, avoiding allergens and eye makeup
Setting	Indoors, outdoors
Timing	Seasonal, intermittent, continuous
5. Dryness	Reduced amount of lubricating secretions in the eye
Associated Manifestations	With systemic disease, redness of the eye, reduced tearing, itching
Aggravating Factors	Decreased humidity, wind, reading
Alleviating Factors	Artificial tears, humidified air
Setting	Outdoors, indoors with decreased humidity
Timing	With aging, during the winter (decreased humidity), postmenopause
PAST HEALTH HISTORY	*The various components of the past health history are linked to eye pathology and eye-related information.*
Medical History	
Eye Specific	Myopia, hyperopia, strabismus, diplopia, astigmatism, glaucoma, cataracts, conjunctivitis, hordeolum, pterygium, blepharitis, chalazion, trachoma, macular degeneration, prosthesis
Non-Eye Specific	Diabetes mellitus, renal disease, atherosclerotic disease, hypertension, thyroid disease, inflammatory processes, infections (viral or bacterial), immunosuppressive disease, nutritional disturbances, collagen vascular diseases, MS, myasthenia gravis
Surgical History	Cataract extraction, lens implant, LASIK (laser-assisted in situ-keratomileusis) [laser vision correction], repair of detached retina, neurosurgery, enucleation of eye, optic nerve decompression, prosthesis insertion
Allergies	Pollen: watery or itchy eyes Insect stings: swelling around the eyes Animal dander: watery or itchy eyes
Medications	Carbonic anhydrase inhibitors, nonselective β-blockers, mast cell stabilizers, antibiotics, antihistamines, decongestants, corticosteroids, artificial tears, mydriatics, myotics
Injuries and Accidents	Foreign bodies; trauma to the eyes
Special Needs	Legal blindness, glasses/contacts for driving/reading
Childhood Illnesses	Rubella and visual sequelae (blindness), congenital syphilis, strabismus

continues

Health History (continued)

FAMILY HEALTH HISTORY	*Eye diseases that are familial are listed.* Myopia, hyperopia, strabismus, color blindness, cataracts, glaucoma, macular degeneration, retinitis pigmentosa, retinoblastoma, neonatal blindness secondary to cataracts from mother contracting rubella in pregnancy
SOCIAL HISTORY	*The components of the social history are linked to eye factors and pathology.*
Tobacco Use	Smoking is associated with macular degeneration and cataracts
Travel History	Prolonged facial exposure to sun; facial exposure to contaminated waste
Work Environment	Exposure to toxins/chemicals, infections, allergens, eye strain from long hours reading/computer use
Stress	Can be linked with decreased vision
Ethnic Background	Trachoma: Middle Easterners, American Indians
HEALTH MAINTENANCE ACTIVITIES	*This information provides a bridge between the health maintenance activities and eye functions.*
Diet	Vitamin deficiencies may affect vision
Use of Safety Devices	Goggles or face shields for sports, job, or home projects; sunglasses in bright ultraviolet light
Health Check-ups	Eye examination, intraocular pressure check

NURSING**TIP**

Prosthetic Eyes

Observe and talk with the patient to determine whether or not a prosthetic eye is worn. If so, determine the reason for the loss of the natural eye. A prosthetic eye may be needed following eye trauma or extensive disease of the eye. Ask the patient if he or she has any difficulties with the eye prosthesis.

EQUIPMENT

- Ophthalmoscope
- Penlight
- Clean gloves
- Snellen chart, Snellen E chart, Rosenbaum near vision pocket screening card
- Vision occluder
- Cotton-tipped applicator

ASSESSMENT OF THE EYE

Assessment of the eyes should be carried out in an orderly fashion, moving from the extraocular structures to the intraocular structures. The eye assessment usually includes testing of associated cranial nerves and can be performed in the following order:

1. Determination of visual acuity
2. Determination of visual fields
3. Assessment of the external eye and lacrimal apparatus
4. Evaluation of extraocular muscle function
5. Assessment of the anterior segment structures
6. Assessment of the posterior segment structures

VISUAL ACUITY

The assessment of visual acuity (cranial nerve II) is a simple, noninvasive procedure that is carried out with the use of a Snellen chart and an occluder to cover

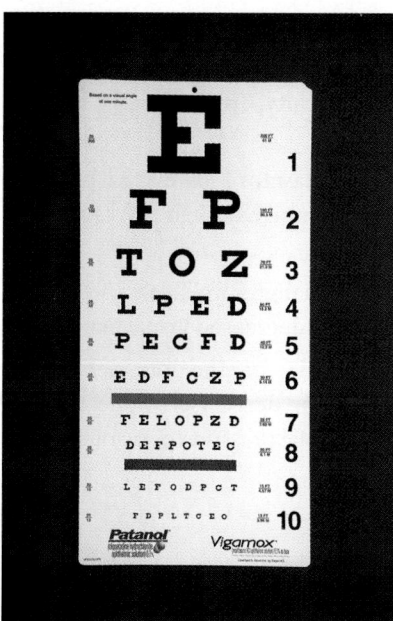

A. Snellen Vision Chart

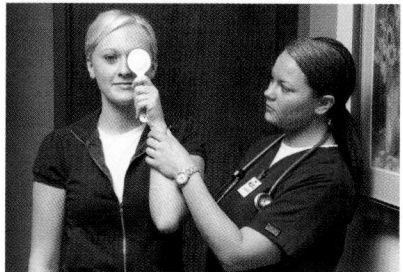

B. Assist the patient in occluding the eye.

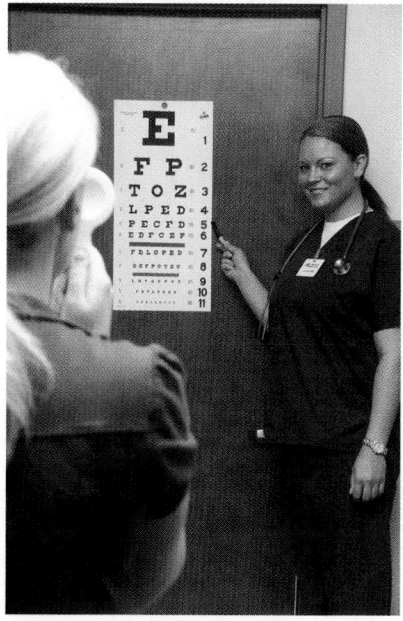

C. Assessing Distance Vision

FIGURE 12-4 Visual Acuity Testing

the patient's eye. The **Snellen chart** contains letters of various sizes with standardized visual acuity numbers at the end of each line of letters (Figure 12-4A). The numbers indicate the degree of visual acuity when the patient is able to read that line of letters at a distance of 20 feet. For instance, a patient who has a visual acuity of 20/70 can read at 20 feet what a patient with 20/20 vision is able to read at 70 feet.

It is sometimes difficult to have a space of 20 feet available for the placement of the chart, but the distance can be simulated with the use of mirrors. For all vision screening, the chart should be illuminated with a diffuse light source to prevent spot lighting or glare.

Distance Vision

E 1. Ask the patient to stand or sit facing the Snellen chart at a distance of 20 feet.

2. If the patient normally wears glasses, ask that they be removed. Contact lenses may be left in the eyes.

3. Instruct the patient to cover the left eye with the occluder (Figure 12-4B) and to read as many lines on the chart as possible.

4. Note the number at the end of the last line the patient was able to read (Figure 12-4C).

5. If the patient is unable to read the letters at the top of the chart, move the patient closer to the chart. Note the distance at which the patient is able to read the top line.

6. Repeat the test, occluding the right eye.

7. Repeat the test, using both eyes.

8. If the patient normally wears glasses, the test should be repeated with the patient wearing the glasses, and it should be so noted (corrected or uncorrected).

N The patient who has a visual acuity of 20/20 is considered to have normal visual acuity.

A The patient is unable to read the chart with an uncorrected visual acuity of 20/30 in one eye, vision in both eyes is different by two lines or more, or acuity is absent.

P The patient may have a refractive error related to a difference in the refractive power of the cornea. Figure 12-5A illustrates how light rays focus on the retina in a normal eye. In **myopia** (nearsightedness), the axial length of the globe is longer than normal, resulting in the image not being focused directly on the retina; this condition can be changed with corrective lenses (see Figure 12-5B). If the patient is amblyopic, no corrective lenses will improve vision. **Amblyopia** is the permanent loss of visual acuity resulting from strabismus that was not corrected in early childhood, or certain medical conditions (alcoholism, uremia, diabetes mellitus).

P The patient may have corneal opacities that are congenital, from lesions that have scarred the cornea (e.g., herpes simplex), from trauma, or from degeneration and dystrophies.

P Visual acuity can be decreased because of opacities of the lens caused by senile or traumatic cataracts.

| **E** Examination | **N** Normal Findings | **A** Abnormal Findings | **P** Pathophysiology |

P Systemic autoimmune diseases such as inflammatory bowel disease, arthritis, or other collagen vascular diseases can be associated with inflammation of the iris (iritis), which will affect visual acuity. Iritis can also be idiopathic.

P Inflammation of the retina caused by toxoplasmosis or by the presence of blood in the vitreous humor following hemorrhage can be responsible for decreased visual acuity.

P Systemic diseases, such as hypertension or diabetes mellitus, and trauma may damage the choroid and retina, causing decreased visual acuity.

P Visual acuity can be impaired by pathology affecting the optic nerve, such as multiple sclerosis, tumors or abscesses of the nerve itself, optic atrophy, papilledema resulting from increased intracranial pressure, optic neuritis, or neovascularization of the optic nerve.

Near Vision

E 1. Use a pocket Snellen chart, Rosenbaum card (see Figure 12-6), or any printed material written at an appropriate reading level.

   2. If the pocket vision card is available, have the patient sit comfortably and hold the card 14 inches from the face without moving it.

   3. Ask the patient to read the smallest line possible. If other printed material is used, you will be able to gain only a general understanding of the patient's near vision.

N Until the patient is in the late 30s to the late 40s, reading is generally possible at a distance of 14 inches.

A A patient in this age range who cannot read at 14 inches is considered **presbyopic**. Younger persons may have difficulty seeing up close because they have **hyperopia**, or farsightedness (Figure 12-5C).

P The normal aging process causes the lens to harden (nuclear sclerosis), decreasing its ability to change shape and therefore focus on near objects.

Color Vision

E Color vision is usually tested in young children. If there is suspicion that the patient has a color vision deficit, have the patient identify the primary colors on the Snellen chart or colors in the examining room. For more specific testing, refer to Chapter 24.

N The patient should be able to identify colors correctly.

A The color vision defect is designated as red/green, blue/yellow, or complete when the patient sees only shades of gray.

P Defects in color vision can result from diseases of the optic nerve, macular degeneration, pathology of the fovea centralis, nutritional deficiency, or heredity.

VISUAL FIELDS

The confrontation technique is used to test visual fields of each eye (CN II). The visual field of each eye is divided into quadrants, and a stimulus is presented in each quadrant.

E 1. Sit or stand approximately 2 to 3 feet away from and opposite the patient, with your eyes at the same level as the patient's (see Figure 12-7A).

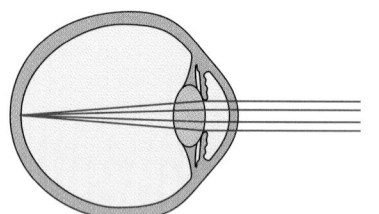

A. Normal eye
Light rays focus on the retina.

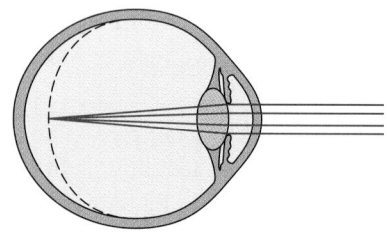

B. Myopia (nearsightedness)
Light rays focus in front of the retina.

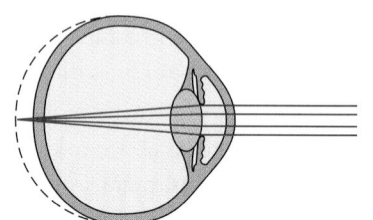

C. Hyperopia (farsightedness)
Light rays focus behind the retina.

FIGURE 12-5 **Eye Refraction**

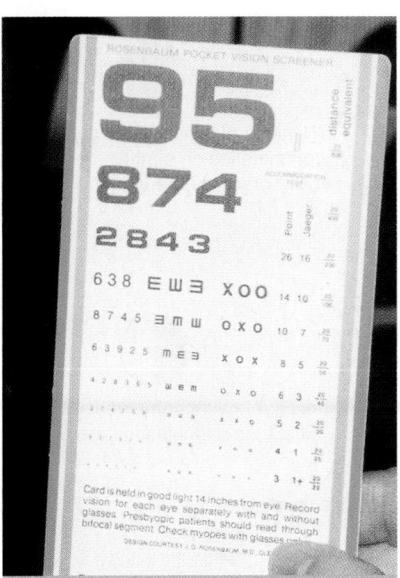

FIGURE 12-6 Near Vision Testing with the Rosenbaum Pocket Vision Screener

2. Have the patient cover the right eye with the right hand or an occluder.

3. Cover your left eye in the same manner.

4. Have the patient look at your uncovered eye with his or her uncovered eye.

5. Hold your free hand at arm's length equidistant from you and the patient and move it or a held object such as a pen into your and the patient's field of vision from nasal, temporal, superior, inferior, and oblique angles.

6. Ask the patient to say "now" when your hand is seen moving into the field of vision. Use your own visual fields as the control for comparison to the patient's.

7. Repeat the procedure for the other eye.

N The patient is able to see the stimulus at about 90° temporally, 60° nasally, 50° superiorly, and 70° inferiorly (Figure 12-7B).

A If the patient is unable to identify movement that you perceive, a defect in the visual field is presumed. The portion of the visual field loss should be noted (see Figure 12-8).

P Defects in the patient's visual field can be associated with tumors, strokes, or neurological diseases such as glaucoma or retinal detachment.

EXTERNAL EYE AND LACRIMAL APPARATUS

The assessment of the external eye includes the eyelids and the lacrimal apparatus. Pathology of the eyelids is among the most common eye complaints of patients seeing a health care provider.

Eyelids, Eyebrows, and Eyelashes

E 1. Ask the patient to sit facing you.

2. Observe the patient's eyelids for drooping, infection, tumors, or other abnormalities.

3. Note the distribution and symmetry of the eyelashes and eyebrows. Note any lesions.

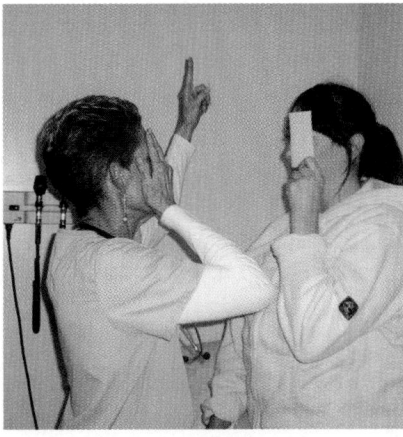

A. The nurse and patient should be approximately at an eye-to-eye level.

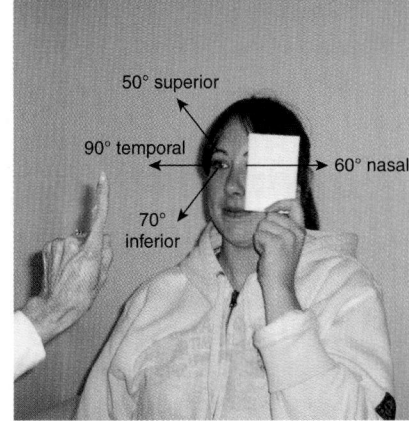

B. Visual Fields Range

FIGURE 12-7 Testing Visual Fields by Confrontation

E Examination   **N** Normal Findings   **A** Abnormal Findings   **P** Pathophysiology

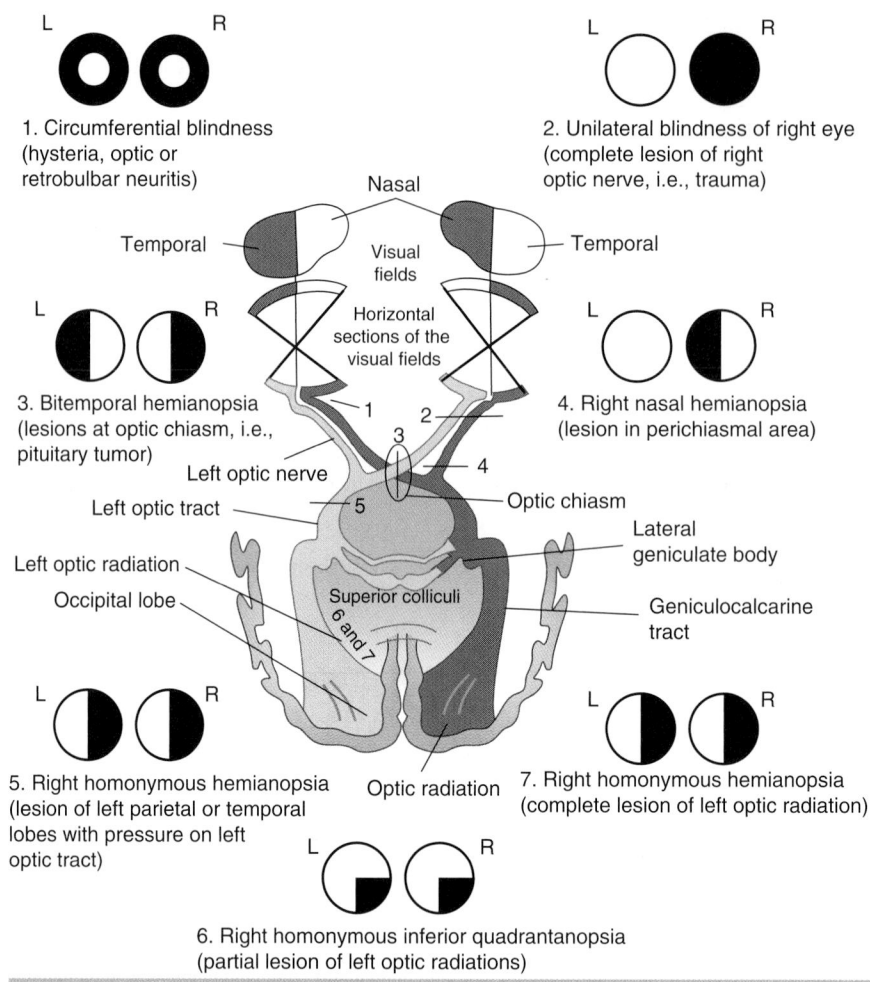

1. Circumferential blindness (hysteria, optic or retrobulbar neuritis)

2. Unilateral blindness of right eye (complete lesion of right optic nerve, i.e., trauma)

Nasal

Temporal — Visual fields — Temporal

Horizontal sections of the visual fields

3. Bitemporal hemianopsia (lesions at optic chiasm, i.e., pituitary tumor)

4. Right nasal hemianopsia (lesion in perichiasmal area)

Left optic nerve

Left optic tract — Optic chiasm

Left optic radiation — Lateral geniculate body

Occipital lobe — Superior colliculi — Geniculocalcarine tract

5. Right homonymous hemianopsia (lesion of left parietal or temporal lobes with pressure on left optic tract)

Optic radiation

7. Right homonymous hemianopsia (complete lesion of left optic radiation)

6. Right homonymous inferior quadrantanopsia (partial lesion of left optic radiations)

FIGURE 12-8 Visual Field Defects

4. Instruct the patient to focus on an object or a finger held about 10 to 12 inches away and slightly above eye level.

5. Move the object or finger slowly downward and observe for a white space of sclera between the upper lid and the limbus.

6. Observe the blinking of the eyes.

7. Ask the patient to elevate the eyelids.

N The eyelids should appear symmetrical with no drooping, infections, or tumors of the lids. Eyelids of Asians normally slant upward. When the eyes are focused in a normal frontal gaze, the lids should cover the upper portion of the iris. The patient can raise both eyelids symmetrically (CN III). Slight **ptosis**, or drooping of the lid, can be normal. When the eye is closed, no portion of the cornea should be exposed. Normal lid margins are smooth, with the lashes evenly distributed and sweeping upward from the upper lids and downward from the lower lids. Eyebrows are present bilaterally and are symmetrical and without lesions or scaling.

A The patient has either unilateral or bilateral, constant or intermittent ptosis of the lid (Figure 12-9). If part of the pupil is occluded, there may be wrinkling of the forehead above the affected eye in an attempt to compensate by using the frontalis muscle to lift the lid.

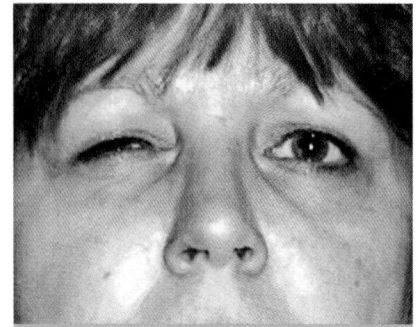

FIGURE 12-9 Ptosis

| **E** Examination | **N** Normal Findings | **A** Abnormal Findings | **P** Pathophysiology |

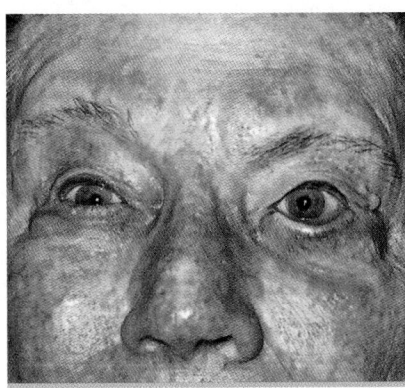

FIGURE 12-10 **Ectropion.** *Courtesy of Mary A. Hitcho.*

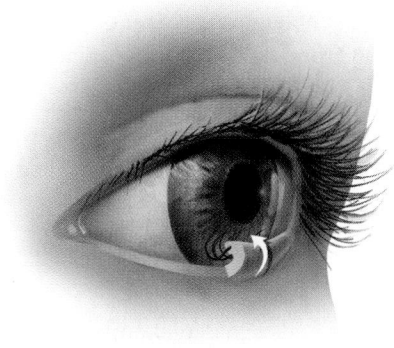

FIGURE 12-11 **Entropion**

P Ptosis can be either congenital or acquired. In congenital ptosis, there is failure of the levator muscle to develop. This condition may be associated with pathology of the superior rectus muscle as well. If the ptosis is acquired, it is related to one of three factors:

1. Mechanical: heavy lids from lesions, adipose tissue, swelling, or edema
2. Myogenic: muscular diseases such as myasthenia gravis or multiple sclerosis
3. Neurogenic: paralysis from damage or interruption of the neural pathways

A An area of white sclera appears between the upper lid and the limbus, widening as the object is moved downward.

P This condition is called lid lag and may indicate the presence of thyrotoxicosis or increased circulating levels of free thyroxine or triiodothyronine.

A The patient is unable to bring about complete lid closure. This is generally a unilateral condition.

P This condition is referred to as **lagophthalmos** and can be associated with Bell's palsy, stroke, trauma, or **ectropion** (everted eyelid) (Figure 12-10).

A During inspection of the lids, a disparity of the palpebral fissure is noted with apparent lid retraction, indicating a protrusion of the globe. This condition may be unilateral or bilateral.

P This abnormality is **exophthalmos** (or proptosis) and can be present unilaterally in orbital tumors, thyroid disease, trauma, or inflammation. Bilateral exophthalmos is related to thyroid disease.

A There is apparent disparity in the size of the globe, manifested by a narrowing of the palpebral fissure.

P Enophthalmos is a backward displacement of the globe in the orbit, generally caused by orbital blowout fracture due to trauma. When this occurs, the orbital contents herniate through the fracture site.

A The turning inward, or inversion, of the lower lid is referred to as **entropion** and can cause severe discomfort to the patient as the eyelashes abrade the cornea (trichiasis) (Figure 12-11). If left untreated, it can cause inflammation, corneal scarring, and eventual ulceration.

P Entropion is caused by spasms or advancing age (senile). In senile entropion, there is a loss of muscle tone, which causes the lid to fold inward.

A The turning outward, or eversion, of the lower lid is referred to as ectropion and may be unilateral or bilateral. With ectropion, the lower lids appear to be sagging outward.

P The normal aging process can cause the muscles to lose their tone and relax, or they may be affected by Bell's palsy.

A The patient exhibits excessive blinking that may or may not be accompanied by increased tearing and pain.

P The causes of excessive blinking are:

1. Voluntary: irritation to the cornea or the conjunctiva, or stress and anxiety (usually disappears when stimulus is removed)
2. Involuntary: tonic spasms of the orbicularis oculi muscle called blepharospasm; often seen in elderly individuals as well as in patients with CN VII lesions, irritation of the eye, fatigue, and stress

A The lids are black and blue, bluish, yellow, or red, depending on race and skin color.

P Color changes in the lids can result from the following:

1. Redness: generalized redness is nonspecific; however, redness in the nasal half of the lid may indicate frontal sinusitis. Redness adjacent to the lower lid can indicate disease of the lacrimal sac or nasolacrimal duct, such as dacryocystitis; and redness in the temporal portion of the lid can result from dacryoadenitis, an inflammation of the lacrimal gland.

2. Bluish: cyanosis can result from orbital vein thrombosis, orbital tumors, or aneurysms in the orbit.

3. Black and blue: ecchymosis is caused by bleeding into the surrounding tissues following trauma (black eye).

A Swelling or edema is noted in the eyelid.

P Swelling or edema may be noted in nonocular conditions such as inflammation associated with allergies, herpes simplex virus, systemic diseases, medications that contribute to swelling from fluid overload, trichinosis, early myxedema, thyrotoxicosis, or contact dermatitis.

A There is an acute localized inflammation, tenderness, and redness, with the patient complaining of pain in the infected area. This is called a **hordeolum**.

P *Staphylococcus* is generally the infecting organism that causes a hordeolum.

There are two types of hordeolum:

1. Internal: affects the meibomian glands, is usually large, and can point either to the skin or to the conjunctival side of the lid.

2. External: often called a "stye," an infection of a sebaceous gland that usually points to the skin side of the lid, and extends to the lid margin.

Infections of the glands of the eyelid can be caused by improper removal of makeup, dry eyes, or seborrhea. There may be some connection between a hordeolum and increased handling of the lids in activities such as inserting and removing contact lenses.

A There is a chronic inflammation of the meibomian gland in either the upper or the lower lid (Figure 12-12). It generally forms over several weeks and, in many cases, points toward the conjunctival side of the lid, usually not on the lid margin. There is no redness or tenderness.

P This inflammation is referred to as a **chalazion** and its cause is unknown.

A The lids are inflamed bilaterally and are red rimmed, with scales clinging to both the upper and the lower lids. The patient complains of itching and burning along the lid margins. There may also be some loss of the eyelashes.

P This is **blepharitis**, which may be either staphylococcal or seborrheic. Often a patient has both types simultaneously. If the patient has seborrheic infections elsewhere (scalp or eyebrows), it is more likely that the blepharitis is of the seborrheic type.

A Raised, yellow, nonpainful plaques are present on upper and lower lids near the inner canthus.

P These lesions are **xanthelasma**, a form of xanthoma frequently associated with hypercholesterolemia.

A The eyebrows have scaling areas.

P This is caused by seborrhea.

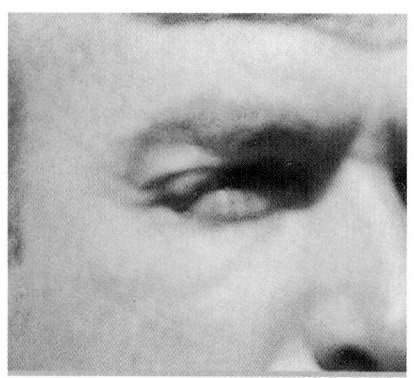

FIGURE 12-12 Chalazion

Lacrimal Apparatus

INSPECTION.

E 1. Have the patient sit facing you.

2. Identify the area of the lacrimal gland. Note any swelling or enlargement of the gland or elevation of the eyelid. Note any enlargement, swelling, redness, increased tearing, or exudate in the area of the lacrimal sac at the inner canthus.

3. Compare to the other eye in order to determine whether there is unilateral or bilateral involvement.

N There should be no enlargement, swelling, or redness; no large amount of exudate; and minimal tearing.

A There is inflammation and swelling in the upper lateral aspect of one or both eyes, and the patient complains of pain in the affected area.

P Acute inflammation of the lacrimal gland is called **dacryoadenitis** and does not occur commonly. Dacryoadenitis may result from trauma or may be found in association with measles, mumps, and mononucleosis.

A There is inflammation and painful swelling beside the nose and near the inner canthus and possibly extending to the eyelid.

P **Dacryocystitis** is caused by inflammatory or neoplastic obstruction of the lacrimal duct.

PALPATION.

E 1. To assess the lacrimal sac for obstruction, don gloves.

2. Gently press the index finger near the inner canthus, just inside the rim of the bony orbit of the eye.

3. Note any discharge from the punctum.

N There should not be excessive tearing or discharge from the punctum.

A Mucopurulent discharge is noted.

P Obstruction anywhere along the system from the lacrimal sac to the point at which the ducts empty below the inferior nasal turbinate can cause mucopurulent discharge.

A There is an overflowing of tears from the eye.

P This condition is epiphora, which is caused by obstruction of the lacrimal duct.

EXTRAOCULAR MUSCLE FUNCTION

Six extraocular muscles control the movement of each eye in relation to three axes: vertical, horizontal, and oblique (see Figure 12-13). Assessing extraocular function is carried out by observing corneal light reflex or alignment, using the

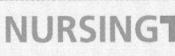

NURSINGTIP

Extraocular Muscles

One method of remembering the names of extraocular muscles and associated cranial nerves is: LR (lateral rectus) VI; SO (superior oblique) IV; all others (superior, inferior, and medial rectus and inferior oblique) are III.

| **E** Examination | **N** Normal Findings | **A** Abnormal Findings | **P** Pathophysiology |

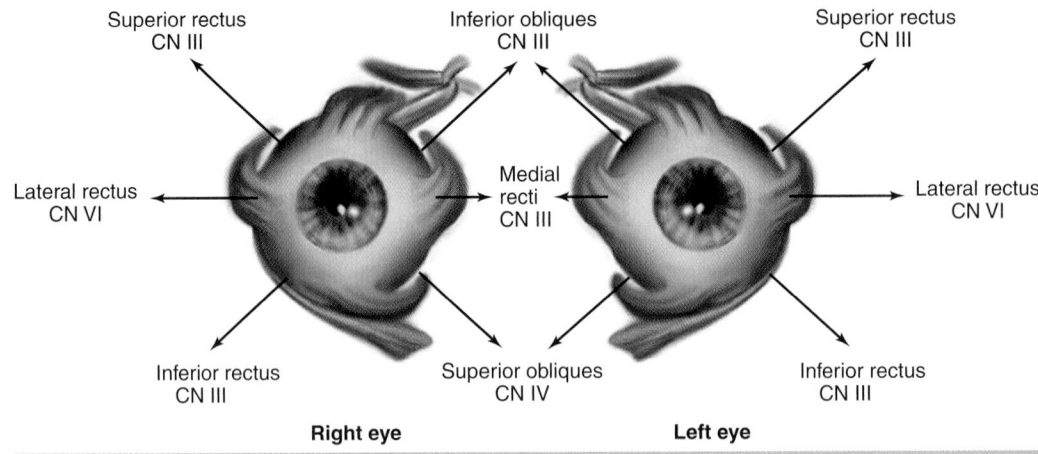

Superior rectus
CN III

Inferior obliques
CN III

Superior rectus
CN III

Lateral rectus
CN VI

Medial
recti
CN III

Lateral rectus
CN VI

Inferior rectus
CN III

Superior obliques
CN IV

Inferior rectus
CN III

Right eye **Left eye**

FIGURE 12-13 Direction of Movement of Extraocular Muscles

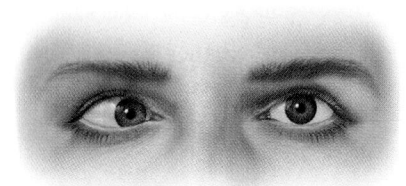

A. Right esotropia

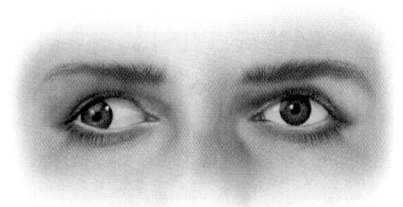

B. Right exotropia

FIGURE 12-14 Strabismus

cover/uncover test, and by testing the six cardinal fields of gaze (cranial nerves III, IV, and VI).

Corneal Light Reflex (Hirschberg Test)

E 1. Instruct the patient to look straight ahead.

2. Focus a penlight on the corneas from a distance of 12 to 15 inches away at the midline.

3. Observe the location of reflected light on the cornea.

N The reflected light (light reflex) should be seen symmetrically in the center of each cornea.

A There is a discrepancy in the placement of one of the light reflections.

P Asymmetrical corneal light reflexes indicate an extraocular muscle imbalance that may be related to a variety of causes, depending on the patient's age and medical condition: neurological, such as myasthenia gravis, multiple sclerosis, stroke, neuropathies of diabetes mellitus; uncorrected childhood strabismus (misalignment); trauma; or hypertension. The condition of one eye constantly being deviated is called **strabismus**, or tropia: **esotropia** is an inward turning of the eye; **exotropia** is an outward turning of the eye (Figure 12-14).

Cover/Uncover Test

E 1. Ask the patient to look straight ahead and to focus on an object in the distance.

2. Place an occluder over the left eye for several seconds and observe for movement in the uncovered right eye.

3. As the occluder is removed, observe the covered eye for movement.

4. Repeat the procedure with the same eye, having the patient focus on an object held close to the eye.

5. Repeat on the other side.

N If the eyes are in alignment, there will be no movement of either eye.

A If the uncovered eye shifts position as the other eye is covered, or if the covered eye shifts position as it is uncovered, a **phoria**, or latent misalignment of an eye, exists.

P This condition is a mild weakness elicited by the cover/uncover test and has two forms: **esophoria**, nasal or inward drift, and **exophoria**, a temporal or outward drift (see Figure 12-15).

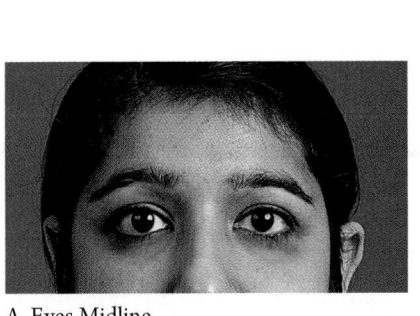

A. Eyes Midline

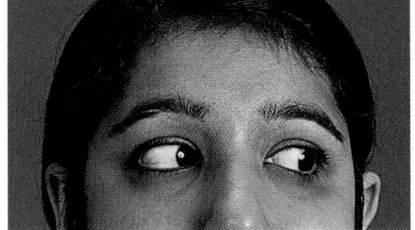

B. Left Lateral Gaze

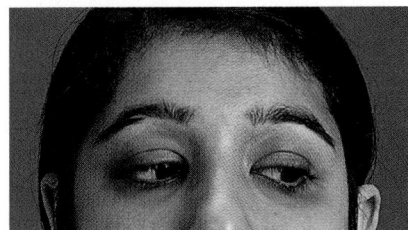

C. Left Lateral Inferior Gaze

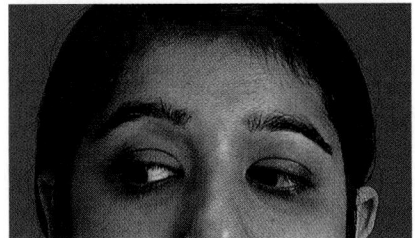

D. Right Lateral Inferior Gaze

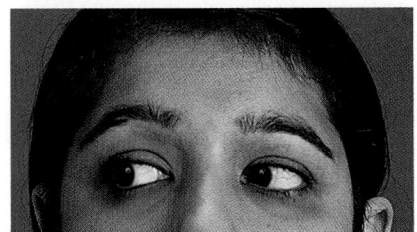

E. Right Lateral Gaze

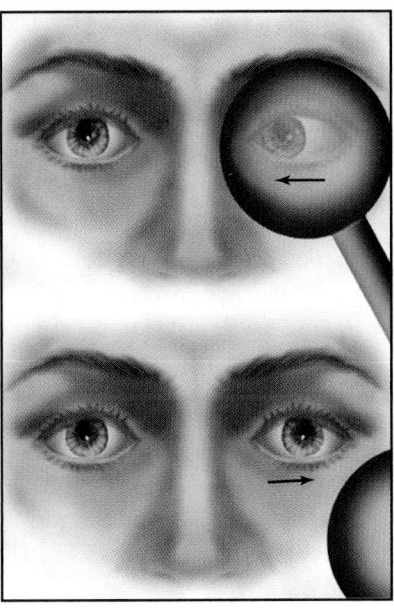

Left covered eye is weaker.
(Left exophoria)

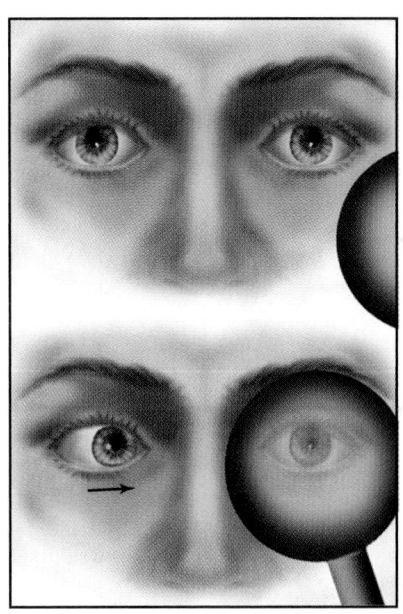

Right uncovered eye is weaker.
(Right esophoria)

FIGURE 12-15 Cover/Uncover Test

Cardinal Fields of Gaze (Extraocular Muscle Movements)

E 1. Place the patient in a sitting position facing you.

2. Place the nondominant hand just under the patient's chin or on top of the patient's head as a reminder to hold the head still.

3. Ask the patient to follow an object (finger, pencil, or penlight) with the eyes.

4. Move the object through the six fields of gaze (Figure 12-16) in a smooth and steady manner, pausing at each extreme position to detect any **nystagmus**, or involuntary movement, and returning to the center after each field is tested.

5. Note the patient's ability to move the eyes in each direction.

6. Move the object forward to about 5 inches in front of the patient's nose at the midline.

7. Observe for convergence of gaze.

N Both eyes should move smoothly and symmetrically in each of the six fields of gaze and converge on the held object as it moves toward the nose. A few beats of nystagmus with extreme lateral gaze can be normal.

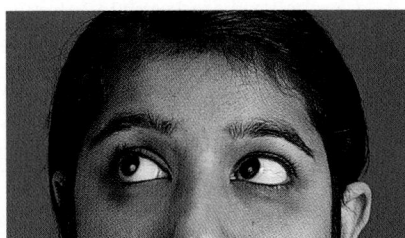

F. Right Lateral Superior Gaze

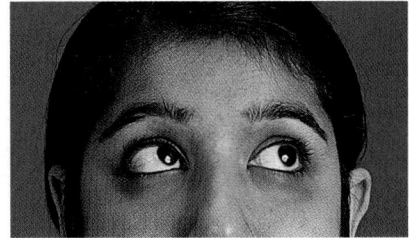

G. Left Lateral Superior Gaze

FIGURE 12-16 Cardinal Fields of Gaze

| **E** Examination | **N** Normal Findings | **A** Abnormal Findings | **P** Pathophysiology |

A There is a lack of symmetrical eye movement in a particular direction.

P Inability to move the eye in a given direction indicates a weakness in the muscle responsible for moving the eye in that direction.

A Abnormal eye movements consist of failure of an eye to move outward (CN VI), inability of an eye to move downward when deviated inward (CN IV), or other defects in movement (CN III).

P Traumatic ophthalmoplegia may be caused by fracture of the orbit near the foramen magnum, causing damage to the extraocular muscles or CN II, III, IV, and VI. Basilar skull fractures that involve the cavernous sinus may also cause extraocular muscle palsy.

P Vitamin deficiency, especially thiamine (which may occur in chronic alcoholism), may cause extraocular muscle palsy and nystagmus. Usually CN VI is affected.

P Herpes zoster, syphilis, scarlet fever, whooping cough, or botulism are infections that may affect CN III, IV, and VI, causing extraocular muscle palsy.

A Ophthalmoplegia is paralysis of one or more of the optic muscles.

P Increased intracranial pressure may cause strangulation of CN VI. CN VI palsy occurs late after the onset of increased intracranial pressure.

P Parasellar meningiomas or tumors in the sphenoid sinus may impinge on the wall of the cavernous sinus and involve one or more cranial nerves (CN III, IV, and VI).

A Vertical gaze is a paralysis of upward gaze and it is abnormal.

P Destruction at the area of the midbrain-diencephalic junction or the medial longitudinal fasciculus, or tumors of the pineal gland that press on the brain stem at the superior colliculus can cause a vertical gaze deviation.

A Paralysis of horizontal gaze is abnormal.

P Damage to the motor areas of the cerebral cortex causes the loss of the ability of both eyes to look to the contralateral side, so the eyes tend to deviate toward the side of the lesion.

A With internuclear ophthalmoplegia, the eyes are unable to look medially, but convergence may be maintained because the pathway for convergence is different from that for conjugate gaze.

P The medial rectus muscle is involved, so the eyes are unable to look medially. Internuclear ophthalmoplegia may be caused by demyelinization due to multiple sclerosis.

A If one eye deviates down and the other eye deviates up, it is called skew deviation.

P Cerebellar disease or a lesion in the pons on the same side as the eye that is deviated down may cause skew deviation.

A There is a rhythmic, beating, involuntary oscillation of the eyes as the object is held at points away from the midline. Movement is usually lateral, vertical, or rotary. Nystagmus can be jerky, with fast and slow components, or rhythmic, similar to the pendulum of a clock.

P Nystagmus may be caused by a lesion in the brain stem, cerebellum, vestibular system, or along the visual pathways in the cerebral hemispheres.

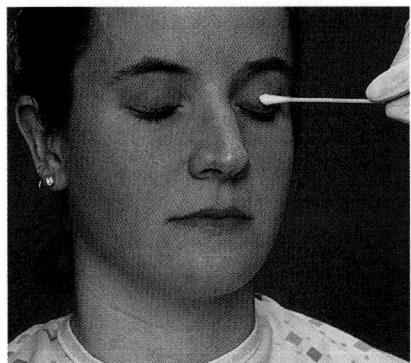

A. Patient Position

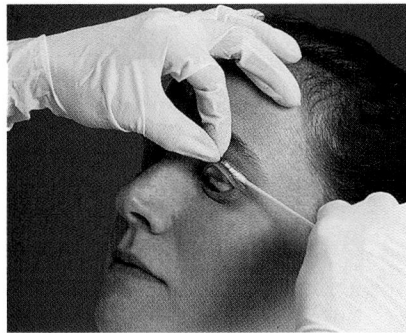

B. Everting the Eyelid

FIGURE 12-17 Assessing Palpebral Conjunctiva

ANTERIOR SEGMENT STRUCTURES

Conjunctiva

To assess the bulbar conjunctiva:

E 1. Separate the lid margins with the fingers.

2. Have the patient look up, down, and to the right and left.

3. Inspect the surface of the bulbar conjunctiva for color, redness, swelling, exudate, or foreign bodies. Note whether **injection** or redness is around the cornea or toward the periphery.

4. With the thumb, gently pull the lower lid toward the cheek and inspect the surface of the bulbar conjunctiva for color, inflammation, edema, lesions, or foreign bodies.

N The bulbar conjunctiva is transparent, with small blood vessels visible in it. It should appear white except for a few small blood vessels, which are normal. No swelling, injection, exudate, foreign bodies, or lesions are noted.

A/P Refer to palpebral conjunctiva.

The palpebral conjunctiva is examined only when there is a concern about its condition. To examine the palpebral conjunctiva of the upper lid:

E 1. Explain the procedure to the patient to alleviate the fear of pain or damage to the eye.

2. Don gloves. Have the patient look down to relax the levator muscle (Figure 12-17A).

3. Gently pull the eyelashes downward and place a sterile, cotton-tipped applicator about 1 cm above the lid margin.

4. Gently exert downward pressure on the applicator while pulling the eyelashes upward to evert the lid (Figure 12-17B).

5. Inspect the palpebral conjunctiva for injection, swelling or **chemosis**, exudate, and foreign bodies.

6. Return the lid to its normal position by instructing the patient to look up and then pulling the eyelid outward and removing the cotton-tipped applicator. Ask the patient to blink.

N The palpebral conjunctiva should appear pink and moist. It is without swelling, lesions, injection, exudate, or foreign bodies.

A Bilateral injected conjunctiva with purulent, sticky discharge and lid edema are noted (Figure 12-18).

P These findings usually indicate the presence of bacterial conjunctivitis.

A Unilateral injection with moderate pain and without purulent discharge is noted, but the patient complains of increased lacrimation.

P These symptoms indicate that the conjunctivitis is viral. Viral conjunctivitis is most commonly due to adenovirus, which may become epidemic. Herpes simplex may also be a viral cause of conjunctivitis. A preauricular node is often felt on palpation.

A Mild inflammation and injection and follicles of palpebral conjunctiva are present with scant discharge. The patient reports an itching and burning sensation, as well as increased lacrimation.

P This is allergic conjunctivitis and is often associated with hay fever.

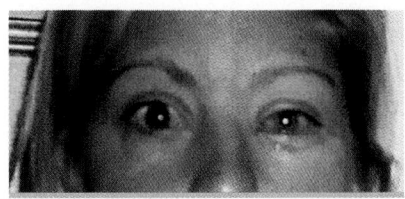

FIGURE 12-18 Bacterial Conjunctivitis

| **E** Examination | **N** Normal Findings | **A** Abnormal Findings | **P** Pathophysiology |

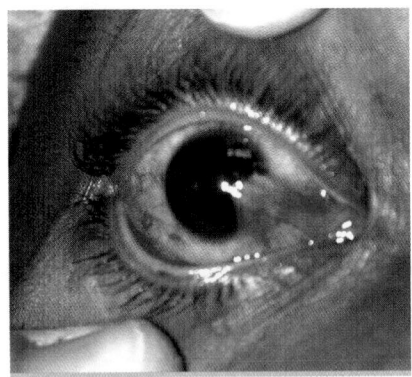

FIGURE 12-19 **Pterygium.** *Courtesy of Salim I. Butrus, M.D., Senior Attending, Department of Ophthalmology, Washington Hospital Center, Washington, DC, & Associate Clinical Professor, Georgetown University Medical Center, Washington, DC.*

A A yellow nodule is noted on the nasal side of the bulbar conjunctiva adjacent to the cornea. It may be on the temporal side as well. This lesion is painless unless it becomes inflamed.

P This lesion is called a **pinguecula**. It is a nodular degeneration of the conjunctiva and is thought to be a result of increased exposure to ultraviolet light.

A A unilateral or bilateral triangle-shaped encroachment onto the conjunctiva is abnormal (Figure 12-19). This lesion always occurs nasally and remains painless unless it becomes ulcerated. If the lesion covers the cornea, loss of vision may occur.

P This lesion is called a **pterygium** and is also caused by excessive ultraviolet light exposure.

A The patient exhibits a sudden onset of a painless, bright red appearance on the bulbar conjunctiva.

P This is a subconjunctival hemorrhage and may result from the pressure exerted during coughing, sneezing, or a Valsalva maneuver. It can also be attributed to anticoagulant medications or uncontrolled hypertension.

Sclera

E While assessing the conjunctiva, inspect the sclera for color, exudate, lesions, and foreign bodies.

N In light-skinned individuals, the sclera should be white with some small, superficial vessels and without exudate, lesions, or foreign bodies. In dark-skinned individuals, the sclera may have tiny brown patches of melanin or a grayish-blue or "muddy" color.

A The color of the sclera is uniformly yellow (Figure 12-20).

P This condition is known as jaundice or scleral icterus and is due to coloring of the sclera with bilirubin, which infiltrates all tissues of the body. This is an early manifestation of systemic conditions such as hepatitis, sickle cell disease, gallstones, and physiological jaundice of the newborn.

A The sclera is blue.

P This finding is a distinctive feature of osteogenesis imperfecta and is due to the thinning of the sclera, which allows the choroid to show through.

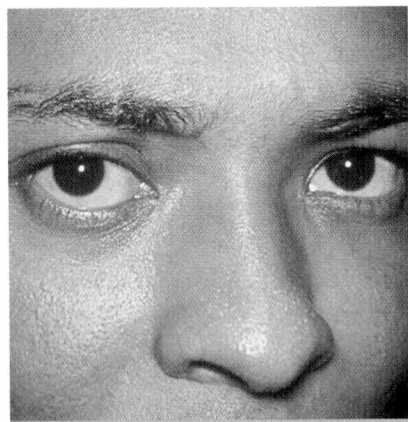

FIGURE 12-20 **Scleral Icterus.** *Courtesy of the Centers for Disease Control and Dr. Thomas F. Sellers, Emory University.*

Cornea

E 1. Stand in front of the patient.

2. Shine a penlight directly on the cornea.

3. Move the light laterally and view the cornea from that angle, noting color, discharge, and lesions.

N The corneal surface should be moist and shiny, with no discharge, cloudiness, opacities, or irregularities.

A A grayish, well-circumscribed ulcerated area on the cornea is abnormal (Figure 12-21).

P The most common cause of this condition is a corneal ulceration resulting from a bacterial invasion.

A A treelike configuration on the corneal surface is identified. The patient complains of mild discomfort, photophobia, and in some cases blurred vision (depending on the location of the lesions).

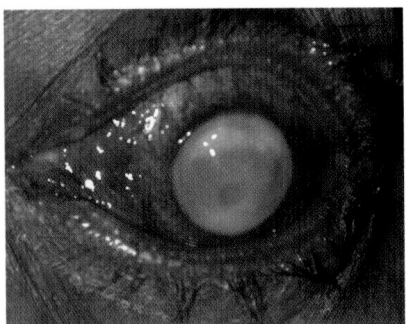

FIGURE 12-21 **Corneal ulceration.** Note the injection and hypopyon (purulent material in the anterior chamber), which frequently occur with corneal ulceration. *Courtesy of Salim I. Butrus, M.D., Senior Attending, Department of Ophthalmology, Washington Hospital Center, Washington, DC, & Associate Clinical Professor, Georgetown University Medical Center, Washington, DC.*

E Examination   **N** Normal Findings   **A** Abnormal Findings   **P** Pathophysiology

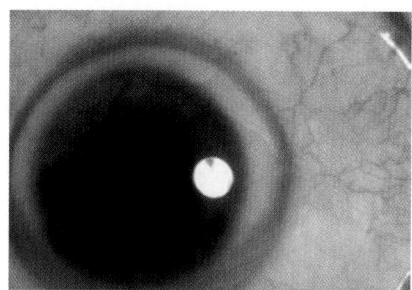

FIGURE 12-22 **Arcus Senilis.** *Courtesy of Salim I. Butrus, M.D., Senior Attending, Department of Ophthalmology, Washington Hospital Center, Washington, DC, & Associate Clinical Professor, Georgetown University Medical Center, Washington, DC.*

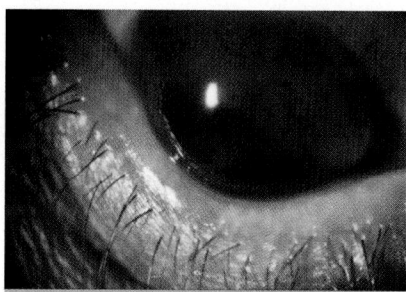

FIGURE 12-23 **Keratoconus.** *Courtesy of Salim I. Butrus, M.D., Senior Attending, Department of Ophthalmology, Washington Hospital Center, Washington, DC, & Associate Clinical Professor, Georgetown University Medical Center, Washington, DC.*

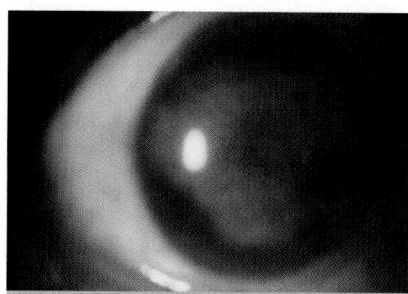

FIGURE 12-24 **Corneal Scar.** *Courtesy of Salim I. Butrus, M.D., Senior Attending, Department of Ophthalmology, Washington Hospital Center, Washington, DC, & Associate Clinical Professor, Georgetown University Medical Center, Washington, DC.*

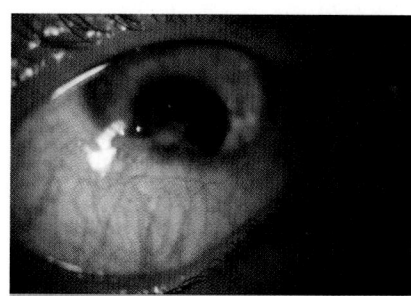

FIGURE 12-25 **Corneal Laceration.** *Courtesy of Salim I. Butrus, M.D., Senior Attending, Department of Ophthalmology, Washington Hospital Center, Washington, DC, & Associate Clinical Professor, Georgetown University Medical Center, Washington, DC.*

P This type of ulceration is caused by the herpes simplex virus. The patient usually has a history of having had a cold sore somewhere on the face.

A There is a hazy gray ring about 2 mm in width just inside the limbus (Figure 12-22).

P This common finding is **arcus senilis,** a bilateral, benign degeneration of the peripheral cornea. It can be found at any age but is most common in older individuals. If found in a young person, it may be associated with hypercholesterolemia.

A A steamy or cloudy cornea is abnormal. The patient also has ocular pain.

P Glaucoma is caused by increased intraocular pressure. Refer to Anterior Chamber assessment.

A Any irregularities in the appearance of the cornea are abnormal.

P Keratoconus (Figure 12-23) is the conical protrusion of the center of the cornea. It is a noninflammatory condition in which the cornea thins, sometimes leading to the need for corneal transplant surgery.

P A corneal scar (Figure 12-24) forms at the site of past injury or inflammation.

P Corneal laceration (Figure 12-25) can occur secondary to trauma.

Anterior Chamber

The anterior chamber is that compartment of the eye found between the cornea and the iris. The space between the flat plane of the iris and the periphery of the cornea must be adequate to allow drainage of aqueous fluid out of the eye. If this angle is too narrow, drainage is inadequate, the pressure of the aqueous fluid in the anterior chamber increases, and **glaucoma** develops. If intraocular fluid pressure remains high, optic nerve damage and visual field loss occur.

To differentiate a normal from a narrowed angle:

E 1. Face the patient and shine a light obliquely through the anterior chamber from the lateral side toward the nasal side (see Figure 12-26).

2. Observe the distribution of light in the anterior chamber (see Figure 12-27).

3. Repeat the procedure with the other eye.

N In a normal eye, the entire iris will be illuminated.

A The eye has a narrow angle, with the decreased space between the iris and the cornea appearing as a crescent-shaped shadow on the far portion of the iris.

REFLECTIVE THINKING

Corneal Abrasion

You are examining a 25-year-old male with severe eye pain, photophobia, and tearing. This is his fourth visit in the past 3 months. His previous three visits were for confirmed corneal abrasions caused by sleeping in his hard contact lenses. While you are examining the patient, he tells you that he got drunk again and fell asleep with his contact lenses in his eyes. What type of physical examination would you perform? List some strategies you could use to promote eye health in this patient.

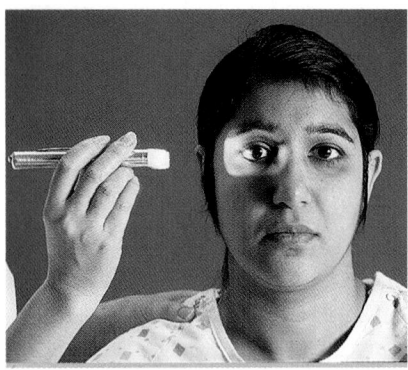

FIGURE 12-26 Examining the Anterior Chamber

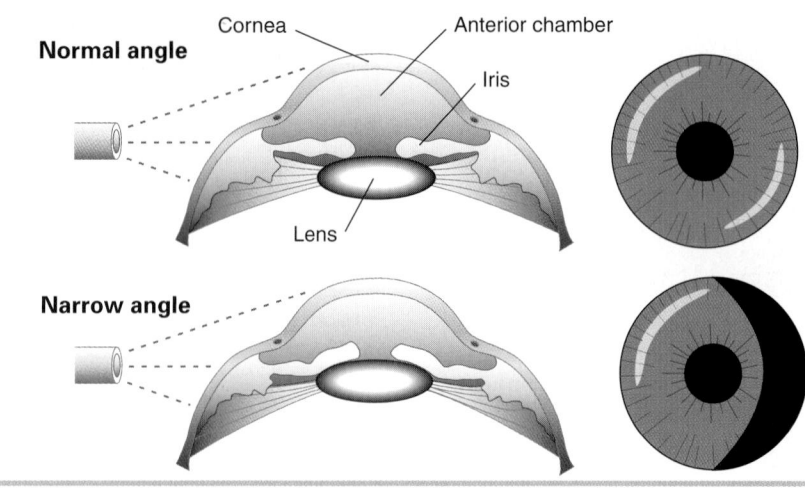

FIGURE 12-27 Evaluating the Angle of the Anterior Chamber

<table>
</table>

NURSING ALERT

Risk Factors for Glaucoma

- Older adults
- Family history of glaucoma
- Ethnicity (especially African Americans, Asians, and Hispanics)
- Elevated intraocular pressure
- Hypertension
- Diabetes mellitus
- Myopia
- Prolonged steroid use

REFLECTIVE THINKING

Pupil Assessment

You are in the physical assessment lab practicing the eye examination. You tell your female partner that her right pupil is smaller than her left. Both pupils react briskly to direct and consensual light. What additional assessments would you perform on your lab partner? What health history questions would you ask?

P The narrow angle is an anatomic variant that can predispose an individual to the development of angle-closure glaucoma. As aging progresses, the lens thickens, which may cause even further narrowing of the angle.

Iris

E With the penlight, inspect the iris for color, nodules, and vascularity.

N Normally, the color is evenly distributed over the iris, although there can be a mosaic variant. It is normally smooth and without apparent vascularity.

A There is a heavily pigmented, slightly elevated area visible in the iris.

P This lesion can be a benign iris nevus or a malignant melanoma. An iris nevus is much more common than melanoma.

A The inferior portion of the iris is obscured by blood.

P This is a **hyphema** and is caused by bleeding from vessels in the iris as a result of direct trauma to the globe. It can also occur as a result of eye surgery.

A An absent wedge portion of the iris is abnormal.

P The shape of the iris changes after surgical removal of a cataract; the pupil may also have an irregular shape.

Pupil

E 1. Stand in front of the patient in a darkened room.

2. Note the shape and size of the pupils in millimeters.

3. Move a penlight from the side to the front of one eye without allowing the light to shine on the other eye (see Figure 12-28).

4. Observe the pupillary reaction in that eye. This is the direct light reflex. Note the size of the pupil receiving light stimulus and the speed of pupillary response to light.

5. Repeat in the other eye.

6. Move the penlight in front of one eye, and observe the other eye for pupillary constriction. This is the consensual light reflex.

7. Repeat the procedure on the other eye.

8. Instruct the patient to shift the gaze to a distant object for 30 seconds.

| **E** Examination | **N** Normal Findings | **A** Abnormal Findings | **P** Pathophysiology |

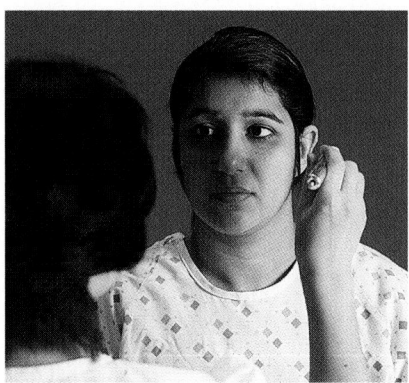

A. Starting Position with Penlight to Side of Pupil

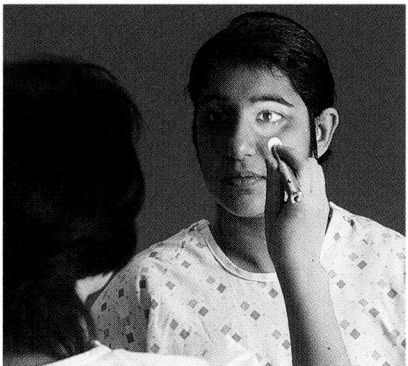

B. Move the penlight directly in front of the pupil.

FIGURE 12-28 **Pupil Assessment**

9. Instruct the patient to then look at your finger or an object held in your hand about 10 cm from the patient.

10. Note the reaction and size of the pupils. **Accommodation** occurs when pupils constrict and converge to focus on objects at close range.

N The pupils should be deep black, round, and of equal diameter, ranging from 2 to 6 mm. Pupils should constrict briskly to direct and consensual light and to accommodation (CN III). Small differences in pupil size (**anisocoria**) may be normal in some people.

A The pupil that constricts to less than 2 mm in diameter is termed miotic. The pupil that dilates to more than 6 mm in diameter is termed mydriatic.

P Abnormal pupillary size can be caused by medications such as sympathomimetics or parasympathomimetics, iritis, or disorders such as CN III paralysis, which can occur as a result of a carotid artery aneurysm. These abnormalities may also be due to nerve damage or trauma (see Table 12-1 for further pathologies).

A The pupil has an irregular shape.

P This is a common finding associated with the surgical removal of cataracts and iridectomy.

A When the direct light reflex is defective, the pupil dilates in response to light, but consensual reaction is appropriate. This is called a Marcus Gunn pupil.

P Optic nerve damage in the optic chiasm, such as in trauma, results in destruction of the afferent pathways of the pupillary light reflex (deafferented pupil).

A The hippus phenomenon occurs after the pupil has been stimulated by direct light. Light causes the pupil to constrict, but then the pupil appears to rhythmically vacillate in size from a larger to a smaller diameter.

P Hippus may be caused by a lesion in the midbrain.

A The presence of midposition, round, regular, and fixed (5 to 6 mm) pupils that may show hippus is abnormal.

P These signs usually indicate midbrain damage that interrupts the light reflex but may leave accommodation intact.

Lens

E 1. Stand in front of the patient.

2. Shine a penlight directly on the pupil. The lens is behind the pupil.

3. Note the color.

N The lens is transparent in color.

A One or more of the pupils are not deep black.

P In an adult, a pearly gray appearance of one or both pupils may indicate an opacity (cloudiness) in the lens (**cataract**) (see Figure 12-29).

NURSING**TIP**

Assessment of the Lens

A detailed assessment of the lens requires the use of a slit lamp by an ophthalmologist. Some lens opacities, however, can be seen with the direct ophthalmoscope.

TABLE 12-1 Pupil Abnormalities

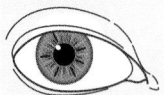 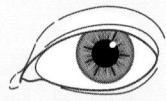

A: The size of pupils is unequal but both pupils react to light and accommodation.
P: Inequality of pupillary size is called **anisocoria** and may be congenital or due to inflammation of ocular tissue or disturbances of neurophthalmic pathways.

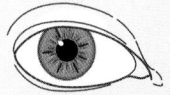 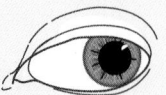

A: A fixed and dilated pupil is observed on one side. The abnormal pupil does not react to direct or consensual light stimulation and does not accommodate. Ptosis and lateral downward deviation may also be noted.
P: This abnormality is caused by **oculomotor nerve damage** due to head trauma and increased intracranial pressure. Atropine-like agents applied topically may cause an even more widely fixed and dilated pupil.

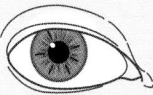 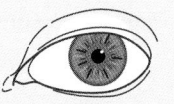

A: A unilateral, small, regularly shaped pupil is observed. Both pupils react directly and consensually and accommodate. Ptosis and diminished or absent sweating on the affected side may also be noted.
P: This finding is **Horner's syndrome,** which is caused by a lesion of the sympathetic nerve pathway.

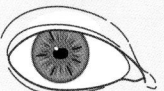 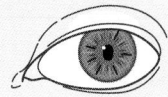

A: Pupils are bilaterally small and irregularly shaped. They react to accommodation but sluggishly or not at all to light.
P: These abnormalities are **Argyll Robertson** pupils and are usually caused by central lesions of neurosyphilis. Other causes include encephalitis, drugs, diabetes, brain tumors, and alcoholism.

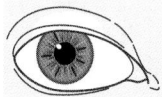 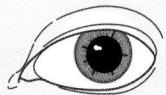

A: A unilateral, large, regularly shaped pupil is noted. The affected pupil's reaction to light and accommodation is sluggish or absent. The patient may report blurred vision because of the slow accommodation. You may observe diminished ankle and knee deep-tendon reflexes.
P: This abnormality, a tonic or **Adie's** pupil, is due to impaired sympathetic nerve supply.

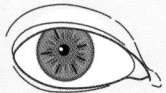 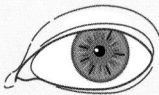

A: Both pupils are **small, fixed,** regularly shaped, and do not react to light or accommodation.
P: This abnormality may be caused by opiate ingestion, topical application of miotic drops, or lesions in the brain.
A: Pupils are small, equal, and reactive.
P: Diencephalic injury or metabolic coma may cause these findings.

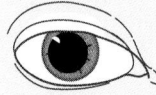 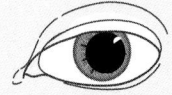

A: Both pupils are **dilated** and **fixed,** and do not react to light or accommodation.
P: Severe head trauma, brain stem infarction, and cardiopulmonary arrest (after 4 to 6 min) can lead to these findings.

Blind eye

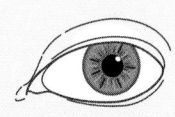

Light

A: Light shone into a blind eye (amaurotic pupil) will cause no reaction (direct or consensual) in either pupil. If light is shone in the other eye, and CN III is intact, both pupils should constrict.
P: Due to a lesion in the retina or the optic nerve, the light stimulus shown in the amaurotic pupil is unable to pass along the sensory pathway; therefore, the oculomotor response in both eyes is absent.

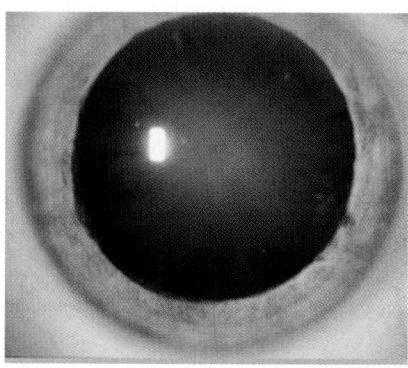

FIGURE 12-29 Cataract. *Courtesy of Salim I. Butrus, M.D., Senior Attending, Department of Ophthalmology, Washington Hospital Center, Washington, DC, & Associate Clinical Professor, Georgetown University Medical Center, Washington, DC.*

NURSINGALERT

Risk Factors for Cataracts

- Increasing age
- Ultraviolet light exposure
- Cigarette use
- Diabetes
- Steroid use (prolonged)

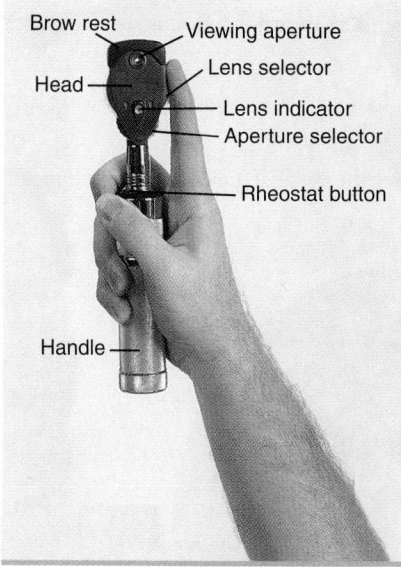

FIGURE 12-30 Ophthalmoscope

P A senile cataract is the most common type. Progressively blurred distance vision is the main symptom, although near vision may be improved because of greater convexity of the lens.

P A unilateral cataract may occur soon after eye injury caused by a foreign body. Along with the lens opacity, there may be intraocular hemorrhage or aqueous or vitreous humor leaking from the globe. The patient reports an immediate blurring of vision.

P Bilateral cataracts found in infants or young children are congenital cataracts. These cataracts are probably genetically determined, although maternal rubella in the first trimester can also be responsible.

POSTERIOR SEGMENT STRUCTURES

The funduscopic assessment (CN II) requires the use of a direct ophthalmoscope to assess the structures in the posterior segment of the eye (Figure 12-30). The ophthalmoscope consists of two parts: the head and the handle. To activate the light source in the head, depress the rheostat button and move it as far as possible. Move the aperture selector to produce the largest beam of light that can be visualized by focusing the beam of light on the palm of the hand. The larger beam is preferred when assessing an average-sized pupil, and the smaller beam makes assessment of a smaller pupil easier. Table 12-2 lists the various apertures of the ophthalmoscope and their uses. The lens selector allows you to choose lenses of varying power for different parts of the assessment. These lenses are marked with red and black numbers, signifying different focal lengths. These numbers are called **diopters**, a unit of refractive measurement. The 0 lens sits between the red- and black-numbered lenses and has no correction. In some ophthalmoscopes, there is no color designation (red or black), and the lens power is signified by + or − signs in front of the numbers. A + sign, or diopter, is equivalent to black and focuses closer to the ophthalmoscope. This is used to correct for farsightedness, or hyperopia. A − sign, or diopter, is equivalent to red and focuses farther from the instrument. This is used to correct for nearsightedness or myopia. These lenses compensate for the refractive error of both the patient and the nurse.

TABLE 12-2 Apertures of the Ophthalmoscope

○	Small round light	Used to examine eyes with small, undilated pupils
◯	Large round light	Used for routine eye examinations and examination of dilated eyes
▦	Grid	Used to assess size and location of funduscopic lesions
▯	Slit light	Assesses anterior eye and determines elevation of funduscopic lesions
●	Green light (red-free filter)	Used to assess retinal hemorrhages (which appear black) and small vessel changes

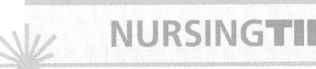

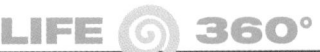

Patient with Potential Multiple Eye Pathologies

Demetrius is a 62-year-old man with a history of severe asthma and type 2 diabetes mellitus. He has taken oral corticosteroids for 5 years to help control his asthma. Today, he presents with shingles of the right scalp and cheek. What questions would you pose to this patient? Knowing his history, describe some possible findings on the physical assessment of his eyes.

Retinal Structures

In a darkened room, ask the patient to remove eyeglasses; contact lenses may be left in place.

E 1. Instruct the patient to look at a distant object across the room. This will help to dilate the eyes.

2. Set the ophthalmoscope on the 0 lens and hold it in front of your right eye with your index finger on the lens selector.

3. From a distance of 8 to 12 inches from the patient and about 15° to the lateral side, shine the light into the patient's right pupil, eliciting a light reflection from the retina; this is called the **red reflex** (Figure 12-31A).

4. While maintaining the red reflex in view, move closer to the patient and move the lens selector from 0 to the +, or black, numbers in order to focus on the anterior ocular structures.

5. For optimum visualization, keep the ophthalmoscope within an inch of the patient's eye (Figure 12-31B).

6. At this point, move the lens selector from the +, or black, numbers, through 0, and into the −, or red, numbers in order to focus on structures progressively more posterior.

7. Focus on the optic disc at the nasal side of the retina by following any retinal vessels centrally (Figure 12-32).

8. You may need to reverse direction along the vessel if the disc does not appear.

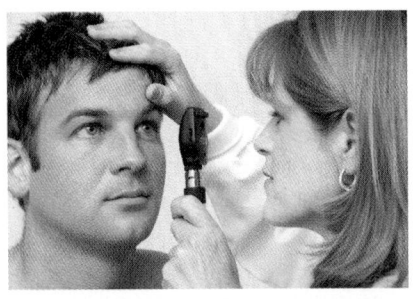

A. Eliciting the Red Reflex

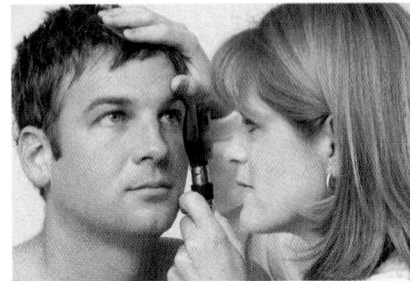

B. Funduscopic Examination

FIGURE 12-31 **Examining Retinal Structures**

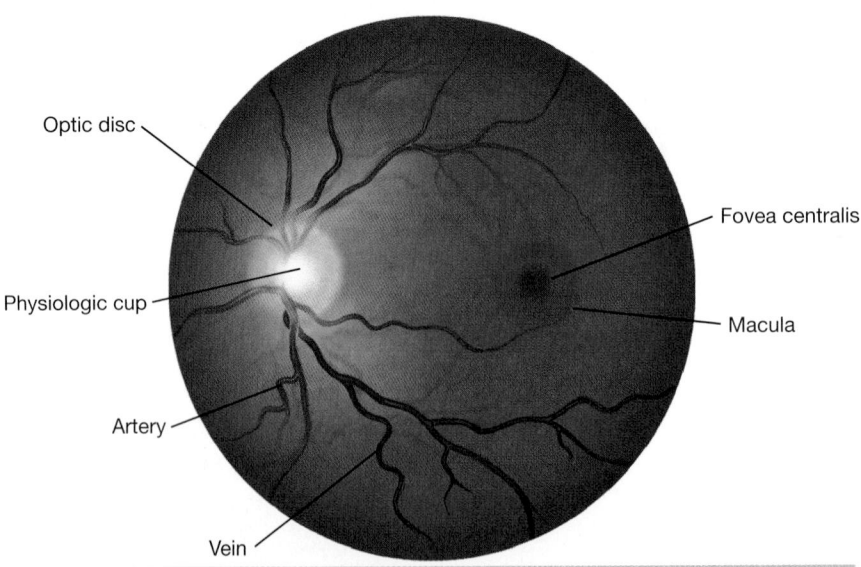

FIGURE 12-32 **Optic Disc of the Left Eye**

9. Observe the retina for color and lesions; the retinal vessels for configuration and characteristics of their crossing; and the optic disc for color, shape, size, margins, and comparison of cup-to-disc ratio.

10. Describe the size, position, and location of any abnormality. Use the diameter of the disc (DD) as a guide to describe the distance of the abnormality from the optic disc. View the optic disc as a clock face for a reference point to describe the location of the abnormality. Describe the size of the abnormality in relation to the size of the optic disc.

11. Repeat on the left side, using the ophthalmoscope in your left hand to examine the patient's left optic fundus.

N Refer to Table 12-3. The red reflex is present. The optic disc is pinkish-orange in color, with a yellow-white excavated center known as the physiologic cup (see Figure 12-32). The ratio of the cup diameter to that of the entire disc is 1:3. The border of the disc may range from a sharp, round demarcation from the surrounding retina to a more blended border, but should be on the same plane as the retina. In general, there are four main vascular branches emanating from the disc, each branch consisting of an arteriole and a venule. The venules are approximately four times the size of the accompanying arterioles and are darker in color. Light often produces a glistening "light reflex" from the arteriolar vessel. Normal arterial-to-venous width is a ratio of 2:3 or 4:5.

A The red reflex is absent.

P The presence of cataracts can prevent the red reflex from being observed due to the opacity of the lens.

A The red reflex is absent and the pupil appears white.

P Leukocoria, or white reflex, is found in retinoblastoma, congenital cataracts, and retinal detachment. This is often referred to as the cat's eye reflex.

A The optic disc is pale.

TABLE 12-3 Retinal Color Variations

FINDINGS	CHARACTERISTICS
Fair-skinned individual	• Retina appears a lighter red-orange color
	• Tessellated appearance of the fundi (pigment does not obscure the choroid vessels)
Dark-skinned individual	• Fundi appear darker in color; grayish-purple to brownish (from increased pigment in the choroid and retina)
	• No tessellated appearance
	• Choroidal vessels usually obscured
Aging individual	• Vessels are straighter and narrower
	• Choroidal vessels are easily visualized
	• Retinal pigment epithelium atrophies and causes the retinal color to become paler

---

| **E** Examination | **N** Normal Findings | **A** Abnormal Findings | **P** Pathophysiology |

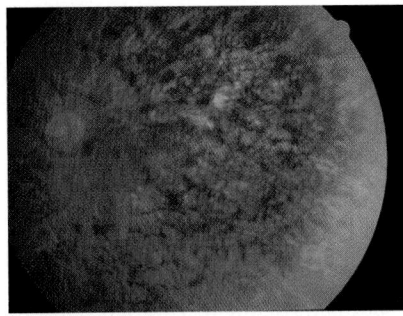

A. Retinitis Pigmentosa. *Courtesy of Salim I. Butrus, M.D., Senior Attending, Department of Ophthalmology, Washington Hospital Center, Washington, DC, & Associate Clinical Professor, Georgetown University Medical Center, Washington, DC.*

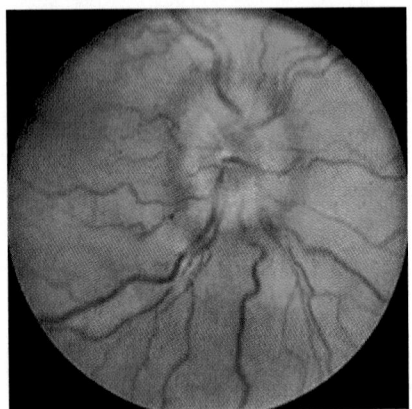

B. Papilledema. *Courtesy of Salim I. Butrus, M.D., Senior Attending, Department of Ophthalmology, Washington Hospital Center, Washington, DC, & Associate Clinical Professor, Georgetown University Medical Center, Washington, DC.*

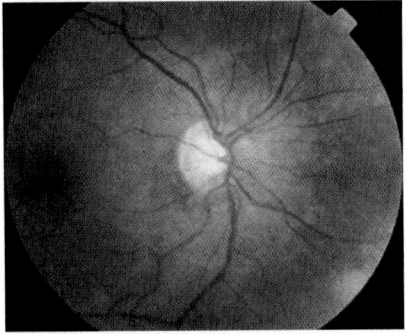

C. Glaucomatous Cupping. *Courtesy of Salim I. Butrus, M.D., Senior Attending, Department of Ophthalmology, Washington Hospital Center, Washington, DC, & Associate Clinical Professor, Georgetown University Medical Center, Washington, DC.*

FIGURE 12-33   Retinal Abnormalities *continues*

P Pallor is due to optic atrophy caused by increased intracranial pressure or from congenital syphilis; an intracranial space-occupying lesion, for example, meningioma; or end-stage glaucoma.

A Optic atrophy is abnormal.

P Optic atrophy occurs in retinitis pigmentosa (Figure 12-33A). Arteriole narrowing and "bone spicule" are also noted on the fundus. There is a loss of central and/or peripheral vision, night blindness, and glare sensitivity in this familial condition.

A The physiologic cup exceeds the normal 1:3 ratio. The disc appears elevated above the plane of the surrounding retina.

P Disc edema and loss of vision are caused by the papillitis resulting from optic neuritis. The disc is hyperemic, the margins are blurred, and the disc surface is elevated.

P Disc edema and an elevated disc without loss of vision are found in papilledema (Figure 12-33B), which is caused by increased intracranial pressure obstructing return blood flow from the eye. This is also called a "choked disc."

P Glaucomatous cupping (Figure 12-33C) occurs due to increased intraocular pressure. The physiologic cup is enlarged and may extend to the edge of the optic disc. Blood vessels are displaced nasally.

A The normal white stripe of retinal arteries appears instead as a copper-colored stripe.

P This copper wire appearance of retinal arteries is characteristic of hypertensive changes.

A At the crossing of retinal arteries over veins, the vein is not seen on either side of the overlying artery.

P This finding is arteriovenous (A-V) nicking, a sign of retinal arteriolar sclerosis that occurs as the walls become thickened and obscure portions of the veins that lie underneath. This can also occur in hypertension.

A Superficial retinal hemorrhages are flame-shaped hemorrhages found in the fundi, or they may appear as red hemorrhages with white centers called Roth's spots. These hemorrhages form a pattern related to the nerve fibers that radiate from the optic disc.

P These hemorrhages may be due to severe hypertension, occlusion of the central retinal vein, and papilledema. Roth's spots are sometimes associated with infective endocarditis.

A Deep retinal hemorrhages, or dot hemorrhages, appear as small red dots or irregular spots in the deep layer of the retina (see Figure 12-33D).

P Deep retinal hemorrhages can be associated with diabetes mellitus.

A Diffuse preretinal hemorrhages occur in the small space between the vitreous and the retina.

P Preretinal hemorrhages may occur in conjunction with a sudden increase in intracranial pressure.

A Microaneurysms are tiny, round, red dots that can be seen in peripheral and macular areas of the retina (see Figure 12-33E).

P These dots are small retinal vessels that dilate in diabetic retinopathy.

A Neovascularization is the formation of new vessels that are very narrow and disorderly in appearance and that may extend into the vitreous (see Figure 12-33F). These vessels may bleed, resulting in a loss of vision.

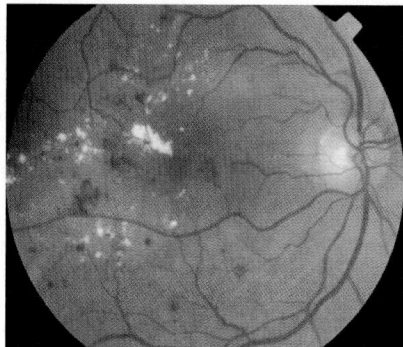

D. Microaneurysms with Exudate and Dot Hemorrhages. *Courtesy of Salim I. Butrus, M.D., Senior Attending, Department of Ophthalmology, Washington Hospital Center, Washington, DC, & Associate Clinical Professor, Georgetown University Medical Center, Washington, DC.*

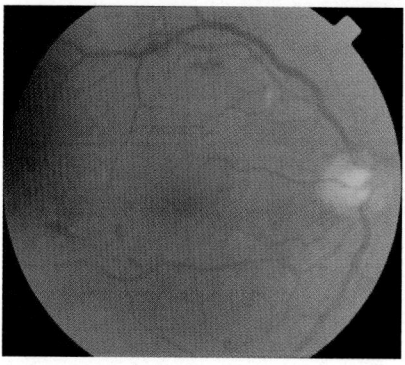

E. Microaneurysms in Diabetic Retinopathy. *Courtesy of Salim I. Butrus, M.D., Senior Attending, Department of Ophthalmology, Washington Hospital Center, Washington, DC, & Associate Clinical Professor, Georgetown University Medical Center, Washington, DC.*

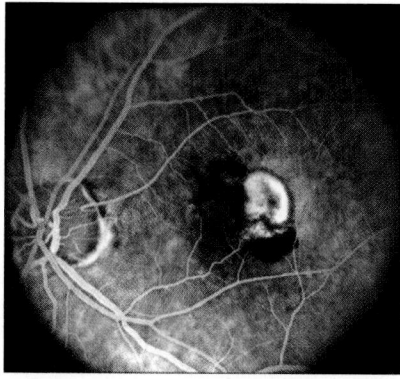

F. Subretinal Neovascularization in Age-Related Exudative Macular Degeneration. *Courtesy of Salim I. Butrus, M.D., Senior Attending, Department of Ophthalmology, Washington Hospital Center, Washington, DC, & Associate Clinical Professor, Georgetown University Medical Center, Washington, DC.*

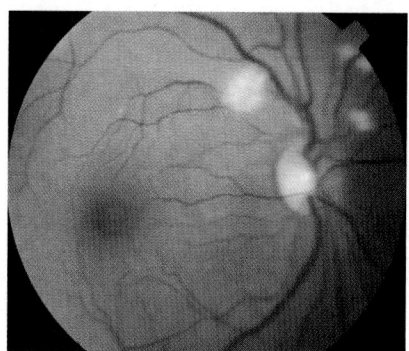

G. Cotton Wool Spots. *Courtesy of Salim I. Butrus, M.D., Senior Attending, Department of Ophthalmology, Washington Hospital Center, Washington, DC, & Associate Clinical Professor, Georgetown University Medical Center, Washington, DC.*

FIGURE 12-33 **Retinal Abnormalities** *continued*

P Neovascularization occurs in proliferative diabetic retinopathy.

A Fluffy white or gray, slightly irregular areas that appear on the retina and are ovoid in shape are abnormal (Figure 12-33G).

P Cotton wool spots represent microscopic infarcts of the nerve fiber layer and are due to diabetic or hypertensive retinopathy.

P Drusen are small white dots in the fundus that are arranged in an irregular pattern. They may also occur on the optic disc, and may become shiny with calcification.

P Drusen are findings of the normal aging process. They may cause loss of vision if they occur in the macular region.

A Hard exudates are yellow with distinct borders, and are small unless they coalesce. They are arranged in round, linear, or star-shaped patterns.

P Hard exudates are associated with diabetes mellitus or hypertension.

E Examination   **N** Normal Findings   **A** Abnormal Findings   **P** Pathophysiology

A A cleft defect of the choroid and retina is abnormal. The size ranges from medium to large.

P **Coloboma** is a congenital, pathological, or surgically induced abnormality.

A The red-orange retinal reflex is absent in the area of a retinal detachment. The area appears pearly gray and is elevated and wrinkled.

P A detached retina may be associated with severe myopia, cataract surgery, or diabetic retinopathy, or it may be caused by trauma.

A Fibrous white bands that obscure the retinal vessels are abnormal. Neovascularization may also be present.

P These findings occur in proliferative diabetic retinopathy.

Macula

When the retinal structures and the optic disc have been assessed:

E 1. Move the ophthalmoscope approximately two disc diameters temporally to view the macula or ask the patient to look at the light. The red-free filter lens of the ophthalmoscope may also be helpful in assessing the macula. Because the macula is not clearly demarcated and because it is very light sensitive, you may have difficulty assessing it.

2. Note the macula's color, shape, and the presence of any lesions.

3. Note the foveal light reflex. This is a small white light in the center of the macula (fovea centralis) that is reflected from the ophthalmoscope's light. The patient tends to turn away when the light strikes the fovea centralis, making it difficult to assess details of the macular area.

4. Repeat with the other eye.

N The macula is a darker, avascular area with a pinpoint reflective center known as the fovea centralis. The fovea centralis is present.

A The retina is pale with the macular region appearing as a cherry red spot.

P This finding is central retinal artery occlusion, an indication of Tay-Sachs disease.

A An enlarged macula is abnormal (Figure 12-34).

P Macular edema is caused by the leakage of fluid from retinal blood vessels. This can occur in diabetes mellitus, hypertension, age-related macular degeneration, and retinal blood vessel obstruction.

A Sharply defined, small red spots are found in and around the macula.

P These microaneurysms are pathognomonic of diabetes mellitus.

A Macular borders are blurred, with a few spots of pigment near the macula; a hole may appear to be present in the center of the region, or a hemorrhage may have occurred.

P This finding is characteristic of age-related macular degeneration. Hemorrhages, patches of retina atrophy, and pigmented areas may also be associated with this condition.

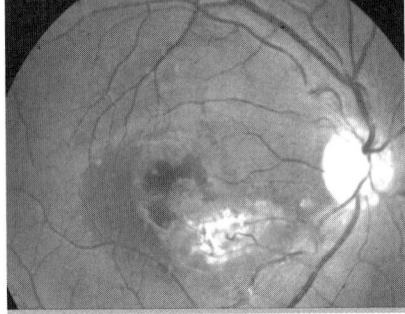

FIGURE 12-34 **Macular Edema with Bleeding.** *Courtesy of Salim I. Butrus, M.D., Senior Attending, Department of Ophthalmology, Washington Hospital Center, Washington, DC, & Associate Clinical Professor, Georgetown University Medical Center, Washington, DC.*

CASE STUDY

The Patient with Bacterial Conjunctivitis

This case study illustrates the application and objective documentation of the eyes assessment.
Shalani comes to the clinic to have her eye evaluated with her 5-month-old baby in her arms.

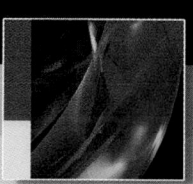

HEALTH HISTORY

PATIENT PROFILE	32 yo Asian MF
CHIEF COMPLAINT	"My eyes are very red and have nasty gunk coming out of them."
HISTORY OF PRESENT ILLNESS	Pt describes herself as healthy x̄ for her current eye complaint. 2 days ago she helped at her daughter's preschool. She noted that her eyelashes were matted together the next morning "like glue." A thick, yellow discharge was washed off her face that AM and today. When pt woke this AM, she also noticed very red eyes and mild swelling around her eyes. Pt wore her contacts yesterday as well as mascara and eyeshadow. Denies fever, itchiness, pain, or change in vision. No new soaps or eye creams. Pt is concerned, as she needs to go on a job interview tomorrow and does not want to look ill.

PAST HEALTH HISTORY

Medical History	Seasonal allergic rhinitis, myopia dx'd age 7
Surgical History	C section '09, wisdom teeth extraction × 4 in '92
Allergies	Sulfa: hives; Bee sting: dyspnea
Medications	Fexofenadine 180 mg po daily prn, MVI c̄ Fe; does not have an EpiPen
Communicable Diseases	Denies
Injuries and Accidents	Fx Ⓛ wrist age 10, s̄ sequelae
Special Needs	Denies
Blood Transfusions	Denies
Childhood Illnesses	Chickenpox age 4
Immunizations	BCG as child, last tetanus '06

continues

CASE STUDY (Continued)

The Patient with Bacterial Conjunctivitis

FAMILY HEALTH HISTORY

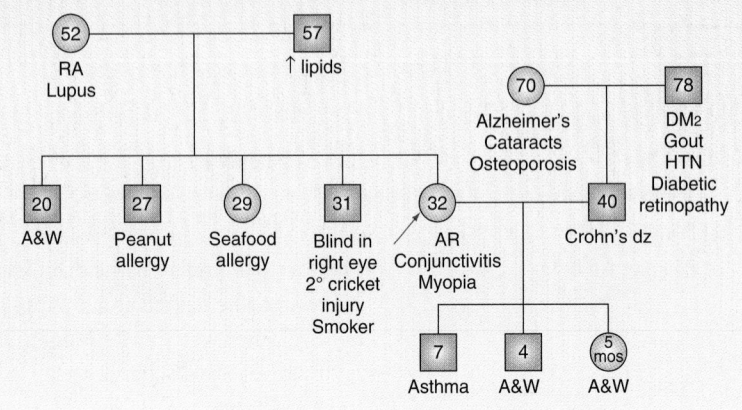

LEGEND

◯ Living female

▢ Living male

／ Points to patient

A&W = Alive & well

AR = Allergic rhinitis

DM = Diabetes mellitus

HTN = Hypertension

RA = Rheumatoid arthritis

52 RA Lupus

57 ↑ lipids

70 Alzheimer's Cataracts Osteoporosis

78 DM2 Gout HTN Diabetic retinopathy

20 A&W

27 Peanut allergy

29 Seafood allergy

31 Blind in right eye 2° cricket injury Smoker

32 AR Conjunctivitis Myopia

40 Crohn's dz

7 Asthma

4 A&W

5 mos A&W

Denies family h/o hyperopia, strabismus, color blindness, glaucoma, retinitis pigmentosa

SOCIAL HISTORY

Alcohol Use	Denies
Tobacco Use	Denies
Drug Use	Denies
Domestic and Intimate Partner Violence	Admits to being pushed around by husband and verbally abused; has not sought help
Sexual Practice	Monogamous c̄ husband
Travel History	Travels to India q yr to see family
Work Environment	Currently unemployed
Home Environment	Lives in Cape Cod house c̄ 3 bedrooms, 1½ baths; in need of much repair, but has not had the money to fix it up; no smoke or CO detectors
Hobbies and Leisure Activities	Enjoys making jewelry
Stress	Pt is mother of 3 children, ages 7 yrs, 4 yrs, 5 mos. Marriage has been difficult for the past few yrs. Husband is American and was becoming less tolerant of her "Indian" ways. He refused to accompany her to India and did not want her to see her American friends from India. Husband grew tired of her "Indian" cooking and complained about how the house smelled p̄ she cooked. Pt had her infant 5 months ago, and last wk her husband left her and the children so he "could get on c̄ his life." Pt does not know what bills need to be paid, and she is currently unemployed. She is unsure how she is going to get through this new life situation.

continues

CASE STUDY ⟩ (Continued)

The Patient with Bacterial Conjunctivitis

Education	High school and AA degree
Economic Status	"I have no idea what I have!"
Military Service	Denies
Religion	Practicing Hindu faith; observes all major holidays
Ethnic Background	Indian
Roles and Relationships	Estranged from husband. Mother to her 3 children. Has friends in America but not sure if any can help her financially. Close to family back in India (e-mails siblings daily), but is too embarrassed about her family situation to tell them what is happening or to ask for their help.
Characteristic Patterns of Daily Living	"It is so hectic. I am up at night c̄ the baby. Then I need to get the other 2 kids up for school and preschool. I cook, I clean. Now I need to find a job."
HEALTH MAINTENANCE ACTIVITIES	
Sleep	Very interrupted due to newborn; tries to get 6 hrs q night
Diet	Vegetarian
Exercise	Not currently
Stress Management	Meditates when she can find the time; practices yoga from videotape
Use of Safety Devices	Wears seat belt; buckles children in appropriate restraining devices
Health Check-ups	Her GYN followed her through the last pregnancy and postpartum; doesn't seek routine hl care
PHYSICAL ASSESSMENT	
Eyes	
Visual Acuity	Distance vision: contacts: 20/20 both eyes; s̄ contacts: 20/40 Ⓡ eye, 20/70 Ⓛ eye Near vision: reads paper c̄/s̄ contacts s̄ errors Color vision: intact
Visual Fields	Intact
External Eye and Lacrimal Apparatus	Eyelids, eyebrows, and eyelashes: eyelids are mildly edematous c̄ dark pink tinge, no lesions or ptosis; eyebrows s̄ lesions; eyelashes c̄ dry discharge Lacrimal apparatus: inner canthus Ⓛ eye c̄ yellow discharge; mild periorbital edema and erythema
Extraocular Muscle Function	Corneal light reflex: symmetric s̄ strabismus Cover/uncover test: no mvt of eyes Cardinal fields of gaze: EOMI s̄ nystagmus

continues

CASE STUDY (Continued)

The Patient with Bacterial Conjunctivitis

Anterior Segment Structures	Conjunctiva: bulbar conjunctiva: peripheral injection of both eyes c̄ and s̄ contacts; palpebral conjunctiva = pink; Ø foreign bodies Sclera: Ø lesions Cornea: s̄ opacities Anterior chamber: iris illuminates Iris: brown Pupils: PERRLA at 4 mm Lens: transparent
Posterior Segment Structures	Retinal structures: ⊕ RR both eyes; discs flat c̄ sharp margins Macula: sharp border s̄ edema or microaneurysms, ⊕ foveal light reflex

ASSESSMENT IN BRIEF

Eye Assessment

Visual Acuity

- Distance vision
- Near vision
- Color vision

Visual Fields

External Eye and Lacrimal Apparatus

- Eyelids, eyebrows, and eyelashes
- Lacrimal apparatus
  - Inspection
  - Palpation

Extraocular Muscle Function

- Corneal light reflex
- Cover/uncover test
- Cardinal fields of gaze

Anterior Segment Structures

- Conjunctiva
- Sclera
- Cornea
- Anterior chamber
- Iris
- Pupil
- Lens

Posterior Segment Structures

- Retinal structures
- Macula

REVIEW QUESTIONS

1. The eye structure that is nonvascular, transparent, and continuous with the conjunctival epithelium is which of the following?
   a. Limbus
   b. Cornea
   c. Sclera
   d. Caruncle

   The correct answer is (b).

2. Reviewing your patient's record, you see that he is on medication to decrease his ocular itchiness. Which class of medications is this patient taking?
   a. Mydriatic
   b. Myotic
   c. Antihistamine

d. Carbonic anhydrase inhibitor
The correct answer is (c).

3. A 40-year-old patient tells you that he is getting headaches from reading. The printed material is being held "almost to my nose." What condition is this patient describing?
   a. Amblyopia   c. Esotropia
   b. Myopia   d. Hyperopia
   The correct answer is (d).

4. A patient presents with a raised, yellow, nonpainful plaque on the upper lid by the inner canthus. What disease process is associated with this assessment finding?
   a. Hypercholesterolemia
   b. Hypothyroidism
   c. *Staphylococcus* infection
   d. Thyrotoxicosis
   The correct answer is (a).

5. You ask a patient to look to the right. Which cranial nerve is the patient using in the right eye?
   a. Cranial nerve II (optic)
   b. Cranial nerve III (oculomotor)
   c. Cranial nerve IV (trochlear)
   d. Cranial nerve VI (abducens)
   The correct answer is (d).

6. If a patient is looking down and to the left, which muscle is the right eye using?
   a. Superior rectus   c. Superior oblique
   b. Inferior rectus   d. Inferior oblique
   The correct answer is (c).

7. The patient's bulbar conjunctiva has a bright red appearance. What condition may have caused this clinical finding?

a. Ultraviolet light
b. Warfarin therapy
c. Osteogenesis imperfecta
d. Cholecystitis
The correct answer is (b).

8. Which of the following physical assessment finding is a patient likely to exhibit in glaucoma?
   a. Steamy, cloudy cornea
   b. Conical protrusion of the center of the cornea
   c. Grayish, well-circumscribed ulcerated area on the cornea
   d. Treelike configuration on the cornea
   The correct answer is (a).

9. Pupils that are fixed, dilated, and unreactive to light and accommodation can be caused by which of the following states?
   a. Congenitally acquired   c. Neurosyphilis
   b. Brain stem infarction   d. Retinal lesion
   The correct answer is (b).

10. Which aperture of the ophthalmoscope is used to examine eyes with small, undilated pupils?
    a. Small round light
    b. Large round light
    c. Grid
    d. Slit lamp
    The correct answer is (a).

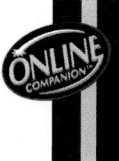

BIBLIOGRAPHY

Albert, D. M., Miller, J. W., Azar, D. T., & Blodi, B. A. (2008). *Albert & Jakobiec's principles & practice of ophthalmology* (3rd ed.). Philadelphia: Saunders.

Bressler, S. B., Munoz, B., Solomon, S. D., & West, S. K. (2008). Racial differences in the prevalence of age-related macular degeneration. *Archives of Ophthalmology, 126*(2), 241–245.

Chung-Jung, C., Milton, R. C., Gensler, G., & Taylor, A. (2007). Association between dietary glycemic index and age-related macular degeneration in nondiabetic participants in the Age-Related Eye Disease Study. *American Journal of Clinical Nutrition, 86*, 180–188.

Doshi, N. R., & Rodriguez, M. L. F. (2007). Amblyopia. *American Family Physician, 75*(3), 361–367.

Ehlers, J. P., Shah, C. P., Fenton, G. L., Hoskins, E. N., Shelsta, H. N., Friedberg, M. A., & Rapuano, C. J. (2008). *The Wills Eye manual: Office and emergency room disease and treatment of eye disease.* Philadelphia: Lippincott Williams & Wilkins.

Galloway, N. R., Amoaku, W. M. K., Galloway, P. H., & Browning, A. C. (2006). *Common eye diseases and their management* (3rd ed.). London: Springer.

Goldblum, K., & Lamb, P. A. (Eds.). (2002). *Core curriculum for ophthalmic nursing* (2nd ed.). Dubuque, IA: Kendall/Hunt.

Kertes, P. J., & Johnson, T. M. (2006). *Evidence-based eye care.* Philadelphia: Lippincott Williams & Wilkins.

LeBlond, R. F., DeGowin, R. L., & Brown, D. D. (Eds.). (2004). *DeGowin's diagnostic examination* (8th ed.). New York: McGraw-Hill.

Mitchell, J. (2007). Investigating the burden of wet macular degeneration [Editorial]. *Archives of Ophthalmology, 125*(9), 1266–1268.

Palay, D. A., & Krachman, J. H. (2006). *Primary care ophthalmology.* St. Louis: Mosby.

Pavan-Langston, D. (2008). *Manual of ocular diseases and therapy* (6th ed.). Philadelphia: Wolters Kluwer.

Peate, W. F. (2007). Work-related eye injuries and illnesses. *American Family Physician, 75*(7), 1017–1022.

Pokhrel, P. K., & Loftus, S. A. (2007). Ocular emergencies. *American Family Physician, 76*(6), 829–836.

Roy, F. H., Fraunfelder, F. W., & Fraunfelder, F. T. (2008). *Roy and Fraunfelder's current ocular therapy* (6th ed.). Philadelphia: Saunders.

Schexnaydre, M., & Carruth, A. K. (2008). My father's experience with macular degeneration. *Home Healthcare Nurse, 26*(1), 8–14.

Tan, J. S. L., Mitchell, P., Kifley, A., Flood, V., Smith, W., & Wang, J. J. (2007). Smoking and the long-term incidence of age-related macular degeneration: The Blue Mountains Eye Study. *Archives of Ophthalmology, 125*(8), 1089–1095.

WEB SITES

All About Vision:
http://www.allaboutvision.com

American Optometric Association:
http://www.aoa.org

American Society of Ophthalmic Registered Nurses:
http://www.webeye.ophth.uiowa.edu/ASORN

National Eye Institute:
http://www.nei.nih/gov

Opticians Association of America:
http://www.oaa.org

U.S. Food and Drug Administration Lasik Eye Surgery:
http://www.fda.gov/CDRH/LASIK

Wills Eye Institute:
http://www.willseye.org

CHAPTER 13

Ears, Nose, Mouth, and Throat

COMPETENCIES

1. Identify the structures of the ears, nose, mouth, and throat.

2. Discuss the system-specific history for the ears, nose, mouth, and throat.

3. Describe normal findings in the physical assessment of the ears, nose, mouth, and throat.

4. Describe common abnormalities found in the physical assessment of the ears, nose, mouth, and throat.

5. Explain the pathophysiology of common abnormalities of the ears, nose, mouth, and throat.

6. Perform the physical assessment of the ears, nose, mouth, and throat.

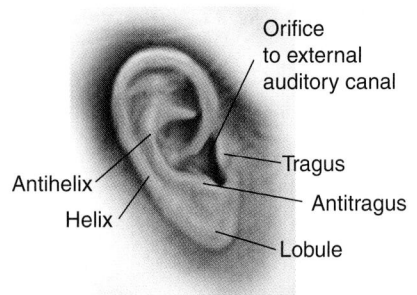

FIGURE 13-1 **External Ear**

Physical examination of the ears, nose, sinuses, mouth, and throat provides a wealth of information about the integrity of many body systems and serves as the foundation for assessment of the neurological, respiratory, endocrine, gastrointestinal, musculoskeletal, and cardiovascular systems.

ANATOMY AND PHYSIOLOGY

EAR

The ear has three sections: the external, the middle, and the inner ear.

External Ear

The external ear, which is also called the **auricle** or pinna, extends through the auditory canal to the tympanic membrane. The auricle receives sound waves and funnels them through the auditory canal to produce vibrations on the tympanic membrane. The auricle is composed of cartilage (Figure 13-1).

The external auditory canal is an S-shaped tube approximately 2.5 cm in length, with the outer third made up of cartilage and the remainder of bone covered by a thin layer of skin (Figure 13-2). The canal is lined with tiny hairs and modified sweat glands that secrete a thick, waxlike substance called **cerumen**, which can vary in consistency from dry and flaky to wet and waxy. Cerumen ranges from a pale, honey color in light-skinned individuals to dark brown or black in dark-skinned people.

Middle Ear

The middle ear is composed of the tympanic membrane, the ossicles, and the tympanic cavity. The cavity is an air-filled compartment that separates the external

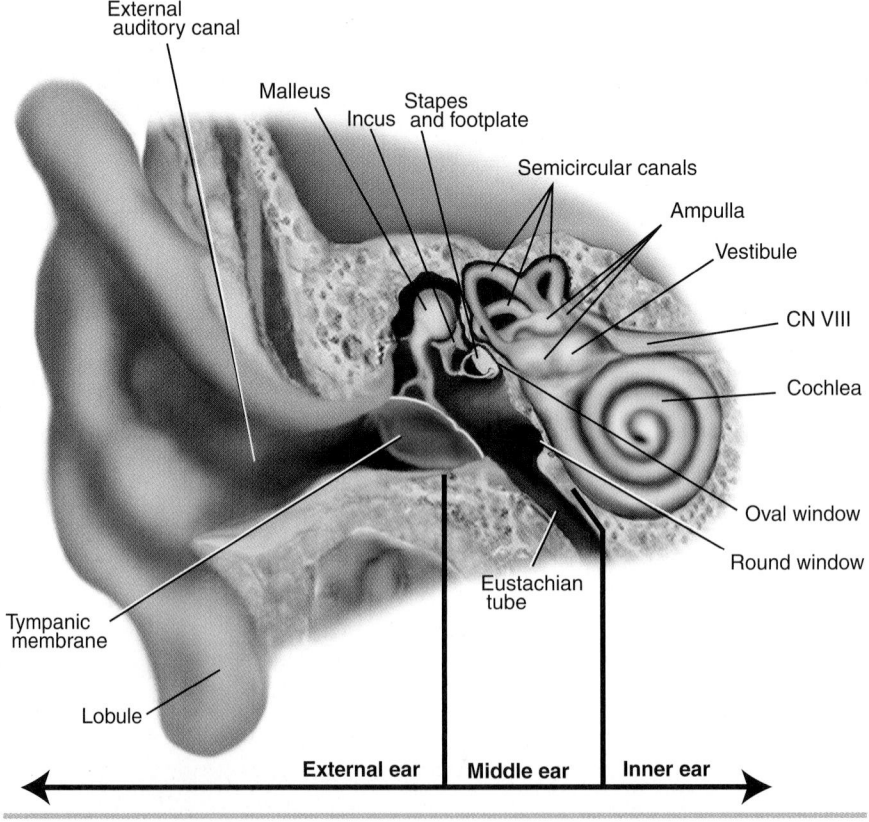

FIGURE 13-2 **Cross Section of the Ear**

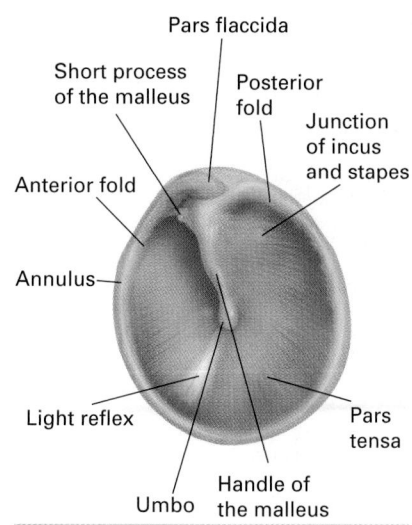

Pars flaccida

Short process
of the malleus

Posterior
fold

Junction
of incus
and stapes

Anterior fold

Annulus—

Light reflex

Pars
tensa

Umbo

Handle of
the malleus

FIGURE 13-3 Landmarks of the Left Tympanic Membrane

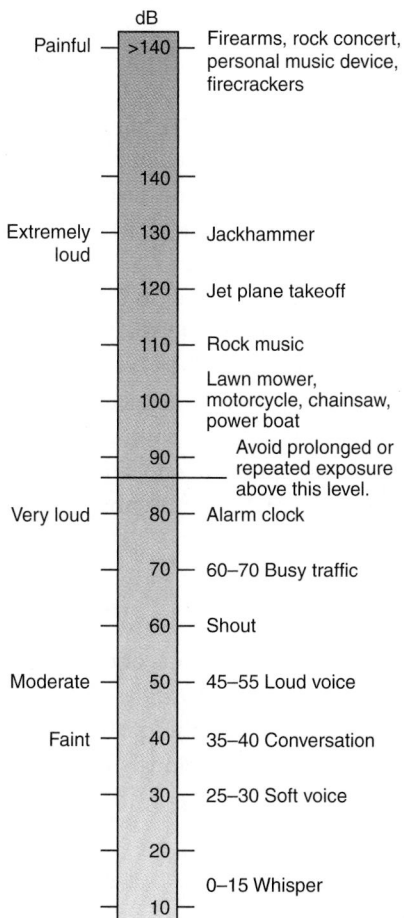

dB	
Painful — >140	Firearms, rock concert, personal music device, firecrackers
— 140	
Extremely loud — 130	Jackhammer
— 120	Jet plane takeoff
— 110	Rock music
— 100	Lawn mower, motorcycle, chainsaw, power boat
— 90	Avoid prolonged or repeated exposure above this level.
Very loud — 80	Alarm clock
— 70	60–70 Busy traffic
— 60	Shout
Moderate — 50	45–55 Loud voice
Faint — 40	35–40 Conversation
— 30	25–30 Soft voice
— 20	
— 10	0–15 Whisper

FIGURE 13-4 Decibel Scale of Frequently Heard Sounds

ear from the internal ear. The tympanic membrane, which is circular or oval and is about an inch in diameter, sits in an oblique position in the external canal so that it leans slightly forward. The rim of the tympanic membrane is called the annulus, the superior portion is the pars flaccida, and the tighter, largest area of the drum is the pars tensa (Figure 13-3).

The **ossicles** are three tiny bones—the malleus (hammer), the incus (anvil), and the stapes (stirrup)—that play a crucial role in the transmission of sound. The long handle, or manubrium, of the malleus extends downward from the short process and meets the tympanic membrane at the umbo. The stapes is held against the wall of the tympanic membrane at the oval window by tiny ligaments. The head of the malleus articulates with the incus, which in turn articulates with the stapes; they work as a unit when the tympanic membrane begins to vibrate. Vibrations set up in the tympanic membrane by sound waves reaching it through the external auditory canal are transmitted to the inner ear by rapid movement of the ossicles.

The tensor tympani and the stapedius are two tiny muscles involved in movement of the ossicles. The tensor tympani maintains the tension of the tympanic membrane and pulls the malleus inward when it contracts. The stapedius works in opposition by pulling the stapes outward. This coordinated movement is an important mechanism in reducing the intensity of loud sounds that might otherwise result in serious damage to hearing receptors in the inner ear.

The middle ear is connected to the nasopharynx by the auditory or **eustachian tube**, which serves as a channel through which air pressure within the cavity can be equalized with air pressure outside to maintain normal hearing. Equalization of pressure is aided by yawning or swallowing, which causes the opening of valvelike flaps that cover the openings of the eustachian tubes.

Inner Ear

The inner ear is a complex, closed, fluid-filled system of interconnecting tubes called the **labyrinth**, which is essential for hearing and equilibrium. The labyrinth has bony and membranous portions. The bony labyrinth is composed of the cochlea, the semicircular canals, and the vestibule. The **vestibule** is located between the cochlea and the **semicircular canals** and is important in both hearing and balance. The three semicircular canals located at right angles to each other provide balance and equilibrium for the body. The **cochlea** is a snail-shaped structure made up of three compartments. The first two compartments contain perilymph, and the third contains endolymph. As sound waves travel through the ear, they cause the perilymph and the endolymph to vibrate, stimulating the thousands of hearing-receptor cells of the organ of Corti. Nearby nerve fibers transmit impulses along the cochlear branch of the vestibulocochlear nerve to the brain, allowing us to hear. The human ear is capable of hearing within a frequency range of 20 to 20,000 Hz, and a decibel range of 0 to 140 (O'Donoghue, Narula, & Bates, 2000). Figure 13-4 illustrates the decibel levels of various commonly heard sounds.

NOSE

The nose consists of the external or outer nose and the nasal fossae, or internal nose (see Figure 13-5). The outer nose is made up of bone and cartilage and is divided internally into two nasal fossae by the nasal septum, and externally by the columella. Anterior openings into the nasal fossae are nostrils, or nares. Each fossa has a lateral extended "wing" portion called the ala nasi on the outside and a vestibule just inside the nostril. Superior, middle, and inferior meatuses or grooves are located on the lateral walls of the nostrils just below the corresponding conchae, or **turbinates**. The nasal turbinates are covered by mucous membranes and greatly

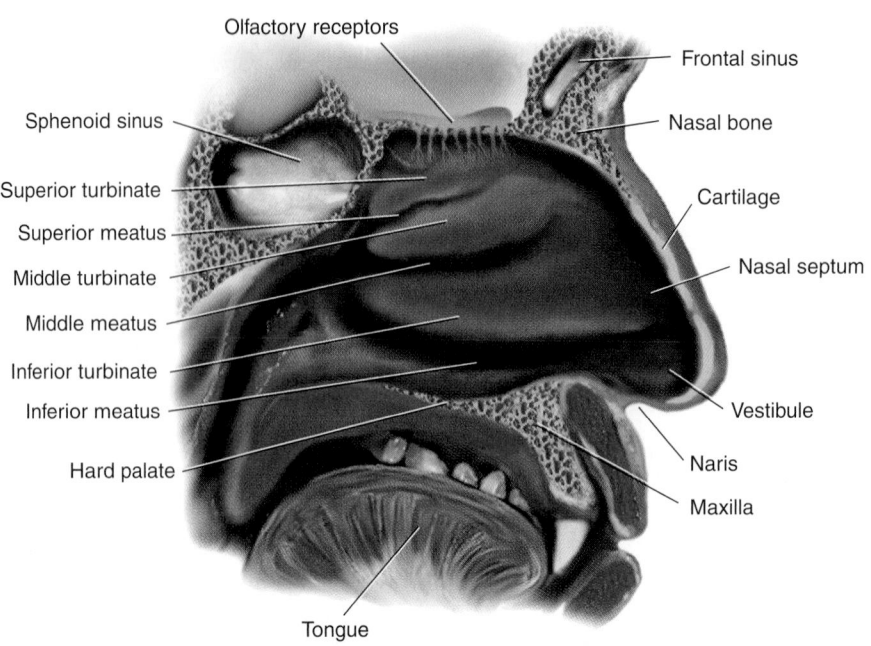

FIGURE 13-5 Lateral Cross Section of the Nose

increase the surface area of mucous membrane in the nose because of their shape. Kiesselbach's plexus is a vascular area on the nasal septum, and a common site of nosebleeds.

Air enters the anterior nares, passes through the vestibule, and enters the fossa. The vestibule contains nasal hairs and sebaceous glands. The fossae have both olfactory and respiratory functions. To protect the lungs from noxious agents, these structures of the nose clean, filter, humidify, and control the temperature of inspired air. The mucous covering in the nose and sinuses traps fine dust particles, and lysosomes kill most of the bacteria. The tiny hairs of the nose (cilia) transport the mucus and the particles to the pharynx to be swallowed.

The nasal mucosa is capable of adding large amounts of water to inspired air through evaporation from its surface. The rich vascular supply to the turbinates radiates heat to the incoming air as it passes through the nasal cavity.

Olfactory receptor cells are located in the upper parts of the nasal cavity, the superior nasal conchae, and on parts of the nasal septum and are covered by hair-like cilia that project into the cavity. The chemical component of odors binds with the receptors, causing nerve impulses to be transmitted to the olfactory cortex, located in the base of the frontal lobe.

SINUSES

Air-filled cavities lined with mucous membranes are present in some of the cranial bones and are referred to as **paranasal sinuses** (see Figure 13-6). These air-filled sinuses lighten the weight of the skull and add resonance to the quality of the voice. The frontal, maxillary, ethmoid, and sphenoid paranasal sinuses open into the nose. Only the frontal and maxillary sinuses can be assessed in the physical examination.

MOUTH AND THROAT

The lips are sensory structures found at the opening of the mouth (see Figure 13-7). The labial tubercle is the small projected area in the midline of the upper lip. The

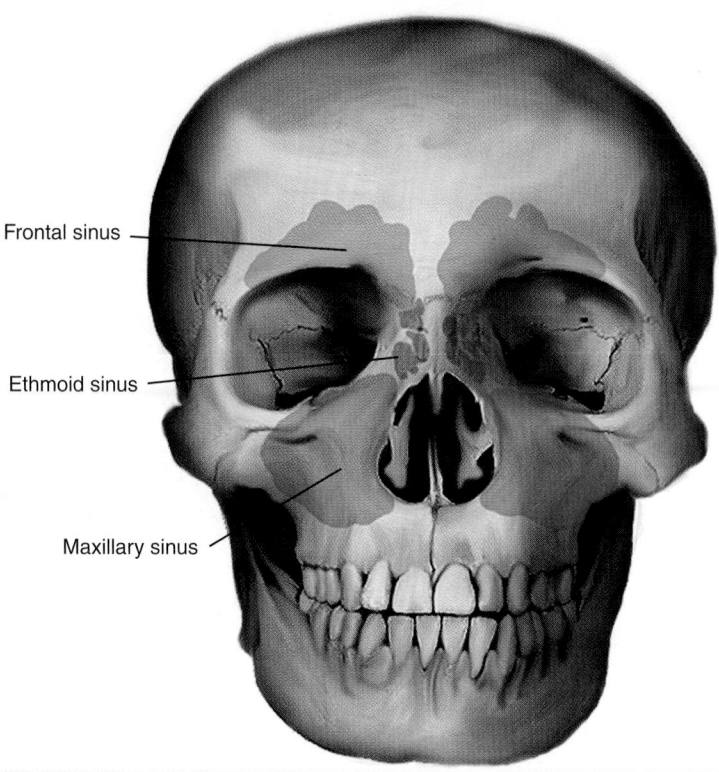

FIGURE 13-6 Location of the Sinuses (Sphenoid sinuses are directly behind ethmoid sinuses.)

area where the upper and lower lips meet is the labial commissure. The vermilion zone is the reddish or reddish-brown area of the lips, and the area where the lips meet the facial skin is called the vermilion border. The median groove superior to the upper lip is called the philtrum. The cheeks form the lateral walls of the mouth and are lined with buccal mucosa. The posterior pharyngeal wall is at the back of the mouth.

The roof of the mouth consists of the hard palate anteriorly and the soft palate posteriorly (see Figure 13-8). The **linear raphe** is a linear ridge in the middle of the hard palate that is formed by two palatine bones and part of the superior maxillary bone. The mucous membrane on either side of the linear raphe is thick, pale, and corrugated, while the posterior mucous membrane is thin, a deeper pink, and smooth.

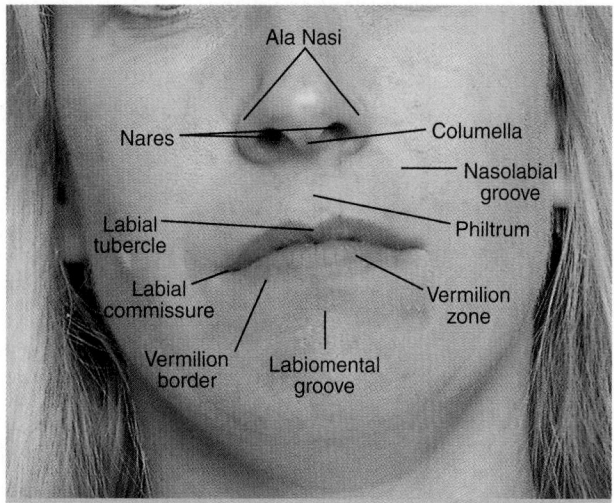

FIGURE 13-7 Landmarks of the Area around the Mouth

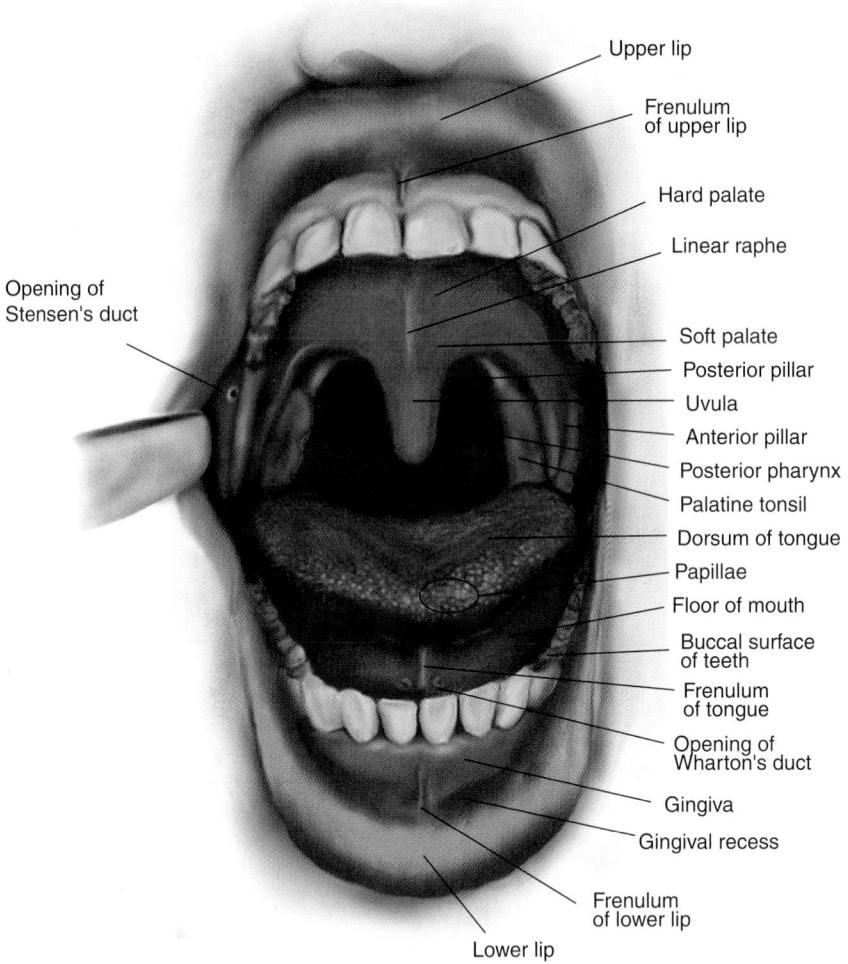

Upper lip

Frenulum of upper lip

Hard palate

Linear raphe

Opening of Stensen's duct

Soft palate

Posterior pillar

Uvula

Anterior pillar

Posterior pharynx

Palatine tonsil

Dorsum of tongue

Papillae

Floor of mouth

Buccal surface of teeth

Frenulum of tongue

Opening of Wharton's duct

Gingiva

Gingival recess

Frenulum of lower lip

Lower lip

FIGURE 13-8 **Structures of the Mouth**

Situated in the floor of the mouth, the tongue is a muscular organ connected to the hyoid bone posteriorly and to the floor of the mouth anteriorly by the **frenulum**. The tongue assists with mastication, swallowing, speech, and mechanical cleansing of the teeth.

The mucous membrane covering the upper surface of the tongue has numerous projections called **papillae**, which assist in handling food and contain taste buds. Four qualities of taste are found in taste buds distributed over the surface of the tongue: bitter is located at the base, sour along the sides, and salty and sweet near the tip. The **sulcus terminalis** is the midline depression that separates the anterior two-thirds of the tongue from the posterior one-third.

Two of the three pairs of salivary glands open into the mouth on the ventral surface of the tongue. Submaxillary glands secrete fluid through **Wharton's ducts**, located on both sides of the frenulum. Sublingual glands open into the floor of the mouth posteriorly to Wharton's ducts. The larger parotid glands are located in the cheeks and secrete their amylase-rich fluid through **Stensen's ducts**, located just opposite the upper second molars.

These salivary glands produce 1,000 to 1,500 mL of saliva per day to assist with digestion of food and maintenance of oral hygiene. Saliva prevents dental caries and bacterial damage of healthy oral tissue by washing away bacteria and destroying it with antibodies and proteolytic enzymes.

Gums, or gingivae, appear pink or coral in light-skinned individuals and brown with a darker melanotic line along the edges in dark-skinned individuals. Gums hold the teeth in place.

Adults have 32 permanent teeth: four incisors, two canines, four premolars, and six molars in each half of the mouth (Figure 13-9). The three parts of the tooth are the top, or the crown, the root, which is embedded in the gum, and the neck, which connects the root and the crown. The teeth are well designed for chewing. Incisors provide strong cutting action, and molars provide strong grinding action.

The soft palate is suspended from the posterior border of the hard palate and extends downward as folds called palatine arches or pillars, forming an incomplete septum between the mouth and the nasopharynx. The **uvula** is a fingerlike projection of tissue that hangs down from the center of the soft palate. Two palatine tonsils containing primarily lymphoid tissue are connected to the palatine arches; they vary greatly in size from one individual to another. Lymphoid tissue in the tonsils plays a role in the control of infection.

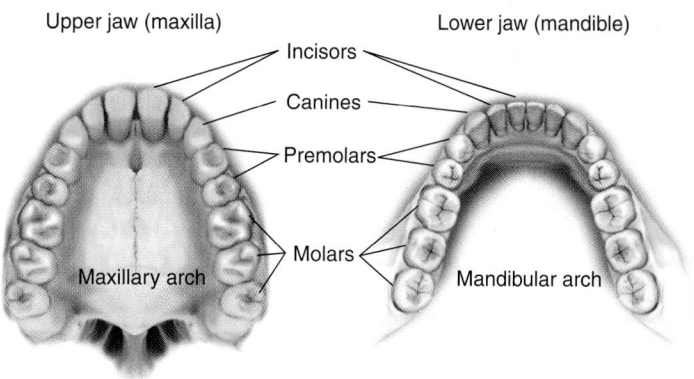

FIGURE 13-9 Permanent Teeth

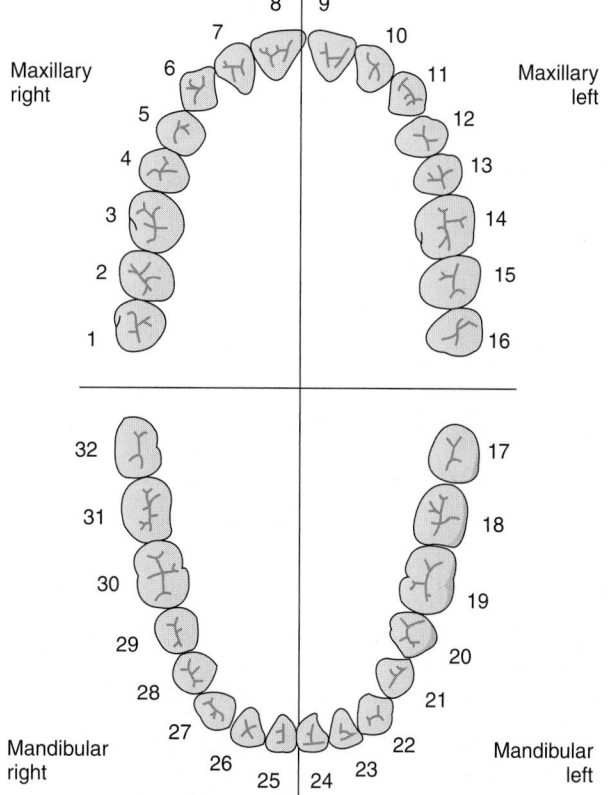

FIGURE 13-10 Tooth Numbering System

NURSINGTIP

Tooth Numbering System

When examining the patient's teeth, it is best to document tooth anomalies using the tooth numbering system. Figure 13-10 illustrates this system in the adult mouth. For example, the left mandibular central incisor is tooth number 24.

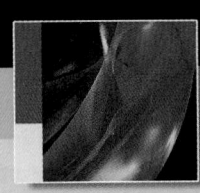

HEALTH HISTORY

The ears, nose, mouth, and throat health history provides insight into the link between a patient's life and lifestyle and ears, nose, mouth, and throat information and pathology.

PATIENT PROFILE

Diseases that are age- and gender-specific for the ears, nose, mouth, and throat are listed.

Age

Ears
Hearing loss related to presbycusis, sensorineural degeneration, or otosclerosis (elderly)
Excessive or impacted cerumen (elderly)

Nose
Decrease in ability to smell (elderly)

Mouth and Throat
Orthodonture (middle age)
Tooth loss and gum disease (elderly)
Thrush related to immunosuppression (elderly)
Decrease in ability to taste (elderly)

Gender

Ears
Female: Calcifications of the ossicles

Nose
Male: Rhinophyma, deviated septum related to trauma, polyps

Mouth and Throat
Male: Singer's nodule on the larynx (over 30), cancer of the larynx, leukoplakia of the tongue, gums, and buccal mucosa

CHIEF COMPLAINT

Common chief complaints for the ears, nose, mouth, and throat are defined, and information on the characteristics of each sign or symptom is provided.

Ear

1. Change in or Loss of Hearing
Reduction in the perception of sound

Location
Unilateral, bilateral

Quality
Loud sounds heard, soft sounds heard

Quantity
Partial or complete

Associated Manifestations
Tinnitus, vertigo, drainage, swelling, fever, ear pain

Aggravating Factors
Loud noises, excessive or impacted cerumen, swimming

Alleviating Factors
Hearing aid, removal of excessive cerumen, turning up volume when possible, cupping the ear, facing the speaker

Setting
Work (jobs with loud background noise or machinery)

Timing
Constant, intermittent, after drug therapy, onset sudden, gradual, or slow

2. Otorrhea
Drainage of liquid from the ear

Location
Unilateral or bilateral

Quality
Painful or nontender, watery, bloody or purulent, foul odor

continues

Health History (continued)

Associated Manifestations	Hearing loss, headache, fever, vertigo, upper respiratory infection
Aggravating Factors	Upright or supine position
Alleviating Factors	Upright or supine position
Timing	Following trauma, continuous, intermittent
3. Otalgia	Discomfort in the ear
Location	Unilateral or bilateral, in jaw region, in pinna region
Quality	Aching, dull, sharp
Associated Manifestations	Drainage, tinnitus, dysphagia, sore throat, vertigo, diminished hearing
Aggravating Factors	Tooth infection, upper respiratory infection, perforated tympanic membrane, insect bites in the ear, upright or supine position, objects in ear, change in air pressure
Alleviating Factors	Analgesics, upright or supine position, avoiding swimming, avoiding pressure changes, removal of objects, change in air pressure
Setting	Outdoors, high altitudes, noisy environments
Timing	Continuous, intermittent, after swimming, following trauma to the head or ear, following loud noises, after pressure changes, flying
4. Tinnitus	"Ringing" in the ears
Location	Unilateral or bilateral
Quality	Pulsatile, buzzing, high-pitched ringing
Associated Manifestations	Vertigo, drainage, pain, nausea, fullness or pressure in the ears, hearing loss, upper respiratory infection, allergies, middle ear infection, inner ear lesions, eustachian tube inflammation
Aggravating Factors	Medications, fluid in the middle ear, perforation of the tympanic membrane, position, pressure on the neck, excessive cerumen
Alleviating Factors	Discontinuing medications, position change, avoiding allergens
Setting	Work (high noise levels), outdoors
Timing	Long-standing, recent, constant, intermittent, following drug therapy, after exposure to loud noises

Nose

1. Pain	Discomfort in the nose
Quality	Aching, throbbing, sharp
Associated Manifestations	Fever, chills, visual changes, swelling, sneezing, nasal discharge
Aggravating Factors	Exposure to allergens, decreased humidity indoors, cocaine use
Alleviating Factors	Use of medications (decongestant or antihistamine), removal of allergens, humidification of the environment, discontinuation of cocaine
Setting	Outdoors, dry heat, low humidity

continues

Timing	Seasonal, in the morning
2. Drainage	Excessive discharge of nasal secretions
Quality	Unilateral or bilateral, amount, viscosity, color, odor, blood-tinged
Associated Manifestations	Fever, sneezing, pain, mouth breathing, swelling, skin irritation around drainage site, itchy eyes
Aggravating Factors	Allergens, infections
Alleviating Factors	Medication, hydration, avoiding allergens
Setting	Outdoors, indoors
Timing	In the morning, seasonal, after trauma
3. Blockage or Congestion	Reduced ability to move air through the nose secondary to obstruction
Quality	Complete, partial
Associated Manifestations	Mouth breathing, snoring, pain, disfigurement, sneezing, itchy eyes, sinus infection
Aggravating Factors	Infection, allergens, medications, objects in nose
Alleviating Factors	Mouth breathing, medications, avoidance of allergens, removal of objects
Setting	Outdoors, indoors
Timing	Following drug therapy, trauma after oral intake, after nasal surgery

Mouth and Throat

1. Halitosis	Unpleasant odor of the breath
Quality	Ammonia, acetone, newly mown grass or old wine odor, foul
Associated Manifestations	Gum disease, caries, systemic disease, sinusitis, pharyngitis, GERD, smoking
Aggravating factors	Poor oral hygiene, poor nutrition, poor diabetic control, alcohol intake, decreased hydration, inadequate renal function
Alleviating Factors	Good oral hygiene, control of systemic diseases, breath mints, good nutrition, adequate dental care, treatment of infection
Timing	Associated with systemic disease or acute infectious process
2. Lesions	Disruptions in the mucosa of the mouth or tongue
Quality	Tender, nontender
Associated Manifestations	Malnutrition, odor, pain, swelling, fever, stress
Aggravating Factors	Eating, drinking, spices, smoking, hot or cold stimuli, alcohol, dehydration
Alleviating Factors	Medications, avoiding eating, hydration, proper nutrition, avoiding smoking and alcohol
Timing	Associated with systemic disease, intermittent, continuous
3. Swelling	Edema of the pharynx

continues

Health History (continued)	
Quality	Mild, moderate, severe
Associated Manifestations	Dysphagia, urticaria, wheezing, pruritus, rhinorrhea, difficulty breathing, lesions, chills, sweats, fever, sneezing, itchy eyes
Aggravating Factors	Exposure to allergens, heat
Alleviating Factors	Medications, avoiding allergens, ice, saltwater gargles
Timing	Following drug therapy, after eating, after an insect bite, after trauma, during or after an infectious process
PAST HEALTH HISTORY	*The various components of the past health history are linked to ears, nose, mouth, and throat pathology and ears-, nose-, mouth-, and throat-related information.*
Medical History	
Ear Specific	Acute otitis media, acute otitis externa, serous otitis media, hearing difficulties
Nose Specific	Polyps, septal deviation, sinus infection, allergic rhinitis, anosmia
Mouth and Throat Specific	Tonsillitis, caries, herpes simplex virus, *Candida* infections, strep throat, frequent upper respiratory infections, tonsillar abscess
Non-Ear, Nose, Mouth, and Throat Specific	Diabetes mellitus, renal disease, atherosclerotic disease, hypertension, inflammatory processes, infections (viral or bacterial), immunosuppressive disease, dental pathology, blood dyscrasias, sexually transmitted diseases, anaphylaxis, nutritional disturbances
Surgical History	Neurosurgery, tonsillectomy, adenoidectomy, tumor removal, cosmetic surgery of head or neck, repair of septal deviation, oral surgery, tympanostomy tube placement
Allergies	Pollen: sneezing, nasal congestion, watery or itchy eyes, cough Insect stings: swelling of the throat, around the eyes Animal dander: sneezing, nasal congestion, watery or itchy eyes, cough
Medications	Antibiotics, antihistamines, decongestants, steroids, chemotherapy, immunotherapy, immunosuppressive drugs
Injuries and Accidents	Foreign bodies; trauma to the ears, nose, mouth, throat; noxious fumes; sports injuries to the face; motor vehicle accidents
Special Needs	Deafness, speech disorders
Childhood Illnesses	Frequent tonsillitis, frequent ear infections
FAMILY HEALTH HISTORY	*Ears, nose, mouth, and throat diseases that are familial are listed.* Hearing loss, otosclerosis, neonatal blindness secondary to cataracts from mother contracting rubella in pregnancy
SOCIAL HISTORY	*The components of the social history are linked to ears, nose, mouth, and throat factors and pathology.*
Alcohol Use	Predisposes the patient to cancer of the oral cavity as well as decreased nutrition leading to cheilosis
Tobacco Use	Snuff or chewing tobacco predisposes the patient to mouth, lip, or throat cancer

continues

Health History (continued)

Drug Use	Snorting cocaine may cause perforation of the nasal septum
Sexual Practice	Herpes simplex viruses I and II and gonorrhea can be contracted from oral sex
Work Environment	Exposure to toxins, chemicals, infections, excess noise, allergens
Home Environment	Exposure to loud music may cause hearing loss
Hobbies and Leisure Activities	Hunting without proper ear protection may cause hearing loss
Stress	Relationship to frequent upper respiratory infections, decreased hearing Brushing—grinding of teeth
Ethnic Background	Nasopharyngeal cancer: Chinese Rhinoscleroma: individuals from Mediterranean countries, Southeast Asians, Indonesians, South Americans
HEALTH MAINTENANCE ACTIVITIES	*This information provides a bridge between the health maintenance activities and ears, nose, mouth, and throat functions.*
Sleep	Deprivation may be associated with frequent upper respiratory infections
Diet	Deficiencies may affect integrity of nasal and oral mucosa
Use of Safety Devices	Use of mouth guard for sports participants; face shields for sports, job, or home projects; ear protection when around loud noise to prevent damage to hearing
Health Check-ups	Hearing assessment, dental examination

EQUIPMENT

- Otoscope with earpieces of different sizes and pneumatic attachment
- Nasal speculum
- Penlight
- Tuning fork, 512 Hz
- Tongue blade
- Watch
- Gauze square
- Clean gloves
- Transilluminator
- Cotton-tipped applicator

ASSESSMENT OF THE EAR

Physical assessment of the ear consists of three parts:
1. Auditory screening (CN VIII)
2. Inspection and palpation of the external ear
3. Otoscopic assessment

✓ NURSING CHECKLIST

General Approach to Ears, Nose, Mouth, and Throat Assessment

1. Greet the patient and explain the assessment techniques that you will be using.
2. Use a quiet room that will be free from interruptions.
3. Ensure that the light in the room provides sufficient brightness to allow adequate observation of the patient.
4. Place the patient in an upright sitting position on the examination table, or for patients who cannot tolerate the sitting position, gain access to the patient's head so that it can be rotated from side to side for assessment.
5. Visualize the underlying structures during the assessment process to allow adequate description of findings.
6. Always compare right and left ears, as well as right and left sides of the nose, sinuses, mouth, and throat.
7. Use a systematic approach that is followed consistently each time the assessment is performed.

Auditory Screening

Voice-Whisper Test

E 1. Instruct the patient to occlude one ear with a finger.

2. Stand 2 feet behind the patient's other ear and whisper a two-syllable word or phrase that is evenly accented.

3. Ask the patient to repeat the word or phrase.

4. Repeat the test with the other ear.

N The patient should be able to repeat words whispered from a distance of 2 feet.

A The patient is unable to repeat the words correctly or states that he or she was unable to hear anything.

P This indicates a hearing loss in the high-frequency range that may be caused by excessive exposure to loud noises.

Tuning Fork Tests

Weber and **Rinne tests** help to determine whether the type of hearing loss the patient is experiencing is conductive or sensorineural. In order to understand how these tests are evaluated, it is important to know the difference between air and bone conduction. Air conduction refers to the transmission of sound through the ear canal, tympanic membrane, and ossicular chain to the cochlea and auditory nerve. Bone conduction refers to the transmission of sound through the bones of the skull to the cochlea and auditory nerve.

Weber Test.

E 1. Hold the handle of a 512 Hz (vibrates 512 cycles per second to create a specific frequency) tuning fork and strike the tines on the ulnar border of the palm to activate it.

2. Place the stem of the fork firmly against the middle of the patient's forehead, on the top of the head at the midline, or on the front teeth (Figure 13-11).

3. Ask the patient if the sound is heard centrally or toward one side.

N The patient should perceive the sound equally in both ears or "in the middle."

A The sound lateralizes to the affected ear.

P This occurs with unilateral conductive hearing loss because the sound is being conducted directly through the bone to the ear. Conductive hearing loss occurs when there are external or middle ear disorders such as impacted cerumen, perforation of the tympanic membrane, serum or pus in the middle ear, or a fusion of the ossicles.

A The sound lateralizes to the unaffected ear.

P This occurs with sensorineural loss related to nerve damage in the impaired ear. Sensorineural hearing loss occurs when there is a disorder in the inner ear, the auditory nerve, or the brain; disorders include congenital defects, effects of ototoxic drugs, and repeated or prolonged exposure to loud noise.

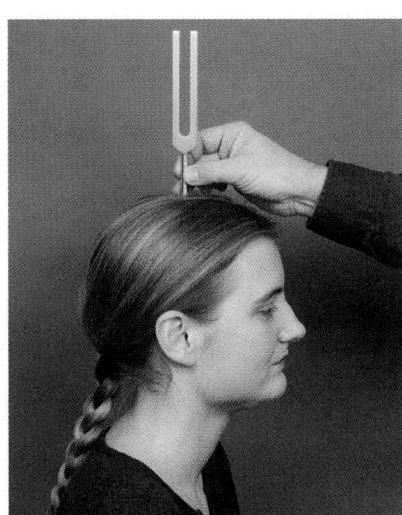

Figure 13-11 Weber Test

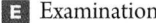

E Examination   **N** Normal Findings   **A** Abnormal Findings   **P** Pathophysiology

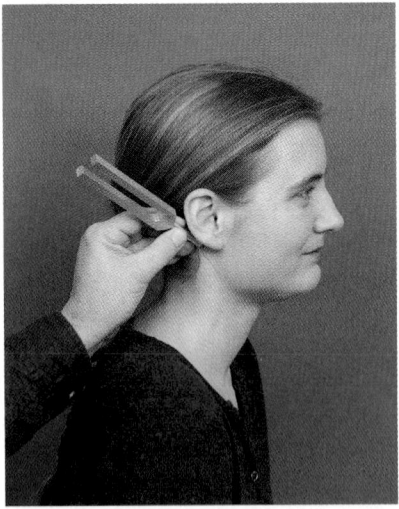

A. Assessing Bone Conduction

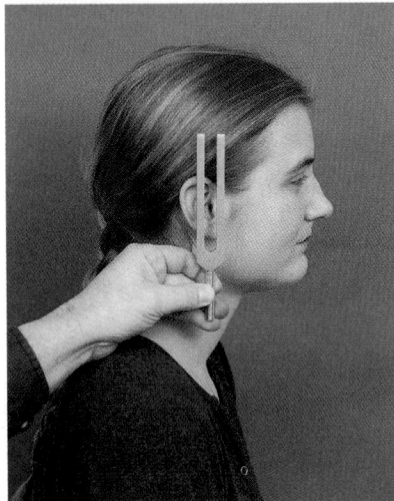

B. Assessing Air Conduction

FIGURE 13-12 Rinne Test

RINNE TEST.

E 1. Stand behind or to the side of the patient and strike the tuning fork.

2. Place the stem of the tuning fork against the patient's right mastoid process to test bone conduction (Figure 13-12A).

3. Instruct the patient to indicate if the sound is heard.

4. Ask the patient to tell you when the sound stops.

5. When the patient says that the sound has stopped, move the tuning fork, with the tines facing forward, in front of the right auditory meatus, and ask the patient if the sound is still heard. Note the length of time the patient hears the sound (testing air conduction) (Figure 13-12B).

6. Repeat the test on the left ear.

N Air conduction is heard twice as long as bone conduction when the patient hears the sound through the external auditory canal (air) after it is no longer heard at the mastoid process (bone). This is denoted as AC > BC, or a ⊕ Rinne.

A The patient reports hearing the sound longer through bone conduction; that is, bone conduction is equal to or greater than air conduction. This is a ⊖ Rinne.

P This occurs when there is a conductive hearing loss resulting from disease, obstruction, or damage to the outer or middle ear.

A Bone conduction is prolonged in the context of a normal tympanic membrane, patent eustachian tube, and middle ear disease.

P These findings are typical of otosclerosis.

EXTERNAL EAR

Inspection

E 1. Inspect the ears and note their position, color, size, and shape.

2. Note any deformities, nodules, inflammation, or lesions.

3. Note color, consistency, and amount of cerumen.

N The ear should match the flesh color of the rest of the patient's skin and should be positioned centrally and in proportion to the head. The top of the ear should cross an imaginary line drawn from the outer canthus of the eye to the occiput (see Figure 13-13). Cerumen should be moist and not obscure the tympanic membrane. There should be no foreign bodies, redness, drainage, deformities, nodules, or lesions.

A The ears are pale, red, or cyanotic.

P Vasomotor disorders, fevers, hypoxemia, and cold weather can account for various color changes.

A The ears are abnormally large or small.

P These abnormalities can be congenitally determined or the result of trauma. Figure 13-14 depicts microtia, or an unusually small external ear. Frequently, this is accompanied by an absent external ear canal and middle ear, but an intact inner ear.

A An ear that is permanently swollen and deformed resembling a "cauliflower" is abnormal.

E Examination   **N** Normal Findings   **A** Abnormal Findings   **P** Pathophysiology

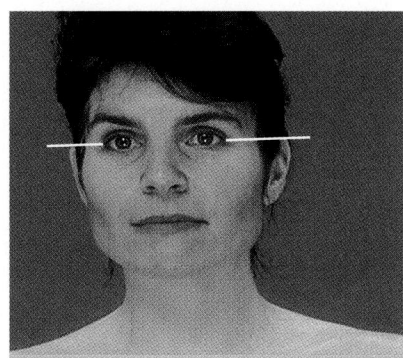

FIGURE 13-13 **Normal Ear Alignment**

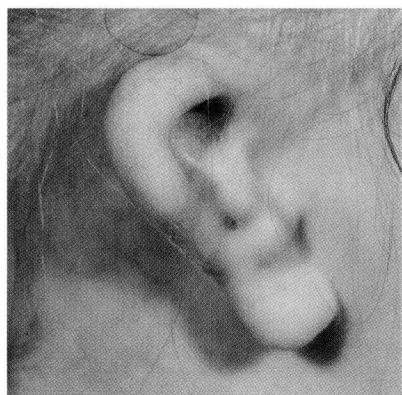

FIGURE 13-14 **Microtia.** *Courtesy of Dr. Andrew B. Silva, Pediatric Otolaryngology.*

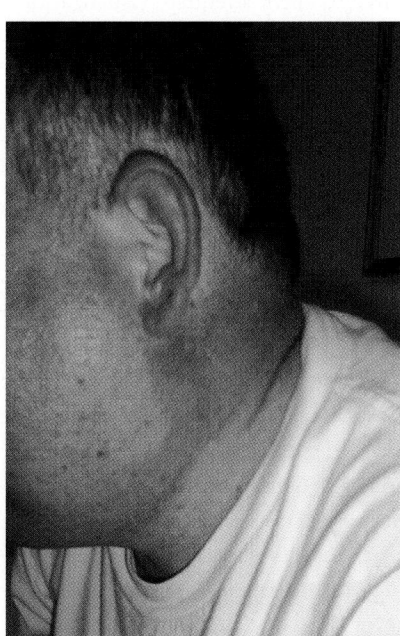

FIGURE 13-15 **Perichondritis**

P Perichondrial hematoma (cauliflower ear) is a condition common among wrestlers and boxers that is caused by blunt trauma to the external ear resulting in a blood clot formation and fluid collection under the perichondrium, which leads to fibrosis and deformity of the external ear.

A An external ear that is erythematous, edematous, warm to the touch, and painful is abnormal.

P Perichondritis is an inflammation of the fibrous connective tissue that overlies the cartilage of the ear (Figure 13-15).

A At umor on the external ear is abnormal.

P Basal cell and squamous cell carcinoma are the most common external ear tumors. Prolonged sunlight exposure is a predisposing factor for these tumors.

A Purulent drainage is abnormal.

P Purulent drainage usually indicates an infection.

A Clear or bloody drainage is present.

P Clear or bloody drainage may be due to cerebrospinal fluid leaking as a result of head trauma or surgery.

A A hematoma behind an ear over the mastoid bone is abnormal.

P This is called Battle's sign and indicates head trauma to the temporal bone of the skull.

A A hard, painless, irregular-shaped nodule on the pinna is abnormal.

P Tophi are uric acid nodules and may indicate the presence of gout. These are usually located near the helix. Many other nodules are benign fibromas.

A Sebaceous cysts are abnormal.

P Sebaceous cysts or retention cysts form as a result of the blockage of the ducts to the sebaceous gland.

A Lymph nodes anterior to the tragus or overlying the mastoid are abnormal.

P Lymph nodes may be enlarged due to a malignancy or an infection such as external otitis.

Palpation

E 1. Palpate the auricle between the thumb and the index finger, noting any tenderness or lesions. If the patient has ear pain, assess the unaffected ear first, then cautiously assess the affected ear.

2. Using the tips of the index and middle fingers, palpate the mastoid tip, noting any tenderness.

3. Using the tips of the index and middle fingers, press inward on the tragus, noting any tenderness.

4. Hold the auricle between the thumb and the index finger and gently pull up and down, noting any tenderness.

N The patient should not complain of pain or tenderness during palpation.

A Auricular pain or tenderness is noted.

P Auricular pain is a common finding in external ear infection and is called acute otitis externa.

A There is tenderness over the mastoid process.

P Mastoid tenderness is associated with middle ear inflammation or mastoiditis.

Ear Cleaning

During the health history your patient stated that he never puts anything in his ears. When you conduct the internal otoscopic examination, you notice a neat "scooped" appearance to the cerumen in the EAC. What would you say to the patient? What health teaching is appropriate?

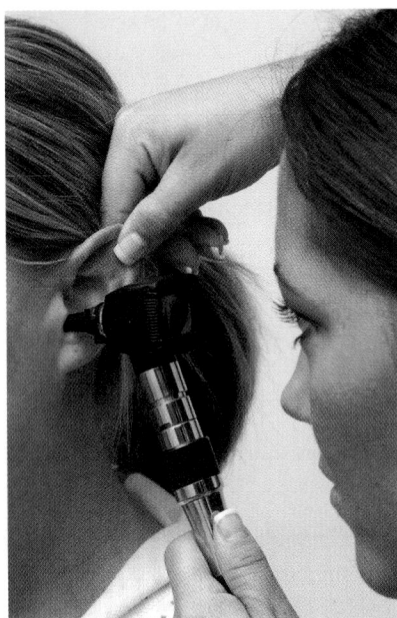

FIGURE 13-16 Position for Otoscopic Examination

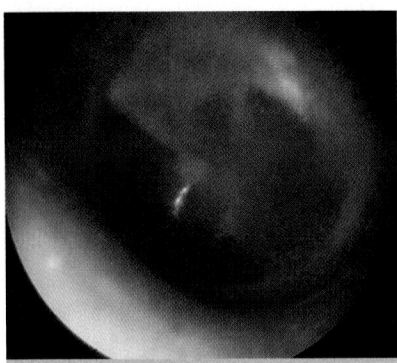

FIGURE 13-17 Normal Tympanic Membrane. *Courtesy of Dr. Andrew B. Silva, Pediatric Otolaryngology.*

A The tragus is edematous or sensitive.

P This finding may indicate inflammation of the external or middle ear.

OTOSCOPIC ASSESSMENT

E 1. Ask the patient to tip the head away from the ear being assessed.

2. Select the largest speculum that will comfortably fit the patient.

3. Hold the otoscope securely in the dominant hand, with the handle held like a pencil between the thumb and the forefinger.

4. Rest the back of the dominant hand on the right side of the patient's head (Figure 13-16).

5. Use the free hand to pull the right ear in a manner that will straighten the canal. In adults and in children over 3 years old, pull the ear up and back. See Chapter 24 for the assessment of children.

6. If hair obstructs visualization, moisten the speculum with water or a water-soluble lubricant.

7. If wax obstructs visualization, it should be removed only by a skilled practitioner, either by curettement (if the cerumen is soft or the tympanic membrane is ruptured) or by irrigation (if the cerumen is dry and hard and the tympanic membrane is intact).

8. Slowly insert the speculum into the canal, looking at the canal as the speculum passes.

9. Assess the canal for inflammation, exudates, lesions, and foreign bodies.

10. Continue to insert the speculum into the canal, following the path of the canal until the tympanic membrane is visualized.

11. If the tympanic membrane is not visible, gently pull the pinna slightly further in order to straighten the canal to allow adequate visualization.

12. Identify the color, light reflex, umbo, the short process, and the long handle of the malleus. Note the presence of perforations, lesions, bulging or retraction of the tympanic membrane, dilatation of blood vessels, bubbles, or fluid.

13. Ask the patient to close the mouth, pinch the nose closed, and blow gently while you observe for movement of the tympanic membrane. A pneumatic attachment may be used to create this movement if one is available.

14. Gently withdraw the speculum and repeat the process with the left ear.

N The ear canal should have no redness, swelling, tenderness, lesions, drainage, foreign bodies, or scaly surface areas. Cerumen varies in amount, consistency, and color. The tympanic membrane should be pearly gray with clearly defined landmarks and a distinct cone-shaped light reflex extending from the umbo toward the anteroinferior aspect of the membrane. This light reflex is seen at 5 o'clock in the right ear and at 7 o'clock in the left ear. Blood vessels should be visible only on the periphery, and the membrane should not bulge, be retracted, or have any evidence of fluid behind it (Figure 13-17). The tympanic membrane should move when the patient blows against resistance.

A A foreign body in the external auditory canal (EAC) is abnormal. See Figure 13-18.

| **E** Examination | **N** Normal Findings | **A** Abnormal Findings | **P** Pathophysiology |

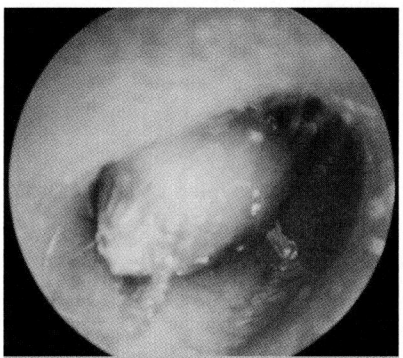

FIGURE 13-18 EAC Foreign Body (a bean). *Courtesy of Dr. Andrew B. Silva, Pediatric Otolaryngology.*

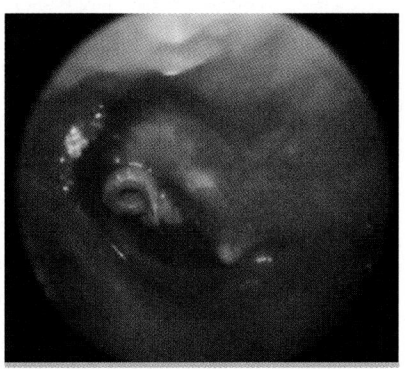

FIGURE 13-19 PE Tube. *Courtesy of Dr. Andrew B. Silva, Pediatric Otolaryngology.*

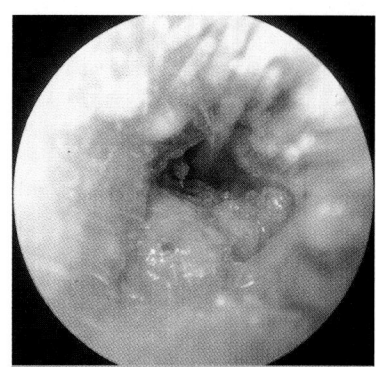

FIGURE 13-20 Furunculosis. *Courtesy of Bruce Black, MD, Brisbane, Australia.*

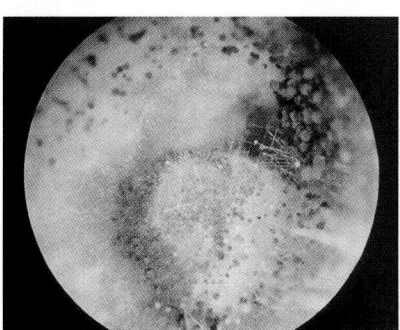

A. Aspergillus Nigra

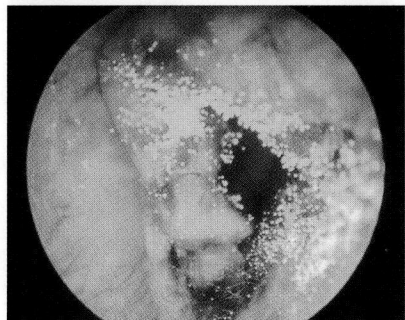

B. Aspergillus Flavum

FIGURE 13-21 Otomycosis. *Courtesy of Bruce Black, MD, Brisbane, Australia.*

P Both adults and children can have foreign bodies in the EAC. Some objects are more difficult to remove than others; for instance, vegetables in the EAC can swell with time and make removal challenging.

P Tympanostomy tubes, or PE tubes (pressure equalization) (Figure 13-19), are surgically placed for prolonged otitis media with effusion (OME). The tubes allow drainage of the effusion, normal vibration of the ossicles, and equalization of pressures across the tympanic membrane. When a myringotomy has been performed with tympanostomy tube placement, the presence of the tubes (or lack of) needs to be documented.

A A painful, boil-like pustule in the EAC is abnormal (Figure 13-20).

P Furunculosis is an infection of a hair follicle. EAC edema and otorrhea may also be present.

A Black or brown spores (Figure 13-21A), yellow or orange spores (Figure 13-21B), or white fluffy hyphae in the EAC are abnormal.

P Prolonged use of aural antibiotics can cause otomycosis, or a fungal infection, in the ear. Different strains of fungi cause the variations in appearance.

A Bony, hard lesions in the deep EAC (see Figure 13-22) are abnormal.

P These are exostoses. Patients who frequently participate in cold-water activities are at risk for developing them. If an exostosis becomes large enough, it can block the EAC and trap debris between it and the tympanic membrane. This can lead to infection.

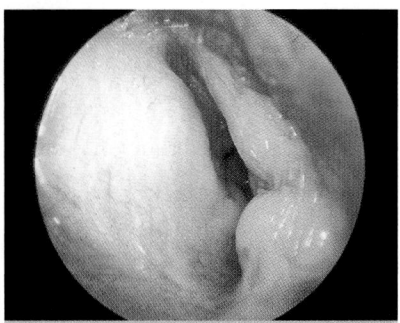

FIGURE 13-22   Exostoses. *Courtesy of Bruce Black, MD, Brisbane, Australia.*

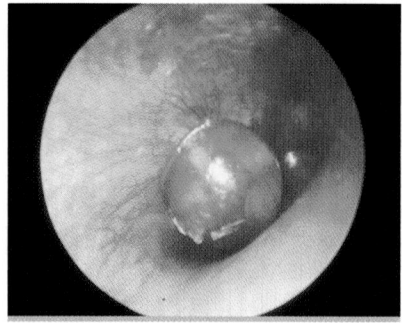

FIGURE 13-23   Bullous Myringitis. *Courtesy of Bruce Black, MD, Brisbane, Australia.*

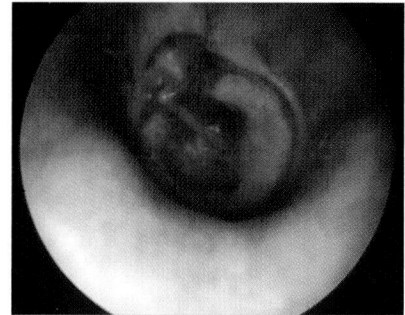

FIGURE 13-24   Myringosclerosis and Otitis Media with Effusion. *Courtesy of Dr. Andrew B. Silva, Pediatric Otolaryngology.*

A   Severe pain accompanied by erythema deep into the EAC and on the tympanic membrane, along with serous-filled blebs (Figure 13-23), is abnormal.

P   This describes viral bullous myringitis. This can easily be mistaken for acute otitis media.

A   The appearance of chalk patches on the tympanic membrane (Figure 13-24) is abnormal.

P   These are calcifications found in myringosclerosis, which can occur after tympanic membrane surgery, infection, or inflammation. Myringosclerosis can be associated with a gradual hearing loss. Involvement of the entire tympanic membrane is called tympanosclerosis.

A   Air bubbles on the tympanic membrane (Figure 13-25) are abnormal.

P   Conditions such as coryza and influenza and changes in extratympanic pressure (such as in scuba diving, airplane travel) can lead to eustachian tube failure.

A   The presence of blood in the middle ear is abnormal (Figure 13-26).

P   Hemotympanum occurs as a result of trauma to the head. The tympanic membrane can have a bluish hue or can be red in appearance.

A   A severely retracted tympanic membrane has exaggerated landmarks (Figure 13-27). Mobility of the tympanic membrane is decreased.

P   Retraction of the tympanic membrane can occur when the intratympanic membrane pressures are reduced, as in eustachian tube blockage caused by otitis media with effusion or allergies. Repeated negative pressure in the middle ear sucks in the tympanic membrane and leads to retractions. Over time, keratinized epithelial debris deposits itself in these retraction pockets and

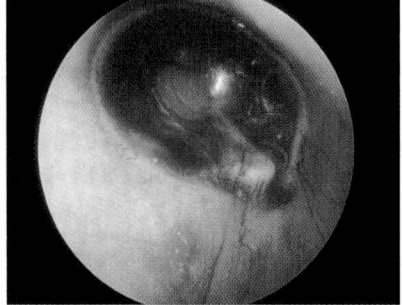

FIGURE 13-25   Barotrauma Caused by Scuba Diving. *Courtesy of Bruce Black, MD, Brisbane, Australia.*

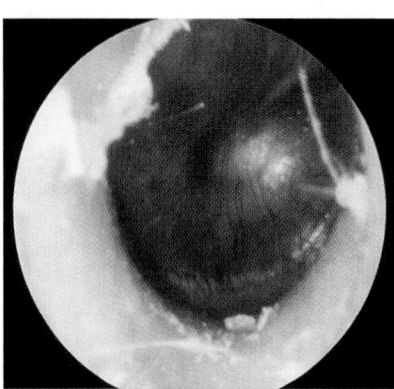

FIGURE 13-26   Hemotympanum. *Courtesy of Dr. Andrew B. Silva, Pediatric Otolaryngology.*

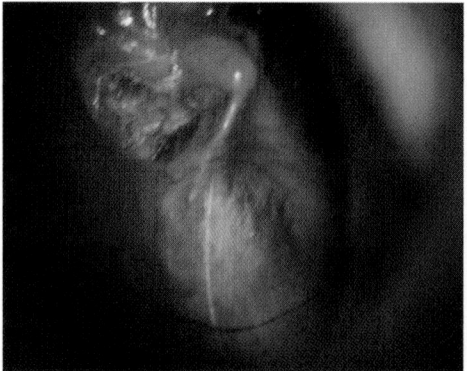

FIGURE 13-27A   Tympanic Membrane Retraction. *Courtesy of Dr. Andrew B. Silva, Pediatric Otolaryngology.*

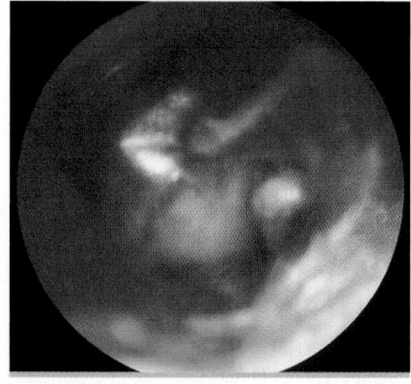

FIGURE 13-27B   Severe Tympanic Membrane Retraction. *Courtesy of Dr. Andrew B. Silva, Pediatric Otolaryngology.*

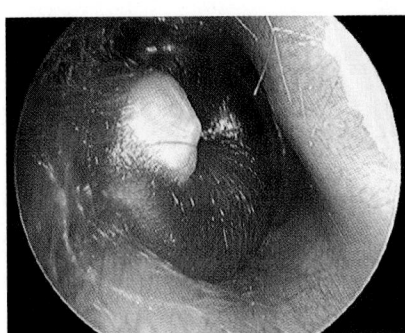

FIGURE 13-28 **Cholesteatoma.**
Courtesy of Dr. Andrew B. Silva, Pediatric Otolaryngology.

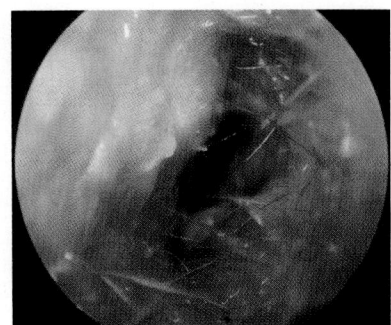

FIGURE 13-29 **Acute Otitis Externa.** *Courtesy of Bruce Black, MD, Brisbane, Australia.*

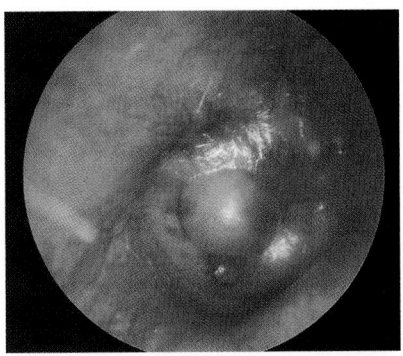

A. Early AOM. Note the bulging TM.

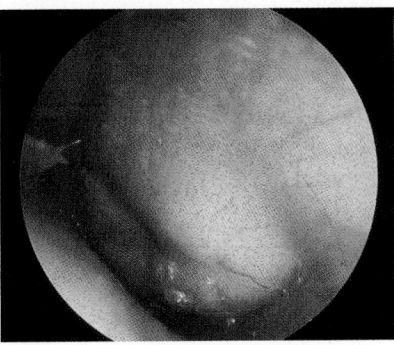

B. More Advanced AOM with Bleb Formation. Note the bulging TM and purulent effusion behind the tympanic membrane. The pressure behind the membrane caused a vesicle to form on the pars tensa.

FIGURE 13-30 **Acute Otitis Media.**
Courtesy of Bruce Black, MD, Brisbane, Australia.

leads to ossicle fixation. This leads to cholesteatoma (Figure 13-28). A foul smelling ear discharge, as well as deafness, may accompany cholesteatoma.

A There is redness, swelling, narrowing, and pain of the external ear (Figure 13-29). Drainage may be present.

P Acute otitis externa is caused by infectious organisms or allergic reactions. Predisposing factors include excessive moisture in the ear related to swimming, trauma from cleansing the ears with a sharp instrument, or allergies to substances such as hairspray.

A Hard, dry, and very dark yellow-brown cerumen is abnormal.

P Old cerumen is harder and drier, and may become impacted if not removed.

A The tympanic membrane is red, with decreased mobility and possible bulging (Figure 13-30).

P This is acute **otitis media** (AOM), or an inflammation of the middle ear. Pain and fever may accompany the ear infection. Otalgia, fever, decreased hearing, irritability, disturbed sleep, and otorrhea may accompany the middle ear infection. *Streptococcus pneumoniae*, *Haemophilus influenzae*, and *Moraxella catarrhalis* are the major pathogens that cause AOM.

NURSING**ALERT**

Risk Factors for Otitis Media

- Less than 2 years of age
- Frequent upper respiratory tract infections
- Cold weather
- Males
- Caucasians, Native Americans, Alaskan natives
- Family history (parents, siblings)
- Pacifier use after 6 months of age
- Smoky environment
- Day care attendance
- Bottle fed
- Down syndrome
- Craniofacial disorders

E Examination   **N** Normal Findings   **A** Abnormal Findings   **P** Pathophysiology

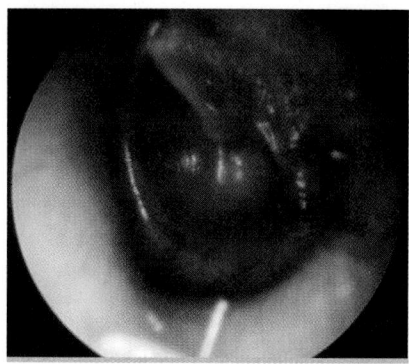

FIGURE 13-31 **Otitis Media with Effusion.** *Courtesy of Dr. Andrew B. Silva, Pediatric Otolaryngology.*

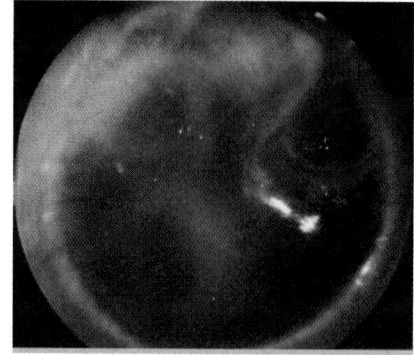

FIGURE 13-32 **Serous Otitis Media.** *Courtesy of Dr. Andrew B. Silva, Pediatric Otolaryngology.*

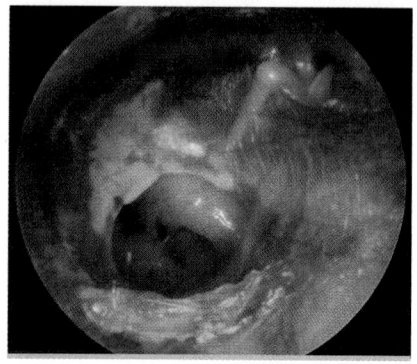

FIGURE 13-33 **Tympanic Membrane Perforation.** *Courtesy of Dr. Andrew B. Silva, Pediatric Otolaryngology.*

A Along with a bulging eardrum and decreased mobility, the landmarks are diffuse, displaced, or absent.

P The late stage of acute otitis media causes landmarks to become progressively obscured.

A Amber-yellow fluid on the tympanic membrane is abnormal. It may be accompanied by a fluid line or bubbles behind the membrane. Bulging may be present and mobility of the eardrum may be decreased (Figures 13-31 and 13-32). The patient may complain of ear popping, pain, and decreased hearing.

P Otitis media with effusion, or serous otitis media, can be caused by allergies, infections, and a blocked eustachian tube. Table 13-1 compares AOM, OME, and otitis externa.

A The tympanic membrane appears to have a darkened area or a hole.

P A perforated eardrum is caused by untreated ear infection secondary to increasing pressure. Trauma to the ear canal can also cause a perforation (Figure 13-33).

A The tympanic membrane is pearly gray and has dark patches.

P These patches are usually old perforations in the tympanic membrane.

A The tympanic membrane is pearly gray and has dense white plaques.

P These plaques represent calcific deposits of scarring of the tympanic membrane from frequent past episodes of otitis media.

TABLE 13-1 Comparison of AOM, OME, and Otitis Externa

	AOM	OME	OTITIS EXTERNA
TM color	Diffuse red, dilated peripheral vessels	Yellowish	WNL
TM appearance	Bulging	Bubbles, fluid line	WNL
TM landmarks	Decreased	Retracted with prominent malleus	WNL
Movement of tragus	Painless	Painless	Painful
Hearing	WNL/decreased	WNL/decreased	WNL
EAC	WNL	WNL	Erythematous, edematous

ASSESSMENT OF THE NOSE

EXTERNAL INSPECTION

E Inspect the nose, noting any trauma, bleeding, lesions, masses, swelling, and asymmetry.

N The shape of the external nose can vary greatly among individuals. Normally, it is located symmetrically in the midline of the face and is without swelling, bleeding, lesions, or masses.

A The nose is misshapen, broken, or swollen.

P The shape of the nose is determined by genetics; however, changes can occur because of trauma or cosmetic surgery.

PATENCY

E 1. Have the patient occlude one nostril with a finger.

2. Ask the patient to breathe in and out through the nose as you observe and listen for air movement in and out of the nostril.

3. Repeat on the other side.

N Each nostril is patent.

A You observe or the patient states that air cannot be moved through the nostril(s).

P Occlusion of the nostrils can occur with a deviated septum, foreign body, upper respiratory infection, allergies, or nasal polyps.

A Nasal drainage is observed from only one side of the nose.

P Unilateral nasal drainage may be a sign of nasal obstruction.

INTERNAL INSPECTION

E 1. Position the patient with the head in an extended position.

2. Place the nondominant hand firmly on top of the patient's head.

3. Using the thumb of the same hand, lift the tip of the patient's nose.

4. Gently insert a nasal speculum or an otoscope with a short, wide nasal speculum (Figure 13-34). If using a nasal speculum, use a penlight to view the nostrils.

5. Assess each nostril separately.

6. Inspect the mucous membranes for color and discharge.

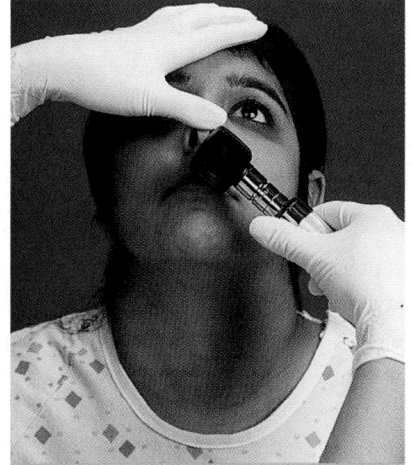

FIGURE 13-34 **Internal Inspection of the Nose**

LIFE ◎ 360°

Suspected Cocaine Abuse in a College Student

Jason, a 19-year-old college student, presents to the student health clinic complaining of recurrent nosebleeds, nasal congestion, and sinus headaches. You note a white powder substance on the nasal hairs and significant edema of the nasal mucosa. Jason appears to be agitated and restless. You suspect cocaine abuse. How should you respond? What questions should you ask? What action would be appropriate at this time?

E Examination   **N** Normal Findings   **A** Abnormal Findings   **P** Pathophysiology

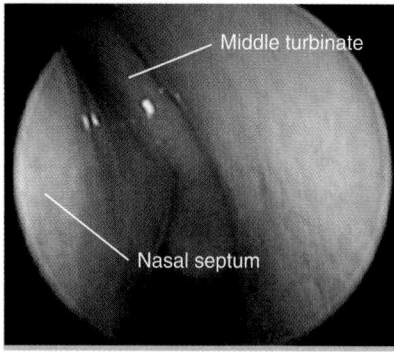

FIGURE 13-35 **Deviated Septum.**
Courtesy of Dr. Andrew B. Silva, Pediatric Otolaryngology.

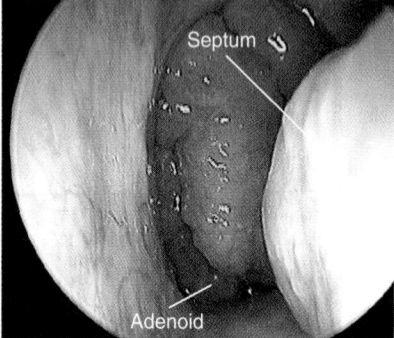

FIGURE 13-36 **Nasal Cavity Blocked by Adenoid.** *Courtesy of Dr. Andrew B. Silva, Pediatric Otolaryngology.*

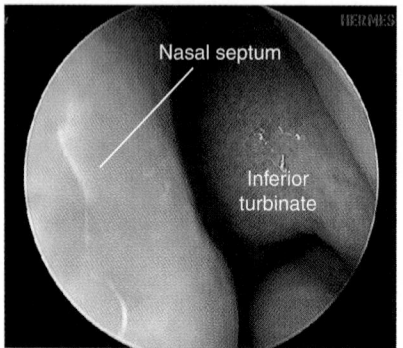

FIGURE 13-37 **Edematous inferior turbinate causing almost total occlusion of the nasal cavity. Note the slight difference in color between the septum and the turbinate. These findings can occur in patients with allergic rhinitis.** *Courtesy of Dr. Andrew B. Silva, Pediatric Otolaryngology.*

7. Inspect the middle and inferior turbinates and the middle meatus for color, swelling, drainage, lesions, and polyps.

8. Observe the nasal septum for deviation, perforation, lesions, and bleeding.

N The nasal mucosa should be pink or dull red without swelling or polyps. The septum is at the midline and without perforation, lesions, or bleeding. A small amount of clear, watery discharge is normal.

A A nasal septum that is "pushed" to one side can be an abnormal finding (Figure 13-35).

P A deviated septum can be a naturally occurring finding, or it can be caused by trauma to the face and nasal area.

A A nasal septum with a hole or fissure is abnormal.

P A perforated nasal septum may be caused by nasal insufflation (snorting) of cocaine, which can lead to necrosis of the septal cartilage. Long-term intrasnasal corticosteroids can also result in a perforated nasal septum if incorrect administration technique is used.

A A nasal cavity that is occluded is abnormal.

P There are many causes of an occluded nasal cavity. Foreign bodies may be present, especially in children. Trauma may induce nasal edema, sinus infection may produce copious discharge, an adenoid may be so large that it occludes the nasal cavity (Figure 13-36), and allergies can lead to edematous turbinates (Figure 13-37).

A The nasal mucosa is red and swollen with copious clear, watery discharge. This is called rhinitis, an inflammation of the nasal mucosa.

P These findings indicate the occurrence of the common cold (coryza) when there is an acute onset of symptoms. Discharge may become purulent if a secondary bacterial infection develops.

A Nasal mucosa is pale and edematous with clear, watery discharge.

P These findings usually indicate the presence of allergies or hay fever.

A Following trauma to the head, there is a clear, watery nasal discharge with normal-appearing mucosa. This discharge tests positive for glucose.

P These findings indicate the presence of cerebrospinal fluid. This may occur following head injury or complications of nose or sinus surgery or dental work. Immediate referral is warranted.

A Nasal mucosa is red and swollen with purulent nasal discharge (see Figure 13-38). These findings are usually worse on one side but may be found bilaterally.

P These are common findings in bacterial sinusitis.

A Smooth, round masses that are pale and shiny are noted protruding from the middle meatus.

P These masses are nasal polyps (see Figure 13-39), which may obstruct air passages. They are often seen in patients who have chronic allergic rhinitis, asthma, and cystic fibrosis. They are usually found bilaterally. A unilateral polyp is suspect for a malignancy until proven otherwise.

A Bleeding is noted from an area of the lower portion of the nasal septum.

P Kiesselbach's plexus, a vascular area on the septum, is the site of most nosebleeds (see Figure 13-40). Repeated nosebleeds warrant attention for blood dyscrasias, environmental causes, medication use (e.g., anticoagulants), and malignancies, among other etiologies.

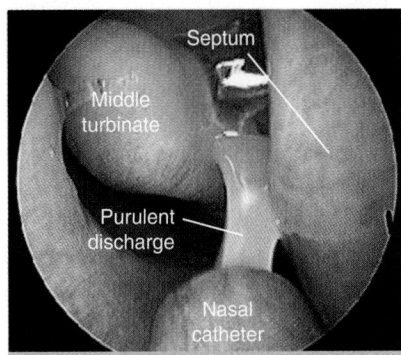

FIGURE 13-38 Purulent Discharge in the Nasal Cavity at the Middle Turbinate. *Courtesy of Dr. Andrew B. Silva, Pediatric Otolaryngology.*

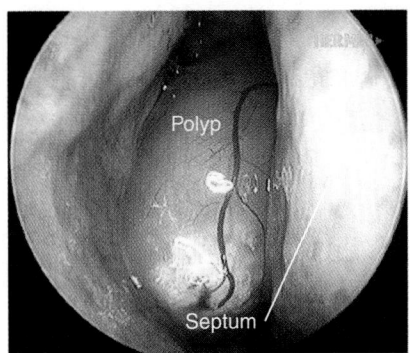

FIGURE 13-39 Nasal Polyp. *Courtesy of Dr. Andrew B. Silva, Pediatric Otolaryngology.*

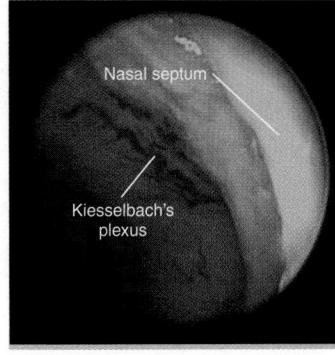

FIGURE 13-40 Kiesselbach's Plexus. *Courtesy of Dr. Andrew B. Silva, Pediatric Otolaryngology.*

A There is unilateral purulent discharge; however, the patient does not experience other symptoms of an upper respiratory infection. Nasal mucosa on the unaffected side appears normal.

P Unilateral purulent discharge without other findings of an upper respiratory infection indicates the development of a local infection. A common cause of localized infection is the presence of a foreign body.

A Nasal mucosa is inflamed and friable with possible septal perforation. There is no infection present.

P These findings may indicate nasal inhalation of cocaine or amphetamines or the overuse of nasal spray.

ASSESSMENT OF THE SINUSES

INSPECTION

E Observe the patient's face for any swelling around the nose and eyes.

N There is no evidence of swelling around the nose and eyes.

A Swelling is noted above or below the eyes.

P Acute sinusitis may result in swelling of the face around the eyes due to inflammation and accumulation of purulent material in the paranasal sinuses.

PALPATION AND PERCUSSION

To palpate and percuss the frontal sinuses:

E 1. Stand facing the patient.

2. Gently press the thumbs under the bony ridge of the upper orbits (see Figure 13-41A). Avoid applying pressure on the globes themselves.

3. Observe for the presence of pain.

4. Percuss the areas using the middle or index finger of the dominant hand (direct percussion).

5. Note the sound.

REFLECTIVE THINKING

Septal Perforation

You note that your patient has a small septal perforation. She adamantly denies snorting cocaine even though her friends do. She admits to using other illegal substances in the past, and you are aware that she was recently released from a drug rehab program. What questions would you ask this patient? What other physical assessments would be appropriate?

| **E** Examination | **N** Normal Findings | **A** Abnormal Findings | **P** Pathophysiology |

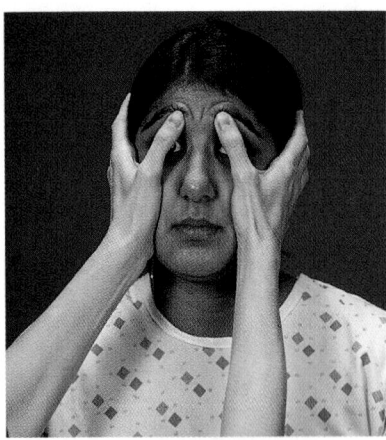

A. Palpation of Frontal Sinuses

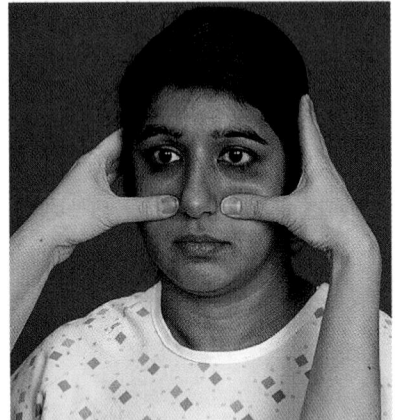

B. Palpation of Maxillary Sinuses

FIGURE 13-41 Palpation of Sinuses

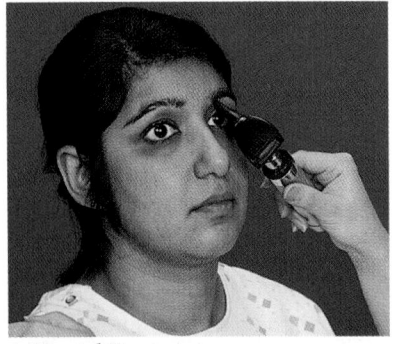

A. Frontal Sinus

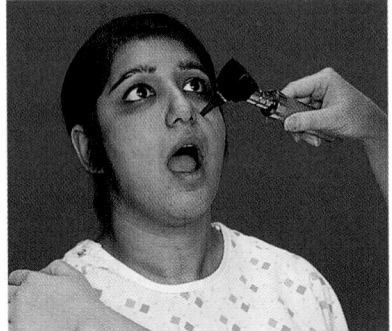

B. Maxillary Sinus

FIGURE 13-42 Transillumination of Sinuses

N/A/P Refer to maxillary sinuses.

To palpate and percuss the maxillary sinuses:

E 1. Stand in front of the patient.

2. Apply gentle pressure in the area under the infraorbital ridge using the thumb or middle finger (Figure 13-41B).

3. Observe for the presence of pain.

4. Percuss the area using the dominant middle or index finger.

5. Note the sound.

N The patient should experience no discomfort during palpation or percussion. The sinuses should be air filled and therefore resonant to percussion.

A The patient complains of pain or tenderness at the site of palpation or percussion.

P Sinusitis can be due to viral, bacterial, or allergic processes that cause inflammation of the mucous membranes and obstruction of the drainage pathways.

A Percussion of the sinuses elicits a dull sound.

P Dullness can be caused by fluid or cells present in the sinus cavity from an infectious or allergic process, or congenital absence of a sinus.

ADVANCED TECHNIQUE

Transillumination of the Sinuses

If palpation and percussion of the sinuses suggest sinusitis, transillumination of the frontal and maxillary sinuses should be performed.

To evaluate the frontal sinuses:

E 1. Place the patient in a sitting position facing you in a dark room.

2. Place a strong light source such as a transilluminator, penlight, or tip of an otoscope with the speculum under the bony ridge of the upper orbits (Figure 13-42A).

3. Observe the red glow over the sinuses and compare the symmetry of the two sides.

To evaluate the maxillary sinuses:

E 1. Place the patient in a sitting position facing you in a dark room.

2. Place the light source firmly under each eye and just above the infraorbital ridge (Figure 13-42B).

3. Ask the patient to open the mouth; observe the red glow on the hard palate.

4. Compare the two sides.

N The glow on each side is equal, indicating air-filled frontal and maxillary sinuses.

A Absence of glow is abnormal.

P Absence of glow suggests sinus congestion or the congenital absence of a sinus.

A An extremely bright glow is abnormal.

P This phenomenon may be present in an elderly patient with decreased subcutaneous fat.

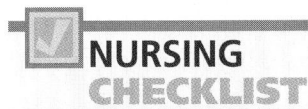

Preparing for the Assessment of the Mouth and Throat

1. Physical assessment of the oral cavity should include the following: breath, lips, tongue, buccal mucosa, gums and teeth, hard and soft palates, throat (oropharynx), and temporomandibular joint (see Chapters 11 and 18).
2. If the patient is wearing dentures or removable orthodontia, ask that they be removed before the examination begins.
3. Use gloves and a good light source such as a penlight for optimum visualization of the oral cavity and pharynx.

ASSESSMENT OF THE MOUTH AND THROAT

ASSESSMENT OF THE MOUTH

Breath

E 1. Stand facing the patient and about 12 inches away.

2. Smell the breath.

N The breath should smell fresh.

A The breath smells foul.

P The foul smell of halitosis can be a symptom of tooth decay, poor oral hygiene, or diseases of the gums, tonsils, or sinuses.

A The breath smells of acetone.

P Acetone or "fruity" breath is common in patients who are malnourished or who have diabetic ketoacidosis. The patient may also be on a low carbohydrate diet.

A The breath smells musty.

P Fetor hepaticus is the musty smell of the breath of a patient in liver failure and is caused by the breakdown of nitrogen compounds.

A The breath smells of ammonia.

P The smell of ammonia can be detected in a patient in end-stage renal failure (uremia) because of the inability to eliminate urea.

Lips

INSPECTION.

E 1. Observe the lips for color, moisture, swelling, lesions, or other signs of inflammation.

2. Instruct the patient to open the mouth.

3. Use a tongue blade to inspect the membranes that connect the upper and lower lips to the gums for color, inflammation, lesions, and hydration.

N The lips and membranes should be pink and moist with no evidence of lesions or inflammation.

A The lips are pale or cyanotic.

P Refer to Chapter 16.

A The lips are dry and cracked.

P Chapping or superficial cracking of the lips may be due to exposure to wind, sun, or a dry environment, dehydration of the patient, or persistent licking of the lips.

A Swelling of the lips is noted.

P Allergic reactions to medications, foods, or other allergens can result in swelling of the lips.

A The skin at the outer corners of the mouth is atrophic, irritated, and cracked (see Figure 13-43A).

P Angular cheilosis may be due to increased accumulation of saliva in the corners of the mouth or constant drooling from the mouth. This occurs in nutritional deficiencies (such as riboflavin), poorly fitting dentures, and deficiencies of the immune system. *Candida* infections may also be present.

| **E** Examination | **N** Normal Findings | **A** Abnormal Findings | **P** Pathophysiology |

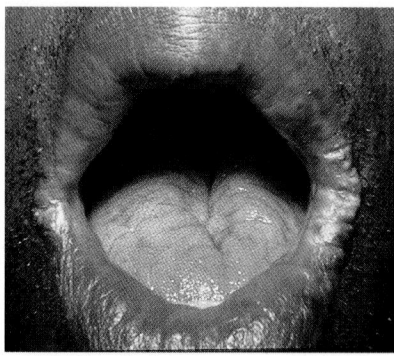

A. Angular Cheilosis. *Courtesy of Dr. Joseph Konzelman, School of Dentistry, Medical College of Georgia.*

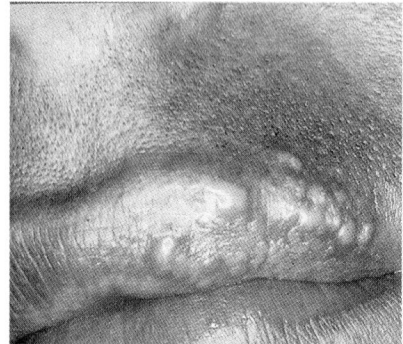

B. Fever Blister (Herpes Simplex Virus). *Courtesy of Dr. Joseph Konzelman, School of Dentistry, Medical College of Georgia.*

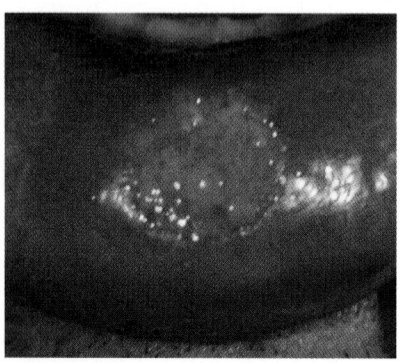

C. Chancre from Primary Syphilis

A Vesicles on erythematous bases with serous fluid are found on the lips, gums, or hard palate, either singly or in clusters. They later rupture, crust over, and become painful (Figure 13-43B).

P These are herpes simplex lesions, which are commonly called cold sores or fever blisters. This common viral infection may be precipitated by febrile illness, sunlight, stress, or allergies.

A A round, painless lesion with central ulceration (Figure 13-43C) is noted. This lesion may become crusted.

P This is a chancre, the primary lesion of syphilis.

A A plaque, wart, nodule, or ulcer is noted, usually on the lower lip.

P This may be squamous cell carcinoma, the most common form of oral cancer, which is more frequent in males (Figure 13-43D).

P Basal cell carcinoma lesions can have pearly borders, crusting, and central ulcerations (Figure 13-43E).

A Persistent, painless, white, painted-looking patches are noted on the lips (Figure 13-43F). They are associated with heavy smoking and the use of chewing tobacco.

P These patches are called leukoplakia and are considered premalignant lesions. They often occur at sites of chronic irritation from dentures, tobacco, or excessive alcohol intake.

PALPATION.

E 1. Don clean gloves.

2. Gently pull down the patient's lower lip with the thumb and index finger of one hand and pull up the patient's upper lip with the thumb and index finger of the other hand.

3. Note the tone of the lips as they are manipulated.

4. If lesions are present, palpate them for consistency and tenderness.

N Lips should not be flaccid and lesions should not be present.

A/P See inspection of the lips for pathologies.

Tongue

E 1. Ask the patient to stick out the tongue (CN XII assesses tongue movement).

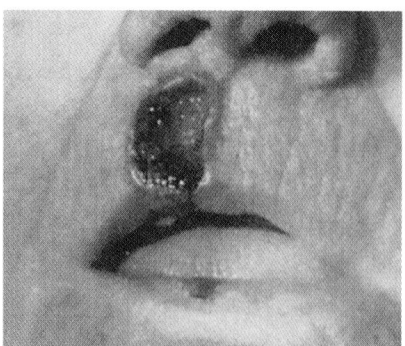

D. Squamous Cell Carcinoma. *Courtesy of Dr. Joseph Konzelman, School of Dentistry, Medical College of Georgia.*

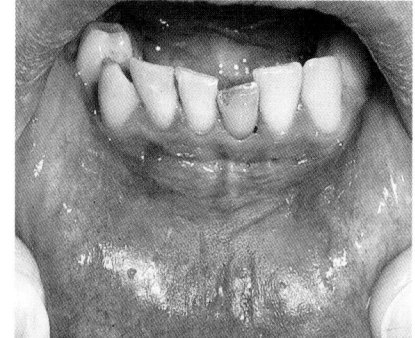

E. Basal Cell Carcinoma

F. Leukoplakia. *Courtesy of Dr. Joseph Konzelman, School of Dentistry, Medical College of Georgia.*

FIGURE 13-43 Lip Abnormalities

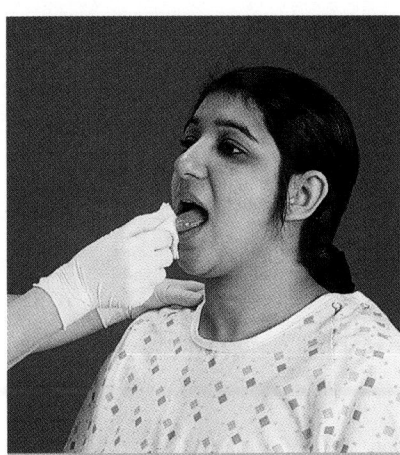

FIGURE 13-44 **Tongue Assessment**

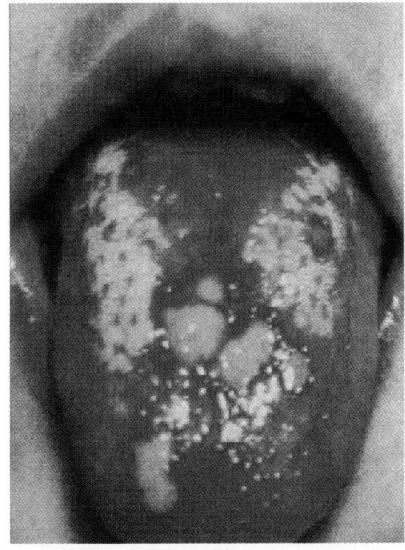

A. Candidiasis (Thrush)

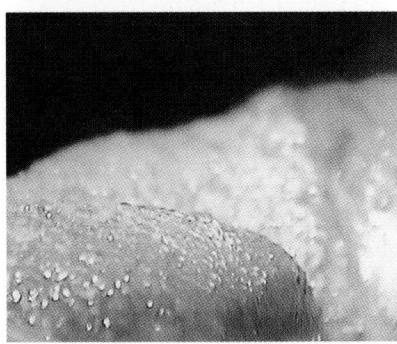

B. Leukoplakia of the Tongue. *Courtesy of Dr. Daniel D. Rooney.*

FIGURE 13-45 **Tongue Conditions**
continues

2. Observe the dorsal surface for color, hydration, texture, symmetry, fasciculations, atrophy, position in the mouth, and the presence of lesions.

3. Ask the patient to move the tongue from side to side and up and down.

4. With the patient's tongue back in the mouth, ask the patient to press it against the cheek. Provide resistance with your finger pads held on the outside of the cheek. Note the strength of the tongue and compare bilaterally.

5. Ask the patient to touch the tip of the tongue to the roof of the mouth. You may also grasp the tip of the tongue with a gauze square held between the thumb and the index finger of the gloved hand (Figure 13-44).

6. Inspect the ventral surface of the tongue, the frenulum, and Wharton's ducts for color, hydration, lesions, inflammation, and vasculature.

7. With the gauze square, pull the tongue to the left and inspect and palpate the tongue using the finger pads.

8. Repeat with the tongue held to the right side.

N The tongue is in the midline of the mouth. The dorsum of the tongue should be pink, moist, rough (from the taste buds), and without lesions. The tongue is symmetrical and moves freely. The strength of the tongue is symmetrical and strong. The ventral surface of the tongue has prominent blood vessels and should be moist and without lesions. Wharton's ducts are patent and without inflammation or lesions. The lateral aspects of the tongue should be pink, smooth, and lesion free.

A The tongue is enlarged.

P An enlarged tongue may be associated with myxedema, acromegaly, Down syndrome, or amyloidosis. Transient enlargement may be associated with glossitis, stomatitis, cellulitis of the neck, angioneurotic edema, hematoma, or abscess.

A The tongue is red and smooth with absent papillae.

P This indicates glossitis caused by a vitamin B_{12}, iron, or niacin deficiency. It may also be a side effect of chemotherapy.

A There is a thick, white, curdlike coating on the tongue that leaves a raw, red surface when it is scraped off (Figure 13-45A).

P This is candidiasis, or thrush, which may also be red in the absence of the coating. Thrush can result from changes in the normal oral flora due to chemotherapy, radiation therapy, disorders of the immune system such as AIDS, antibiotic therapy, or excessive use of alcohol, tobacco, or cocaine.

A Thin, pearly white lesions that coalesce and become thick and palpable are noted on the sides of the tongue. These white lesions are firmly attached to the underlying tissue and will not scrape off.

P This is leukoplakia. It is considered a premalignant lesion. Some leukoplakia progresses from dysplasia to a malignancy. Refer to Figure 13-45B.

A A painful, small, round white ulcerated lesion with erythematous borders is abnormal (see Figure 13-45C).

P This is an aphthous ulcer (canker sore), which can be associated with stress, extreme fatigue, food allergies, and oral trauma.

A A short lingual frenulum is observed (see Figure 13-45D).

| **E** Examination | **N** Normal Findings | **A** Abnormal Findings | **P** Pathophysiology |

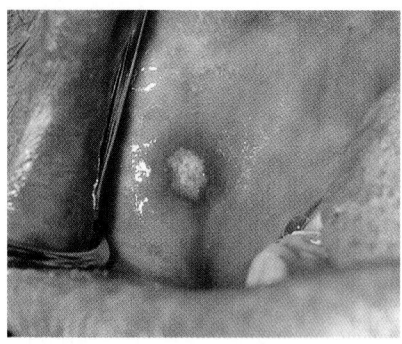

C. Aphthous Ulcer (Canker Sore). *Courtesy of Dr. Joseph Konzelman, School of Dentistry, Medical College of Georgia.*

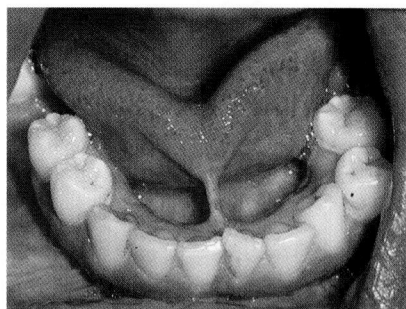

D. Ankyloglossia. *Courtesy of Dr. Joseph Konzelman, School of Dentistry, Medical College of Georgia.*

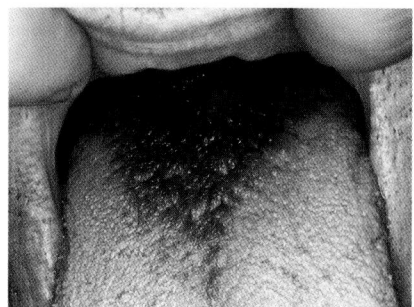

E. Oral Hairy Leukoplakia. *Courtesy of Dr. Joseph Konzelman, School of Dentistry, Medical College of Georgia.*

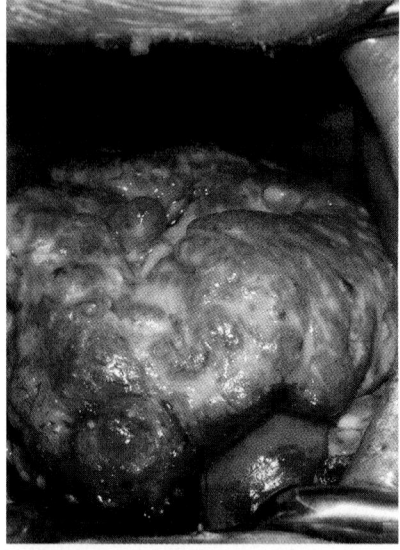

F. Carcinoma of the Tongue. *Courtesy of Dr. Daniel D. Rooney.*

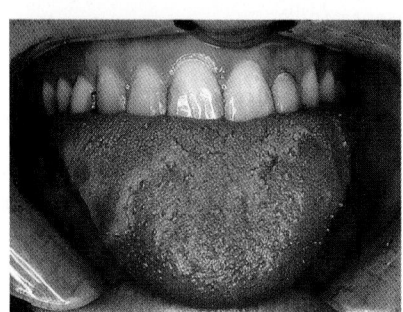

G. Geographic Tongue. *Courtesy of Dr. Joseph Konzelman, School of Dentistry, Medical College of Georgia.*

FIGURE 13-45 **Tongue Conditions**
continues

P Ankyloglossia is a congenital abnormality.

A The tongue has a hairy appearance and is yellow, black, or brown (Figure 13-45E).

P This is known as oral hairy leukoplakia, or hairy tongue, a benign condition that can result from antibiotic therapy. The hairy appearance is caused by elongated papillae.

A Lesions are noted on the ventral surface of the tongue.

P The ventral surface of the tongue is an area where malignancies are likely to develop, especially in patients who drink alcohol and smoke or use smokeless tobacco.

A Indurations, or ulcerations (Figure 13-45F) are present on the lateral surfaces of the tongue.

P Most lingual cancers are located in this area and are associated with use of alcohol and tobacco.

A Patches of red denuded areas on the lingual surface of the tongue, frequently at the papillae, surrounded by ridges of pale yellow epithelium are abnormal (Figure 13-45G).

P This harmless condition, known as geographic tongue, has no known cause. Its name is derived from the patterns of regular and irregular surfaces on the tongue that resemble a map.

A Numerous furrows or grooves are observed, often radiating horizontally from the midline of the dorsal surface of the tongue (see Figure 13-45H).

P This is a harmless and often inherited condition known as fissured or scrotal tongue. It is different from syphilitic glossitis, which is characterized by longitudinal furrows.

A Engorged blood vessels of the tongue are abnormal (see Figure 13-45I).

P A hemangioma of the tongue is a benign overgrowth of vascular tissue.

A Deviation of the tongue toward one side (see Figure 13-45J), atrophy, and asymmetrical shape of the tongue are abnormal.

P Unilateral paralysis of the tongue muscles will cause the tongue to deviate toward the affected side because the muscles on the paralyzed side are unable to oppose the strong muscles of the unaffected side. The patient is unable to push the tongue toward the nonparalyzed side. Lesions of the hypoglossal nucleus or nerve fiber cause these unilateral symptoms.

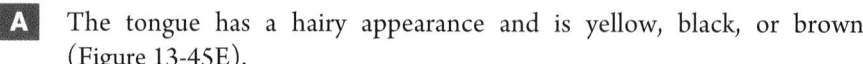

E Examination   **N** Normal Findings   **A** Abnormal Findings   **P** Pathophysiology

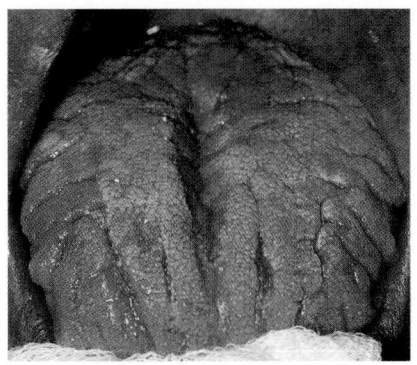

H. Fissured Tongue (Scrotal Tongue). *Courtesy of Dr. Joseph Konzelman, School of Dentistry, Medical College of Georgia.*

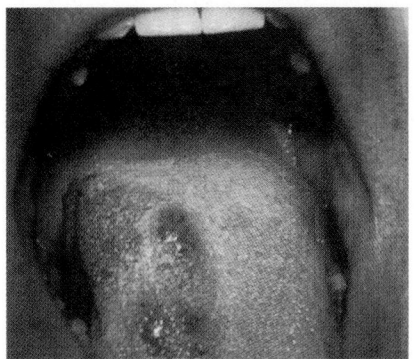

I. Hemangioma. *Courtesy of Dr. Joseph Konzelman, School of Dentistry, Medical College of Georgia.*

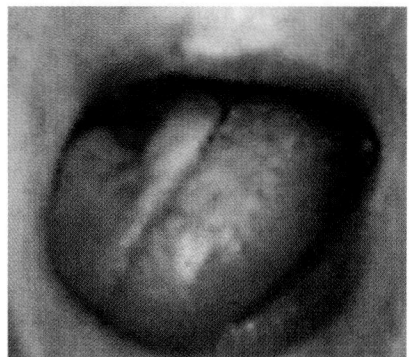

J. Cranial Nerve XII (Hypoglossal) Palsy

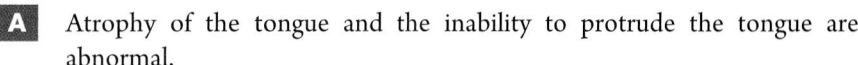

FIGURE 13-45 **Tongue Conditions** *continued*

A Atrophy of the tongue and the inability to protrude the tongue are abnormal.

P Bilateral paralysis of the tongue muscles will prevent the patient from protruding the tongue. Syringobulbia or trauma to CN XII may cause hypoglossal nerve paralysis.

Buccal Mucosa

E 1. Ask the patient to open the mouth as wide as possible.

2. Use a tongue depressor and a penlight to assess the inner cheeks and the openings of Stensen's ducts (Figure 13-46).

3. Observe for color, inflammation, hydration, and lesions.

N The color of the oral mucosa on the inside of the cheek may vary according to race. African Americans have a bluish hue; Caucasians have pink mucosa. Freckle-like macules may appear on the inside of the buccal mucosa. The buccal mucosa should be moist, smooth, and free of inflammation and lesions. Some patients may have torus mandibularis (see Figure 13-47A), which are bony nodules in the mandibular region.

A Leathery, painless, white, painted-looking patches are noted.

P Leukoplakia may be found in the buccal mucosa. Figure 13-47B shows leukoplakia caused by snuff.

A Yellow patches on the buccal mucosa are present.

P Fordyce's spots are small sebaceous glands (see Figure 13-47C).

A The orifice of Stensen's duct is erythematous and edematous. It may be tender to palpation.

P This is seen in parotitis, an inflammation of the parotid gland. The area between the ear lobule and angle of the mandible may not be visible due to the swelling of the parotid gland (see Figure 13-47D). Acute unilateral swelling may be seen in mumps.

A Small, round, white ulcers, each surrounded by a halo of reddened mucosa are found on the mucosa.

P These are aphthous ulcers. Refer to Figure 13-45C.

A The mucosa is pale.

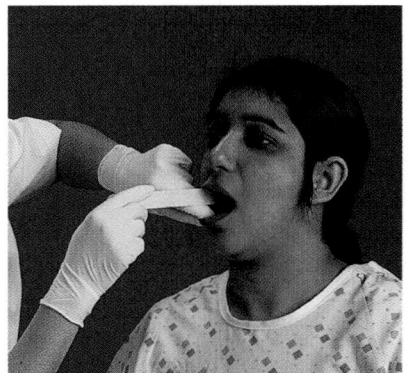

FIGURE 13-46 **Assessment of the Buccal Mucosa**

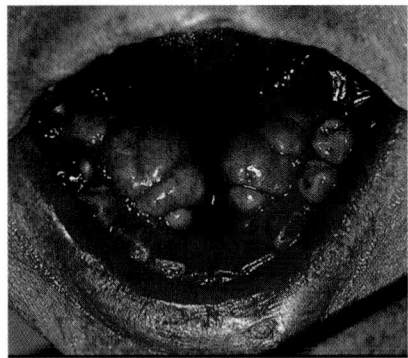

A. Torus Mandibularis. *Courtesy of Dr. Joseph Konzelman, School of Dentistry, Medical College of Georgia.*

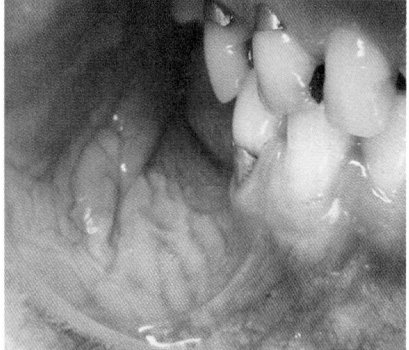

B. Leukoplakia Caused by Snuff. *Courtesy of Dr. Joseph Konzelman, School of Dentistry, Medical College of Georgia.*

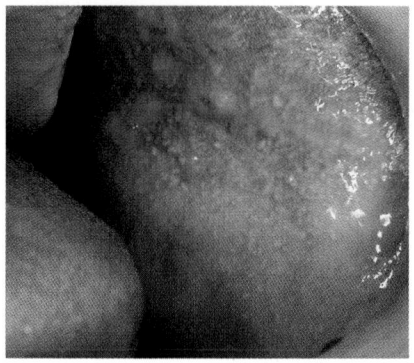

C. Fordyce's Spots. *Courtesy of Dr. Joseph Konzelman, School of Dentistry, Medical College of Georgia.*

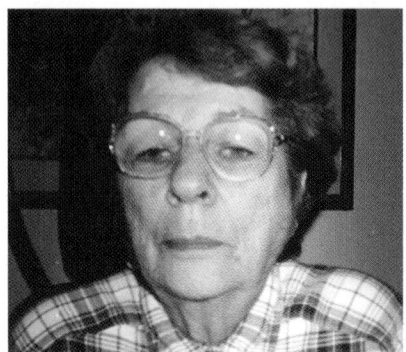

D. Left Parotitis

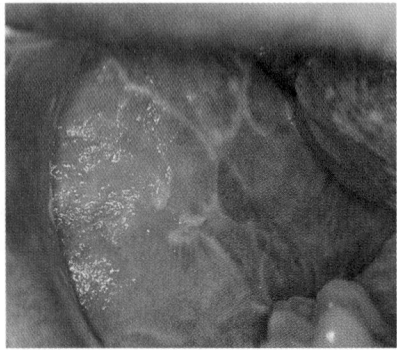

E. Lichen Planus. *Courtesy of Dr. Joseph Konzelman, School of Dentistry, Medical College of Georgia.*

FIGURE 13-47 **Buccal Mucosa Conditions**

NURSINGTIP

Examining the Patient with Dentures

Before examining the oral cavity, it is essential that dentures or other dental appliances be removed so that the gums can be fully visualized and palpated.

P This can be caused by anemia or vasoconstriction that may occur when the sympathetic nervous system is stimulated, such as in shock.

A The mucosa is cyanotic.

P Cyanosis can indicate systemic hypoxemia. See Chapters 10 and 16.

A The mucosa is erythematous.

P Erythema can be associated with stomatitis.

A There is excessive dryness of the mucosa.

P This is xerostomia, which occurs when salivary gland activity is decreased, when the patient is hypovolemic, or with mouth breathing, Sjögren's syndrome, or salivary gland obstruction.

A Excessive moisture is noted in the mouth.

P This condition may be noted in the early stages of inflammation or when the patient is hypervolemic.

A Flat-topped papules with thin, bluish-white spider-web lines (Figure 13-47E) resembling leukoplakia are noted on the mucosa or tongue.

P Wickham's striae are the lesions of lichen planus, which is an inflammatory and pruritic disease of the skin and mucous membranes. It is usually a benign disease and the cause is unknown.

Gums

E 1. Instruct the patient to open the mouth.

2. Observe dentures or orthodontics for fit.

3. Remove any dentures or removable orthodontia.

4. Shine the penlight in the mouth.

5. Use the tongue depressor to move the tongue to visualize the gums.

6. Observe for redness, swelling, bleeding, retraction from the teeth, or discoloration.

N In light-skinned individuals, the gums have a pale red, stippled surface. Patchy brown pigmentation may be present in dark-skinned patients. The gum margins should be well defined with no pockets existing between the gums and the teeth and no swelling or bleeding.

A The gingiva are red, tender, and swollen and bleed easily (see Figure 13-48).

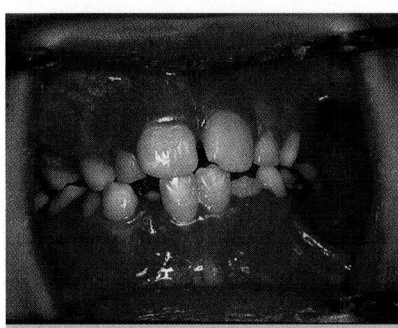

FIGURE 13-48 **Gingivitis with Herpes Simplex.** *Courtesy of Dr. Joseph Konzelman, School of Dentistry, Medical College of Georgia.*

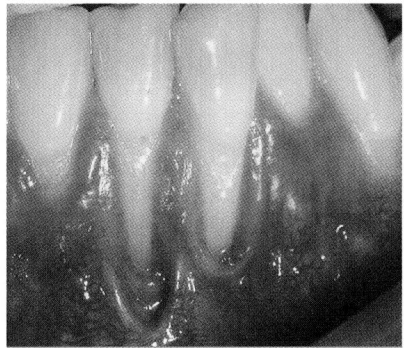

FIGURE 13-49 **Gingival Recession.** *Courtesy of Gary Shellerud, DDS.*

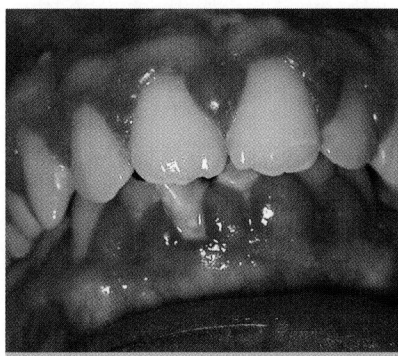

FIGURE 13-50 **Gingival Hyperplasia.** *Courtesy of Dr. Joseph Konzelman, School of Dentistry, Medical College of Georgia.*

P This describes gingivitis, which may be caused by poor dental hygiene, improperly fitted dentures, and scurvy. Gingivitis can also occur with stomatitis that occurs in mouth infections and upper respiratory tract infections.

A Gingival borders are red and there is infection of the pockets formed between receding gums and teeth. Purulent drainage may be present.

P This is periodontitis, which is an inflammation of the periodontium due to chronic gingivitis. This condition is caused by infrequent brushing of the teeth and poor oral hygiene.

A Blue lines are noted approximately 1 mm from the gingival margin.

P These are lead bismuth lines caused by chronic exposure to lead or bismuth.

A The gums are brownish.

P This occurs in association with Addison's disease.

A A grayish membrane is noted over an inflamed and ulcerated area of the mucosa.

P This condition is Vincent's stomatitis, or trench mouth, a bacterial infection of the gums that may extend into pharyngeal structures and bones.

A A nontender, immobile tumor lighter than the gums is noted on the gum.

P This lesion is epulis, a fibrous tumor of the gums.

A The gums are retracted from the teeth (Figure 13-49), sometimes exposing the roots of the teeth.

P This recession of the gums often occurs in older individuals due to poor oral hygiene.

A Hypertrophy of gum tissue is abnormal (Figure 13-50).

P This is called gingival hyperplasia and is usually painless; it occurs in pregnancy, in wearers of orthodontic braces, by dental plaque, or with the use of some medications such as phenytoin.

A Small ulcers or folds of excess tissue are noted on the gums under an ill-fitting denture. Inflamed and swollen nodules may be seen in the area of the palate.

P Continued irritation of the gums by ill-fitting dentures results in hyperplasia.

Teeth

E 1. Instruct the patient to open the mouth.

2. Count the upper and lower teeth.

3. Observe the teeth for discoloration, loose or missing teeth, caries, malocclusion, and malformation.

N The adult normally has 32 teeth, which should be white with smooth edges, in proper alignment, and without caries.

A Teeth are absent.

P This problem may be due to loss or failure of development. The patient's nutritional status may be seriously impaired when the teeth are insufficient.

A There are white or black patches on the surface of a tooth. These patches may become eroded as damage progresses.

P These are dental caries, or cavities, resulting from poor oral hygiene.

E Examination   **N** Normal Findings   **A** Abnormal Findings   **P** Pathophysiology

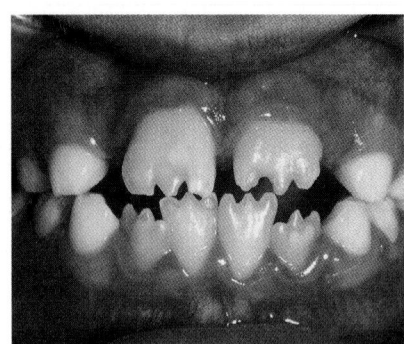

FIGURE 13-51 Hutchinson's Incisors.
Courtesy of Dale Ruemping, DDS, MSD.

A The teeth are worn at an angle.

P Biting surfaces of the teeth may become worn down by repetitive biting on hard substances or objects or grinding of teeth, called bruxism, especially at night.

A A tooth is dark in color and the patient reports insensitivity to cold.

P This is usually a dead tooth, which results in a darkening of the enamel.

A Teeth that have serrated edges (Figure 13-51) are abnormal.

P These are called Hutchinson's incisors. Pregnant women with syphilis can have abnormal fetal dentition because of the effects of the disease on tooth development.

Palate

E 1. Ask the patient to tilt the head back and open the mouth as wide as possible.

2. Shine the penlight in the patient's mouth.

3. Observe both the hard and the soft palates.

4. Note their shape and color, and the presence of any lesions or malformations.

N The hard and soft palates are concave and pink. The hard palate has many ridges; the soft palate is smooth. No lesions or malformations are noted.

A The palates are red, swollen, tender, or with lesions.

P These findings are symptoms of infection.

A There is a bony ridge in the midline of the hard palate (Figure 13-52).

P This is a benign condition called torus palatinus, which develops in adulthood.

A A fibrous, encapsulated tissue growth on the palate is abnormal (Figure 13-53).

P A fibroma may be idiopathic or neoplastic in origin. Chronic trauma can also lead to fibroma formation.

A A lesion that has become eroded is noted on the palate.

P This may be a cancerous lesion in the epithelium of the hard palate.

A The palate is highly arched.

P This finding is associated with Turner's syndrome and Marfan's syndrome.

A There is a hole in the hard palate.

P Palatine perforation is related to syphilis or radiation therapy.

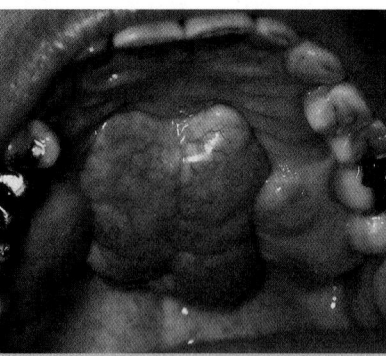

FIGURE 13-52 Torus Palatinus.
Courtesy of Dr. Joseph Konzelman, School of Dentistry, Medical College of Georgia.

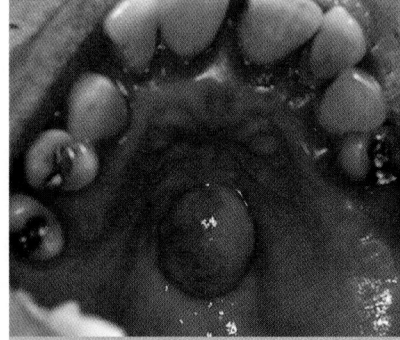

FIGURE 13-53 Fibroma. *Courtesy of Dr. Joseph Konzelman, School of Dentistry, Medical College of Georgia.*

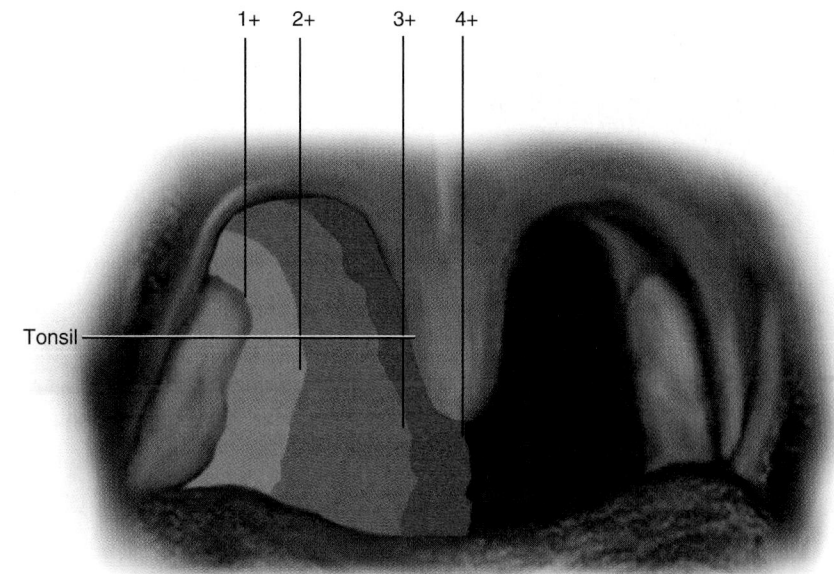

FIGURE 13-54 Grading of Tonsils: 1+ tonsils are visible, 2+ tonsils are between the pillars and uvula, 3+ tonsils are touching the uvula, 4+ tonsils extend to the midline of the oropharynx.

INSPECTION OF THE THROAT

P 1. Ask the patient to tilt the head back and to open the mouth widely. The patient can either stick out the tongue or leave it resting on the floor of the mouth.

2. With the right hand, place the tongue blade on the middle third of the tongue.

3. With the left hand, shine a light at the back of the patient's throat.

4. Ask the patient to say "ah."

5. Observe the position, size, color, and general appearance of the tonsils and uvula.

6. Touch the posterior third of the tongue with the tongue blade.

7. Note movement of the palate and the presence of the gag reflex.

8. Assess the color of the oropharynx. Note the presence of swelling, exudate, or lesions.

N When the patient says "ah," the soft palate and the uvula should rise symmetrically (CN IX and X). The uvula is midline. The throat is normally pink and vascular and without swelling, exudate, or lesions. Normal tonsillar size is evaluated as 1+ to 2+. (See Figure 13-54 for grading scale.) This indicates that both tonsils are behind the pillars. The patient's gag reflex should be present but is congenitally absent in some patients (CN IX and X).

A The posterior pharynx is red with white patches. The tonsils are large and red with white patches, and the uvula is red and swollen.

P Viral pharyngitis and tonsillitis are common illnesses with these findings.

A Tonsils, pillars, and uvula are very red and swollen, with patches of white or yellow exudate on the tonsils (Figure 13-55). The posterior pharynx is bright red. The patient reports soreness of the throat with swallowing.

P These findings are typical of streptococcal pharyngitis and tonsillitis and are usually associated with significant lymphadenopathy. However, diagnosis requires throat culture or rapid strep test.

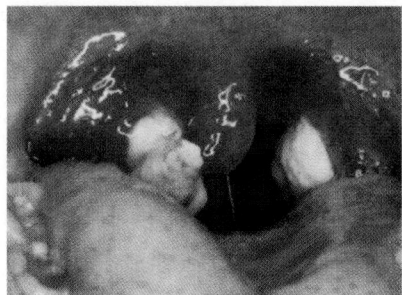

FIGURE 13-55 **Streptococcal Pharyngitis**

E Examination   **N** Normal Findings   **A** Abnormal Findings   **P** Pathophysiology

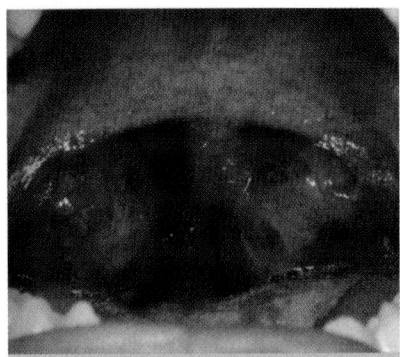

FIGURE 13-56 **Left tonsil is 4+ and right tonsil is 3+.**

A There is a grayish membrane covering the tonsils, uvula, and soft palate.

P These findings are typical of diphtheria, acute tonsillitis, or infectious mononucleosis.

A The patient speaks with a hoarse voice and the oropharynx is red.

P Causes of hoarseness are varied and may include overuse of the voice, inflammation due to viral or bacterial infection, lesions of the larynx, foreign bodies, and pressure on the larynx from masses or an enlarged thyroid gland.

A The patient has difficulty opening the mouth (trismus) and is noted to have unilateral tonsillar swelling. Unusual phonation is also observed.

P These findings are associated with peritonsillar abscess, which is most commonly seen in older children and young adults with a history of frequent tonsillitis.

A Chronic 3+ or 4+ tonsils (Figure 13-56) are abnormal.

P Large tonsils frequently lead to loud snoring and obstructive sleep apnea.

A The patient has a small oropharynx and history of snoring.

P Obstructive sleep apnea occurs when muscles in the nasopharynx and pharynx relax during sleep, resulting in pauses in breathing. Typically patients are overweight, middle-aged men who complain of excessive daytime sleepiness.

CASE STUDY

The Patient with Acute Rhinosinusitis

This case study illustrates the application and the objective documentation of the ears, nose, mouth, and throat assessment.

Margaret is a 47-year-old schoolteacher who is complaining of facial pain and frontal headache.

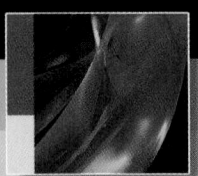

HEALTH HISTORY

PATIENT PROFILE	47-year-old Caucasian female
CHIEF COMPLAINT	"I have had a headache and facial pressure for over 10 days."
HISTORY OF PRESENT ILLNESS	Pt was in her usual state of health until 10 days ago, when she developed an upper respiratory infection that seems to have gotten worse. Her sx started with nasal congestion, PND, and mild facial pressure. After 5 days, she developed thick, green, purulent nasal discharge, bilateral frontal headache (4/10 intensity), maxillary facial pain, and bilateral maxillary toothache. She has had a low-grade fever (100.1°F) without chills, sweats, ear pain, sore throat, chest congestion, wheezing, or dyspnea. The sx seem to get worse when she leans over. She has been taking decongestants every 6 hrs and ibuprofen 400 mg at bedtime without relief for 3 days. Pt has been tearing down wallpaper in her 52-year-old house for the past week.

continues

CASE STUDY (Continued)

The Patient with Acute Rhinosinusitis

PAST HEALTH HISTORY

Medical History	Hypertension since age 40
Surgical History	Cholecystectomy age 41
Allergies	Penicillin: hives, urticaria
Medications	Hydrochlorothiazide 25 mg every AM Ibuprofen for headaches 200–600 mg BID PRN Phenylephrine PRN for nasal stuffiness (does not know dose)
Communicable Diseases	Denies
Injuries and Accidents	Denies
Special Needs	Denies
Blood Transfusions	Denies
Childhood Illnesses	Chickenpox age 5 without sequelae
Immunizations	UTD; completed hepatitis A series last year; annual flu vaccine

FAMILY HEALTH HISTORY

LEGEND

◯ Living female
▢ Living male
⊗ Deceased female
⊠ Deceased male
↗ Points to patient

COPD = Chronic obstructive pulmonary disease
CVA = Cerebrovascular accident
DM = Diabetes mellitus
HTN = Hypertension
IBS = Irritable bowel disease

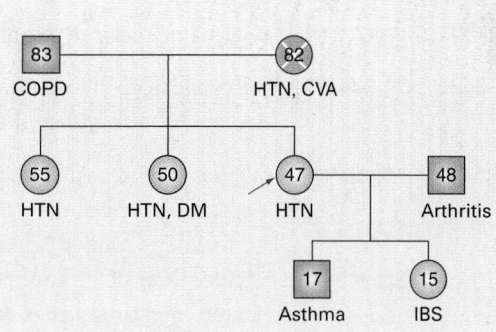

Denies FH of otosclerosis

SOCIAL HISTORY

Alcohol Use	1–2 glasses of wine per week
Tobacco Use	Quit smoking age 22; smoked ½ PPD X 6 years (3 yr pack hx); denies use of chewing tobacco, pipes, cigars, snuff
Drug Use	Denies

continues

Domestic and Intimate Partner Violence	Denies
Sexual Practice	Monogamous relationship with husband
Travel History	Denies recent travel more than 100 miles from home in the past 10 years
Work Environment	Teaches high school English in rural area
Home Environment	Lives with husband and 2 teenagers in a single-family home that was purchased 2 mos ago, a "real fixer-upper" per pt, "after all, it is a beautiful old farmhouse but it is in need of much repair after 52 years"; no smoke detectors or carbon monoxide detectors in home at present—needs to buy them
Hobbies and Leisure Activities	Reading, playing golf, swimming
Stress	New work environment, repairing home
Education	Master's degree in education
Economic Status	Middle class; husband works with computers
Military Service	None
Religion	Lutheran
Ethnic Background	German American; would like to visit German cousins someday
Roles and Relationships	Very close to her husband and children; several close friends from her book club and neighborhood
Characteristic Patterns of Daily Living	Wakes at 5:45 AM, skips breakfast, drives 45 minutes to get to school; school day starts at 7:30 AM; brings lunch and eats in teacher's lounge; classes end at 2:30 PM; usually stays after school for 1–1 ½ hours to talk with colleagues or participate in faculty meetings; goes to the gym 3 times a week after school; arrives home around 6:30 PM, prepares dinner for family; grades papers and watches TV and goes to bed around 10 PM.
HEALTH MAINTENANCE ACTIVITIES	
Sleep	7–8 hours of sleep during the week; 8–9 hours on the weekends; feels well rested
Diet	No special diet
Exercise	Walks on the treadmill three times weekly for 45 minutes followed by stretching; occasional spinning class
Stress Management	Talks openly with her friends and exercises regularly

continues

CASE STUDY (Continued)

The Patient with Acute Rhinosinusitis

Use of Safety Devices	Uses seat belt in car; not taking any precautions with home remodeling
Health Check-ups	Annual well-woman exam; sees primary care provider every 4 months for hypertension; has not visited dentist or eye MD in years; last mammogram was WNL 2 years ago; does not perform BSE

PHYSICAL ASSESSMENT

Ears

Auditory Screening	Voice-whisper test—intact
	Tuning fork tests
	  Weber—midline without lateralization
	  Rinne—⊕

External Ear	Nontender, EAC clear without inflammation, no mastoid tenderness
Otoscopic Assessment	Both TMs are shiny pink and mobile with visible light reflexes; without bulging or perforation

Nose

External Inspection	Midline without swelling, bleeding, lesions, or masses
Patency	Each nare is patent
Internal Inspection	Mucosa is red and swollen with purulent nasal discharge bilaterally; septum deviated to the left

Sinuses

Inspection	Swelling noted below eyes bilaterally
Palpation and Percussion	Tenderness over right maxillary sinus; dullness to percussion noted over right maxillary
Transillumination of the Sinuses	Absence of glow noted over right maxillary sinus

Mouth and Throat

Breath	Foul smell noted
Lips	Pink, moist without lesions
Tongue	Midline, pink, well papillated without fasciculations, lesions, swelling, or bleeding
Buccal Mucosa	Pink, moist without lesions

continues

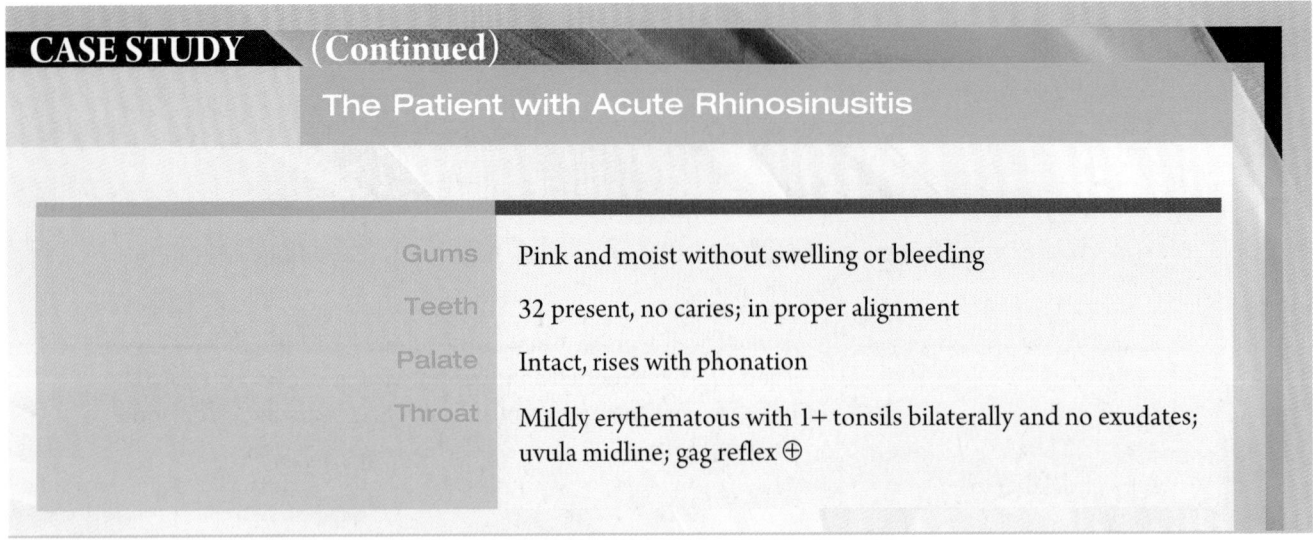

CASE STUDY (Continued)

The Patient with Acute Rhinosinusitis

Gums	Pink and moist without swelling or bleeding
Teeth	32 present, no caries; in proper alignment
Palate	Intact, rises with phonation
Throat	Mildly erythematous with 1+ tonsils bilaterally and no exudates; uvula midline; gag reflex ⊕

ASSESSMENT IN BRIEF

Ears, Nose, Mouth, and Throat Assessment

Ears
- Auditory screening
  - Voice-whisper test
  - Tuning fork tests
    Weber test
    Rinne test
- External ear
  - Inspection
  - Palpation
- Otoscopic Assessment

Nose
- External inspection
- Patency
- Internal inspection

Sinuses
- Inspection
- Palpation and percussion

Mouth and Throat
- Mouth
  - Breath
  - Lips
    Inspection
    Palpation
  - Tongue
  - Buccal mucosa
  - Gums
  - Teeth
  - Palate
- Throat

Advanced Technique
- Transillumination of the sinuses

REVIEW QUESTIONS

1. Which statement describes a positive Rinne test?
   a. BC > AC
   b. The sound lateralizes to the affected ear.
   c. AC > BC
   d. AC is equal to BC.
   The correct answer is (c).

2. Acute otitis externa is a common infection among children and adults. Which describes a typical exam finding of otitis externa?
   a. Thickening and clouding of the TM
   b. Erythema and edema of the EAC
   c. Bubbles and air-fluid levels are visible
   d. Retraction and immobility of TM
   The correct answer is (b).

3. Risk factors for hearing loss are noise exposure, aging, and:
   a. Male gender
   b. Cocaine use
   c. Excessive alcohol use
   d. Recurrent infections
   The correct answer is (d).

4. During examination of the nasal mucosa, you note that the nasal mucosa is pale and edematous with clear, watery discharge. These findings are most consistent with:
   a. The common cold
   b. Acute sinusitis
   c. Allergies or hay fever
   d. Presence of cerebrospinal fluid
   The correct answer is (c).

5. Leukoplakia is considered to be a premalignant lesion that may appear on the tongue and buccal mucosa. It can best be described as:
   a. Thin, pearly white lesions that coalesce
   b. Pearly borders, crusting, and central ulcerations
   c. Thick, white, adherent, curdlike
   d. Painful, small, round, white, and ulcerated
   The correct answer is (a).

6. The paranasal sinuses are air-filled cavities lined with mucous membranes that lighten the weight of the skull and add resonance to the quality of the voice. The sinuses that can be assessed on physical examination include:
   a. Frontal and sphenoid sinuses
   b. Frontal and ethmoid sinuses
   c. Maxillary and frontal sinuses
   d. Maxillary and sphenoid sinuses
   The correct answer is (c).

7. Which structure can be found under the tongue on either side of the frenulum?
   a. Sublingual glands   c. Sulcus terminalis
   b. Stensen's ducts   d. Wharton's ducts
   The correct answer is (d).

8. During examination of your patient's throat, you note that the patient has difficulty opening her mouth and has 3+ swelling of the right tonsil with exudate. These findings are commonly associated with:
   a. Infectious mononucleosis
   b. Peritonsillar abscess
   c. Viral pharyngitis
   d. Diphtheria
   The correct answer is (b).

9. During your assessment of a 17-year-old male, you note that his breath smells of acetone and has a "fruity" odor. Acetone breath is most commonly associated with the following condition:
   a. Fetor hepaticus   c. Diabetic ketoacidosis
   b. Uremia   d. Halitosis
   The correct answer is (c).

10. During examination of your patient's buccal mucosa, you note several yellow patches on the inside of the cheek. This finding is known as:
    a. Fordyce's spots   c. Lichen planus
    b. Aphthous ulcers   d. Xerostomia
    The correct answer is (a).

Visit the Estes online companion resource at
www.delmar.cengage.com
for additional content and study aids.
Click on Online Companions, then select
the Nursing discipline.

REFERENCE

O'Donoghue, G. M., Narula, A. A., & Bates, G. J. (2000). *Clinical ENT: An illustrated textbook.* San Diego, CA: Singular.

BIBLIOGRAPHY

Collins, R. D. (2008). *Differential diagnosis in primary care* (4th ed.). Philadelphia: Lippincott Williams & Wilkins.

Daugherty, J. (2007). The latest buzz on tinnitus. *The Nurse Practitioner: The American Journal of Primary Healthcare, 32*(10), 42–47.

Goolsby, M., & Grubbs, L. (2006). *Advanced assessment: Interpreting findings and formulating differential diagnosis.* Philadelphia: F.A. Davis.

Hart, A. (2007). An evidence-based approach to the diagnosis & management of acute respiratory infections. *The Journal for Nurse Practitioners, 3*(9), 607–611.

Hayden, M. L., & Womack, C. R. (2007). Caring for patients with allergic rhinitis. *Journal of the American Academy of Nurse Practitioners, 19*(6), 290–298.

Kamienski, M. (2007). When sore throat gets serious: Three different cases, three very different causes. *American Journal of Nursing, 107*(10), 35–38.

Labuguen, R. (2006). Initial evaluation of vertigo. *American Family Physician, 73*(2), 244–251, 254.

McCarter, D., Courtney, U., & Pollart, S. (2007). Cerumen impaction. *American Family Physician, 75*(10), 1523–1528, 1530.

Rabago, D., Barrett, B., Marchand, L., Maberry, R., & Mundt, M. (2006). Qualitative aspects of nasal irrigation use by patients with chronic sinus disease in a multimethod study. *Annals of Family Medicine, 4*(4), 295–301.

Ramakrishnan, K., Sparks, R., & Berryhill, W. (2007). Diagnosis and treatment of otitis media. *American Family Physician, 76*(10), 1650–1660.

Salvador, S. L., & Figueiredo, L. C. (2005). Halitosis and periodontal disease in subjects with mental disabilities. *Oral Diseases, 11*(Suppl. 1), 108–108(1).

Uphold, C., & Graham, M. (2003). *Clinical guidelines in family practice* (4th ed.). Gainesville, FL: Barmarrae Books, Inc.

Williamson, I. G., Rumsby, K., Benge, S., Moore, M., Smith, P. W., Cross, M., & Little, P. (2007). Antibiotics and topical nasal steroids for treatment of acute maxillary sinusitis. *JAMA, 298*(21), 2487–2496.

Woodson, B. T., & Han, J. K. (2005). Relationship of snoring and sleepiness as presenting symptoms in a sleep clinic population. *Annals of Otology, Rhinology, and Laryngology, 114*(10), 762–767.

Zitelli, B., & Davis, H. (2007). *Atlas of pediatric physical diagnosis* (5th ed.). Philadelphia: Mosby.

WEB SITES

American Academy of Otolaryngology—Head and Neck Surgery:
http://www.ent.net.org

American Academy of Periodontology:
http://www.perio.org

American Dental Association:
http://www.ada.org

American Sleep Apnea Association:
http://www.sleepapnea.org

American Tinnitus Association:
http://www.ata.org

League for the Hard of Hearing:
http://www.lhh.org

Society of Otorhinolaryngology and Head-Neck Nurses, Inc.:
http://www.sohnnurse.com

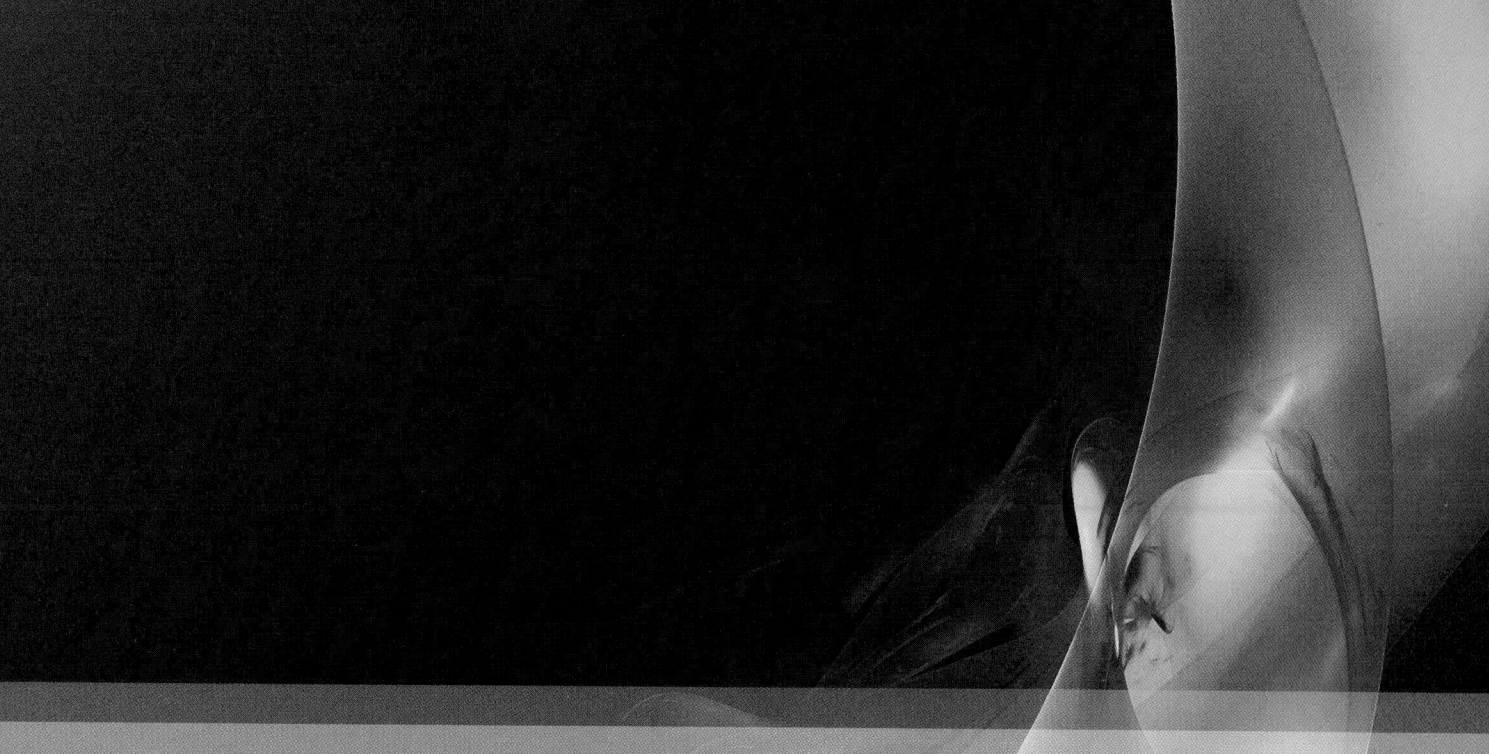

CHAPTER 14
Breasts and Regional Nodes

COMPETENCIES

1. Describe the anatomy and physiology of the breasts and regional lymphatics, including age-related variations.

2. Demonstrate assessment techniques for the evaluation of the breasts and regional lymphatics.

3. Distinguish common variations and abnormal changes of the breasts.

4. Discuss methods of teaching breast self-examination to patients.

5. Identify risk factors for breast cancer.

The breasts hold significant symbolism in our society. In women, they are an external symbol of sexuality, femininity, and nurturance. In men, they symbolize strength, fitness, and masculinity. Breast disease and its devastating effects have come to the forefront of public attention in recent years. Breast cancer incidence rates have increased significantly over the past 50 years; however, survival rates remain constant despite increased research dollars and public attention.

Long-term survival rates have a direct correlation to early detection of breast cancer. Nurses can have a major impact on women's health by teaching women breast self-examination techniques and by supporting women in achieving healthier lifestyles, which are believed to diminish breast cancer risk.

This chapter focuses primarily on the female breast because it is a more complicated structure than the male gland and because of the higher incidence of breast disease in women.

ANATOMY AND PHYSIOLOGY

The breasts and regional nodes are discussed as is the development of the breasts during adolescence.

BREASTS

The female **breasts** are a pair of mammary glands located on the anterior chest wall, extending vertically from the second to the sixth rib and laterally from the sternal border to the axilla. Anatomically, the breast may be divided into four quadrants: the upper inner quadrant, the lower inner quadrant, the upper outer quadrant, and the lower outer quadrant (Figure 14-1). The upper outer quadrant, which extends into the axilla, is known as the **tail of Spence**. The breasts are supported by a bed of muscles: the pectoralis major and minor, latissimus dorsi, serratus anterior, rectus abdominus, and external oblique muscles, which extend vertically from the deep fascia (Figure 14-2). **Cooper's ligaments**, which extend vertically from the

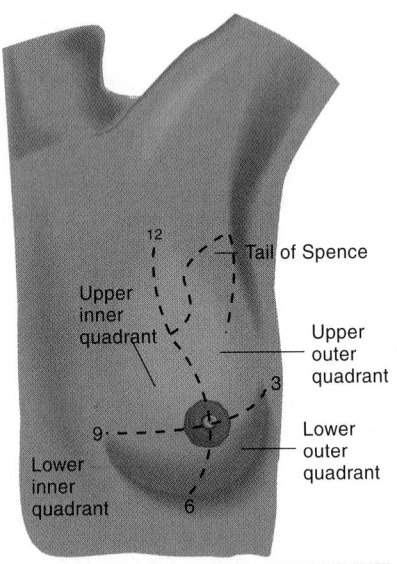

FIGURE 14-1 **Quadrants of the Left Breast. Note the numbers on the breast. They represent the hours of a clock face that can be used to specify the location of a finding on the circular breast. The right breast clock notation is a mirror image of the left breast.**

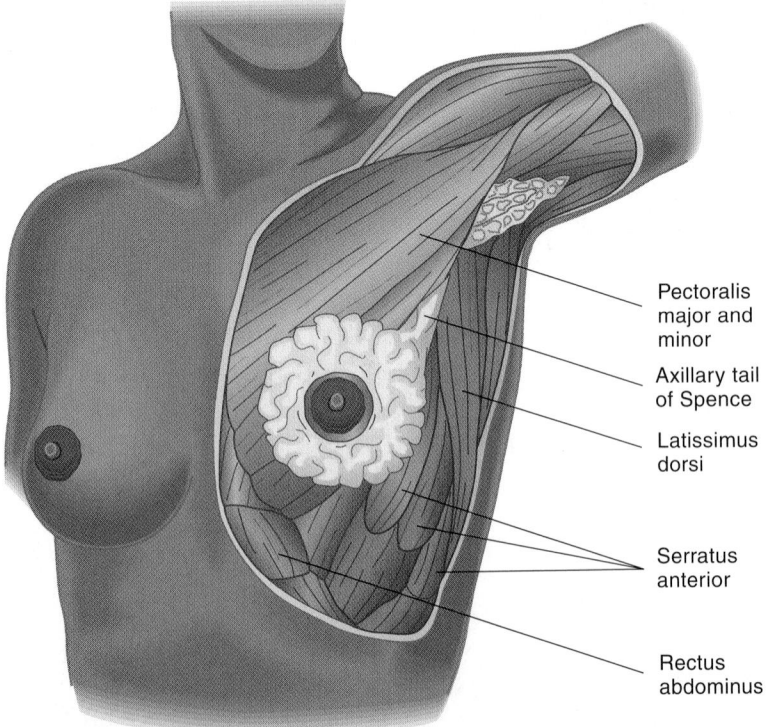

Pectoralis major and minor

Axillary tail of Spence

Latissimus dorsi

Serratus anterior

Rectus abdominus

FIGURE 14-2 **Muscles Supporting the Breast**

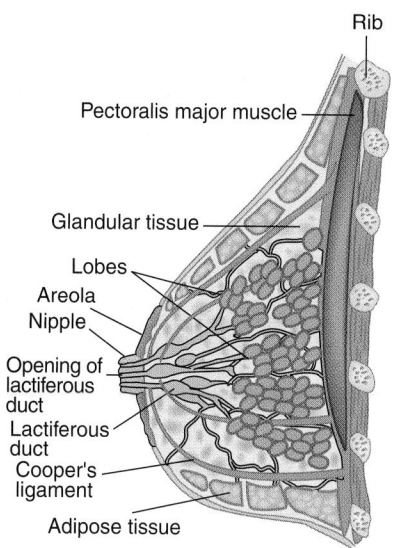

FIGURE 14-3 **Cross Section of the Left Breast**

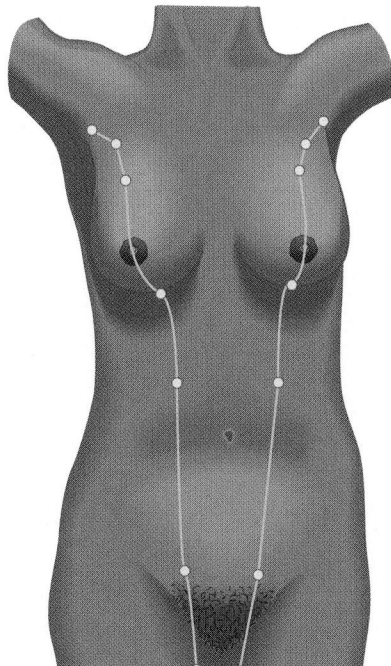

A. These bands develop in utero and later atrophy.

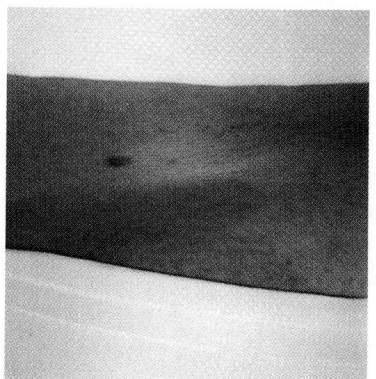

B. Supernumerary Nipple

FIGURE 14-4 **Ectodermal Galactic Bands**

deep fascia through the breast to the inner layer of the skin, provide support for the breast tissue (Figure 14-3).

In the center of each breast is the **nipple,** a round, hairless pigmented protrusion of erectile tissue approximately 0.5 to 1.5 cm in diameter. The nipple becomes more erect during sexual excitement, pregnancy, lactation, cold temperatures, and certain phases of the menstrual cycle. There are 12 to 20 minute openings on the surface of the nipple. These are openings of the **lactiferous ducts** through which milk and colostrum are excreted.

The **milk line,** or **ectodermal galactic band,** shown in Figure 14-4A, develops from the axilla to the groin during the fifth week of fetal development. Most of the band atrophies except in the thoracic area, where it forms a mammary ridge. Incomplete atrophy of the galactic band results in the development of extra nipples or breast tissue known as **supernumerary nipples,** shown in Figure 14-4B. The additional nipples or mammary tissue develop along the milk lines and are a normal variant in a small percentage of adult women.

Surrounding the nipple is the **areola,** a pigmented area approximately 2.5 to 10 cm in diameter. The size and pigmentation vary from woman to woman. Several sebaceous glands (**Montgomery's tubercles**) are present on the surface of the areola. These glands lubricate the nipple, helping to keep it supple during lactation. Hair follicles punctuate the border of the areola.

The breast is composed of glandular, connective (Cooper's ligaments), and adipose tissue. The glandular tissue is arranged radially in the form of 12 to 20 **lobes.** This disbursement is similar to a bicycle wheel; each lobe represents a spoke of the wheel and extends from a central point (the nipple) to the outermost border (Figure 14-5). Each lobe is composed of 20 to 40 **lobules** that contain milk producing glands called **alveoli** or **acini.** The lobules are arranged in grapelike bunches and are clustered around several ducts. These ducts gradually form one main lactiferous (excretory) duct per lobe. Each lactiferous duct widens to form a sinus that acts as a reservoir for milk during lactation. The duct opens onto the surface of the nipple.

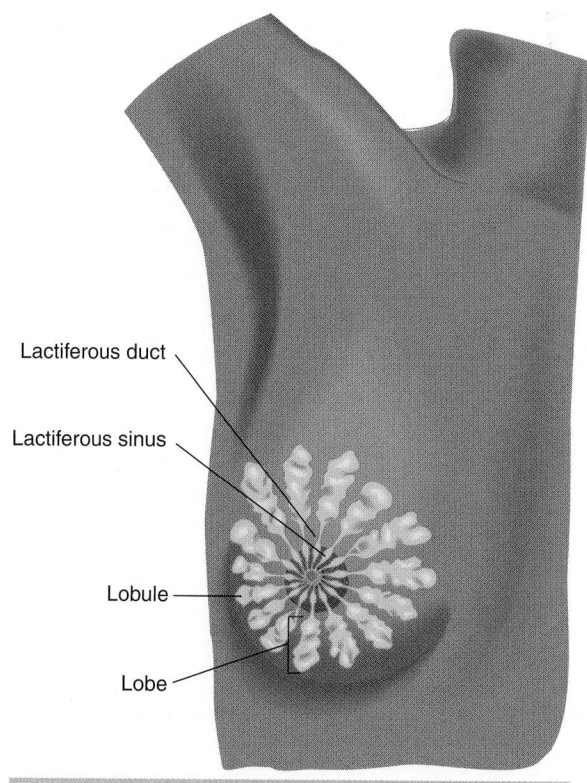

FIGURE 14-5 **Glandular Tissue of the Right Breast**

The lobes are lodged in tissue composed of subcutaneous and **retromammary adipose tissue**, and it is this tissue that composes the bulk of the breast.

The function of the female breast is to produce milk for the nourishment and protection of neonates and infants. In many cultures, breasts provide sensual pleasure during sexual foreplay and breastfeeding. The breasts also provide some protection to the anterior thoracic chest wall.

TABLE 14-1 Sexual Maturity Rating (SMR) for Female Breast Development

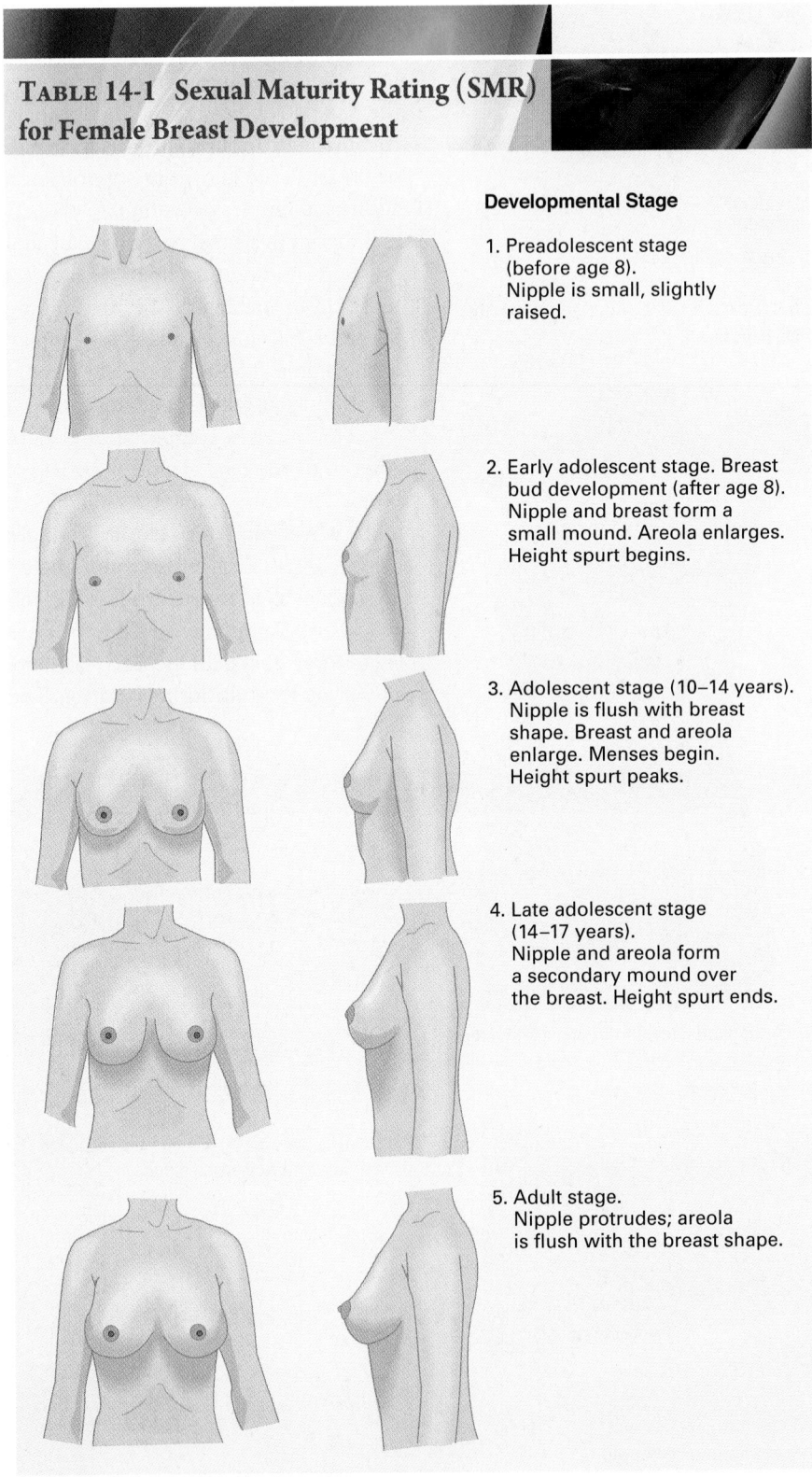

Developmental Stage

1. Preadolescent stage (before age 8). Nipple is small, slightly raised.

2. Early adolescent stage. Breast bud development (after age 8). Nipple and breast form a small mound. Areola enlarges. Height spurt begins.

3. Adolescent stage (10–14 years). Nipple is flush with breast shape. Breast and areola enlarge. Menses begin. Height spurt peaks.

4. Late adolescent stage (14–17 years). Nipple and areola form a secondary mound over the breast. Height spurt ends.

5. Adult stage. Nipple protrudes; areola is flush with the breast shape.

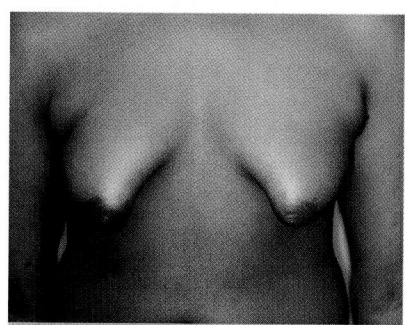

FIGURE 14-6 Gynecomastia. *Courtesy of Steven M. Lynch, M.D.*

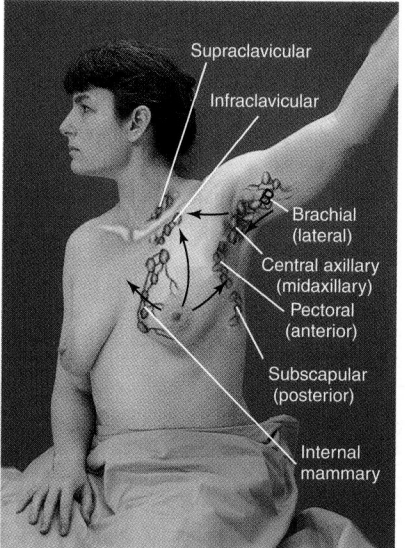

FIGURE 14-7 Regional Lymphatics and Drainage Patterns of the Left Breast

The male breast is composed of a well-developed areola and a small nipple that has immature tissue underneath. **Gynecomastia**, the enlargement of male breast tissue (Figure 14-6), may occur normally in adolescent and in elderly males. The condition is normally unilateral and temporary.

REGIONAL NODES

The **lymphatic drainage** (the yellow alkaline drainage composed primarily of lymphocytes) of the breast is via a complex network of lymph vessels and nodes. It is estimated that a majority of the lymph from the breast flows to the axillary nodes. The **axillary nodes** are composed of four groups: brachial nodes (lateral), central axillary nodes (midaxillary), pectoral nodes (anterior), and subscapular nodes (posterior). The central axillary nodes receive lymph from the three other nodal groups. The lymph is then channeled from the central axillary nodes to the infraclavicular and supraclavicular nodes. The remainder of the lymph flows into the internal mammary chain or directly to the infraclavicular chain via the Rotter's nodes, deep into the chest or abdominal cavity, or to the other breast. The pattern of lymph drainage is illustrated in Figure 14-7.

The axillary nodes are easily accessible by palpation because of their superficial location. The internal mammary nodes are very deep in the chest wall and are inaccessible by palpation.

BREAST DEVELOPMENT

Female breast development usually begins at 8 to 10 years of age and is stimulated by estrogen release during puberty. Enhanced fat deposition increases the size of the breasts, while the ductal system, lobes, and lobules increase in number and in size. Asymmetry in breast development is not abnormal. Tanner staging, or sexual maturity ratings, describe the pattern of adolescent breast development for females (see Table 14-1).

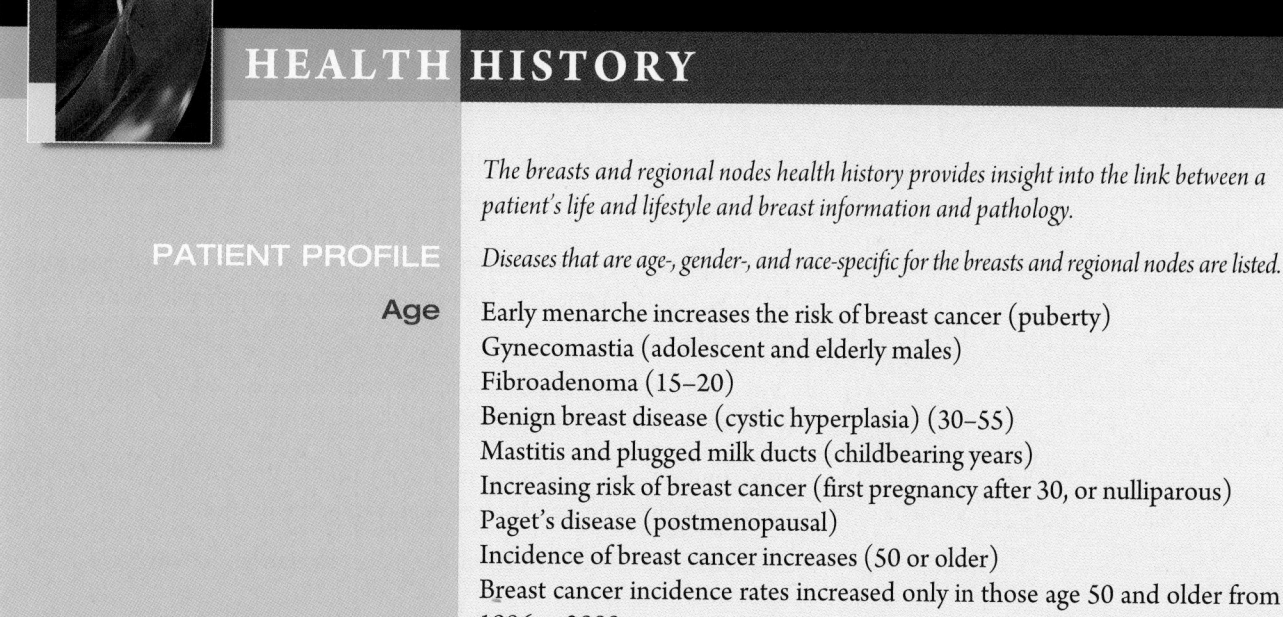

HEALTH HISTORY

The breasts and regional nodes health history provides insight into the link between a patient's life and lifestyle and breast information and pathology.

PATIENT PROFILE

Diseases that are age-, gender-, and race-specific for the breasts and regional nodes are listed.

Age
Early menarche increases the risk of breast cancer (puberty)
Gynecomastia (adolescent and elderly males)
Fibroadenoma (15–20)
Benign breast disease (cystic hyperplasia) (30–55)
Mastitis and plugged milk ducts (childbearing years)
Increasing risk of breast cancer (first pregnancy after 30, or nulliparous)
Paget's disease (postmenopausal)
Incidence of breast cancer increases (50 or older)
Breast cancer incidence rates increased only in those age 50 and older from 1986 to 2000.

continues

Health History (continued)

Gender	
Female	An estimated 178,480 new cases of breast cancer were expected to occur among women in the United States during 2007. 99% of all breast disease is in women: see Table 14-2 for additional breast cancer risk factors. One in every eight women in the United States will develop breast cancer; breast cancer is second only to skin cancer in new cases in women; it's the second leading cause of cancer death.
Male	1,450 new cases of breast cancer are expected in men in 2007 (American Cancer Society, 2007). Gynecomastia (adolescent and elderly men)
Race	African American breast cancer death rate is higher than that of Caucasian women in the United States.
CHIEF COMPLAINT	*Common chief complaints for the breasts and regional nodes are defined and information on the characteristics of each sign or symptom is provided.*
1. Breast Mass	Presence of a lump in the breast
Location	Anywhere in the breast or axilla; usually in the upper outer quadrant, unilateral or bilateral
Quality	Size, size in relationship to menstrual cycle, shape, consistency, mobility, delineation of borders
Quantity	Number of masses
Associated Manifestations	Tenderness, presence of dimpling, nipple retraction, nipple discharge, tender palpable lymph nodes
Aggravating Factors	Methylxanthines, recent injury to breast
Alleviating Factors	Aspiration, biopsy, surgery, radiation, chemotherapy
Timing	Incidence rises with age, in relation to menses and ovulation
2. Breast Tenderness	Sensation of discomfort in the breast
Location	Pinpoint, discrete, generalized, unilateral or bilateral
Quality	Sharp, dull, pulling
Associated Manifestations	Mass, dimpling, nipple retraction, breast swelling, premenstrual syndrome symptoms (see Chapter 20), induration, discharge, palpable nodes, fever, breastfeeding
Aggravating Factors	Recent injury to breast, palpation, vigorous exercise, oral contraceptives, chlorpromazine, or alpha-methyldopa
Alleviating Factors	Warm compresses, analgesics, massage, support bras, aspiration, biopsy, surgery, breastfeeding, cessation of aggravating medications
Timing	In relation to menses or ovulation, pregnancy, lactation, activity

continues

Health History (continued)

3. Breast Discharge	Abnormal substance expressed from the breast
Location	From the nipple or sebaceous gland, unilateral or bilateral
Quality	Color, odor, consistency
Associated Manifestations	Redness, swelling, induration, mass, dimpling, nipple retraction, breast swelling, palpable nodes, lactation, headaches, history of pituitary disorders, fever
Aggravating Factors	Trauma to breast, breastfeeding, pituitary tumor, hyperthyroidism, chlorpromazine, alpha-methyldopa, digitalis, diuretics, oral contraceptives, papillomas, carcinomas of the ducts
Alleviating Factors	Breastfeeding, biopsy, surgery, cessation of medications
Timing	In relation to pregnancy, menses, lactation, ovulation
PAST HEALTH HISTORY	*The various components of the past health history are linked to breasts and regional nodes pathology and related information.*
Medical History	
Breast Specific	Benign breast disease, cysts, fibroadenomas, intraductal papillomas, mammary duct ectasia, mastitis, areas of greater density, breast cancer, masses, breast abscess, Paget's disease, inflammatory breast disease
Non-breast Specific	Thyroid disorders, pituitary tumor, chest radiation, cancer of ovary or endometrium, obesity, and lifetime weight gain associated with increased risk of postmenopausal breast cancer
Surgical History	Breast biopsy, lumpectomy, quadrantectomy, partial mastectomy, radical mastectomy, breast reduction or augmentation
Allergies	Localized rashes of breast, contact dermatitis
Medications	Oral contraceptives, chlorpromazine, alpha-methlydopa, diuretics, digitalis, steroids, and tricyclics may precipitate nipple discharge; use of hormone replacement therapy has been linked with increased incidences of some breast cancers.
Injuries and Accidents	May cause hematoma or edema; lumps may result from previous trauma to soft tissue
Childhood Illnesses	Varicella scarring of cutaneous tissue
FAMILY HEALTH HISTORY	*Breasts and regional nodes diseases that are familial are listed.*
	8% to 20% of breast cancers are thought to have a familial link via a primary relative, for example, mother, sister, grandmother. The link is stronger if the family history includes bilateral breast cancer. *BRCA 1* or *BRCA 2* gene mutation, Cowden or Hamartoma syndrome (PTEN gene mutation), Li-Fraumeni (TP53 and CHEK 2 gene mutations), Peutz-Jeghers syndrome (STK 11 gene mutation), ataxia telangiectasia (ATM) Benign breast disease
SOCIAL HISTORY	*The components of the social history are linked to breasts and regional nodes factors and pathology.*

continues

Health History (continued)

Alcohol Use	More than two drinks per day is associated with some risk; recurrent/current use increases risk rather than past use; research shows a dose response relationship.
Tobacco Use	Cigarette smoking of long duration poses a role in breast cancer.
Work Environment	Radiation exposure
Home Environment	Increased incidence of breast cancer noted in urban dwellers
Economic Status	Increased incidence of breast cancer in women of upper socioeconomic status
Ethnic Background	Incidence of breast cancer among American and European women is higher than that of Japanese and Middle Eastern women; it is estimated that 1 in 100 women of Ashkenazi Jewish origin are at greater risk of breast cancer due to a mutation of the *BRCA 1* gene.
HEALTH MAINTENANCE ACTIVITIES	*This information provides a bridge between the health maintenance activities and breasts and regional nodes function.*
Diet	No longer a correlation between high-fat diet and incidence of breast cancer; increased incidence of benign breast disease with caffeine use
Exercise	Strong correlation between obesity and incidence of breast cancer, in multiple studies there is a breast cancer reduction with increased activity
Use of Safety Devices	Use of restraining devices in motor vehicles to prevent chest trauma
Health Check-ups	Monthly breast self-examination starting in their 20s Clinical breast examination every 3 years for women aged 20–39 Clinical breast examination every year for women starting at the age of 40 Baseline mammography and annual mammography screening starting at age 40 in asymptomatic women Women at high risk (greater than a 20% lifetime risk) should get an MRI and mammogram annually. Annual MRI screening is not recommended for women whose lifetime risk of breast cancer is less than 15%. (American Cancer Society, 2007)

TABLE 14-2 Breast Cancer Risk Factors

NONMODIFIABLE FACTORS

Female gender

Age greater than 50

Personal history of breast cancer

Family history of breast cancer

Prior thoracic radiation (e.g., Hodgkin's disease)

Number and result of prior breast biopsies (e.g., atypical hyperplasia)

continues

TABLE 14-2 (Continued)

Hereditary breast cancer syndromes:

- BRCA1 and BRCA2 are the majority of breast cancer syndromes

- Cowden or Hamartoma syndrome (PTEN gene mutation)

- Li-Fraumeni (TP53 and CHEK2 gene mutations)

- Peutz-Jeghers syndrome (STK11 gene mutation)

- Ataxia telangiectasia (ATM)

Reproductive history (earlier age at menarche, nulliparity, first child after age 30, late onset of menopause)

African American/Ashkenazi Jewish heritage

MODIFIABLE FACTORS

Increased alcohol consumption

High-fat diet

Obesity

Physical inactivity

Cigarette smoking

Postmenopausal hormonal therapy

RED FLAGS FOR HIGH RISK FACTORS

Early age of onset of breast cancer (< 50 in patient or family member)

Multiple family members with breast cancer

Autosomal dominant pattern

Individual with more that one primary breast cancer

Male breast cancer at any age

Family member with known hereditary mutation (e.g., BRCA1, BRCA2, TP53, PTEN)

Family history of breast cancer and ovarian cancer on same side of family

EQUIPMENT

- Towel
- Drape
- Centimeter ruler
- Teaching aid for breast self-examination

ASSESSMENT OF THE FEMALE BREASTS AND REGIONAL NODES

Physical assessment produces feelings of fear, anxiety, embarrassment, and loss of control in many women. These feelings may be reduced by the sensitivity of the nurse before, during, and after assessment of the breasts. Assessment of the female breasts and regional nodes includes inspection and palpation.

INSPECTION

 1. Position the patient uncovered to the waist, seated at the edge of the examination table, and facing you.

2. Instruct the patient to let her arms relax by her sides as shown in Figure 14-8.

3. Inspect the breasts, axillae, areolar areas, and nipples for color, vascularity, thickening, edema, size, symmetry, contour, lesions or masses, and exudates.

4. Repeat the above inspection sequence with the patient's arms raised over her head (see Figure 14-9). This will accentuate any retraction (tissue drawn back) if present.

E Examination   **N** Normal Findings   **A** Abnormal Findings   **P** Pathophysiology

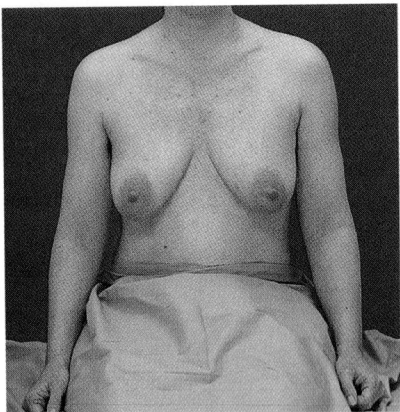

FIGURE 14-8 Position of Patient for Breast Inspection: Arms at Side

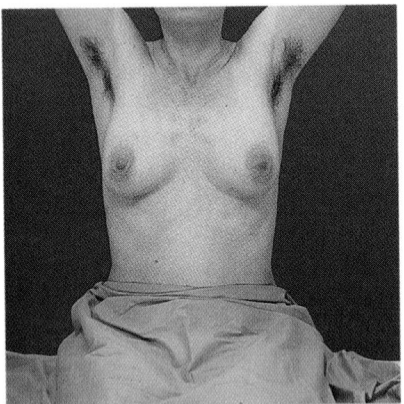

FIGURE 14-9 Position of Patient for Breast Inspection: Arms Overhead

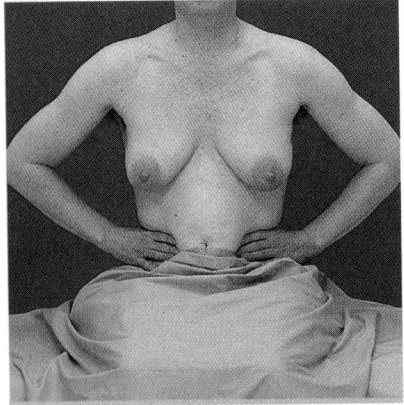

FIGURE 14-10 Position of Patient for Breast Inspection: Hands Pressed against Hips

NURSINGCHECKLIST

General Approach to Breast Assessment

Prior to the assessment

1. When possible, instruct the patient to neither use creams, lotions, or powders, nor shave her underarms 24 to 48 hours before the scheduled examination. Application of toiletry products may mask or alter the nature of the surface integument of the breasts, and shaving the underarms may cause folliculitis, which may result in pain upon palpation.

2. Encourage the patient to express any anxieties and concerns about the physical examination. Acknowledge anxieties and validate concerns. Many women avoid having their breasts assessed because they fear abnormal findings. Assure the patient that she has taken a positive step in her own health care by having her breasts assessed.

3. Inform the patient that the examination should not be painful but may be uncomfortable at times. This is especially true if the patient is currently experiencing menses, ovulation, or pregnancy.

4. Adopt a nonjudgmental and supportive attitude.

5. Be aware of the impact of culture on breast assessment and breast self-examination. In Asian cultures, breast self-examination may be considered a form of masturbation. In some Middle Eastern cultures, baring the breasts to a male is taboo, even if the male is a health care provider.

6. Instruct the patient to remove any jewelry that might interfere with the assessment.

7. Ensure that the room is warm enough to prevent chilling, and provide additional draping material as necessary.

8. Warm your hands with warm water or by rubbing them together prior to the assessment.

9. Ensure that privacy will be maintained during the examination. Provide screens, closed doors, and door sign stating that an examination is in progress.

During the assessment

1. Inform the patient of what you are going to do before you do it.

2. Use this time to educate the patient about her body.

3. Offer the patient the opportunity to ask questions about her body and sexuality.

4. Keep areas not being assessed appropriately draped.

5. Always compare right and left breasts.

6. Wear gloves if the patient has any discharge from the breast.

After the assessment

1. Assess whether the patient needs assistance in dressing.

2. After the patient is dressed, discuss the experience with her, invite questions and comments, listen carefully, and provide her with information regarding the examination.

5. Repeat inspection sequence with patient pressing hands into hips, which will contract the pectoral muscles (Figure 14-10). Once again, if retraction is present, it will be more pronounced with this maneuver.

6. Have the patient lean forward to allow the breasts to hang freely away from the chest wall as shown in Figure 14-11, and repeat the inspection sequence. Provide support to the patient as necessary.

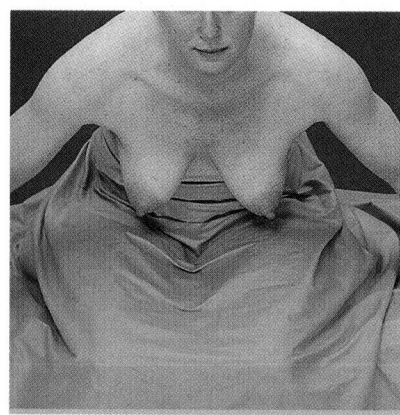

FIGURE 14-11 **Position of Patient for Breast Inspection: Leaning Forward**

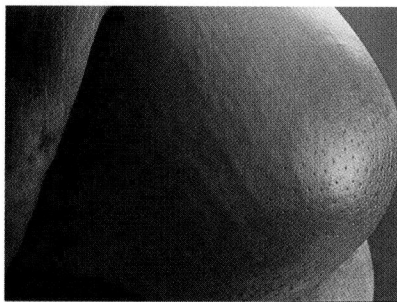

FIGURE 14-12 **Striae Secondary to Inflammatory Breast Cancer. Also note peau d'orange.** *Courtesy of Dr. S. Eva Singletary, University of Texas, M.D. Anderson Cancer Center.*

Color

E Inspect the breasts, areolar areas, nipples, and axillae for coloration.

N The breasts and axillae are flesh-colored and the areolar areas and nipples are darker in pigmentation. This pigmentation is normally enhanced during pregnancy. Moles and nevi are normal variants, and terminal hair may be present on the areolar areas.

A Reddened areas of the breasts, nipples, or axillae need further assessment.

P Redness may be an indication of inflammation, an infection such as mastitis, or inflammatory carcinoma (See Table 14-3 for a description of the five major types of breast cancer.)

A Striae (Figure 14-12) are streaks over the breasts or axillae and are abnormal. In light-skinned individuals, new striae are red and become silver to white in coloration with age. In dark-skinned individuals, new striae are a ruddy, dark brown color, and older striae become lighter than the skin color.

P Striae are caused by rapid stretching of the skin, which damages the elastic fibers found in the dermis. Though normal in pregnancy, striae are often observed with obesity.

Vascularity

E Observe the entire surface of each breast for superficial vascular patterns.

N Normal superficial vascular patterns are diffuse and symmetrical.

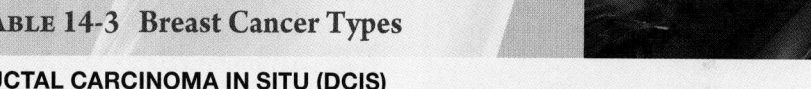

TABLE 14-3 Breast Cancer Types

DUCTAL CARCINOMA IN SITU (DCIS)
Cancer cells confined to the milk ducts. DCIS may present as microcalcifications on mammography. There is no invasion to outlying tissue or lymph nodes.

INFILTRATING (INVASIVE) DUCTAL CARCINOMA (IDC)
Cancer cells that have invaded tissues beyond the milk ducts. Constitutes 85–90% of all breast cancers. IDC will usually present as a discrete, solid breast mass on mammography.

INFILTRATING (INVASIVE) LOBULAR CARCINOMA (ILC)
Cancer cells that started in the lobules and milk ducts, and have invaded outlying tissue. ILC represents 10% of breast cancers that may be more easily diagnosed from an MRI than mammography. This cancer may present as a thickened area rather than a mass.

INFLAMMATORY BREAST CANCER (IBC)
Cancer cells that have rapid tumor growth with an erythemic, thickened skin or diffuse edema (peau d'orange). IBC represents 1–6% of breast cancers. It is diagnosed via core biopsy or punch biopsy.

PAGET'S DISEASE
Presents as an eczematous rash on the nipple. Represents 1–3% of breast cancers. Pruritus, erythema, and nipple discharge may be present. Paget's disease can coexist with DCIS or IDC.

E Examination   **N** Normal Findings   **A** Abnormal Findings   **P** Pathophysiology

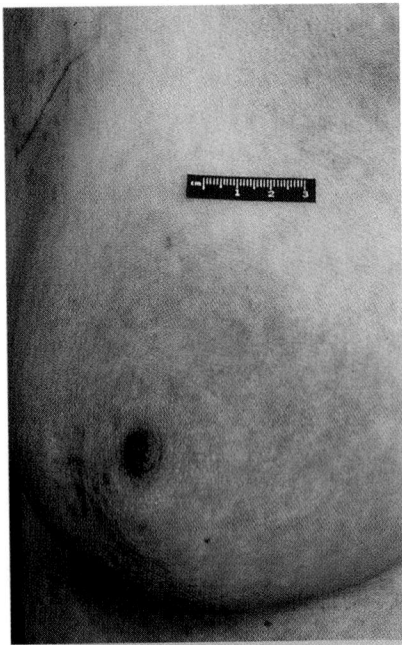

FIGURE 14-13 **Erythema with Abnormal Vascular Pattern Secondary to Inflammatory Breast Cancer.** *Courtesy of Dr. S. Eva Singletary, University of Texas, M.D. Anderson Cancer Center.*

A Abnormal patterns of vascularity are focal or unilateral.

P Focal or unilateral superficial vascular patterns (Figure 14-13) occur as the result of an increased blood supply and may indicate tumor formation, which requires increased vascularization and an increased blood supply.

Thickening or Edema

E Observe the breasts, axillae, and nipples for thickening or edema.

N Normally, thickening or edema is not found in the breasts, axillae, or nipples.

A Thickening or edema of the breast tissue or nipple may present itself as enlarged skin pores that give the appearance of an orange rind (**peau d'orange**). It may be more prevalent in the dependent or inferior portions of the breast (Figure 14-14).

P This peau d'orange appearance may be indicative of obstructed lymphatic drainage due to a tumor, or inflammatory breast cancer.

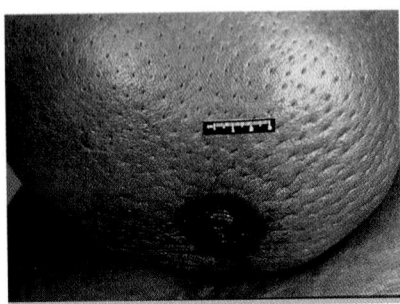

FIGURE 14-14 **Peau d'Orange.** *Courtesy of Dr. S. Eva Singletary, University of Texas, M.D. Anderson Cancer Center.*

Size and Symmetry

E Observe the breasts, axillae, areolar areas, and nipples for size and symmetry.

N It is not unusual for there to be some difference in the size of the breasts and areolar areas, with the breast on the side of the dominant arm being larger. Bilateral hypertrophy of the breasts may be normal for some patients (Figure 14-15). Nipple inversion, which is present from puberty, is a normal variant and is of no clinical consequence except for difficulty in breastfeeding. Nipples should point upward and laterally, or they may point outward and downward (Figure 14-16A). Supernumerary nipples are a variant of normal and have no pathological significance in either males or females.

A Asymmetry in the directions in which the nipples are pointed is an abnormal finding (Figure 14-16B).

P Asymmetrical nipple direction is suggestive of an underlying invasive process that is contorting nipple tissue. Often the direction of nipple deviation is toward the underlying process.

A Significant differences in the size or symmetry of the breasts, axillae, areolar areas, or nipples are abnormal (see Figure 14-17).

P Significant enlargement of one breast, axilla, or areola may be indicative of tumor formation.

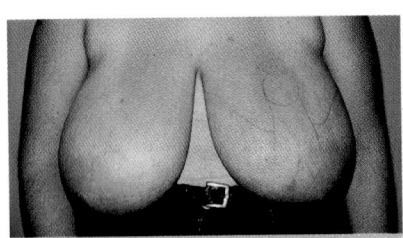

FIGURE 14-15 **Massive Hypertrophy of Breasts.** *Courtesy of Steven M. Lynch, M.D.*

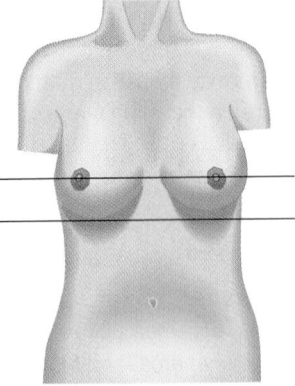

A. Symmetrical without Deviation

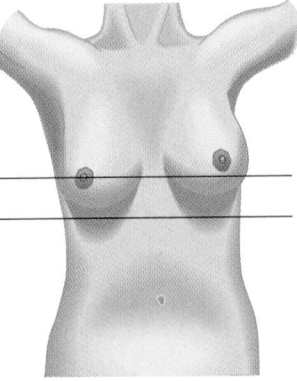

B. Asymmetrical with Deviation

FIGURE 14-16 **Deviation of Nipples**

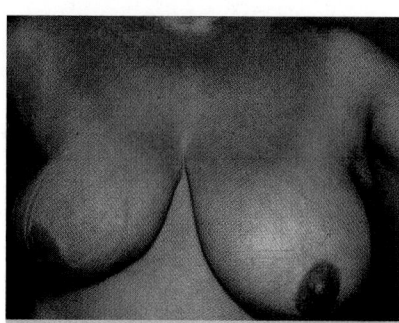

FIGURE 14-17 **Asymmetry of Breasts Due to Cancer.** *Courtesy of Dr. S. Eva Singletary, University of Texas, M.D. Anderson Cancer Center.*

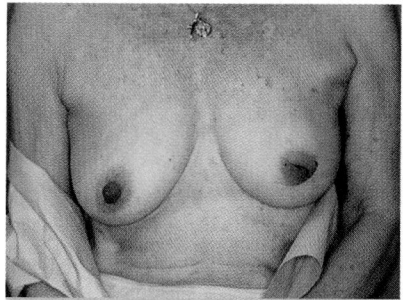

FIGURE 14-18 **Nipple Retraction of Left Breast.** *Courtesy of Steven M. Lynch, M.D.*

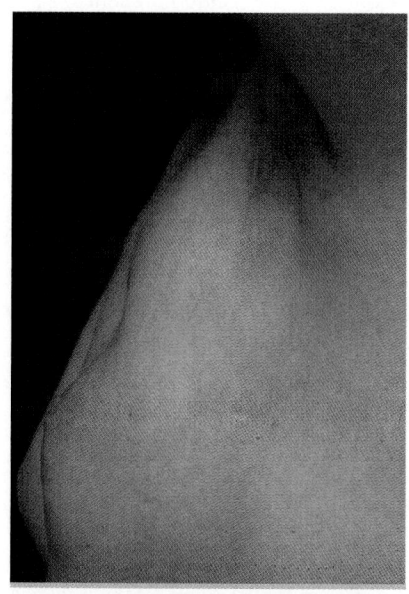

FIGURE 14-19 **Dimpling of Left Breast Tissue.** *Courtesy of Dr. S. Eva Singletary, University of Texas, M.D. Anderson Cancer Center.*

A Recent inversion, flattening, or depression of a nipple is abnormal.

P A sudden onset of nipple inversion, flattening, or depression is indicative of nipple retraction, which is suggestive of an underlying cancer (Figure 14-18).

A Nipples that have been inverted since puberty and become broader or thicker are abnormal.

P Additional broadening or thickening of a previously inverted nipple may be indicative of tumor formation.

A Lack of breast tissue unilaterally is abnormal.

P Unilateral reduction of breast tissue or structures may result from trauma, mastectomy, or breast reduction.

Contour

E 1. Assess the breasts for contour.

2. Compare the breasts to each other.

N The breast is normally convex, without flattening, retractions, or dimpling.

A Dimpling, retractions, flattening (Figure 14-19), or other changes in breast contour are abnormal.

P Changes in contour are highly suggestive of cancer. The invasive process that causes the contour changes is the result of fibrotic shortening and disablement of the Cooper's ligament. Fat necrosis and mammary duct ectasia may also cause retraction, dimpling, and puckering.

Lesions or Masses

E Inspect the breasts, axillae, areolar areas, and nipples for lesions or masses.

N The breasts, axillae, areolar areas, and nipples are free of masses, tumors, and primary or secondary lesions.

A Breast masses, tumors, nodules, or cysts of any kind are abnormal.

P See Table 14-4 for common pathologies of breast masses.

A A scaly, eczema-like erosion of the nipple, or persistent dermatitis of the areola and nipple, is abnormal.

P Persistent eczematous dermatitis of the areola and nipple region is suggestive of **Paget's disease**, a malignant neoplasm, which is usually unilateral in its involvement.

Discharge

E Observe for spontaneous discharge from the nipples or other areas of the breast.

N In the nonpregnant, nonlactating female, there should be no discharge. During pregnancy and up through the first week after birth, there may be a yellow discharge known as **colostrum**. During lactation, there is a white discharge of breast milk.

A The presence of a nipple discharge in the nonpregnant, nonlactating woman is abnormal.

P Nipple discharge may be caused by the use of medications such as tranquilizers and oral contraceptives, manual stimulation, pituitary tumor, or infection. It may also be indicative of malignant or benign breast disease.

E Examination   **N** Normal Findings   **A** Abnormal Findings   **P** Pathophysiology

TABLE 14-4 Characteristics of Common Breast Masses

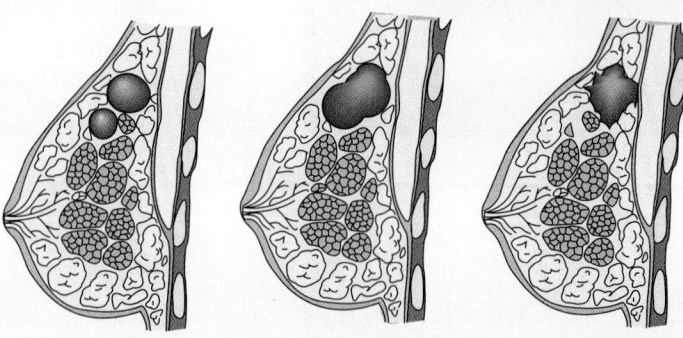

	GROSS CYST	FIBROADENOMA	CARCINOMA
Age	30–50; diminishes after menopause	Puberty to menopause; peaks between ages 20–30	Most common after 50 years
Shape	Round	Round, lobular, or ovoid	Irregular, stellate, or crab-like
Consistency	Soft to firm	Usually firm	Firm to hard
Discreteness	Well defined	Well defined	Not clearly defined
Number	Single or grouped	Most often single	Usually single
Mobility	Mobile	Very mobile	May be mobile or fixed to skin, underlying tissue, or chest wall
Tenderness	Tender	Nontender	Usually nontender
Erythema	No erythema	No erythema	May be present
Retraction/ dimpling	Not present	Not present	Often present

PALPATION

Palpation is performed in a sequential manner:

1. Supraclavicular and infraclavicular lymph node areas
2. Breasts, with the patient in sitting position
   a. Arms at side
   b. Arms raised over head
3. Axillary lymph node regions
4. Breasts, with the patient in supine position

Supraclavicular and Infraclavicular Lymph Nodes

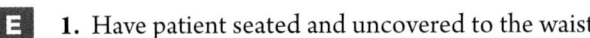

E 1. Have patient seated and uncovered to the waist.
   2. Encourage the patient to relax the muscles of the head and neck because this pulls the clavicles down and allows a thorough exploration of the supraclavicular area.
   3. Flex the patient's head to relax the sternocleidomastoid muscle.

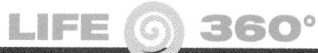

LIFE 360°

Cultural Influences on Breast Examination

The women's health nurse practitioner is to conduct a well-woman examination on a new 28-year-old patient. She made this appointment at the insistence of her husband, who wants to start a family. The woman has been in the United States two years and has never had a well-woman check. She comes from a culture that highly respects women's privacy and modesty. The female nurse spends 10 minutes explaining the exam and what the patient will experience. The equipment that will be used is shown to the patient. The patient has no questions so the nurse leaves the room to let the patient undress in privacy. The nurse returns a few minutes later to find the woman wearing the paper gown. The nurse tells the patient that the breast examination will be performed first. The nurse inspects the patient's breasts. The patient allows the female nurse to complete the palpation of the breast. The nurse finds a small area she would like her "male" colleague to assess. The patient refuses, stating, "Only women may see me in a state of undress in my culture." What might the nurse say to the patient? What action would be taken?

4. Standing in front of the patient, in a bilateral and simultaneous motion, place the finger pads over the patient's clavicles, lateral to the tendinous portion of the sternocleidomastoid muscles.

5. Using a rotary motion of the palmar surfaces of the fingers, probe deeply into the scalene triangles in order to palpate the supraclavicular lymph nodes (Figure 14-20).

6. Palpate the infraclavicular nodes using the same rotary motion of the palmar surfaces of the fingers (Figure 14-21).

N Palpable lymph nodes less than 1 cm in diameter are usually considered normal and clinically insignificant, provided that there are no additional enlarged lymph nodes found in other regions such as the axilla. Palpation should not elicit pain.

A Fixed, firm, immobile, irregular lymph nodes more than 1 cm in diameter are considered abnormal.

P These nodes are considered suspicious for metastasis from a variety of sources or primary lymphoma.

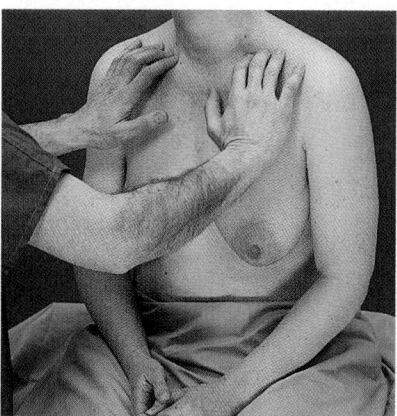

FIGURE 14-20 Palpation of Supraclavicular Nodes

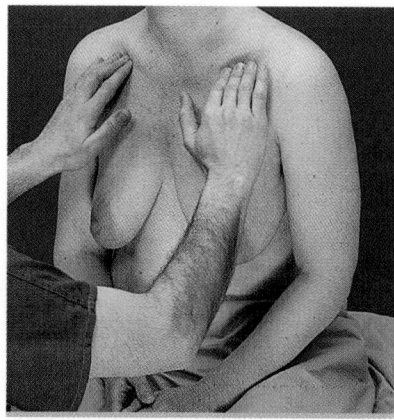

FIGURE 14-21 Palpation of Infraclavicular Nodes

E Examination   **N** Normal Findings   **A** Abnormal Findings   **P** Pathophysiology

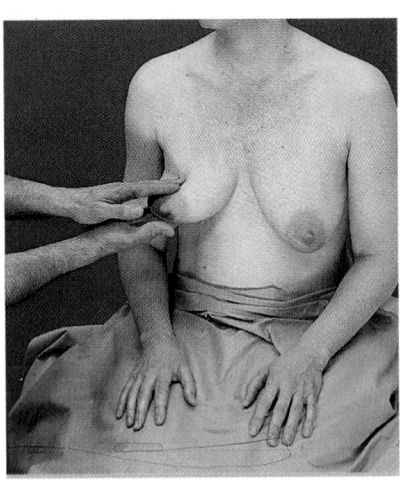

FIGURE 14-22 Bimanual Palpation of the Breasts while Patient Is Sitting

A Enlarged, painful, or tender nodes that are matted together are abnormal.

P Tender, enlarged nodes may indicate systemic infection or carcinoma.

Breasts: Patient in Sitting Position

E 1. Place the patient in a sitting position with arms at sides.

2. Stand to the patient's right side, facing the patient.

3. Using the palmar surfaces of the fingers of the dominant hand, begin the palpation at the outer quadrant of the patient's right breast.

4. Use the other hand to support the inferior aspect of the breast.

5. In small-breasted patients, the dominant hand can palpate the tissue against the chest wall, but if the breasts are pendulous, use a bimanual technique of palpation as shown in Figure 14-22.

6. Palpate in a downward fashion, sweeping from the outer quadrants to the sternal border of each breast.

7. Repeat this sequence on the other breast.

8. Repeat the entire assessment with the patient's arms raised over her head to enhance any potential retraction.

N The consistency of the breasts is widely variable, depending on age, time in menstrual cycle, and proportion of adipose tissue. The breasts may have a nodular or granular consistency that may be enhanced prior to the onset of menses. The inferior aspect of the breast will be somewhat firmer due to a transverse inframammary ridge. Palpation should not elicit significant tenderness, although the breasts and especially the nipples may become full and slightly tender premenstrually. Breasts that feel fluid-filled or firm throughout with accompanying inferior suture-line scars are indicative of breast augmentation.

A The presence of any lump, mass, thickening, or unilateral granulation that is noticeably different from the rest of the breast tissue should be considered suspicious and abnormal.

P For a description of breast masses and their pathologies, see Table 14-4.

A Significant breast tenderness is abnormal and may indicate mammary duct ectasia.

P This is a benign condition in which lactiferous ducts become inflamed.

A Erythema and swelling of the breast with possible pitting edema is abnormal and usually indicates mastitis.

NURSING**TIP**

Lowering the Risk of Breast Cancer

- Breastfeeding
- Moderate to vigorous physical activity
- Healthy body weight
- Stop smoking
- Low alcohol consumption

NURSING**ALERT**

Risk Factors for Benign Breast Disease

The following risk factors enhance a woman's potential for benign breast disease:
- Caffeine use
- Imbalance between estrogen and progesterone
- Estrogen excess
- Hyperprolactinemia
- Ages 20–50 years

E Examination　　**N** Normal Findings　　**A** Abnormal Findings　　**P** Pathophysiology

P This condition is usually seen postpartum and is an inflammation of the breast usually caused by *Staphylococcus aureus*.

Axillary Lymph Node Region

E
1. Stand at the patient's right side, facing the patient.
2. Tell the patient to take a deep breath and relax the shoulders and arms (this relaxes the areas to be palpated).
3. Using your left hand, adduct the patient's right arm so that it is close to the chest wall. This maneuver relaxes the muscles.
4. Support the patient's right arm with your left hand.
5. Using the palmar surfaces of the finger pads of your right hand, place your fingers into the apex of the axilla. Your fingers will be positioned behind the pectoral muscles.
6. Gently roll the tissue against the chest wall and axillary muscles as you work downward.
7. Locate and palpate the four axillary lymph node groups:
    a. Brachial (lateral) at the inner aspect of the upper part of the humerus, close to the axillary vein.
    b. Central axillary (midaxillary) at the thoracic wall of the axilla.
    c. Pectoral (anterior) behind the lateral edge of the pectoralis major muscle.
    d. Subscapular (posterior) at the anterior edge of the latissimus dorsi muscle.
8. Repeat this method of palpation with the patient's arm abducted, i.e., instruct the patient to remain in the same position and lift the upper arm and elbow away from the body. Support the patient's abducted arm on your left shoulder, as shown in Figure 14-23.
9. Palpate the patient's left axilla using the same technique.

N Palpable lymph nodes less than 1 cm in diameter are usually considered normal and clinically insignificant provided that there are no additional enlarged lymph nodes found in other regions. Palpation should not elicit pain.

A Fixed, firm, immobile, irregular lymph nodes more than 1 cm in diameter are clinically significant.

P These nodes are considered suggestive of metastasis from a variety of sources or primary lymphoma.

A Enlarged, painful, or tender nodes that are matted together are abnormal.

P Tender, enlarged nodes may be indicative of a systemic infection or carcinoma.

Breasts: Patient in Supine Position

E
1. Keep the patient uncovered to the waist.
2. Instruct the patient to assume a supine position. This position spreads the breast tissue thinly and evenly over the chest wall. Palpation is more accurate when there is the least amount of breast tissue between the skin and the chest wall.
3. If the breasts are large, place a small towel or folded sheet under the patient's right shoulder. This helps to flatten the breast more.
4. Stand at the right side of the patient. Palpation can be performed with the patient's arms at her sides or with her right arm above her head.

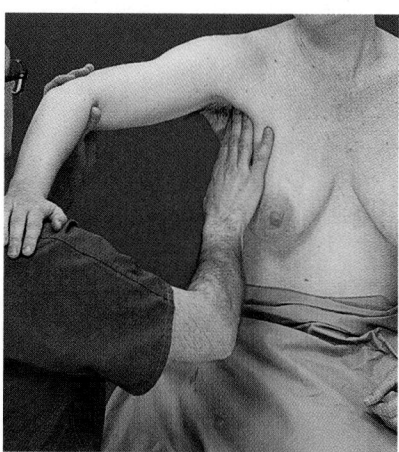

FIGURE 14-23 **Palpation of Axillary Nodes**

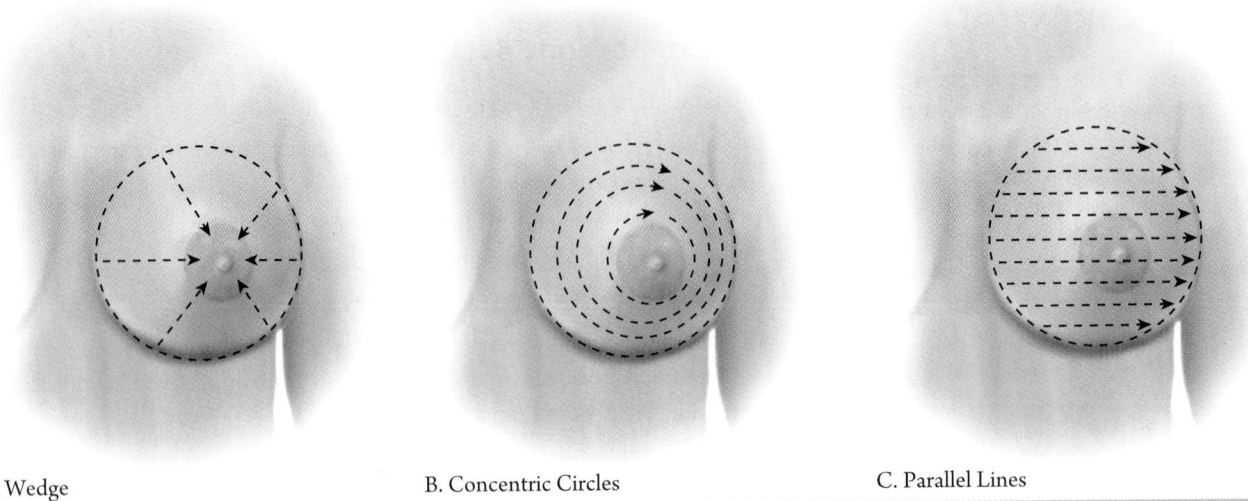

A. Wedge   B. Concentric Circles   C. Parallel Lines

FIGURE 14-24 **Breast Palpation Methods**

5. Using the palmar surfaces of the fingers, palpate the right breast by compressing the mammary tissues gently against the chest wall. Do not press too hard. You may mistake a rib for a hard breast mass. Palpation may be performed in either wedge sections, concentric circles, or parallel lines (Figure 14-24). Using two out of the three palpation methods is acceptable, in order to ensure thoroughness of palpation.

6. Palpation must include the tail of Spence, periphery (Figure 14-25A), and areola (Figure 14-25B).

7. Finally, don gloves and compress the nipple to express any discharge, as shown in Figure 14-25C. If discharge is noted, palpate the breast along the wedge radii to determine from which lobe the discharge is originating.

8. Repeat procedure on opposite breast.

N See previous section on normal breast tissue findings upon palpation. The nipple should be elastic and return readily to its previous shape. No discharge should be expressed in the nonpregnant, nonlactating patient.

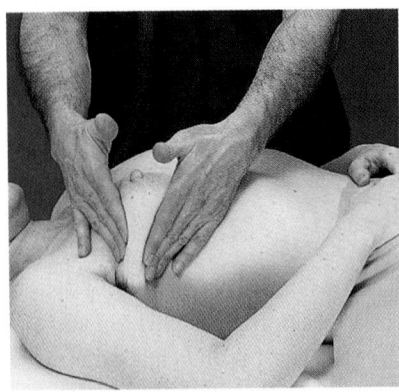
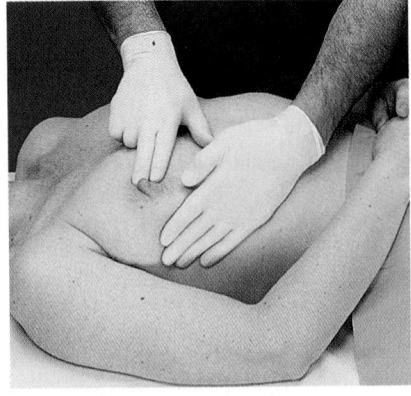
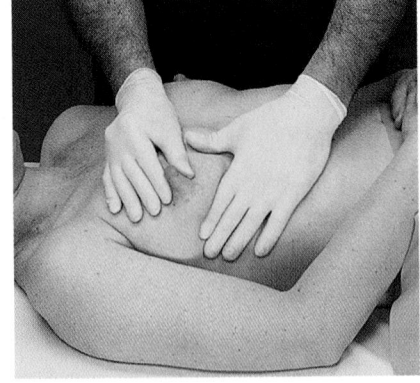

A. Palpation of the Glandular Tissue   B. Palpation of the Areola   C. Compression of the Nipple

FIGURE 14-25 **Palpation of the Breasts while Patient Is Supine**

E Examination   **N** Normal Findings   **A** Abnormal Findings   **P** Pathophysiology

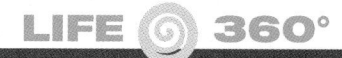

Attitude of Older Women and Breast Cancer

You are conducting a seminar on female health to residents of an assisted living community. You review the importance of breast examination and how to perform a BSE. Some of the women start to laugh and you hear comments such as:

"My breasts are so saggy, no need to worry."

"I had one breast removed for cancer and the other breast is OK."

"Breast cancer only occurs in young women."

How might you respond to these comments?

Refer to Table 14-4 for a description of breast masses. Table 14-5 offers a list of breast mass characteristics that are used to evaluate abnormal findings.

A Loss of nipple elasticity or nipple thickening is abnormal.

P Loss of elasticity in the nipple may indicate tumor formation.

A Milky-white discharge in a nonpregnant, nonlactating patient may be non-puerperal galactorrhea.

P Nonpuerperal galactorrhea is either hormonally induced from lesions of the anterior pituitary gland or drug induced.

A Nonmilky discharge from the nipple, which may be green, brown, straw colored, or gray, is abnormal.

P Nonmilky discharge may be indicative of benign or malignant breast disease such as duct ectasia.

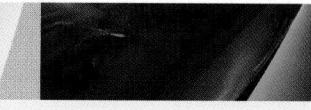

TABLE 14-5 Evaluation of Breast Mass Characteristics

If a mass is noted during palpation, the following information should be obtained regarding the mass. Always note if one or both breasts are involved.

LOCATION

Identify the quadrant involved or visualize the breast with the face of a clock superimposed upon it. The nipple represents the center of the clock. Note where the mass lies in relation to the nipple, e.g., 3 cm from the nipple in the 3 o'clock position.

SIZE

Determine size in centimeters in all three planes (height, width, and depth).

SHAPE

Masses may be round, ovoid, matted, or irregular.

NUMBER

Note if mass is singular or multiple. Note if one or both breasts are involved.

CONSISTENCY

Masses may be firm, hard, soft, fluid, or cystic.

DEFINITION

Note if the mass borders are discrete or irregular.

MOBILITY

Determine if the mass is fixed or freely movable in relation to the chest wall.

TENDERNESS

Note if palpation elicits pain.

ERYTHEMA

Note any redness over involved area.

DIMPLING OR RETRACTION

Observe for dimpling or retraction as the patient raises arms overhead and presses her hands into her hips.

LYMPHADENOPATHY

Note if the mass involves any of the regional lymph nodes, and indicate whether there is associated lymphadenopathy.

REFLECTIVE THINKING

The Patient with a New Breast Mass

What nursing care would you offer to a patient who has a newly diagnosed breast mass? How would you answer her questions about cancer, death, or cure rates? Would you just refer her to a physician to answer her questions? How could you provide positive support, education, and information while working within the framework of nursing practice? Ask yourself how you would want to be treated.

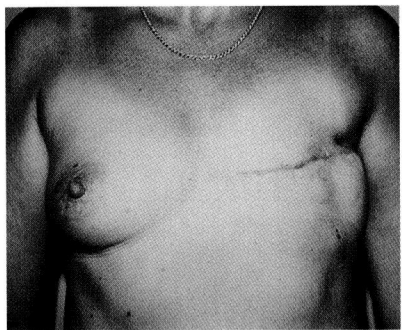

A. Modified Radical

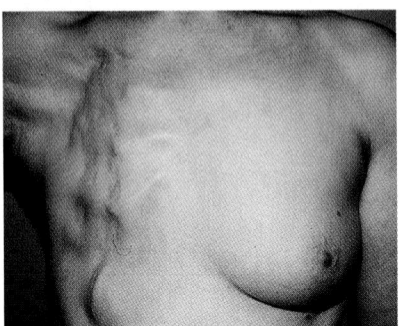

B. Radical

FIGURE 14-26 **Mastectomy Patients.**
Courtesy of Steven M. Lynch, M.D.

NURSING**TIP**

The Mastectomy Patient

There are four types of **mastectomy** (excision of the breast) procedures. In a simple mastectomy, only the breast is removed. In a modified radical procedure, the breast and lymph nodes from the axilla are removed (Figure 14-26A). In a radical mastectomy, the breast, lymph nodes from the axilla, and pectoral muscles are removed (Figure 14-26B). This procedure is rarely performed. In a subcutaneous mastectomy, the skin and nipple are left intact, but the underlying breast tissue and lymph nodes are removed. The patient who has undergone a simple, modified radical, or radical mastectomy literally has had the breast amputated from the chest wall.

Reconstruction techniques include synthetic implants, tissue expansion techniques (in which a temporary device is placed in a subpectoralis-subserratus position between the anterior chest wall and skin and is then inflated with saline over a period of weeks), and latissimus dorsi myocutaneous flap breast reconstruction. A myocutaneous flap reconstruction involves transferring skin from the back or the abdomen to the anterior chest wall.

Assessment of the mastectomy patient will be guided by the type of mastectomy and the presence or absence of reconstructive surgery. Follow the standard assessment procedures and modify your technique to suit the amount of breast tissue and the presence, if any, of a nipple. Always begin the assessment on the unaffected breast. Mastectomy patients should continue to perform monthly breast self-examinations to determine if masses have returned to the excised area. Annual clinical evaluations and mammography are also recommended.

NURSING**TIP**

Breast Augmentation and Reduction

Breast augmentation, or **augmentation mammoplasty**, is the second most popular surgical procedure among women in the United States. There are three types of synthetic implants: the gel-filled implant, the saline inflatable implant, and the polyurethane-covered implant filled with silicone. When assessing a patient, ask if the breasts have been augmented and what type of implant was used.

Incision sites can be found in the axillae, circumareolar areas, and inframammary creases. Potential complications from augmentation include hematoma; infection; scarring; loss of nipple sensation or skin sensation; pain from engorgement; asymmetry; malpositioning; and breakage of the implant, which can lead to **granulomatous reaction** in the breasts in which small, nodular, inflammatory lesions develop, and a capsular membrane forms over the breasts. The augmented breast will feel firmer upon palpation and remain more erect when the patient is supine.

Breast reduction is usually performed on women who complain of back, neck, or shoulder pain caused by breast hypertrophy. Two types of procedures may be performed to reduce the breasts: free nipple graft and dermal pedicles. The type of procedure can be ascertained from the postoperative scarring. A free nipple graft leaves scars around the nipple and at the inferior mammary fold. A dermal pedicles procedure leaves "keyhole" scars over the breasts. Recently, breast liposuction has become popular.

Potential complications from these breast reduction procedures include hematoma, infection, nipple or skin necrosis, fat necrosis, and asymmetry. Palpation results will depend on the type of procedure performed and the amount of scar tissue formed.

For both breast augmentation and breast reduction, a baseline mammogram should be performed to provide a reference for future mammography. Otherwise, the guidelines for breast self-examination, clinical assessment, and mammography are the same as for women who have not undergone breast surgeries.

Monthly BSE and Mammography

Your mother states that she questions the value of monthly BSE and serial mammography in light of recent publicity of their value. What health teaching is appropriate?

Breast Self-Examination (BSE)

Teaching BSE can be quick and simple.

- BSE should be performed once a month, 8 days following menses or on any given fixed date. Advise the patient to avoid the time when her breasts might be tender due to menstruation or ovulation. Encourage her to put the BSE on her calendar and include her significant other in the process.
- **B** (bed): Show the patient how to palpate her breast while supine in bed using the palmar surfaces of her fingers. She should start by placing her right arm over her head and palpating the right breast with the left hand, moving in concentric circles from the periphery inward, including the periphery, tail of Spence, and areola (Figure 14-27A). Finally, instruct her to squeeze the nipple to examine for discharge. Using the reverse procedure, she should examine the other breast.
- **S** (standing): Instruct the patient to repeat the above palpation method while standing, as shown in Figures 14-27B and 14-27C.
- **E** (examination before a mirror): The patient should stand in front of a mirror with her arms at her sides (see Figure 14-27D), then with her arms raised over her head (see Figure 14-27E), and finally with her hands pressed into her hips (see Figure 14-27F). She should examine her breasts for symmetry, retractions, dimpling, inverted nipples, or nipple deviation.

A Bleeding from the nipple is abnormal.

P Bleeding from the nipple is often seen in the benign condition of intraductal papilloma.

INSPECTION AND PALPATION OF THE MALE BREASTS

Assessment of the male breasts is completed in essentially the same manner as that of the female breast. Modify your technique for a smaller breast with less tissue bulk. Having the patient lean forward is usually not necessary unless gynecomastia is present. Males should perform breast self-examinations every month and have clinical examinations of the breast every 1 to 3 years because 1% of all breast cancer is found in men.

DIAGNOSTIC TECHNIQUES

Etiologic determination of breast or lymphatic masses can be accurately assessed only via a combination of the diagnostic techniques listed below.

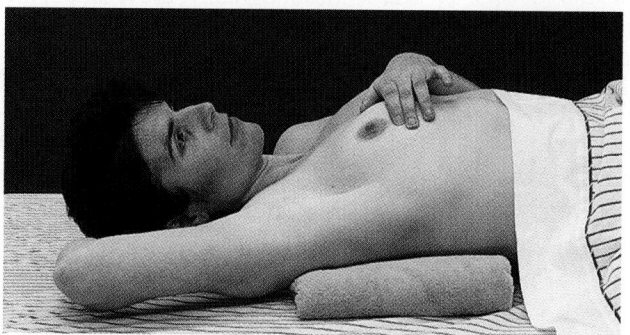

A. In Bed

FIGURE 14-27 **Breast Self-Examination** *continues*

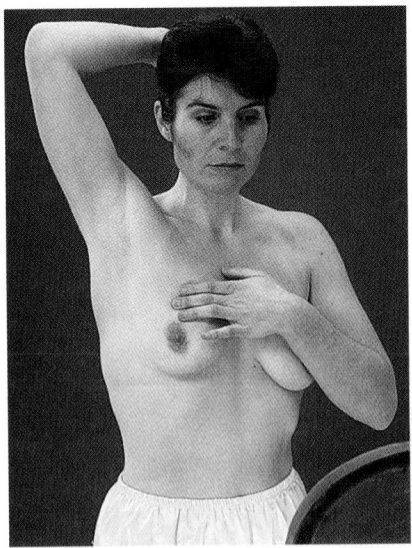

B. Standing

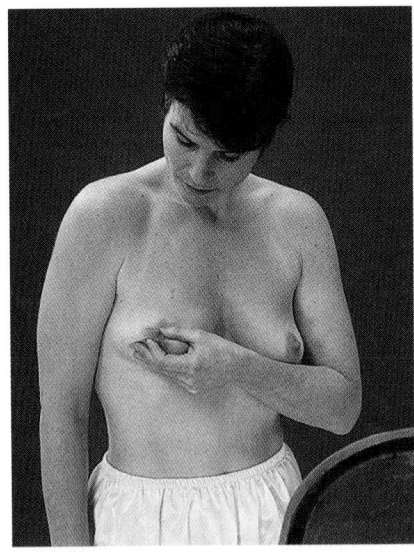

C. Compression of the Nipple

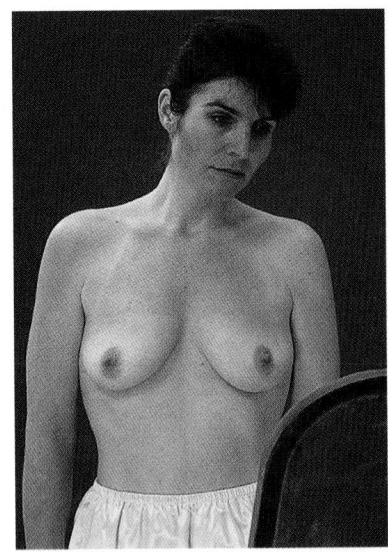

D. Before a Mirror: Arms at Side

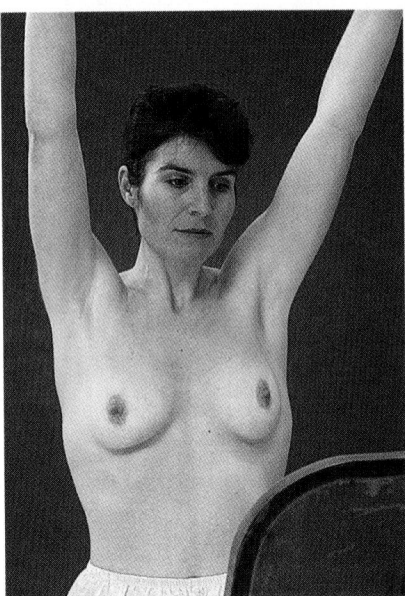

E. Before a Mirror: Arms Overhead

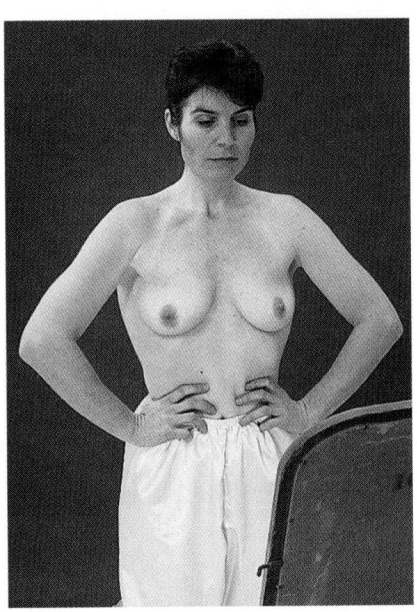

F. Before a Mirror: Hands Pressed into Hips

FIGURE 14-27 **Breast Self-Examination** *continued*

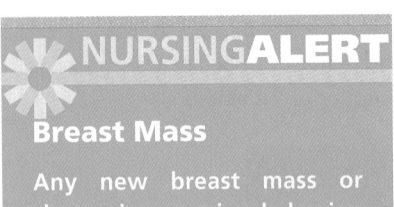

NURSINGALERT

Breast Mass

Any new breast mass or change in a previously benign breast mass must be referred for evaluation.

1. Mammography: roentgenographic examination of the breasts by means of X-rays, ultrasound, or magnetic resonance imaging (MRI). There is contradictory evidence as to whether mammography saves lives.

2. Ultrasonography: the location, measurement, and delineation of deep structures by measuring the reflection of ultrasonic waves.

3. Needle aspiration: the withdrawal of fluid or tissue from a cavity via a hollow needle with an aspirator tube attached to one end.

4. Biopsy: the process of removing tissue from a suspicious area for examination. Methods include needle biopsy, punch biopsy, excisional biopsy, core biopsy, and stereotactic biopsy.

5. Thermography: measuring the regional temperature of a body part or organ. Malignant lesions are often warmer than nonmalignant areas and are called "hot spots."

6. Ductal lavage: a method of rinsing the milk duct to obtain cells for analysis of atypia.

The Patient with Erythematous Changes to the Right Breast

This case study illustrates the application and objective documentation of the breasts and regional nodes assessment.

Ms. McCray came to the family practice clinic with a complaint of redness and erythema of the right breast.

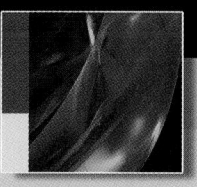

HEALTH HISTORY

PATIENT PROFILE	52 yo MBF
CHIEF COMPLAINT	"I'm scared I have an infection or cancer. My insurance will only pay for 80% of my medical costs. I can't afford to be seriously ill."
HISTORY OF PRESENT ILLNESS	Ms. McCray states that she has noticed a reddened, thickened area of the Ⓡ breast for approximately 2 wks. She reports that the area is warm to the touch and somewhat tender when palpated or wearing a bra. Pt states the skin has a slightly puckered appearance. She denies any nipple discharge and any breast masses/retractions/nipple changes. Pt has been in menopause for 1 yr and started HRT 6 mos ago.
PAST HEALTH HISTORY	
Medical History	Ⓡ stereotactic breast biopsy 2 yrs ago: benign. Yearly mammograms: WNL since. Denies hx of fibrotic breast dz, breast cysts, fibroadenomas, mastitis, breast cancer, endometrial or ovarian cancer. Denies HTN, dyslipidemia, thyroid dz, exposure to chest radiation; onset of menarche age 9
Surgical History	1st trimester SAB, which required a D&C at age 36
Allergies	PCN (rash and throat swelling)
Medications	Prempro .45/1.5 po daily, MVI PRN, Calcium 1200 mg plus Vit. D 800 IU in 2 divided doses PRN
Communicable Disease	Hepatitis A as a child, no sequelae
Injuries and Accidents	Fractured Ⓡ wrist at age 18, no sequelae
Special Needs	Denies
Blood Transfusions	Denies
Childhood Illnesses	Mumps age 5, chickenpox age 5
Immunizations	dT 2000, flu vaccine 2008

continues

CASE STUDY (Continued)
The Patient with Erythematous Changes to the Right Breast

FAMILY HEALTH HISTORY

LEGEND

 Living female

 Living male

 Deceased female

 Deceased male

⟋ Points to patient

⫫ Divorced

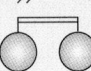 Twin girls

CA = Cancer
CVA = Cerebrovascular accident
DM = Diabetes mellitus
HTN = Hypertension
IBC = Inflammatory breast cancer

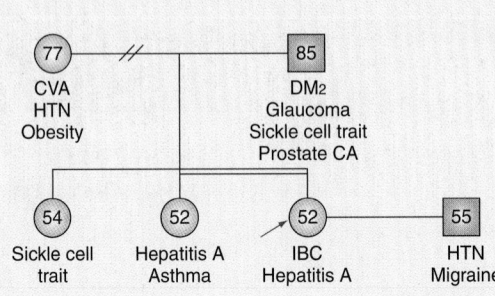

Denies family hx of breast dz

SOCIAL HISTORY

Alcohol Use	1–3 glasses wine per wk
Tobacco Use	Quit smoking 7 yrs ago; previously 1 PPD for 10 yrs
Drug Use	Denies $\bar{x}$ experimentation as a teenager
Domestic and Intimate Partner Violence	Denies
Sexual Practice	Heterosexual, sexually active $\bar{c}$ spouse for 25 yrs; 3 lifetime partners
Travel History	Goes to Bermuda q yr on vacation
Work Environment	Quality assurance coordinator for insurance company
Home Environment	5-yr-old colonial in a suburban neighborhood; little upkeep; meets code regulations for everything; recent basement radon check was WNL
Hobbies and Leisure Activities	Scrapbooking
Stress	Bills and insurance concerns
Education	High school grad $\bar{c}$ some college credits
Economic Status	Middle socioeconomic status
Military Service	Denies
Religion	Raised Southern Baptist, converted to Jehovah's Witnesses 7 yrs ago

continues

CASE STUDY (Continued)
The Patient with Erythematous Changes to the Right Breast

Ethnic Background	African American; attends local extended-family reunions every few years
Roles and Relationships	Wife, employee; she is close to her family and sisters
Characteristic Patterns of Daily Living	Wakes at 7 AM, no breakfast, at work by 8 AM, works until 4:30 PM, eats lunch at fast food or convenience store, arrives home by 6 PM, eats dinner c̄ spouse, occasionally walks p̄ dinner, watches TV until 10 PM, in bed by 11 PM
HEALTH MAINTENANCE ACTIVITIES	
Sleep	7 hrs/night; wakens c̄ an occasional hot flash
Diet	High-fat/high-calorie diet, average calories greater than 2,800/day
Exercise	Occasional walking p̄ dinner for 20 minutes
Stress Management	Prayer, walking, talking to spouse
Use of Safety Devices	Wears seat belts, smoke detector and CO detector in home, alarm system in home
Health Check-ups	Last gyn exam and mammogram 8 mos ago, performs BSE sporadically
PHYSICAL ASSESSMENT	
Inspection	
Color	Ⓡ breast c̄ thickened erythemic area at tail of Spence approximately 4 cm × 6 cm, irregular in shape. Ⓛ breast and axillae are cocoa-flesh-colored c̄ striae over breasts and axillae bilaterally; areolar areas and nipples are dark in pigmentation; no nevi
Vascularity	No enhanced vascular pattern
Thickening or Edema	Lesion of Ⓡ breast is thickened c̄ puckering of skin and hair follicles, peau d'orange appearance
Size and Symmetry	Large, pendulous breasts. Asymmetrical due to Ⓡ breast edema; no nipple inversion or distortion of nipples
Contour	Convex in shape but asymmetrical on Ⓡ due to flattening of tail of Spence
Lesions or Masses	Thickened erythemic area around tail of Spence approximately 4 cm × 6 cm, irregular in shape
Discharge	∅

continues

CASE STUDY (Continued)
The Patient with Erythematous Changes to the Right Breast

Palpation	
Supraclavicular and Infraclavicular Lymph Nodes	Nonpalpable
Breasts: Patient in Sitting Position	Palpable thickness at right tail of Spence c̄ warmth and pain
Axillary Lymph Node Region	Slight matting of midaxillary nodes approximately 2 cm, tender, but mobile
Breasts: Patient in Supine Position	Palpable thickness at Ⓡ tail of Spence c̄ warmth and pain; no nipple discharge
DIAGNOSTIC DATA	
Mammography	Shows questionable asymmetry, a possible Ⓡ lobular mass
MRI	Inconclusive
Stereotactic Biopsy	Confirms inflammatory breast cancer (IBC)

ASSESSMENT IN BRIEF

Breasts and Regional Nodes Assessment

Inspection

- Color
- Vascularity
- Thickening or edema
- Size and symmetry
- Contour
- Lesions or masses
- Discharge

Palpation

- Supraclavicular and infraclavicular lymph nodes
- Breasts: Patient in sitting position
- Axillary lymph node region
- Breasts: Patient in supine position

REVIEW QUESTIONS

1. Camilla, a 14-year-old female, is having a school physical for her high school entrance requirement. She tells you that she began her menses at age 10 and she is 62 inches tall. On examination you see that her nipple is flush with the breast. The areola and breast are larger than a small mound. What is Camilla's Sexual Maturity Rating stage for breast development?

   a. 1   c. 3
   b. 2   d. 4
   The correct answer is (c).

2. Which breast structure is a sebaceous gland that lubricates the nipple and helps to keep it supple during lactation?

   a. Montgomery's tubercles
   b. Ectodermal galactic band

c. Cooper's ligaments

d. Tail of Spence

The correct answer is (a).

3. Which of the following conditions is usually found in postmenopausal women?

a. Mastitis

b. Paget's disease

c. Fibroadenoma

d. Cystic hyperplasia

The correct answer is (b).

4. A patient visits the health clinic because she has been experiencing nipple discharge for a few weeks. You review her health history. Which of the following medications may have a link to breast discharge?

a. Theophylline

b. Chemotherapy

c. Hormone replacement

d. Chlorpromazine

The correct answer is (d).

5. Which of the following recommendations by the American Cancer Society is true for breast health checks in a 35-year-old woman?

a. Bimonthly breast self-examination

b. Clinical breast examination every 3 years

c. Annual mammogram

d. Baseline breast MRI

The correct answer is (b).

6. Which of the following women is at the highest risk for breast cancer?

a. A 72-year-old who smokes and has a BMI of 21

b. A 25-year-old with malignant melanoma of the foot

c. A 40-year-old who had radiation therapy 10 years ago for Hodgkin's disease

d. A 50-year-old who is obese and has Down syndrome

The correct answer is (c).

7. Which type of breast cancer starts in the lobules and milk ducts and has invaded outlying tissue?

a. Ductal carcinoma in situ

b. Invasive ductal carcinoma

c. Infiltrating lobular carcinoma

d. Paget's disease

The correct answer is (c).

8. A breast cancer that results in fibrotic shortening and disablement of Cooper's ligaments may be manifested in which clinical finding?

a. Eczematous dermatitis

b. Dimpling

c. Breast edema

d. Nipple discharge

The correct answer is (b).

9. An 81-year-old woman is found to have an irregularly shaped mass in the upper outer quadrant of the left breast. The mass is nontender and not clearly delineated. This mass is most likely which of the following?

a. A gross cyst

b. A fibroadenoma

c. A furuncle

d. A carcinoma

The correct answer is (d).

10. Breast self-examination is best performed:

a. The first of every month

b. Eight days after menses

c. During ovulation

d. The last day of menses

The correct answer is (b).

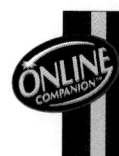

Visit the Estes online companion resource at
www.delmar.cengage.com
for additional content and study aids.
Click on Online Companions and then select the Nursing discipline.

REFERENCE

American Cancer Society. (2007). *Cancer facts and figures 2005.* Retrieved May 16, 2008, from http://www.cancer.org/docroot/STT/stt_0.asp

---

BIBLIOGRAPHY

Brody, J. G., Rudel, R. A., Michels, K. B., Moysich, K. P., Bernstein, L., Attfield, K. R., & Gray, S. (2007). Environmental pollutants, diet, physical activity, body size, and breast cancer: Where do we stand in research to identify opportunities for prevention? *Cancer, 109*(12 suppl), 2627–2634.

Cox, C. L., Montgomery, M., Rai, S. N., McLaughlin, R., Steen, B. D., & Hudson, M. M. (2008). Supporting breast self-examination in female childhood cancer survivors: A secondary analysis of behavioral interventions. *Oncology Nursing Forum, 35*(3), 423–430.

Croce, C. M. (2008). Oncogenes and cancer. *The New England Journal of Medicine, 358*(5), 502–511.

Daniels, R., Nosek, L., & Nicoll, L. H. (2007). *Contemporary medical-surgical nursing.* Clifton Park, NY: Delmar Cengage Learning.

Ferri, F. (2008). *Ferri's clinical advisor, 2008.* St. Louis: Mosby.

Giordano, S. H. (2005). A review of the diagnosis and management of male breast cancer. *Oncologist, 10*(7), 471–479.

Green, F., & Newbell, B. (2007). Inflammatory breast cancer. *The Journal for Nurse Practitioners, 3*(6), 385–388.

Hampton, T. (2007). Breast cancer prevention in Limbo. *JAMA, 297*(18), 1968–1969.

Hanby, A. M. (2005). The pathology of breast cancer and the role of the histopathology laboratory. *Clinical Oncology, 17*(4), 234–239.

Harvey, J. A. (2007). Unusual breast cancers: Useful clues to expanding the differential diagnosis. *Radiology, 242*(3), 683–694.

Klein, S. (2005). Evaluation of palpable breast masses. *American Family Physician, 71*(9), 1731–1738.

Lipsky, M. S., Koenigs, M., Nora, R., Peralta, E., & Zahasky, K. M. (2008). Breast cancer prevention for rural healthcare practitioners. *The American Journal for Nurse Practitioners, 12*(1), 49–58.

Mellington, T. E., & Fields, M. M. (2008). Targeting breast cancer: With hormonal treatment options. *The Nurse Practitioner, 33*(5), 16–21.

Michels, K. B., Terry, K. L., & Willett, W. C. (2006). Longitudinal study on the role of body size in premenopausal breast cancer. *Archives of Internal Medicine, 166*(21), 2395–2402.

Newman, L. (Ed.). (2007). Breast cancer. *Surgical Clinics of North America, 87*(2), 279–574.

Parkin, D. M., & Fernandez, L. M. G. (2006). Use of statistics to access the global burden of breast cancer. *The Breast Journal, 12*(s1), s70–s80.

Rubin, E., & Reisner, H. M. (2008). *Essentials of Rubin's pathology* (5th ed.). Philadelphia: Lippincott Williams & Wilkins.

Sellers, R. (2007). *Differential diagnosis of common complaints* (5th ed.). Philadelphia: Saunders.

Shockney, L. (2008). *The Johns Hopkins breast cancer handbook for health care professionals.* Sudbury, MA: Jones and Bartlett.

Smith-Bindman, R., Miglioretti, D. L., Lurie, N., Abraham, L., Barbash, R. B., Strzelczyk, J., Dignan, M., Barlow, W. E., Beasley, C. M., & Kerlikowske, K. (2006). Does utilization of screening mammography explain racial and ethnic differences in breast cancer? *Annals of Internal Medicine, 144*(8), 541–553.

WEB SITES

American Cancer Society:
http://www.cancer.org

Breastcancer.org:
http://www.breastcancer.org

Breast Cancer Support:
http://www.bcsupport.org

Cancer News on the Net:
http://www.cancernews.com

Inflammatory Breast Cancer Research Foundation:
http://www.ibcresearch.org

National Cancer Institute:
http://www.cancer.gov

National Library of Medicine:
http://www.nlm.nih.gov

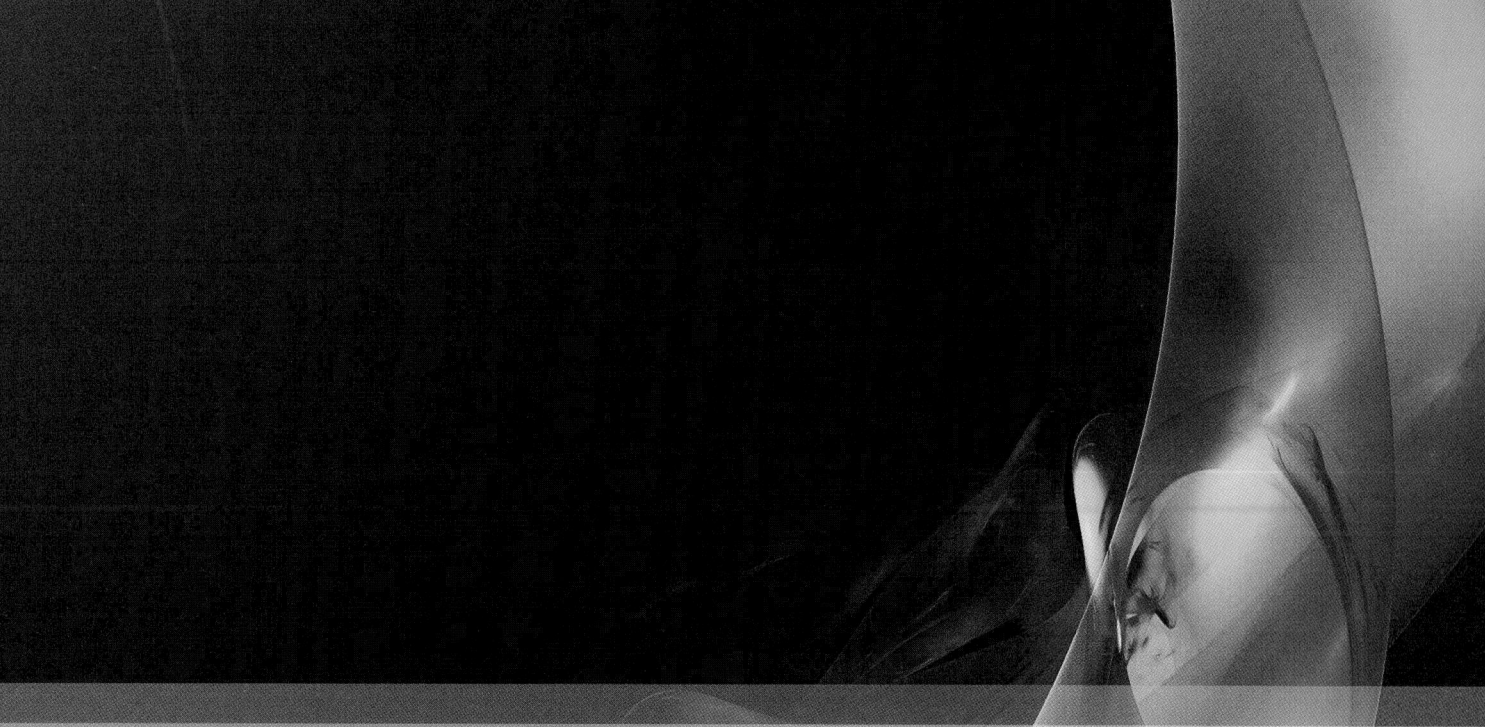

CHAPTER 15

Thorax and Lungs

COMPETENCIES

1. Identify the anatomic landmarks of the thorax.

2. Describe the characteristics of the most common respiratory complaints.

3. Perform inspection, palpation, percussion, and auscultation on a healthy adult and on a patient with pulmonary pathology.

4. Explain the pathophysiology for abnormal findings.

5. Document respiratory assessment findings.

The respiratory system extends from the nose to the alveoli (Figure 15-1). The normal air pathway is nose, pharynx, larynx, trachea, mainstem bronchus, right and left main bronchi, lobar/secondary bronchi, tertiary/segmental bronchi, terminal bronchioles, respiratory bronchioles, alveolar ducts, alveolar sacs, and alveoli.

The respiratory system is divided into the upper and lower tracts. The upper respiratory tract comprises the nose, pharynx, larynx, and the upper trachea. The nose and pharynx are discussed in Chapter 13. The lower respiratory tract is composed of the lower trachea to the lungs. This chapter deals only with those components of the respiratory system that are located in the thorax.

ANATOMY

THORAX

The thorax is a cone-shaped structure (narrower at the top and wider at the bottom) that consists of bones, cartilage, and muscles. Of these, the bones are the supportive structure of the thorax. On the anterior thorax, these bones are the 12 pairs of ribs and the sternum. Posteriorly, there are the 12 thoracic vertebrae and the spinal column.

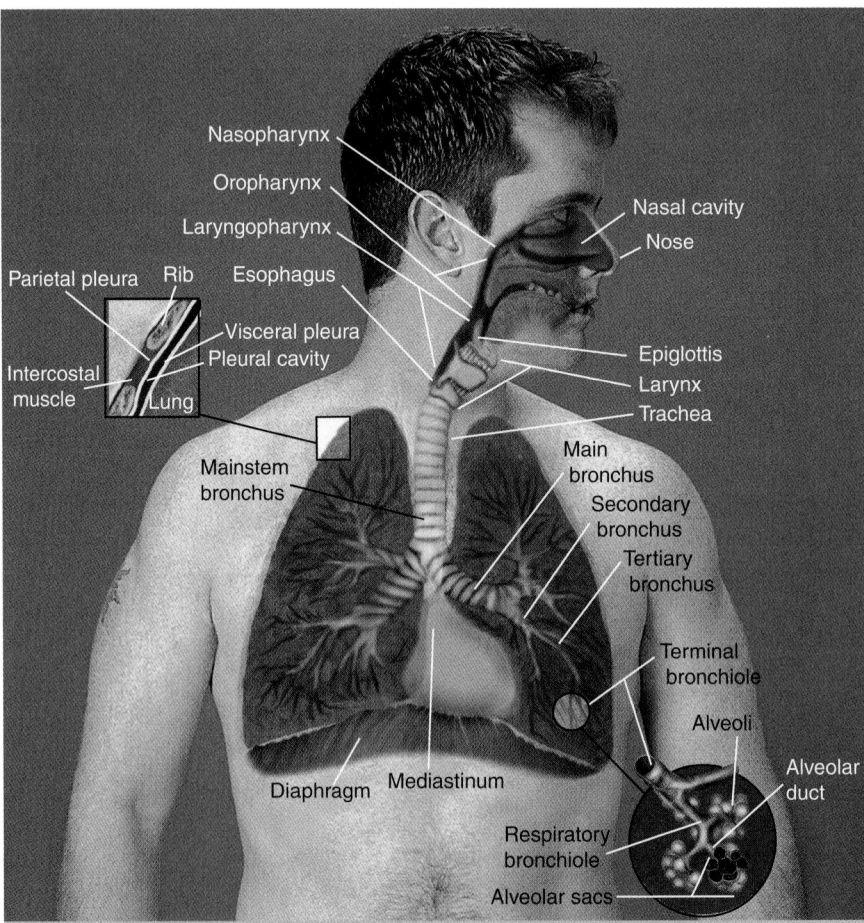

FIGURE 15-1 The Respiratory Tract

STERNUM

The sternum, or breastbone, is a flat, narrow bone approximately 15 cm long. It is located at the median line of the anterior chest wall and is divided into three sections: the **manubrium** (the upper bone of the sternum that articulates with the clavicles and the first pair of ribs), the body, and the **xiphoid process** (a cartilaginous process at the base of the sternum that does not articulate with the ribs).

RIBS

The first seven pairs of ribs are articulated to the sternum via the costal cartilages and are called the **vertebrosternal** or **true ribs**. The **false ribs**, or rib pairs 8–10, articulate with the costal cartilages just above them. The remaining two pairs of ribs (11 and 12) are termed **floating ribs** and do not articulate at their anterior ends. The 10th rib is the lowest rib that can be palpated anteriorly. The 11th rib is palpated on the lateral thorax, and the 12th rib is palpated on the posterior thorax. All ribs articulate posteriorly to the vertebral column. When a rib is palpated, the costal cartilage cannot be distinguished from the rib itself (Figure 15-2).

INTERCOSTAL SPACES

Each area between the ribs is called an **intercostal space** (ICS). There are 11 ICSs.

LUNGS

The lungs are cone-shaped organs that fill the lateral chamber of the thoracic cavity. The lower outer surface of each lung is concave where it meets the convex diaphragm. Likewise, the medial aspect is concave to allow room for the heart, with the left lung having a more pronounced concavity (cardiac notch). The lungs lie against the ribs anteriorly and posteriorly.

The right lung is broader than the left lung because of the position of the heart. Inferiorly, the right lung is about 2.5 cm shorter than the left lung because of

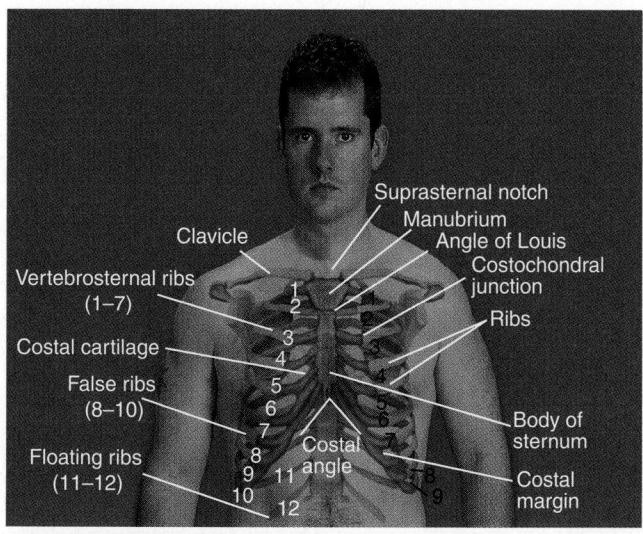

A. Anterior View

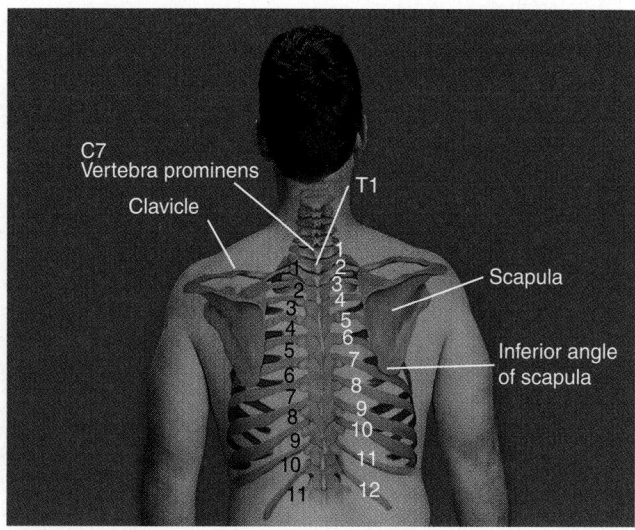

B. Posterior View

FIGURE 15-2 Thorax: Rib number is shown on the patient's right; intercostal space number is shown on the patient's left.

NURSING**TIP**

Identifying Thoracic Landmarks

Anterior

- Sternum
- Clavicles
- Nipples
- **Suprasternal notch:** With the finger pad of the index finger, feel in the midsternal line above the manubrium; the depression is the suprasternal notch.
- **Angle of Louis** (or **manubriosternal junction** or **sternal angle**): With the finger pads, feel for the suprasternal notch and move your finger pads down the sternum until they reach a horizontal ridge (the junction of the manubrium and the body of the sternum); this is the angle of Louis (or sternal angle); the second rib articulates with this landmark and serves as a convenient reference point for counting the ribs and ICSs (the first rib is difficult to palpate).
- **Costal angle:** Place your right finger pads on the bottom of the patient's anterior left rib cage (10th rib); place your left finger pads on the bottom of the anterior right rib cage (10th rib); move both hands horizontally toward the sternum until they meet in the midsternal line; the angle formed by the intersection of the ribs creates the costal angle.

Posterior

- **Vertebra prominens:** Flex the neck forward; palpate the posterior spinous processes; if two processes are palpable, the superior process is C7 (vertebra prominens) and the inferior is T1; this landmark is useful in counting ribs to the level of T4; beyond T4 the spinous processes project obliquely and no longer correspond to the rib of the same number as the vertebral process.
- **Inferior angle of scapula:** Locate the inferior border of the scapula; this level corresponds to the seventh rib or seventh ICS.
- Spine
- **Twelfth rib:** Palpate the lower thorax in the scapular line. Move your hand laterally to palpate the free tip of the 12th rib.

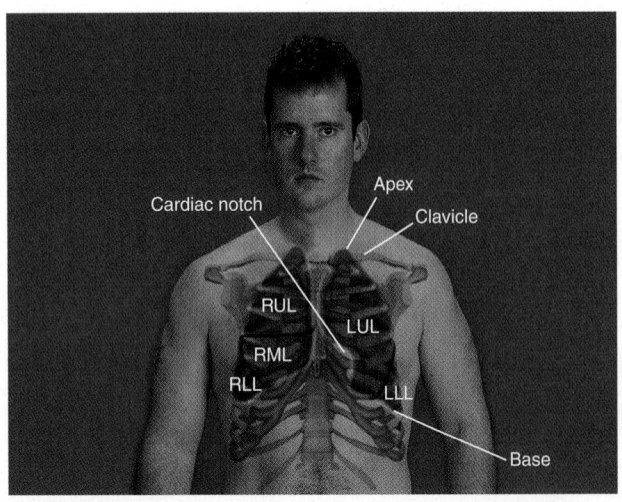

A. Anterior View

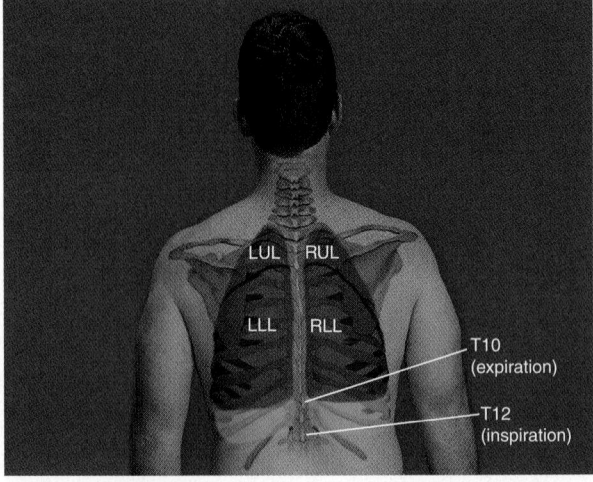

B. Posterior View

FIGURE 15-3 Lungs: RUL = Right Upper Lobe, RML = Right Middle Lobe, RLL = Right Lower Lobe, LUL = Left Upper Lobe, LLL = Left Lower Lobe

the upward displacement of the diaphragm by the liver. The right lung consists of three lobes (upper, middle, and lower) while the left lung has two lobes (upper and lower). In the lung, the **apex** denotes the top of the lung while the **base** refers to the bottom of the lung. Anteriorly, the apices of the lung extend 2.5 to 4 cm superior to the inner third of the clavicles, and posteriorly, the apices lie near the T1 process. On deep inspiration posteriorly, the lower lung border extends to the level of T12, and to T10 on deep expiration. The anterior inferior border of the lungs is at the sixth rib at the **midclavicular line** (MCL: vertical line drawn from the midpoint of the clavicle) and at the eighth rib at the **midaxillary line** (MAL: vertical line drawn from the apex of the axillae and lying midway between the anterior and the posterior axillary lines) (see Figure 15-3).

The lobes of the right and left lungs are divided by grooves called fissures. It is important to know the locations of the fissures to describe clinical findings. Figure 15-4 illustrates the right oblique (or diagonal) fissure, the right horizontal fissure, and the left oblique (or diagonal) fissure.

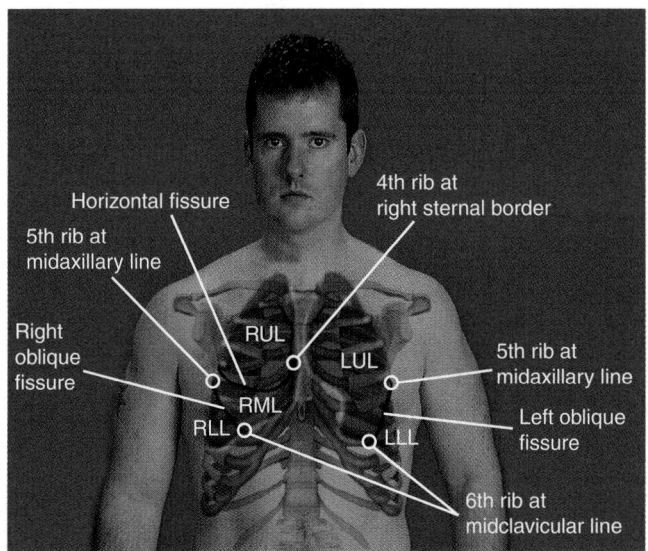

A. Anterior View

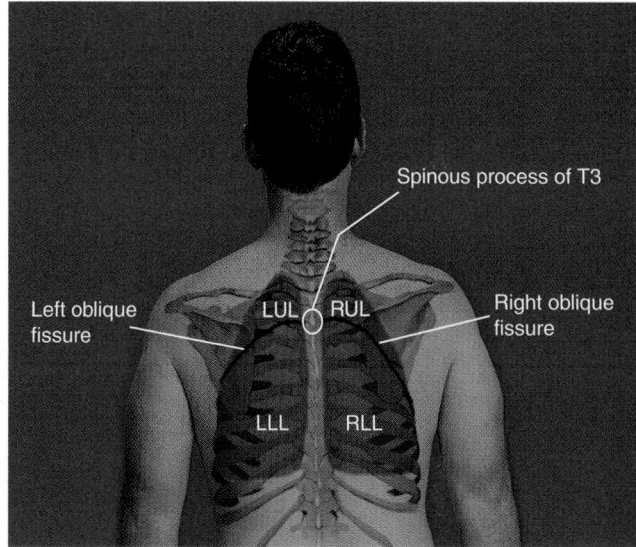

B. Posterior View

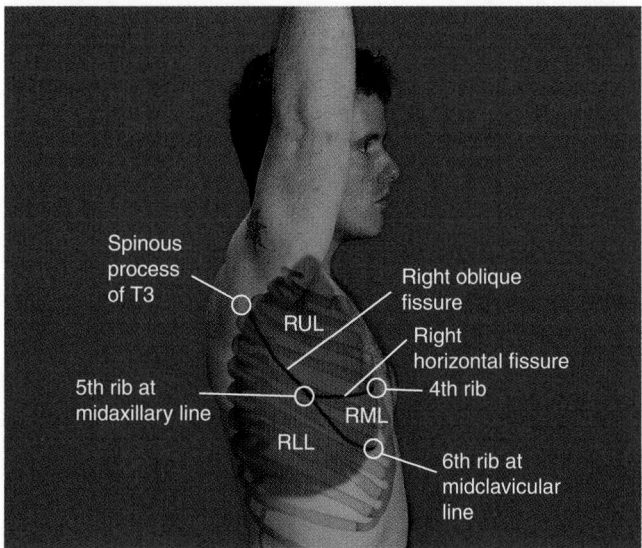

C. Right Lateral View

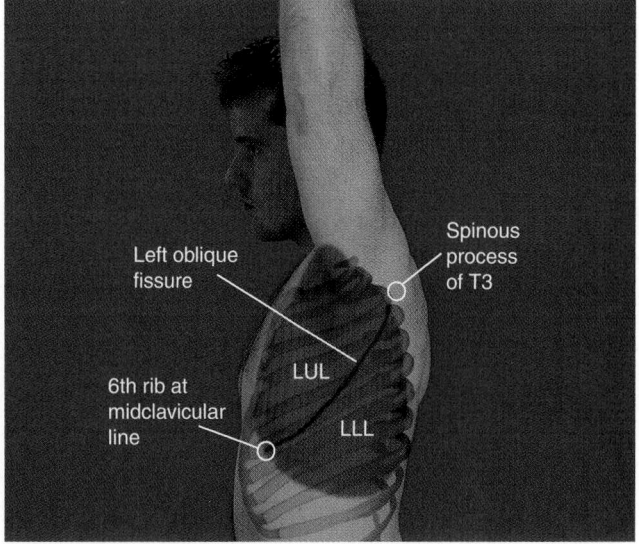

D. Left Lateral View

FIGURE 15-4 Lung Fissures

NURSING**TIP**

Thoracic Anatomic Topography

Additional landmarks that are useful when describing assessment findings are:
- **Anterior axillary line:** vertical line drawn from the origin of the anterior axillary fold and along the anterolateral aspect of the thorax.
- **Midspinal (vertebral) line:** vertical line drawn from the midpoint of the spinous process.
- **Midsternal line:** vertical line drawn from the midpoint of the sternum.
- **Posterior axillary line:** vertical line drawn from the posterior axillary fold.
- **Scapular line:** vertical line drawn from the inferior angle of the scapula.

When assessing the thorax, it is helpful to envision it as a rectangular box, with the four sides being the anterior, posterior, right lateral, and left lateral thoraxes. Figure 15-5 illustrates the imaginary thoracic lines on each of the four sides. These landmarks are helpful in discussing clinical findings.

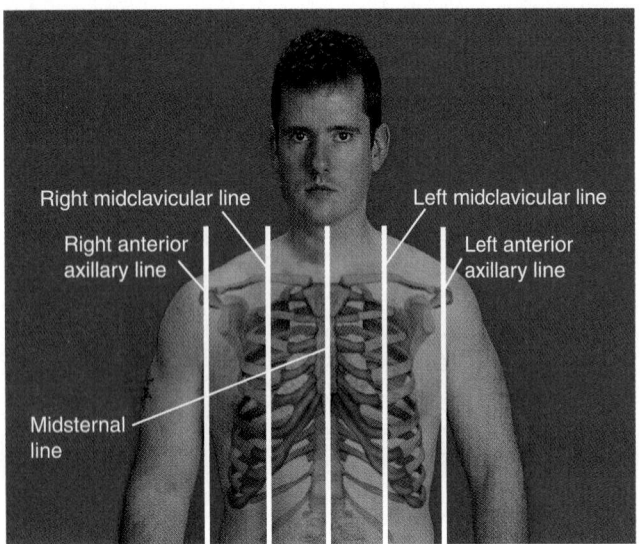

A. Anterior View

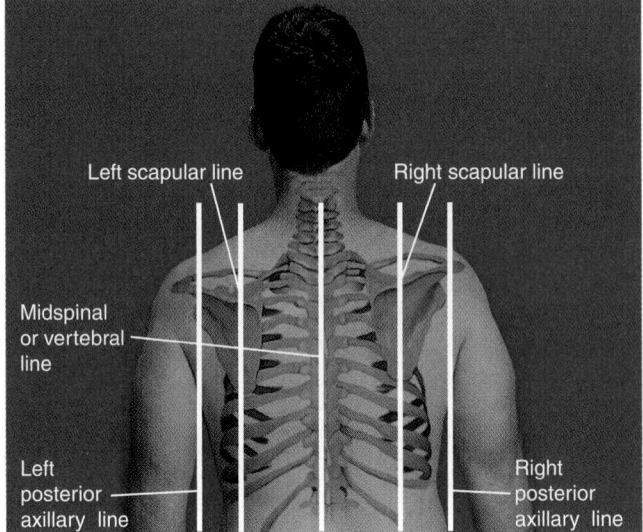

B. Posterior View

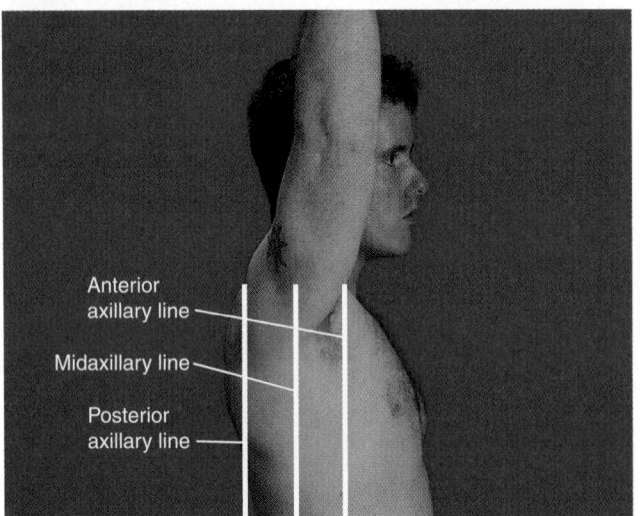

C. Right Lateral View

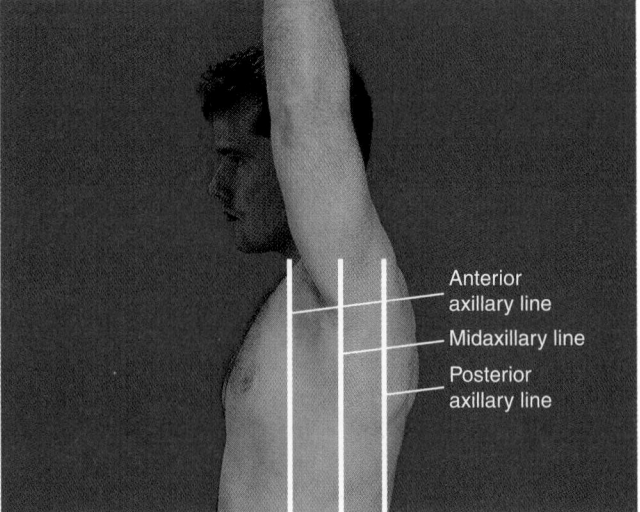

D. Left Lateral View

FIGURE 15-5 **Imaginary Thoracic Lines**

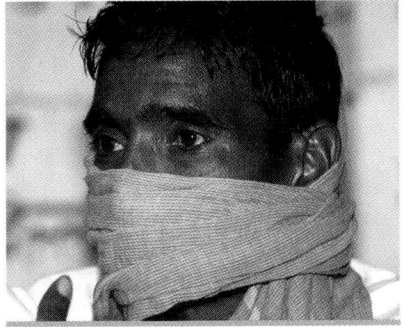

FIGURE 15-6 Since TB is spread via droplet nuclei, the infected person needs to wear a mask or other barrier device. *Courtesy of WHO/P. Virot.*

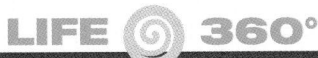

Assessing for Tuberculosis Exposure

A recent college graduate comes to your clinic for a purified protein derivative (PPD) test and physical examination in order to start his new teaching job. He returns 48 hours later and is found to have a positive PPD. He informs you that 1 year ago, he lived in Haiti teaching in a school. How would you proceed with this patient's history and physical examination?

PLEURA

Each lung is encased in a serous sac, or **pleura**. The **parietal pleura** lines the chest wall and the superior surface of the diaphragm. The **visceral pleura** lines the external surface of the lungs. Usually, a small amount of fluid is found in the space between these two pleurae; this fluid prevents the pleurae from rubbing against each other and acts as a cushioning agent for the lungs.

MEDIASTINUM

The **mediastinum**, or **interpleural space**, is the area between the right and left lungs. It extends from the sternum to the spinal column and contains the heart, great vessels, trachea, esophagus, and lymph vessels. The only respiratory structures in the mediastinum are the trachea and the pulmonary vasculature. The trachea is a fibromuscular hollow tube located in the anterior thorax in the median plane. It is 11 to 13 cm in length and 2 to 3 cm in width. The trachea lies anterior to the esophagus.

BRONCHI

The trachea bifurcates into the left and right mainstem bronchi at the level of the fourth or fifth vertebral process posteriorly and the sternal angle anteriorly. The right mainstem bronchus is wider, shorter, and more vertical than the left. This anatomic difference is critical because it makes the right mainstem bronchus more susceptible to aspiration and endotracheal intubation. The mainstem bronchi further divide into lobar or secondary bronchi. Each lobar bronchus supplies a lobe of the lung. The bronchi transport gases as well as trap foreign particles in their mucus. Cilia aid in sweeping the foreign particles upward in the respiratory tract for possible elimination. Culmination of the tracheobronchial tree is in the alveoli.

ALVEOLI

The **alveoli** are the smallest functional units of the respiratory system. It is here that gas exchange occurs. It is estimated that approximately 300 million alveoli are present in each lung. This aerating surface is about equal to 100 times the body surface area of an adult. Each alveolus has its own blood supply and lymphatic drainage. Branches of the pulmonary artery carry blood to the capillaries surrounding the alveoli to be oxygenated. Branches of the pulmonary vein transport oxygenated blood from the alveoli to the heart.

DIAPHRAGM

The diaphragm, which is innervated by the phrenic nerve, is a dome-shaped muscle that forms the inferior border of the thorax. Anteriorly, its right edge is located at the fifth rib—fifth ICS at the MCL. The left dome of the diaphragm is at the sixth rib—sixth ICS at the MCL. The presence of the liver below the right dome of the diaphragm accounts for the elevated border on that side. On expiration posteriorly, the diaphragm is located at the level of the 10th vertebral process, and at T12 on inspiration. Laterally, the diaphragm is found at the eighth rib at the midaxillary line. The diaphragm is the principal muscle of respiration. Contraction of the diaphragm leads to an increase in volume in the thoracic cavity.

EXTERNAL INTERCOSTAL MUSCLES

The external intercostal muscles are located in the ICS. During inspiration, the external intercostal muscles elevate the ribs, thus increasing the size of the thoracic cavity. The internal intercostal muscles draw adjacent ribs together, thereby decreasing the size of the thoracic cavity during expiration.

ACCESSORY MUSCLES

Accessory respiratory muscles are used to accommodate increased oxygen demand. Exercise and some diseases lead to the use of accessory muscles. The accessory muscles are the scalene, sternocleidomastoid, trapezius, and abdominal rectus.

PHYSIOLOGY

VENTILATION

The primary function of the respiratory system is to deliver oxygen to the lungs and to remove carbon dioxide from the lungs. The breathing process includes inspiratory and expiratory phases. During inspiration, the pressure inside the lungs becomes subatmospheric when the diaphragm and external intercostal muscles contract. The diaphragm lowers and the ribs elevate, thus increasing the intrapulmonic volume. As a result of the negative intra-alveolar pressure, atmospheric air is pulled into the respiratory tract until intra-alveolar pressure equals atmospheric pressure. The lungs increase in size with the air.

Expiration is a passive process and occurs more rapidly than inspiration. During expiration, the diaphragm and external intercostal muscles relax, decreasing the volume of the thoracic cavity. The diaphragm rises. The intrapulmonic volume decreases and the intrapulmonic pressure increases above the atmospheric pressure. The lungs possess elastic recoil capabilities that allow air to be expelled until intrapulmonic pressure equals atmospheric pressure.

LIFE 360°

Tobacco Use

- How do you feel about others who smoke? Are you a smoker?
- How do you feel about patients who have pathology related to tobacco use?
- Do you treat patients who smoke any differently from non-smoking patients? If so, what interventions can you implement to deal with this bias?
- How do you feel about health care professionals who smoke?

External Respiration

External respiration is the process by which gases are exchanged between the lungs and the pulmonary vasculature. Oxygen diffuses from the alveoli into the blood, and carbon dioxide diffuses from the blood to the alveoli. Diffusion is a passive process in which gases move across a membrane from an area of higher concentration to an area of lower concentration. In the lungs, the membrane is the alveolar-capillary network.

Internal Respiration

Internal respiration is the process by which gases are exchanged between the pulmonary vasculature and the body's tissues. Oxygen from the lungs diffuses from the blood into body tissue. Carbon dioxide diffuses from the tissue into the blood. This blood is then carried back to the right side of the heart for reoxygenation.

Control of Breathing

Control of breathing is influenced by neural and chemical factors. The pons and medulla are the central nervous system structures primarily responsible for involuntary respiration. The stimulus for breathing is an increased carbon dioxide level, a decreased oxygen level, or an increased blood pH level.

HEALTH HISTORY

	The thorax and lungs health history provides insight into the link between a patient's life and lifestyle and thorax and lungs information and pathology.
PATIENT PROFILE	*Diseases that are age-, gender-, and race-specific for the thorax and lungs are listed.*
Age	Bronchiectasis (birth–20) Cystic fibrosis (birth–30) Pneumothorax (20–40) Sarcoidosis (30–40) Chronic bronchitis (> 35) Pneumonia (> 60) Emphysema (50–60) Idiopathic pulmonary fibrosis (60–70)
Gender	
Female	Sarcoidosis
Male	Mesothelioma, idiopathic pulmonary fibrosis, pneumothorax
Race	
African American	Sarcoidosis
Caucasian	Cystic fibrosis
CHIEF COMPLAINT	*Common chief complaints for the thorax and lungs are defined and information on the characteristics of each sign or symptom is provided.*

continues

1. Dyspnea	Subjective feeling of shortness of breath (SOB)
Quantity	The number of steps that can be climbed before SOB occurs; distance that can be walked; number of pillows needed to sleep comfortably
Associated Manifestations	Palpitations, leg pain, faintness, anxiety, fatigue, cough, sputum, wheezing, diaphoresis, cyanosis, pain, fever
Aggravating Factors	Smoking, exercise, poorly ventilated rooms
Alleviating Factors	Pillow orthopnea, side-lying position, tripod position, fresh air, medications (e.g., bronchodilators), supplemental oxygen, resting
Timing	Nighttime (paroxysmal nocturnal dyspnea)
2. Cough	Stimulation of afferent vagal endings, which helps clean the airway of extraneous material by producing a sudden, forceful, and noisy expulsion of air from the lungs
Quality	Dry, wet, hacking, barking, congested, harsh, brassy, high pitched, whooping, bubbling
Associated Manifestations	SOB, wheezing, sputum, pleuritic pain, chest pain, fever, hemoptysis, coryza, anxiety, diaphoresis, GERD symptoms, postnasal drip, hoarseness
Aggravating Factors	Position of patient, exposure to noxious stimuli, exercise
Alleviating Factors	Medications (e.g., nebulizer, inhaler, cough suppressant medications, steroids), humidity, cool air, cool liquids
Setting	Temperature and humidity of environment, exertion
Timing	Winter, early morning, bedtime, middle of the night, after eating, prior to fainting, continuous
3. Sputum	Substance produced by the respiratory tract that can be expectorated or swallowed; it is composed of mucus, blood, purulent material, microorganisms, cellular debris, and, occasionally, foreign objects
Quality	Color: white or clear, purulent, blood-tinged, yellow or green, mucoid, rust, black, pink Consistency: thick, thin, moderate; frothy—separates into layers Odor: malodorous
Quantity	Normal daily sputum production is 60 to 90 mL (normally this is not expectorated); small, moderate, copious
Associated Manifestations	Cough, fever, dyspnea
Aggravating Factors	Exposure to allergens, smoking
Alleviating Factors	Medications (e.g., guaifenesin), liquids
Setting	Sleep, exposure to allergen
Timing	Early morning
4. Chest Pain	Pain can have a pulmonary, cardiac, gastrointestinal, or musculoskeletal etiology. Chapter 16 differentiates the types of chest pain.

continues

Health History (continued)

PAST HEALTH HISTORY	*The various components of the past health history are linked to thorax and lung pathology and thorax- and lung-related information.*
Medical History	
Respiratory Specific	Asthma, bronchitis, croup, frequent coryza, cystic fibrosis, emphysema, epiglottitis, pleurisy, pneumonia, pneumothorax, pulmonary edema, pulmonary embolus, lung cancer, tuberculosis
Non-respiratory Specific	Lupus, drug-induced respiratory pathology, rheumatoid arthritis, congenital musculoskeletal chest defects, severe scoliosis, multiple sclerosis, amyotrophic lateral sclerosis
Surgical History	Lobectomy, pneumonectomy, tracheostomy, wedge resection, bronchoscopy
Allergies	Asthma is the predominant manifestation of allergies in the respiratory patient. Hypersensitivity to drugs, food, pets, dust, cigarette smoke, perfume, or pollen should be closely scrutinized. In addition, any common signs of allergies, such as cough, sneeze, and sinusitis, should be closely evaluated.
Medications	Antibiotics, bronchodilators, cough expectorant, cough suppressant, oxygen, steroids
Communicable Diseases	Coryza: sneezing, coughing Tuberculosis (TB): pulmonary fibrosis and calcification Flu: pneumonia AIDS: *Pneumocystis carinii* pneumonia Hantavirus: bilateral pulmonary infiltrates, respiratory failure
Injuries and Accidents	Chest trauma, near drowning
Special Needs	Oxygen dependent, phrenic pacer dependent, ventilator dependent
Childhood Illnesses	Pertussis and measles: bronchiectasis
FAMILY HEALTH HISTORY	*Thorax and lung diseases that are familial are listed.*
	Allergies, alpha$_1$-antitrypsin deficiency, asthma, bronchiectasis, cancer, cystic fibrosis, emphysema, sarcoidosis, TB
SOCIAL HISTORY	*The components of the social history are linked to thorax and lung factors and pathology.*
Alcohol Use	Decreases efficiency of lung defense mechanisms, predisposes to aspiration pneumonia; patients with carbon dioxide retention are more sensitive to alcohol's depressant effect
Tobacco Use	Cigarette smoking is the primary risk factor for chronic bronchitis, emphysema, and lung cancer, as well as other disorders.
Drug Use	Heroin: pulmonary edema Barbiturates or narcotic overdose: respiratory depression Cocaine: tachypnea
Travel History	Prolonged exposure to confined space with recirculated air (e.g., airplane) TB (Haiti, Southeast Asia): poor sanitation and rural conditions San Joaquin Valley fever or coccidioidomycosis (Southwest United States and Mexico): agent is in dirt and dusty winds Pneumonic plague (India): carried by nuclei droplets

continues

Health History (continued)

Work Environment	Repeated exposure to materials in the workplace can create respiratory complications that range from minor problems to life-threatening events. Numerous categories of respiratory diseases have been identified, from repeated exposure to toxic substances. These diseases are listed along with the industries and agents related to them.

Silicosis: glassmaking, tunneling, stonecutting, mineral mining, insulation work, quarrying, cement work, ceramics, foundry work, semiconductor manufacturing

Asbestosis: mining, shipbuilding, construction

Coal worker's pneumoconiosis: coal mining

Pneumoconioses: tin and aluminum production, welding, insecticide manufacturing, rubber industry, fertilizer industry, ceramics, cosmetic industry

Occupational asthma: electroplating, grain working, woodworking, photography, printing, baking, painting

Chronic bronchitis: coal mining, welding, firefighting

Byssinosis: cotton mill dust, flax

Extrinsic allergic alveolitis (hypersensitivity pneumonia): animal hair, contamination of air conditioning or heating systems, moldy hay, moldy grains, moldy dust, sugarcane

Toxic gases and fumes: welding, cigarette smoke, auto exhaust, chemical industries, firefighting, hair spray

Pulmonary neoplasms: radon gas, mustard gas, printing ink, asbestos, chromium (from chrome plating, stainless steel welding)

Pneumonitis: furniture polish, gasoline, or kerosene ingestion; mineral oil, olive oil, and milk aspiration

Home Environment	Air pollution, cigarette smoke, wood-burning stoves, gas stoves and heaters, kerosene heaters, radon gas, pet hair and dander
Hobbies and Leisure Activities	Birds (bird breeder's lung), mushroom growers (mushroom grower's lung), scuba diving (lung rupture, oxygen toxicity, decompression sickness), high-altitude activities (skiing, climbing: pulmonary edema and pulmonary embolus)
Stress	Asthma can be exacerbated by stress.
Economic Status	Poor sanitation and densely populated areas are ideal conditions for the spread of TB.
HEALTH MAINTENANCE ACTIVITIES	*This information provides a bridge between the health maintenance activities and thorax and lung function.*
Sleep	Obstructive sleep apnea: absence of inspiratory muscle activation; upper airway occlusion Chronic obstructive pulmonary disease (COPD) or neuromuscular disease: nocturnal oxygen desaturation caused by hypoventilation without apnea
Diet	Obesity: chronic hypoventilation, obstructive sleep apnea (Pickwickian syndrome)
Exercise	Regular exercise improves pulmonary function.
Use of Safety Devices	Mask worn when exposed to toxic substances, other occupational precautions as mandated by OSHA; knowledge of Heimlich maneuver
Health Check-ups	Respiratory rate, lung auscultation, chest X-ray, sputum culture and sensitivity, pulmonary function test, purified protein derivative (tuberculin, PPD), influenza and pneumococcal vaccines, immunotherapy (allergy shots)

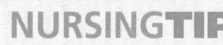

NURSINGTIP

Reducing Exposure to Respiratory Hazards in the Workplace

- Always wear a mask if exposed to substances that cause respiratory disease.
- Avoid respiratory irritants when possible.
- Maintain proper ventilation of the environment to ensure minimal breathing of dangerous substances.
- Follow Occupational Safety and Health Administration (OSHA) and employer's safety guidelines.

NURSINGCHECKLIST

Maintaining Respiratory Health

- Avoid smoking; encourage those living with you to stop.
- Never smoke around infants and children.
- Never smoke in bed.
- If you must live with a smoker, ask that smoking be confined to one well-ventilated room, or preferably outside.
- If dust and mold are allergy triggers or aggravating factors for other respiratory ailments, clean house frequently, avoid wall-to-wall carpeting, use easily washed curtains, and avoid having a cluttered room.
- Change filters on furnace, heaters, air conditioners, exhaust systems, and range hoods as frequently as the manufacturer specifies.
- Have chimneys cleaned at the beginning of each season and more frequently if used heavily.
- Have home inspected for radon and take remedial steps as needed.
- Check carbon monoxide and smoke detectors on a monthly basis.
- If oxygen is used in the home, use and store away from heat; avoid contact with open flames and cigarettes.

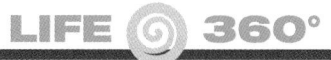
Inhalants

You are conducting a history on a new 18-year-old patient in the student health center of the local college. The patient has a history of asthma and needs a refill on her short-acting bronchodilator. The patient denies using tobacco but admits to inhaling some substances at recent parties. You ask her to tell you more about this practice when she says, "I have said too much. I never should have brought it up. I just want a prescription for my asthma medication and I will leave." How should you proceed?

NURSINGCHECKLIST

General Approach to Thorax and Lung Assessment

1. Greet the patient and explain the assessment techniques that you will be using.
2. Ensure that the examination room is at a warm, comfortable room temperature to prevent patient chilling and shivering.
3. Use a quiet room that will be free from interruptions.
4. Ensure that the light in the room provides sufficient brightness to adequately observe the patient.
5. Instruct the patient to remove all street clothes from the waist up and to don an examination gown.
6. Place the patient in an upright sitting position on the examination table.
7. Expose the entire area being assessed. Provide a drape that women can use to cover their breasts (if desired) when the posterior thorax is assessed.
8. When palpating, percussing, or auscultating the anterior thorax of female or obese patients, ask them to displace the breast tissue. Assessing directly over breast tissue is not an accurate indicator of underlying structures.
9. Visualize the underlying respiratory structures during the assessment process in order to accurately describe the location of any pathology.
10. Always compare the right and the left sides of the anterior thorax and the posterior thorax to one another, as well as the right lateral thorax to the left lateral thorax.
11. Use a systematic approach every time the assessment is performed. Proceed from the lung apices to the bases, right to left to lateral.

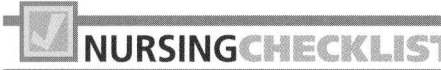

NURSING CHECKLIST

Influenza Vaccine

Annual vaccination against influenza is recommended for:

- All persons, including school-age children, who want to reduce the risk of becoming ill with influenza or of transmitting influenza to others
- All children aged 6–59 months (i.e., 6 months–4 years)
- All persons aged 50 years and older
- Children and adolescents (aged 6 months–18 years) receiving long-term aspirin therapy who therefore might be at risk for experiencing Reye syndrome after influenza virus infection
- Women who will be pregnant during the influenza season
- Adults and children who have chronic pulmonary (including asthma), cardiovascular (except hypertension), renal, hepatic, hematological, or metabolic disorders (including diabetes mellitus)
- Adults and children who have immunosuppression (including immunosuppression caused by medications or by human immunodeficiency virus)
- Adults and children who have any condition (e.g., cognitive dysfunction, spinal cord injuries, seizure disorders, or other neuromuscular disorders) that can compromise respiratory function or the handling of respiratory secretions or that can increase the risk for aspiration
- Residents of nursing homes and other chronic-care facilities
- Health care personnel
- Healthy household contacts (including children) and caregivers of children aged <5 years and adults aged 50 years and older, with particular emphasis on vaccinating contacts of children aged <6 months
- Healthy household contacts (including children) and caregivers of persons with medical conditions that put them at higher risk for severe complications from influenza

From Prevention & Control of Influenza—Recommendations of the Advisory Committee on Immunization Practices (ACIP). (2007, July 13). *MMWR, 56*(RR06), 1–54.

EQUIPMENT

- Stethoscope
- Centimeter ruler or tape measure
- Washable marker
- Watch with second hand

ASSESSMENT OF THE THORAX AND LUNGS

INSPECTION

Shape of Thorax

E 1. Stand in front of the patient.

2. Estimate visually the transverse diameter of the thorax.

3. Move to either side of the patient.

4. Estimate visually the width of the anteroposterior (AP) diameter of the thorax.

5. Compare the estimates of these two visualizations.

N In the normal adult, the ratio of the AP diameter to the transverse diameter is approximately 1:2 to 5:7. In other words, the normal adult is wider from side to side than from front to back. The normal thorax is slightly elliptical in shape. A barrel chest is normal in infants and sometimes in the older adult. Chapter 24 for a discussion of the pediatric patient. Figure 15-7 illustrates the normal and abnormal configurations of the thorax.

A In **barrel chest**, the ratio of the AP diameter to the transverse diameter is approximately 1:1. The patient's chest is circular or barrel shaped in appearance.

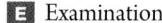

E Examination   **N** Normal Findings   **A** Abnormal Findings   **P** Pathophysiology

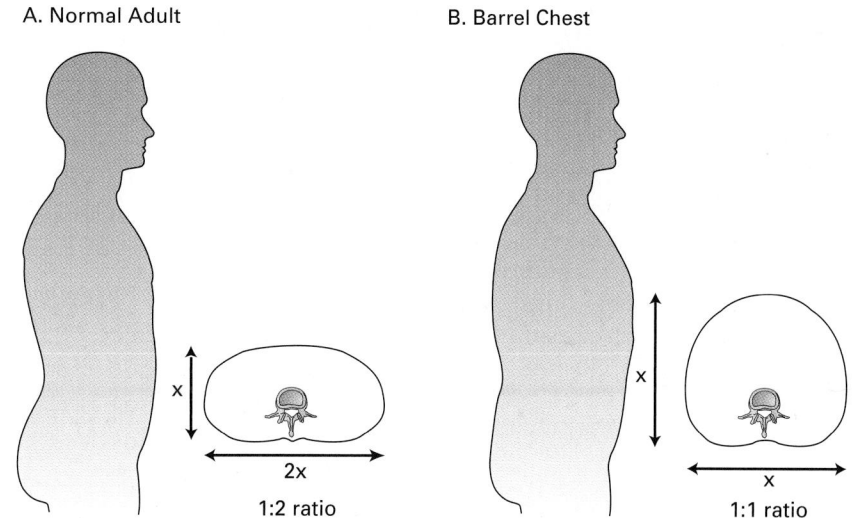

A. Normal Adult

B. Barrel Chest

x

$2x$

1:2 ratio

x

x

1:1 ratio

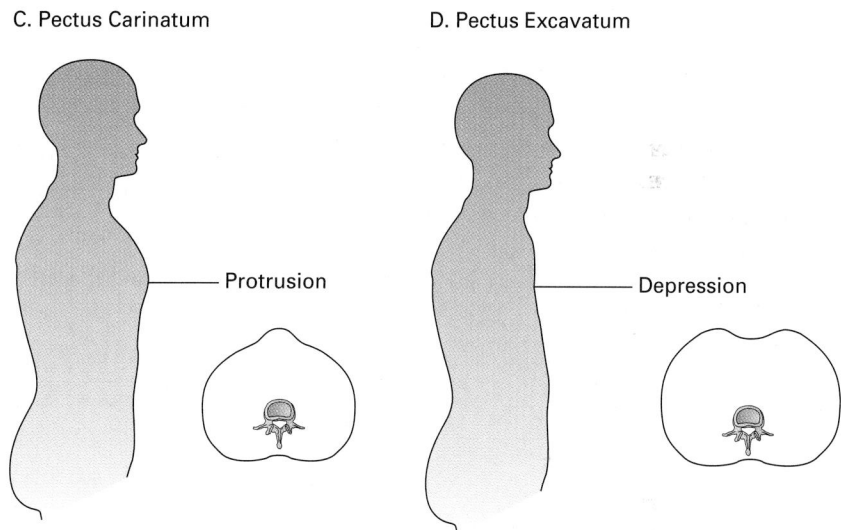

C. Pectus Carinatum

D. Pectus Excavatum

Protrusion

Depression

FIGURE 15-7 **Chest Configurations**

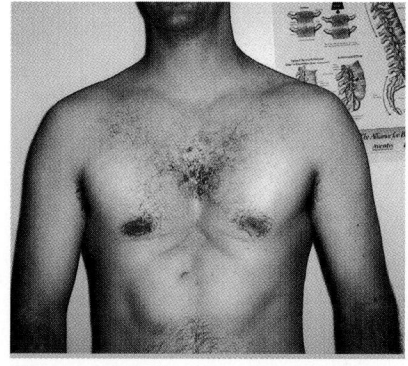

FIGURE 15-8 **Pectus Excavatum**

P The patient with COPD has a barrel chest due to air trapping in the alveoli and subsequent lung hyperinflation. Lung volume thus increases and the diaphragm flattens over time. The ribs are forced upward and outward. Collectively these changes result in the barrel chest appearance.

A **Pectus carinatum,** or pigeon chest, is a marked protrusion of the sternum. This increases the AP diameter of the thorax.

P Pectus carinatum can result from a congenital anomaly. A patient with severe pectus carinatum will exhibit respiratory difficulty.

P Rickets results from a vitamin D deficiency. In this condition, the bones become demineralized and weak. The loss of bone strength allows the intercostal muscles to pull the ribs and sternum forward, resulting in pectus carinatum.

A **Pectus excavatum,** or funnel chest (Figure 15-8), is a depression in the body of the sternum. This indentation can compress the heart and cause myocardial disturbances. The AP diameter of the chest decreases.

P Pectus excavatum results from a congenital anomaly. Respiratory insufficiency can ensue from the compression of the lungs in marked pectus excavatum.

A **Kyphosis,** or humpback, is an excessive convexity of the thoracic vertebrae. Gibbus kyphosis is an extreme deformity of the spine.

P The majority of kyphosis cases are idiopathic. Respiratory compromise is manifested only in severe cases.

A **Scoliosis** is a lateral curvature of the thorax or lumbar vertebrae. See Chapter 18 for further discussion.

P The majority of the cases of scoliosis are idiopathic, although scoliosis can also result from neuromuscular diseases, connective tissue diseases, and osteoporosis. Marked scoliosis can interfere with normal respiratory function. The total lung capacity and vital capacity decline in proportion to the severity of the scoliosis.

Symmetry of Chest Wall

E
1. Stand in front of the patient.
2. Inspect the right and the left anterior thoraxes.
3. Note the shoulder height. Observe any differences between the two sides of the chest wall, such as the presence of masses.
4. Move behind the patient.
5. Inspect the right and the left posterior thoraxes, comparing right and left sides.
6. Note the position of the scapula.

N The shoulders should be at the same height. Likewise, the scapula should be the same height bilaterally. There should be no masses.

A Having one shoulder or scapula higher than the other is abnormal.

P The presence of scoliosis can lead to a shoulder or a scapula that is higher than its corresponding part. Marked scoliosis impairs lung function.

A The presence of a visible mass is abnormal.

P A visible chest mass is always abnormal. Likely etiologies are mediastinal tumors or cysts. If large enough, they can compress lung tissue and impair normal lung function.

Presence of Superficial Veins

E
1. Stand in front of the patient.
2. Inspect the anterior thorax for the presence of dilated superficial veins.

N In the normal adult, dilated superficial veins are not seen.

A The presence of dilated superficial veins on the anterior chest wall is an abnormal finding.

P Dilated veins on the anterior thorax may be indicative of superior vena cava obstruction. Due to the obstruction, the superficial veins and collateral vessels become engorged with blood and dilate. Venous return to the heart is diminished, compromising oxygenation. A patient may present with dyspnea.

Costal Angle

E   1. Stand in front of the patient.

2. In a patient whose thoracic skeleton is easily viewed, visually locate the **costal margins** (medial borders created by the articulation of the false ribs).

3. Estimate the angle formed by the costal margins during exhalation and at rest. This is the costal angle.

4. In a heavy or obese patient, place your fingertips on the lower anterior borders of the thoracic skeleton.

5. Gently move your fingertips medially to the xiphoid process.

6. As your hands approach the midline, feel the ribs as they meet at the apex of the costal margins. Visualize the line that is created by your fingers as they move up the floating ribs toward the sternum. This is the costal angle (see Figure 15-9A). Approximate this angle.

N   The costal angle is less than 90° during exhalation and at rest. The costal angle widens slightly during inhalation due to the expansion of the thorax.

A   A costal angle greater than 90° is abnormal.

P   Processes where hyperinflation of the lungs (emphysema) or dilation of the bronchi (bronchiectasis) occurs also result in a costal margin angle greater than 90°. The diaphragm flattens out and the ribs are forced upward and outward, leading to the change in the costal margin angle.

Angle of the Ribs

E   1. Stand in front of the patient.

2. In a patient whose thoracic skeleton is easily viewed, visually locate the midsternal area.

3. Estimate the angle at which the ribs articulate with the sternum.

4. In a heavy or obese patient, place your fingertips on the midsternal area.

5. Move your fingertips along a rib laterally to the anterior axillary line. Visualize the line that is created by your hand as it traces the rib. Approximate this angle. See Figure 15-9B.

N   The ribs articulate at a 45° angle with the sternum.

A   An angle greater than 45° is considered abnormal. Patients with particular respiratory pathology may have ribs that are nearly horizontal and perpendicular to the sternum.

P   Conditions characterized by an increased AP diameter, such as emphysema, bronchiectasis, and cystic fibrosis, result in an angle greater than 45° because the lungs are forced out due to hyperinflation or dilation of the bronchi.

Intercostal Spaces

E   1. Stand in front of the patient.

2. Inspect the ICS throughout the respiratory cycle.

3. Note any bulging of the ICS and any retractions.

N   There should be an absence of retractions and of bulging of the ICS.

| **E** Examination | **N** Normal Findings | **A** Abnormal Findings | **P** Pathophysiology |

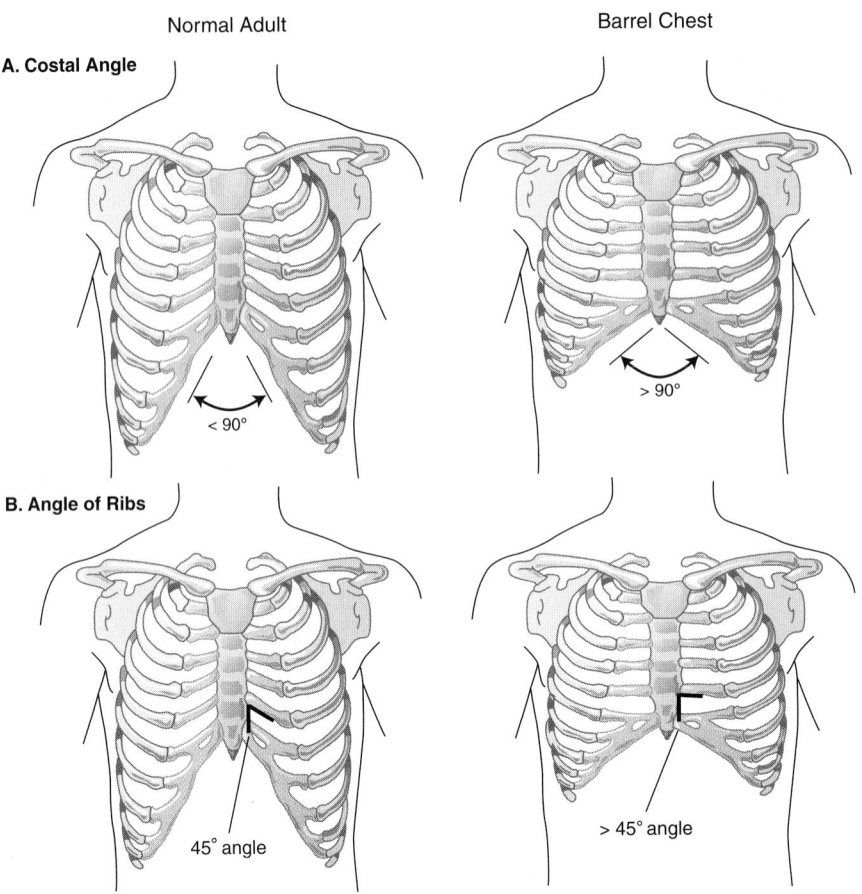

FIGURE 15-9 Rib Cage Angles

A The presence of retractions is abnormal. Retractions occur during inspiration.

P Conditions that obstruct the free inflow of air may lead to retractions. These include emphysema, asthma, tracheal or laryngeal obstruction, and the presence of a foreign body or tumor that compresses the respiratory tract.

A The presence of bulging of the ICS is abnormal. Bulging of the ICS tends to occur during expiration.

P Abnormal bulging of the ICS occurs when there is an obstruction to the free exhalation of air, such as in emphysema, asthma, an enlarged heart, aortic aneurysm, massive pleural effusion, tension pneumothorax, and tumors.

Muscles of Respiration

E 1. Stand in front of the patient.

2. Observe the patient's breathing for a few respiratory cycles, paying close attention to the anterior thorax and the neck.

3. Note all of the muscles that are being used by the patient.

N No accessory muscles are used in normal breathing.

A The use of the accessory muscles is a pathological finding.

P Any condition that creates a state of hypoxemia or hypermetabolism may lead to the use of accessory muscles. Accessory muscles are attempting to create an extra respiratory effort to inhale needed oxygen. Patients experiencing hypermetabolic states such as exercise, fever, or infection, or hypoxic events such as COPD, pneumonia, pneumothorax, pulmonary edema, or pulmonary embolus usually present with accessory muscle use.

Respirations

The inspection of the respiration process includes seven components: rate, pattern, depth, symmetry, audibility, patient position, and mode.

RATE.

E
1. Stand in front of the patient or to the right side.

2. Observe the patient's breathing without stating what you are doing, because the patient may change the respiratory rate (increase or decrease it) if aware that you are watching the chest rising and falling. This assessment can be conducted simultaneously with the pulse rate assessment.

3. Count the number of respiratory cycles that the patient has for one full minute. A respiratory cycle consists of one inhaled and one exhaled breath.

N In the resting adult, the normal respiratory rate is 12 to 20 breaths per minute. This type of breathing is termed eupnea, or normal breathing.

A A respiratory rate greater than 20 breaths per minute is termed **tachypnea**.

P Tachypnea is frequently present in hypermetabolic and hypoxic states. By increasing the respiratory rate, the body is trying to supply additional oxygen to meet the body's demands. Tachypnea occurs in many disease states, such as pneumonia, bronchitis, asthma, and pneumothorax.

P Tachypnea is often a sign of stress. In stressful situations, the body releases catecholamines that elevate the respiratory rate to supply sufficient oxygen.

A A respiratory rate lower than 12 breaths per minute is termed **bradypnea**.

P Injury to the brain may cause bradypnea because of excessive intracranial pressure applied to the respiratory center in the medulla oblongata.

P In drug overdoses (barbiturates, alcohol, and opiates), bradypnea is a sign of the drug's depressant effect on the respiratory center.

P Bradypnea occurs in sleep because of the lowered metabolic state of the body. The respiratory rate also slows in non-REM sleep due to changes in the response of the respiratory center to chemical signals.

A **Apnea** is the lack of spontaneous respirations for 10 or more seconds.

P Traumatic brain injury may lead to apnea because of herniation of the brain stem.

P Sleep apnea can be central or obstructive in nature. In central sleep apnea, the respiratory drive is altered, leading to periods of respiratory cessation. In obstructive sleep apnea, enlarged upper airway anatomy leads to a physical blockage in the oropharynx.

| **E** Examination | **N** Normal Findings | **A** Abnormal Findings | **P** Pathophysiology |

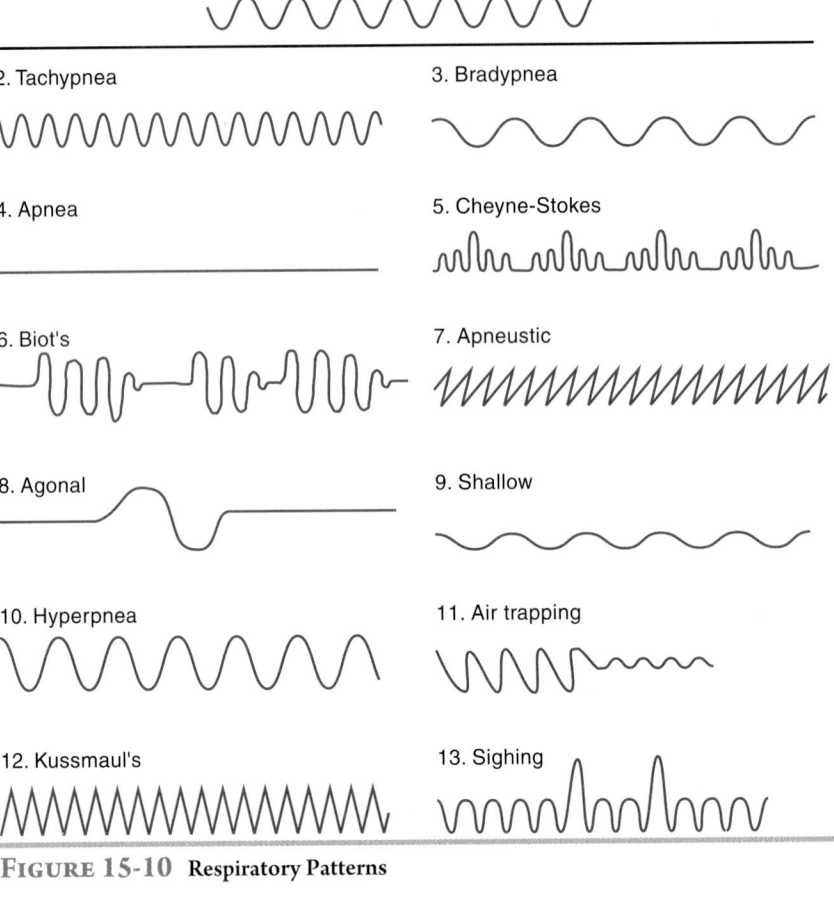

FIGURE 15-10 Respiratory Patterns

PATTERN.

E 1. Stand in front of the patient.

2. While counting the respiratory rate, note the rhythm or pattern of the breathing for regularity or irregularity (Figure 15-10).

N Normal respirations are regular and even in rhythm.

A **Cheyne-Stokes respirations** occur in crescendo and decrescendo patterns interspersed between periods of apnea that can last 15 to 30 seconds. This can be a normal finding in elderly patients and in young children. Cheyne-Stokes respiration is an example of a regularly irregular respiratory pattern, that is, the respirations predictably or regularly become irregular.

P Central cerebral or high brain-stem lesions that occur in brain injury produce Cheyne-Stokes respirations.

P Cheyne-Stokes respirations can also appear in sleep due to alterations in the respiratory center's ability to accurately perceive chemical and mechanical stimuli.

A **Biot respirations**, or **ataxic respirations**, is an example of an irregularly irregular respiratory pattern. In an irregularly irregular rhythm, there is no identifiable pattern to the respiratory cycle. There is an absence of a crescendo and decrescendo pattern. Deep and shallow breaths occur at random intervals interspersed with short and long pauses. Periods of apnea can be long and frequent.

P Biot's breathing indicates damage to the medulla.

A **Apneustic respirations** are characterized by a prolonged gasping during inspiration followed by a very short, inefficient expiration. These pauses can last 30 to 60 seconds.

P Injury to the upper portion of the pons can lead to apneustic breathing.

A **Agonal respirations** are irregularly irregular respirations. They are of varying depths and patterns.

P Impending death, where there is little or no oxygen supplying the brain, or compression of the respiratory center may lead to agonal breaths.

DEPTH.

E 1. Stand in front of the patient.

2. Observe the relative depth with which the patient draws a breath during inspiration.

N The normal depth of inspiration is nonexaggerated and effortless.

A In hypoventilation, or shallow respirations, the chest wall is moved minimally during inspiration and expiration. A small tidal volume is being inspired.

P Obese patients frequently have small tidal volumes due to the sheer weight of the chest wall and the effort it takes to move it with each breath.

P The patient in pain or with a recent abdominal or thoracic incision has shallow respirations due to the discomfort of moving the rib cage, the integument, and the respiratory muscles with each breath.

P Shallow respirations are also seen in conditions where lung pathology exists and breathing is painful: pulmonary embolus, pneumonia, pneumothorax.

A **Hyperpnea** is a breath that is greater in volume than the resting tidal volume. The respiratory rate is normal and the pattern is even in hyperpnea.

P In the warm-up and cool-down periods of exercise, hyperpnea is present. The deep breath is drawn to meet the increased metabolic needs of the body.

P Patients in highly emotional states exhibit hyperpnea as the body attempts to meet the increased oxygen demand.

P Patients who are thrust into high-altitude regions will become hyperpneic due to the decreased partial pressure of oxygen. Deep breaths and slight tachypnea represent an attempt to supply the oxygen needs of the body.

A **Air trapping** is an abnormal respiratory pattern with rapid, shallow respirations and forced expirations.

P Patients with COPD have difficulty with exhaling. When these patients exercise or experience increased heart rate, they have insufficient time to fully exhale. As a result, air is trapped in the lungs, and, over time, the chest overexpands. Likewise, an asthmatic patient experiencing an acute attack has difficulty exhaling due to increased mucus and bronchial constriction. Air trapping ensues.

A **Kussmaul's respirations** are characterized by extreme increased depth and rate of respirations. These respirations are regular and the inspiratory and expiratory processes are both active.

| **E** Examination | **N** Normal Findings | **A** Abnormal Findings | **P** Pathophysiology |

P Diabetic ketoacidosis and metabolic acidosis may result in Kussmaul's respirations. The body is lowering its $PaCO_2$ level, thereby raising the pH and attempting to correct the acidosis.

A **Sighing** is characterized by normal respirations interrupted by a deep inspiration and followed by a deep expiration. It may be accompanied by an audible sigh. Sighing is pathological if it occurs frequently.

P Excessive sighing can occur in central nervous system lesions.

SYMMETRY.

E 1. Stand in front of the patient.

2. Observe the symmetry with which the chest rises and falls during the respiratory cycle.

N The healthy adult's thorax rises and falls in unison in the respiratory cycle. There is no paradoxical movement.

A Unilateral expansion of either side of the thorax is abnormal.

P Conditions where the lung is absent or collapsed (pneumonectomy, pneumothorax) are characterized by unilateral thoracic expansion secondary to the lack of active alveolar expansion on inspiration.

P Absence of expansion is evident on the affected lung side in a patient with pulmonary fibrosis due to the thickening of the lung and decreased elasticity.

P Acute pleurisy and massive atelectasis are pathologies where pain and collapsed alveoli, respectively, interfere with the respiratory process and prevent adequate bilateral and equal chest symmetry.

A Paradoxical, or seemingly contradictory, chest wall movement is always abnormal. In paradoxical chest wall movement, the unaffected part of the thorax will rise during inspiration while the affected area will fall. Conversely, during expiration the unaffected part of the thorax will fall while the affected area will rise.

P Broken ribs from trauma to the chest wall or flail chest interferes with the normal rib cage dynamics during the respiratory process and may lead to paradoxical chest wall movement.

A Hoover's sign is the paradoxical inward movement of the lower ICS during inspiration. This occurs when the diaphragm is flat instead of its normal dome shape. Muscle fibers are horizontal, and diaphragmatic contraction pulls the rib cage inward rather than down.

P Broken ribs from trauma to the chest wall or flail chest interferes with the normal rib cage dynamics during the respiratory process and may lead to the presence of Hoover's sign.

AUDIBILITY.

E 1. Stand in front of the patient.

2. Listen for the audibility of the respirations.

N A patient's respirations are normally heard by the unaided ear a few centimeters from the patient's nose or mouth.

A It is abnormal to hear audible breathing when standing a few feet from the patient. Upper airway sounds may also be heard. These should not be confused with pulmonary sounds.

LIFE ◎ 360°

Respiratory Distress

You are attending a concert at your town's community center. Just as the concert is about to begin, the person sitting next to you grabs your hand and says, "Help me! I can't breathe." What questions would you ask the patient? What assessments could you make? How would you proceed?

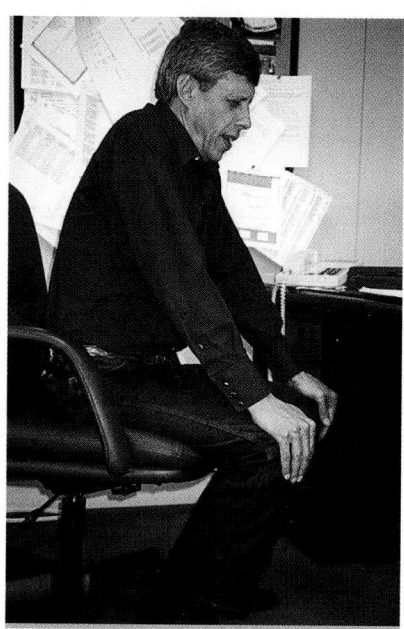

FIGURE 15-11 Tripod Position

P Any condition where air hunger exists has the potential to create audible and noisy breathing. The body is attempting to meet its oxygen demands. Examples of these states are exercise, COPD, pneumonia, and pneumothorax.

PATIENT POSITION.

E 1. Ask the patient to sit upright for the respiratory assessment.

2. View the patient either before or after the assessment and note the assumed position for breathing. Ask if the assumed position is required for respiratory comfort.

3. Note if the patient can breathe normally when in a supine position.

4. Note if pillows are used to prop the patient upright to facilitate breathing.

N The healthy adult breathes comfortably in a supine, prone, or upright position.

A Orthopnea is difficulty breathing in positions other than upright.

P COPD, congestive heart failure, and pulmonary edema exemplify conditions where orthopnea may be present. The upright position maximizes the use of the respiratory muscles in patients who might otherwise be unable to breathe in a supine position, secondary to fluid in the lungs. Patients with COPD may assume the tripod position to breathe easier and make breathing look natural (Figure 15-11). The tripod position allows for easier use of accessory muscles.

MODE OF BREATHING.

E 1. Stand in front of the patient.

2. Note whether the patient is using the nose, the mouth, or both, to breathe.

3. Note for which part of the respiratory cycle each is used.

N Normal findings vary among individuals but, generally, most patients inhale and exhale through the nose.

A Continuous mouth breathing is usually abnormal.

P Any type of nasal or sinus blockage obstructs the normal breathing passageway and leads to mouth breathing.

A Pursed-lip breathing is performed by patients who need to prolong the expiration phase of the respiratory cycle. It appears that the patient is trying to blow out a candle or is preparing for a kiss.

P Pursed-lip breathing is performed by patients with COPD. It is the patient's innate mechanism to apply positive-pressure breathing to prevent total alveolar collapse with every breath. Less energy is expended with each breath because the alveoli do not completely collapse after expiration.

A Patients may breathe through a stoma or tracheostomy (Figure 15-12).

P Patients with laryngeal cancer who have had a surgical removal of the larynx breathe initially through a tracheostomy and then through a stoma. This is their normal mode of breathing.

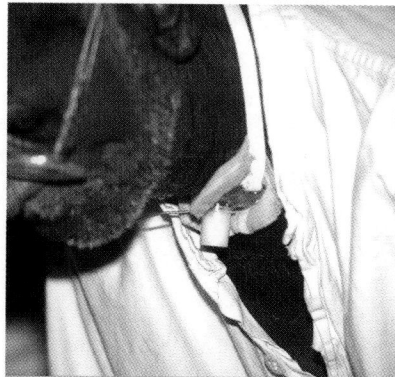

FIGURE 15-12 Tracheostomy. *Courtesy of WHO/P. Virot.*

E Examination   **N** Normal Findings   **A** Abnormal Findings   **P** Pathophysiology

TABLE 15-1 Pathologies Associated with Different Colors of Sputum

SPUTUM COLOR	PATHOLOGY
Mucoid	Tracheobronchitis, asthma, coryza
Yellow or green	Bacterial infection
Rust or blood-tinged	Pneumococcal pneumonia, pulmonary infarction, tuberculosis, lung cancer
Black	Black lung disease
Pink	Pulmonary edema

Sputum

E 1. Ask the patient to expectorate a sputum sample.

2. If the patient is unable to expectorate, ask the patient for a recent sputum sample from a handkerchief or tissue.

3. Note the color, odor, amount, and consistency of the sputum.

N A small amount of sputum is normal in every individual. The color is light yellow or clear. Normal sputum is odorless. Depending on the hydration status of the patient, the sputum can be thick or thin.

A Colors of sputum that are abnormal are mucoid, yellow or green, rust or blood-tinged, black, and pink (and frothy).

P Table 15-1 lists the pathologies that are associated with different colors of sputum.

A Foul-smelling sputum is always abnormal.

P Anaerobic infections produce foul-smelling sputum.

A A large amount of sputum can be pathological.

P Chronic bronchitis produces a large amount of sputum as a result of the irritation to the respiratory tract.

P Patients with pneumonia expectorate large quantities of sputum. The sputum is produced in reaction to the infectious process.

P An excessive amount of sputum is found in pulmonary edema, from the fluid that has leaked from pulmonary capillary membranes into large airways.

A Very thick sputum can be abnormal.

P Water is a normal component of the sputum. Therefore, when a patient is dehydrated, the sputum will be thicker because the mucus, blood, purulent material, and cellular debris form the bulk of the sputum.

A Sputum that has a thin consistency can be abnormal.

P In overhydration, the extra fluid tends to dilute the remaining components of the sputum. In pulmonary edema, the sputum is thin, pink, and frothy.

PALPATION

General Palpation

General palpation assesses the thorax for pulsations, masses, thoracic tenderness, and crepitus.

To perform anterior palpation:

E 1. Stand in front of the patient.

2. Place the finger pads of the dominant hand on the apex of the right lung (above the clavicle).

3. Using light palpation, assess the integument of the thorax in that area.

4. Move the finger pads down to the clavicle and palpate.

5. Proceed with the palpation, moving down to each rib and ICS of the right anterior thorax. Palpate any area(s) of tenderness last.

6. Repeat the procedure on the left anterior thorax.

E Examination	**N** Normal Findings	**A** Abnormal Findings	**P** Pathophysiology

To perform posterior palpation:

E 1. Stand behind the patient.

2. Place the finger pads of the dominant hand on the apex of the right lung (approximately at the level of T1).

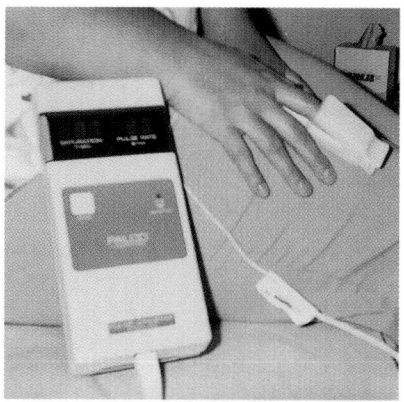

A. Pulse Oximeter

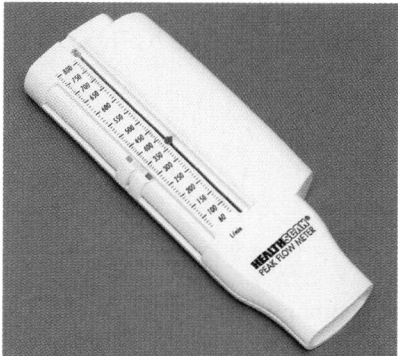

B. Peak Flow Meter

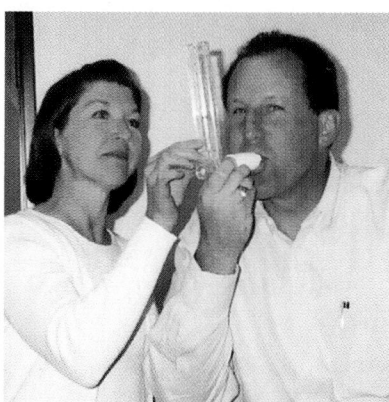

C. Patient Using Another Type of Peak Flow Meter

FIGURE 15-13 Respiratory Assistive Devices

☑ASSISTIVE DEVICES CHECKLIST

Assessing Patients with Respiratory Assistive Devices

Oxygen

- Mode of delivery (e.g., nasal cannula, face mask)
- Percentage of oxygen that is being delivered (e.g., 25%, 40%)
- Flow rate of the oxygen (e.g., 2 liters per minute, 4 liters per minute)
- Humidification provided and oxygen warmed

Incentive Spirometer

- Frequency of use
- Volume achieved (e.g., 1,000 mL, 1,500 mL)
- Number of times patient reaches goal with each use
- Endotracheal Tube
- Size of endotracheal tube
- Nasal or oral insertion
- Tube secured to the patient
- Length of the endotracheal tube as it exits the nose or the mouth (e.g., 24 cm at the lips or 27 cm at the tip of the left nare)
- Cuff inflated or deflated

Tracheostomy Tube

- Size of tracheostomy tube
- Cuff present; if yes, cuff inflated or deflated
- Tracheostomy ties secure the tube

Mechanical Ventilation

- Type of ventilator (e.g., Servo, Bear, Emerson)
- FiO_2 setting
- Mode used (e.g., assist, intermittent mandatory ventilation)
- Amount of positive end-expiratory pressure
- Rate and tidal volume
- Peak inspiratory pressure
- Temperature of the humidification
- Alarms set

Pulse Oximeter (Figure 15-13A)

- Determine the monitor's settings.
- The monitor's alarms are on. The appropriate limits are set.
- If using the probe on a nail, the patient's nail polish has been removed.
- If using the probe on the ear, the skin is intact and earrings are not interfering. Peak Flow Meter (Figure 15-13B)
- Patient is seated while performing the maneuver.
- Indicator line is lowered to the baseline level.
- Patient exhales as deeply as possible while maintaining a firm seal with the lips around the mouthpiece (Figure 15-13C).
- Patient does not obstruct the exhalation outlet.

ADVANCED TECHNIQUE

Locating the Site of a Fractured Rib

To locate the site of a fractured rib:

E 1. Tell the patient what you are going to do and that some pain may be involved.

2. Place the patient in a supine or upright position. In the latter position, support the patient's back with one hand.

3. Place your hand over the middle of the sternum and depress lightly.

4. Quickly remove your hand from the sternum.

Outcome: The patient will complain of pain at the fracture site. Have the patient point to the site of pain. This technique is not effective for the 11th and 12th pairs of ribs because of their anatomic nature and location.

3. Using light palpation, assess the integument of the thorax in that area.

4. Move the finger pads down to the first thoracic vertebra and palpate.

5. Proceed with the palpation, moving down to each thoracic vertebra and ICS of the right posterior thorax.

6. Repeat the procedure on the left posterior thorax.

To perform lateral palpation:

E 1. Stand to the patient's right side.

2. Have the patient lift the arms overhead.

3. Place the finger pads of the dominant hand beneath the right axillary fold.

4. Using light palpation, assess the integument of the thorax in that area.

5. Move the finger pads down to the first rib beneath the axillary fold.

6. Proceed with the palpation, moving down to each rib and ICS of the right lateral thorax.

7. Move to the patient's left side.

8. Repeat steps 2–6 for the left lateral thorax.

PULSATIONS.

N No pulsations should be present.

A The presence of pulsations on the thorax is abnormal.

P A thoracic aortic aneurysm that is large may be seen pulsating on the anterior chest wall.

MASSES.

N No masses should be present.

A The presence of a thoracic mass is abnormal.

P The presence of a thoracic tumor or cyst should be closely evaluated and malignancy ruled out.

THORACIC TENDERNESS.

N No thoracic tenderness should be present.

A Fractured ribs may cause thoracic tenderness.

P Blunt chest trauma can affect any component of the respiratory tract, as well as the heart and great vessels. The region involved, the type of injury, and the impact of the injury dictate the amount of internal damage.

CREPITUS.

N Crepitus should be absent.

A The presence of **crepitus**, also referred to as subcutaneous emphysema, is always an abnormal finding. Fine beads of air escape the lung and are trapped in the subcutaneous tissue. As this area is palpated, a crackling sound may be heard. This air is slowly absorbed by the body. Crepitus is usually felt earliest in the clavicular region, but it can easily be found in the neck, face, and torso. It can also be described as feeling similar to bubble packing material that can be palpated and popped.

P Any condition that interrupts the integrity of the pleura and the lungs has the potential to lead to crepitus. Pathologies where crepitus is frequently found are pneumothorax, chest trauma, thoracic surgery, mediastinal emphysema, alveolar rupture, and tearing of pleural adhesions.

NURSINGTIP

Assessing the Thoracic Skin

When palpating the thorax, remember to assess temperature, turgor, moisture, texture, and edema. See Chapter 10.

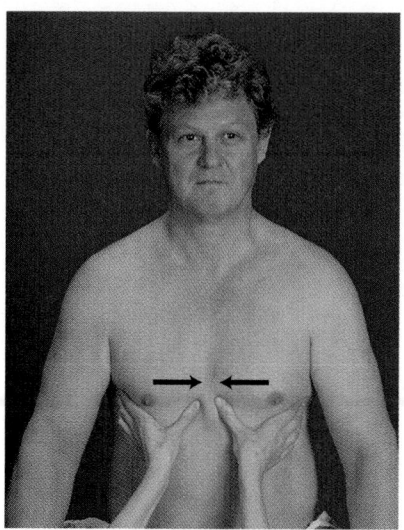

A. Anterior

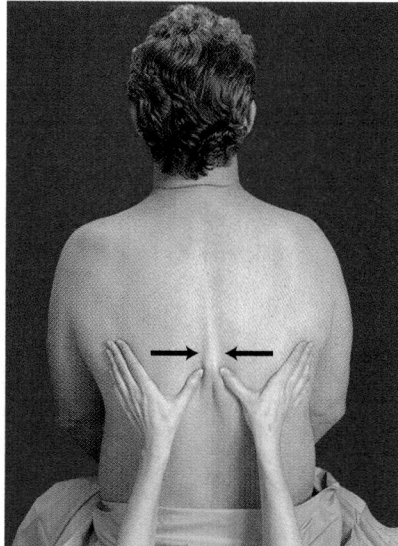

B. Posterior

FIGURE 15-14 **Thoracic Expansion**

Thoracic Expansion

Thoracic expansion assesses the extent of chest expansion and the symmetry of chest wall expansion. Anterior and posterior thoracic expansions can be assessed (Figure 15-14).

To perform anterior thoracic expansion:

E 1. Stand directly in front of the patient. Place the thumbs of both hands on the costal margins and pointing towards the xiphoid process. Gather a small fold of skin between the thumbs to assist with the visualization of the results of this technique.

2. Lay your outstretched palms on the anterolateral thorax.

3. Instruct the patient to take a deep breath.

4. Observe the movement of the thumbs, both in direction and in distance.

5. Ask the patient to exhale.

6. Observe the movement of the thumbs as they return to the midline.

To perform posterior thoracic expansion:

E 1. Stand directly behind the patient. Place the thumbs of both hands at the level of the 10th spinal vertebra, equidistant from the spinal column and approximately 1 to 3 inches apart. Gather a small amount of skin between the thumbs as directed for anterior expansion.

2. Place your outstretched palms on the posterolateral thorax.

3. Instruct the patient to take a deep breath.

4. Observe the movement of the thumbs, both in direction and in distance.

5. Ask the patient to exhale.

6. Observe the movement of the thumbs as they return to the midline.

N The thumbs separate an equal amount from the spinal column or xiphoid process (distance) and remain in the same plane of the 10th spinous vertebra or costal margin (direction). The normal distance for the thumbs to separate during thoracic expansion is 3 to 5 cm.

A Unilateral decreased thoracic expansion is abnormal.

P Unilateral decreased thoracic expansion on the affected or pathological side occurs in pneumothorax, pneumonia, atelectasis, lower lobe lobectomy, pleural effusion, and bronchiectasis. In these conditions, the alveoli are either not present or not fully expanding on the affected side due to pathology inside or external to the lung.

A Bilateral decreased thoracic expansion is an abnormal finding.

P Bilateral disease external or internal to the lungs must be present in order for bilateral decreased thoracic expansion to be present. Hypoventilation, emphysema, pulmonary fibrosis, and pleurisy exemplify diseases where the alveoli do not fully expand.

A Displacement of thumbs from the 10th spinal vertebra region (thumbs will not meet in the midline when the patient exhales) is abnormal.

P In scoliosis, the spine is laterally deviated to a particular side. Thus, when the patient takes a deep breath, there can be a slight or marked expansion of the lungs in an unequal fashion due to the compression of the lungs by the spine.

| **E** Examination | **N** Normal Findings | **A** Abnormal Findings | **P** Pathophysiology |

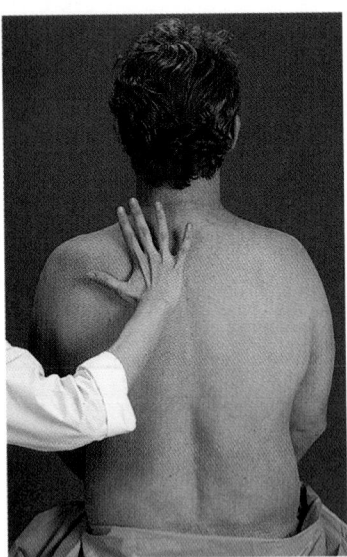

A. Using Palmar Base of Fingers

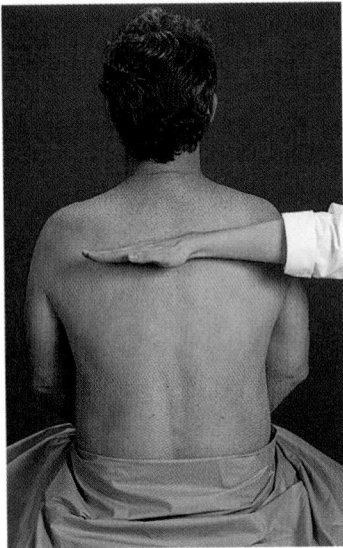

B. Using Ulnar Aspect of Hand

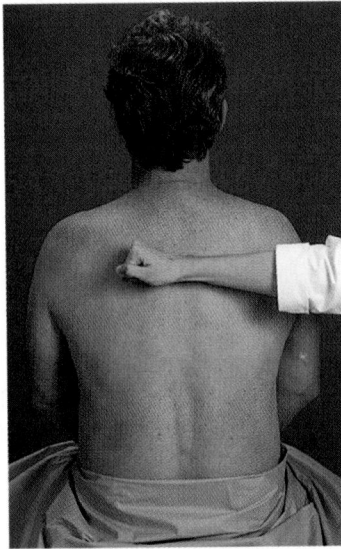

C. Using Ulnar Aspect of Closed Fist

FIGURE 15-15 **Tactile Fremitus**

Tactile Fremitus

Tactile or vocal fremitus is the palpable vibration of the chest wall that is produced by the spoken word. This technique is useful in assessing the underlying lung tissue and pleura. The anterior, posterior, and lateral chest walls are assessed. Three different aspects of the hand can be used to perform this skill: the palmar bases of the fingers, the ulnar aspect of the hand, and the ulnar aspect of a closed fist (Figure 15-15). The beginning nurse may wish to experiment with each technique and decide which is the most comfortable. It is recommended that the ulnar aspect of the hand be used initially because this exposes the least amount of surface area, and, therefore, more discrete areas can be assessed.

To perform tactile fremitus:

1. Firmly place the ulnar aspect of an open hand (or palmar base of the fingers or ulnar aspect of a closed fist) on the patient's right anterior apex (remember that this is above the clavicle).

2. Instruct the patient to say the words "99" or "1, 2, 3" with the same intensity every time you place your hand on the thorax.

3. Feel any vibration on the ulnar aspect of the hand as the patient phonates. If no fremitus is palpated, you may need to have the patient speak more loudly.

4. Move your hand to the same location on the left anterior thorax.

5. Repeat steps 2 and 3.

6. Compare the vibrations palpated on the right and left apices.

7. Move the hand down 2 to 3 inches and repeat the process on the right and then on the left. Ensure that your hand is in the ICS in order to avoid the bony structures. Minimal or no fremitus will be felt over the ribs because they lie on top of the lungs.

8. Continue this process down the anterior thorax to the base of the lungs.

9. Repeat this procedure for the lateral chest wall and compare symmetry. Either do the entire right then the entire left thorax, or alternate right and left at each ICS.

10. Repeat this procedure for the posterior chest wall. Figure 15-16 illustrates the progression of the assessment.

N Normal fremitus is felt as a buzzing on the ulnar aspect of the hand. The fremitus will be more pronounced near the major bronchi (second ICS anteriorly, and T1 and T2 posteriorly) and the trachea, and will be less palpable in the periphery of the lung. The diaphragm is approximately at the level of T10–T12 posteriorly and it is slightly higher on the right because of the presence of the liver.

A Increased tactile fremitus is abnormal.

P Diseases that involve consolidation, such as pneumonia, atelectasis, and bronchitis, also involve increased tactile fremitus in the affected area. A compressed lung will also exhibit increased tactile fremitus because solids conduct sound better than does air.

A Decreased or absent tactile fremitus is a pathological finding.

P Because porous materials conduct vibrations less effectively than do fluids and solids, decreased tactile fremitus will be present in pneumothorax, emphysema, and asthma.

P In a pleural effusion, the exudate is external to the alveoli and therefore acts as a blockade to the transmission of sound waves. This results in decreased tactile fremitus.

P A patient with a large chest wall or the obese patient will have decreased tactile fremitus because the sound waves are dampened as they pass through a greater distance.

A A high diaphragm level is abnormal.

P The diaphragm level is abnormally high in a patient with a lower lobe lobectomy. Tactile fremitus will be present above the surgical site.

A There are three additional findings that can be revealed during tactile fremitus: pleural friction fremitus, tussive fremitus, and rhonchal fremitus.

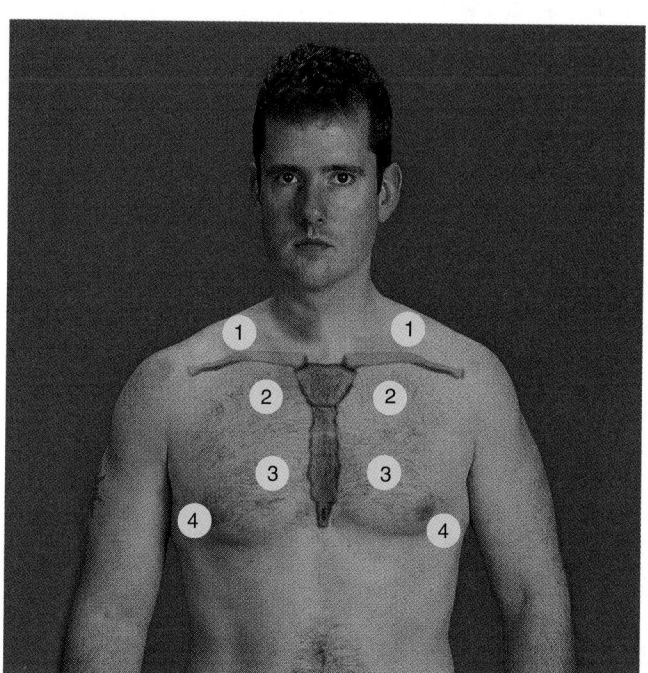

A. Anterior Thorax

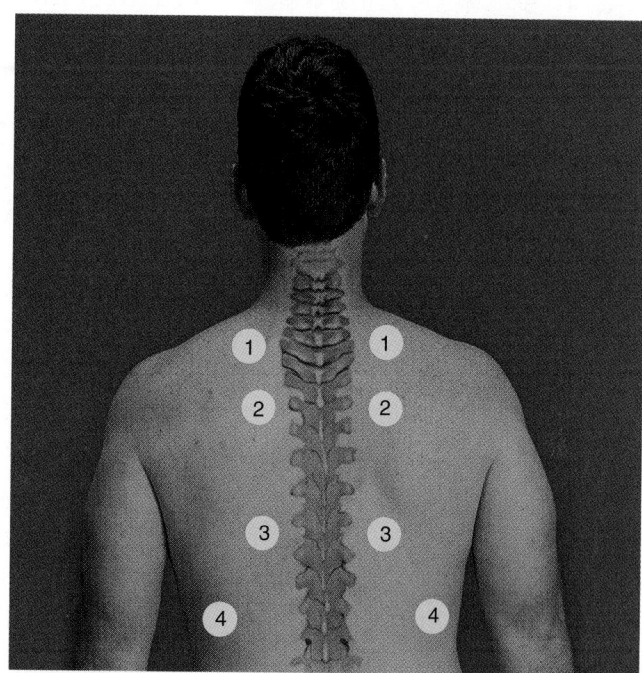

B. Posterior Thorax

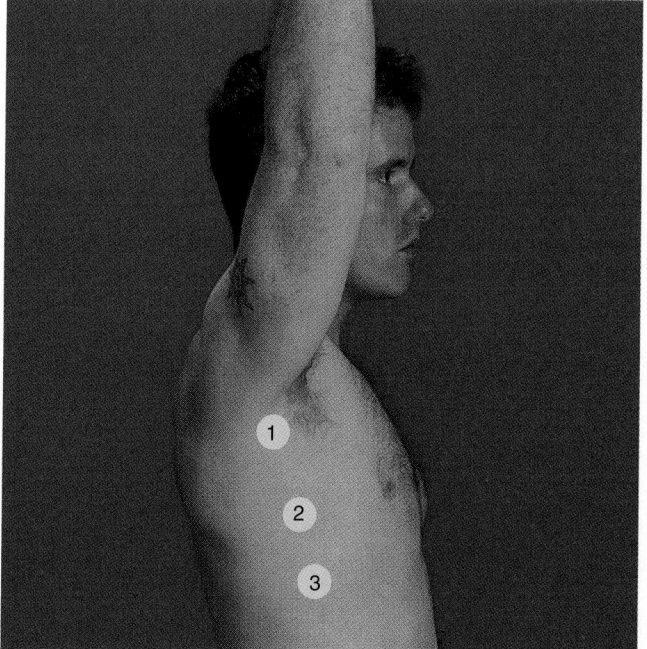

C. Right Lateral Thorax

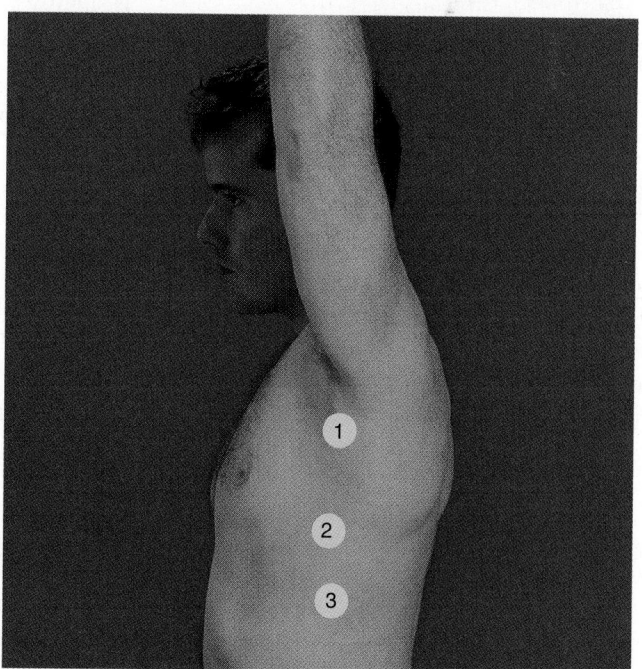

D. Left Lateral Thorax

FIGURE 15-16   **Pattern for Tactile Fremitus**

E Examination   **N** Normal Findings   **A** Abnormal Findings   **P** Pathophysiology

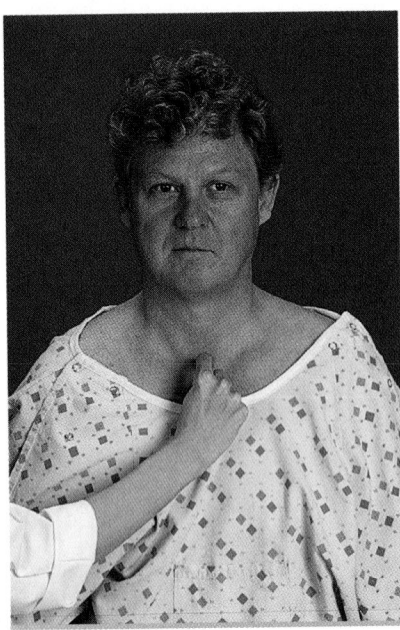

FIGURE 15-17 Assessing Tracheal Position

NURSINGTIP

Percussion Strategy

The patient may use a drape to cover the anterior thorax during posterior percussion. The entire chest must be exposed for anterior and lateral percussions.

There is no harm in repeating the percussion strike in a given area if you are uncertain about the sound that was produced or if you would like to compare it to the sound from another area. Remember to always visualize the underlying structures that are being assessed.

P **Pleural friction fremitus** is a palpable grating sensation that feels more pronounced on inspiration when there is an inflammatory process between the visceral and the parietal pleuras.

P **Tussive fremitus** is the palpable vibration produced by coughing.

P **Rhonchal fremitus** is the coarse palpable vibration produced by the passage of air through thick exudate in large bronchi or the trachea. This can clear with coughing.

Tracheal Position

To assess the position of the trachea:

E 1. Place the finger pad of the index finger on the patient's trachea in the suprasternal notch (Figure 15-17).

2. Move the finger pad laterally to the right and gently move the trachea in the space created by the border of the inner aspect of the sternocleido-mastoid muscle and the clavicle.

3. Move the finger pad laterally to the left and repeat the procedure.

Another method by which the trachea can be palpated is:

E 1. Gently place the finger pad of the index finger in the midline of the suprasternal notch.

2. Palpate for the position of the trachea.

N The trachea is midline in the suprasternal notch.

A Tracheal deviation to the affected side is abnormal.

P The normal midline position of the trachea is maintained by the counterbalancing forces of the air in the alveoli in the right and left lungs. In atelectasis and pneumonia, alveoli are closed to some degree or filled with exudate. Fewer aerating alveoli are present and therefore the trachea is slightly pushed by the healthy lung to the affected side, which contains less air.

P The mechanical pulling force of ventilator tubing that is attached to an endotracheal tube or tracheostomy for a prolonged period of time can cause tracheal deviation toward the side of the pulling.

A Tracheal deviation to the unaffected side is abnormal.

P A tension pneumothorax, pleural effusion, and a tumor may each generate sufficient pressure to force the trachea toward the unaffected side.

P An enlarged thyroid may also deviate the trachea via its space-occupying capacity.

PERCUSSION

Indirect or mediate percussion is used to further assess the underlying structures of the thorax. Remember that percussion reverberates a sound that is generated from structures approximately 5 cm below the chest wall. Deep pathological conditions will not be revealed during the percussion process.

General Percussion

Figure 15-18 demonstrates the percussion pattern for the anterior, posterior, right lateral, and left lateral thoraxes.

E Examination	**N** Normal Findings	**A** Abnormal Findings	**P** Pathophysiology

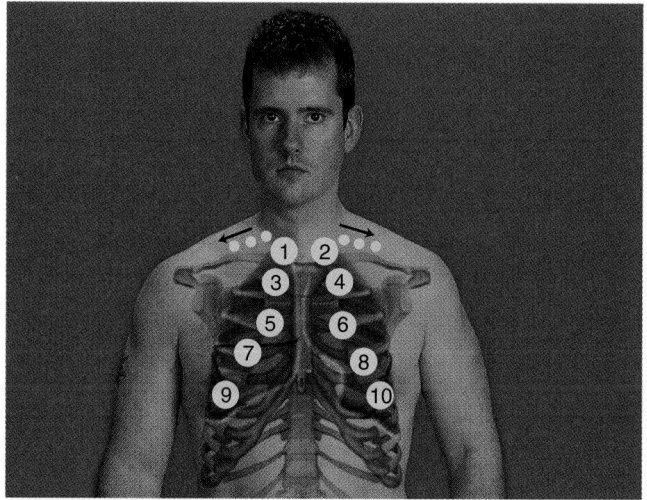

A. Anterior Thorax

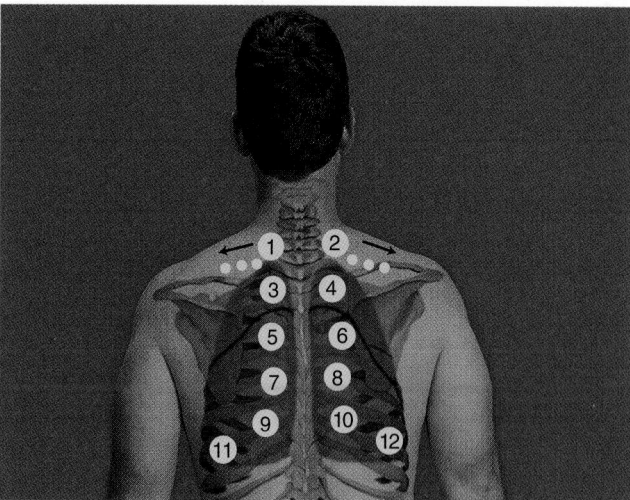

B. Posterior Thorax

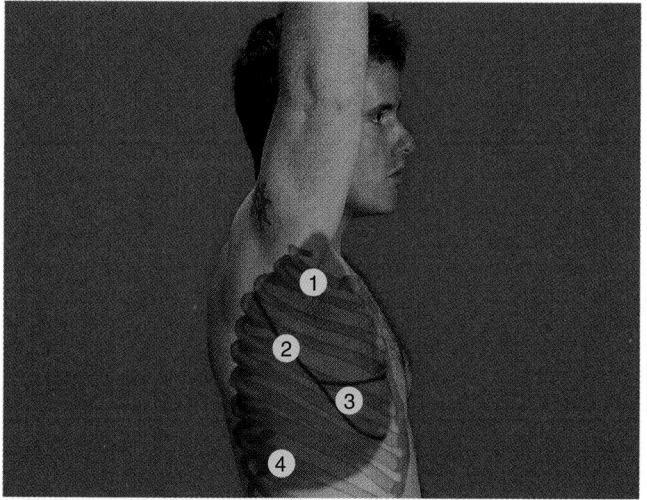

C. Right Lateral Thorax

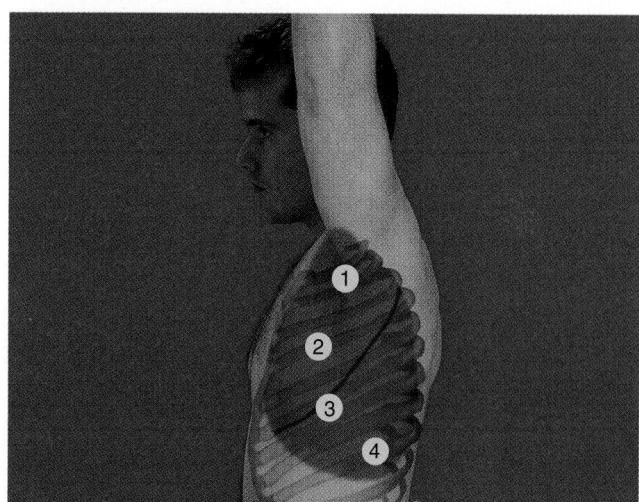

D. Left Lateral Thorax

FIGURE 15-18 **Percussion Patterns**

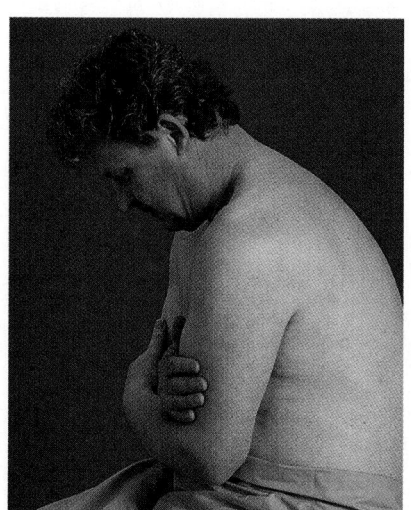

FIGURE 15-19 **Patient Position for Posterior Percussion**

To perform anterior thoracic percussion:

E 1. Place the patient in an upright sitting position with the shoulders back.

2. Percuss two or three strikes along the right lung apex.

3. Repeat this process at the left lung apex.

4. Note the sound produced from each percussion strike and compare the sounds from each. If different sounds are produced or if the sound is not resonant, then pathology is suggested.

5. Move down approximately 5 cm, or every other ICS, and percuss in that area.

6. Percuss in the same position on the contralateral side.

7. Continue to move down until the entire lung has been percussed.

To perform posterior thoracic percussion:

E 1. Place the patient in an upright sitting position with a slight forward tilt. Have the patient bend the head down and fold the arms in front at the waist. These actions move the scapula laterally and maximize the lung area that can be percussed (Figure 15-19).

2. Percuss the right lung apex located along the top of the shoulder. Approximately three percussion strikes should be struck along this area.

3. Repeat the process on the left lung apex.

4. Note the sound produced from each percussion strike and compare the sounds from each. If different sounds are produced or if the sound is not resonant, then pathology is suggested.

5. Move down approximately 5 cm, or every other ICS, and percuss in that area.

6. Percuss in the same position on the contralateral side.

7. Continue to move down the thorax until the entire posterior lung field has been percussed.

To perform lateral thoracic percussion:

E 1. Place the patient in an upright sitting position, with hands and arms raised directly overhead. This position allows for the greatest exposure of the thorax.

2. Either percuss the entire right lateral thorax and then the entire left lateral thorax, or alternate right and left sides. Start to percuss in the ICS directly below the axilla.

3. Note the sound produced from that strike.

4. Percuss approximately 5 cm below the original location, or about every other ICS.

5. Percuss down to the base of the lung.

N Normal lung tissue produces a resonant sound. The diaphragm and the cardiac silhouette emit dull sounds. Rib sounds are flat. Hyperresonance is normal in thin adults and in patients with decreased musculature.

A The presence of hyperresonance in the majority of adults is abnormal.

P Hyperresonance is percussed in air-filled spaces. It can be elicited in pneumothorax, emphysema, asthma, and an emphysematous bulla.

A The healthy human lung never produces a dull sound.

P Dullness is found in solid or fluid-filled structures. Pneumonia, atelectasis, pulmonary edema, pleural effusion, pulmonary fibrosis, hemothorax, empyema, and tumors are dull to percussion.

Diaphragmatic Excursion

Diaphragmatic excursion provides information on the patient's depth of ventilation. This is accomplished by measuring the distance the diaphragm moves during inspiration and expiration.

To perform diaphragmatic excursion:

E 1. Position the patient for posterior thoracic percussion.

2. With the patient breathing normally, percuss the right lung from the apex (resonance in healthy adults) to below the diaphragm (dull). Note the level at which the percussion note changes quality to orient your assessment to the patient's percussion sounds. If full posterior thoracic percussion has already been performed, then this step can be eliminated.

3. Instruct the patient to inhale as deeply as possible and hold that breath.

4. With the patient holding the breath, percuss the right lung in the scapular line from below the scapula to the location where resonance changes to dullness.

5. Mark this location and tell the patient to exhale and breathe normally.

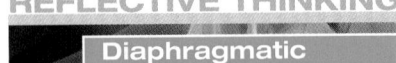

REFLECTIVE THINKING

Diaphragmatic Excursion Technique

You are performing diaphragmatic excursion on a patient. Midway through performing this assessment, the patient states, "Are you sure you know what you are doing? You keep tapping me and I keep breathing over and over." How would you respond to the patient? Would you alter your assessment any after this comment? Why?

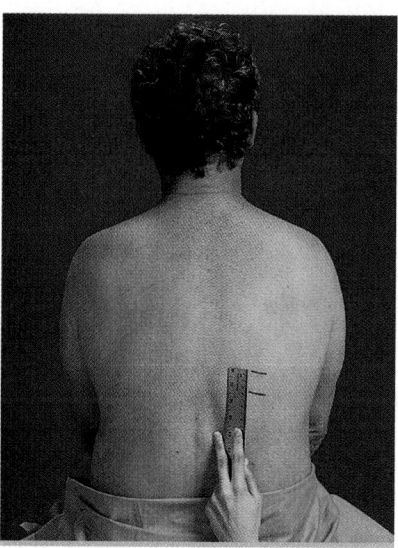

FIGURE 15-20 Diaphragmatic Excursion

6. When the patient has recovered, instruct the patient to inhale as deeply as possible, exhale fully, and hold this exhaled breath.

7. Repercuss the right lung below the scapula in the scapular line in a caudal direction. Mark the spot where resonance changes to dullness.

8. Measure the distance between the two marks.

9. Repeat steps 1–8 for the left posterior thorax. Figure 15-20 illustrates diaphragmatic excursion.

N The measured distance for diaphragmatic excursion is normally 3 to 5 cm. The level of the diaphragm on inspiration is T12, and T10 on expiration. The right side of the diaphragm is usually slightly higher than the left.

A A diaphragmatic excursion that is less than 3 cm is abnormal.

P Conditions involving hypoventilation, where the patient is unable to inhale deeply or hold that breath, can lead to a reduction in the diaphragmatic excursion. Pain, obesity, lung congestion, emphysema, asthma, and pleurisy are examples.

A A high diaphragm level suggests lung pathology.

P Surgical intervention can elevate the diaphragm. If a lower lobe lobectomy is performed, the diaphragm will move upward to partially fill the empty space. Likewise, after a pneumonectomy the paralyzed diaphragm will move upward, leading to a high diaphragm level.

P Space-occupying states such as ascites and pregnancy will lead to an elevated diaphragm due to the upward displacement of the lungs and diaphragm.

P If atelectasis or a pleural effusion is present in a lower lobe, then the diaphragm will seem abnormally high, because these conditions are dull to percussion as is the diaphragm. The border between the diaphragm and the dull lung will thus be indistinguishable.

AUSCULTATION

The aim of respiratory auscultation is to identify the presence of normal breath sounds, abnormal lung sounds, adventitious (or added) lung sounds, and adventitious pleural sounds. The anterior, posterior, and lateral aspects of the chest are auscultated. A stethoscope is required for this assessment. If an acoustic stethoscope is used, the diaphragm, which transmits high-pitched sounds, is the headpiece of choice.

General Auscultation

To perform anterior thoracic auscultation:

E 1. Place the patient in an upright sitting position with the shoulders back.

2. Instruct the patient to breathe only through the mouth. Mouth breathing, when compared to nasal breathing, decreases air turbulence, which can interfere with the interpretation of breath sounds. Have the patient inhale and exhale deeply and slowly every time the stethoscope is felt or when instructed to do so.

3. Place the stethoscope on the apex of the right lung and listen for one complete respiratory cycle (one inhalation and one exhalation).

| **E** Examination | **N** Normal Findings | **A** Abnormal Findings | **P** Pathophysiology |

4. Note the sound that is auscultated.

5. Repeat on the left apex.

6. Note the breath sound auscultated in each area and compare one side to the other.

7. Continue to move the stethoscope down approximately 5 cm, or every other ICS, comparing contralateral sides. Remember to visualize the anatomic topography of the chest during auscultation.

To perform posterior thoracic auscultation:

E 1. Place the patient as shown in Figure 15-19, in an upright sitting position with a slight forward tilt, head bent down, and arms folded in front at the waist. These actions move the scapula laterally and maximize the lung area that can be auscultated.

2. Place the stethoscope firmly on the patient's right lung apex. Ask the patient to inhale and exhale deeply and slowly every time the stethoscope is felt on the back.

3. Repeat this process on the left lung apex.

4. Move the stethoscope down approximately 5 cm, or every other ICS, and auscultate in that area.

5. Auscultate in the same position on the contralateral side.

6. Continue to move inferiorly with the auscultation until the entire posterior lung has been assessed. See Figure 15-18 from the percussion section for the recommended stethoscope location for each auscultation.

To perform lateral thoracic auscultation:

E 1. Place the patient in an upright sitting position with the hands and arms directly overhead.

2. Auscultate the entire right thorax first, then the entire left thorax, or auscultate the right and left lateral thoraxes by comparing side to side. The stethoscope should initially be placed in the ICS directly below the axilla.

3. Instruct the patient to breathe only through the mouth. Have the patient inhale and exhale deeply and slowly every time the stethoscope is felt on the lateral thorax.

4. Note the sound that is auscultated and continue to move the stethoscope inferiorly approximately every 5 cm, or every other ICS, until the entire thorax has been auscultated.

Breath Sounds

N Air rushing through the respiratory tract during inspiration and expiration generates different breath sounds in the normal patient. There are three distinct types of normal breath sounds (see Figure 15-21):

1. Bronchial (or tubular)

2. Bronchovesicular

3. Vesicular

Each breath sound is unique in its pitch, intensity, quality, relative duration in the inspiratory and expiratory phases of respiration, and location. Table 15-2 depicts this information. It is abnormal to auscultate these breath sounds in locations other than where they are usually found. For example, a patient with emphysema may have bronchial breath sounds in the peripheral lung

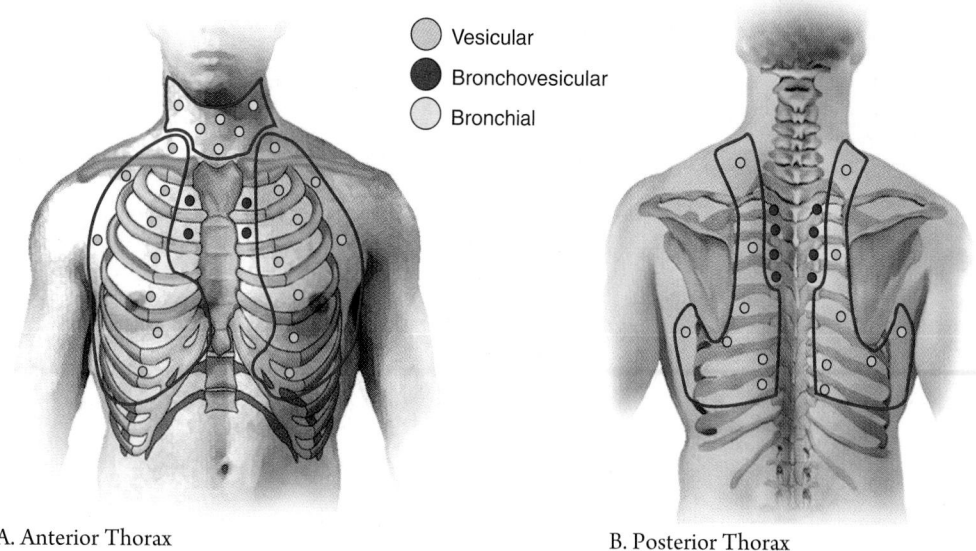

A. Anterior Thorax   B. Posterior Thorax

FIGURE 15-21 Location of Breath Sounds

parenchyma, where vesicular sounds are expected to be found. Also keep in mind that heart sounds may obscure some of the breath sounds during the anterior chest auscultation.

Breath sounds that are not normal can be classified as either abnormal or adventitious breath sounds. Abnormal breath sounds are characterized by decreased or absent breath sounds. **Adventitious breath sounds** are superimposed sounds on the normal bronchial, bronchovesicular, and vesicular breath sounds. There are six adventitious breath sounds:

1. Fine crackle
2. Coarse crackle
3. Sonorous wheeze

4. Sibilant wheeze
5. Pleural friction rub
6. Stridor

Table 15-3 depicts general characteristics of adventitious breath sounds.

TABLE 15-2 Characteristics of Normal Breath Sounds

BREATH SOUND	PITCH	INTENSITY	QUALITY	RELATIVE DURATION OF INSPIRATORY AND EXPIRATORY PHASES	LOCATION
Bronchial	High	Loud	Blowing or hollow	I < E	Trachea
Bronchovesicular	Moderate	Moderate	Combination of bronchial and vesicular	I = E	Between scapulae, first and second ICS lateral to the sternum
Vesicular	Low	Soft	Gentle rustling or breezy	I > E	Peripheral lung

E Examination   N Normal Findings   A Abnormal Findings   P Pathophysiology

TABLE 15-3 Characteristics of Adventitious Breath Sounds

BREATH SOUND	RESPIRATORY PHASE	TIMING	DESCRIPTION	CLEAR WITH COUGH	ETIOLOGY	CONDITIONS
Fine crackle (rale)	Predominantly inspiration	Discontinuous	Dry, high-pitched crackling, popping, short duration; roll hair near ears between your fingers to simulate this sound	No	Air passing through moisture in small airways that suddenly reinflate	COPD, congestive heart failure (CHF), pneumonia, pulmonary fibrosis, atelectasis
Coarse crackle (coarse rale)	Predominantly inspiration	Discontinuous	Moist, low-pitched crackling, gurgling; long duration	Possibly	Air passing through moisture in large airways that suddenly reinflate	Pneumonia, pulmonary edema, bronchitis, atelectasis
Sonorous wheeze (rhonchi)	Predominantly expiration	Continuous	Low pitched; snoring	Possibly	Narrowing of large airways or obstruction of bronchus	Asthma, bronchitis, airway edema, tumor, bronchiolar spasm, foreign body obstruction
Sibilant wheeze (wheeze)	Predominantly expiration	Continuous	High pitched; musical	Possibly	Narrowing of large airways or obstruction of bronchus	Asthma, chronic bronchitis, emphysema, tumor, foreign body obstruction
Pleural friction rub	Inspiration and expiration	Continuous	Creaking, grating	No	Inflamed parietal and visceral pleura; can occasionally be felt on thoracic wall as two pieces of dry leather rubbing against each other	Pleurisy, tuberculosis, pulmonary infarction, pneumonia, lung abscess
Stridor	Predominantly inspiration	Continuous	Crowing	No	Partial obstruction of the larynx, trachea	Croup, foreign body obstruction, large airway tumor

A Decreased breath sounds are abnormal.

P Decreased breath sounds may be noted when auscultating a large chest because of the distance between the lungs, where the sounds are generated, and the chest wall.

P An emphysematous patient may have decreased breath sounds due to the inability to inhale and exhale deeply.

P Conditions such as bronchial obstruction and atelectasis may lead to decreased breath sounds because a foreign object or sputum occludes some portion of the respiratory tract, thus blocking the passage of air.

A Absent breath sounds are always a pathological finding.

P A pleural effusion, tumor, pulmonary fibrosis, empyema, hemothorax, and hydrothorax lead to absent breath sounds. These states occupy or displace normal aerating lung space internally or externally to the lungs.

P A patient with a large pneumothorax can present with absent breath sounds due to the collapse of the lung.

P Absent breath sounds occur when the lung has been removed (pneumonectomy).

P Blocked passageways in the respiratory tract explain the etiology for absent breath sounds in pulmonary edema, massive atelectasis, and complete airway obstruction.

Voice Sounds

The assessment of **voice sounds** will reveal whether the lungs are filled with air, with fluid, or are solid. This auscultation need be performed only if an abnormality is detected during the general auscultation, percussion, or palpation. There are three techniques by which voice sounds can be assessed:

1. Bronchophony
2. Egophony
3. Whispered pectoriloquy

Only one of these assessments needs to be performed because they all are variations of the same physical principle and assessment technique, and they all provide the same information. The voice sound findings will parallel those obtained during tactile fremitus. Thus, voice sounds will be heard loudest over the trachea and softest in the lung's periphery.

To perform **bronchophony**:

E 1. Position the patient for posterior, lateral, or anterior chest auscultation. The area to be auscultated will be that in which an abnormality was found during percussion or palpation or in which adventitious breath sounds were heard.

2. Place the stethoscope in the appropriate location on the patient's chest.

3. Instruct the patient to say the words "99" or "1, 2, 3" every time the stethoscope is placed on the chest or when told to do so.

4. Auscultate the transmission of the patient's spoken word.

ADVANCED TECHNIQUE

Forced Expiratory Time

Forced expiratory time is a gross measurement of the forced expiratory volume (FEV).

To perform this assessment:

E 1. Place your stethoscope over the patient's trachea.

2. Instruct the patient to inhale as deeply as possible and then exhale forcefully through the mouth (as if blowing out a candle).

3. Time the exhalation phase.

N Normal exhalation occurs in less than 4 seconds.

A The forced expiratory time is abnormal if it is greater than 4 seconds.

P Patients with COPD have a prolonged forced expiratory time and FEV because of the air trapping in the lungs. A complete exhalation is difficult to achieve.

To perform **egophony**:

E 1. Repeat steps 1 and 2 from the bronchophony procedure.

2. Instruct the patient to say the sound "ee" every time the stethoscope is placed on the chest or when told to do so.

3. Auscultate the transmission of the patient's spoken word.

To perform **whispered pectoriloquy**:

E 1. Repeat steps 1 and 2 from the bronchophony procedure.

2. Instruct the patient to whisper the words "99" or "1, 2, 3" every time the stethoscope is placed on the chest or when told to do so.

3. Auscultate the transmission of the patient's spoken word.

N The normal finding when performing tests for bronchophony, egophony, and whispered pectoriloquy is an unclear transmission or muffled sounds.

A Positive (or present) voice sounds are:

Bronchophony: clear transmission of "99" or "1, 2, 3" with increased intensity.

Egophony: transformation of "ee" to "ay" with increased intensity; the voice has a nasal or bleating quality.

Whispered pectoriloquy: clear transmission of "99" or "1, 2, 3" with increased intensity.

P Any type of consolidation process, such as pneumonia, will produce positive voice sounds. Remember the principle that sound is transmitted reasonably well by a fluid medium.

A Voice sounds are absent or even more decreased than in the normal lung in conditions where the lung is more air filled than usual.

P Air conducts sound poorly. Therefore, air-filled lungs (emphysema, asthma, pneumothorax) will produce absent voice sounds.

Figure 15-22 illustrates these conditions. Table 15-4 compares physical assessment findings for 12 respiratory conditions.

NURSING ALERT

Risk Factors for Pneumonia

- Smoking
- Advanced age
- Underlying lung disease
- Malnutrition
- Intoxication
- Bedridden status
- Postoperative status
- Immunosuppressed status
- Decreased cough reflex
- Sedated or decreased consciousness
- Oxygen therapy that is harboring bacteria

E Examination   **N** Normal Findings   **A** Abnormal Findings   **P** Pathophysiology

Left lung: depicts healthy lung
Right lung: depicts pathology

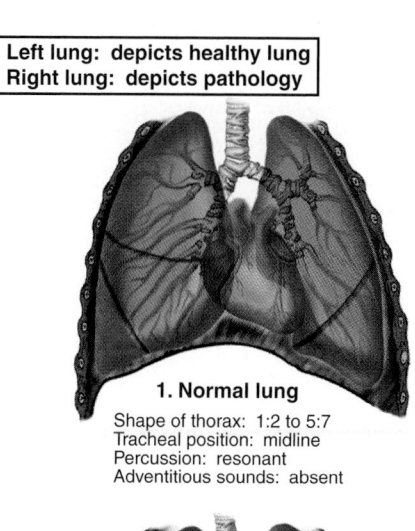

1. Normal lung

Shape of thorax: 1:2 to 5:7
Tracheal position: midline
Percussion: resonant
Adventitious sounds: absent

Bronchial edema with
increased production of thick mucus

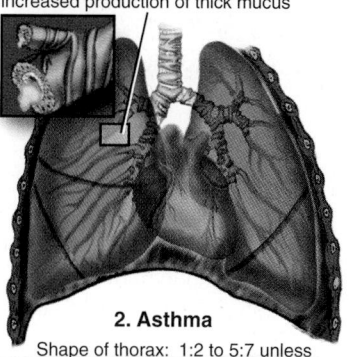

2. Asthma

Shape of thorax: 1:2 to 5:7 unless
chronic may have barrel chest
Tracheal position: midline
Percussion: hyperresonant
Adventitious sounds: wheezes

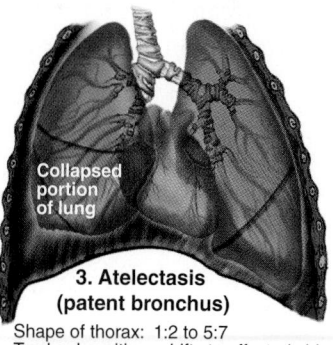

Collapsed
portion
of lung

**3. Atelectasis
(patent bronchus)**

Shape of thorax: 1:2 to 5:7
Tracheal position: shifts to affected side
Percussion: dull
Adventitious sounds: crackles or wheezes

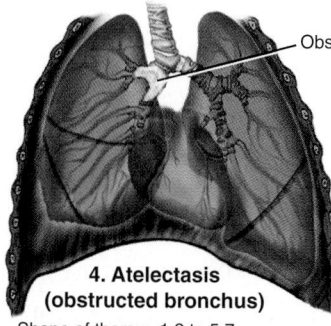

Obstruction

**4. Atelectasis
(obstructed bronchus)**

Shape of thorax: 1:2 to 5:7
Tracheal position: shifts to affected side
Percussion: dull
Adventitious sounds: absent

Dilated
bronchi

5. Bronchiectasis

Shape of thorax: 1:1
Tracheal position: midline or
deviated toward affected side
Percussion: resonant to dull
Adventitious sounds: crackles
or wheezes

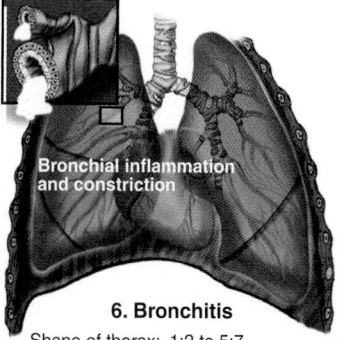

Bronchial inflammation
and constriction

6. Bronchitis

Shape of thorax: 1:2 to 5:7
Tracheal position: midline
Percussion: resonant
Adventitious sounds: crackles or
wheezes

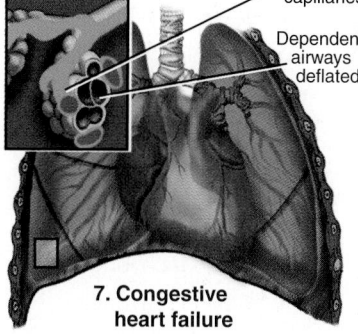

Engorged
pulmonary
capillaries

Dependent
airways
deflated

**7. Congestive
heart failure**

Shape of thorax: 1:2 to 5:7
Tracheal position: midline
Percussion: resonant
Adventitious sounds: crackles

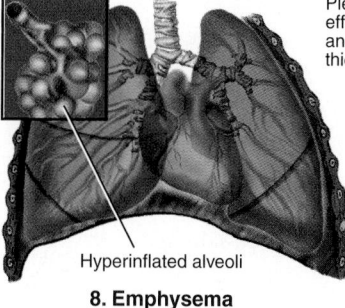

Hyperinflated alveoli

8. Emphysema

Shape of thorax: 1:1
Tracheal position: midline
Percussion: hyperresonant
Adventitious sounds: wheezes

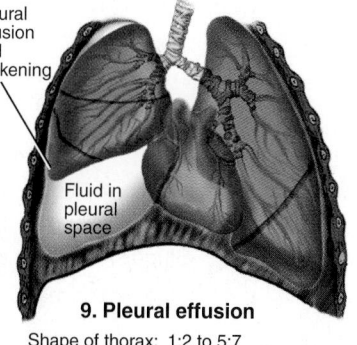

Pleural
effusion
and
thickening

Fluid in
pleural
space

9. Pleural effusion

Shape of thorax: 1:2 to 5:7
Tracheal position: shifts to unaffected side
Percussion: dull
Adventitious sounds: possible friction rub

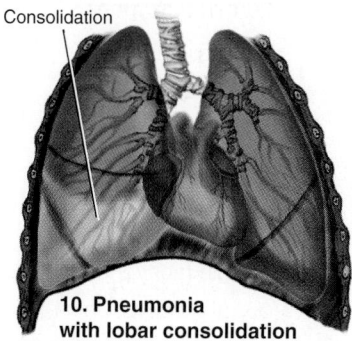

Consolidation

**10. Pneumonia
with lobar consolidation**

Shape of thorax: 1:2 to 5:7
Tracheal position: shifts to affected side
Percussion: dull
Adventitious sounds: crackles or
occasional friction rub

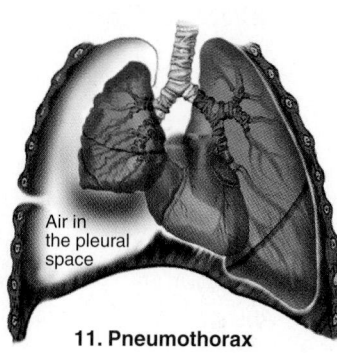

Air in
the pleural
space

11. Pneumothorax

Shape of thorax: 1:2 to 5:7
Tracheal position: shifts to
unaffected side
Percussion: hyperresonant
Adventitious sounds: absent

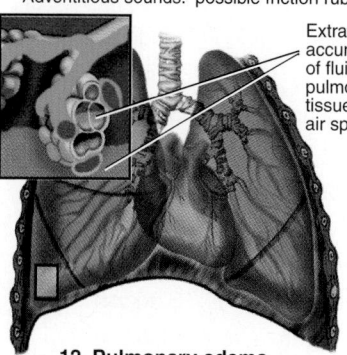

Extravascular
accumulation
of fluid in the
pulmonary
tissues and
air spaces

12. Pulmonary edema

Shape of thorax: 1:2 to 5:7
Tracheal position: midline
Percussion: dull
Adventitious sounds: crackles

FIGURE 15-22 **Comparison of Selected Respiratory Conditions**

TABLE 15-4 Comparison of Physical Assessment Findings in Selected Respiratory Conditions

	INSPECTION		
CONDITION	*SHAPE OF THORAX*	*SKIN COLOR: LIPS AND NAILS*	*CLUBBING, ANGLE OF RIBS*
A. Normal lung	1:2 to 5:7	Pink in light-skinned individuals; darker than normal in dark-skinned individuals	No clubbing, rib angle 45°
B. Asthma	If chronic, may have barrel chest	Pale or cyanotic in acute attack	No clubbing, rib angle 45°
C. Atelectasis (patent bronchus)	1:2 to 5:7	Pale or cyanotic	No clubbing, rib angle 45°
D. Atelectasis (obstructed bronchus)	1:2 to 5:7	Pale or cyanotic	No clubbing, rib angle 45°
E. Bronchiectasis	1:1 (barrel chest)	Pale or cyanotic if severe	Clubbing possible, rib angle > 45°
F. Bronchitis	1:2 to 5:7	Possibly pale	No clubbing, rib angle 45°
G. Congestive heart failure	1:2 to 5:7	Pale or cyanotic	Clubbing possible, rib angle 45°
H. Emphysema	1:1 (barrel chest)	Pale	Clubbing, rib angle > 45°
I. Pleural effusion	1:2 to 5:7	Pale or cyanotic	No clubbing, rib angle 45°
J. Pneumonia with lobar consolidation	1:2 to 5:7	Pale or cyanotic	No clubbing, rib angle 45°
K. Pneumothorax	1:2 to 5:7	Pale or cyanotic	No clubbing, rib angle 45°
L. Pulmonary edema	1:2 to 5:7	Pale or cyanotic	No clubbing, rib angle 45°

	INSPECTION		
CONDITION	*CAPILLARY REFILL*	*RETRACTIONS OR BULGING OF ICS*	*RESPIRATORY RATE*
A. Normal lung	Brisk	Absent	12–20/min eupnea
B. Asthma	Sluggish in acute attack	Retractions	> 20/min tachypnea
C. Atelectasis (patent bronchus)	Sluggish to moderate	Absent	> 20/min tachypnea
D. Atelectasis (obstructed bronchus)	Sluggish	Absent	> 20/min tachypnea
E. Bronchiectasis	Sluggish if severe	Retractions if severe	> 20/min tachypnea
F. Bronchitis	Sluggish to moderate	Absent	> 20/min tachypnea
G. Congestive heart failure	Sluggish	Retractions	> 20/min tachypnea
H. Emphysema	Sluggish	Both present	> 20/min tachypnea
I. Pleural effusion	Sluggish	Bulging	> 20/min tachypnea
J. Pneumonia with lobar consolidation	Sluggish	Absent	> 20/min tachypnea
K. Pneumothorax	Sluggish	Bulging	> 20/min tachypnea
L. Pulmonary edema	Sluggish	Absent	> 20/min tachypnea

continues

TABLE 15-4 (Continued)

PALPATION

CONDITION	THORACIC EXPANSION	TACTILE FREMITUS	TRACHEAL POSITION
A. Normal lung	3–5 cm	Moderate (normal)	Midline
B. Asthma	Decreased in attack	Decreased	Midline
C. Atelectasis (patent bronchus)	Decreased	Increased	Shifts to affected side
D. Atelectasis (obstructed bronchus)	Decreased	Increased	Shifts to affected side
E. Bronchiectasis	Decreased on affected side	Increased	Midline or deviated toward affected side
F. Bronchitis	Possibly decreased	Moderate or increased	Midline
G. Congestive heart failure	May be decreased	Moderate	Midline
H. Emphysema	Decreased	Decreased	Midline
I. Pleural effusion	Decreased	Decreased	Shifts to unaffected side
J. Pneumonia with lobar consolidation	Decreased	Increased	Shifts to affected side
K. Pneumothorax	Decreased	Absent or decreased	Shifts to unaffected side
L. Pulmonary edema	Decreased	Increased	Midline

PERCUSSION

CONDITION	GENERAL PERCUSSION	DIAPHRAGMATIC EXCURSION
A. Normal lung	Resonant	3–5 cm
B. Asthma	Hyperresonant	Decreased
C. Atelectasis (patent bronchus)	Dull	Decreased
D. Atelectasis (obstructed bronchus)	Dull	Decreased
E. Bronchiectasis	Resonant to dull	Decreased
F. Bronchitis	Resonant	Decreased if severe
G. Congestive heart failure	Resonant	Decreased
H. Emphysema	Hyperresonant	Decreased
I. Pleural effusion	Dull	Decreased
J. Pneumonia with lobar consolidation	Dull	Decreased
K. Pneumothorax	Hyperresonant	Decreased
L. Pulmonary edema	Dull	Decreased

AUSCULTATION

CONDITION	BREATH SOUNDS	ADVENTITIOUS SOUNDS	VOICE SOUNDS
A. Normal lung	Vesicular in periphery	Absent	Muffled
B. Asthma	Decreased or absent in severe obstruction	Wheezes	Decreased
C. Atelectasis (patent bronchus)	Bronchial	Crackles or wheezes	Increased or muffled
D. Atelectasis (obstructed bronchus)	Absent or decreased	Absent	Absent or muffled
E. Bronchiectasis	Vesicular or bronchial if severe	Crackles or wheezes	Muffled or decreased

continues

TABLE 15-4 (Continued)

	AUSCULTATION (continues)		
CONDITION	BREATH SOUNDS	ADVENTITIOUS SOUNDS	VOICE SOUNDS
F. Bronchitis	Vesicular or bronchial	Crackles or wheezes	Increased of muffled
G. Congestive heart failure	Vesicular	Crackles	Muffled
H. Emphysema	Bronchial and decreased	Wheezes	Decreased
I. Pleural effusion	Absent or decreased	Possible friction rub	Decreased or absent
J. Pneumonia with lobar consolidation	Bronchial	Crackles or occasional friction rub	Increased
K. Pneumothorax	Absent or decreased	Absent	Decreased or absent
L. Pulmonary edema	Absent or decreased	Crackles	Increased

CASE STUDY

The Patient with Asthma

This case study illustrates the application and objective documentation of the thorax and lungs assessment. Mel Yenouskas visits an Urgent Care center for an illness while on vacation.

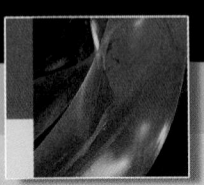

HEALTH HISTORY

PATIENT PROFILE   25 yo MWF

CHIEF COMPLAINT   "I feel so tight in my chest and I can't catch my breath."

HISTORY OF PRESENT ILLNESS   Pt was in her usual state of hl until 3 days ago, when she came to an East Coast beach community for vacation. She reports that this is the 3rd year in a row that she has been in the same rental unit and has been "sick." She reports clear rhinorrhea, frequent throat clearing, itchy ears, and itchy hard palate. The sx seem to be worse p̄ spending time in the family room of the vacation home. When she goes to bed she feels "tight" in her chest and winded, requiring the use of 2 pillows to get through the night. Pt denies fever, H/A, tooth pain, sputum, facial pressure, otalgia, and wheezing. She normally swims 1 mile freestyle daily but has been unable to do that today due to sx. Pt denies tobacco use and secondhand smoke exposure. Pt recalls she has felt like this in the past when she has visited her in-laws, who have a cat. On those occasions she reports hanging out the window to get fresh air so she can breathe. Denies allergies or ever being allergy tested.

continues

CASE STUDY (Continued)

The Patient with Asthma

PAST HEALTH HISTORY

Medical History	ITP age 4 (followed for a few yrs by an MD and then discharged); ⊖ sequelae
	Pneumonia requiring hospitalization ages 4/5, ⊖ sequelae
	Reports bronchitis and frequent colds growing up
Surgical History	Plantar wart excision bilat, age 15 (local anesthesia)
Allergies	Erythromycin (dx'd in childhood, doesn't know rx)
Medications	BCP and MVI daily
Communicable Diseases	Denies TB exposure; PPD skin test earlier this yr was ⊖
Injuries and Accidents	"No broken bones"
Special Needs	Denies
Blood Transfusions	Denies
Childhood Illnesses	Chickenpox age 3 s̄ sequelae; no other information
Immunizations	UTD; denies influenza and pneumococcal vaccines; last tetanus 2 yrs ago; completed Gardasil series last yr

FAMILY HEALTH HISTORY

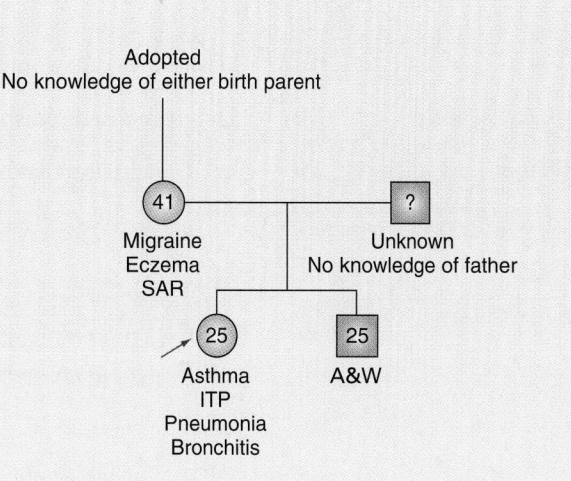

LEGEND

○ Living female
□ Living male
⊗ Deceased female
⊠ Deceased male
↗ Points to patient

A&W = Alive & well
ITP = Idiopathic thrombocytopenia purpura
SAR = Seasonal allergic rhinitis

Adopted
No knowledge of either birth parent

(41) Migraine Eczema SAR

(?) Unknown No knowledge of father

(25) Asthma ITP Pneumonia Bronchitis

(25) A&W

Denies family hx of asthma, TB

SOCIAL HISTORY

Alcohol Use	1–2 glasses of wine on wkends

continues

CASE STUDY (Continued)

The Patient with Asthma

Tobacco Use	Denies
Drug Use	Denies
Domestic and Intimate Partner Violence	Denies
Sexual Practice	Monogamous relationship
Travel History	Goes to East Coast beach q summer for past 3 yrs
Work Environment	Elementary school art teacher
Home Environment	Lives in suburban condo c̄ all modern appliances; has security guard at front desk of housing complex
Hobbies and Leisure Activities	Knits, crochets, active in women's book club; likes to paint c̄ watercolors in her spare time
Stress	During the school yr her job is stressful; summer is less stressful as she teaches only a 3-wk art class
Education	College educated, working on Master's degree
Economic Status	"My husband and I are trying to save up to buy a house, so we are watching our spending."
Military Service	Denies
Religion	Roman Catholic attending Mass q Sunday and 1–2 days during the wk
Ethnic Background	Polish American, would like to visit relatives in Poland
Roles and Relationships	Happily married c̄ husband of 2 yrs
Characteristic Patterns of Daily Living	"Let's not go into that now."
HEATH MAINTENANCE ACTIVITIES	
Sleep	Usually sleeps s̄ difficulty at home; tends to have trouble sleeping at other people's homes and hotels
Diet	Vegan
Exercise	Swims 1 mile freestyle daily p̄ work
Stress Management	Swimming/painting
Use of Safety Devices	Uses seat belt
Health Check-ups	"I only come when I am sick and that seems to be more often lately."

continues

CASE STUDY (Continued)

The Patient with Asthma

PHYSICAL ASSESSMENT

Inspection

Shape of Thorax	AP diameter/transverse diameter = 5:7, ⊖ barrel chest/pectus carinatum/pectus excavatum/kyphoscoliosis
Symmetry of Chest Wall	Shoulder and scapula ht =; ∅ masses
Presence of Superficial Veins	∅
Costal Angle	less than 90°
Angle of the Ribs	45° c̄ sternum
Intercostal Spaces	∅ bulging/retractions
Muscles of Respiration	Minimal use of SCM muscles
Respirations	Rate: 30/min Pattern: reg Depth: nonexaggerated and effortless Symmetry: no paradoxical mvt Audibility: heard upon entering room Patient position: sitting upright Mode of breathing: predominantly mouth
Sputum	Dark yellow

Palpation

General Palpation	Pulsations: ∅
	Masses: ∅
	Thoracic tenderness: ∅
	Crepitus: ∅
Thoracic Expansion	Ant and post expansion: 2.5 cm
Tactile Fremitus	⊕ throughout; ⊕ rhoncal fremitus
Tracheal Position	Midline

Percussion

General Percussion	Hyperresonant
Diaphragmatic Excursion	2 cm ant and post thorax

continues

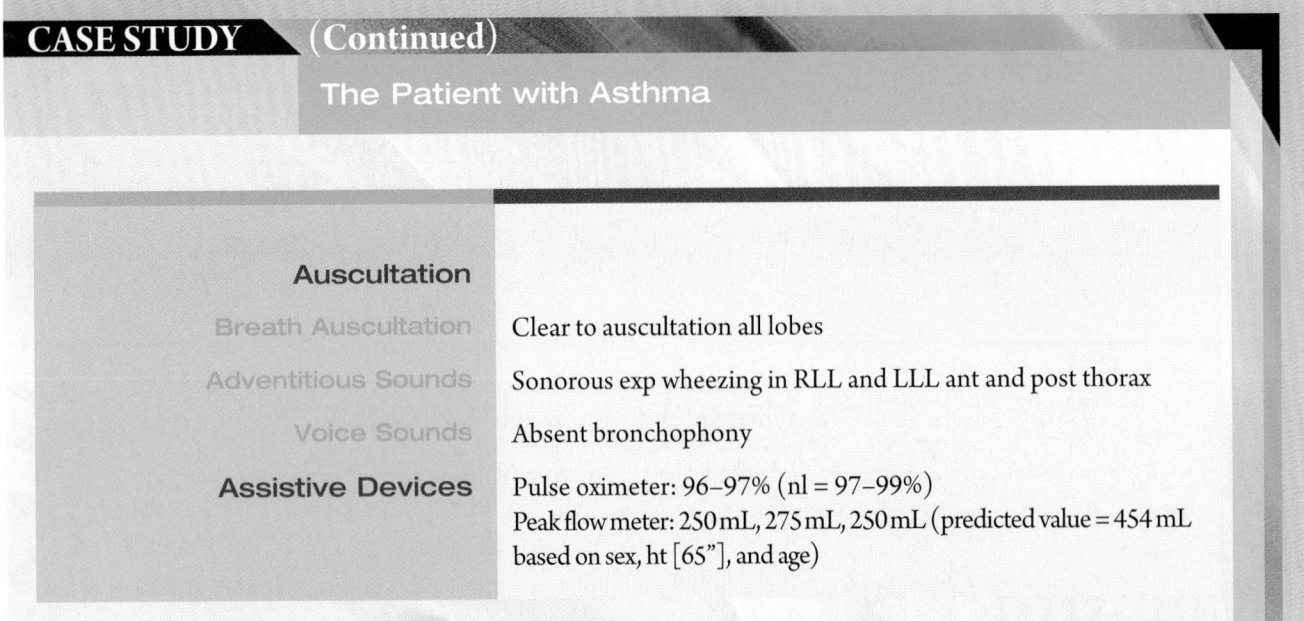

Auscultation	
Breath Auscultation	Clear to auscultation all lobes
Adventitious Sounds	Sonorous exp wheezing in RLL and LLL ant and post thorax
Voice Sounds	Absent bronchophony
Assistive Devices	Pulse oximeter: 96–97% (nl = 97–99%) Peak flow meter: 250 mL, 275 mL, 250 mL (predicted value = 454 mL based on sex, ht [65"], and age)

ASSESSMENT IN BRIEF

Thorax and Lung Assessment

Inspection

- Shape of thorax
- Symmetry of chest wall
- Presence of superficial veins
- Costal angle
- Angle of the ribs
- Intercostal spaces
- Muscles of respiration
- Respirations
  - Rate
  - Pattern
  - Depth
  - Symmetry
  - Audibility
  - Patient position
  - Mode of breathing
- Sputum

Palpation

- General palpation
  - Pulsations
  - Masses
  - Thoracic tenderness
  - Crepitus
- Thoracic expansion

- Tactile fremitus
- Tracheal position

Percussion

- General percussion
- Diaphragmatic excursion

Auscultation

- Breath sounds
- Adventitious sounds
- Voice sounds

Advanced Techniques

- Locating the site of a fractured rib
- Forced expiratory time

Assistive Devices

- Oxygen
- Incentive spirometer
- Endotracheal tube
- Tracheostomy tube
- Mechanical ventilation
- Pulse oximeter
- Peak flow meter

REVIEW QUESTIONS

1. Which of the following patients has the highest risk of contracting tuberculosis?
   a. A 19-year-old anorexic patient who spends a lot of time with her grandmother in a nursing home
   b. A 48-year-old patient who grows corn and milks cows who presents with a cough
   c. A 75-year-old patient with pneumonia and shingles
   d. A 33-year-old patient with a history of alcoholism who recently moved to the United States from Sicily

   The correct answer is (a).

2. Which of the following clinical assessment findings indicates that a patient may be experiencing immediate respiratory distress?
   a. A respiratory rate of 19
   b. Use of sternocleidomastoid muscles to breathe
   c. The presence of dilated superficial veins on the chest
   d. A costal angle of 110°

   The correct answer is (b).

3. A patient reports that he was climbing Mount Hood and noted an increase in the depth of his respirations. This physical assessment finding is called:
   a. Biot's respirations
   b. Apneustic respirations
   c. Hyperpnea
   d. Air trapping

   The correct answer is (c).

4. Kussmaul's respirations are respirations that:
   a. Have an increased depth and slow rate
   b. Are the body's attempt to raise its $PaCO_2$ level
   c. Are regularly irregular
   d. Are tachypneic and hyperpneic

   The correct answer is (d).

5. The nurse suctions the patient's endotracheal tube and notes that the secretions are rust colored. What is a possible etiology of this patient's pathology?
   a. Asthma
   b. Pulmonary edema
   c. Viral infection
   d. Pneumococcal pneumonia

   The correct answer is (d).

6. While performing diaphragmatic excursion, you measure a distance of 1.5 cm. This finding suggests:
   a. A normal distance
   b. Pneumonectomy
   c. Hypoventilation
   d. High diaphragm level

   The correct answer is (c).

7. A breath sound that is high in pitch, loud in intensity, has a blowing quality, and has a longer expiratory than inspiratory phase is called:
   a. Vesicular
   b. Bronchial
   c. Bronchovesicular
   d. Adventitious

   The correct answer is (b).

8. During inspection of a patient's thorax, you note that the patient's ribs attach to the sternum at a 45° angle. This patient has:
   a. A normal finding
   b. Pleural effusion
   c. Cystic fibrosis
   d. Chronic bronchitis

   The correct answer is (a).

9. You auscultate abnormal breath sounds on the patient's right chest at the fifth rib in the midclavicular line. In which lobe of the lung are you auscultating this sound?
   a. Right upper lobe
   b. Right middle lobe
   c. Right lower lobe
   d. Right oblique fissure

   The correct answer is (b).

10. In which condition might you expect to see a barrel chest, clubbing, a rib angle greater than 45°, tachypnea, decreased tactile fremitus, and decreased voice sounds?
    a. Pneumothorax
    b. Emphysema
    c. Pulmonary edema
    d. Atelectasis

    The correct answer is (b).

 Visit the Estes online companion resource at **www.delmar.cengage.com** for additional content and study aids. Click on Online Companions and then select the Nursing discipline.

REFERENCES

Food and Drug Administration. (2007) First "bird flu" vaccine for humans approved. Retrieved November 23, 2007, from www.fda.gov/consumer/updates/birdflu043007.html

Prevention & Control of Influenza-Recommendations of the Advisory Committee on Immunization Practices (ACIP). (2007). *MMWR,* *56*(RR06), 1–54. Retrieved November 23, 2007, from http://www.cdc.gov/flu/professionals/acip/persons.htm

BIBLIOGRAPHY

Baik, I., Kim, J., Abbott, R. D., Joo, S., Jung, K., Lee, S., Shim, J., In, K., Kang, K., Yoo, S., & Shin, C. (2007). Association of snoring with chronic bronchitis. *Archives of Internal Medicine, 168*(2), 167–173.

Baldi, F., Cappiello, R., Cavoli, C., Ghersi, S., Torresan, F., & Roda, E. (2006). Proton pump inhibitor treatment of patients with gastroesophageal reflux-related chronic cough: A comparison between two different doses of lansoprazole. *World Journal of Gastroenterology, 12*(1), 82–88.

Brown J. W. (2007). One flu over the cuckoo's nest: Is concern for Avian flu warranted in a busy clinic. *The Journal for Nurse Practitioners, 3*(9), 598–605.

CDC. (2007). Corrected: Investigation of U.S. traveler with extensively drug resistant tuberculosis (XDR TB). Retrieved November 23, 2007, from www2a.cdc.gov/HAN/ArchiveSys/ViewMsgV.asp?AlertNum=00262

Collins, L. G., Haines, C., Perkel, R., & Enck, R. E. (2007). Lung cancer: Diagnosis and management. *American Family Physician, 75*(1), 56–63.

Curry, K. (2007). Pertussis: A reemerging threat. *The Journal for Nurse Practitioners, 3*(2), 97–100.

Dicpinigaitis, P. V., & Alva, R. V. (2008). Chronic cough: Seeking the cause and the solution. *Consultant, 48*(2), 130–143.

Downs, C. A., & Appel, S. J. (2007). Chronic obstructive pulmonary disease: Diagnosis and management. *Journal of the American Academy of Nurse Practitioners, 19*(3), 126–132.

Erickson, S. E., Iribarren, C., Tolstykh, I. V., et al. (2007). Effect of race on asthma management and outcomes in a large, integrated managed care organization. *Archives of Internal Medicine, 167*(17), 1846–1852.

GlaxoSmithKline (1998) Asthma in America: A landmark survey. Retrieved May 28, 2008, from http://www.asthmainamerica.com

Jani, A. L., & Hamilos, D. L. (2005). Current thinking on the relationship between rhinosinusitis and asthma. *Journal of Asthma, 1*, 1–7.

Jeffries, M., Townsend, R., & Horrigan, E. (2007). Helping your patient combat lung cancer. *Nursing 2007, 37*(12), 36–41.

Kass, S. M., Williams, P. M., & Reamy, B. V. (2007). Pleurisy. *American Family Physician, 75*(9), 1357–1364.

Martinez, F. J., Curtis, J. L., Sciurba, F., et al. (2007). Sex differences in severe pulmonary emphysema. *American Journal of Respiratory and Critical Care Medicine, 176*(3), 243–252.

Michaels, D., Lurie, P., & Monforton, C. (2006). Lung cancer mortality in the German chromate industry, 1958–1998 [Letter to the Editor]. *Journal of Occupational and Environmental Medicine, 48*(10), 995–997.

Mintz, M. L. (2006). *Disorders of the respiratory tract: Common challenges in primary care.* Totowa, NJ: Humana Press.

National Heart, Lung, and Blood Institute, National Asthma Education and Prevention Program. (2007) Expert Panel Report 3: Guidelines for the Diagnosis and Management of Asthma (EPR-3). Retrieved January 8, 2008, from www.nhlbi.nih.gov/guidelines/asthma/index.htm

Platts-Mills, T., Leung, D. Y. M., & Schatz, M. (2007). The role of allergies in asthma. *American Family Physician, 76*(5), 675–680.

Schlossberg, D. (2006). *Tuberculosis & nontuberculosis mycobacterial infections* (5th ed.). New York: McGraw-Hill.

Shaughnessy, K. (2007). Massive pulmonary embolus. *Critical Care Nurse, 27*(1), 39–50.

Stockley, R., Rennard, S., Rabe, K., & Celli, B. (Eds.). (2007). *Chronic obstructive pulmonary disease.* Oxford: Blackwell Publishing.

Shaw, K. (2006). The 2003 SARS outbreak and its impact on infection control practices. *Public Health, 120*, 8–14.

Wong, S. S., & Yuen, K. Y. (2006). Avian influenza virus infections in humans. *Chest, 129*, 156–168.

World Health Organization. Summary of probable SARS cases with onset of illness from 1 November 2002 to 31 July 2003. Retrieved November 26, 2007.

WEB SITES

American Cancer Society:
http://www.cancer.org

American Lung Association:
http://www.lungusa.org

Asthma and Allergy Foundation of America:
http://www.aafa.org

Centers for Disease Control and Prevention:
http://www.cdc.gov

EFFORTS—Emphysema Foundation for Our Right to Survive:
http://www.emphysema.net

Mayo Clinic:
http://www.mayoclinic.com

National Heart, Lung, and Blood Institute:
http://www.nhlbi.nih.gov

The R.A.L.E. Repository:
http://www.rale.ca

CHAPTER 16

Heart and Peripheral Vasculature

COMPETENCIES

1. Identify the anatomic landmarks of the chest and periphery.

2. Describe the characteristics of the most common cardiovascular chief complaints.

3. Elicit a health history from a patient with cardiovascular pathology.

4. Perform a cardiovascular assessment on a healthy adult.

5. Perform a cardiovascular assessment on a patient with cardiovascular pathology.

6. Provide scientific rationale for abnormal cardiovascular assessment findings.

The heart's primary function is to pump blood to all parts of the body. The circulating blood not only brings oxygen and nutrients to the body's tissues but also helps to take away the body's waste products. The body's activities determine the amount of blood that is pumped. The heart will beat faster or slower and the blood vessels will expand or relax in order to properly distribute the blood that the body demands.

ANATOMY AND PHYSIOLOGY

HEART

In a resting, healthy adult, the heart contracts 60 to 100 times while pumping 4 to 5 liters of blood per minute. An individual's heart is about the size of a clenched fist. The human heart is remarkably efficient considering its size in relation to the rest of the body.

The heart is located in the thoracic cavity between the lungs and above the diaphragm in an area known as the mediastinum (Figure 16-1). The **base** of the heart is the uppermost portion, which includes the left and right atria as well as the aorta, pulmonary arteries, and the superior and inferior venae cavae. These structures lie behind the upper portion of the sternum. The **apex**, or lower portion of the heart, extends into the left thoracic cavity, causing the heart to appear as if it is lying on its right ventricle.

Pericardium

The heart and roots of the great vessels lie within a sac called the pericardium, which is composed of fibrous and serous layers. The fibrous layer is the outermost

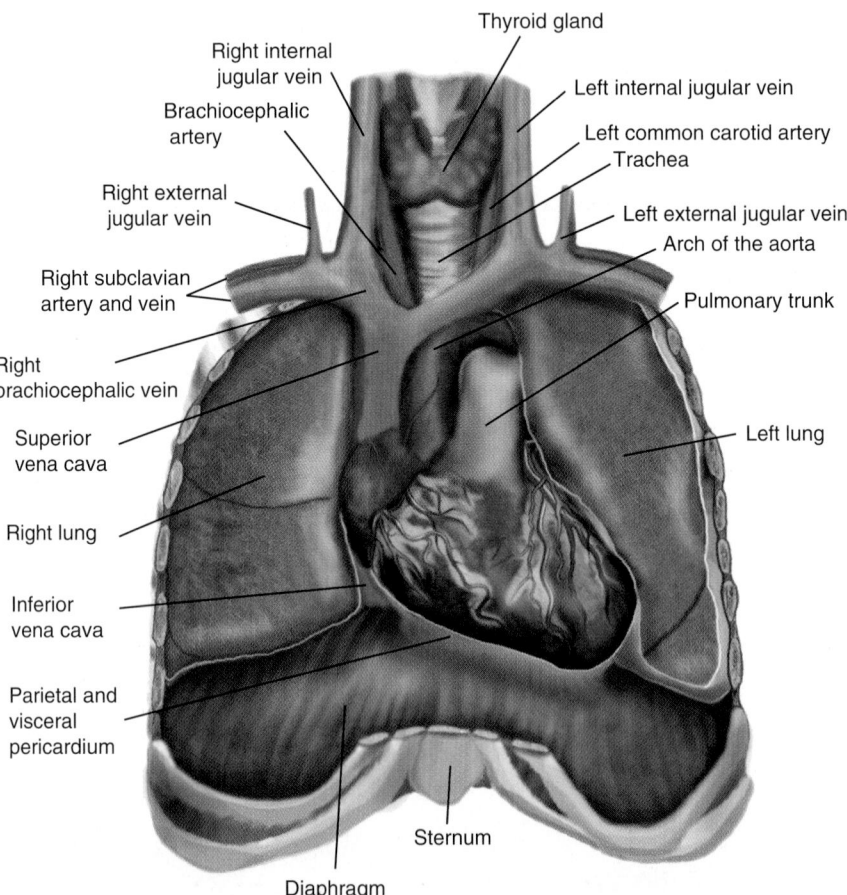

FIGURE 16-1 Position of the Heart in the Thoracic Cavity

layer and is connected to the diaphragm and sternum by ligaments and tendons. Its major role is to limit the stretching of the myocardial muscle, especially in the setting of strenuous activity or hypervolemia.

There are two serous layers of the pericardium: the **parietal** layer, which lies close to the fibrous tissues, and the **visceral** layer, which lies against the actual heart muscle. This visceral layer is often referred to as the epicardium. Between the two serous layers is a small space that contains approximately 20 to 50 mL of pericardial fluid. This pericardial fluid serves to facilitate the movement of the heart muscle and protect it via its lubricant effect.

Chambers of the Heart

The heart is divided into four chambers, which are separated laterally by walls known as the vertical **septa.** These vertical septa divide the heart into the right and the left atria (interatrial septum) and the right and the left ventricles (interventricular septum). The right atrium is the collection point for the blood returning from the systemic circulation for reoxygenation in the lungs. The left atrium receives its freshly oxygenated blood via the four pulmonary veins, which are the only veins in the body that carry oxygenated blood.

The walls of the left ventricle are three times thicker than those of the right ventricle because of its greater workload as it pumps blood through the high-pressure systemic arterial system. Left ventricular pressures are five times greater than those in the right ventricle. Figure 16-2 shows the configuration of the heart's chambers, the pressures, and normal oxygen content of the blood contained therein.

Heart Valves

As blood empties into the two atria, the **atrioventricular (A-V) valves** prevent it from prematurely entering the ventricles. The A-V valve between the right atrium and the right ventricle is known as the tricuspid valve, named for its three flaps or cusps. The A-V valve between the left atrium and the left ventricle is the bicuspid valve, named for its two flaps or cusps; it is commonly known as the mitral valve. When the tricuspid and mitral valves are closed, blood cannot flow from the atria into the ventricles. In a normal heart, they open only as atrial pressures increase with progressive filling.

The semilunar valves are also known as outflow valves because blood exits the heart through them. Blood flows from the right ventricle to the pulmonary vasculature for oxygenation by way of the pulmonic valve. Blood is pumped from the left ventricle into the systemic and coronary circulation through the aortic valve.

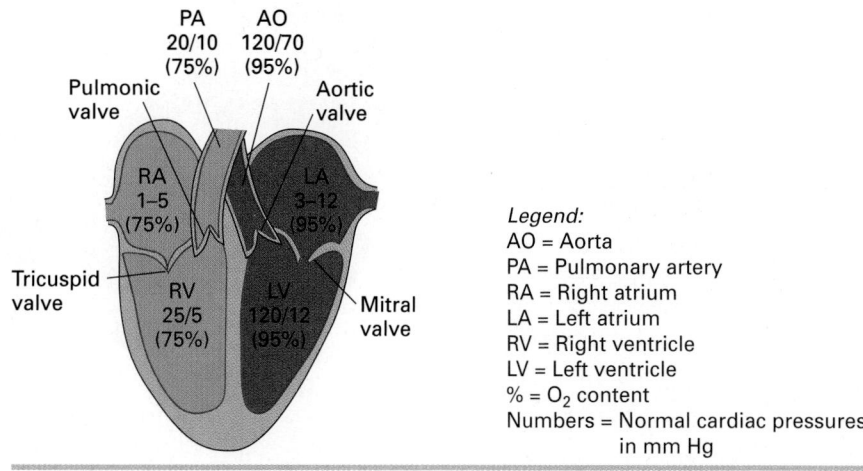

FIGURE 16-2 The Configuration, Normal Pressures, and Oxygen Content of the Heart Chambers

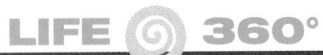
NURSING ALERT

Warning Signs of Potential Cardiovascular Problems

- Change in color of lips, face, or nails
- Chest discomfort (e.g., uncomfortable pressure, squeezing, fullness, or pain)
- Breaking out in a cold sweat
- Lightheadedness
- Shortness of breath
- Edema
- Extremity pain
- Fatigue
- Feeling of doom
- Numbness in the extremities
- Pain that limits self-care
- Palpitations
- Syncope
- Tingling in the extremities

CORONARY CIRCULATION

The exterior surface of the heart muscle contains a very important and intricate blood supply. Two major coronary arteries arise from the small openings in the aorta known as the sinuses of Valsalva, located just behind the aortic valve. Figure 16-3 demonstrates the position of the coronary arteries as they exit from the aorta to cover the myocardium with an arterial network. The left and right coronary arteries run superficially across the heart muscle, but the smaller branches of these two main arteries actually penetrate deeply into the myocardium, carrying with them a rich, nutritive blood supply. Blood flow to the coronary arteries is greatest during diastole because the force of the ventricular contraction during systole actually impedes flow through the sinuses of Valsalva.

The myocardium is extremely dependent on a constant supply of oxygen that is delivered through the coronary arterial system. The heart's oxygen requirements increase when it is stimulated by conditions such as exercise. If the coronary blood supply is not sufficient to meet the needs of the heart, the result may be **ischemia** (local and temporary lack of blood supply to the heart), injury (beyond ischemia but still reversible), or an **infarction** (necrosis) of the heart muscle itself. Myocardial ischemia is often manifested as chest, neck, or arm pain known as **angina.**

The left main coronary artery branches into the left circumflex coronary artery and the left anterior descending (LAD) coronary artery. The left main coronary artery may be referred to as the "widowmaker" because of the lethal effect of any obstruction to blood flow prior to its branch point.

The LAD supplies blood to the anterior wall and apex of the left ventricle as well as to the anterior portion of the interventricular septum. The smaller arterial branches that supply the septum also nourish the ventricular conduction system, including the bundle of His and the right and left bundle branches. The left circumflex (LCX) branch supplies arterial blood to the left atrium and to the lateral and posterior portions of the left ventricle. In some individuals, the sinoatrial (S-A) node and the A-V node are also supplied by this branch.

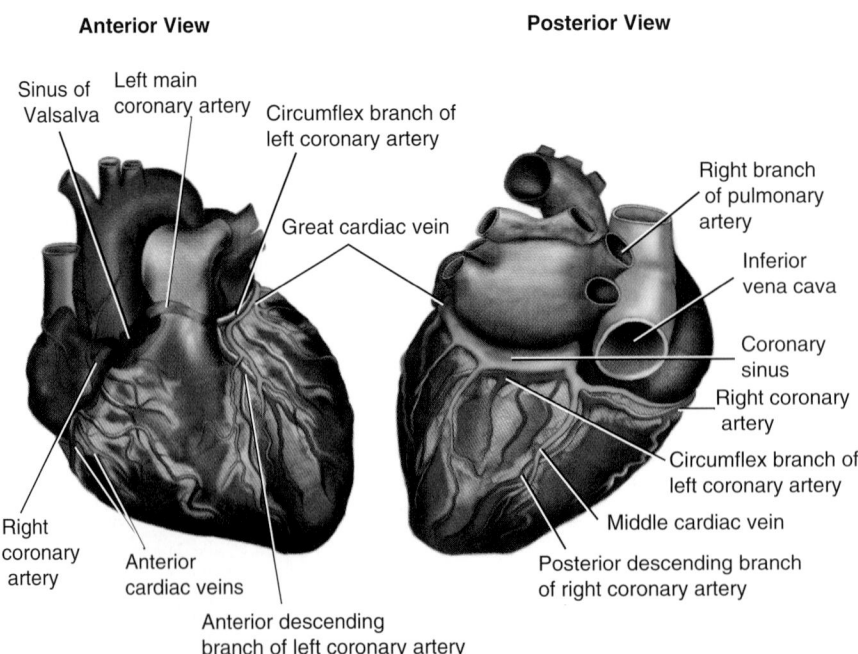

FIGURE 16-3 **The Coronary Arteries and Major Veins of the Heart (Anterior and Posterior Views)**

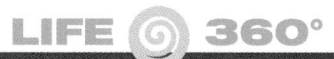

Nurses Who Use Tobacco

Suppose you smoke cigarettes, knowing the side effects smoking has on cardiovascular status. How can you instruct your patients not to smoke when you don't "practice what you preach"? What if your patient smells cigarette smoke on you after your break and asks you if you smoke? How would you respond?

The right coronary artery (RCA) supplies nutrients and oxygen to the right atrium, the right ventricle, and the inferior wall of the left ventricle. In most individuals, the RCA supplies the S-A and the A-V nodes as well as the posterior portion of the interventricular septum. With an inferior wall infarction, the RCA is most likely the vessel that has been occluded. With an anterior wall infarction, the LAD branch would be the most likely source of occlusion, with resulting complications in the ventricular conduction system, such as bundle branch blocks or ventricular dysrhythmias.

Venous drainage from the myocardium is carried by the coronary sinus, anterior cardiac veins, and thebesian veins. About 75% of the venous blood empties into the right atrium via the coronary sinus. The thebesian veins carry only a small portion of the unoxygenated blood that is emptied directly into all four chambers of the heart.

CARDIAC CYCLE

Figure 16-4 illustrates the electrical and mechanical events in the heart. Physical assessment findings can be correlated with these electrophysiological mechanisms.

The cardiac cycle consists of two phases: systole and diastole. In **systole**, the myocardial fibers contract and tighten to eject blood from the ventricles (for the purpose of this chapter, any mention of systole will mean ventricular systole unless specifically called atrial systole). **Diastole** is a period of relaxation and reflects the pressure remaining in the blood vessels after the heart has pumped.

Systole is divided into three phases, beginning with the isovolumic (or isometric) contraction phase, which marks the onset of a ventricular contraction. During this phase, the pressure is increasing but no blood is entering or leaving the ventricle. As the pressure rises in the left ventricle, the mitral valve closes (similar events occur in the right ventricle with the tricuspid valve). Closure of these A-V valves produces the first heart sound, known as S_1 (depicted as "1st" on the phonocardiogram [a recording of the heart sounds] curve in Figure 16-4).

Once the pressure in the left ventricle exceeds that in the aorta, and the pressure in the right ventricle exceeds that in the pulmonary artery, the semilunar (aortic and pulmonic) valves open and blood is rapidly ejected. This rapid ejection phase is also referred to as early systole. It is followed by a third phase of reduced ejection, which is also known as late systole.

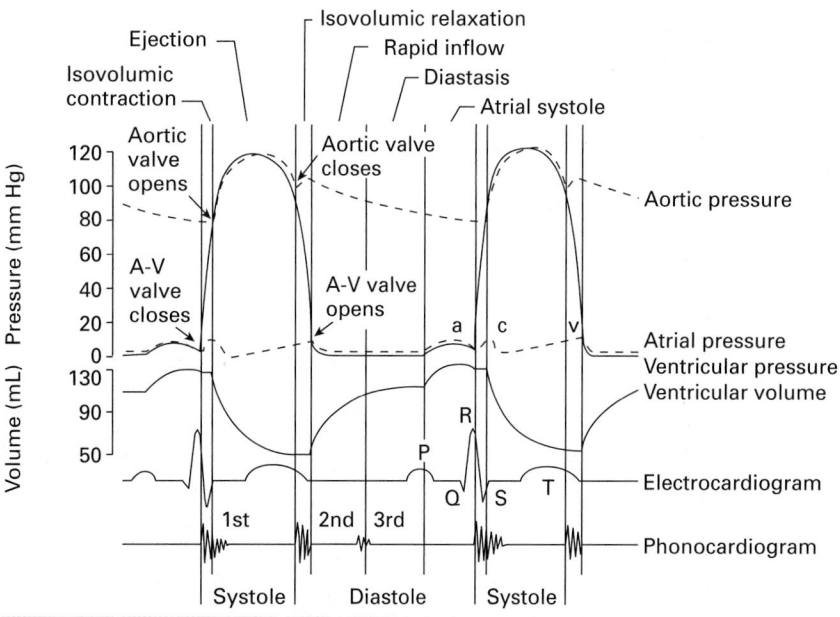

FIGURE 16-4   Events of the Cardiac Cycle. *Reproduced with permission from Textbook of Medical Physiology (11th ed.), by A. C. Guyton and J. E. Hall, 2005, Philadelphia: W. B. Saunders Company.*

Ventricular diastole begins with the isovolumic, or isometric, relaxation phase. During this phase, ventricular ejection ceases and the pressure in the left ventricle is reduced to less than that in the aorta. This permits a backflow of blood from the aorta to the left ventricle, causing the aortic valve to close (similar events occur in the pulmonary artery to cause the pulmonic valve to close). The closure of the semilunar valves produces the second heart sound, known as S_2 (depicted as "2nd" on the phonocardiogram curve in Figure 16-4). When the A-V and semilunar valves are closed, the pressure in the left ventricle falls rapidly.

Atrial pressures then rise as a result of the large amount of blood accumulating in the atria because of the closed A-V valves. When systole is over and the ventricular pressures fall, the high pressure in the atria forces the A-V valves to open to allow for rapid ventricular filling (rapid inflow) during early diastole. Filling then slows during a phase called diastasis or mid-diastole. Seventy percent of ventricular filling occurs in a passive manner during these early and mid-diastolic filling periods.

The final phase of diastole is known as atrial systole. The atria contract to complete the remaining 20% to 30% of ventricular filling, which is often referred to as **atrial kick.** After atrial systole, the cardiac cycle starts all over again.

The electrocardiogram (abbreviated as either **ECG** or **EKG**, from the German word "Elektrokardiogramm") in Figure 16-4 shows the P, Q , R, S, and T waves. These waves are electrical voltages produced by the heart and recorded by EKG leads placed on the body. When the atria depolarize, the P wave is produced on the EKG. During this period, the pressure in the atria exceeds that in the ventricles, thus forcing the blood from the atria into the ventricles. Approximately 0.16 second after the appearance of the P wave, the QRS complex on the EKG occurs as the ventricles

NURSING**TIP**

Sexual Activity following Cardiac Compromise

Teach your patients the following about sex after cardiac surgery or myocardial infarction (MI), as recommended by the American Heart Association (AHA):

1. Resume sexual activity as soon as you feel ready; however, check with your health care provider first. Most patients who have had an MI are able to resume sex after 4 weeks; heart surgery patients usually resume sex 2 to 3 weeks after leaving the hospital.
2. Although most patients resume sex with the same frequency as before the hospitalization, others may be less active. Begin with lower-energy forms of sexual expression, such as touching, holding, and caressing, if this will raise your comfort level. Avoid strenuous positions.
3. Seek medical care or sexual counseling if you are afraid to resume sex because of anxiety, depression, cardiac symptoms, or lack of desire.
4. Medications such as those used for chest pain, irregular heart beats, high blood pressure, edema, anxiety, and depression can affect sexual desire and performance. If a sexual problem occurs, continue taking the medication and consult your health care provider.
5. If recovering from an MI, you may be more aware of your breathing, heart beat, muscle tightening, or tension; this awareness is normal.
6. Two psychological factors that can affect sexual interest are fears about performance and general depression. After recovery, heart patients may feel depressed. This depression is normal, and in a majority of cases it will disappear after 3 months.
7. Wait 1 to 3 hours after eating a full meal to allow time for digestion prior to sex.
8. Patients who use nitrate drugs should not take phosphodiesterase type 5 inhibitor medications (sildenafil citrate, tadalafil, vardenafil).

are electrically depolarized. As the ventricles begin to repolarize, the T wave appears on the EKG. The downslope of the T wave indicates the end of ventricular repolarization and the beginning of a relaxation period. Note that the EKG contains an **isoelectric line**, or flat line, after the T wave, indicating a period of electrical rest.

CONDUCTION SYSTEM OF THE HEART

The **sinoatrial (S-A) node** is the normal pacemaker of the heart and is located about 1 mm below the right atrial epicardium at its junction with the superior vena cava. It initiates a rhythmic impulse approximately 70 times per minute. The infranodal atrial pathways conduct the impulse initiated in the S-A node to the **atrioventricular (A-V) node** via the myocardium of the right atrium. The three infranodal pathways are the anterior, the middle, and the posterior tracts. Meanwhile, the Bachmann's bundle conducts the impulse from the S-A node to the left atrium. In the absence of a signal from the S-A node, the A-V node has its own intrinsic rate of 40 to 60 impulses per minute. The A-V node, also known as the A-V junction, delays the impulse received from the atria before transmitting it to the ventricles in order to give them time to fill prior to the next systole. The impulse then travels very rapidly from the A-V node to the bundle branch system via the bundle of His. The bundle branch system is composed of the right bundle branch (RBB) and the left bundle branch (LBB). The RBB carries the impulse down the right side of the interventricular septum into the right ventricle. The LBB separates into three fascicles that relay the impulse to the left ventricle. Finally, the Purkinje fibers arising from the distal portions of the bundle branches transmit the impulse into the subendocardial layers of both ventricles. Barring interference with the connections described above, the final transmission of the impulse allows depolarization of the ventricles to occur followed by a normal systole. Figure 16-5 depicts the normal conduction pathways of the heart. If A-V node disease causes transmission of the electrical signal to be blocked, the intrinsic rate of the ventricles kicks in at a rate of fewer than 40 beats per minute.

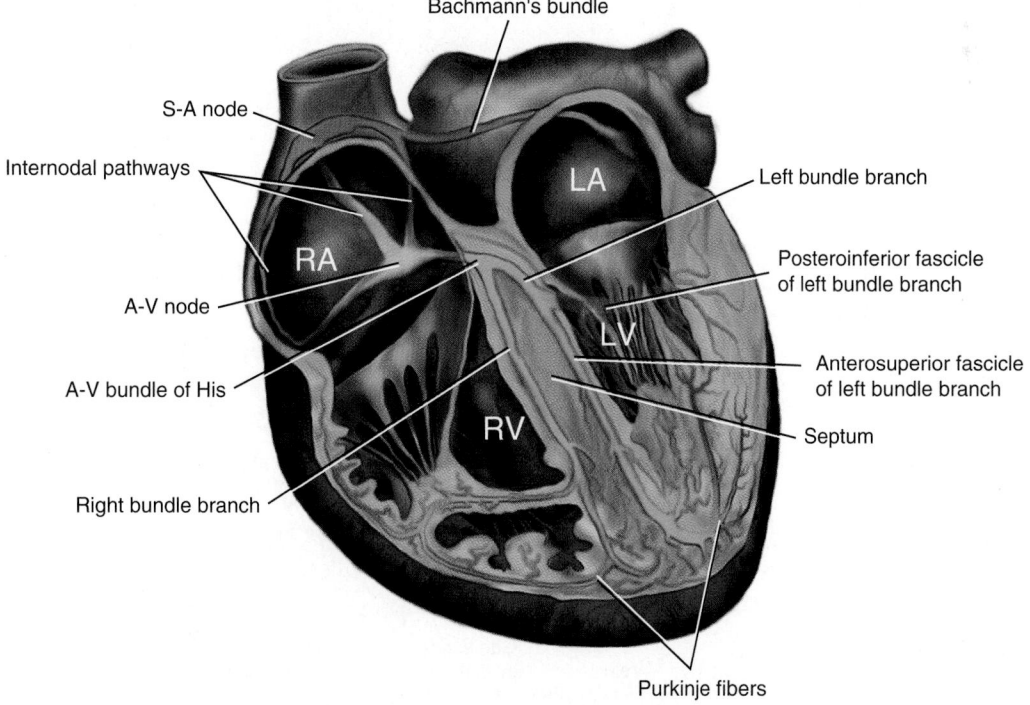

FIGURE 16-5 Conduction System of the Heart. **The cardiac impulse is transmitted from the S-A node to the A-V node via the internodal pathways and Bachmann's bundle, and then on to the bundle of His and down the left and right bundle branches to the Purkinje fibers, which distribute the impulse to the rest of the ventricles.**

PERIPHERAL VASCULATURE

The circulatory system consists of arterial pathways, which are the distribution routes, and venous pathways, the collection system that returns the blood to the central pumping station, the heart. Figure 16-6 demonstrates the journey of the blood through the systemic and pulmonary circuits.

Arterial walls are composed of three coats or linings. The innermost lining is known as the tunica intima and is composed of the endothelium and some connective tissue. The tunica media is the middle layer and is composed of both smooth muscle and an elastic type of connective tissue. The outer layer, the tunica externa or adventitia, has a more fibrous connective tissue that is arranged longitudinally.

As the arterial system branches and subdivides on its way to the periphery, the diameters of the vessels decrease. Arterioles are the smallest group of arteries, with a diameter of less than 0.5 mm. It is here that the rapid velocity of blood flow found

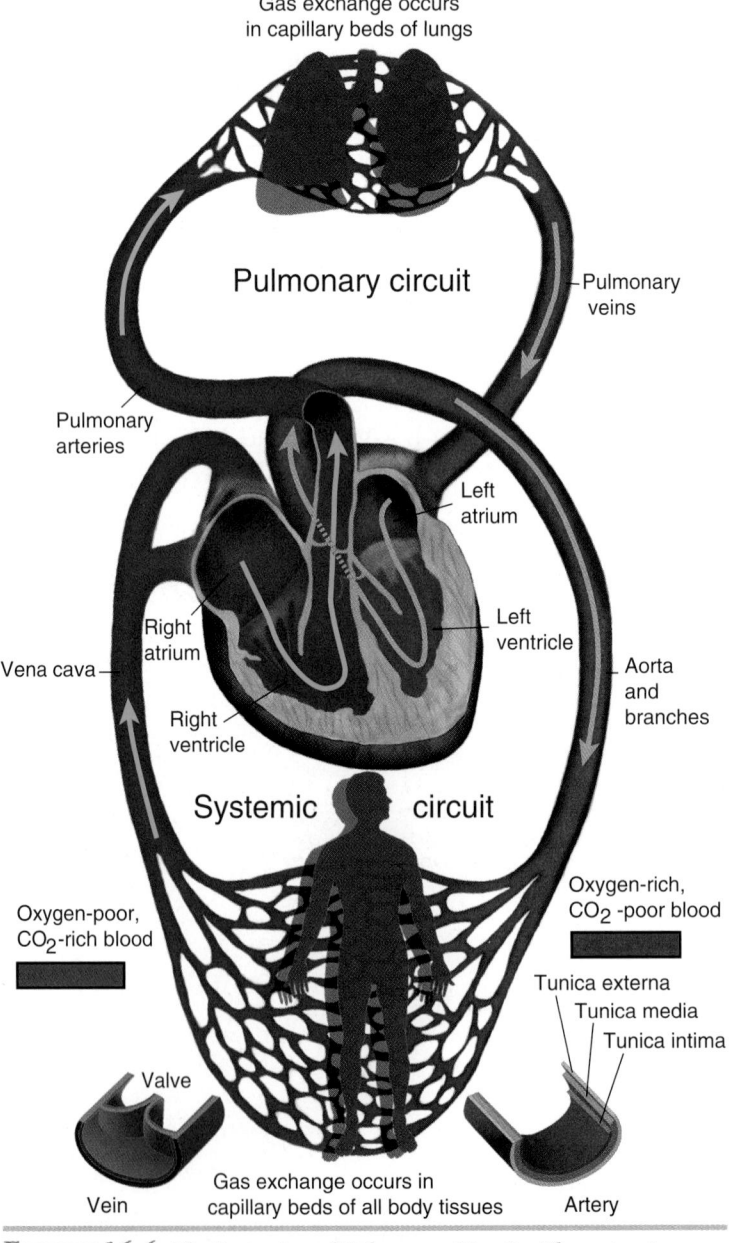

FIGURE 16-6 **The Systemic and Pulmonary Circuits. The systemic pump consists of the left side of the heart, and the pulmonary circuit pump represents the right side of the heart.**

NURSING**TIP**

Calculating Target Heart Rate Zone

1. Subtract the patient's age in years from 220 to calculate the patient's maximum heart rate.
2. The low end of the patient's target heart rate (THR) zone is 50% of the value obtained in step 1. The high end of the patient's THR zone is 85% of the value obtained in step 1. For example, a 48-year-old's THR zone would be calculated as follows:

$$(220 - 48) \times 0.50 = 86 \text{ (low end)}$$
$$(220 - 48) \times 0.85 = 146 \text{ (high end)}$$

Thus, the patient's THR zone (range) would be 86–146 beats per minute.
3. If the patient's goal is weight management and/or to burn fat, then the patient should train to 50–65% of the maximum heart rate determined in step 1. If the patient's goal is purely aerobic exercise, then the patient should train to 65–85% of the maximum heart rate calculated in step 1.

in the larger arteries begins to decrease. Blood flow becomes even slower in the capillaries arising from each arteriole. The walls of the capillaries are only one cell thick, which, coupled with the slow rate of blood flow, provides optimal conditions for the exchange of nutrients and wastes and the transfer of fluid volume between the plasma and the interstitium.

After leaving the capillaries, the blood flows into the low-pressure venous system beginning with vessels known as venules. Veins are similar in construction to arteries, but they have much less elasticity, thinner walls, and greater diameters. One-way valves are found in most veins where blood is carried against the force of gravity, such as in the lower extremities. Arteries do not have valves.

As blood passes from the arterial system through the capillaries, there is a change from the pulsatile character of arterial flow to a steady flow in the venous system. Arterial pulsations are caused by the intermittent contractions of the left ventricle. Figures 16-7 and 16-8 illustrate the arterial and venous networks of blood flow.

EPITROCHLEAR NODES

The epitrochlear nodes are located 3 cm proximal to the medial humeral epicondyle, in the groove between the biceps and triceps brachii. The nodes drain afferently from the ulnar aspect of the forearm and hand, the little and ring fingers, and the ulnar part of the middle finger.

NURSING**ALERT**

Risk Factors for Cardiovascular Disease

Fixed (patient cannot alter)
Age, gender, race, family history
Major Modifiable (patient can significantly reduce risk of cardiovascular disease by controlling these factors)
HTN, hyperlipidemia, tobacco use, glucose intolerance, physical inactivity, diet, lack of estrogen in postmenopausal women
Minor Modifiable (patient can decrease risk of cardiovasculardisease to a lesser degree)
Psychophysiological stress, sedentary living, obesity

NURSING**TIP**

Managing Anger

When confronted with a stressful situation, teach your patients to:
- Always keep things in perspective.
- Learn to "cool off" when confronted with a stressful situation (e.g., count to 10).
- Walk away from potentially stressful situations if they feel that they may lose control.
- Use humor liberally in situations that would otherwise lead to exasperation.
- Consider the consequences: letting it out and clearing the air once in a while may be better than keeping anger and frustration bottled up inside.

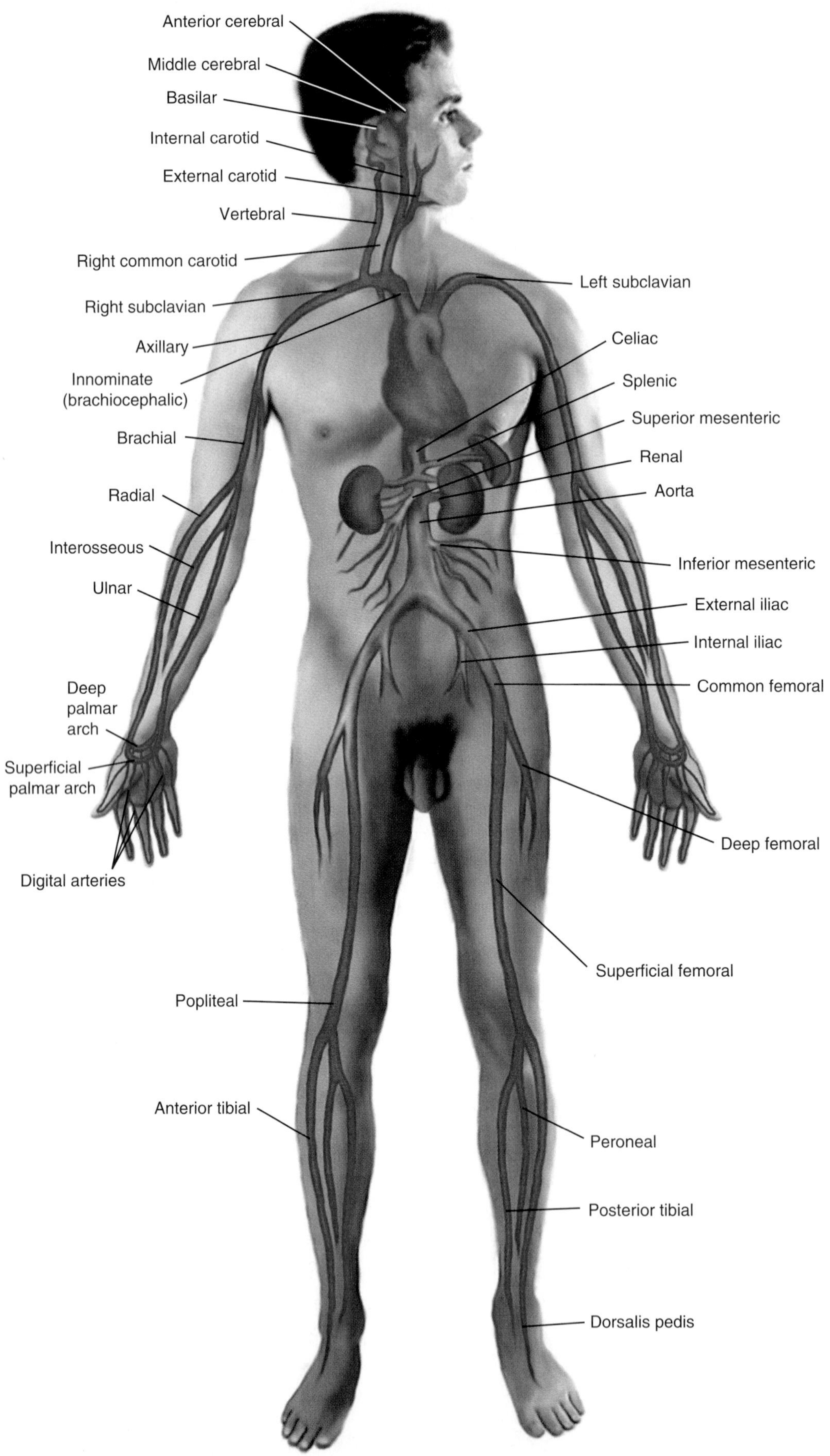

Anterior cerebral
Middle cerebral
Basilar
Internal carotid
External carotid
Vertebral
Right common carotid
Right subclavian
Axillary
Innominate (brachiocephalic)
Brachial
Radial
Interosseous
Ulnar
Deep palmar arch
Superficial palmar arch
Digital arteries

Left subclavian
Celiac
Splenic
Superior mesenteric
Renal
Aorta
Inferior mesenteric
External iliac
Internal iliac
Common femoral
Deep femoral
Superficial femoral
Popliteal
Anterior tibial
Peroneal
Posterior tibial
Dorsalis pedis

FIGURE 16-7 **Arterial System Anatomy**

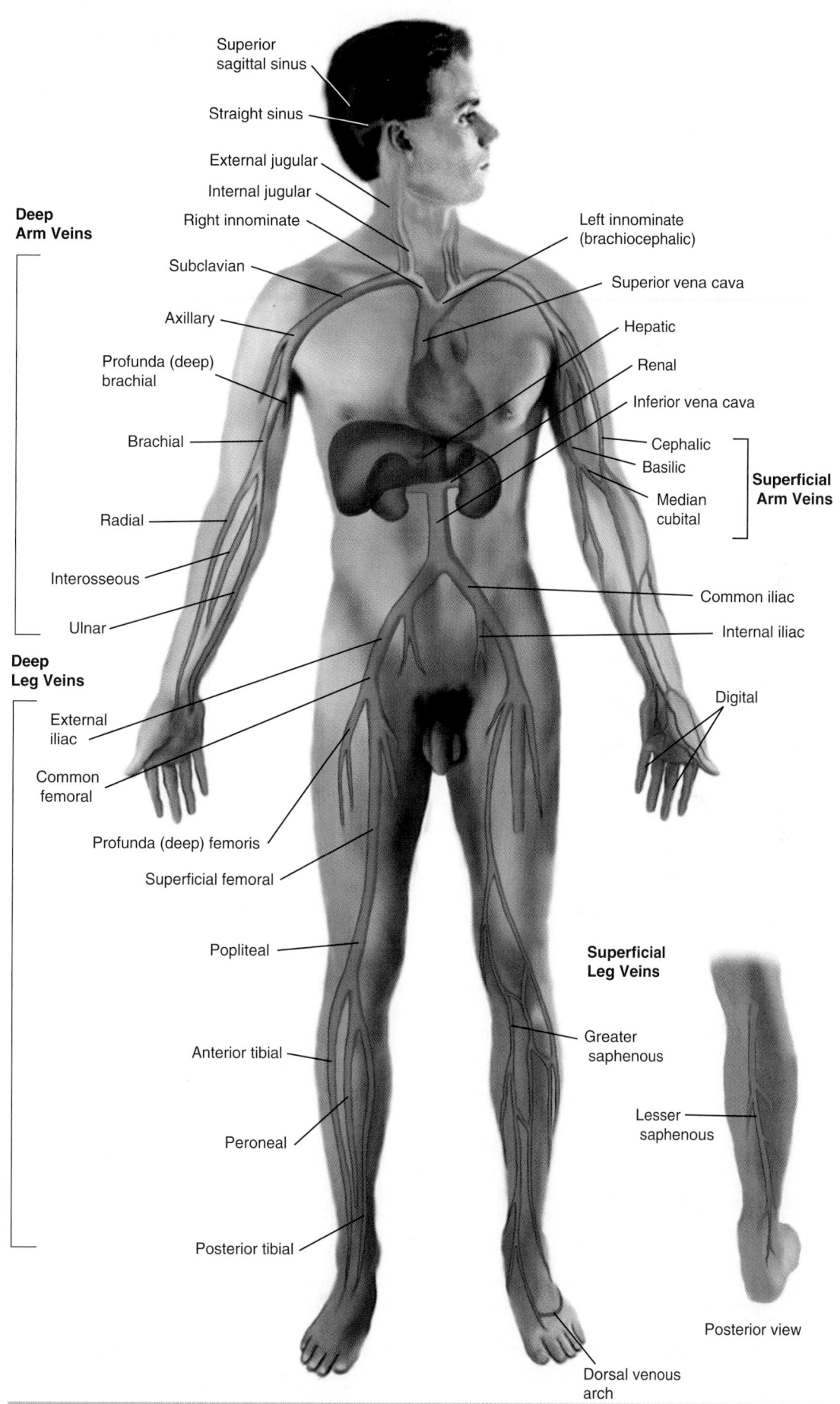

FIGURE 16-8 Venous System Anatomy

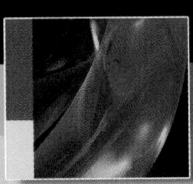

HEALTH HISTORY

The heart and peripheral vasculature health history provides insight into the link between a patient's life and lifestyle and heart and peripheral vasculature information and pathology.

PATIENT PROFILE

Diseases that are age-, gender-, and race-specific for the heart and peripheral vasculature are listed. Table 16-1 (see page 535) differentiates the common cardiovascular disorders. Table 16-2 (see page 537) differentiates congenital cardiovascular defects.

Age

Rheumatic fever (5–15)
Raynaud's disease (18–50)
Mitral valve prolapse (20–50)
Hypertension (HTN) (20–70)
Valve **stenosis** (narrowing or constriction of a diseased heart valve) or **regurgitation** (backward flow of blood through a heart valve) (30–50)
Coronary artery disease (CAD) (40–60)
Dilated or congestive cardiomyopathy (40–60)
Myocardial infarction (MI) (40–70)
Arteriosclerosis (50–70)
Cerebrovascular accident (CVA) (50–70)
Abdominal aortic aneurysm (AAA) (60–70)

Gender

Female

Higher mortality rate after a severe MI; marked rise in CAD after menopause; atrial septal defect (ASD); Raynaud's disease.

Women experiencing an MI may not have the classic warning signs experienced by men. Instead, they may complain of unusual fatigue, sleep disturbance, and/or shortness of breath.

Combination hormone therapy is no longer used to prevent cardiovascular disease in healthy, postmenopausal women. If hormone therapy is used for the symptoms of menopause, it should be taken only in the smallest dose over the shortest feasible time period.

Male

Marked predisposition to CAD; ventricular septal defect (VSD)

Race

African American

CVA, CAD, HTN

Hispanic and Filipino

HTN

American Indian

CVA, CAD

CHIEF COMPLAINT

Common chief complaints for the heart and peripheral vasculature are defined and information on the characteristics of each sign or symptom is provided.

1. Chest Pain

Subjective sense of discomfort in the thorax; also referred to as angina if it is caused by myocardial ischemia; all chest pain is not angina; Table 16-3 differentiates different origins of chest pain

Radiation

Arm, shoulder, neck, jaw, teeth

continues

Quality	Crushing, heavy, tight, stabbing, burning, squeezing, aching, smothering, or perceived as indigestion
Associated Manifestations	Nausea and vomiting, shortness of breath (SOB), restlessness, anxiety, weakness, feeling of impending doom, diaphoresis, faintness, dizziness
Aggravating Factors	Exercise, stress
Alleviating Factors	Medication (e.g., nitroglycerin), rest, position change
Setting	While dreaming, eating, excited, stressed, exercising, or resting; hot or cold environment
Timing	Early morning is more common but can be any time of the day
2. Syncope	Fainting caused by a transient decrease in cerebral blood flow
Associated Manifestations	Nausea, perspiration, palpitations, yawning, seizures, flushed face, cessation of breathing during episode, aura prior to episode
Aggravating Factors	Exercise, medications, fever, lack of food
Alleviating Factors	Rest
Setting	Heavy activity, hot environment, buttoning the collar of a shirt
Timing	Early morning, after medication, after exercise, arising from a supine or sitting position
3. Palpitations	Irregular heart beats; the sensation of a rapidly throbbing or fluttering heart
Quality	Skipped heart beats, throbbing, pounding, fluttering
Associated Manifestations	Anxiety, weakness, nausea, SOB, chest pain, perspiration, fainting
Aggravating Factors	Smoking, caffeine, exercise
Alleviating Factors	Rest
Setting	Resting, smoking, exercising, drinking or eating food containing caffeine
Timing	After exercise or at rest
4. Peripheral Edema	Swelling of the extremities, usually the feet and hands
Quality	Imprints on swollen areas after applying pressure
Associated Manifestations	Recent weight gain, pain in upper right half of abdomen, swollen abdomen, shoes tighter, rings difficult to remove from fingers
Aggravating Factors	Continuous standing, high salt intake
Alleviating Factors	Lying down or elevating the feet
5. Extremity Pain	Sense of discomfort usually occurring in the legs or feet; claudication
Quality	Temperature change in feet or leg
Associated Manifestations	Swelling in the affected extremity, discoloration of the skin, tenderness, change in skin temperature
Aggravating Factors	Continual standing, walking, exercise, cold weather, smoking, stress

continues

Health History (continued)

Alleviating Factors	Rest, elevation, dangling the extremity to a dependent position if the pain is caused by arterial insufficiency (but pain actually worsens with venous insufficiency)
Setting	Walking, exercise
Timing	Late night, early morning
PAST HEALTH HISTORY	*The various components of the past health history are linked to heart and peripheral vasculature pathology and heart- and peripheral-vasculature-related information.*
Medical History	
Cardiac Specific	AAA, angina, cardiogenic shock, cardiomyopathy, chest trauma, congenital anomalies, congestive heart failure (CHF), CAD, endocarditis, hyperlipoproteinemia, HTN, MI, myocarditis, pericarditis, peripheral vascular disease (PVD), rheumatic fever, valvular disease
Non-cardiac Specific	Bleeding or blood disorder, diabetes mellitus, gout, Marfan's syndrome, pheochromocytoma, primary aldosteronism, renal artery disease, CVA, thyroid disease
Surgical History	Ablation of accessory pathways, aneurysm repair, cardiac catheterization, chest surgery for trauma, congenital heart repair, coronary artery bypass graft (CABG), coronary stents, directional coronary atherectomy (DCA), electrophysiology studies (EPS), heart transplant, implantable or internal cardioverter/defibrillator (ICD) placement, myotomy or myectomy, percutaneous laser myoplasty, pacemaker insertion, percutaneous transluminal coronary angioplasty (PTCA), pericardial window, pericardiectomy, pericardiotomy, peripheral vascular grafting and bypass, valve replacement
Allergies	Aspirin (most patients who are recovering from an MI receive aspirin), intravenous pyelogram (IVP) dye and seafood (both contain iodine compounds used in the dye that is injected during a cardiac catheterization), latex (found in gloves used for procedures), betadine (which is used as a skin surface prep for cardiac and vascular procedures)
Medications	Antianginals, antidysrhythmics, anticoagulants, antihypertensives, antilipemics, diuretics, inotropics, thrombolytic enzymes, vasodilators
Communicable Diseases	Rheumatic fever (valvular dysfunction), untreated syphilis (aortic regurgitation, aortitis, and aortic aneurysm), viral myocarditis (cardiomyopathy)
Injuries and Accidents	Chest trauma (falls, motor vehicle accidents, blunt force)
Childhood Illnesses	Rheumatic fever (valvular dysfunction)
FAMILY HEALTH HISTORY	*Heart and peripheral vasculature diseases that are familial are listed.*
	Aneurysm, CVA, CAD, HTN, hypertrophic cardiomyopathy, Marfan's syndrome, mitral valve prolapse (MVP), MI, Raynaud's disease, rheumatic fever, sudden cardiac death
SOCIAL HISTORY	*The components of the social history are linked to heart and peripheral vasculature factors and pathology.*

continues

Alcohol Use	Prolonged use of alcohol can interfere with the normal pumping function and electrical activity of the heart, leading to **cardiomegaly** (enlargement of the heart), poor left ventricular contractility, ventricular dilatation, palpitations, peripheral edema, fatigue, and SOB.
	Thiamine deficiencies that usually occur concurrently with alcohol abuse may contribute to dysrhythmias and heart failure.
	Excessive alcohol intake may play a role in the pathogenesis of dilated cardiomyopathy, angina, CAD, hypertension, dysrhythmias, stroke, and beriberi heart disease. On the other hand, the use of alcohol in moderation, up to 2 ounces a day, is inversely related to the development of CAD due to the protective effect of the increased HDL cholesterol.
Tobacco Use	Nicotine increases catecholamine release, leading to elevated cardiac output, heart rate, and blood pressure. Nicotine also inhibits the development of collateral circulation, causes peripheral vasoconstriction, thickens cardiac arterioles, causes platelet aggregation, leads to dysrhythmias, and neutralizes heparin, thus increasing the risk of thrombus formation. The tobacco habit contributes to the pathogenesis of CAD, angina, and atherosclerosis.
Drug Use	Intravenous drug use: Increased risk for contracting infective endocarditis because of the use of nonsterile needles and the embolization of localized infections from the injection site
	Amphetamines, cocaine, and heroin: Tachycardia, severe hypertension, hypotension, coronary vasospasm, MI, dysrhythmias, aortic rupture or dissection, coronary artery dissection, stroke, and dilated cardiomyopathy
Sexual Practice	Effect of intercourse on the heart (such as exertional chest pain) or eliciting a vagal response (which may occur with anal intercourse), thus making the patient prone to syncope and other sequelae
	Patients who use nitrate drugs should never take phosphodiesterase type 5 inhibitors.
Travel History	Arsenic poisoning: Systemic arterial disease, including gangrene and PVD; traced to the elevated arsenic content in drinking water and soil in Taiwan and Chile
	Chagas' disease: Severe dysrhythmias, mitral regurgitation or insufficiency, and cardiomegaly; caused by a protozoan parasite endemic to Central America, South America, and the Southwestern United States
Work Environment	Table 16-4 (see page 543) lists toxic substances that can cause profound cardiac pathology.
Home Environment	A dirty fireplace may cause a smoky environment that leads to the worsening of chest pain.
Hobbies and Leisure Activities	Any activity that involves exertion may contribute to a decline in status in a patient with cardiovascular pathology.
Stress	Atherosclerosis, tachycardia, HTN, dysrhythmias, sudden death

continues

Health History (continued)

HEALTH MAINTENANCE ACTIVITIES

This information provides a bridge between the health maintenance activities and heart and peripheral vasculature function.

Sleep

Dyspnea, orthopnea, or paroxysmal nocturnal dyspnea (PND)

Diet

Eating disorders (e.g., bulimia) and liquid protein diets have been associated with sudden death due to electrolyte imbalances (e.g., hypokalemia).

Foods high in vitamin K may reduce the effectiveness of anticoagulants.

Awareness of the sodium content of the tap water in your area (home water softeners often contain sodium)

Caffeine (in coffee, tea, soft drinks, chocolate, over-the-counter medications) is a sympathomimetic amine that increases the blood pressure and heart rate, elevates the serum catecholamine level, and can lead to dysrhythmias (especially premature atrial contractions).

BMI score should be 20–24.9 (see Chapter 7).

Exercise

Physical exercise may have either deleterious or beneficial effects on the heart, depending on the type of activity performed, the amount, and the condition of the exerciser. The aim of an individual's cardiovascular fitness program should be the attainment of the THR (also known as perceived rate of exertion) to increase cardiovascular tone. In general, it is believed that aerobic exercise or sustained physical activity for at least 20 to 30 minutes per day, three to five times per week, positively affects one's cardiovascular conditioning.

Stress Management

Exercise, time management, pet therapy, reading, listening to music, eating, biofeedback, yoga, imagery, massages, transcendental meditation, and participation in a variety of support groups

Use of Safety Devices

Patients with older pacemakers should avoid areas with microwaves; cellular phones (especially digital cellular phones) may cause interference with pacemakers.

Health Check-ups

EKG, chest X-ray, blood pressure, pulse, serum triglyceride, serum cholesterol

PATIENT CLASSIFICATION

The New York Heart Association (NYHA) has outlined four classifications for patients with cardiac pathologies. Class I indicates that the patient has no symptoms with ordinary physical activity. Class II means that the patient has some symptoms with normal activity and may have a slight limitation of activity. Class III states that a patient has symptoms with less than ordinary activity and has a marked limit of activity. Class IV indicates that the patient has symptoms with any physical activity or even at rest.

A consensus report sponsored by four cardiology societies defined myocardial infarction (MI) as "myocardial cell death due to prolonged ischemia" and recognizes five clinical classifications of MI. Type 1 is a spontaneous MI related to ischemia due to a primary coronary event such as plaque erosion and/or rupture, fissuring, or dissection. Type 2 is an MI where the ischemia is related to either increased oxygen demand or decreased supply (e.g., coronary artery spasm, coronary embolism, anemia, dysrhythmias, hypertension, or hypotension). Type 3 is sudden, unexpected cardiac death, including cardiac arrest. Type 4a is an MI associated with a percutaneous coronary intervention (PCI), while Type 4b is associated with stent thrombosis. Finally, Type 5 is an MI associated with coronary artery bypass grafting (CABG).

TABLE 16-1 Cardiovascular Disorders

DISORDER	DEFINITION	COMMON FINDINGS
Acute coronary syndrome (ACS)	An umbrella term used to describe a constellation of events associated with an acute myocardial ischemic episode, ranging from unstable angina to myocardial infarction	Chest pain that is similar to angina except that it is more intense and more persistent (>30 minutes); not fully relieved by rest or nitroglycerin; and accompanied by systemic symptoms (e.g., nausea, sweating, or apprehension)
Aneurysm	Localized abnormal dilation of a blood vessel	AAA: dulled abdominal or lower back pain; nausea and vomiting; ruptured AAA—severe, sudden, and continuous pain that radiates to back
		Thoracic aortic aneurysm (TAA): sudden, tearing pain in chest radiating to shoulders, neck, and back; dysphagia; dyspnea
Aortic regurgitation or insufficiency	Backflow of blood from the aorta to the left ventricle during diastole because of an incompetent valve	Dyspnea; PND; orthopnea; palpitations; angina; fatigue; syncope; diastolic murmur
Aortic stenosis	A narrowing or constriction of the aortic valve causing an obstruction to the ejection of blood from the left ventricle during systole	Syncope; fatigue; weakness; palpitations; angina; systolic murmur
Atherosclerosis (coronary artery disease)	A type of arteriosclerosis; localized accumulations of lipid-containing material within the blood vessels	Angina; MI; CHF; sudden cardiac death; dysrhythmias
Cardiac tamponade	Compression of the heart resulting from the accumulation of excess fluid in the pericardium	Beck's triad (hypotension, distended neck veins, and distant heart sounds); pulsus paradoxus
Cardiogenic shock	A shock of cardiac origin caused by pump failure	Pulmonary congestion; peripheral edema; hypotension; tachycardia; decreased pulse pressure; cool, pale, and clammy skin
Cardiomyopathy • congestive or dilated • hypertrophic • restrictive	Heart muscle disease	CHF-type symptoms; cardiomegaly with dilated or congestive form; familial history with hypertrophic form
Cerebrovascular accident (CVA)	Brain damage that results from decreased blood flow; a CVA can have an embolic, thrombotic, or hemorrhagic cause	Decreased neurological function; headaches; hemiparesis; hemiplegia; aphasia; coma; abnormal cranial nerve findings
Congestive heart failure	A condition whereby pump failure makes the heart unable to maintain a cardiac output sufficient to meet the metabolic needs of the body; the left ventricle, the right ventricle, or both may fail	Left-sided: anxiety, diaphoresis, rales, S_3, cough, PND, fatigue; right-sided: dependent pitting edema, hepatomegaly, weight gain, hepatojugular reflux
Deep vein thrombosis (DVT) and thrombophlebitis	The formation of a blood clot in a deep vein (most commonly in the leg or pelvis); inflammation of a vein due to a blood clot	Unilateral edema; calf pain or tenderness; temperature and color changes in the affected leg; cyanosis in the foot
Endocarditis (bacterial)	Infection of the endocardial surface or the heart valves	Fever; chills; fatigue; anorexia; nausea and vomiting; arthralgia; back pain; dyspnea; splinter hemorrhages of the nails; petechiae

continues

TABLE 16-1 (Continued)

DISORDER	DEFINITION	COMMON FINDINGS
Hypertension	Elevated blood pressure	Systolic blood pressure (SBP) >140 mm Hg; diastolic blood pressure (DBP) >90 mm Hg; most often asymptomatic; headaches or epistaxis; see Chapter 9 for further clarification
Marfan's syndrome (annuloaortic ectasia)	A syndrome of congenital collagen deficiency affecting the connective tissues	Patient may be tall and thin with hyper-extensive joints and long arms, legs, and fingers; aortic dissection; aortic regurgitation; mitral regurgitation; dysrhythmias
Metabolic syndrome (insulin-resistance syndrome)	Characterized by a group of metabolic risk factors that place patients at greater risk for coronary artery disease, stroke, and/or peripheral vascular disease as well as type 2 diabetes	Abdominal obesity and insulin resistance or glucose intolerance are the predominant risk factors associated with this disorder. Others include hyperlipidemia; hypertension; a prothrombotic state; and/or a proinflammatory state.
Mitral regurgitation or insufficiency	The backflow of blood from the left ventricle to the left atrium during systole and resulting from an incompetent valve	CHF-type symptoms; history of rheumatic fever, infection, trauma, or mitral valve prolapse; systolic murmur
Mitral stenosis	A narrowing or constriction of the mitral valve causing an obstruction of blood flow from the left atrium to the left ventricle during diastole	CHF-type symptoms; history of rheumatic heart disease or congenital heart defect; diastolic murmur; thrill at apex
Myocardial infarction	Myocardial cell death due to prolonged ischemia	Nausea and vomiting; diaphoresis; shortness of breath; abnormal heart and lung sounds; angina; dysrhythmias; CHF; cardiogenic shock
Myocarditis	Inflammation of the heart's muscular tissue	History of rheumatic fever; viral or parasitic infection; irregular pulse; tenderness over the pericardium; may lead to dilated cardiomyopathy
Pericarditis	An inflammation of the pericardium; origin may be viral, malignant, or autoimmune	Precordial pain that increases with inspiration or in the supine position; pain may be relieved by leaning forward; fever; fatigue; pulsus paradoxus; pericardial friction rub
Peripheral vascular disease	Vascular disorders of the arteries and veins that supply the extremities (usually refers to arterial disease)	Intermittent claudication; pain in the toes; ulcers that don't heal; impotence; loss of pulses; severe extremity pain; paresthesia
Pulmonary regurgitation or insufficiency	The backflow of blood from the pulmonary artery to the right ventricle because of an incompetent valve	Dyspnea on exertion (DOE); fatigue; diastolic murmur
Pulmonary stenosis	A narrowing or constriction of the pulmonary artery causing an obstruction to the ejection of blood from the right ventricle	DOE; fatigue; right-sided heart failure symptoms; systolic murmur
Raynaud's disease	A condition caused by abnormal blood vessel spasms in the extremities, especially in response to cold temperatures	Finger or toe becomes pale, cold, and numb, then becomes red, hot, and tingling
Tricuspid regurgitation or insufficiency	The backflow of blood from the right ventricle to the right atrium because of an incompetent valve	Dyspnea; fatigue; systolic murmur
Tricuspid stenosis	A narrowing or constriction of the tricuspid valve causing an obstruction of blood flow from the right atrium to the right ventricle	Dyspnea; fatigue; diastolic murmur; right-sided CHF
Ventricular aneurysm	The dilatation of a portion of necrosed ventricular wall after an MI	Tachydysrhythmias; CHF-type symptoms; clot formation; arterial emboli; rupture: cardiac tamponade; systolic murmur

TABLE 16-2 Congenital Cardiovascular Defects

A congenital cardiovascular defect (CCD), also known as congenital heart disease, occurs when the heart or blood vessels near the heart do not develop normally before birth. CCDs occur in about 1% of live births. Although there are few cures for CCD, more patients are now surviving to adulthood. Often the cause of the defect is unknown but it may be related to teratogenic, genetic, or random factors. The majority of patients with CCDs require long-term follow-up for the management of persistent problems such as electrophysiologic sequelae, myocardial changes, ventricular failure, prosthetic materials, or endocarditis.

Most CCDs either obstruct blood flow in the heart or vessels near the heart, or cause blood to flow through the heart in an abnormal pattern. Another rare defect occurs when the right or left side of the heart is not completely formed.

CLASSIFICATION	DISORDER	DEFINITION	COMMON FINDINGS	TREATMENT OPTIONS	SPECIAL CONSIDERATIONS
Obstruction Defects	Pulmonary stenosis (PS)	Occurs when a defective pulmonary valve does not open properly. Thus, the right ventricle must pump harder than normal to overcome the obstruction.	If stenosis is severe, especially in babies, then cyanosis may occur. Older children may not have symptoms. A pulmonic systolic ejection click, murmur, and/or a diminished S_2, possibly with a wide split, may be auscultated. Patient may also have a thrill.	Required when the pressure in the right ventricle is higher than normal. Obstruction can be relieved by balloon valvuloplasty or open-heart surgery.	Patients need subacute bacterial endocarditis (SBE) prophylaxis: Before and after treatment for their CCD, patients need to take antibiotics before certain dental and surgical procedures to prevent endocarditis.
	Aortic stenosis (AS)	Occurs when the aortic valve is narrowed. This makes it hard for the heart to pump blood to the body.	Chest pain, DOE, unusual tiring, dizziness, or fainting may occur. A systolic ejection murmur may be auscultated. Patient may also have a thrill.	The need for surgery depends on how bad the stenosis is. The stenosis may be relieved by enlarging the valve opening. Eventually, the valve may need to be replaced with an artificial valve.	• Patients need SBE prophylaxis. • Lifelong follow-up is required.
	Coarctation of the aorta (COA)	When the aorta is constricted, blood flow to the lower part of the body is obstructed. Also, the blood pressure above the obstruction is increased.	Symptoms of CHF and hypertension may develop in the week after birth. Blood pressure that is higher in the upper extremities than the lower extremities is suggestive of COA. A systolic murmur will often be present. Absent or weak femoral pulses are another hallmark sign. A heave over the left ventricle may be observed. In adulthood, the upper body may be more developed than the lower body.	Balloon angioplasty or surgery, or both.	• Patients need SBE prophylaxis. • Defect may reoccur. • Hypertension may ensue even after repair. • Lifelong follow-up is required.

continues

TABLE 16-2 (Continued)

CLASSIFICATION	DISORDER	DEFINITION	COMMON FINDINGS	TREATMENT OPTIONS	SPECIAL CONSIDERATIONS
Obstruction Defects *continued*	Bicuspid aortic valve	Occurs when the bicuspid valve has only two cusps, rather than the normal three.	There may be no symptoms in childhood but by adulthood, the valve can become stenotic or regurgitant. Thus, a diastolic or systolic murmur may be auscultated depending on the condition of the valve.	Treatment depends on how well the valve works.	Patients need SBE prophylaxis.
	Subaortic stenosis	Refers to a narrowing of the left ventricle just below the aortic valve. Thus, blood flow out of the left ventricle is limited. This condition may be congenital or it may be the result of a type of cardiomyopathy known as idiopathic hypertrophic subaortic stenosis (IHSS).	Patient may have an ejection murmur and thrill.	Treatment depends on the cause and severity of the narrowing and may include drugs or surgery.	Patients need SBE prophylaxis.
	Ebstein's anomaly	Occurs when the tricuspid valve is displaced downward into the right ventricle. It is usually associated with an atrial septal defect (ASD).	In mild cases, there are no symptoms. Later, patients may complain of tiredness, palpitations, or an abnormal heart beat. In severe cases, children may turn cyanotic and have CHF.	Medications for mild cases and surgery for severe cases.	Patients need SBE prophylaxis.
Septal Defects	Atrial septal defect (ASD)	Occurs when there is an opening between the heart's upper chambers. Thus, blood from the left atrium flows into the right atrium instead of flowing through the left ventricle, out of the aorta, and through the rest of the body.	Many children have few, if any, symptoms. A systolic ejection murmur, a diastolic murmur, a fixed widely split S_2, or a heave may be auscultated. Signs of CHF may occur in older patients.	Open-heart surgery in some cases.	None
	Ventricular septal defect (VSD)	Occurs when there is an opening between the heart's lower chambers. Thus, blood that has returned from the lungs and has been pumped into the left ventricle flows into the right ventricle instead of being pumped	Patient may have high pulmonary pressures. A lift is often observed, a thrill may be palpated, and a harsh holosystolic murmur may be auscultated. Children with VSDs may have poor weight gain,	Open-heart surgery for a large defect.	• Patients need SBE prophylaxis. • After a VSD has been successfully fixed with surgery, prophylactic antibiotics are usually not required.

continues

TABLE 16-2 (Continued)

CLASSIFICATION	DISORDER	DEFINITION	COMMON FINDINGS	TREATMENT OPTIONS	SPECIAL CONSIDERATIONS
Septal Defects *continued*		directly through the aorta. The heart may enlarge because it has to pump extra blood and thus may become overworked.	slow growth, feeding difficulties, DOE, and failure to thrive (FTT).		• Lifelong follow-up is required.
	Eisenmenger's complex or syndrome	Consists of both a VSD and pulmonary hypertension. Therefore, blood shunts from the right side of the heart to the left, causing the right ventricle to enlarge. It may also include an overriding aorta whereby a malpositioned aorta receives ejected blood from both ventricles.	Severe CHF and cyanosis with a right to left shunt. Patients may have healthy childhoods but become progressively cyanotic in adulthood, with poor exercise tolerance. Syncope may occur. Problems might not arise until pregnancy or some other type of cardiovascular stress occurs.	Surgery followed by a possible heart or heart-lung transplant.	• Patients need SBE prophylaxis. • Lifelong follow-up is required.
	Atrioventricular canal defect (also known as endocardial cushion defect or atrioventricular septal defect)	Consists of both a large hole in the center of the heart plus a single, large valve (which is a combination of the tricuspid and mitral valves) that crosses the defect. Eventually, the heart may enlarge because it has to pump extra blood and thus may become overworked. The defect may be complete, intermediate, or partial (the most common form).	Babies may become undernourished because they don't grow normally. Pulmonary hypertension occurs because there is increased blood flowing to the lungs. Patients may present with CHF. S_2 may be widely split. Diastolic and systolic murmurs may be auscultated.	Surgery	• Patients need SBE prophylaxis. • A reconstructed valve may not work normally. • About 40% to 50% of patients with this defect have Down syndrome.
Cyanotic Defects	Tetralogy of Fallot	Has four components: 1. VSD 2. Stenosis at or beneath the pulmonic valve 3. Right ventricular hypertrophy 4. Dextroposition of the aorta (the aorta now lies directly over the VSD)	Cyanosis may occur soon after birth or with rapid breathing. Older children may faint during exercise because not enough blood flows to the lungs to supply the body with oxygen. Subsequently, clubbing of the fingers and toes may occur. Patients may have a heave as well as a systolic ejection murmur, a loud S_2, and a thrill.	Surgery	Patients need SBE prophylaxis.

continues

TABLE 16-2 (Continued)

continues

CLASSIFICATION	DISORDER	DEFINITION	COMMON FINDINGS	TREATMENT OPTIONS	SPECIAL CONSIDERATIONS
Cyanotic Defects *continued*	Transposition of the great arteries	Occurs when the positions of the pulmonary artery and the aorta are reversed. The aorta is connected to the right ventricle, so most of the blood returning to the heart from the body has not gone through the lungs to be oxygenated. The pulmonary artery is connected to the left ventricle, so most of the blood returning from the lungs goes back to the lungs again.	Cyanosis, tachypnea without respiratory distress, loud S_2, poor feeding in infants	Surgery	• Patients need SBE prophylaxis. • Lifelong follow-up is required. • This defect is rare (<1% of all congenital heart defects).
	Tricuspid atresia	With this defect, there is no tricuspid valve; therefore, blood cannot flow from the right atrium to the right ventricle. Thus, the right ventricle is small and underdeveloped. The child's survival depends on whether there is both an ASD and a VSD.	Cyanosis	If left untreated, patients will die. Thus, surgery is required.	• Patients need SBE prophylaxis. • Lifelong follow-up is required.
	Pulmonary atresia	With this defect, there is no pulmonary valve; therefore, blood cannot flow from the right ventricle into the pulmonary artery and on into the lungs. The right ventricle may be small and underdeveloped. The tricuspid valve may also be abnormal. An ASD allows blood to exit the right side of the heart. A coexisting PDA is the only source of lung blood flow.	Cyanosis, clubbing, dyspnea, or tachypnea	Medications and surgery	• Patients need SBE prophylaxis. • Lifelong follow-up is required.

TABLE 16-2 (Continued)

CLASSIFICATION	DISORDER	DEFINITION	COMMON FINDINGS	TREATMENT OPTIONS	SPECIAL CONSIDERATIONS
Cyanotic Defects continued	Truncus arteriosus	Consists of only one artery, which arises from the heart and forms the aorta and the pulmonary artery. May also have a VSD. There are four types of this defect depending on how the pulmonary arteries originate from the single arterial vessel.	Cyanosis, CHF, tachypnea, or poor feeding. A systolic ejection click is often heard, as well as a harsh pansystolic murmur.	Medications and surgery	• Patients need SBE prophylaxis. • Lifelong follow-up is required.
	Total anomalous pulmonary venous connection	Occurs when the pulmonary veins do not connect to the left atrium. Instead, they drain through abnormal connections to the right atrium.	Cyanosis	Surgery	Lifelong follow-up is required.
Miscellaneous	Hypoplastic left heart syndrome	Results in an underdeveloped left side of the heart. May also have an ASD, PDA, or both.	Babies become ashen within days of birth, sometimes cyanotic. They will also have rapid breathing and difficulty in feeding. CHF, shock, and multisystem organ failure may be present.	Compassionate care, medications, surgery, and/or possibly a heart transplant.	• This heart defect is usually fatal without treatment. • Patients need SBE prophylaxis. • Lifelong follow-up is required.
	Patent ductus arteriosus (PDA)	This defect occurs when the ductus, which is patent in utero, fails to close after birth. This allows blood to mix between the pulmonary artery and aorta. Consequently, the right ventricle has to work harder and pulmonary hypertension may ensue.	If ductus is large, children may tire quickly, grow slowly, breathe rapidly, and catch pneumonia easily. A continuous, harsh, loud, and machine-like murmur is often heard throughout systole and diastole.	Surgery	

TABLE 16-3 Differentiating Chest Pain

All of these conditions (excluding musculoskeletal) are life threatening and require immediate attention.

CARDIAC ISCHEMIA (also known as acute coronary syndrome)

Pain: burning, squeezing or aching, heaviness, smothering

- Not reproducible by palpation of the chest wall, may be relieved with rest or oxygen, and may or may not be accompanied by EKG changes.
- Myocardial ischemia may lead to myocardial infarction; when in doubt, assume a cardiac cause and follow your institution's chest pain protocol.

AORTIC (THORACIC) DISSECTION

Pain: sudden, sharp, and tearing, and radiates to shoulders, neck, back, and abdomen

- Neurological complications: hemiplegia, sensory deficits secondary to carotid artery occlusion.
- May present with a new murmur, bruits, or unequal blood pressure in upper extremities.

PERICARDITIS

Pain: positional ache, dyspnea

- May also present with a pericardial friction rub or distended neck veins.

PULMONARY EMBOLUS

Pain: sudden onset, sharp or stabbing, varies with respiration

- May also present with dyspnea, tachypnea, fever, tachycardia, diaphoresis, or DVT.

PNEUMOTHORAX

Pain: sudden onset, tearing or pleuritic, worsened by breathing

- May also have dyspnea, tachycardia, decreased breath sounds, and a deviated trachea. Refer to Chapter 15 for further information.

PNEUMONIA

Pain: stabbing that is exacerbated by coughing and deep breathing

- Presents with fever, chills, productive cough, tachypnea. Refer to Chapter 15 for further information.

ESOPHAGEAL RUPTURE

Pain: sudden onset upon swallowing or constant retrosternal, epigastric pain

- May mimic signs and symptoms of a pneumothorax.
- Consider esophageal rupture when a patient has experienced penetrating trauma, a severe epigastric blow, or a first or second rib fracture.

MISCELLANEOUS: MUSCULOSKELETAL

Pain: reproducible by chest wall palpation

- May be relieved by position changes.

MISCELLANEOUS: RECREATIONAL DRUG USE (cocaine, amphetamines, or stimulants)

Pain: Cardiac ischemia pain (as listed above)

- May produce a direct, toxic effect on the myocardium.

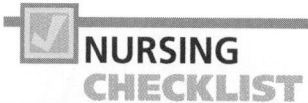

NURSING CHECKLIST

General Approach to Heart Assessment

1. Explain to the patient what you are going to do.
2. Ensure that the room is warm, quiet, and well lit.
3. Expose the patient's chest only as much as is needed for the assessment.
4. Position the patient in a supine or sitting position.
5. Stand to the patient's right side. The light should come from the opposite side of where you are standing so that shadows can be accentuated.

EQUIPMENT

- Stethoscope
- Sphygmomanometer
- Watch with second hand
- Tape measure

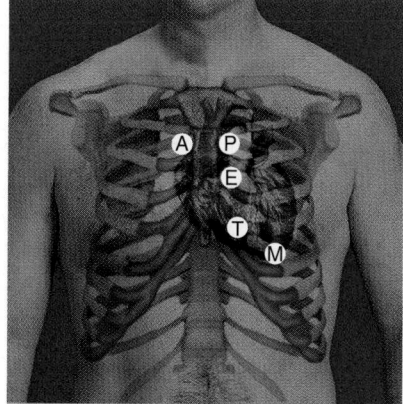

FIGURE 16-9 The Cardiac Landmarks. A = Aortic Area; P = Pulmonic Area; E = Erb's Point; T = Tricuspid Area; M = Mitral Area

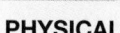

TABLE 16-4 Work-Related Exposures to Cardiotoxic Substances

PHYSICAL

- Extremes of oxygen pressure, barometric pressure, gravity, acceleration, noise, temperature, and humidity

BIOLOGICAL

- Laboratory-acquired infections
- Work in endemic areas

CHEMICAL

- Arsenic
- Carbon disulfide
- Carbon monoxide
- Cobalt
- Fibrogenic dust found in asbestos
- Fluorocarbons found in solvents and propellants
- Halogenated hydrocarbons
- Heavy metals such as lead

ASSESSMENT OF THE PRECORDIUM

The cardiovascular physical assessment has two major components:

1. Assessment of the **precordium** (the area on the anterior surface of the body overlying the heart, great vessels, pericardium, and some pulmonary tissue) and
2. Assessment of the periphery.

Inspection, palpation, and auscultation should be performed in a systematic manner, using certain cardiac landmarks. Percussion has limited usefulness in the cardiovascular assessment because X-rays and other diagnostic tests provide the same information in a much more accurate manner. The cardiac landmarks (Figure 16-9) are defined as follows:

1. The aortic area is the second intercostal space (ICS) to the right of the sternum.
2. The pulmonic area is the second ICS to the left of the sternum.
3. The midprecordial area, Erb's point, is located in the third ICS to the left of the sternum.
4. The tricuspid area is the fifth ICS to the left of the sternum. Other terms for this area are the right ventricular area or the septal area.
5. The mitral area is the fifth ICS at the left midclavicular line. Other terms for this area are the left ventricular area or the apical area.

These cardiac landmarks are the locations where the heart sounds are heard best, not where the valves are actually located. The mitral area correlates anatomically with the apex of the heart; the aortic and pulmonic areas correlate anatomically with the base of the heart. Assessment of the heart should proceed in an orderly fashion from the base of the heart to the apex, or from the apex of the heart to the base.

INSPECTION

Aortic Area

E 1. Lightly place your index finger on the angle of Louis.

2. Move your finger laterally to the right of the sternum to the rib. This is the second rib.

3. Move your finger down beneath the second rib to the ICS. The aortic area is located in the second ICS to the right of the sternum.

N No pulsations should be visible.

A A pulsation in the aortic area is abnormal.

P A pulsation in the aortic area may indicate the presence of an aortic root aneurysm. The aneurysm's dilation may become bigger when the patient experiences hypertension. A rupture can occur at any time but the risk is greater when the aneurysm becomes 5 cm or more in diameter.

Pulmonic Area

E 1. Lightly place your index finger on the left second ICS.

2. The pulmonic area is located at the second ICS to the left of the sternum.

N No pulsations should be visible.

A A pulsation or bulge in the pulmonic area is an abnormal finding.

P Pulmonary stenosis, which is usually congenital, impedes blood flow from the right ventricle into the lungs, causing a bulge. The right side of the heart then dilates and the right ventricle becomes hypertrophied in order to accommodate the load.

Midprecordial Area

E 1. Lightly place your index finger on the left second ICS.

2. Continue to move your finger down the left rib cage, counting the third rib and the third ICS.

3. The midprecordial area, or Erb's point, is located at the third ICS, left sternal border. Both aortic and pulmonic murmurs may be heard here.

N No pulsations should be visible.

A The presence of a pulsation or a systolic bulge in the midprecordial area is not normal.

P A left ventricular aneurysm can produce a midprecordial pulsation. Ventricular aneurysms can develop several weeks following an acute MI. With an MI, the hydraulic stress on the infarcted area may cause the damaged ventricular wall to bulge and become extremely thin during systole.

A A retraction in the midprecordial area is abnormal.

P Pericardial disease can produce retractions in this area (retractions occur when there is a pulling in some of the tissues of the precordium, depending on the activities of the heart).

| **E** Examination | **N** Normal Findings | **A** Abnormal Findings | **P** Pathophysiology |

Tricuspid Area

E   1. Lightly place your index finger on the left third ICS.

2. Continue to move your finger down the left rib cage, counting the fourth rib, the fourth ICS, and the fifth rib followed by the fifth ICS.

3. The tricuspid area is located at the fifth ICS, left of the sternal border.

N   No pulsations should be visible.

A   A visible systolic pulsation in the tricuspid area is abnormal.

P   A visible systolic pulsation can result from right ventricular enlargement secondary to an increased stroke volume. Anxiety, hyperthyroidism, fever, and pregnancy are clinical situations that produce an increased stroke volume.

Mitral Area

E   1. Lightly place your index finger on the left fifth ICS.

2. Move your finger laterally to the midclavicular line. This is the mitral landmark. In a large-breasted patient, have the patient displace the left breast upward and to the left so you can locate the mitral landmark.

N   Normally, there is no movement in the precordium except at the mitral area, where the left ventricle lies close enough to the skin's surface that it visibly pulsates during systole. The apical impulse at the mitral landmark is generally visible in about half of the adult population. This pulsation is also known as the point of maximal impulse (PMI) and occurs simultaneously with carotid pulsation.

A   Hypokinetic (decreased movement) pulsations at the mitral area are considered abnormal.

P   Conditions that place more fluid between the left ventricle and the chest wall, such as a pericardial effusion or cardiac tamponade, produce a hypokinetic or absent pulsation. In obese individuals, excess subcutaneous tissue dampens the apical impulse. Low-output states such as shock produce a less palpable apical impulse from the reduced blood volume and decreased myocardial contractility. Keep in mind that absent pulsations are normal in half of the adult population.

A   Hyperkinetic (increased movement) pulsations are always abnormal when located at the mitral area.

P   High-output states such as mitral regurgitation, thyrotoxicosis, severe anemia, and left-to-right heart shunts are potential causes of hyperkinetic pulsations.

PALPATION

Inspection and palpation of the heart go hand in hand. Again, you must be systematic in this part of the assessment and palpate the cardiac landmarks starting at either the base or the apex of the heart. During palpation, assess for the apical impulse, pulsations, **thrills** (vibrations that feel similar to what one feels when a hand is placed on a purring cat), and **heaves** (lifting of the cardiac area secondary to an increased workload and force of left ventricular contraction; also referred to as lift). The patient should be in a supine position for this portion of the assessment.

NURSING**TIP**

PMI versus Apical Impulse

The term *PMI* has fallen out of favor because it can be a misnomer if cardiac pathology causes a stronger impulse in a different region. Any movement other than the apical impulse is abnormal and should be described in terms of type, location, and timing in relation to the cardiac cycle.

CARDIOVASCULAR ASSISTIVE DEVICESCHECKLIST

Assessing Patients with Cardiovascular Assistive Devices

The patient with cardiovascular disease may need the assistance of special equipment to maintain an optimal cardiovascular system. The presence of cardiovascular assistive devices must be noted during the inspection process. Consider the following to assist you in observing these devices:

1. Artificial cardiac pacemakers (e.g., temporary external chest pacing, temporary internal pacing, permanent pacemaker); ICD
   - The pacemaker is on. Check the settings.
   - The ICD is on. Check the settings.
   - Check for external pacer wires. Wires should be protected from electrical hazards per your facility's policy.
   - The insertion site is free of infection.
   - Check your facility's policy for verifying and controlling the settings.

2. Hemodynamic monitoring (e.g., arterial pressure line [a-line]; central venous pressure [CVP] line; right atrial pressure [RAP] line; left atrial pressure [LAP] line; pulmonary artery [PA] catheter [Swan-Ganz])
   - Check the goal of the line (e.g., fluid, monitoring).
   - The monitor's alarms are on. The appropriate limits are set.
   - The transducer level is at the patient's right atrium (phlebostatic axis—fourth ICS, midaxillary line).
   - The pressure bag(s) is pumped to 300 mm Hg.
   - Change the flush bag(s) per your facility's policy.
   - The line is safely secured to the patient or the bed (it is not just dangling).
   - The insertion site is free of infection.

3. Antiembolic stockings
   - Determine whether the stockings are knee-high or thigh-high.
   - Ensure that they are the correct size (see the manufacturer's directions for correct sizing).
   - The patient has palpable or audible pulses in the lower extremities.
   - The stockings have been removed at least once per day to assess the patient's skin.

4. Chest tubes
   - Determine where the chest tube is.
   - Determine whether the chest tube is for air or fluid.
   - Ascertain if drainage system is wet suction or dry suction.
   - Determine whether the chest tube is on wall suction or water seal.
   - If the chest tube is on suction, the chest drainage system is bubbling and the water-seal chamber is fluctuating.
   - The chest tube connections are secured.
   - The chest tube is kink-free.
   - The insertion site is free of subcutaneous emphysema.
   - The insertion site is free of infection.

5. EKG monitoring
   - The patient's skin is intact where the EKG pads are located.
   - The leads are placed correctly.
   - The monitor's alarms are on. The appropriate limits are set.

6. Intravenous (IV) catheters
   - Determine whether the catheter is inserted peripherally or centrally.
   - The insertion site is free of infection, infiltration, or thrombophlebitis.
   - Determine what the fluid is.
   - Determine whether there are any additives in the fluid.
   - Determine the rate of the IV.
   - Determine when the IV can be discontinued.
   - Rotate IV site per your facility's policy.

7. Pneumatic compression stockings
   - Determine whether the patient has some sort of stocking between the legs and the plastic enclosures.
   - The device is on.
   - The stockings have been removed at least once per day to assess the patient's skin.

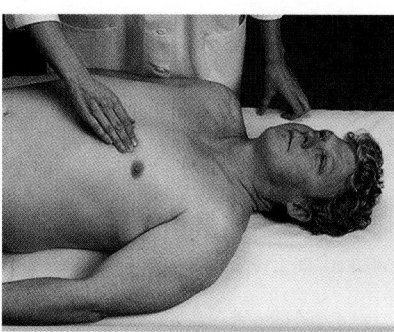

FIGURE 16-10 Palpating for Pulsations

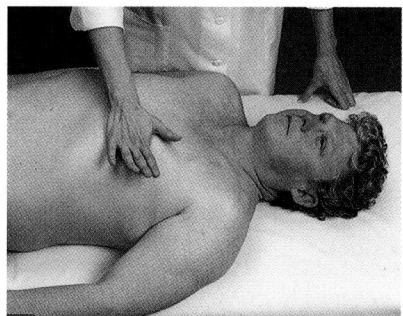

FIGURE 16-11 Palpating for Thrills

E Palpate the cardiac landmarks for:

1. Pulsations: Using the finger pads, locate the cardiac landmark and palpate the area for pulsations (Figure 16-10).
2. Thrills: Using the palmar surface of the hand at the base of the fingers (also known as the ball of the hand), locate the cardiac landmark and palpate the area for thrills (Figure 16-11).
3. Heaves: Follow step 2 and palpate the area for heaves.

Aortic Area

E Palpate the aortic area for pulsations, thrills, and heaves.

N No pulsations, thrills, or heaves should be palpated.

A Palpation of a thrill in the aortic area is abnormal.

P Aortic stenosis and aortic regurgitation create turbulent blood flow in the left ventricle, which may be palpated as a thrill.

Pulmonic Area

E Palpate the pulmonic area for pulsations, thrills, and heaves.

N No pulsations, thrills, or heaves should be palpated.

A Palpation of a thrill in the pulmonic area is abnormal.

P Pulmonic stenosis and pulmonic regurgitation create turbulent blood flow in the right ventricle, which may be palpated as a thrill.

Midprecordial Area

E Palpate the midprecordial area for pulsations, thrills, and heaves.

N No pulsations, thrills, or heaves should be palpated.

A Palpation of pulsations in the midprecordial area is abnormal.

P Both a left ventricular aneurysm and an enlarged right ventricle can produce a pulsation in the midprecordial area.

Tricuspid Area

E Palpate the tricuspid area for pulsations, thrills, and heaves.

N No pulsations, thrills, or heaves should be felt.

A Palpation of a thrill in the tricuspid area is abnormal.

P Tricuspid stenosis and tricuspid regurgitation create turbulent blood flow in the right atrium, which may be palpated as a thrill.

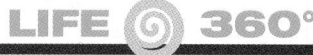

Assessing Assistive Devices

You are starting a new shift in the cardiovascular intensive care unit. You are assigned to a patient who returned from the operating room 2 hours ago after undergoing a mitral valve replacement. The patient has been having hypotensive episodes since arriving in the unit and is receiving a dopamine infusion. You conduct your physical assessment of the patient and include the patient's assistive devices. You find that an antibiotic infusion is infusing into the line that is marked dopamine. What would you do in this situation?

| **E** Examination | **N** Normal Findings | **A** Abnormal Findings | **P** Pathophysiology |

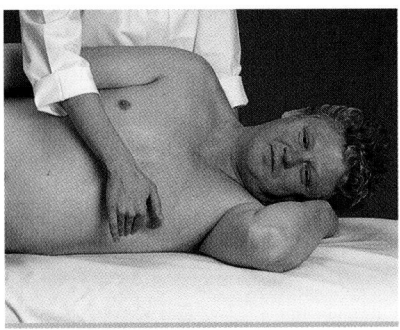

FIGURE 16-12 Palpating the Apical Impulse with the Patient on the Left Side

A Palpation of a heave in the tricuspid area is abnormal.

P Right ventricular enlargement may produce a heave in the tricuspid area secondary to an increased workload.

Mitral Area

E Palpate the mitral area for pulsations, thrills, and heaves. If a pulsation (apical impulse) is not palpable, turn the patient to the left side and palpate in this position (Figure 16-12). This position facilitates palpation because the heart shifts closer to the chest wall.

N The apical impulse is palpable in approximately half of the adult population. It is felt as a light, localized tap that is 1 to 2 cm in diameter. The amplitude is small and it can be felt immediately after the first heart sound, lasting for about one-half of systole. This impulse may be exaggerated in young patients. A thrill is not found in the normal adult population. A heave is absent in the healthy adult.

A A thrill palpated at the fifth ICS at the left midclavicular line is considered abnormal.

P Mitral stenosis and mitral regurgitation may produce a thrill from the turbulent blood flow found in the left atrium.

A A visible heave, or sustained apex beat, displaced laterally to the left sixth ICS at the anterior axillary line is abnormal. It is usually more than 3 cm in diameter and has a large amplitude.

P Left ventricular hypertrophy produces a laterally displaced apical impulse because of the increased size of the left ventricle in the thorax and the subsequent shifting of the heart. In addition, the hypertrophied muscle works harder during a contraction to produce a heave or sustained apex beat. This frequently occurs in conditions such as aortic stenosis, systemic hypertension, and idiopathic hypertrophic subaortic stenosis (which is a form of hypertrophic cardiomyopathy).

A Hypokinetic pulsations, usually less than 1 to 2 cm in diameter and of small amplitude, are abnormal.

P Conditions that place more fluid between the left ventricle and the chest wall, such as a pericardial effusion or cardiac tamponade, produce a hypokinetic or absent pulsation. In obesity, the excess subcutaneous tissue dampens the apical impulse. Low-output states such as shock produce a less palpable apical impulse from the reduced blood volume and decreased myocardial contractility.

A Hyperkinetic pulsations, usually greater than 1 to 2 cm in diameter and of increased amplitude, are abnormal.

P High-output states such as mitral regurgitation, thyrotoxicosis, severe anemia, and left-to-right heart shunts are potential causes of hyperkinetic pulsations.

AUSCULTATION

Aortic Area

E Place the diaphragm of the stethoscope on the aortic landmark and listen for S_2.

N S_2 is caused by the closure of the semilunar valves. S_2 corresponds to the "dub" sound in the phonetic "lub-dub" representation of heart sounds.

NURSING**TIP**

Heart Auscultation Practice

In addition to practicing auscultation in the clinical setting, it is possible to refine auscultation skills on the Internet. Web sites—such as Auscultation Assistant at www.wilkes.med. ucla.edu/intro.html—allow the listener to hear a variety of normal and pathological heart sounds.

E Examination   **N** Normal Findings   **A** Abnormal Findings   **P** Pathophysiology

☑**NURSING**CHECKLIST

General Approach to Heart Auscultation

1. Explain to the patient what you are going to do.
2. Expose the patient's chest only as much as is needed for the assessment. Never auscultate through any type of clothing.
3. Position the patient in a supine or sitting position. The left lateral position may be used for auscultation of the mitral and tricuspid areas. Also, the upright, leaning-forward position may be used for thorough auscultation of the aortic area.
4. Stand to the patient's right side.
5. Use the correct headpiece of the stethoscope. The diaphragm transmits high-frequency sounds, whereas the bell is used for low-pitched sounds. Keep in mind when using the bell that it should rest lightly on the skin. If too much pressure is applied, the bell will act like a diaphragm.
6. Warm the headpiece in your hands prior to touching it to the patient.
7. Listen to all four of the valvular cardiac landmarks at least twice. During the first auscultation, identify S_1 and S_2, and then listen for a possible S_3 and S_4. During the second auscultation, listen for murmurs and friction rubs. As you gain expertise, you may be able to listen for S_1, S_2, S_3, S_4, murmurs, and friction rubs all at the same time.
8. Listen for at least a few cardiac cycles (10 to 15 seconds) in each area. It may be helpful to close your eyes when you auscultate heart sounds to facilitate increased auditory concentration.

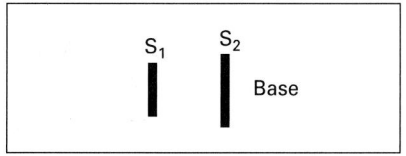

A. Normal S_2

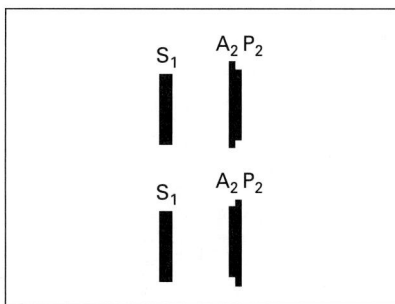

B. Intensified A_2, Diminished A_2

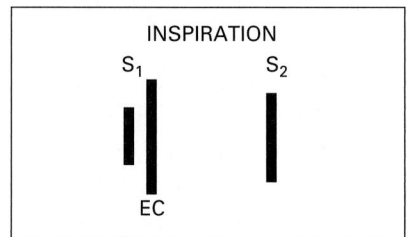

C. Aortic Ejection Click

FIGURE 16-13 **Summation of Heart Sounds** *continues*

S_2 heralds the onset of diastole. S_2 is louder than S_1 at this landmark (Figure 16-13A).

A The components of S_2 are A_2 (aortic) and P_2 (pulmonic). A greatly intensified or diminished A_2 is considered abnormal (Figure 16-13B).

P Arterial hypertension, which increases the pressure in the aorta, may be suspected in the case of a greatly intensified A_2. Aortic stenosis, where the aortic valve is calcified or thickened, may be the cause of a diminished A_2.

A An ejection **click** is an abnormal systolic sound that is high pitched and can radiate in the chest wall. It is created by the opening of the damaged valve and it does not vary with the respiratory cycle. An ejection click follows S_1 (Figure 16-13C).

P An ejection click can be auscultated in aortic stenosis, where the calcified valve produces this sound on opening.

Pulmonic Area

E Place the diaphragm of the stethoscope on the chest wall at the pulmonic landmark and listen for S_2.

N S_2 is also heard in the pulmonic area. S_2 is louder than S_1 at this landmark as depicted in Figure 16-13A. It is softer than the S_2 auscultated in the aortic area because the pressure on the left side of the heart is greater than that on the right. There is a normal physiological splitting of S_2 that is heard best at the pulmonic area. The components of a split S_2 are A_2 (aortic) and P_2 (pulmonic) (see Figure 16-13D). The aortic component occurs slightly before the pulmonic component during inspiration. The physiology of a split S_2 is that during inspiration, because of

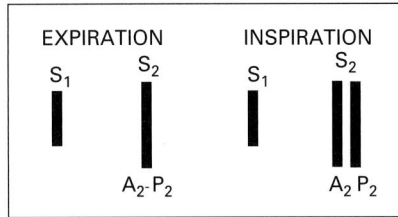

D. Normal Physiological Split of S_2

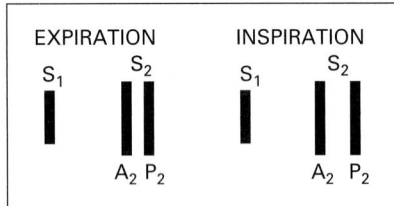

E. Wide Splitting of S_2

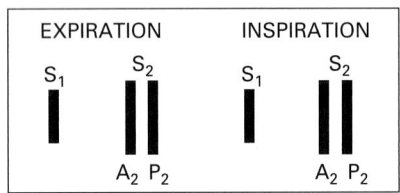

F. Fixed Splitting of S_2

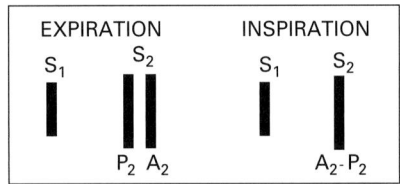

G. Paradoxical Splitting of S_2

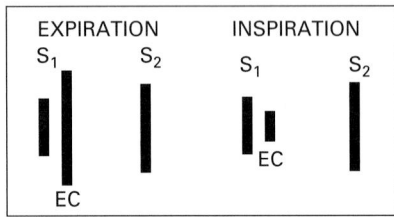

H. Pulmonic Ejection Click

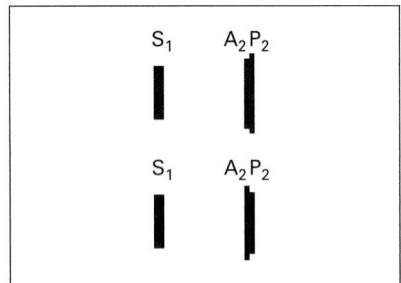

I. Intensified P_2, Diminished P_2

FIGURE 16-13 **Summation of Heart Sounds** *continues*

the more negative intrathoracic pressure, the venous return to the right side of the heart increases. Thus, pulmonic closure is delayed because of the extra time needed for the increased blood volume to pass through the valve. Normally, the A_2 component of the split S_2 is louder than the P_2 component because of the greater pressures in the left side of the heart.

A When a split S_2 occurs that is abnormally wide, the aortic valve closes early and the pulmonic valve closes late. There is a split on both inspiration and expiration, but a wider split on inspiration, as shown in Figure 16-13E.

P Delayed closure of the pulmonic valve may be due to a delay in the electrical stimulation of the right ventricle, as seen with right bundle branch block.

A Fixed splitting, a wide splitting that does not change with inspiration or expiration, is abnormal (Figure 16-13F). The pulmonic valve consistently closes later than the aortic valve. The right side of the heart is already ejecting a large volume, so filling cannot be increased during inspiration.

P Right ventricular failure that results in a prolonged right ventricular systole or a large atrial septal defect can lead to fixed splitting.

A In paradoxical splitting, the aortic valve closes after the pulmonic valve because of the delay in left ventricular systole. This occurs during expiration and disappears with inspiration. It is considered abnormal (Figure 16-13G).

P Left bundle branch block, aortic stenosis, patent ductus arteriosus, severe hypertension, and left ventricular failure are conditions in which paradoxical splitting may be auscultated.

A A pulmonic ejection click always indicates an abnormality (Figure 16-13H).

P A pulmonic ejection click is caused by the opening of a diseased pulmonic valve. It is heard loudest on expiration and is quieter on inspiration. It occurs early in systole and it does not radiate.

A A P_2 that is louder than or equal in volume to A_2 is abnormal, as is a greatly diminished P_2 (Figure 16-13I).

P A loud P_2 is expected in pulmonary hypertension, where the pressures in the pulmonary artery are abnormally high; pulmonic stenosis, where the pulmonic valve is calcified or thickened, may be the cause of a diminished P_2.

Midprecordial Area

Erb's point is where both aortic and pulmonic murmurs may be auscultated. Refer to the discussion on murmurs later in this chapter for additional information.

Tricuspid Area

E Place the diaphragm of the stethoscope on the chest wall at the tricuspid landmark to listen for S_1.

N S_1 in the tricuspid area is softer than the S_1 auscultated in the mitral area because the pressure in the left side of the heart is greater than that in the right. S_1 is louder than S_2 at this landmark (see Figure 16-13J). There is a normal physiological splitting of S_1 that is best heard in the tricuspid area (see Figure 16-13K). This split occurs because the mitral valve closes slightly before the tricuspid valve due to greater pressures in the left side of the heart.

| **E** Examination | **N** Normal Findings | **A** Abnormal Findings | **P** Pathophysiology |

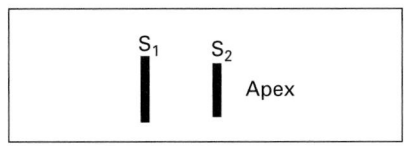

J. Normal S_1

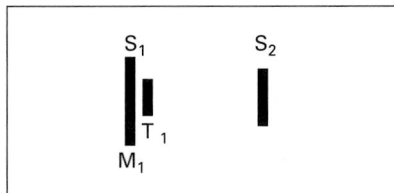

K. Normal Physiological Split of S_1

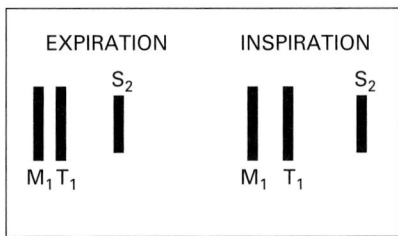

L. Wide Split of S_1

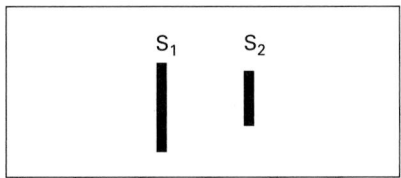

M. Loud S_1

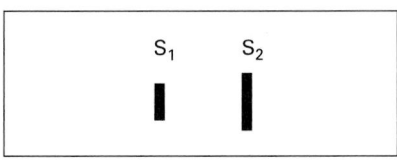

N. Soft S_1

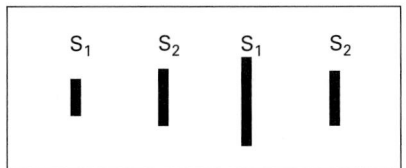

O. Variable S_1

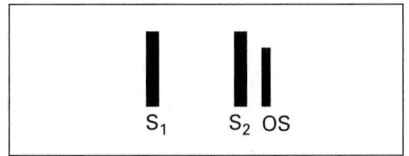

P. Opening Snap

FIGURE 16-13 **Summation of Heart Sounds** *continues*

The components of a split S_1 are M_1 (mitral) and T_1 (tricuspid). Physiological splitting disappears when the patient holds his or her breath.

A A split S_1 with an abnormally wide split is pathological (Figure 16-13L). The split is wider than usual during inspiration and is still heard on expiration.

P A split S_1 is usually due to electrical malfunctions such as right bundle branch block or mechanical problems such as mitral stenosis. In mitral stenosis, the tricuspid valve can close before the mitral valve closes because of calcification of the diseased mitral valve.

Mitral Area

E 1. Place the diaphragm of the stethoscope over the mitral area to identify S_1.

2. If you are unable to distinguish S_1 from S_2, palpate the carotid artery with the hand closest to the head while auscultating the mitral landmark. You will hear S_1 with each carotid pulse beat.

N S_1 is heard the loudest in the mitral area. S_1 is caused by the closure of the mitral and tricuspid valves. S_1 corresponds to the "lub" sound in the phonetic "lub-dub" representation of heart sounds. S_1 is louder than S_2 at this landmark (Figure 16-13J). S_1 also heralds the onset of systole. At normal or slow heart rates, systole (the time occurring between S_1 and S_2) is usually shorter than diastole. Diastole constitutes two-thirds of the cardiac cycle, with systole being the other third. The intensity of S_1 depends on:

   1. The adequacy of the A-V cusps in halting the ventricular blood flow

   2. The mobility of the cusps

   3. The position of the cusps and the rate of ventricular contraction

A An abnormally loud S_1 occurs when the mitral valve is wide open when systolic contraction begins, then slams shut (Figure 16-13M).

P A loud S_1 occurs in mitral stenosis, short PR interval syndrome (0.11 to 0.13 second), or in high-output states such as tachycardia, hyperthyroidism, and exercise.

A A soft S_1 is abnormal (Figure 16-13N).

P A soft S_1 can occur as a result of rheumatic fever, where the mitral valve has only limited motion.

A A variable abnormal S_1 occurs when diastolic filling time varies. Both a soft and a loud S_1 can be auscultated (Figure 16-13O).

P A variable S_1 can occur with complete heart block, where the atria and the ventricles are beating independently, and in atrial fibrillation, where the ventricles are beating irregularly.

A An opening **snap** is an early diastolic sound that is high-pitched. It is abnormal (Figure 16-13P).

P An opening snap is caused by the opening of a diseased valve and can be auscultated in mitral stenosis. The sound does not vary with respirations and can radiate throughout the chest. It follows S_2 and can be differentiated from an S_3 because it occurs earlier than an S_3.

A In tachycardia, the heart rate increases, diastole shortens, and systole and diastole become increasingly difficult to distinguish. Tachycardia is abnormal.

P Tachycardia can occur in exercise, fever, anxiety, pregnancy, and conditions that lead to hypertrophy, such as heart failure.

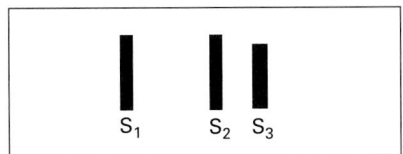

Q. S₃

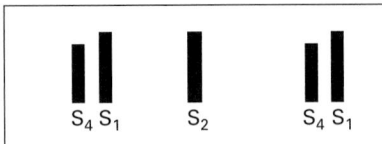

R. S₄

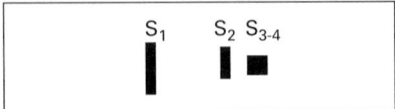

S. Summation Gallop

FIGURE 16-13 **Summation of Heart Sounds** *continued*

Mitral and Tricuspid Areas (S₃)

Auscultation of the mitral and tricuspid areas is repeated for low-pitched sounds, specifically an S₃ (otherwise known as a ventricular diastolic **gallop**, or extra heart sound). An S₃ is an early diastolic filling sound that originates in the ventricles and is therefore heard best at the apex of the heart. A right-sided S₃ (tricuspid area) is heard louder during inspiration because the venous return to the right side of the heart increases with a more negative intrathoracic pressure. An S₃ sound occurs just after an S₂ (Figure 16-13Q).

E   1. Place the bell of the stethoscope lightly over the mitral landmark. When the S₃ originates in the left ventricle, it is heard best with the patient in a left lateral decubitus position and exhaling.

2. When originating in the right ventricle, an S₃ can best be heard by placing the bell of the stethoscope lightly over the third or fourth ICS at the left sternal border.

3. Auscultate for 10 to 15 seconds for a left- or right-sided S₃.

N   An S₃ heart sound can be a normal physiological sound in children and in young adults. After the age of 30, a physiological S₃ is very infrequent. An S₃ can also be normal in high-output states such as the third trimester of pregnancy.

A   In an adult, an S₃ heart sound may be one of the earliest clinical findings of cardiac dysfunction. A loud, persistent S₃ can be an ominous sign. The average life expectancy after a persistent S₃ sound is detected is approximately 4 to 5 years.

P   An S₃ is caused by rapid ventricular filling. An S₃ sound may occur with ventricular dysfunction, excessively rapid early diastolic ventricular filling, and restrictive myocardial or pericardial disease. It often indicates congestive heart failure and fluid overload.

Mitral and Tricuspid Areas (S₄)

An S₄ heart sound, or atrial diastolic gallop, is a late diastolic filling sound associated with atrial contraction. An S₄ can be either left- or right-sided and is therefore heard best in the mitral or tricuspid areas. An S₄ is a late diastolic filling sound that occurs just before S₁ (Figure 16-13R).

Sometimes, the S₃ and the S₄ heart sounds can occur simultaneously in middiastole, thus creating one loud diastolic filling sound. This is known as a summation gallop (Figure 16-13S).

E   1. Place the bell of the stethoscope lightly over the mitral area.

2. Place the bell of the stethoscope lightly over the tricuspid area.

3. Auscultate for 10 to 15 seconds for a left- or right-sided S₄.

N   An S₄ heart sound may occur with or without any evidence of cardiac decompensation. A left-sided S₄ is usually louder on expiration. A right-sided S₄ is usually louder on inspiration.

A   The presence of an S₄ can be indicative of cardiac decompensation.

P   An S₄ heart sound can be auscultated in conditions that increase the resistance to filling because of a poorly compliant ventricle (e.g., MI, CAD, CHF, and cardiomyopathy) or in conditions that result in systolic overload (e.g., HTN, aortic stenosis, and hyperthyroidism).

NURSING**TIP**

S₃ Heart Sound

Phonetically, an S₃ heart sound is thought to resemble the pronunciation of the word *Kentucky:*

S₁	S₂	S₃
Ken	túc	ky

NURSING**TIP**

S₄ Heart Sound

Phonetically, an S₄ heart sound is thought to resemble the pronunciation of the word *Tennessee:*

S₄	S₁	S₂
Ten	nes	sée

| **E** Examination | **N** Normal Findings | **A** Abnormal Findings | **P** Pathophysiology |

TABLE 16-5 Grading Heart Murmurs

GRADE	CHARACTERISTICS
I	Very faint; heard only after a period of concentration
II	Faint; heard immediately
III	Moderate intensity
IV	Loud; may be associated with a thrill
V	Loud; stethoscope must remain in contact with the chest wall in order to hear; thrill palpable
VI	Very loud; heard with stethoscope off of chest wall; thrill palpable

A. Crescendo

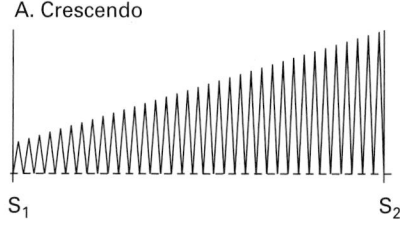

B. Decrescendo

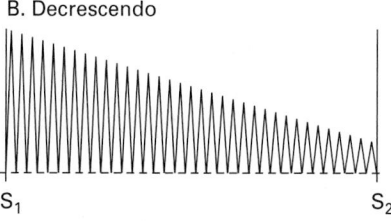

C. Crescendo-decrescendo

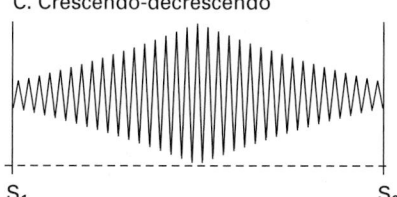

D. Plateau

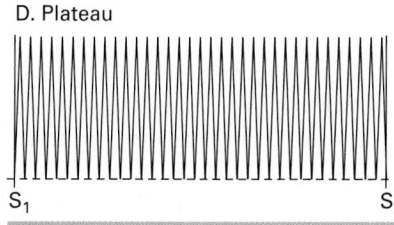

FIGURE 16-14 **Characteristic Patterns of Murmurs**

Murmurs

Murmurs are distinguished from heart sounds by their longer duration. Murmurs may be classified as innocent (which are always systolic and are not associated with any other abnormalities), functional (which are associated with high-output states), or pathological (which are related to structural abnormalities). Murmurs are produced by turbulent blood flow in the following situations:

1. Flow across a partial obstruction
2. Increased flow through normal structures
3. Flow into a dilated chamber
4. Backward or regurgitant flow across incompetent valves
5. Shunting of blood out of a high-pressure chamber or artery through an abnormal passageway

When assessing for a murmur, analyze the murmur according to the following seven characteristics:

1. Location: area where the murmur is heard the loudest (e.g., mitral, pulmonic, etc.).
2. Radiation: transmission of sounds from the specific valves to other adjacent anatomic areas. For example, mitral murmurs can often radiate to the axilla.
3. Timing: phase of the cardiac cycle in which the murmur is heard. Murmurs can be either systolic or diastolic. If the murmur occurs simultaneously with the pulse, it is a systolic murmur. If it does not, it is a diastolic murmur. Murmurs can further be characterized as **pansystolic** or **holosystolic**, meaning that the murmur is heard throughout all of systole. Murmurs can also be characterized as early, mid-, or late systolic or diastolic murmurs.
4. Intensity: See Table 16-5 for the six grades of loudness or intensity. The murmur is recorded with the grade over the roman numeral "VI" to show the scale being used (e.g., III/VI).
5. Quality: harsh, rumbling, blowing, or musical.
6. Pitch: high, medium, or low. Low-pitched murmurs should be auscultated with the bell of the stethoscope whereas high-pitched murmurs should be auscultated with the diaphragm of the stethoscope.
7. Configuration: pattern that the murmur makes over time (Figure 16-14). The configuration of a murmur can be described as **crescendo** (soft to loud), **decrescendo** (loud to soft), crescendo-decrescendo (soft to loud to soft), and plateau (sound is sustained).

E
1. The patient should be in the same position for murmur auscultation as for the first auscultation (i.e., supine or sitting).

2. Auscultate each of the following cardiac landmarks for 10 to 15 seconds:
   a. Aortic and pulmonic areas, with the diaphragm of the stethoscope
   b. Mitral and tricuspid areas, with the diaphragm of the stethoscope
   c. Mitral and tricuspid areas, with the bell of the stethoscope

3. Label the murmur using the characteristics of location, radiation, timing, intensity, quality, pitch, and configuration. See Table 16-5 for information on grading heart murmurs.

4. You may also have the patient sit up, lean forward, completely exhale, and hold his or her breath while you listen at the right and left second and third ICSs for aortic murmurs (especially aortic regurgitation).

N No murmur should be heard; however, a physiological or functional murmur in children and adolescents may be innocent. These murmurs are usually systolic, short, grade I or II, vibratory, heard at the left sternal border, and do not radiate. No cardiac symptoms accompany the murmur.

A Abnormal murmurs of stenosis can be found in each of the four valvular cardiac landmarks.

P Stenosis occurs when a valve that should be open remains partially closed. It produces an increased **afterload**, or pressure overload. Stenosis may develop from rheumatic fever, congenital defects of the valves, or calcification associated with the aging process.

A Abnormal murmurs of regurgitation or insufficiency can be auscultated in each of the four valvular cardiac landmarks.

P Regurgitation or insufficiency occurs when a valve that should be closed remains partially open. An insufficient valve causes volume overload, or increased **preload**. Regurgitation frequently results from the effects of rheumatic fever and congenital defects of the valves.

Pericardial Friction Rub

E 1. Position the patient so that he or she is reclining in the sitting position, in the knee-chest position, or leaning forward.

2. Auscultate from the sternum (third to fifth ICS) to the apex (mitral area) with the diaphragm of the stethoscope for 10 to 15 seconds.

3. Characterize any sound according to its location, radiation, timing, quality, and pitch.

N No pericardial friction rub should be auscultated.

A A pericardial friction rub is always an abnormal finding. It is heard best during held inspiration or expiration. It does not change with the respiratory cycle. See Table 16-6 for additional information on pericardial friction rubs.

P Pericardial friction rubs are caused by the rubbing together of the inflamed visceral and parietal layers of the pericardium. They may be present in conditions such as **pericarditis** (inflammation of the pericardium) and renal failure.

Prosthetic Heart Valves

E/N Prosthetic heart valves can be located in any of the four heart valves, although mitral and aortic valve replacements are the most common. Refer to the aortic and mitral valve auscultation discussions.

A Prosthetic heart valves produce abnormal heart sounds. Furthermore, mechanical prosthetic valve sounds can sometimes be heard without the use of a stethoscope.

P Mechanical prosthetic valves (caged-ball, tilting disk, and bileaflet valves) produce "clicky" opening and closing sounds. Homograft (human tissue) and heterograft (animal tissue) valves produce sounds that are similar to those of the human valves; however, they usually produce a murmur.

NURSING**TIP**

Pericardial Friction Rub versus Pleural Friction Rub

- A pericardial friction rub produces a *high*-pitched, multiphasic, and scratchy (may be leathery or grating) sound that *does not* change with respiration. It is a sign of pericardial inflammation.

- A pleural friction rub produces a *low*-pitched, coarse, and grating sound that *does* change with respiration. When the patient holds his or her breath, the sound disappears. The patient may also complain of pain upon breathing. It is a sign of visceral and parietal pleurae inflammation.

| **E** Examination | **N** Normal Findings | **A** Abnormal Findings | **P** Pathophysiology |

TABLE 16-6 Murmurs and Pericardial Friction Rub

HEART SOUND	LOCATION/RADIATION	QUALITY/PITCH	CONFIGURATION
Systolic Murmurs			
Aortic stenosis	Second right ICS; may radiate to neck or left sternal border	Harsh/medium	Crescendo/decrescendo
Pulmonic stenosis	Second or third left ICS; radiates toward shoulder and neck	Harsh/medium	Crescendo/decrescendo
Mitral regurgitation	Apex; fifth ICS, left midclavicular line; may radiate to left axilla and back	Blowing/high	Holosystolic/plateau
Tricuspid regurgitation	Lower left sternal border; may radiate to right sternum	Blowing/high	Holosystolic/plateau
Diastolic Murmurs			
Aortic regurgitation	Second right ICS and Erb's point; may radiate to left or right sternal border	Blowing/high	Decrescendo
Pulmonic regurgitation	Second left ICS; may radiate to left lower sternal border	Blowing/high	Decrescendo
Mitral stenosis	Apex; fifth ICS, left midclavicular line; may get louder with patient on left side; does not radiate	Rumbling/low	Crescendo/decrescendo
Tricuspid stenosis	Fourth ICS, at sternal border	Rumbling/low	Crescendo/decrescendo
Pericardial Friction Rub	Third to fifth ICS, left of sternum; does not radiate	Leathery, scratchy, grating/high	Three components: 1. Ventricular systole 2. Ventricular diastole 3. Atrial systole

Timing is described as systolic or diastolic; intensity is described in Table 16-5.

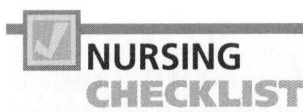

NURSING CHECKLIST

General Approach to Peripheral Vasculature Assessment

1. Explain to the patient what you are going to do.
2. Use a drape and uncover only those areas that are necessary as the assessment is done.
3. Position the patient in a supine or sitting position.

ASSESSMENT OF THE PERIPHERAL VASCULATURE

Assessment of the periphery is the second major component of a comprehensive cardiovascular assessment. The components of the assessment of the periphery include:

1. Inspection of the jugular venous pressure (JVP)
2. Inspection of the hepatojugular reflux
3. Palpation and auscultation of the arterial pulses
4. Inspection and palpation of peripheral perfusion
5. Palpation of the epitrochlear node

INSPECTION OF THE JUGULAR VENOUS PRESSURE

Identify the internal and external jugular veins (see Figure 16-15) with the patient in a supine position with the head elevated to 30° or 45° so that the jugular veins are visible. Tangential lighting (lighting across the veins rather than on top of the veins) will facilitate the assessment. Both sides of the neck should be assessed. The external jugular veins are more superficial than the internal jugular (IJ) veins and

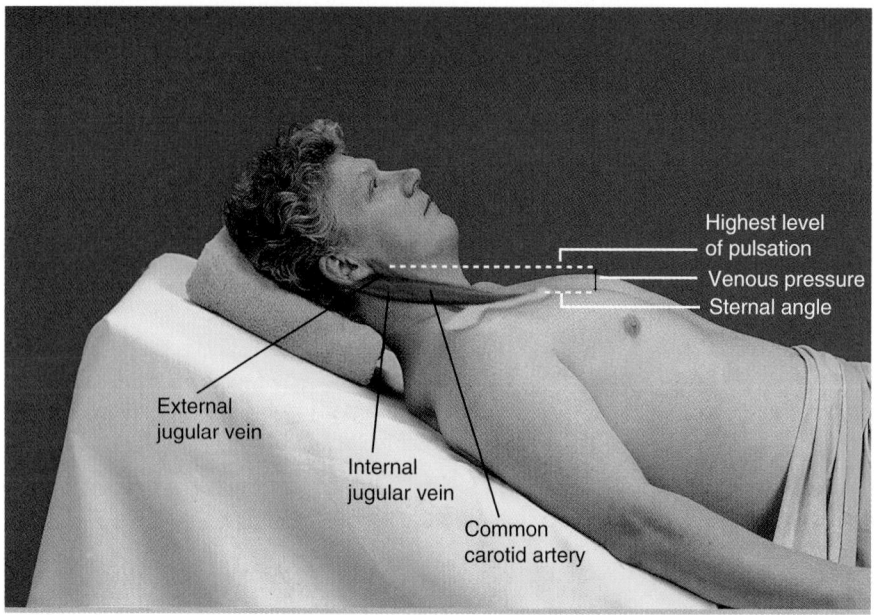

FIGURE 16-15 Inspection of Jugular Venous Pressure

traverse the neck diagonally from the center of the clavicle to the angle of the jaw. The IJ veins are larger and are located deep below the sternocleidomastoid muscle adjacent to the carotid arteries. The pulsations of the IJ veins can be difficult to identify visually because the veins are deep and the pulsations can be confused with the adjacent carotid arteries.

Jugular vein pulsations consist of two or three waves (Figure 16-16). These waves are called the *a, c,* and v waves. The *a* wave is produced by the contraction of the right atrium and it reflects the backflow of blood into the vena cava as the right atrium ejects blood into the right ventricle. The *a* wave occurs just before S_1.

The *c* wave occurs at the end of S_1 and is produced when the right ventricle begins to contract. The *c* wave is caused by both the slight backflow of blood into the right atrium when the ventricular contraction occurs and the bulging of the tricuspid valve backward toward the right atrium because of increased right ventricular pressure.

The *v* wave results from the slow buildup of blood in the right atrium during the ventricular contraction (when the tricuspid valve is closed) and occurs during late systole. The *v* wave disappears when the tricuspid valve opens and blood flows rapidly into the right ventricle.

Two negative slopes, the *x* and *y* descents, also occur in the jugular venous pulse. The *x* descent occurs after the *c* wave and reflects the fall of the right atrial pressure when the tricuspid valve closes and the right atrium relaxes. The *y* descent follows the *v* wave and occurs when the tricuspid valve opens and blood flows rapidly from the right atrium into the right ventricle.

These waves and descents are clearly noted when the patient has a direct central venous pressure (CVP) line and the right atrial pressure waves are depicted on an oscilloscope.

Information about the CVP can be obtained directly via a catheter inserted into one of the jugular veins (the IJ veins are the veins of choice for cannulation because they do not have valves and they provide a more direct route to the right atrium) or indirectly as discussed below.

E 1. To indirectly estimate a patient's CVP, estimate the JVP (Figure 16-15):
 a. Place the patient at a 30° to 45° angle (the highest position where the neck veins remain visible).

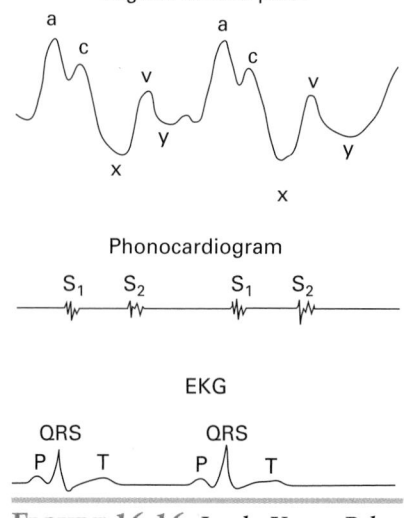

FIGURE 16-16 Jugular Venous Pulse Waves in Relation to the Phonocardiogram and Electrocardiogram

  b. Measure the vertical distance in centimeters from the patient's sternal angle to the top of the distended neck vein. This will give you the JVP.

  c. Knowing that the sternal angle is roughly 5 cm above the right atrium, take the JVP measurement obtained in the previous step and add 5 cm to get an estimate of the CVP. For example, a JVP of 2 cm at a 45° angle estimated on a patient's right side is equivalent to a CVP of 5 + 2, or 7, cm.

2. Direct CVP measurements in the patient with a central venous cannula should be obtained with the patient in the supine position or reclining at no more than a 45° angle.

  a. Do not forget to level the transducer at the patient's right atrium (phlebostatic axis—fourth ICS, midaxillary line) prior to obtaining any CVP reading.

  b. When recording CVP measurements, chart the angle of the patient when the measurement was taken.

N A JVP reading less than 4 cm is considered normal. Normally, the jugular veins are:

  1. Most distended when the patient is flat because gravity is eliminated and the jugular veins fill

  2. 1 to 2 cm above the sternal angle when the head of the bed is elevated to a 45° angle

  3. Absent when the head of the bed is at a 90° angle

  Normal direct CVP readings are 3–8 cm H2O or 0–8 mm Hg.

A A JVP greater than 4 cm is considered abnormal.

P An elevated JVP can be due to an increased right ventricular pressure, increased blood volume, or an obstruction to right ventricular flow.

A Bilateral jugular venous distension (JVD) is abnormal.

P JVD indicates an increased JVP.

A Unilateral JVD is abnormal.

P Unilateral JVD indicates a local vein blockage.

A JVD with the head of the bed elevated to a 90° angle is abnormal.

P JVD at a 90° angle indicates more serious pathology such as severe right ventricular failure, constrictive pericarditis, or cardiac tamponade.

A An increased *a* wave is abnormal.

P An increased *a* wave can occur with stenosis of the tricuspid valve (because the right atrium has difficulty emptying blood into the right ventricle) or when the right ventricle is enlarged and the right atrium needs to more forcefully contract to fill it. An increased *a* wave can also occur in complete heart block because the right atrium contracts at its own pace against a closed tricuspid valve.

A An enlarged *v* wave is abnormal.

P An enlarged *v* wave can occur with tricuspid regurgitation or insufficiency. It is exaggerated when the tricuspid valve allows blood to flow back from the right ventricle to the right atrium during systole, thus causing the *x* slope to be replaced by a large *c–v* wave. It can also occur with right-sided heart failure, where the right ventricle becomes so enlarged that it forces the tricuspid valve to stretch and allow blood back into the right atrium.

E Examination   **N** Normal Findings   **A** Abnormal Findings   **P** Pathophysiology

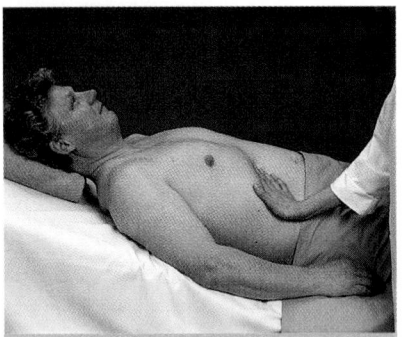

FIGURE 16-17 Hepatojugular Reflux

INSPECTION OF THE HEPATOJUGULAR REFLUX

Hepatojugular reflux is a test that is very sensitive in detecting right ventricular failure. This procedure is performed if the CVP is normal but right ventricular failure is suspected.

 1. Place the patient flat in bed, or elevated to a 30° angle if the jugular veins are visible. Remind the patient to breathe normally.

2. Using single or bimanual deep palpation, press firmly on the right upper quadrant for 30 to 60 seconds. Press on another part of the abdomen if this area is tender.

3. Observe the neck for an elevation in JVP (Figure 16-17).

N Normally, this pressure should not elicit any change in the jugular veins.

A A rise of more than 1 cm in JVP is abnormal.

P A rise in JVP that occurs with this technique is suggestive of right-sided congestive heart failure or fluid overload. The heart simply cannot accept the increase in venous return.

PALPATION AND AUSCULTATION OF ARTERIAL PULSES

Information concerning the function of the right ventricle is gained via the assessment of the venous pulses; however, assessment of the arterial pulses provides information about the left ventricle. The pulses to be evaluated are the temporal, carotid, brachial, radial, femoral, popliteal, posterior tibial, and the dorsalis pedis. The arteries that are most frequently examined are the radial arteries due to their easy accessibility. In a cardiac arrest situation, the carotid pulse is the artery of choice for palpation.

 1. The arterial pulse assessment is best facilitated with the patient in a supine position with the head of the bed elevated at 30° to 45°. If the patient cannot tolerate such a position, then the supine position alone is acceptable.

2. Using your dominant hand, palpate the pulses with the pads of the index and middle fingers. The number of fingers used will be determined by the amount of space where the pulse is located.

3. Evaluate the pulse in terms of:
   a. Rate
   b. Rhythm: If there is an irregularity in the pulse rate, then auscultate the heart.
   c. Amplitude: Refer to Chapter 9 for grading scales.
   d. Symmetry: Palpate the pulses on both sides of the patient's body simultaneously (with the exception of the carotid pulses).

4. If a peripheral pulse cannot be palpated, an amplification device can be used to detect the presence, rate, and rhythm at that location (Figure 16-18).

5. Using the bell of the stethoscope, auscultate the temporal, carotid, and femoral pulses for **bruits**, which are blowing sounds heard when blood flow becomes turbulent as it rushes past an obstruction. Ask the patient to hold his or her breath during auscultation of the carotid pulse because respiratory sounds can interfere with auscultation.

N Refer to Chapter 9 for normal pulse rate, rhythm, and amplitude. When assessing symmetry, the pulses should be equal bilaterally. No bruits should be auscultated in the temporal, carotid, or femoral pulses.

A/P Figure 16-19 illustrates abnormal pulses with possible etiologies.

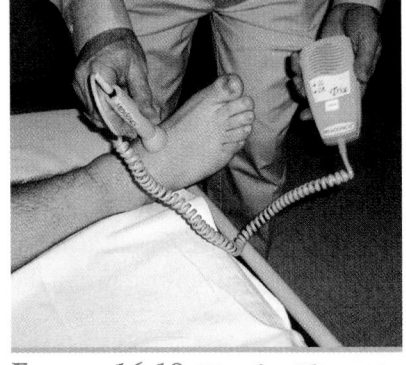

FIGURE 16-18 Use of an Ultrasonic Stethoscope to Detect a Dorsalis Pedis Pulse

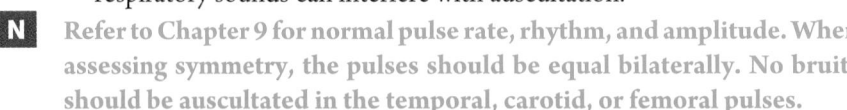

E Examination   **N** Normal Findings   **A** Abnormal Findings   **P** Pathophysiology

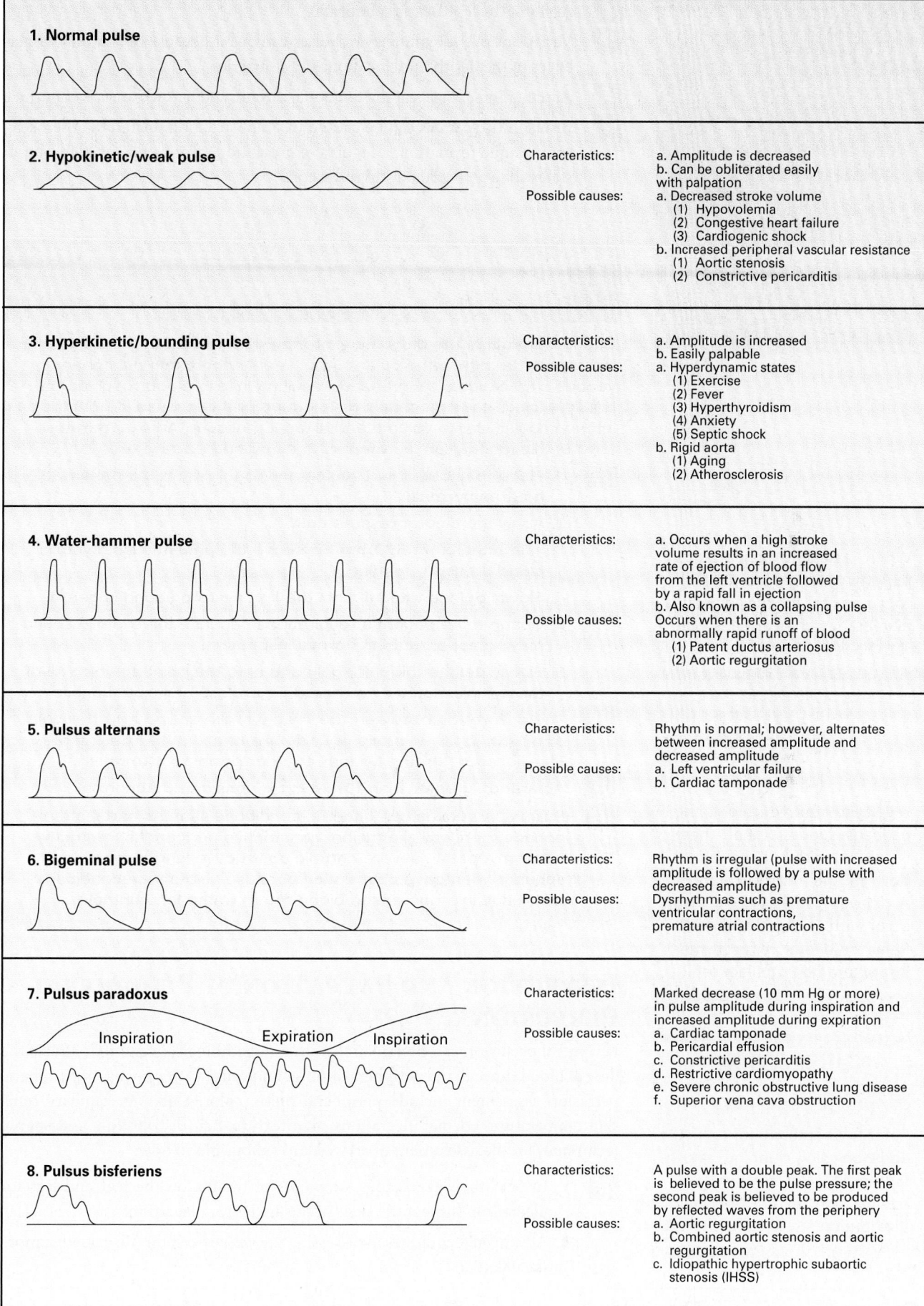

1. Normal pulse

2. Hypokinetic/weak pulse

Characteristics:
a. Amplitude is decreased
b. Can be obliterated easily with palpation

Possible causes:
a. Decreased stroke volume
   (1) Hypovolemia
   (2) Congestive heart failure
   (3) Cardiogenic shock
b. Increased peripheral vascular resistance
   (1) Aortic stenosis
   (2) Constrictive pericarditis

3. Hyperkinetic/bounding pulse

Characteristics:
a. Amplitude is increased
b. Easily palpable

Possible causes:
a. Hyperdynamic states
   (1) Exercise
   (2) Fever
   (3) Hyperthyroidism
   (4) Anxiety
   (5) Septic shock
b. Rigid aorta
   (1) Aging
   (2) Atherosclerosis

4. Water-hammer pulse

Characteristics:
a. Occurs when a high stroke volume results in an increased rate of ejection of blood flow from the left ventricle followed by a rapid fall in ejection
b. Also known as a collapsing pulse

Possible causes:
Occurs when there is an abnormally rapid runoff of blood
   (1) Patent ductus arteriosus
   (2) Aortic regurgitation

5. Pulsus alternans

Characteristics:
Rhythm is normal; however, alternates between increased amplitude and decreased amplitude

Possible causes:
a. Left ventricular failure
b. Cardiac tamponade

6. Bigeminal pulse

Characteristics:
Rhythm is irregular (pulse with increased amplitude is followed by a pulse with decreased amplitude)

Possible causes:
Dysrhythmias such as premature ventricular contractions, premature atrial contractions

7. Pulsus paradoxus

Inspiration   Expiration   Inspiration

Characteristics:
Marked decrease (10 mm Hg or more) in pulse amplitude during inspiration and increased amplitude during expiration

Possible causes:
a. Cardiac tamponade
b. Pericardial effusion
c. Constrictive pericarditis
d. Restrictive cardiomyopathy
e. Severe chronic obstructive lung disease
f. Superior vena cava obstruction

8. Pulsus bisferiens

Characteristics:
A pulse with a double peak. The first peak is believed to be the pulse pressure; the second peak is believed to be produced by reflected waves from the periphery

Possible causes:
a. Aortic regurgitation
b. Combined aortic stenosis and aortic regurgitation
c. Idiopathic hypertrophic subaortic stenosis (IHSS)

FIGURE 16-19 Alterations in Arterial Pulses

A Asymmetrical pulses are abnormal.

P Variations in the symmetry of pulses can occur because of anatomic differences in the depths and locations of the arteries.

A Auscultation of bruits at the temporal, carotid, and femoral areas is abnormal.

P Bruits in these areas can be caused by an obstruction related to atherosclerotic plaque formation, a jugular vein-carotid artery fistula, or high-output states such as anemia or thyrotoxicosis.

ADVANCED TECHNIQUE

Assessing for Pulsus Paradoxus

During inspiration, the blood flow into the right side of the heart is increased, the right ventricular output is enhanced, and pulmonary venous capacitance is increased, resulting in less blood reaching the left ventricle. These mechanisms account for a decrease in both the left ventricular stroke volume and arterial pressure. An exaggerated form of this mechanism is referred to as **pulsus paradoxus**.

E
1. Place the patient in a supine position. Instruct the patient to breathe normally.
2. Apply the blood pressure cuff.
3. Inflate the cuff to 20 mm Hg above the patient's last systolic blood pressure reading.
4. Slowly deflate the cuff until the first systolic sound is heard.
5. Observe the patient's respirations because the systolic sound may disappear during normal inspiration.
6. Slowly deflate the cuff again and note the point at which all of the systolic sounds are heard regardless of respirations.

N The difference between the first systolic sound and the point at which all the systolic sounds are heard is the paradox. The paradox should be less than or equal to 10 mm Hg.

A A paradox greater than 10 mm Hg is considered abnormal.

P Pulsus paradoxus can occur in conditions such as cardiac tamponade, pericardial effusion, constrictive pericarditis, restrictive cardiomyopathy, severe chronic obstructive lung disease, and superior vena cava obstruction because all of these conditions can result in a decreased blood return to the left ventricle.

INSPECTION AND PALPATION OF PERIPHERAL PERFUSION

Peripheral perfusion can be impaired with any pathological state that affects the flow of blood through the peripheral arteries and veins. Components of peripheral perfusion assessment include peripheral pulse, color, clubbing, capillary refill, skin temperature, edema, ulcerations, skin texture, hair distribution, and special techniques for the assessment of arterial and venous blood flow.

E
1. Inspect the fingers, toes, or points of trauma on the feet and legs for ulceration. Inspect the sides of the ankles for ulceration.
2. Advanced techniques for assessing the venous system (discussed in more detail later):

| **E** Examination | **N** Normal Findings | **A** Abnormal Findings | **P** Pathophysiology |

ADVANCED TECHNIQUE

Orthostatic Hypotension Assessment

When an individual stands, blood pools in the lower part of the body and the blood pressure falls transiently. However, in the healthy individual, baroreceptors (receptors located in the walls of most of the great arteries) located in the carotid sinus area sense the decrease in blood pressure and initiate reflex vasoconstriction and increase the heart rate. These mechanisms bring the blood pressure back to normal. When this mechanism fails, orthostatic hypotension may ensue and an evaluation must be made. When assessing for orthostatic hypotension, take the patient's blood pressure and heart rate with the patient in supine, sitting, and standing positions. This set of orthostatic vital signs is commonly referred to as tilts.

E 1. First check the blood pressure in a supine position. In this position, the patient should be flat for at least 5 minutes. (This time ensures that no reflex mechanisms from the upright position are influencing the blood pressure.) Record the blood pressure and the heart rate as the first set of tilts.

2. Next, assist the patient to a sitting position with the feet dangling. Wait 1 to 3 minutes. (There is no consensus in the literature regarding how long to wait after a position change before obtaining the next set of vital signs.) Retake the blood pressure and heart rate. This waiting period allows time for the reflex mechanisms to activate and ensure a normal blood pressure. Record the blood pressure and the heart rate as the second set of tilts. Also, ask the patient about any symptoms of weakness or dizziness related to the position change. If the patient becomes weak or dizzy, assist the patient back to a supine position.

3. Finally, assist the patient to a standing position. Measure the blood pressure and heart rate again after 1 to 3 minutes. Again, ask the patient about any symptoms of weakness or dizziness related to the position change. If the patient becomes weak or dizzy, assist the patient back to a supine position.

N Wide discrepancies in the literature exist regarding the magnitude of the orthostatic response. The latest studies reveal that there is no relationship between orthostatic vital signs and volume status, yet tilts are still frequently used as indicators of intravascular volume status. Many normal patients may have what has been considered in the past to be positive tilts consistent with hypovolemia even though they are not hypovolemic.

A Orthostatic vital signs that have been considered positive in the past include a systolic or a diastolic blood pressure decrease of more than 10 mm Hg or a heart rate increase of more than 20 beats per minute. However, tilts have fallen out of favor with many for the reason previously stated.

P Orthostatic hypotension can occur in patients who are hypovolemic, have a neurogenic problem, or are experiencing side effects from a prescribed medication.

NURSING**TIP**

Peripheral Vascular Disease (PVD)

Caution patients that the single most important thing they can do to slow PVD is to stop smoking.

NURSING**ALERT**

Risk Factors for Chronic Arterial Insufficiency

- Age (> 60 years old)
- Smoking
- Gender (men more than women)
- Hypertension
- Diabetes mellitus
- Hyperlipidemia

a. Homan's sign
b. Manual compression
c. Retrograde filling or Trendelenburg test

3. Advanced techniques for examining the arterial system (discussed in more detail later):
   a. Pallor
   b. Color return (CR) and venous filling time (VFT)
   c. Allen Test

N Ulcerations: No ulcerations should be noted.

A Arterial ulcerations are abnormal.
1. Location: occurs at toes or points of trauma on the feet or the legs.
2. Characteristics: well-defined edges; black or necrotic tissue; a deep, pale base and lack of bleeding; hairlessness or disruption of the hair along with shiny, thick, waxy skin.

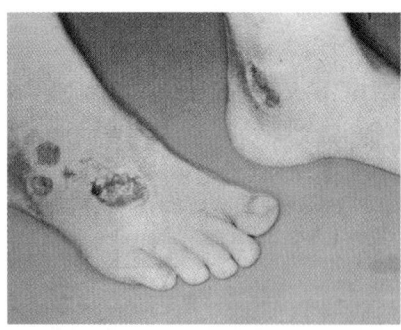

A. Note the ulcerations at the side of the ankle.

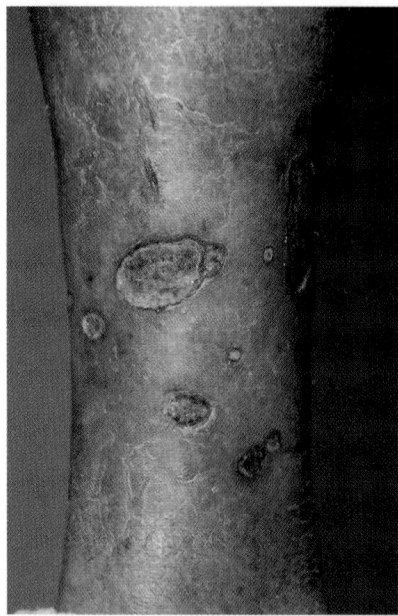

B. Note the thin, shiny skin of this venous stasis ulcer.

FIGURE 16-22 Venous Ulcerations

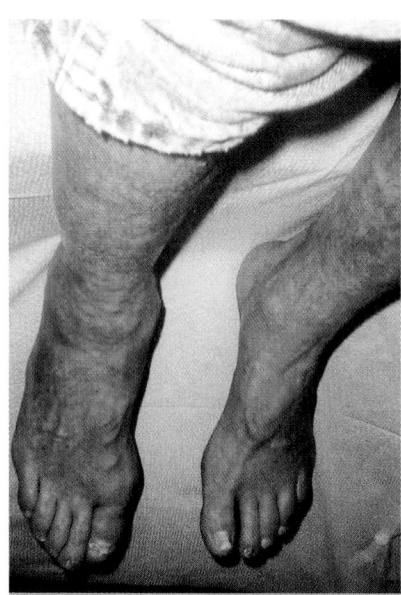

FIGURE 16-23 Varicose Veins

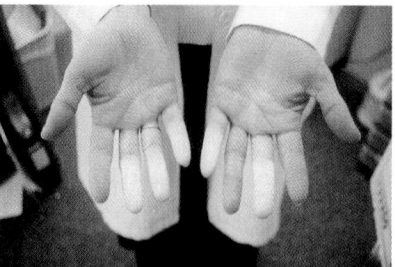

FIGURE 16-20 Raynaud's Disease in the Early Stage. Note the pallor in the distal half of some of the fingers.

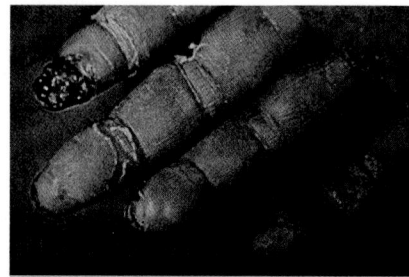

FIGURE 16-21 Raynaud's Disease in the Late Stage. Note the necrotic digit.
Courtesy of Marvin Ackerman, M.D., Scarsdale, NY.

3. Pain: exceedingly painful; claudication related to chronic arterial insufficiency is relieved by rest; pain at rest is relieved by dependency.

P The location and characteristics of ulceration are due to inadequate arterial flow, such as in peripheral vascular disease and diabetes mellitus. Most distal arterial beds are prone to ulceration. The pain is caused by ischemia.

P Arterial ulcers on the tips of the fingers, toes, or nose can be caused by Raynaud's disease (Figure 16-20). Arteriolar spasms lead to pallor and pain in the affected area, followed by cyanosis, with numbness, tingling, and burning; rubor also develops. Over time, the affected area may develop an ulcer (Figure 16-21). Attacks occur bilaterally and last minutes to hours.

A Venous ulcerations are abnormal (Figure 16-22):

1. Location: occurs at the sides of the ankles.

2. Characteristics: uneven edges and ruddy granulation of tissue; thin, shiny skin that lacks the support of subcutaneous tissue; disruption of hair pattern, or hairlessness.

3. Pain: deep muscular pain (associated with inadequate venous flow) with acute DVT; aching and cramping are relieved with elevation.

P Ulcers are due to inadequate venous flow that results when communication between the superficial and deep veins is compromised. Both the characteristics and the pain are related to inadequate venous blood flow.

❊ NURSING**ALERT**

Risk Factors for Varicose Veins

Varicose veins affect approximately 10% of the adult population and occur four times more often in women than in men. The pathogenesis of varicose veins remains unknown; however, it is not uncommon to find varicose veins in patients:
- Who have a family history of varicose veins
- Whose occupation requires long periods of standing
- Who are obese
- Who are pregnant

Measures to prevent unnecessary pressure on the leg veins include:
- Avoid heavy lifting
- Avoid excessive weight gain
- Do not cross legs
- Wear support panty hose
- Stop smoking
- Elevate feet while sitting
- Exercise

ADVANCED TECHNIQUE

Assessing the Venous System

Homan's Sign

It is important to note that because a Homan's sign has a low sensitivity (an indication of the frequency of a positive test result in a population with the disease) for thrombophlebitis, the use of this test has fallen out of favor with some health care providers. The Homan's test is also controversial because there have been reports of the dislodging of deep vein thromboses (DVT) with the performance of the maneuver. In addition, conditions other than DVT could yield positive results from this test. A positive Homan's sign is present in less than 20% of all DVT cases.

E   1. With the patient's knee slightly bent, sharply dorsiflex the patient's foot and ask the patient if this maneuver elicits pain in the calf.

2. Repeat this technique with the other foot.

N   There should be no complaints of calf pain when this is evaluated.

A   A positive Homan's sign may be abnormal.

P   A positive Homan's sign may indicate thrombophlebitis or DVT. Early detection of thrombophlebitis is essential because it can lead to life-threatening complications such as pulmonary emboli, which occurs when a thrombus breaks loose from the vein and travels to the lung. Three factors can disrupt the balance between blood-clotting activators and inhibitors. Known as Virchow's triad, they are stasis of blood flow, an injured venous wall, and hypercoagulability. All three of these factors can predispose a patient to thrombosis. Thrombosis can occur in either deep or superficial veins.

Manual Compression

Manual compression tests the competency of the saphenous vein's valves.

E   1. Palpate the dilated vein with one hand.

2. Use the other hand to compress the same vein 20 cm higher in the leg.

3. Note if an impulse is felt.

N   If the valves are competent, you will not feel the impulse because competent valves block transmission of the impulse.

A   An impulse felt with manual compression is abnormal.

P   Varicose veins are dilated, tortuous veins that are caused by incompetent valves (see Figure 16-23). They are most prevalent in the saphenous veins of the lower extremities.

Retrograde Filling, or Trendelenburg Test

The retrograde filling, or Trendelenburg test, assesses the competency of the valves in the communicating and saphenous veins (evaluating varicose veins).

E   1. Raise the patient's leg 90° to drain the venous blood.

2. Place a tourniquet or your hands around the upper thigh to occlude the patient's saphenous vein.

3. Instruct the patient to stand so that venous filling can be noted.

4. Release the compression and watch venous filling again.

N   Normal veins fill from below the occlusion and within 35 seconds as blood flows down from the arteries to the veins. Following release of the hands or tourniquet, there should be no additional filling because competent valves prevent the backflow of blood.

A   A varicose vein that fills from above is abnormal.

P   This occurs in varicose veins because of the backward flow of blood through incompetent valves. Ifsudden, additional filling occurs when the hands or tourniquet are removed, it is another indication that varicosities occur because of incompetent valves.

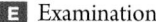			
E Examination	**N** Normal Findings	**A** Abnormal Findings	**P** Pathophysiology

ADVANCED TECHNIQUE

Assessing the Arterial System

Pallor

E 1. Instruct the patient to raise the extremities.

2. Note the time it takes for pallor, or lack of color, to develop.

N Normally no pallor develops within 60 seconds.

A Pallor that develops quickly in the extremities when the extremities are lifted is abnormal.

P Pallor that develops quickly is indicative of arterial insufficiency. The quicker the pallor develops, the more severe the disease.

Color Return and Venous Filling Time

E 1. To drain the patient's feet of venous blood, elevate the supine patient's legs approximately 12 inches and ask the patient to move his or her feet up and down at the ankles for approximately 1 minute.

2. Next, place the patient in a sitting position on the edge of the bed, with the legs dangling over the side.

3. Note the time it takes for the color to return to the legs and for the superficial veins to refill.

N Normal color return (CR) is 10 seconds and venous filling time (VFT) is 15 seconds.

A A delayed CR of 15 to 25 seconds or a VFT of 20 to 30 seconds is abnormal.

P These scores indicate moderate ischemia.

A A delayed CR of 40 seconds or more or a VFT of 40 seconds or more is abnormal.

P These scores indicate severe ischemia.

Allen Test

The Allen test is used to assess the patency of the radial and ulnar arteries (see Figure 16-24). This test is usually performed prior to radial artery cannulation because radial artery cannulation can be associated with radial artery thrombosis. If the radial artery becomes occluded with a thrombus, continued viability of the hand depends on collateral blood flow from the ulnar artery.

E 1. Ask the patient to make a tight fist. If the patient is unresponsive, raise the arm above the heart for several seconds to force blood to leave the hand.

2. Apply direct pressure on the radial and ulnar arteries to obstruct blood flow to the hand as the patient opens and closes the fist.

3. Instruct the patient to open the hand, with the radial artery remaining compressed. If the patient is unresponsive, keep the arm above the heart level.

4. Examine the palmar surface of the hand for a blush or pallor within 15 seconds.

N If the radial artery is compressed, the blood flow through the ulnar artery should be sufficient to maintain the normal palm color after the patient unclenches the fist. Also, if the ulnar artery is compressed, the blood flow through the radial artery should be sufficient to maintain the normal palm color. This is a positive Allen test.

A If the color does not return to normal within 6 seconds after the patient unclenches the fist, then obstruction of either the radial or the ulnar arteries may be present. This is a negative Allen test. Thus, the radial artery should not be punctured for an arterial blood gas or invasive arterial line.

P Atherosclerosis or a thrombus can cause either artery to be not patent.

E Examination   **N** Normal Findings   **A** Abnormal Findings   **P** Pathophysiology

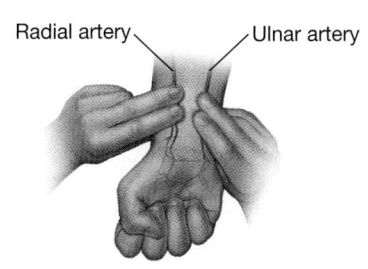

A. Pallor is initiated by compressing the radial and ulnar arteries with the fist clenched.

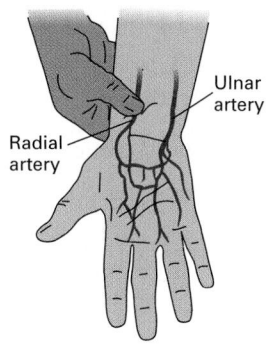

B. A patent ulnar artery reveals the return of palm perfusion despite radial artery compression.

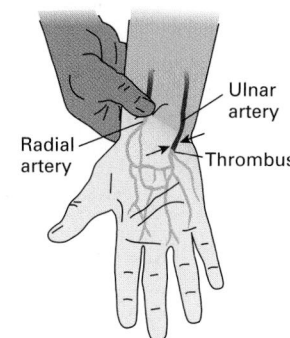

C. An occluded ulnar artery results in continued pallor of the hand while the radial artery is still compressed.

FIGURE 16-24 The Allen Test

ADVANCED TECHNIQUE

Ankle-Brachial Index (ABI)

The ABI is an easy, dependable, and inexpensive test used in the assessment of peripheral arterial disease (PAD). Patients are evaluated annually, to note the progression of the disease as well as their response to treatment.

E
1. Have patient remove socks and shoes, as well as roll up sleeves and/or pants' legs (but do not obstruct blood flow).
2. Patient should rest in a supine position for 5 minutes prior to taking the readings.
3. Place blood pressure (BP) cuffs snuggly on the patient's arms and above the ankles.
4. Apply a small amount of gel to the first brachial artery site and place the Doppler probe at the point with the loudest signal.
5. Inflate the BP cuff 20 mm Hg above the occlusion pressure.
6. Deflate the cuff at approximately 2 mm Hg per second, listening for the blood flow sound to return (this is the systolic pressure). Rapidly deflate the cuff after auscultating this systolic pressure and record the results.
7. Repeat this process for the other arm and record the results.
8. Use either the posterior tibial (PT) or dorsalis pedis (DP) for auscultation when obtaining the ankle pressures. Again, apply a small amount of gel to the first site and place the Doppler probe at the point with the loudest signal.
9. Inflate the BP cuff 20 mm Hg above the occlusion pressure.
10. Deflate the cuff at approximately 2 mm Hg per second, listening for the blood flow sound to return. Rapidly deflate the cuff after auscultating the systolic pressure and record the results.
11. Repeat this process for the other ankle and record the results.
12. For the left-side ABI, divide the left ankle systolic pressure by the higher of the two brachial systolic pressures and record the results. Repeat this process for the right-side ABI, using the right ankle systolic pressure divided by the higher of the two brachial systolic pressures. For example, if the left ankle systolic pressure was 148 and the higher brachial systolic pressure was 152, then the ABI is 0.97 (148÷152).

N
An ABI range of 0.95 to 1.2 is considered normal.

A
An ABI less than 0.90 is abnormal. An ABI greater than 0.80 but less than 0.90 indicates mild PAD. An ABI between 0.50 and 0.80 signals moderate PAD. An ABI less than 0.50 denotes severe PAD, with ischemia noted in an ABI less than 0.25.

P
These abnormal values indicate PAD. Note that the ABI reading may not be accurate for patients who have diabetes, kidney disease, or some elderly patients since they may have rigid blood vessels, which make it difficult to compress the BP cuff to get accurate readings.

PALPATION OF THE EPITROCHLEAR NODE

The epitrochlear node drains lymph from the ulnar surface of the forearm and hand and from the middle, ring, and little fingers.

E 1. Place the patient in a sitting position.

2. Support the patient's hand with your hand.

3. With the other hand, reach behind the elbow and place your finger pads in the groove between the biceps and the triceps muscles, superior to the medial condyle of the humerus.

4. Palpate the epitrochlear node for size, shape, consistency, tenderness, and mobility.

N Normally, the epitrochlear node is not palpable.

A An enlarged lymph node is abnormal.

P An infection (e.g., cat scratch disease) in the forearm or hand can lead to a palpable and tender epitrochlear node.

P Malignancies can cause an enlarged, hard, and nontender epitrochlear node.

CASE STUDY

The Patient with Hypertension

This case study illustrates the application and objective documentation of the heart and peripheral vasculature assessment.

Aiko Takahashi recently moved to a new city and needs a new primary care provider.

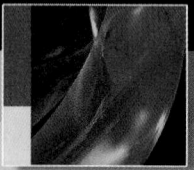

HEALTH HISTORY

PATIENT PROFILE	75 yo Asian female
CHIEF COMPLAINT	"I need to get my blood pressure checked."
PRESENT HEALTH	Patient is feeling well and has no complaints. She has recently relocated to the area, and this is her first appointment with her new primary care provider.
PAST HEALTH HISTORY	
Medical History	Hypertension for 40 yrs Diabetes mellitus type 2 for 20 yrs Degenerative joint disease (DJD) for 10 yrs
Surgical History	Left knee repair 10 years ago (pt not sure what was done, but it feels better) Right knee repair last year (pt not sure what was done, feels a little better than before surgery)
Allergies	Shellfish: hives, difficulty breathing

continues

E Examination **N** Normal Findings **A** Abnormal Findings **P** Pathophysiology

CASE STUDY (Continued)

The Patient with Hypertension

Medications	Hydrochlorothiazide 25 mg every AM Metformin 500 mg BID Glyburide 2.5 mg once daily Acetaminophen for DJD 1300 mg extended-relief caplets every 8 hours
Communicable Diseases	Denies
Injuries and Accidents	Denies
Special Needs	No longer needs a cane now that her right knee has been repaired; still finds it hard to ascend and descend stairs
Blood Transfusions	Denies
Childhood Illnesses	Measles, mumps, chickenpox
Immunizations	Last tetanus booster was 7 years ago. Has never received influenza, pneumococcal, or shingles immunizations

FAMILY HEALTH HISTORY

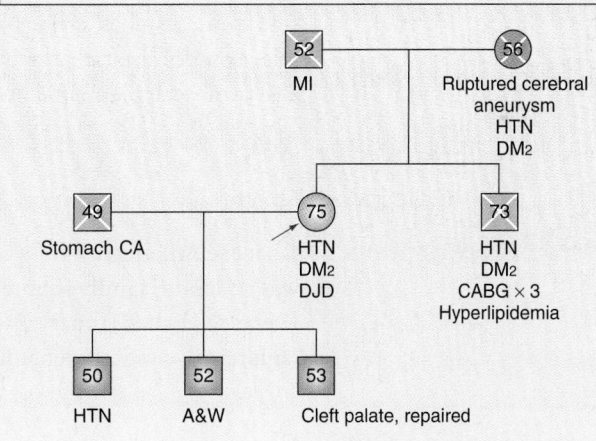

LEGEND

- ◯ Living female
- ☐ Living male
- ⊗ Deceased female
- ⊠ Deceased male
- ↗ Points to patient

A&W = Alive & Well
CA = Cancer
CABG = Coronary artery bypass graft
DM = Diabetes mellitus
DJD = Degenerative joint disease
HTN = Hypertension
MI = Myocardial infarction

52 — MI

56 — Ruptured cerebral aneurysm HTN DM2

49 — Stomach CA

75 — HTN DM2 DJD

73 — HTN DM2 CABG × 3 Hyperlipidemia

50 — HTN

52 — A&W

53 — Cleft palate, repaired

Denies family hx of CVA, MVP, rheumatic fever, hypertrophic cardiomyopathy

SOCIAL HISTORY

Alcohol Use	Denies
Tobacco Use	Denies
Drug Use	Denies
Domestic and Intimate Partner Violence	Denies

continues

Sexual Practice	Denies an active sex life. Has been widowed for 18 years.
Travel History	Until recent move, traveled frequently throughout the United States to visit children and grandchildren. Visit to Japan 15 years ago.
Work Environment	Retired journalist
Home Environment	Relates that she was unable to keep up with the day-to-day management of her own home. Recently relocated to the area to live with her son's family; family built an in-law suite for her; family relieved to have her with them so they do not have to worry about her living on her own, so far away from them.
Hobbies and Leisure Activities	Reads books and watches a lot of television. Misses her lifelong friends in her previous home town.
Stress	Denies, but appears resentful that she left her home of 45 years and had to relocate to a different area of the United States.
Education	Completed junior college
Economic Status	States she is financially comfortable and that her income is derived from her social security benefits and her husband's pension fund; also has savings based on the proceeds of her home sale. Son does not charge her rent. Receives Medicare benefits and carries supplemental health insurance.
Military Service	None
Religion	Shinto
Ethnic Background	Japanese American, family emigrated to United States when she was an infant; family suppressed Shinto faith during World War II era; celebrates January 1 with a big family party annually (her children always visited her in her old house and typically stayed a week)
Roles and Relationships	Cares for granddaughters two afternoons a week; cooks dinner for family once a week. Otherwise, her meals are provided for her.
Characteristic Patterns of Daily Living	Rises at noon and eats breakfast. Spends day in recliner watching television. Eats a snack in the late afternoon, followed by dinner with the family. Retreats to recliner for evening television shows. Retires to bed around 1 AM.
HEALTH MAINTENANCE ACTIVITIES	
Sleep	Sleeps from 1 AM to noon every day; however, has to "go to the bathroom" several times throughout the night. Will sometimes nap in the recliner prior to dinner. "I'm always tired."

continues

CASE STUDY   (Continued)

The Patient with Hypertension

Diet	Coffee and a muffin when she wakes. Bag of chips and a diet soda in the afternoon. Dinner meal provided by son's family: consists of pasta, meat, poultry, fish, cooked vegetables, and/or salad every evening. Snacks on cookies and candy at night. "I have a sweet tooth."
Exercise	None
Stress Management	Loves her cat
Use of Safety Devices	None
Health Check-ups	3–4 times per year and as needed
RISK FACTORS	
Fixed	Age, family history
Major Modifiable	HTN, glucose intolerance, diet, physical inactivity, postmenopausal
Minor Modifiable	Sedentary living, obesity
PATIENT CLASSIFICATION	NYHA I
PHYSICAL ASSESSMENT	
Assessment of the Precordium	
Inspection	Aortic area: Neg Pulmonic area: Neg Midprecordial area: Neg Tricuspid area: Neg Mitral area: Neg
Palpation	Aortic area: Neg Pulmonic area: Neg Midprecordial area: Neg Tricuspid area: Neg Mitral area: Neg
Auscultation	Aortic area: $\oplus$ S_2 Pulmonic area: $\oplus$ S_2 Midprecordial area: Neg for murmurs Tricuspid area: $\oplus$ S_1, $\ominus$ S_3, questionable S_4 Mitral area: $\oplus$ S_1, $\ominus$ S_3, $\oplus$ S_4

continues

CASE STUDY (Continued)

The Patient with Hypertension

Assessment of the Peripheral Vasculature

Inspection of JVP (indirect)

No distention

Inspection of Hepatojugular Reflux

No change in jugular veins

Palpation and Auscultation of Arterial Pulses

Rate: 82
Rhythm: Regular
Amplitude:

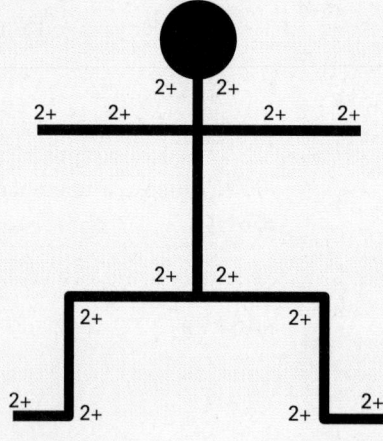

Scale = 3+

Symmetry: All symmetrical
Bruits: None

Inspection and Palpation of Peripheral Perfusion

Color: Normal for race
Clubbing: None
Capillary refill: Less than 2 seconds
Skin temperature: Warm
Edema: 1+ pedal edema
Ulcerations: None
Skin texture: Smooth, even. No varicose veins noted.
Hair distribution: Even

Palpation of Epitrochlear Node

Not palpable

Advanced Techniques

None required for this visit

DIAGNOSTIC DATA

Chest X-ray

Normal

EKG

Normal

Echocardiogram

Normal

continues

CASE STUDY (Continued)

The Patient with Hypertension

Height, Weight, Body Mass Index (BMI)	Height: 170 cm (66.9 inches) Weight: 89.6 kg (197 lbs) BMI: 31.2 (nl = 20–24.9)
LABORATORY	Baseline laboratory values unremarkable except for the following: • HbA1c: 8.4% (nl = less than 6%) • Fasting blood glucose level: 198 mg/dL (nl = 70–110 mg/dL) • Serum cholesterol: 301 mg/dL (nl = less than 200 mg/dL) • LDL cholesterol: 151 mg/dL (nl = less than 100 mg/dL) • HDL cholesterol: 37 mg/dL (nl = greater than 40 mg/dL) • Triglycerides: 346 mg/dL (nl = less than 150 mg/dL) • Serum creatinine: 1.6 mg/dL (nl = 0.5–1.5 mg/dL) • Urinalysis: 1+ proteinuria (nl = 0), 3+ glucose (nl = 0)

ASSESSMENT IN BRIEF

Heart and Peripheral Vasculature Assessment

Assessment of the Precordium

- Inspection
  - Aortic area
  - Pulmonic area
  - Midprecordial area
  - Tricuspid area
  - Mitral area
- Palpation
  - Aortic area
  - Pulmonic area
  - Midprecordial area
  - Tricuspid area
  - Mitral area
- Auscultation
  - Aortic area
  - Pulmonic area
  - Midprecordial area
  - Tricuspid area
  - Mitral area
  - Mitral and tricuspid areas (S_3)
  - Mitral and tricuspid areas (S_4)

  - Murmurs
  - Pericardial friction rub
  - Prosthetic heart valves

Assessment of the Peripheral Vasculature

- Inspection of the jugular venous pressure
- Inspection of the hepatojugular reflux
- Palpation and auscultation of arterial pulses
- Inspection and palpation of peripheral perfusion
  - Peripheral pulse
  - Color
  - Clubbing
  - Capillary refill
  - Skin temperature
  - Edema
  - Ulcerations
  - Skin texture
  - Hair distribution
- Palpation of the epitrochlear node

Advanced Techniques

- Orthostatic hypotension assessment
- Assessing for pulsus paradoxus

continues

ASSESSMENT IN BRIEF *Continued*

- Assessing the venous system
  - Homan's sign
  - Manual compression
  - Retrograde filling, or Trendelenburg test
- Assessing the arterial system
  - Pallor
  - Color return and venous filling time
  - Allen test
  - Ankle-Brachial Index

Assistive Devices

- Artificial cardiac pacemakers
- Hemodynamic monitor
- Antiembolic stockings
- Chest tubes
- EKG monitor
- Intravenous catheters
- Pneumatic compression stockings

REVIEW QUESTIONS

1. Which of the following heart chambers pumps oxygenated blood to the body?
   a. Left atrium
   b. Right atrium
   c. Left ventricle
   d. Right ventricle
   The correct answer is (c).

2. What is the average adult heart rate per minute when the impulse is initiated by the sinoatrial node of the heart?
   a. 50
   b. 60
   c. 70
   d. 90
   The correct answer is (c).

3. Assessment of aortic heart sounds should be checked:
   a. On the left side of the sternum, fifth intercostal space, midclavicular line
   b. On the left side of the sternum, fifth intercostal space
   c. Within 2 inches of the xyphoid process
   d. On the right side of the sternum, second intercostal space
   The correct answer is (d).

4. What is the best location to auscultate the mitral valve of the heart?
   a. On the left side of the sternum, fifth intercostal space, midclavicular line
   b. On the left side of the sternum, fifth intercostal space
   c. Within 2 inches of the xyphoid process
   d. On the right side of the sternum, second intercostal space
   The correct answer is (a).

5. An S_3 heart sound is often associated with which of the following conditions?
   a. Congestive heart failure
   b. Myocardial infarction
   c. Congenital cardiovascular defects
   d. Tachycardia
   The correct answer is (a).

6. A systolic blowing/high heart murmur auscultated on the left side of the sternum, fifth intercostal space, midclavicular line is indicative of:
   a. Aortic stenosis
   b. Pulmonic regurgitation
   c. Tricuspid stenosis
   d. Mitral regurgitation
   The correct answer is (d).

7. Which of the following is a modifiable risk factor for cardiovascular disease?
   a. Family history
   b. Smoking
   c. Race
   d. Gender
   The correct answer is (b).

8. What is a tear in the lining of the thoracic aorta called?
   a. Dissection
   b. Friction rub
   c. Aneurysm
   d. Bleed
   The correct answer is (a).

9. When checking carotid pulses, it is important to check them:
   a. Simultaneously
   b. One at a time
   c. Along with the apical pulse
   d. For 90 seconds
   The correct answer is (b).

10. The Allen Test is a technique used to assess the arterial system by testing for:
    a. The development of pallor in the extremities
    b. The return of color to the patient's legs
    c. The patency of the radial and ulnar arteries
    d. Thrombophlebitis
    The correct answer is (c).

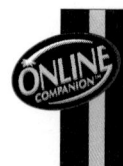

REFERENCES

Guyton, A. C., & Hall, J. E. (2005). *Textbook of medical physiology* (11th ed.). Philadelphia: W. B. Saunders.

McSweeney, J. C., Cody, M., O'Sullivan, P., Elberson, K., Moser, D. K., & Garvin, B. J. (2003). Women's early warning symptoms of acute myocardial infarction. *Circulation, 108,* 2619–2623.

Summit Doppler. (2008). *ABI diagnostic examination guide.* Retrieved March 7, 2008, from http://www.summitdoppler.com

Thygesen, K., Alpert, J. S., & White, H. D. (2007). Joint ESC/ACCF/AHA/WHF task force for the redefinition of myocardial infarction. Universal definition of myocardial infarction. *Journal of the American College of Cardiology, 50*(22), 2173–2195.

Vascular Disease Foundation. (2008). *The Ankle-Brachial index.* Retrieved March 7, 2008, from http://www.vdf.org/diseaseinfo/pad/anklebrachial.php

BIBLIOGRAPHY

Alspach, J. (Ed.). (2005). *Core curriculum for critical care nursing* (6th ed.). Philadelphia: W. B. Saunders.

Baliga, R. R., Eagle, K. A., Armstrong, W. F., & Bach, D. S. (2008). *Practical cardiology: evaluation and treatment of common cardiovascular disorders* (2nd ed.). Philadelphia: Lippincott Williams & Wilkins.

Caboral, M. F. (2008). Guidelines update on the prevention of heart disease in women. *Journal of the American Academy of Nurse Practitioners, 20*(4), 191–193.

Davis, L. (2004). *Cardiovascular nursing secrets.* St. Louis: Mosby.

Dodson, K. J. (2008). Cardiovascular effects of sleep apnea. *The Journal for Nurse Practitioners, 4*(6), 439–444.

Fahey, V. A. (2003). *Vascular nursing* (4th ed.). Philadelphia: W. B. Saunders.

Fauci, A. S., Kasper, D. L., Braunwald, E., Hauser, S. L., Longo, D. L., Jameson, J. L., & Loscalzo, J. (Eds.). (2008). *Harrison's principles of internal medicine* (17th ed.). New York: McGraw-Hill Professional Publishing.

Feinstein, J. (2008). *Practical pediatrics: Cardiology.* New York: McGraw-Hill Professional Publishing.

Field, J., Hazinski, M. F., & Gilmore, D. (Eds.). (2008). *Handbook of emergency cardiovascular care for healthcare providers.* Dallas, TX: American Heart Association.

Fuster, V., O'Rourke, R. A., Walsh, R., Poole-Wilson, P., King, S. B., Prystowsky, E., Roberts, R., & Nash, I. S. (2007). *Hurst's the heart* (12th ed.). New York: McGraw-Hill Professional Publishing.

Levy, M. N., & Pappano, A. J. (2006). *Cardiovascular physiology: Mosby physiology monograph series* (9th ed.). St. Louis: Mosby.

Libby, P., Bonow, R. O., Zipes, D. P., & Mann, D. L. (2007). *Braunwald's heart disease: A textbook of cardiovascular medicine* (8th ed.). Philadelphia: W. B. Saunders.

Lilly, L. S. (Ed.). (2006). *Pathophysiology of heart disease: A collaborative project of medical students and faculty* (4th ed.). Philadelphia: Lippincott Williams & Wilkins.

Reddy, K. S. (2004). Cardiovascular disease in non-Western countries. *New England Journal of Medicine, 350*(24), 2438–2440.

Springhouse: Cardiovascular care made incredibly easy! (2nd ed.). (2008). Philadelphia: Lippincott Williams & Wilkins.

Woods, S. L., Sivarajan Froelicher, E. S., & Motzer, S. A. (2004). *Cardiac nursing* (4th ed.). Philadelphia: Lippincott Williams & Wilkins.

WEB SITES

American Heart Association:
http://www.americanheart.org

Anatomy Atlases:
http://www.anatomyatlases.org

The Auscultation Assistant:
http://www.wilkes.med.ucla.edu

Mayo Clinic:
http://www.mayoclinic.com

National Heart, Lung, and Blood Institute:
http://www.nhlbi.nih.gov

National Institute of Nursing Research:
http://www.ninr.nih.gov

National Institutes of Health:
http://www.nih.gov

U.S. National Library of Medicine:
http://www.nlm.nih.gov

U.S. National Library of Medicine/National Institutes of Health:
http://www.medlineplus.gov

WebMD:
http://www.webmd.com

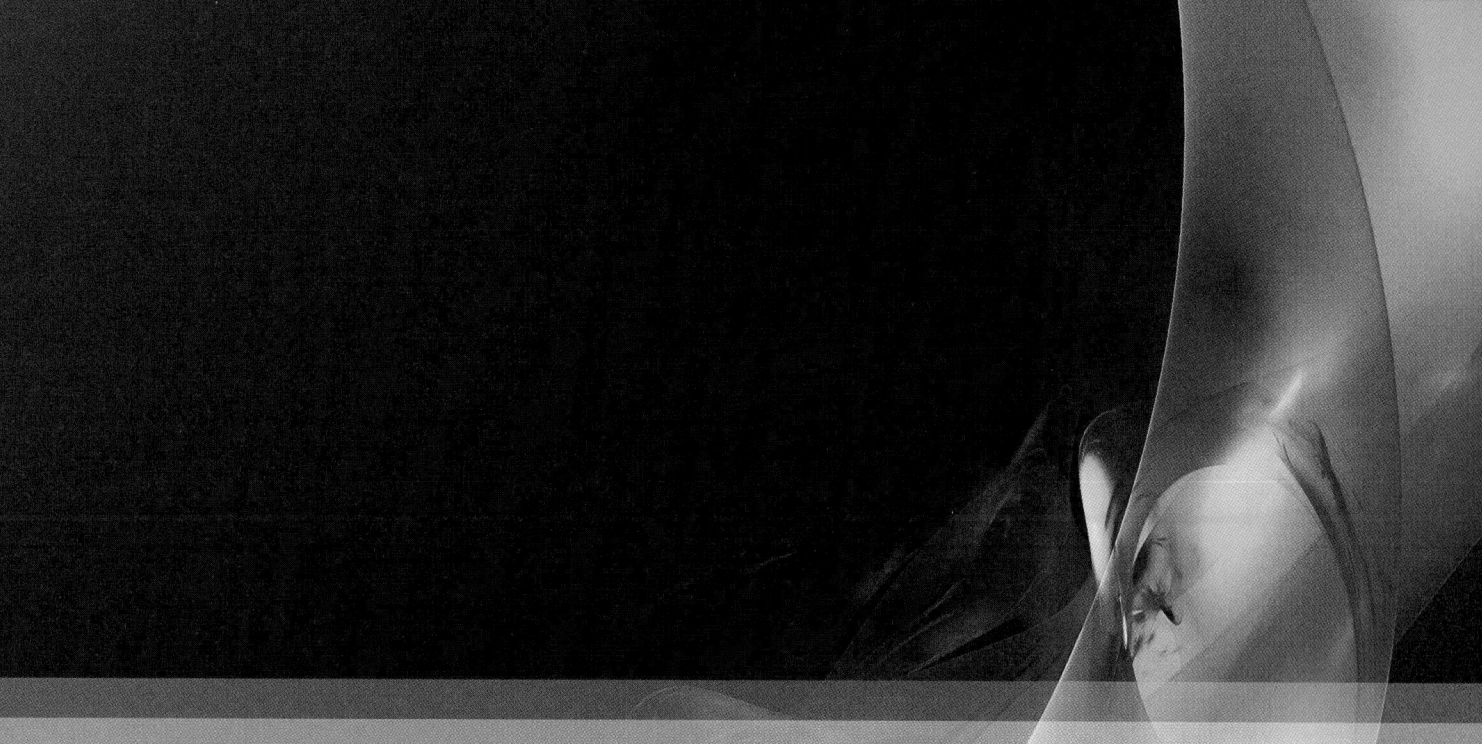

CHAPTER 17

Abdomen

COMPETENCIES

1. Identify the physiological function of the abdominal organs.

2. Obtain the health history of a patient with an abdominal complaint.

3. Demonstrate the techniques of abdominal assessment.

4. Relate abnormal physical assessment findings to pathological processes.

5. Describe assessment techniques of a patient with suspected appendicitis and ascites.

6. Document physical assessment findings of the abdomen.

Assessing the abdomen requires a complete understanding of anatomic and abdominal assessment norms. Examination of the abdomen provides significant information about the various functions of the gastrointestinal, cardiovascular, and genitourinary systems.

ANATOMY AND PHYSIOLOGY

ABDOMINAL CAVITY

The abdomen is the largest cavity of the body. It is located between the diaphragm and the symphysis pubis. It is oval-shaped and contains several vital organs. The posterior wall of the cavity includes the lumbar vertebrae, the sacrum, and the coccyx. The iliac bones and the lateral portion of the ribs shape the sides of the abdominal cavity (Figures 17-1 and 17-2). These bony structures are held together by muscular tissue that surrounds the entire abdominal cavity. The muscles of the abdomen include the rectus abdominis, transversus abdominis, external oblique, and internal oblique. The **linea alba**, a tendinous tissue that extends from the sternum to the symphysis pubis in the midline of the abdomen, is situated between the rectus abdominis muscles (see Figure 17-3).

Peritoneum

The endothelial lining of the abdominal cavity consists of membranes called peritoneal serous membranes. The serous layer that lines the walls of the cavity itself is called the parietal peritoneum and that which covers the organs is called the visceral peritoneum. The potential space between the two layers is referred to as

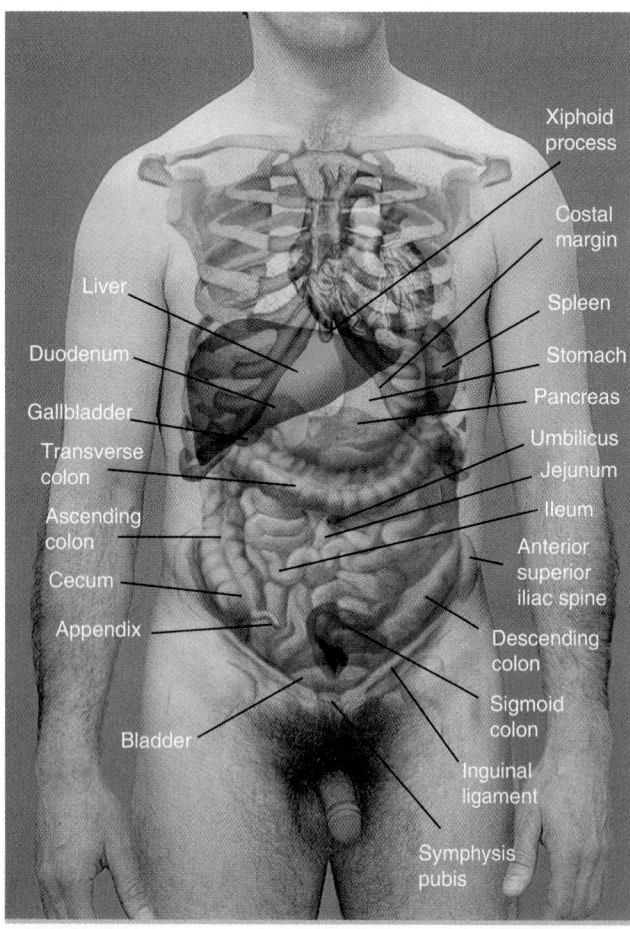

FIGURE 17-1 Structures of the Abdomen: Anterior View

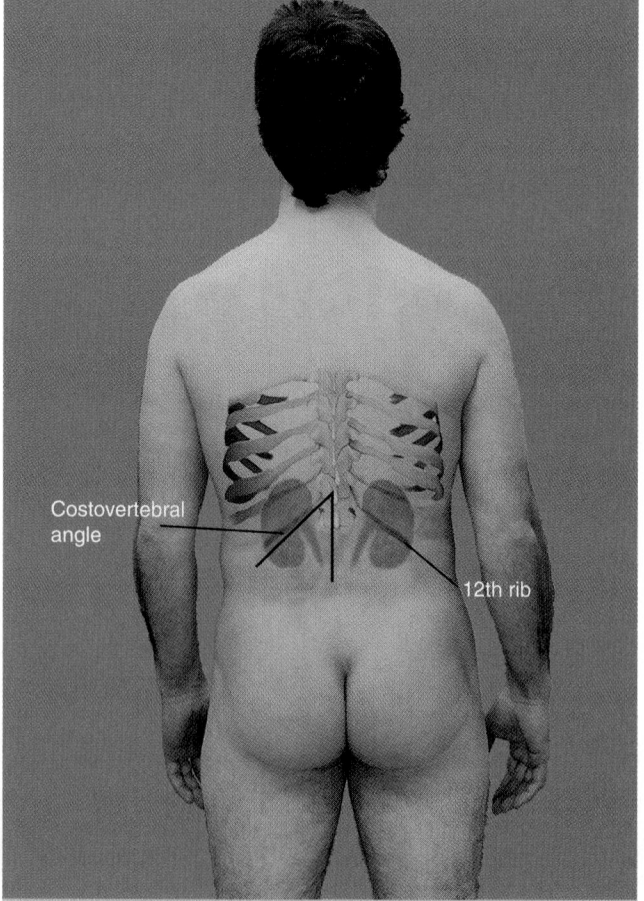

FIGURE 17-2 Structures of the Abdomen: Posterior View

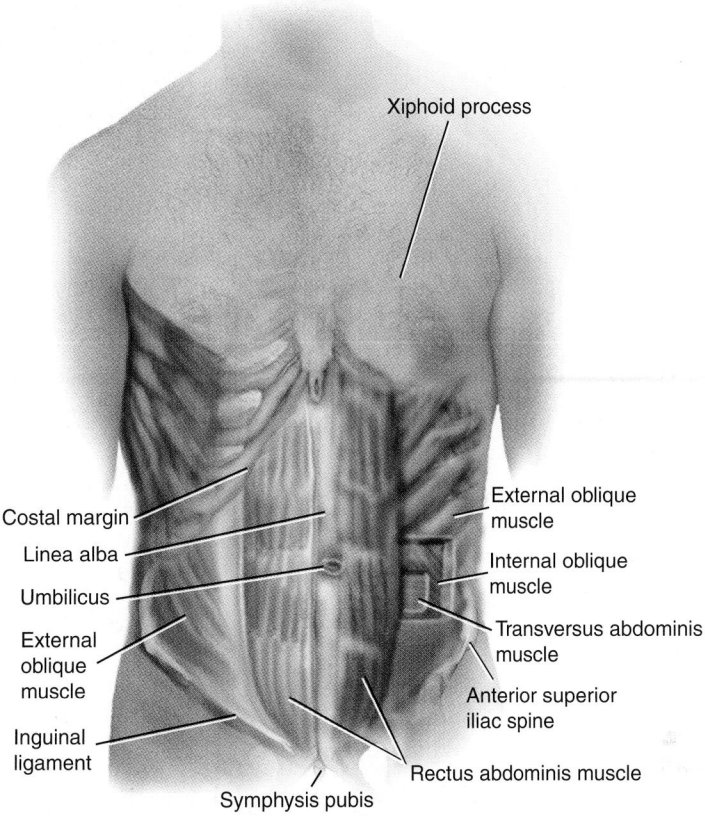

FIGURE 17-3 **Abdominal Musculature**

the peritoneal cavity. In the male, this cavity is completely closed, whereas in the female, openings exist for the fallopian tubes.

The organs covered with peritoneum and held in place by mesentery are referred to as intraperitoneal organs. The intraperitoneal organs are the spleen, gallbladder, stomach, liver, bile duct, small intestine, and large intestine. In contrast, the organs situated behind the peritoneum and without mesenteric attachment are known as retroperitoneal organs. The retroperitoneal organs are the pancreas, kidneys, ureters, and bladder.

Abdominal Vasculature

The aorta is the largest artery in the body. Below the level of the diaphragm, the descending aorta becomes the abdominal aorta, giving rise to arterial vessels that supply the abdominal wall and gastrointestinal organs with blood (see Figure 17-4). At about the fourth lumbar vertebra, the aorta bifurcates to become the right and left common iliac arteries.

Anatomic Mapping

Anatomic maps serve as a frame of reference during assessment of the abdomen. The abdominal cavity can be subdivided using two methods: quadrants or nine regions.

The most commonly used assessment approach in clinical practice is the four-quadrant technique (see Figure 17-5). For accuracy in documentation, the abdominal surface is divided into four sections by imaginary vertical and horizontal lines intersecting at the umbilicus. Commit to memory the location of abdominal organs according to quadrants (see Table 17-1). Table 17-2 lists pathologies by the quadrant or region where the pain is perceived.

Another strategy for pinpointing the location of abdominal assessment findings is via nine abdominal anatomic regions (see Figure 17-6). You can also use the anatomic landmarks in Figure 17-7.

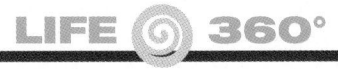

Abdominal Pathologies

Many abdominal pathologies such as pancreatitis, cirrhosis, and portal hypertension can be caused by excessive alcohol intake. Reflect on the last time you provided care to a patient who had an alcohol-induced illness. Did you find it difficult to provide care for that patient? Did you treat that patient in a manner that was different from the way you treat patients without histories of alcohol abuse?

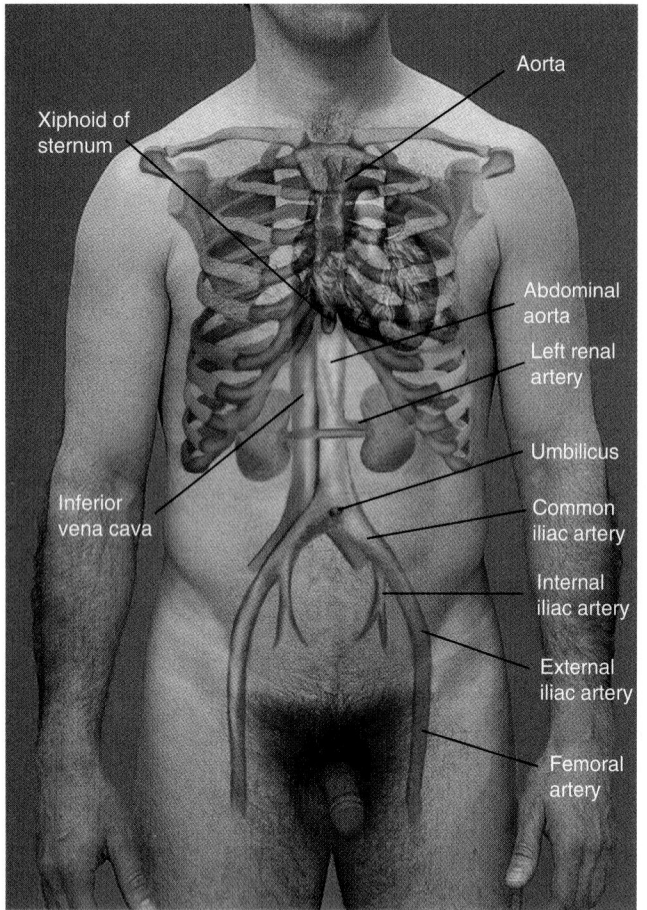

FIGURE 17-4 Abdominal Vasculature

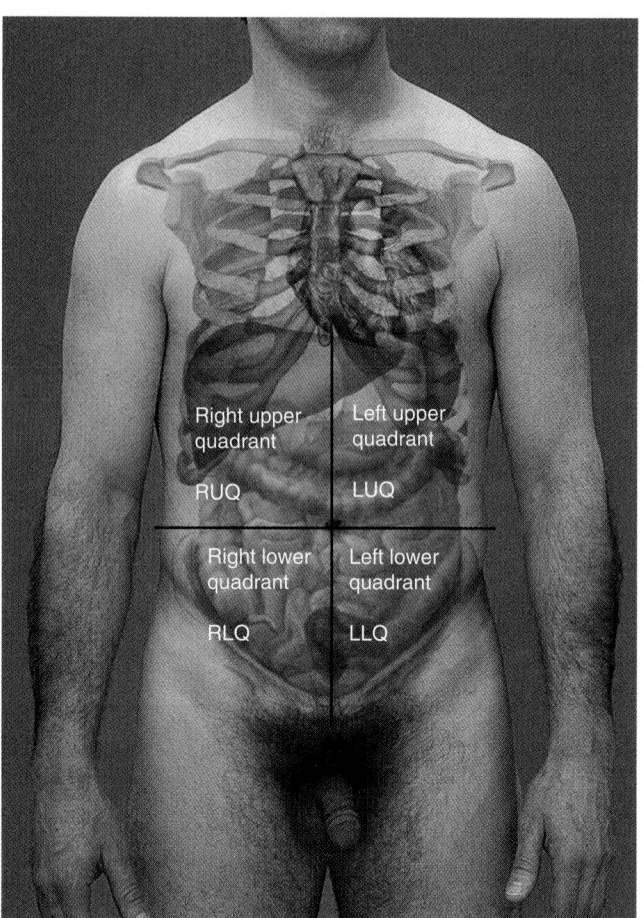

FIGURE 17-5 Abdominal Quadrants

TABLE 17-1 Four-Quadrant Anatomic Map

RIGHT UPPER QUADRANT (RUQ)	LEFT UPPER QUADRANT (LUQ)
Liver	Left lobe of liver
Gallbladder	Stomach
Pylorus	Spleen
Duodenum	Pancreas (body)
Pancreas (head)	Portion of left kidney and adrenal gland
Portion of right kidney and adrenal gland	Splenic flexure of colon
Hepatic flexure of colon	Sections of transverse and descending colons
Section of ascending and transverse colons	

RIGHT LOWER QUADRANT (RLQ)	LEFT LOWER QUADRANT (LLQ)
Appendix	Sigmoid colon
Cecum	Section of descending colon
Lower pole of right kidney	Lower pole of left kidney
Right ureter	Left ureter
Right ovary (female)	Left ovary (female)
Right spermatic cord (male)	Left spermatic cord (male)

TABLE 17-2 Etiologies of Abdominal Pain: Anatomical Regions Where They Are Perceived

RIGHT UPPER QUADRANT	EPIGASTRIUM	LEFT UPPER QUADRANT
Biliary stone	Abdominal aortic	Colitis
Cholecystitis	aneurysm	Gastric ulcer
Cholelithiasis	Appendicitis (early)	Gastritis
Colitis	Biliary stone	Myocardial infarction
Duodenal ulcer	Cholecystitis	Nephrolithiasis
Gastric ulcer	Cholelithiasis	Pneumonia
Hepatic abscess	Diverticulitis	Pulmonary embolus
Hepatitis	Gastroesophageal	Pyelonephritis
Hepatomegaly	reflux disease/gastritis	Splenic enlargement
Nephrolithiasis	Hiatal hernia	Splenic rupture
Pancreatitis	Myocardial infarction	
Pneumonia	Pancreatitis	
Pulmonary embolus	Peptic ulcer disease	
Pyelonephritis		

	PERIUMBILICAL	
	Abdominal aortic aneurysm and	
	dissection	
	Appendicitis (early)	
	Diverticulitis	
	Intestinal obstruction	
	Irritable bowel syndrome	
	Mesenteric ischemia	
	Pancreatitis	
	Peptic ulcer	
	Recurrent abdominal pain (in children)	
	Small bowel obstruction	
	Volvulus	

RIGHT LOWER QUADRANT		LEFT LOWER QUADRANT
Appendicitis		Diverticulitis
Diverticulitis		Ectopic pregnancy (ruptured)
Ectopic pregnancy (ruptured)		Endometriosis
Endometriosis		Hernia (strangulated)
Hernia (strangulated)		Inflammatory bowel disease
Inflammatory bowel disease		Irritable bowel syndrome
Irritable bowel syndrome		Mittelschmerz
Mittelschmerz		Ovarian cyst
Ovarian cyst		Pelvic inflammatory disease
Pelvic inflammatory disease		Renal calculi
Renal calculi		Salpingitis
Salpingitis		Uterine fibroids
Uterine fibroids		

	DIFFUSE	
	Gastroenteritis	
	Herpes zoster	
	Muscle strain	
	Peritonitis	

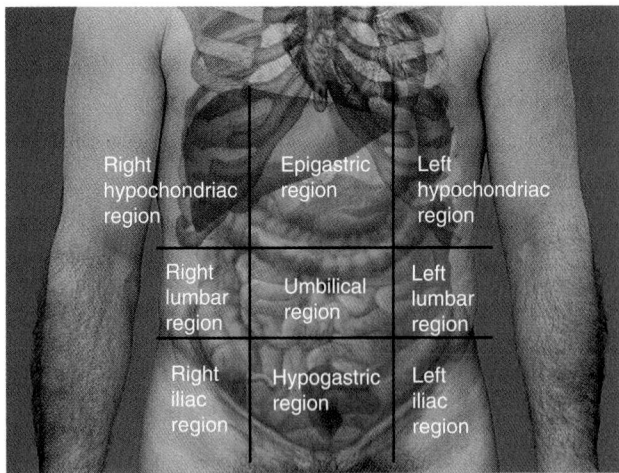

FIGURE 17-6 Nine Abdominal Anatomic Regions

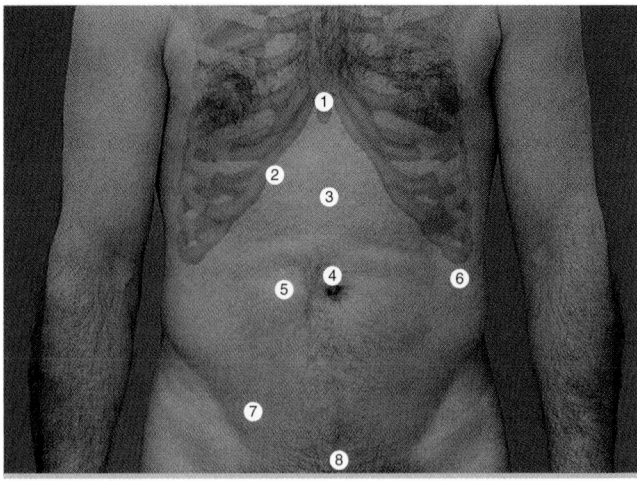

FIGURE 17-7 Abdominal Assessment Landmarks. When describing pathology of the abdomen, it is useful to use these anatomic landmarks: 1. Xiphoid Process; 2. Costal Margin; 3. Abdominal Midline; 4. Umbilicus; 5. Rectus Abdominis Muscle; 6. Anterior Superior Iliac Spine; 7. Inguinal Ligament (Poupart's Ligament); 8. Symphysis Pubis.

NURSING**ALERT**

Risk for Fluid Imbalance

Patients with persistent debilitating diarrhea require fluid and electrolyte replacement therapy to restore homeostasis to the body. If the patient is vomiting, there is a risk of dehydration and electrolyte imbalance.

Remember to assess skin turgor, mucous membranes, and orthostatic blood pressure. See Chapters 10, 13, and 16.

NURSING**ALERT**

Bloody Vomitus

Hematemesis, or the vomiting of blood, may be attributed to gastrointestinal ulcers or esophageal varices. Active bleeding is a medical emergency, and the patient should be promptly treated.

ABDOMINAL VISCERA (ORGANS)

Stomach

The stomach is a J-shaped, pouchlike organ located in the left upper quadrant of the abdomen beneath the diaphragm; it lies to the right of the spleen and is partially covered by the liver.

The stomach functions as a reservoir where the complex mechanical and chemical processes of digestion occur. Hydrochloric acid and digestive enzymes are secreted by the stomach to aid digestion. Little absorption of foodstuffs occurs in the stomach. Foodstuffs are liquified via gastric secretions into a semisolid substance called chyme. The usual capacity of the stomach is 1 to 1.5 L. In a regulated manner, chyme is released into the small intestine's duodenum for further digestion and absorption.

Small Intestine

The small intestine is a tubular-shaped organ extending from the pyloric sphincter to the ileocecal valve at the opening of the large intestine. The majority of foodstuffs are digested and absorbed in the small intestine. The convoluted loops of intestine are relatively mobile and can measure from 10 feet to 30 feet, depending on the degree of muscular relaxation of the intestinal wall and the size of the individual. Portions of the small intestine can be found in all four abdominal quadrants. The three segments of the small intestine are the duodenum, the jejunum, and the ileum. The duodenum is the first and shortest section. It plays a significant role in digestion because hormonal secretions are released and both the common bile and main pancreatic ducts open into the duodenum. The jejunum, the second component, is composed of circular mucosal folds that provide surface area for nutrient absorption. The ileum absorbs bile salts and vitamin B_{12}. The ileum terminates at the ileocecal valve.

Large Intestine

The large intestine is a tubular-shaped organ extending from the ileocecal valve to the anus. It has a greater diameter than the small intestine and can vary considerably in length, depending on the size of the individual, but generally is 5 feet in length.

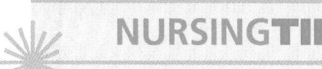

The four segments of the large intestine are the ascending, transverse, descending, and sigmoid colons. The cecum is the blind pouch that is continuous with the ascending colon, the large intestine located in the lower right quadrant of the abdomen.

The work of the large intestine is to form stool from cellulose, indigestible fibers, fat, bacteria, cellular debris, and inorganic materials, and then carry these intestinal contents to the end of the gastrointestinal tract. An additional function of the large intestine is the absorption of water and electrolytes. Water absorption occurs primarily in the ascending colon under the influence of the osmotic pressure gradient produced by sodium ions. The large intestine has limited digestive function.

Liver

The liver is the largest solid organ in the body. It lies directly below the diaphragm. The liver is located in the right upper quadrant, but extends across the midline into the left upper quadrant. In the right upper quadrant, the superior aspect of the liver is at the fifth rib, or at the nipples. The lower border does not extend more than 1 to 2 cm below the right costal margin.

The functions of the liver are complex and varied, and can be divided into:

- Storage (carbohydrates, amino acids, vitamins, minerals, and blood)
- Detoxification and filtration (drugs, hormones, and bacteria)
- Metabolism (carbohydrates, proteins, fat, ammonia to urea)
- Synthesis and secretion (bile production—600 to 1,000 mL/day, formation of lymph, bile salts, plasma proteins, fibrinogen, blood-clotting substances, and antibodies)

Gallbladder

The gallbladder is a pear-shaped sac located in the right upper quadrant of the abdomen. It is attached to the inferior surface of the liver.

The primary role of the gallbladder is to store and concentrate the bile produced by the liver. Bile contributes to fat digestion and absorption. The gallbladder stores approximately 30 to 50 mL of bile and releases bile in the presence of cholecystokinin, pancreozymin, and parasympathetic stimulation. As the gallbladder contracts, bile is released through the cystic duct into the common bile duct, which drains into the duodenum.

Pancreas

The pancreas is an elongated accessory organ of digestion. It lies in a transverse position along the posterior abdominal wall. It is located in the upper right and upper left quadrants of the abdomen. The pancreas is both an exocrine gland that secretes bicarbonate and pancreatic enzymes (which aid in digestion), and an endocrine gland that secretes the hormones insulin, glucagon, and gastrin.

Spleen

The spleen is the largest lymph organ in the body. It is oval in shape and is composed of white, pulpy lymphoid tissue and red pulp containing capillaries and venous sinuses. It is located behind the fundus of the stomach, below the diaphragm and above the left kidney and splenic flexure. The spleen is found in the left upper quadrant of the abdomen.

The spleen is part of the reticuloendothelial system and serves the body as a filter and a reservoir for red blood cell mass. During events that can cause vasoconstriction, such as hemorrhage or exercise, the spleen contributes needed blood to

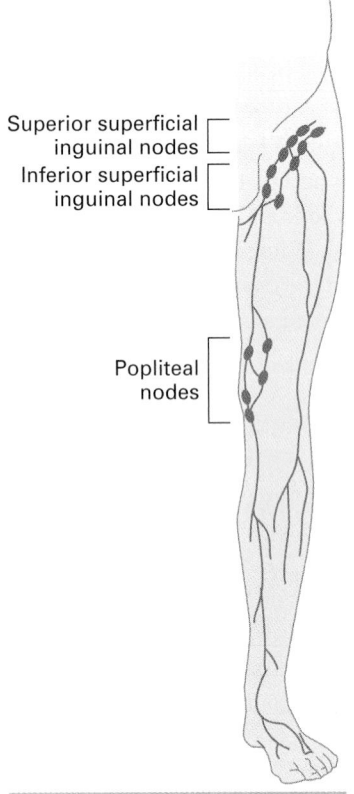

Superior superficial inguinal nodes
Inferior superficial inguinal nodes

Popliteal nodes

FIGURE 17-8 **Inguinal Lymph Nodes**

the general circulation. As a filter, the spleen rids the body of old or deformed red blood cells and platelets.

Vermiform Appendix

The vermiform appendix extends off the lower cecum in the right lower quadrant. This fingerlike appendage fills with digestive materials from the cecum. The vermiform appendix frequently does not empty completely, causing obstruction and subsequent infection.

Kidneys, Ureters, and Bladder

The kidneys are bean-shaped organs that lie tucked against the posterior abdominal wall. The left kidney is slightly larger in some individuals. Because of the superior placement of the liver over the right kidney, that kidney tends to hang about a half inch lower than the left, between T12 and L3.

The primary function of the kidneys is to rid the body of waste products and to maintain homeostasis through regulation of the acid-base balance, fluid and electrolyte balance, and arterial blood pressure.

Urine leaves the kidneys via the ureters. Peristaltic waves move the waste products to the bladder. The bladder stores the urine. Normally the bladder holds 200 to 400 mL of urine; however, its capacity is greater.

Lymph Nodes

The inguinal area contains deep and superficial lymph nodes. Only the superficial nodes are palpable. These lymph nodes are grouped into superior and inferior chains. The superior chain of lymph nodes is located horizontally near the inguinal ligament. The inferior chain of lymph nodes lies vertically below the junction of the saphenous and femoral veins (Figure 17-8).

HEALTH HISTORY

The abdominal health history provides insight into the link between a patient's life and lifestyle and abdominal information and pathology.

PATIENT PROFILE

Diseases that are age- and gender-specific for the abdomen are listed.

Age

Recurrent abdominal pain (2–15)
Appendicitis (young child–30)
Peptic ulcer disease (> 30, with an increased incidence in the elderly)
Cholecystitis (40–50)
Diabetes mellitus (type 2 > 45)
Diverticulosis (> 50)
Bladder cancer (50–70)
Pancreatic cancer (60–70s)
Mesenteric arterial insufficiency or infarct (more prevalent in the elderly, especially those with arteriosclerotic or atherosclerotic disease)

Gender

Female

Gallbladder disease, mittelschmerz (ovulatory pain)

continues

Male	Pancreatic cancer, gastric cancer, cancer of the kidney and bladder, cirrhosis, duodenal ulcer, diverticulosis
CHIEF COMPLAINT	*Common chief complaints for the abdomen are defined and information on the characteristics of each sign or symptom is provided.*
1. Nausea	An uncomfortable sensation in the stomach and abdominal region
Quality	Retching (dry heaves)
Associated Manifestations	Vomiting, medication use, fever, chills, foods eaten, fluids consumed, diarrhea, pregnancy
Aggravating Factors	Noxious odors
Alleviating Factors	Flat soda, dry crackers, sleep, antiemetics
Timing	Early morning, bedtime, middle of the night, after eating, after missed menstrual period
2. Vomiting	Expulsion of contents from the upper gastrointestinal tract via contraction of abdominal wall muscles and relaxation of the esophageal sphincter
Quality	Color (bright red: fresh blood; coffee grounds appearance: "old" blood that has had time to mix with digestive juices; dark brown or black: bile; other colors may occur secondary to food intake), projectile
Associated Manifestations	Nausea, medications, fever, chills, abdominal pain, headache, foods eaten, fluids consumed, diarrhea, pregnancy
Aggravating Factors	Noxious odors
Alleviating Factors	Flat soda, dry crackers, sleep, antiemetic medications
Timing	Early morning, bedtime, middle of the night, after eating, after missed menstrual period
3. Diarrhea	Frequent watery stools resulting in the loss of essential electrolytes
Quality	Color; presence of blood, mucus, or fat; odor
Associated Manifestations	Abdominal cramping, pain, physical weakness, weight loss, fever, stress
Aggravating Factors	Food, medications, stress
Alleviating Factors	Diet (bananas, rice, apples, toast), medications, fluids with electrolyte supplement, physical rest
Timing	Recent travel, especially areas with unpotable water; recent antibiotic use
4. Constipation	Infrequent stools resulting in the passage of dry, hard fecal waste
Quality	Color, odor, appearance of blood
Associated Manifestations	Physical discomfort, rectal fullness, nausea, bloating, pain with defecation
Aggravating Factors	Food, medications (e.g., iron, narcotics), stress
Alleviating Factors	High-fiber diet, medications (e.g., laxatives, stool softeners, enemas), physical activity, increased fluid intake

continues

5. Abdominal Distension	Protuberance of the abdomen
Quantity	Degree of distension and frequency (may need to measure abdomen)
Associated Manifestations	Constipation, abdominal discomfort, ascites, enlarged liver, enlarged spleen
Aggravating Factors	Food, medications, stress
Alleviating Factors	Diet, medications, physical activity
6. Abdominal Pain	Discomfort in the abdomen; may be visceral, parietal, or referred pain (see Table 17-3)
Quality	Dull, burning, sharp, gnawing, stabbing, cramping (severe cramping is referred to as colic pain), aching
Associated Manifestations	Bleeding, flank pain, weight loss, nausea and vomiting, eructation, fever or chills, changes in bowel habits, flatus, prolonged immobility, menstrual cycle
Aggravating Factors	Position, stress, eating, smoking, medications (e.g., aspirin, steroids, NSAID), alcohol or drug use
Alleviating Factors	Antacids, proton pump inhibitors (PPI), histamine-2 antagonists, rest, diet, stress management, position change
Setting	Home environment, work environment, mealtimes, social occasions involving alcohol or drug use
Timing	Pre- or postprandial, nighttime, seasonal, stressful situations, menstruation, gradual, sudden
7. Increased Eructation	Belching, or the oral expression of air (gas) from the stomach
Quantity	Marked increase over patient's normal status
Associated Manifestations	Ingestion of milk products, certain foods, carbonated beverages, beer
8. Increased Flatulence	Passage of excess gas via the rectum
Quantity	Marked increase over patient's normal status
Associated Manifestations	Ingestion of certain foods (onions, cabbage, beans, cauliflower, corn, wheat, barley, rye)
Aggravating Factors	Food or medications
Alleviating Factors	Avoidance of particular foods that are fermentable
Timing	Following meals
9. Dysuria	Painful urination
Location	Suprapubic, near urinary meatus, costovertebral angle
Quality	Burning, stabbing
Associated Manifestations	Abdominal/flank/testicular pain, fever, chills, current bacterial infection, hematuria, dribbling, urethral discharge, decreased urinary flow, urgency, hesitancy, nocturia, recent sexual intercourse
Aggravating Factors	Presence of prostatic stones or renal calculi, decreased oral intake

continues

Health History (continued)	
Alleviating Factors	Medications (antibiotics, pyridium, analgesics), passage or surgical removal of stone, transurethral resection of the prostate, increased oral intake
Setting	New sexual partner in the last 6 months, a sexual partner known to have other sexual partners, unprotected intercourse, wiping genitalia back to front (female)
Timing	At start of urination, midstream, throughout stream, sense of urgency, pregnancy
10. Nocturia	Night arousal to void
Associated Manifestations	Hesitancy, decrease in force of urinary stream, postvoid dribbling, urge incontinence
Aggravating Factors	Enlarged prostate, diabetes mellitus, diuretics, urinary tract infection, alcohol ingestion, anticholinergic medications, diuretics, decongestants and cough medicines
Alleviating Factors	Adrenergic antagonists, 5–alpha-reductase inhibitors, transurethral resection of prostate, elimination of causative medications
11. Urinary Incontinence	
Quality	Constant, intermittent, dribbling, large volumes, hesitancy
Quantity	Frequency, urgency, number of pads used
Associated Manifestations	Recent surgery, coughing, sneezing, crying, laughing, heavy lifting, activity, medications, urinary tract infection, constipation, spinal cord lesions, neurological disease
Aggravating Factors	Medications, caffeine intake, alcohol intake
Alleviating Factors	Pelvic floor muscle rehabilitation, bladder training, biofeedback, anti-incontinence devices, medications
Setting	Accessibility of toilet, distance to toilet, adequate lighting to toilet, grab bars by toilet, height of toilet seat
Timing	Nocturia
PAST HEALTH HISTORY	*The various components of the past health history are linked to abdominal pathology and abdomen-related information.*
Medical History	
Abdomen Specific	Malignancies, peritonitis, cholecystitis, appendicitis, pancreatitis, small bowel obstruction, ulcerative colitis, hepatitis, hiatal hernia, diverticulitis, diverticulosis, peptic ulcer disease, Crohn's disease, acute renal failure, chronic renal failure, gallstones, kidney stone, irritable bowel syndrome, gastroesophageal reflux disease, urinary tract infection, parasitic infections, food poisoning, cirrhosis, infectious mononucleosis, hyper- or hypoadrenalism, malabsorption syndromes
Non-abdomen Specific	Pulmonary tuberculosis, malaria, heart disease, thyroid or parathyroid disease, pneumonia, upper respiratory infections, allergies, postnasal discharge, sinusitis, stress, sexually transmitted disease (STD), puberty, menopause, diabetes, ketoacidosis, ectopic pregnancy, cystic fibrosis, endometriosis, lupus, sickle cell anemia

continues

Health History (continued)

Surgical History	Cholecystectomy, gastrectomy, Billroth I or II, ileostomy, colostomy, appendectomy, colectomy, nephrectomy, pancreatectomy, ileal conduit, portal caval shunt, splenectomy, hiatal hernia repair, umbilical hernia repair, femoral or inguinal hernia repair, removal of renal calculi, liver transplant, renal transplant, bariatric surgery
Allergies	Ingestion of certain food types or medications may cause gastric irritation, nausea, and vomiting; lactose intolerance.
Medications	Histamine-2 antagonists, PPI, antibiotics, lactulose, antacids, vitamins, anti-parasitics, anticholinergics, tranquilizers, steroids, antidiarrheals, electro-lytes, laxatives, stool softeners, insulin, antiemetics, antiflatulents
Communicable Diseases	STD, HIV infection, hepatitis, tuberculosis, infectious mononucleosis, and intestinal parasites
	HIV-opportunistic infections: enteric pathogens—*Cryptosporidium* causes weight loss from malabsorption syndrome and persistent debilitating diarrhea. Kaposi's sarcoma lesions can cause bowel occlusion, leading to constipation.
Injuries and Accidents	Abdominal trauma such as ruptured or bruised organs, gunshot wounds, or knife stabbings; swallowing of foreign bodies
Immunizations	Hepatitis A and Hepatitis B vaccines
FAMILY HEALTH HISTORY	*Abdominal diseases and disorders that are familial are listed.*
	Malignancies of the stomach, liver, pancreas, or colon, peptic ulcer disease, diabetes mellitus, familial polyposis, inflammatory bowel disease, irritable bowel syndrome, polycystic kidney disease, colitis, malabsorption syndromes (celiac disease), cystic fibrosis
SOCIAL HISTORY	*The components of the social history are linked to abdomen factors and pathology.*
Alcohol Use	Altered nutrition, impaired gastric absorption, at risk for upper and lower gastrointestinal bleeding, cirrhosis of liver
Drug Use	Opioids reduce peristalsis and are associated with the development of constipation.
Travel History	Infectious diarrhea may be produced by bacteria such as *Escherichia coli*, and parasites that may not be indigenous to the patient's usual environment.
Home Environment	Public water versus well water; lead-based paint used
Work Environment	Improper food preparation and handling, water contamination, and poor sanitation can lead to hepatitis and *Escherichia coli* infections.
Hobbies and Leisure Activities	Sports such as lacrosse, football, and boxing often associated with traumatic injuries
Economic Status	Bacterial and parasitic diseases from poor sanitation

continues

Health History (continued)

HEALTH MAINTENANCE ACTIVITIES	*This information provides a bridge between the health maintenance activities and abdominal function.*
Sleep	Nocturnal pain with peptic ulcer disease; hiatal hernia discomfort in recumbent position
Diet	Healthy diet as a means of avoiding problems (fruits, vegetables, fiber, alcohol in moderation, decreased intake of fat and prepared foods); gallbladder attacks after fatty meals; caffeinated beverages, coffee, tea, and alcohol exacerbate GERD
Exercise	Regular exercise facilitates gastrointestinal functioning.
Stress Management	High stress levels are associated with stress ulcers.
Use of Safety Devices	Shoulder and lap restraints in automobiles to prevent abdominal injuries; appropriate sports safety equipment to protect abdominal region
Health Check-ups	Blood chemistry: Elevated glucose and HbA1c might indicate onset of diabetes mellitus Blood count: Anemia could reflect silent gastrointestinal bleeds Urinalysis: Dark color may signify bilirubin in urine Stool guaiac: Results need to be investigated Colonoscopy: Reason for procedure, results

TABLE 17-3 Differentiating Abdominal Pain

	VISCERAL PAIN	PARIETAL PAIN	REFERRED PAIN
Origin	Originates in the abdominal organs	Originates in the parietal peritoneum	Originates from abdominal organs to nonabdominal locations (e.g., chest, spine, or pelvis); refer path to abdominal region
Cause	Hollow structures become painful when they contract forcefully or when distended (e.g., intestines); solid organs become painful when stretched	Inflammation	Nerve innervation
Characteristics	Deep, dull, poorly localized; usually begins as dull pain, but when it becomes intense, is associated with nausea, vomiting, pallor, and diaphoresis	Sharp, precisely localized; usually severe from the onset and intensifies with movement	Well localized; pain is from a disorder in another site, for example: Duodenal pain: back and right shoulder Pancreatic pain: back and left shoulder

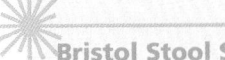

NURSING**TIP**

Bristol Stool Scale

It can be difficult for a patient to describe the exact nature of stools. To assist in identifying stool, it is practical to show the patient the Bristol Stool Scale. This can provide the nurse with clues on colon transit time. Types 1 and 2 can be classified as constipation and the patient usually needs to strain with defecation. Types 3 and 4 are the most comfortable stools to pass. Stool types 5, 6, and 7 are associated with urgency, with 7 constituting diarrhea. Type 1 stool spends the most time in the colon and type 7 the least.

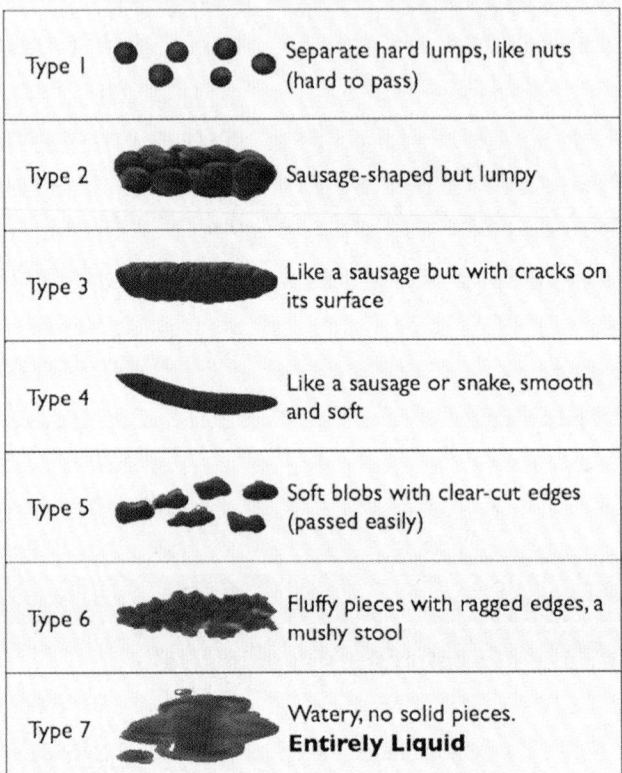

Bristol Stool Chart

Type 1	Separate hard lumps, like nuts (hard to pass)
Type 2	Sausage-shaped but lumpy
Type 3	Like a sausage but with cracks on its surface
Type 4	Like a sausage or snake, smooth and soft
Type 5	Soft blobs with clear-cut edges (passed easily)
Type 6	Fluffy pieces with ragged edges, a mushy stool
Type 7	Watery, no solid pieces. **Entirely Liquid**

Lewis, S. J., & Heaton, K. W. (1997). Stool form scale as a useful guide to intestinal transit time. *Scandinavian Journal of Gastroenterology, 32*(9), 920–924.

NURSING**TIP**

Referred Abdominal Pain

Abdominal pain can be difficult to assess because the location of the abdominal pain may not be directly attributive to the area of the causative factors. In referred pain, the sensory cortex perceives pain via nerve fibers where the internal abdominal organs were located in fetal development. Pain originating from the liver, spleen, pancreas, stomach, and duodenum may be referred (see Figure 17-9).

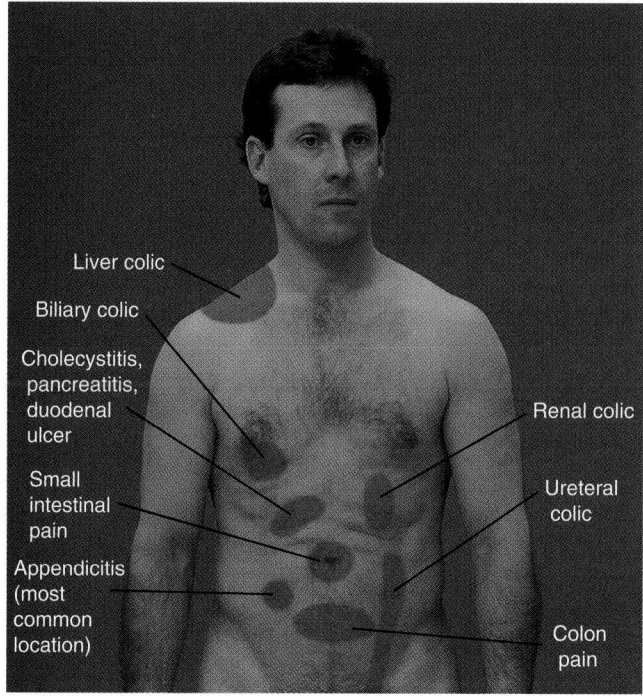

A. Anterior View

Liver colic
Biliary colic
Cholecystitis, pancreatitis, duodenal ulcer
Small intestinal pain
Appendicitis (most common location)
Renal colic
Ureteral colic
Colon pain

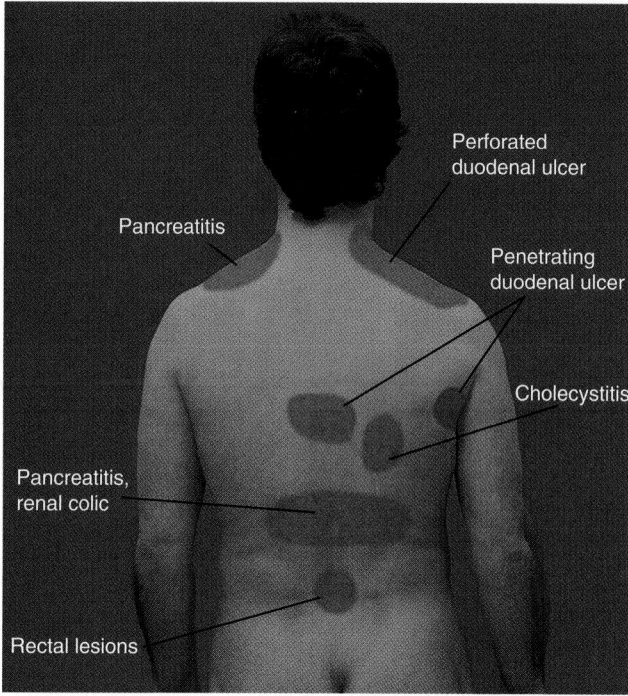

B. Posterior View

Pancreatitis
Perforated duodenal ulcer
Penetrating duodenal ulcer
Cholecystitis
Pancreatitis, renal colic
Rectal lesions

FIGURE 17-9 Areas of Referred Pain

EQUIPMENT

- Drapes
- Small pillow for under knees.
- Tape measure or small ruler with centimeter markings
- Marking pencil
- Gooseneck lamp for tangential lighting
- Stethoscope
- Sterile safety pin or sterile needle

ASSESSMENT OF THE ABDOMEN

The order of abdominal assessment is inspection, auscultation, percussion, and palpation. Auscultation is performed second because palpation and percussion can alter bowel sounds.

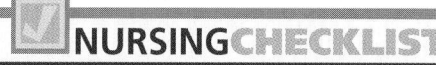
NURSING**CHECKLIST**

General Approach to Abdominal Assessment

1. Greet the patient and explain the assessment technique.
2. Ensure that the room is at a warm, comfortable temperature to prevent patient chilling and shivering.
3. Use a quiet room that will be free from interruptions.
4. Utilize an adequate light source. This includes both a bright overhead light and a freestanding lamp for tangential lighting.
5. Ask the patient to urinate before the exam.
6. Drape the patient from the xiphoid process to the symphysis pubis, then expose the patient's abdomen.
7. Position the patient comfortably in a supine position with knees flexed over a pillow or position the patient so that the arms are either folded across the chest or at the sides to ensure abdominal relaxation.
8. Stand to the right side of the patient for the examination.
9. Visualize the underlying abdominal structures during the assessment process in order to accurately describe the location of any pathology.
10. Have the patient point to tender areas; assess these last. Mark these and other significant findings (scars, dullness, and so on) on the body diagram in the patient's chart.
11. Watch the patient's face closely for signs of discomfort or pain.
12. Help the patient relax by using an unhurried approach, diverting attention with questions, and so on.
13. Ensure that your hands and the stethoscope are warm to promote patient comfort.

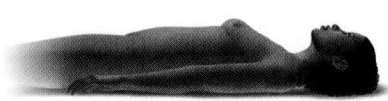

Flat

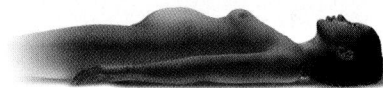

Rounded

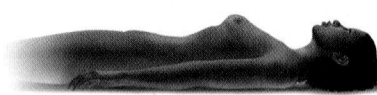

Scaphoid

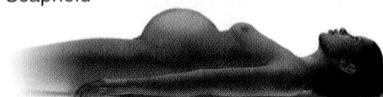

Protuberant

FIGURE 17-10 Abdominal Configurations

INSPECTION

Contour

E View the contour of the patient's abdomen from the costal margin to the symphysis pubis.

N In the normal adult, the abdominal contour is flat (straight horizontal line from costal margin to symphysis pubis) or rounded (convexity of abdomen from costal margin to symphysis pubis). See Figure 17-10.

A Assessment reveals a large convex symmetrical profile from the costal margin to the symphysis pubis.

P A large convex abdomen can result from one of the 7 F's. Refer to the Nursing Tip on this page.

A A convex abdomen that has a marked increase at the height of the umbilicus is abnormal.

P A protuberant abdomen results from a wide range of disorders. Taut stretching of the skin across the abdominal wall may occur. Refer to the Nursing Tip on this page.

A A concave symmetrical profile from the costal margin to the symphysis pubis is abnormal.

P A scaphoid abdomen reflects a decrease in fat deposits, a malnourished state, or flaccid muscle tone.

Symmetry

E 1. View the symmetry of the patient's abdomen from the costal margin to the symphysis pubis.

2. Move to the foot of the examination table and recheck the symmetry of the patient's abdomen.

N The abdomen should be symmetrical bilaterally.

A Assessment reveals an asymmetrical abdomen.

P Asymmetry may be caused by a tumor, cysts, bowel obstruction, enlargement of abdominal organs, or scoliosis. Bulging at the umbilicus can indicate an umbilical hernia.

P If the abdomen is asymmetrical at the site of a surgical incision or scar, suspect an incisional hernia.

Rectus Abdominis Muscles

E 1. Instruct the patient to raise the head and shoulders off the examination table.

2. Observe the rectus abdominis muscles for separation.

N The symmetry of the abdomen remains uniform; no ridge is observed parallel to the umbilicus or between the rectus abdominis muscles.

A A ridge between the rectus abdominis muscles is observed.

P This abnormality is known as diastasis recti abdominis and is attributed to marked obesity or past pregnancy. The observed separation of rectus abdominis muscles is caused by increased intra-abdominal pressure and is not considered to be harmful or ominous.

E Examination   **N** Normal Findings   **A** Abnormal Findings   **P** Pathophysiology

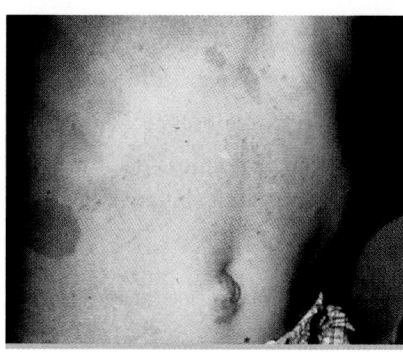

FIGURE 17-11   von Recklinghausen's Disease. *Courtesy of the Armed Forces Institute of Pathology.*

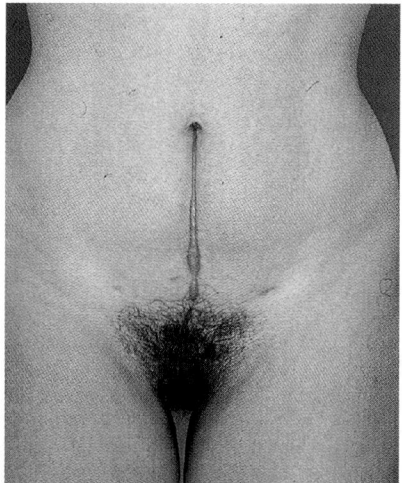

FIGURE 17-12   Abdominal Scar from a Hysterectomy

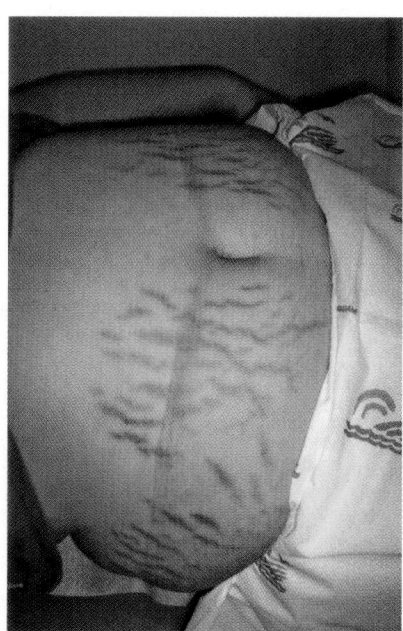

FIGURE 17-13   Abdominal Striae

Pigmentation and Color

E View the color of the patient's abdomen from the costal margin to the symphysis pubis.

N The abdomen should be uniform in color and pigmentation.

A Uneven skin color or pigmentation is abnormal.

P The presence of jaundice suggests liver dysfunction. The yellow discoloration of the skin in light-skinned patients is due to the accumulation of bilirubin in the blood. The average level for visible jaundice is 2 mg/dL.

P In light-skinned individuals, the observation of a blue tint at the umbilicus suggests free blood in the peritoneal cavity, known as **Cullen's sign.** Such bleeding can occur either following rupture of a fallopian tube secondary to an ectopic pregnancy or with acute hemorrhagic pancreatitis.

P Irregular patches of tan skin pigmentation (café au lait spots) may be attributed to von Recklinghausen's disease (Figure 17-11), a familial condition associated with the formation of neurofibromas.

A Engorged abdominal veins are abnormal.

P The appearance of engorged or dilated veins around the umbilicus is called **caput medusae.** It is associated with circulatory obstruction of the superior or the inferior vena cava. In some instances, this condition is related to obstruction of the portal vein or to emaciation.

A A network of dilated veins on the abdomen is abnormal.

P This occurs in portal hypertension, cirrhosis, and vena cava obstruction secondary to increased venous pressures.

Scars

E Inspect the abdomen for scars from the costal margin to the symphysis pubis.

N There should be no abdominal scars present.

A Scars are present (Figure 17-12).

P The site of the scars discloses useful information about the patient's surgical history. Dense, irregular, collagenous scars are keloids, which are more common in dark-skinned individuals and may be associated with traumatic injuries or burns. The presence of surgical scars may indicate internal adhesions.

Striae

E Observe the abdominal skin for **striae,** or abdominal atrophic lines or scars.

N No evidence of striae is present.

A Striae are present (Figure 17-13).

P Striae, atrophic lines or streaks, occur when there has been rapid or prolonged stretching of the skin. Abdominal striae may be caused by Cushing's syndrome, abdominal tumors, obesity, ascites, or pregnancy. Following pregnancy, striae are a normal finding.

Respiratory Movement

E Observe the abdomen for smooth, even respiratory movement.

N There is no evidence of respiratory retractions. Normally, the abdomen rises with inspiration and falls with expiration.

A Abnormal respiratory movements and retractions are observed.

P The origin of abnormal respirations due to an abdominal disorder may include appendicitis with local peritonitis, pancreatitis, biliary colic, or a perforated ulcer.

Masses or Nodules

E Observe the abdominal skin for nodules or masses.

N No masses or nodules are present.

A Abdominal masses or nodules are present.

P The presence of abdominal masses or nodules may indicate tumors, metastases of an internal malignancy, or pregnancy.

P A bulge over an abdominal incision could possibly indicate an incisional hernia.

Visible Peristalsis

E Observe the abdominal wall for surface motion.

N Ripples of peristalsis may be observed in thin patients. Peristalsis movement slowly traverses the abdomen in a slanting, downward direction.

A Strong peristaltic contractions are observed.

P Peristaltic waves may indicate intestinal obstruction.

Pulsation

E Inspect the epigastric area for pulsations.

N In the patient with a normal build, a nonexaggerated pulsation of the abdominal aorta may be visible in the epigastric area. In heavier patients, pulsation may not be visible.

A Marked, strong abdominal pulsations are observed.

P Widened pulse pressure and strong epigastric pulsations may indicate an aortic aneurysm. An exaggerated pulsation can also occur in aortic regurgitation and in right ventricular hypertrophy.

Umbilicus

E 1. Observe the umbilicus in relation to the abdominal surface.

2. Ask the patient to flex the neck and perform the valsalva maneuver.

3. Observe for protrusion of the intestine through the umbilicus.

N The umbilicus is depressed and beneath the abdominal surface.

A The umbilicus protrudes above the abdominal surface (Figure 17-14).

P Umbilical hernia in the adult is the protrusion of part of the intestine through an incomplete umbilical ring. Umbilical hernia is confirmed by inserting the index finger into the navel and feeling an opening in the fascia. It can often be seen when the patient's intra-abdominal pressure increases when coughing, sneezing, laughing, and straining occur.

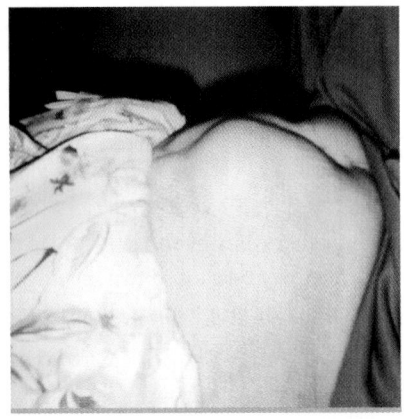

FIGURE 17-14 Umbilical Hernia

| **E** Examination | **N** Normal Findings | **A** Abnormal Findings | **P** Pathophysiology |

P The umbilicus that appears as a nodule may be the manifestation of abdominal carcinoma with metastasis to the umbilicus. This physical finding is known as Sister Mary Joseph's nodule.

P Intra-abdominal pressure from ascites, masses, or pregnancy can cause the umbilicus to protrude.

REFLECTIVE THINKING

Assessing for Hepatitis

A 21-year-old college student visits the student health center. The student recently returned from a 10-day humanitarian trip to Central America. She presents with anorexia, abdominal discomfort, and icteric sclera. What questions would you ask this student?

REFLECTIVE THINKING

Hepatitis Risks

A 29-year-old man who recently emigrated from a third-world country is seeking follow-up care for abdominal pain. On the first visit you completed his health history and physical examination, and obtained laboratory data. Your clinical suspicion is confirmed with the results of the lab tests: he has hepatitis B. This man is sexually active with his wife. You inform him of the importance of his wife being clinically evaluated. He tells you that he will not have health care insurance for her through his job until next year, and it is too expensive for her to be seen until then. How would you respond? What information would you give to him?

NURSING**ALERT**

Risk Factors for Hepatitis A Virus (HAV)

- Overcrowded living quarters
- Poor personal hygiene (poor hand washing, especially after defecation)
- Poor sanitation (sewage disposal)
- Food and water contamination
- Ingestion of shellfish caught in contaminated water
- Travel to endemic area (many third-world countries)
- Those in close personal contact with infected individual
- Native Americans, Alaskan natives
- Day care centers, especially those with children wearing diapers

Risk Factors for Hepatitis B Virus (HBV)

- IV drug use with shared needles
- Receipt of multiple transfusions of blood and blood products (oncology and hemodialysis patients, hemophiliacs)
- Frequent contact with blood (health care workers such as nurses, doctors, phlebotomists, and laboratory personnel)
- Sexual contact with infected individual
- Homosexual activity
- Perinatal transmission
- Travel to endemic areas (e.g., China)

Risk Factors for Hepatitis C Virus (HCV)

- Exposure to blood and blood products
- IV drug users
- High-risk sexual activity
- Sexual contact with infected individual
- Household contact with infected individual
- Contact with contaminated body fluids

Risk Factors for Hepatitis D Virus (HDV)

- Coinfection with hepatitis B or superinfection with chronic hepatitis B virus infection
- Blood and blood products
- IV drug users
- Individuals from endemic areas
- Sexual contact with infected individual
- Perinatal transmission (rare)

Risk Factors for Hepatitis E Virus (HEV)

- Fecal-oral route transmission
- Prevalence in India, Middle East, South Central Asia; rare in the United States

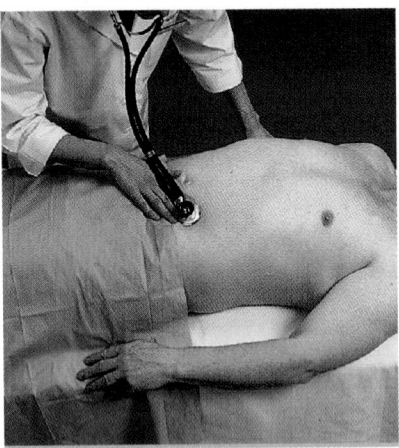

FIGURE 17-15 Technique of Abdominal Auscultation

AUSCULTATION

Bowel Sounds

 1. Place the diaphragm lightly on the abdominal wall beginning at the RLQ.

2. Listen to the frequency and character of the bowel sounds. It is necessary to listen for at least 5 minutes in an abdominal quadrant before concluding that bowel sounds are absent.

3. Move diaphragm to RUQ, LUQ, LLQ (Figure 17-15).

✳ NURSING**ALERT**

Risk Factors for Colorectal Cancer

- Over 50 years of age
- Family history of colorectal cancer or polyps
- Family history of a hereditary colorectal cancer syndrome (familial adenomatous polyposis or hereditary nonpolyposis colon cancer)
- Personal history of adenomatous polyps, colorectal cancer
- Personal history of chronic inflammatory bowel disease (ulcerative colitis, Crohn's disease)
- Personal history of endometrial, ovarian, or breast cancer
- Ashkenazi Jewish descent
- Lack of physical activity
- Low fruit and vegetable intake, high-fat diet
- Obesity
- Alcohol consumption (moderate to heavy)
- Tobacco use

✳ NURSING**ALERT**

American Cancer Society Guidelines for the Early Detection of Colon and Rectal Cancer

- Yearly fecal occult blood test (FOBT)* or fecal immunochemical test (FIT)
- Flexible sigmoidoscopy every 5 years
- Yearly FOBT* or FIT, plus flexible sigmoidoscopy every 5 years**
- * For FOBT, the take-home multiple-sample method should be used.
- ** The combination of yearly FOBT or FIT plus sigmoidoscopy every 5 years is preferred over either of these options alone.

All positive tests should be followed up with colonoscopy.

Patients should talk to their health care provider about starting colorectal cancer screening earlier and/or undergoing screening more often if they have any of the following colorectal cancer risk factors:
- A personal history of colorectal cancer or adenomatous polyps
- A strong family history of colorectal cancer or polyps (cancer or polyps in a first-degree relative [parent, sibling, or child] younger than 60 or in two first-degree relatives of any age
- A personal history of chronic inflammatory bowel disease
- A family history of a hereditary colorectal cancer syndrome (familial adenomatous polyposis or hereditary nonpolyposis colon cancer)

From American Cancer Society Guidelines for the Early Detection of Cancer. Retrieved June 24, 2008, from www.cancer.org/docroot/PED/content/PED_2_3X_ACS_Cancer_Detection_Guidelines_36.asp

---

 Examination   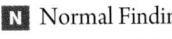 Normal Findings   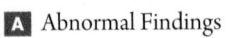 Abnormal Findings   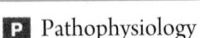 Pathophysiology

NURSINGTIP

Nasogastric Tube Suction

Prior to assessing the abdomen, if the patient has a nasogastric tube that is connected to suction, discontinue the suction in order to avoid interfering with auscultation findings. Remember to turn the suction back on after your assessment.

✓ ABDOMINAL ASSISTIVE DEVICESCHECKLIST

Assessing Patients with Abdominal Tubes and Drains

For all tubes, drains, and intestinal and urinary diversions, note color, odor, amount, consistency, and the presence of blood in any drainage. Check for an obstruction if there is no drainage. The skin around the device should be intact without excoriation.

Tubes

1. Enteral Tubes
   * Nasogastric, nasoduodenal, or nasojejunal
   * Check the residual amount on a frequent basis. If greater than 100 mL, stop the feeding; restart the feeding based on further inspection of residual amounts.

2. Nasogastric Suction Tubes
   * Levin or Salem sump
   * Ensure that the suction setting (intermittent or continuous) is set at the appropriate suction level.

3. Intestinal Tubes
   * Miller-Abbott, Cantor, Johnston, or Baker
   * Ensure that the tube is advancing with peristalsis as expected.
   * Ensure that the suction setting is at the appropriate suction level.

4. Gastrostomy
   * Continuous versus intermittent feeding
   * With intermittent feedings, clamp is applied when not in use.
   * Tube should be secured to abdomen.
   * Check that dressing is applied.

Drains

1. Abdominal Cavity Drain (Jackson-Pratt, Hemovac)
   * To self-suction or wall suction; if wall suction, ensure that it is set at appropriate level.

2. Biliary Drain (T-Tube)
   * Tube is below insertion site.

Intestinal Diversions

1. Colostomy
   * Stoma is pink.
   * Skin barrier should be used around stoma if appliance is worn.
   * Evacuation method: natural or irrigation.

2. Ileostomy
   * Stoma is pink.
   * Skin barrier is used and appliance is worn.
   * If patient has Kock pouch, nipple valve is pink; frequency of drainage.

Urinary Diversions

1. Ileal Conduit
   * Stoma is pink.
   * Skin barrier is used with appliance.

2. Ureteral Stents
   * Stent is secured to collection bag.
   * No bleeding from insertion site.

3. Indwelling Catheter
   * Balloon inflated.
   * Catheter secured to patient to prevent dislodgement.
   * Urinary collecting bag is closed.
   * Drainage tube is below level of bladder and without kinks.

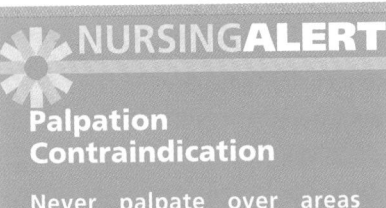

REFLECTIVE THINKING

Bowel Sounds

You auscultate Ms. Enriquez's bowel sounds and do not hear any after listening for 30 seconds in the RLQ. You are aware that you should auscultate the abdomen for 5 minutes in each quadrant if necessary. How would you proceed? What assessment findings would you document?

N Bowel sounds are heard as intermittent gurgling sounds throughout the abdominal quadrants. Usually, they are high-pitched sounds and occur 5 to 30 times per minute. Bowel sounds result from the movement of air through the gastrointestinal tract. Normally, bowel sounds are always present at the ileocecal valve area (RLQ).

Normal hyperactive bowel sounds are called **borborygmi**. They are loud, audible, gurgling sounds. Borborygmi may be due to hyperperistalsis ("stomach growling") or the sound of flatus in the intestines.

A Absent bowel sounds are abnormal.

P Absent bowel sounds are indicative of late intestinal obstruction, both mechanical and nonmechanical in nature. Mechanical obstruction of the bowel may result from extraluminal lesions such as adhesions, hernias, and masses. In nonmechanical obstruction, the gastrointestinal lumen remains unobstructed, but the muscles of the intestinal wall cannot move its contents. This type of obstruction can be caused by physiological, neurogenic, or chemical imbalances that result in paralytic ileus.

A Hypoactive bowel sounds are abnormal.

P Hypoactive or diminished bowel sounds indicate decreased motility of the bowel and can occur with peritonitis and nonmechanical obstruction. Other causes include inflammation, gangrene, electrolyte imbalances, and intraoperative manipulation of the bowel.

A Hyperactive bowel sounds are abnormal.

P Hyperactive or increased bowel sounds signify increased motility of the bowel and can result from gastroenteritis, diarrhea, laxative use, and subsiding ileus.

P Auscultation of high-pitched, tinkling hyperactive bowel sounds is indicative of partial obstruction. These sounds are caused by the powerful peristaltic action of the bowel segment attempting to eject its contents through a narrow, constricted area. Frequently, patients complain of abdominal cramping.

Vascular Sounds

E 1. Place the bell of the stethoscope over the abdominal aorta, renal arteries, iliac arteries, and femoral arteries (see Figure 17-16).

2. Listen for bruits over each area (see Figure 17-17).

N No audible bruits are auscultated.

A Audible bruits are auscultated.

P A bruit over an abdominal vessel indicates turbulence of blood flow and suggests a partial obstruction. Bruits can occur with abdominal aortic aneurysm, renal stenosis, and femoral stenosis.

Venous Hum

E Using the bell of the stethoscope, listen for a **venous hum**, or a continuous, medium-pitched sound, in all four quadrants.

N Venous hums are normally not present in adults.

A A continuous pulsing or fibrillary sound is auscultated.

P A venous hum in the periumbilical area is usually due to obstructed portal circulation. Portal hypertension caused by cirrhosis of the liver impedes portal circulation.

NURSING**ALERT**

Palpation Contraindication

Never palpate over areas where bruits are auscultated. Palpation may cause rupture. Refer the patient immediately.

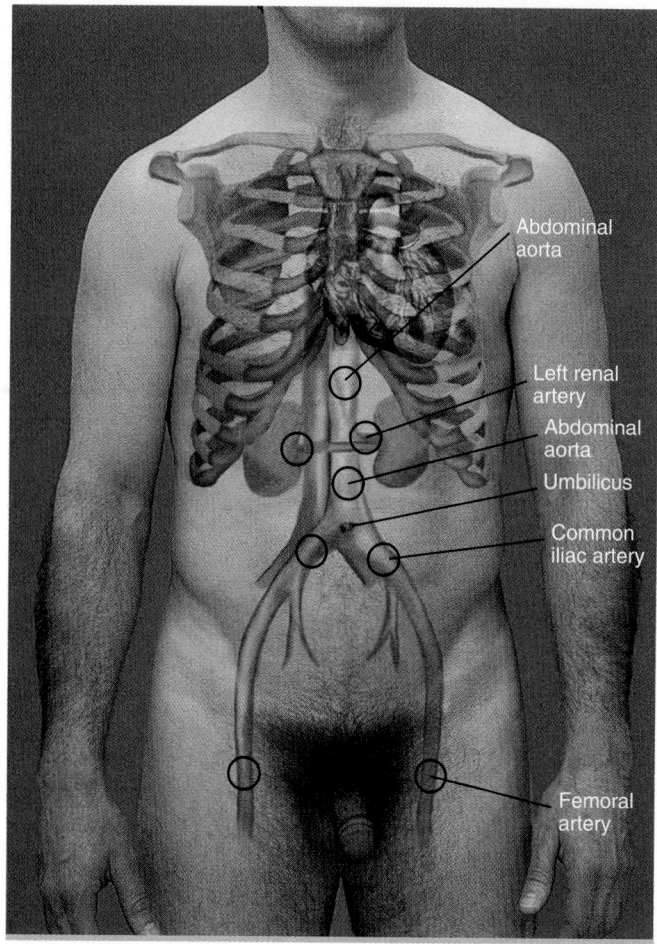

FIGURE 17-16 Stethoscope Placement for Auscultating
Abdominal Vasculature

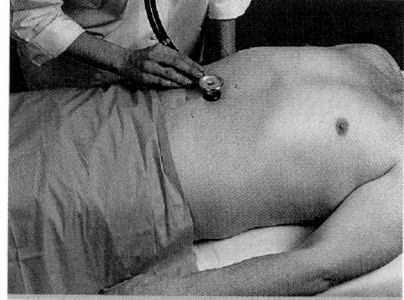

FIGURE 17-17 Auscultation of
Aortic Bruits with Bell of Stethoscope

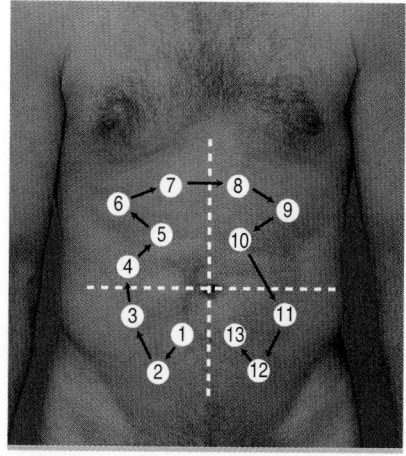

FIGURE 17-18 Direction of Pattern
of Abdominal Percussion

Friction Rubs

E 1. Using the diaphragm of the stethoscope, listen for friction rubs over the right and left costal margins, the liver, and the spleen.

2. Listen for friction rubs in all four quadrants.

N No friction rubs should be present.

A Friction rubs are high-pitched sounds that resemble the sound produced by two pieces of sandpaper being rubbed together. The sound increases with inspiration.

P Friction rubs occur when tumors, inflammation, or infarct cause the visceral layers of the peritoneum to rub together over the liver and the spleen.

PERCUSSION

General Percussion

E 1. Percuss all four quadrants in a systematic manner. Begin percussion in the RLQ, moving upward to the RUQ, crossing over to the LUQ, and moving down to the LLQ (Figure 17-18).

2. Visualize each organ in the corresponding quadrant; note when tympany changes to dullness.

E Examination   **N** Normal Findings   **A** Abnormal Findings   **P** Pathophysiology

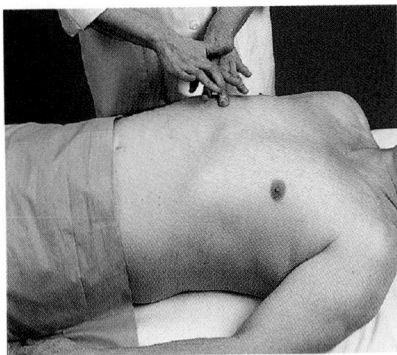

A. Determining Lower Liver Border

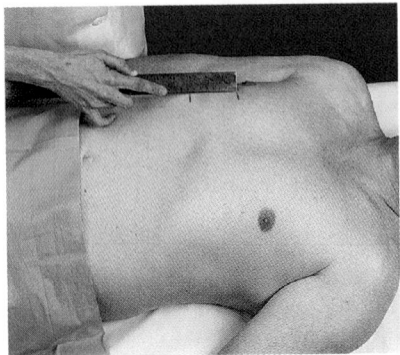

B. Measuring Liver Span

FIGURE 17-19 Percussing Liver Span

N Tympany is the predominant sound heard because air is present in the stomach and in the intestines. It is a high-pitched sound of long duration. In obese patients it may be difficult to elicit tympany due to the quantity of adipose tissue. Dullness is normally heard over organs such as the liver or a distended bladder. Dull sounds are high-pitched and of moderate duration.

A Dullness over areas where tympany normally occurs, such as over the stomach and intestines, is considered abnormal.

P Dullness may be caused by a mass or tumor, pregnancy, ascites, or a full intestine.

Liver Span

E 1. Stand to the right side of the patient.

2. Begin at the right midclavicular line below the umbilicus and percuss upward to determine the lower border of the liver (Figure 17-19A).

3. With a marking pen, mark where the sound changes from tympany to dullness.

4. Then, at the right midclavicular line, percuss downward from an area of lung resonance to one of dullness.

5. With a tape measure or ruler, measure the two marks in centimeters (Figure 17-19B).

N Normally, the distance between the two marks is 6 to 12 cm in the midclavicular line. There is a direct correlation between body size and the size of the liver. The mean span for a man is 10.5 cm and for a woman is 7.0 cm.

A A liver span greater than 12 cm or less than 6 cm is considered abnormal.

P The liver span is increased when the liver becomes enlarged. Hepatomegaly can occur with various liver diseases such as hepatitis, cirrhosis, cardiac or renal congestion, cysts, or metastatic tumors.

P The liver span can be falsely increased when the upper border is obscured by the dullness of lung consolidation with pneumonia or pleural effusion.

P The liver span can be decreased in the later stages of cirrhosis when the disease causes liver atrophy.

P The liver span can be falsely decreased when gas in the colon, tumors, or pregnancy pushes the lower border of the liver upward.

ADVANCED TECHNIQUE

Assessing the Liver Border: Liver Scratch Test

It can be difficult to palpate the liver border if a patient's abdomen is distended or if the muscles are tense. An alternative method to determine the lower edge of the liver is the liver scratch test.

E 1. Place your stethoscope in the right midclavicular line at the lower rib cage.

2. With your other hand scratch short strokes in the right midclavicular line starting in the right lower quadrant of the abdomen.

3. Continue to scratch with short strokes every 1 to 2 cm toward the stethoscope.

4. The scratching sound will be louder when you reach the lower liver border.

| **E** Examination | **N** Normal Findings | **A** Abnormal Findings | **P** Pathophysiology |

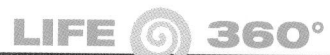
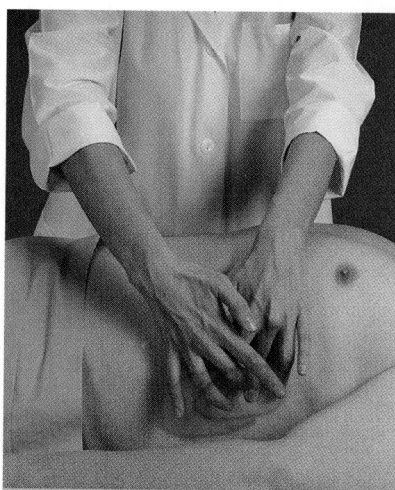

FIGURE 17-20 Percussion of the Spleen

Liver Descent

E 1. Percuss the liver descent by asking the patient to take a deep breath and to hold it (because on inspiration, the diaphragm moves downward).

2. Again, percuss the lower border of the liver at the right midclavicular line by percussing from tympany to dullness. Have the patient exhale.

3. Repercuss the liver-lung border.

4. Mark where the change in sound takes place.

5. Measure the difference in centimeters between the two lower borders of the liver.

N Normally, the area of lower border dullness descends 2 to 3 cm.

A The liver descent is considered abnormal if it is greater or less than 2 to 3 cm.

P The liver descent is greater than 2 to 3 cm due to hepatomegaly, as in cirrhosis.

P The liver descent is less than 2 cm due to abdominal tumors, pregnancy, or ascites.

Spleen

E 1. Percuss the lower level of the left lung slightly posterior to the midaxillary line and continue downward (Figure 17-20).

2. Percuss downward until dullness is ascertained. In some individuals, the spleen is positioned too deeply to be discernable by percussion.

N Normally, the upper border of dullness is found 6 to 8 cm above the left costal margin. Splenic dullness may be heard from the 6th to the 10th rib.

A Dullness beyond the 8 cm line is indicative of splenic enlargement. However, a full stomach or a feces-filled intestine may mimic the dullness of splenic enlargement. Moreover, gastric or colonic air may obscure the dullness of the spleen.

P Splenic enlargement can be due to portal hypertension resulting from liver disease; other potential causes are mononucleosis, thrombosis, stenosis, atresia, angiomatous deformities of the portal or splenic vein, cysts, or aneurysm of the splenic artery.

Stomach

E Percuss for a gastric air bubble in the LUQ at the left lower anterior rib cage and left epigastric region.

N The tympany of the gastric air bubble is lower in pitch than the tympany of the intestine.

A An increase in size of the gastric air bubble is abnormal.

P This increase in size accompanied by gastric distension can suggest gastric dilation.

Fist Percussion

Fist percussion is done over the kidneys and liver to check for tenderness.

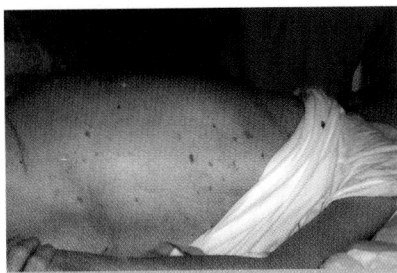

FIGURE 17-21 Ascites

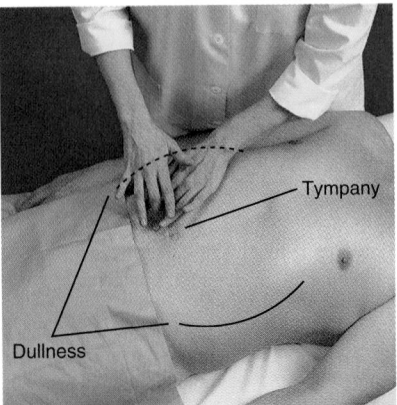

A. Patient Supine

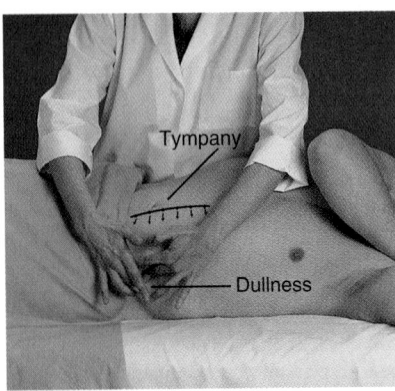

B. Patient on Left Side

FIGURE 17-22 Percussion for
Ascites: Shifting Dullness

ADVANCED TECHNIQUE

Assessing for Ascites: Shifting Dullness and Puddle Sign

Assess the patient for ascites (Figure 17-21), or excess accumulation
of fluid in the abdominal cavity. There are two methods for this assessment: shifting dullness and puddle sign.

Shifting Dullness

E
1. Standing to the right, with the patient supine, percuss over
   the top of the abdomen, beginning at the midline.
2. Percuss outward toward the right side of the patient,
   following a downward direction (Figure 17-22A).
3. Mark on the abdomen where percussion changes from
   tympany to dullness because this change is indicative of
   settled fluid in the flanks of the abdominal cavity.
4. Turn the patient onto the right side.
5. Repercuss the upper side of the abdomen, moving downward.
6. If the percussion sound changes from tympany to dullness
   above the prior-marked fluid line, this shifting dullness is
   positive for ascites.
7. Repeat the same assessment technique on the left side of
   the patient. Change the patient's position from the right to the
   left side (Figure 17-22B).
8. Mark where the percussion changes from tympany to dullness.

N There should be no change from tympany to dullness.

A There is a marked change from tympany to dullness as you percuss outward and downward. Ascites is present in the abdominal
cavity.

P Ascitic fluid sinks with gravity, which accounts for the dullness in
dependent areas. Ascites is found in cirrhosis and in other liver
diseases.

Puddle Sign

E
1. Ask the patient to kneel and assume the knee-chest position
   for several minutes.
2. Percuss the umbilical area (Figure 17-23).

N The umbilical area should remain tympanic.

A The umbilical area percusses dull.

P The ascitic fluid pools in the dependent area of the umbilicus
because of gravity.

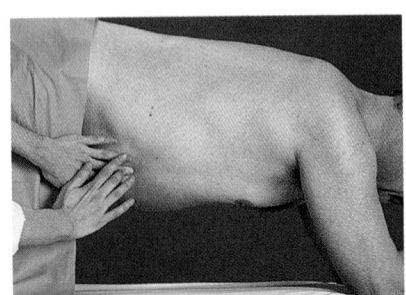

FIGURE 17-23 Percussion for
Ascites: Puddle Sign

KIDNEY.

E
1. Place the patient in a sitting position.
2. Strike the costovertebral angle with a closed fist (direct fist percussion,
   see Figure 17-24A) or

   Place the palmar surface of one hand over the costovertebral angle
   (CVA). Strike that hand with the ulnar surface of the fist of the other
   hand (indirect fist percussion, see Figure 17-24B).
3. Ask the patient what was felt. Observe the patient's reaction.
4. Repeat on the other side.

N No tenderness should be elicited.

NURSING**TIP**

Monitoring Ascites

It is often helpful to monitor the amount of ascites by measuring the patient's abdomen at its largest diameter. In order for there to be consistency among nurses, it is advised that marks be drawn on the patient's abdomen showing placement of the tape measure.

A Tenderness or pain over the costovertebral angle is abnormal.

P Costovertebral angle tenderness can occur in pyelonephritis.

LIVER.

E 1. Place the patient in a supine position.

2. Place the palmar surface of one hand over the lower right rib cage (where the liver was percussed).

3. Strike that hand with the ulnar surface of the fist of the other hand (see Figure 17-25).

4. Ask the patient what was felt. Observe the patient's reaction.

N No tenderness should be elicited.

A Tenderness or pain that can be elicited over the liver is abnormal.

P Liver tenderness can occur in conjunction with cholecystitis or hepatitis.

BLADDER.

E 1. Percuss upward from the symphysis pubis to the umbilicus.

2. Note where the sound changes from dullness to tympany.

N A urine-filled bladder is dull to percussion. A recently emptied bladder should not be percussable above the symphysis pubis.

A It is abnormal to percuss a bladder that has recently been emptied. The urine that remains in the bladder after urination is called residual urine. A bladder may also be dull to percussion when the patient has difficulty voiding.

P The inability to completely empty the bladder occurs in the elderly; in postoperative, bedridden, and acutely ill patients; and in patients with neurogenic bladder dysfunction.

P Difficult voiding can occur in conjunction with benign prostatic hypertrophy (see Chapter 22 for additional information), urethral pathology, and some medications (antipsychotics: phenothiazine; anticholinergics: atropine; antihypertensives: hydralazine).

PALPATION

Light Palpation

E 1. With your hands and forearm on a horizontal plane, use the pads of the approximated fingers to depress the abdominal wall 1 cm (see Figure 17-26).

2. Avoid short, quick jabs.

3. Lightly palpate all four quadrants in a systematic manner.

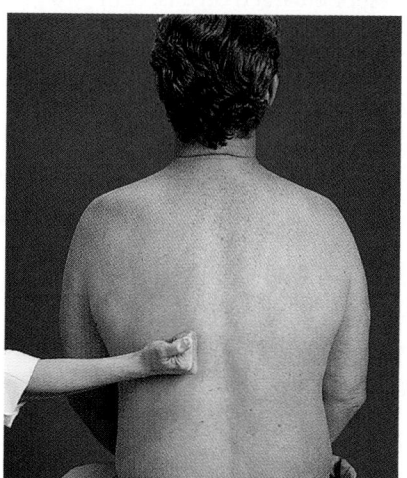

A. Direct Fist Percussion

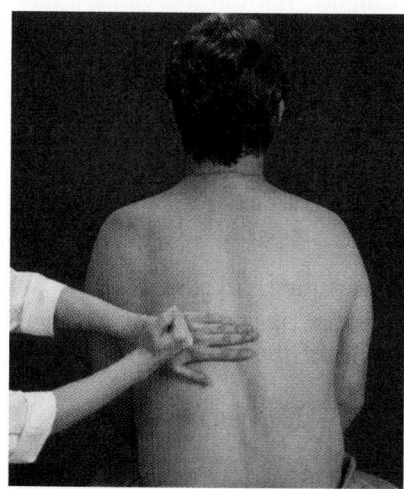

B. Indirect Fist Percussion

FIGURE 17-24 **Fist Percussion of the Left Kidney**

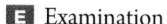 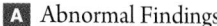

| **E** Examination | **N** Normal Findings | **A** Abnormal Findings | **P** Pathophysiology |

NURSINGTIP

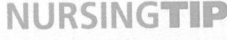

Abdominal Pain Assessment

Before beginning the palpation, ask the patient to cough. Coughing can elicit a sharp twinge of pain in the involved area if peritoneal irritation is present. Palpate the involved area last.

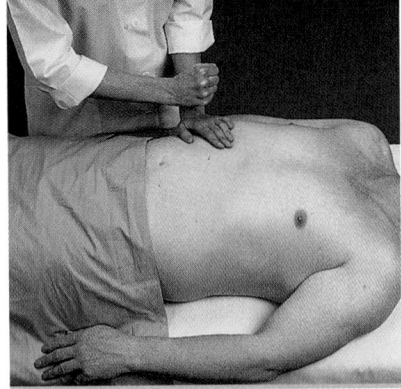

FIGURE 17-25 Indirect Fist Percussion of the Liver

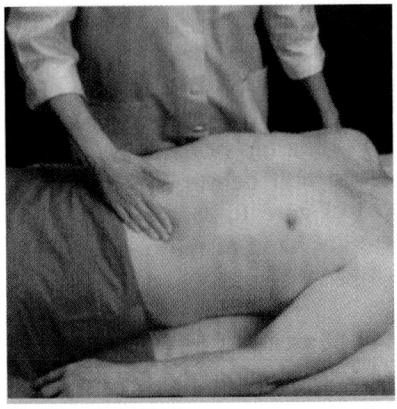

FIGURE 17-26 Light Palpation of the Abdomen

N The abdomen should feel smooth with consistent softness.

A Light palpation reveals changes in skin temperature, tenderness, or large masses.

P Tenderness and elevated skin temperature can be due to inflammation. Large masses can be due to tumors, feces, or enlarged organs.

Abdominal Muscle Guarding

To determine whether muscle guarding is involuntary:

E 1. Perform light palpation of the rectus muscles during expiration.

2. Note muscle tensing.

N Muscle guarding, or tensing of the abdominal musculature, is absent during expiration. The abdomen is soft. Normally during expiration, the patient cannot exercise voluntary muscle tensing.

A Muscle guarding of the rectus muscles occurs during expiration.

P Involuntary muscle guarding suggests irritation of the peritoneum, as in peritonitis.

Deep Palpation

In performing deep palpation of all four quadrants, you can use either a one-handed or a two-handed method.

E 1. With the one-handed method, use the palmar surface of the extended fingers to depress the skin approximately 5 to 8 cm (2 to 3 inches) in the RLQ (see Figure 17-27A).

2. A two-handed approach is used when palpation is difficult because of obesity or muscular resistance. With the bimanual technique, the nondominant hand is placed on top of the dominant hand. The bottom hand is used for sensation, and the top hand is used to apply pressure (see Figure 17-27B).

3. Identify any masses and note location, size, shape, consistency, tenderness, pulsation, and degree of mobility.

4. Continue palpation of RUQ, LUQ, and LLQ.

N No organ enlargement should be palpable, nor should there be any abnormal masses, bulges, or swelling. Normally, only the aorta and the edge of the liver are palpable. When the large colon or the bladder is full, palpation is possible.

E Examination   **N** Normal Findings   **A** Abnormal Findings   **P** Pathophysiology

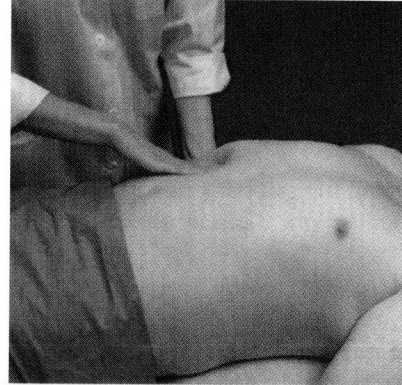 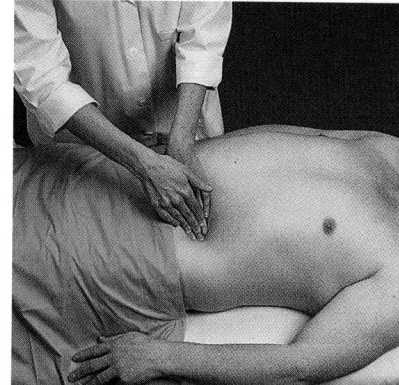

A. One-Handed Method   B. Bimanual Method

FIGURE 17-27 **Deep Palpation**

A The gallbladder, liver, spleen, fecal-filled colon, or flatus-filled cecum should not be palpable. Masses, bulges, and swellings are also considered abnormal.

P Organomegaly can be caused by many pathological states such as cholecystitis, hepatitis, or cirrhosis; masses, bulges, or swelling can be due to tumors, fluids, feces, flatus, or fat.

Liver

Liver palpation can be performed by one of two methods: the bimanual method or the hook method.

BIMANUAL METHOD.

E 1. Stand at th.e patient's right side, facing the patient's head.

2. Place the left hand under the patient's right flank at about the 11th or 12th rib.

ADVANCED TECHNIQUE

Assessing for Ascites: Fluid Wave

E 1. With the patient in a supine position, stand at the patient's right side.

2. Have the patient or a second nurse firmly place the ulnar side of the right hand midline on the abdomen to prevent displacement of fat.

3. Place your right hand on the patient's right hip or flank area. Reach across the patient with your left hand and deliver a blow to the patient's left hip or flank area (Figure 17-28).

4. Assess if a fluid wave is felt on the right hand of the patient or the other nurse.

N No fluid wave should be felt.

A A fluid wave is easily felt if a large amount of ascites is present. This sign is often negative until the ascites is obvious. In addition, the fluid wave is sometimes positive in people without ascites.

P The factors that contribute to the development of ascites are outlined in the Nursing Alert on page 601.

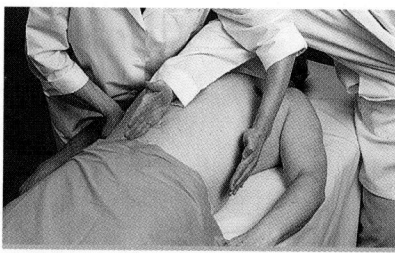

FIGURE 17-28 **Palpation for Ascites: Fluid Wave**

NURSING**ALERT**

Risk Factors for Liver Cancer

- Cirrhosis
- Hepatitis B
- Cigarette smoking
- Alcohol use
- Exposure to toxic substances such as arsenic or vinyl chloride
- Primary malignancy

NURSING**ALERT**

Liver Encephalopathy

Early recognition of signs and symptoms of liver encephalopathy may minimize complications.
- Slowed mentation or mental confusion
- Asterixis (liver flap)
- Uncoordinated muscle movements
- Elevated values for serum BUN, ammonia, liver enzymes, and osmolarity. Increased values reflect systemic effects of liver dysfunction.

3. Press upward with the left hand to elevate the liver toward the abdominal wall.

4. Place the right hand parallel to the midline at the right midclavicular line below the right costal margin or below the level of liver dullness.

5. Instruct the patient to take a deep breath.

6. Push down deeply and under the costal margin with your right fingers. On inspiration, the liver will descend and contact the hand (Figure 17-29A).

7. Note the level of the liver.

8. Note the size, shape, consistency, and any masses.

HOOK METHOD.

E 1. Stand at the patient's right side, facing the patient's feet.

2. Place both hands side by side on the right costal margin below the border of liver dullness.

3. Hook the fingers in and up toward the costal margin and ask the patient to take a deep breath and hold it.

4. Palpate the liver's edge as it descends (Figure 17-29B).

5. Note the level of the liver.

6. Note the size, shape, consistency, and any masses.

N A normal liver edge presents as a firm, sharp, regular ridge with a smooth surface. Normally, the liver is not palpable, although it may be felt in extremely thin adults.

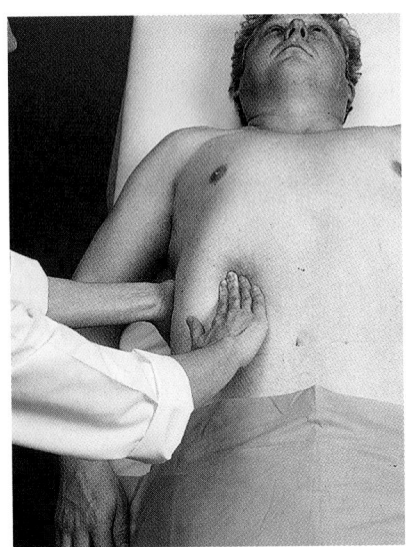

A. Bimanual Method

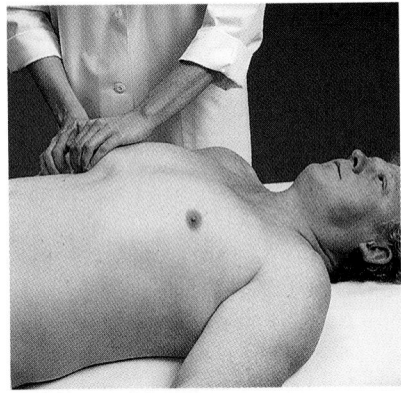

B. Hook Method

FIGURE 17-29 Palpation of the Liver

ADVANCED TECHNIQUE

Assessing for Cholecystitis: Murphy's Sign

E 1. With the patient supine, stand at the patient's right side.

2. Palpate below the liver margin at the lateral border of the rectus muscle.

3. Have the patient take a deep breath.

N No pain is elicited.

A Pain is present with palpation. The patient may stop inhaling to guard against the pain. This is known as Murphy's sign.

P Murphy's sign is positive in inflammatory processes of the gallbladder, such as cholecystitis.

NURSING ALERT

Risk for Spleen Rupture

Palpate the spleen gently because an enlarged spleen will be very tender and may rupture.

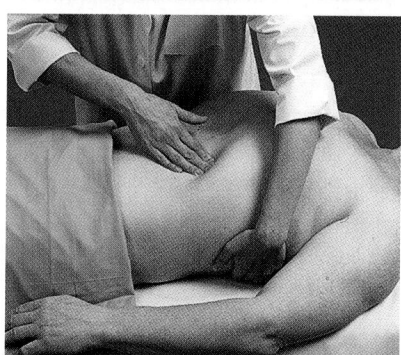

FIGURE 17-30 Palpation of the Spleen

FIGURE 17-31 Palpation of the Right Kidney

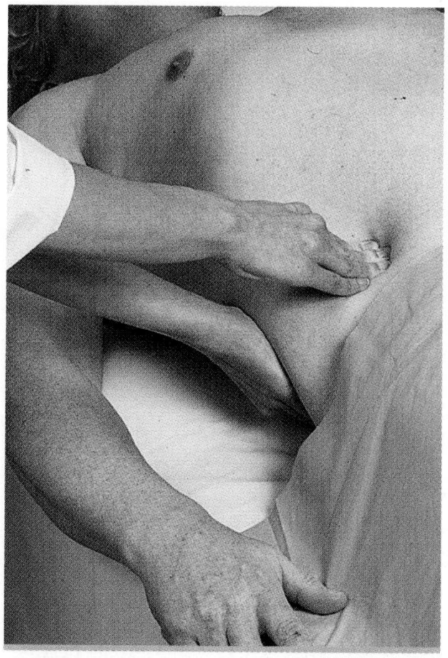

A If the liver is palpable below the costal margin both medially and laterally, it is abnormal.

P An enlarged liver can be due to congestive heart failure, hepatitis, encephalopathy, cirrhosis, cysts, or cancer.

A A liver that is enlarged, has an irregular border and nodules, and is hard is abnormal.

P These findings suggest liver malignancy. Tenderness may or may not be present.

Spleen

Use the bimanual technique to palpate the spleen.

E

1. Stand at the patient's right side.
2. Reach across and place the left hand beneath the patient and over the left costovertebral angle. Press upward to lift the spleen anteriorly toward the abdominal wall.
3. With the right hand, press inward along the left costal margin while asking the patient to take a deep breath (Figure 17-30).

3A. The procedure can be repeated with the patient lying on the right side, with the hips and knees flexed. This position will facilitate the spleen coming forward and to the right because the spleen is located retroperitoneally.

4. Note the size, shape, consistency, and any masses.

N **The spleen should not be palpable.**

A Because of its retroperitoneal position in the body, the spleen becomes palpable only when it has become enlarged to three times its normal size. An enlarged spleen is usually very tender.

P Splenomegaly can be due to inflammation, congestive heart failure, cancer, cirrhosis, or mononucleosis.

Kidneys

E

1. Stand at the patient's right side.
2. Place one hand on the right costovertebral angle on the patient's back.
3. Place the other hand below and parallel to the costal margin.
4. As the patient takes a deep breath, press hands firmly together and try to feel the lower pole of the kidney (Figure 17-31).
5. At the peak of inspiration, press the fingers together with greater pressure from above than from below.
6. Ask the patient to exhale and to hold the breath briefly.
7. Release the pressure of your fingers.
8. If the kidney has been "captured," it can be felt as it slips back into place.
9. Note the size, shape, and consistency. Note any masses.
10. For the left kidney, reach across the patient and place the left hand under the patient's left flank.
11. Apply downward pressure with the right hand below the left costal margin and repeat steps 4 through 9.

N The kidneys should not be palpable in the normal adult. However, the lower pole of the right kidney may be felt in very thin individuals. Kidneys are more readily palpable in the elderly due to loss of muscle tone and muscle bulk.

A Enlarged kidneys are abnormal. The right kidney may be difficult to distinguish from an enlarged liver. Left kidney enlargement may be difficult to distinguish from an enlarged spleen.

P Enlarged, palpable kidneys can be caused by hydronephrosis, neoplasms, or polycystic kidney disease.

Aorta

E 1. Press the upper abdomen with one hand on each side of the abdominal aorta, slightly to the left of the midline.
2. Assess the width of the aorta (Figure 17-32).

N The aorta width is 2.5 to 4.0 cm, and the aorta pulsates in an anterior direction.

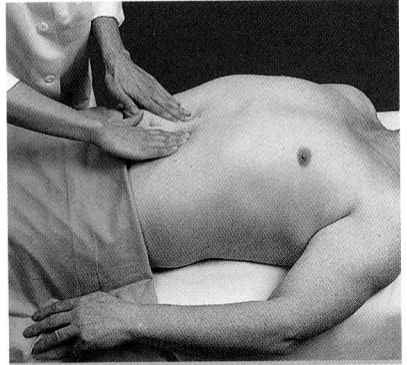

FIGURE 17-32 Palpation of the Aorta

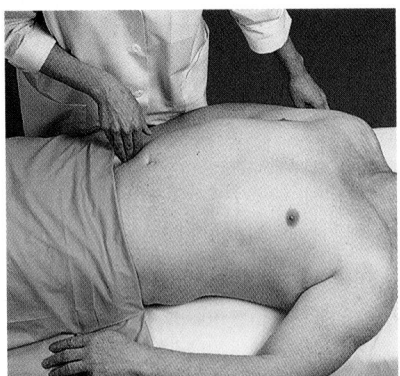

A. Apply firm pressure to the abdomen.

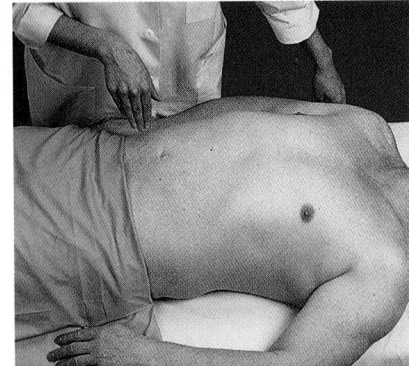

B. Quickly release the pressure.

FIGURE 17-33 Rebound Tenderness

| 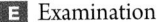 Examination | **N** Normal Findings | **A** Abnormal Findings | **P** Pathophysiology |

ADVANCED TECHNIQUE

Assessing for Abdominal Inflammation: Rebound Tenderness

Rebound tenderness is assessed if pain has been elicited during palpation, or the patient has reported pain. Rebound tenderness is an abnormal finding frequently associated with peritoneal inflammation or appendicitis. Be prepared to recognize that rebound tenderness assessment could elicit a strong pain response from the patient. It is imperative to test for rebound tenderness away from the site where pain is initially determined and to conclude abdominal assessment with this test. If other tests are positive, omit this assessment.

E   1. Apply several seconds of firm pressure to the abdomen, with the hand at a 90° angle (perpendicular to the abdomen) and the fingers extended (Figure 17-33A).

    2. Quickly release the pressure (Figure 17-33B).

N   Pain is not elicited.

A   As the abdominal wall returns to its normal position, the patient complains of pain at the pressure site (direct rebound tenderness) or at another site (referred rebound tenderness).

P   Rebound tenderness may indicate peritoneal irritation. The rebound effect of the internal structures indented by this technique causes sharp pain in the area of inflammation.

P   Pain in the RLQ can indicate appendicitis. This location is known as **McBurney's point.**

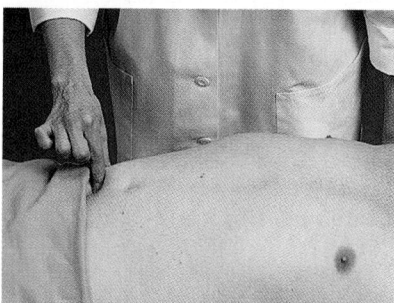

A. Lift a fold of skin away from the underlying muscle.

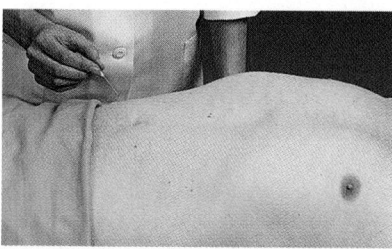

B. Stimulate the skin with a sterile needle.

FIGURE 17-34 Assessment of Cutaneous Hypersensitivity

ADVANCED TECHNIQUE

Assessing for Appendicitis: Rovsing's Sign

Rovsing's sign is a differential technique to elicit referred pain, reflective of peritoneal inflammation secondary to appendicitis.

E   1. Press deeply and evenly in the LLQ for 5 seconds.

    2. Note the patient's response.

N   No pain should be elicited.

A   Abdominal pain felt in the RLQ is abnormal and is a positive Rovsing's sign.

P   This sign is based on the concept that changes in intraluminal pressure will be transmitted through the intestine when the ileocecal valve is competent. Pressing the LLQ traps air within the large intestine and increases the pressure in the cecum. When the appendix is inflamed, this increase in pressure causes pain.

ADVANCED TECHNIQUE

Assessing for Abdominal Inflammation: Cutaneous Hypersensitivity

On stimulation with a sterile pin or by lifting a fold of skin away from the musculature, **cutaneous hypersensitivity** zones of sensory nerves initiate a painful response. The irritative stimulus detects specific zones of peritoneal irritation.

E   1. Lift a fold of skin away from the underlying muscle (Figure 17-34A) or stimulate the skin by gently jabbing the abdominal surface with a sterile pin (Figure 17-34B).

    2. Observe for pain response.

N   No adverse reaction should be noted.

A   The patient experiences an exaggerated sense of pain.

P   Cutaneous hypersensitivity indicates a zone of peritoneal irritation. Localized pain in all or part of the RLQ may accompany appendicitis. Midepigastrium pain could signal a peptic ulcer.

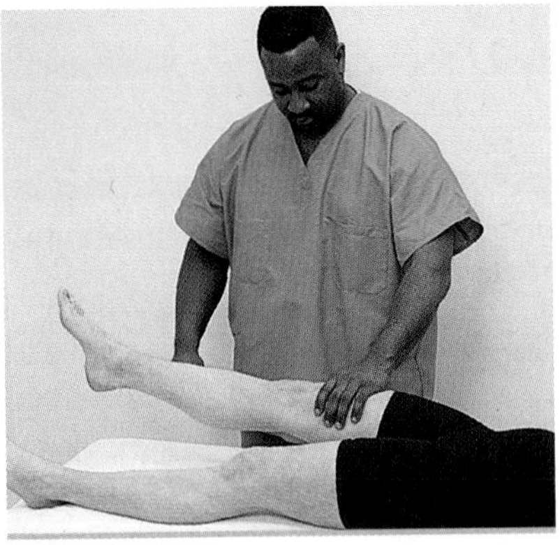

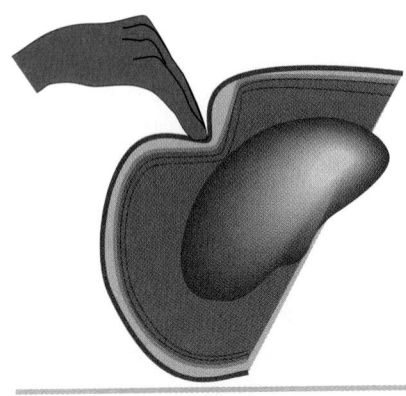

FIGURE 17-35 Iliopsoas Muscle Test

ADVANCED TECHNIQUE

Assessing for Appendicitis: Iliopsoas Muscle Test

When a patient presents with acute abdominal pain, an inflamed or perforated appendix may be distinguished via irritation of the lateral iliopsoas muscle.

E
1. Place your hand over the right thigh and push downward as the patient raises the leg, flexing at the hip (Figure 17-35).
2. Observe for pain response in the RLQ as described by the patient.

N Normally, the patient should experience no pain.

A The patient experiences pain in the RLQ.

P This pain indicates an inflammation of the iliopsoas muscle in the groin and is caused by an inflamed appendix.

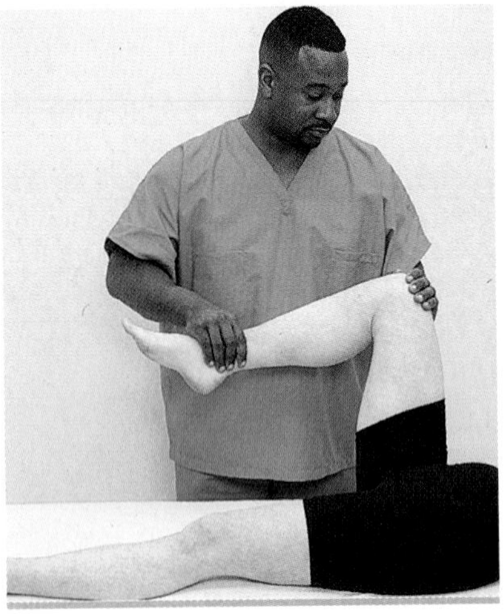

ADVANCED TECHNIQUE

Assessing for Appendicitis or Pelvic Abscess: Obturator Muscle Test

Another differential technique used to help determine if the patient is experiencing appendicitis is eliciting the **obturator sign**. This test can be used when pelvic abscess is suspected. Both conditions may cause irritation of the obturator internus muscle.

E
1. Flex the right leg at the hip and knee at a right angle.
2. Rotate the leg both internally and externally (Figure 17-36).
3. Observe for pain response.

N No pain is elicited with this maneuver.

A Pain is elicited in the hypogastric area.

P This pain indicates irritation of the obturator muscle and can be caused by a ruptured appendix or pelvic abscess.

FIGURE 17-36 Obturator Muscle Test

ADVANCED TECHNIQUE

Assessing for Abdominal Mass: Ballottement

Ballottement is a palpation technique used to displace excess fluid in the abdominal cavity in order to locate an organ or mass.

E
1. Extend the fingers of the right hand in a straight line, perpendicular to the abdominal surface.
2. Stiffen the fingers.
3. Jab the abdominal surface in the desired area (Figure 17-37).
4. Determine if the intended organ is felt at the fingertips.

N Excluding during pregnancy, internal organs are not felt during this assessment technique.

A Internal masses, or organs such as the liver or spleen, are palpated.

P The presence of ascites transmits external pressure to an internal organ or mass. The resulting impact felt on palpation is known as ballottement. It determines the presence of a free-floating abdominal mass, which can indicate a cancerous process in the abdominal cavity. Pain should not be elicited. A painful response would indicate inflammation and require further investigation.

FIGURE 17-37 Abdominal Ballottement

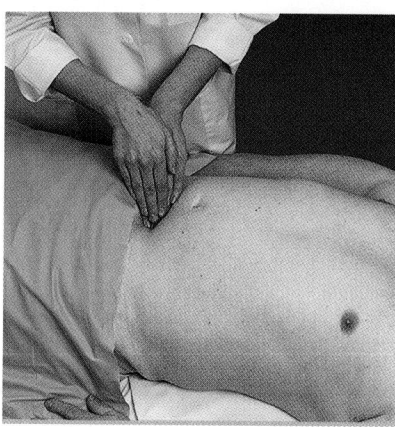

FIGURE 17-38 Palpation of the Bladder

A Aorta width greater than 4.0 cm is abnormal. Lateral pulsation of the aorta is also abnormal.

P A widened aorta and lateral pulsations suggest an abdominal aortic aneurysm.

Bladder

E 1. Using deep palpation, palpate the abdomen at the midline, starting at the symphysis pubis and progressing upward to the umbilicus (Figure 17-38).

2. If the bladder is located, palpate the shape, size, and consistency.

N An empty bladder is not usually palpable. A moderately full bladder is smooth and round, and it is palpable above the symphysis pubis. A full bladder is palpated above the symphysis pubis, and it may be close to the umbilicus.

A A bladder that is nodular or asymmetrical to palpation is abnormal.

P A nodular bladder may indicate a malignancy. An asymmetrical bladder may result from a tumor in the bladder or an abdominal tumor that is compressing the bladder.

A It is abnormal to palpate a bladder that has been recently emptied.

P Men with benign prostatic hypertrophy may be unable to completely empty their bladder because of the pressure that the enlarged prostate places on the bladder.

P Various types of urinary incontinence, due to altered mental status, muscle function, medications, and other causes, can lead to incomplete bladder emptying. See Table 17-4 for additional information on urinary incontinence.

Inguinal Lymph Nodes

E 1. Place the patient in a supine position, with the knees slightly flexed.

2. Drape the genital area.

3. Using the finger pads of the second, third, and fourth fingers, apply firm pressure and palpate with a rotary motion in the right inguinal area.

4. Palpate for lymph nodes in the left inguinal area.

N It is normal to palpate small, movable nodes less than 1 cm in diameter. Palpable nodes are nontender.

A Presence of inguinal lymph nodes greater than 1 cm in diameter or elicitation of nonmovable, tender lymph nodes is abnormal.

P Large, palpable nodes can be attributed to localized or systemic infections. More serious pathology includes processes associated with cancer or lymphomas.

Urinary Incontinence

Can you remember the last time that you sneezed or coughed and experienced some loss of bladder control? How did that make you feel? Did you soil your clothes? Now imagine what it must be like for a patient who has urinary incontinence on a regular basis. Interview a patient with urinary incontinence and ask him or her how it affects his or her life. Does the patient perform "bathroom mapping" when out in public?

E Examination   **N** Normal Findings   **A** Abnormal Findings   **P** Pathophysiology

NURSING**TIP**

Urinary Incontinence

Use the acronym "DIAPPERS" to guide your thought processes when considering nonbladder etiologies of urinary incontinence, especially in the older adult:

D = delirium

I = infection

A = atrophic vaginitis

P = pharmacological agents: diuretics, alcohol, benzodiazepines, anticholinergics, calcium channel blockers, alpha adrenergics, caffeine

P = psychological disorder: depression, Parkinson's disease

E = endocrine disorder: diabetes mellitus, diabetes insipidus; excessive urinary output, heart failure

R = restricted mobility

S = stool impaction; stroke

Adapted from Resnick, N. M. (1984). Urinary incontinence in the elderly. *Medical Grand Rounds, 3,* 281–290.

TABLE 17-4 Types of Urinary Incontinence

TYPE	DEFINITION	ETIOLOGY
Stress	Involuntary loss of urine with activities that increase abdominal pressure (e.g., sneezing, coughing, laughing, heavy lifting, physical activity)	Childbirth, pregnancy, previous abdominal surgery, prostate surgery, radiation therapy
Urge	Involuntary loss of urine due to detrusor hyperactivity; usually associated with a strong desire to void with a larger volume of urine	Stroke, dementia, multiple sclerosis, Parkinson's disease, brain tumor, urinary tract tumors, urinary tract infections
Overflow	Involuntary loss of urine due to an overextended bladder; incontinence occurs when bladder pressure exceeds urethral pressure; usually small amount of urine occurs during dribbling; may be some hesitancy and frequency	Fecal impaction, diabetic neuropathy, obstruction of the bladder or urethra (due to prostate cancer, benign prostatic hypertrophy)
Functional	Involuntary loss of urine due to the inability to reach the toilet because of physical, cognitive, or environmental impairments	Immobility, dementia, inaccessible toilet, inappropriate lighting, physical restraints

CASE STUDY

The Patient with Diverticulitis

This case study illustrates the application and objective documentation of the abdominal assessment.
Jay is away from home on vacation and is experiencing acute abdominal pain.

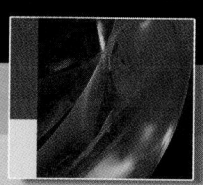

HEALTH HISTORY

PATIENT PROFILE	48 yo WM
CHIEF COMPLAINT	"I have a fever of 102° and my stomach is killing me."
HISTORY OF PRESENT ILLNESS	Pt was in his usual state of good health until 11 AM yesterday. He was skiing c̄ his family at a local resort when he began to feel bad. He left the ski slopes and returned to his hotel room and took his temp. At that time his temp was 101°F. About the same time he started with a "tummy ache." Despite this he met his family for lunch and ate half of his hamburger and fries. His family returned to their skiing and the pt retired to his hotel room. Ibuprofen 400 mg was taken at 2 PM. His abd pain gradually increased over the next few hrs as he rested in bed. He denies N/V/D. At 5 PM his family returned to the hotel and the pt's temp was 102°F. He was unable to eat dinner. At 10 PM the family went to bed for the evening. At 1 AM the pt woke his wife c̄ excruciating (8/10), stabbing LLQ pain, and now he presents at the local community hospital.

PAST HEALTH HISTORY	
Medical History	Denies
Surgical History	2007 Ⓡ eye extracapsular cataract removal c̄ intraocular lens implant; no sequelae
	1999 Ⓛ knee meniscus repair
	1989 Ⓡ knee MCL repair
Allergies	Denies allergies to medications, bee stings/insect bites, food allergies, seasonal allergies
Medications	MVI when he remembers
Communicable Diseases	Denies
Injuries and Accidents	No major injuries but has repeated musculoskeletal issues related to his physical activity
Special Needs	Denies
Blood Transfusions	Denies

continues

CASE STUDY (Continued)

The Patient with Diverticulitis

Health History (continued)

Childhood Illnesses	Chickenpox age 7, frequent strep throat as a child until the age of 10
Immunizations	UTD; has never received influenza vaccine; dT 2006; hepatitis A series completed June 2000

FAMILY HEALTH HISTORY

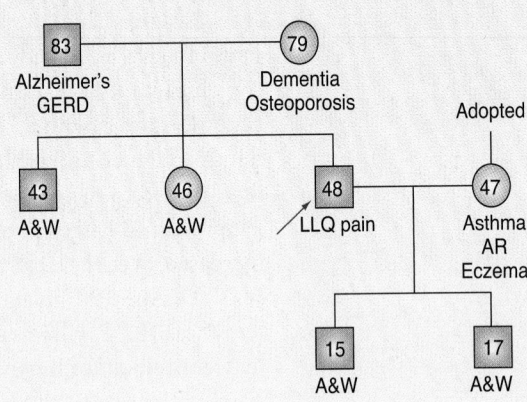

LEGEND

◯ Living female

◻ Living male

⊗ Deceased female

⊠ Deceased male

↗ Points to patient

A&W = Alive & well

AR = Allergic rhinitis

GERD = Gastroesophageal reflux disease

LLQ = Left lower quadrant

Denies family hx of malignancies of stomach, liver, or pancreas, DM, familial polyposis, inflammatory bowel dz, polycystic kidney dz, colitis, PUD, IBS, malabsorption syndromes

SOCIAL HISTORY

Alcohol Use	1 beer q PM p̄ work; 3–4 glasses of wine on the wkend
Tobacco Use	Cigars c̄ monthly poker game
Drug Use	Denies
Domestic and Intimate Partner Violence	Refuses to answer
Sexual Practice	Monogamous relationship c̄ wife × 25 yrs
Travel History	Lived in Colombia, South America 1965–1968; travel for business and pleasure to Puerto Rico, Caribbean, South Africa, and Europe; no travel in past 6 mos
Work Environment	Attorney for major law firm × 22 yrs; enjoys work and colleagues; safe inner-city environment c̄ security in office bldg and parking garage
Home Environment	Lives in gated community c̄ full-time security staff; feels safe

continues

CASE STUDY (Continued)

The Patient with Diverticulitis

Health History (continued)

Hobbies and Leisure Activities	Playing sports; likes to listen to books on tape as he drives to work; watches sporting events on TV on wkend
Stress	Work, especially when a brief is due
Education	College graduate c̄ JD
Economic Status	"Comfortable lifestyle"
Military Service	Denies
Religion	Jewish, observes major holidays
Ethnic Background	No affiliation
Roles/Relationships	Husband/father: feels he is a good provider for family
Characteristic Patterns of Daily Living	Wakes at 6 AM, goes to gym and works out; eats bagel p̄ gym; at office by 8 AM; salad for lunch; arrives home by 8 PM; has family dinner and catches up c̄ teenage children (wife prepares meals); reads paper/watches TV until MN
HEALTH MAINTENANCE ACTIVITIES	
Sleep	6 hrs q night, doesn't feel rested in AM
Diet	Infrequent fast food; caffeine 3–4/d; no particular diet; has tried low-carb diet in past
Exercise	Plays basketball 2 d/wk, soccer 2 d/wk, runs on treadmill 2 d/wk for 30 min followed by weights at gym
Stress Management	Sleeping/eating
Use of Safety Devices	Wears seat belts; no goggles with basketball
Health Check-ups	2 yrs ago had complete physical examination c̄ labs—WNL
PHYSICAL ASSESSMENT	
Inspection	
Contour	Flat
Symmetry	Symmetrical
Rectus Abdominis Muscles	Intact, Ø separation
Pigmentation and Color	Uniform pigmentation
Scars	Ø

continues

CASE STUDY (Continued)

The Patient with Diverticulitis

Health History (continued)

Striae	Ø
Respiratory Movement	Ø retractions
Masses or Nodules	Ø
Visible Peristalsis	Ø
Pulsation	Sl visible in epigastrium
Umbilicus	Ø hernia

Auscultation

Bowel Sounds	⊕ in 4 quads
Vascular Sounds	Ø
Venous Hum	Ø
Friction Rub	Ø

Percussion

General Percussion	Tympany
Liver Span	9 cm in Ⓡ MCL
Liver Descent	↓ 2 cm
Spleen	Unable to percuss
Stomach	Tympany
Fist Percussion	Not performed
Bladder	Dull to symphysis pubis

Palpation

Light Palpation	Smooth, warm, generalized tenderness
Abdominal Muscle Guarding	⊕ guarding
Deep Palpation	Exquisitely tender LLQ
Liver	Ø hepatomegaly
Spleen	Ø splenomegaly
Kidneys	Nonpalpable
Aorta	3 cm c̄ ant pulsation
Bladder	Nonpalpable
Inguinal Lymph Nodes	Ø lymphadenopathy

continues

CASE STUDY (Continued)

The Patient with Diverticulitis

Health History (continued)

Advanced Techniques

Rebound Tenderness: ⊕ in LLQ

Rovsing's Sign: ⊖

Iliopsoas and Obturator Muscles Tests: Mildly ⊕ on Ⓛ

Cutaneous Hypersensitivity: ⊖

SMA 12, amylase, lipase, urinalysis: WNL

LABORATORY DATA

	PT'S VALUES	NORMAL RANGE
RBC	4.7 M/mm³	4.0–5.2 M/mm³
HCT	44%	39–51%
HGB	14 g/dL	12–16 g/dL
MCV	91 fL	81–99 fL
MCH	30 pg	27–34 pg
MCHC	33 g/dL	32–36 g/dL
PLT	400 k/mm³	140–440 k/mm³
WBC	15.2 k/mm³	4–11 k/mm³
Neutrophils	80%	4–74%
Lymphocytes	35%	14–46%
	10% Atypical lymphocytes seen	
ESR	38 mm/hr	0–20 mm/hr (Westergren method)

Abdominal CT with Contrast

1. Diverticulitis with probable contained perforation at the posterior aspect of the descending colon sigmoid junction. No diffuse pneumoperitoneum or abscess.
2. Small, 1.5 cm nonspecific hypodense anterior liver lesion.

ASSESSMENT IN BRIEF

Abdominal Assessment

Inspection
- Contour
- Symmetry
- Rectus abdominis muscles
- Pigmentation and color
- Scars
- Striae
- Respiratory movement
- Masses or nodules
- Visible peristalsis
- Pulsation
- Umbilicus

Auscultation
- Bowel sounds
- Vascular sounds
- Venous hum
- Friction rub

Percussion
- General percussion
- Liver span
- Liver descent
- Spleen
- Stomach
- Fist percussion
  - Kidney
  - Liver
- Bladder

Palpation
- Light palpation
- Abdominal muscle guarding
- Deep palpation
- Liver
  - Bimanual method
  - Hook method
- Spleen
- Kidneys
- Aorta
- Bladder
- Inguinal lymph nodes

Advanced Techniques
- Liver scratch test
- Assessing for ascites
  - Shifting dullness
  - Puddle sign
- Fluid wave
- Murphy's sign
- Rebound tenderness
- Rovsing's sign
- Cutaneous hypersensitivity
- Iliopsoas muscle test
- Obturator muscle test
- Ballottement

Abdominal Tubes and Drains
- Tubes
  - Enteral tube
  - Nasogastric suction tube
  - Intestinal tube
  - Gastrostomy
- Drains
  - Abdominal cavity drain
  - Biliary drain
- Intestinal diversions
  - Colostomy
  - Ileostomy
- Urinary diversions
  - Ileal conduit
  - Ureteral stent
  - Indwelling catheter

REVIEW QUESTIONS

1. While palpating a patient's abdominal LLQ, you visualize the underlying organs, which include:
   a. Stomach, body of pancreas, splenic flexure of colon
   b. Spermatic cord, sigmoid colon, ovary
   c. Hepatic flexure of colon, duodenum, cecum
   d. Appendix, lower pole of kidney, adrenal gland
   The correct answer is (b).

2. After assessing a patient's abdomen, you suspect that she may be experiencing cholecystitis. In which abdominal area is the patient most likely experiencing pain?
   a. Epigastrium
   b. Right upper quadrant
   c. Periumbilical
   d. Left lower quadrant
   The correct answer is (b).

3. Mr. Ahmed is a 44-year-old man who is concerned about colorectal cancer because of his change in bowel habits. Which of the following is a risk factor for colorectal cancer?
   a. Alcohol intake of one beer every night
   b. Vegetarian diet
   c. Middle Eastern ethnicity
   d. Body Mass Index of 32
   The correct answer is (d).

4. An infectious disease nurse investigates an outbreak of a viral illness. The common vector in the investigation is people who ate hot dogs from a vendor in an inner-city location of a large metropolitan area. Which viral illness can most directly be traced to this vector?
   a. Hepatitis A   c. Hepatitis C
   b. Hepatitis B   d. Hepatitis D
   The correct answer is (a).

5. Mrs. T is a 51-year-old grandmother who has been experiencing an increase of involuntary loss of urine with physical activity and sneezing. Her past medical history is positive for ovarian and uterine cancer that required surgery and radiation therapy. What type of incontinence is Mrs. T most likely experiencing?
   a. Functional incontinence
   b. Overflow incontinence
   c. Urge incontinence
   d. Stress incontinence
   The correct answer is (d).

6. A patient with pancreatitis complains of pain in the back and left shoulder. This abdominal pain is best described as:
   a. Visceral pain   c. Referred pain
   b. Parietal pain   d. Nociceptive pain
   The correct answer is (c).

7. As you inspect the patient's abdomen from the costal margin to the symphysis pubis, you note a network of dilated veins. This physical assessment finding can occur in which condition?
   a. Diastasis recti
   b. Portal hypertension
   c. von Recklinghausen's disease
   d. Umbilical hernia
   The correct answer is (b).

8. When auscultating a patient's abdomen, you hear a high-pitched sound that resembles two pieces of sandpaper being rubbed together. What clinical condition might this patient have?
   a. Abdominal aortic aneurysm
   b. Diverticulosis
   c. Splenic inflammation
   d. Renal calculi
   The correct answer is (c).

9. You ask the patient to kneel and assume the knee-chest position for several minutes. Upon percussion you note dullness around the umbilicus. What pathological process is this patient experiencing?
   a. Duodenal ulcer
   b. Ruptured ovarian cyst
   c. Ectopic pregnancy
   d. Ascites
   The correct answer is (d).

10. Which of the following patients is at risk for developing an urinary tract infection?
   a. A circumcised male with hemorrhoids
   b. A woman with an IUD who is sexually active
   c. A male with a CD4+ T-lymphocyte cell count of 2,000
   d. A postmenopausal woman who voids every 6 hours
   The correct answer is (d).

Visit the Estes online companion resource at
www.delmar.cengage.com
for additional content and study aids.
Click on Online Companions and then select the Nursing discipline.

REFERENCES

American Cancer Society Guidelines for the Early Detection of Cancer. Retrieved June 24, 2008, from www.cancer.org/docroot/PED/content/PED_2_3X_ACS_Cancer_Detection_Guidelines_36.asp

Lewis, S. J., & Heaton, K. W. (1997). Stool form scale as a useful guide to intestinal transit time. *Scandinavian Journal of Gastroenterology,* *32*(9), 920–924.

Resnick, N. M. (1984). Urinary incontinence in the elderly. *Medical Grand Rounds, 3,* 281–290.

BIBLIOGRAPHY

Anger, J. T., Saigal, C. S., & Litwin, M. S. (2006). The prevalence of urinary incontinence among community dwelling adult women: Results from the National Health and Nutrition Examination Survey. *Journal of Urology, 175* (2), 601–604.

Brady, A. (2008). Managing the patient with dysphagia. *Home Healthcare Nurse, 26*(1), 42–46.

Burns, R. B. (2006). A 59-year-old woman with gastroesophageal reflux disease and Barrett esophagus, 4 years later. *JAMA, 296*(17), 2140.

Carl, L. L., & Johnson, P. R. (2006). *Drugs and dysphagia: How medications can affect eating and swallowing.* Austin, TX: Pre-ed.

Carroll, J. K., Herrick, B., Gipson, T., & Lee, S. P. (2007). Acute pancreatitis: Diagnosis, prognosis, and treatment. *American Family Physician, 75*(10), 1513–1520.

Cartwright, S. L., & Knudson, N. P. (2008). Evaluation of acute abdominal pain reviewed. *American Family Physician, 77*(7), 971–978.

Chand, N., & Mihas, A. A. (2006). Celiac disease: Current concepts in diagnosis and treatment. *Journal of Clinical Gastroenterology, 40*(1), 3–14.

Drossman, D. A. (2006). The functional gastrointestinal disorders and the Rome III process. *Gastroenterology, 130*(5), 1377–1390.

Farag, N., Reynolds, E., & Lembo, A. (2008). Update: A 54-year-old woman with constipation-predominant irritable bowel syndrome. *JAMA, 299*(1), 88.

Fenoglio-Preiser, C. M., Noffsinger, A. E., Stemmermann, G. N., Lanz, P. E., & Isaacson, P. C. (2008). *Gastrointestinal pathology: An atlas and text* (3rd ed.). Philadelphia: Wolters Kluwer.

Gruber, S. B. (2006). New developments in Lynch syndrome (hereditary nonpolyposis colorectal cancer) and mismatch repair gene testing. *Gastroenterology, 130*(2), 577–587.

Heck, B. N. (2007). Interstitial cystitis: Enhancing early identification in primary care settings. *The Journal for Nurse Practitioners, 3*(8), 509–519.

Jeter, J. M., Kohlmann, W., & Gruber, S. B. (2006). Genetics of colorectal cancer. *Oncology, 20*(3), 269–276.

Lamps, L. W., & Knapple, W. L. (2007). Diverticular disease-associated segmented colitis. *Clinical Gastroenterology and Hepatology, 5*(1), 27–31.

Liao, Y. M., Dougherty, M. C., Liou, Y. S., & Tseng, I. J. (2006). Pelvic floor muscle training effect on urinary incontinence knowledge, attitudes, and severity: An experimental study. *International Journal of Nursing Studies, 43*(1), 29–37.

Martin, S. (2008). Against the grain: An overview of celiac disease. *Journal of the American Academy of Nurse Practitioners, 20*(5), 243–250.

Menon, U., Belue, R., Skinner, C. S., Rothwell, B. E., & Champion, U. (2007). Perceptions of colon cancer screening by stage of screening test adoption. *Cancer Nursing, 30*(3), 178–185.

Molzahn, A., & Butera, E. (Eds.). (2006). *Contemporary nephrology nursing: Principles and practice* (2nd ed.). Pitman, NJ: Anthony J. Jannetti, Inc.

Presutti, R. J., Cangemi, J. R., Cassidy, H. D., & Hill, D. A. (2007). Celiac disease. *American Family Physician, 76*(12), 1795–1802.

Rennke, H. G., & Denker, B. M. (2007). *Renal pathophysiology: The essentials* (2nd ed.). Philadelphia: Lippincott Williams & Wilkins.

Riehl, M. (2007). Help your patient cope with pancreatic cancer. *Nursing 2007, 37*(4), 54–57.

Ruthruff, B. (2007). Clinical review of Crohn's disease. *Journal of the American Academy of Nurse Practitioners, 19*(8), 392–397.

U.S. Preventive Services Task Force. (2007). Routine aspirin or nonsteroidal anti-inflammatory drugs for the primary prevention of colorectal cancer: U.S. Preventive Services Task Force recommendation statement. *Annals of Internal Medicine, 146*(5), 361–364.

Ward, M. M. (2007). Laboratory abnormalities at the onset of treatment of end-stage renal disease. Are there racial or socioeconomic disparities in care? *Archives of Internal Medicine, 167*(10), 1083–1091.

Wexner, S. D., & Stollman, N. (Eds.). (2006). *Diseases of the colon.* New York: Informa Healthcare.

Wong, S. N., & Lok, A. S. F. (2006). Treatment of hepatitis B: Who, when, and how? *Archives of Internal Medicine, 166*(1), 9–12.

WEB SITES

American Gastroenterological Association:
http://www.gastro.org

American Urological Association:
http://www.auanet.org

Celiac.com:
http://www.glutenfreeforum.com

Centers for Disease Control and Prevention:
http://www.cdc.gov/hepatitis

The Cochrane Collaboration:
http://www.cochrane.org

Crohn's & Colitis Foundation of America:
http://www.ccfa.org

Gastrointestinal Nursing:
http://www.gastrointestinalnursing.co.uk

Society of Gastroenterology Nurses and Associates, Inc.:
http://www.sgna.org

Society of Urologic Nurses and Associates:
http://www.suna.org

UrologyHealth.org:
http://www.urologyhealth.org

CHAPTER 18
Musculoskeletal System

COMPETENCIES

1. Elicit a health history from a patient with a musculoskeletal chief complaint.

2. Perform inspection and palpation of the musculoskeletal system.

3. Describe the range of motion movements of the major joints.

4. Measure range of joint motion with a goniometer.

5. Assess muscle strength of the arms and legs using the Muscle Strength Grading Scale.

6. Document the findings of the musculoskeletal assessment.

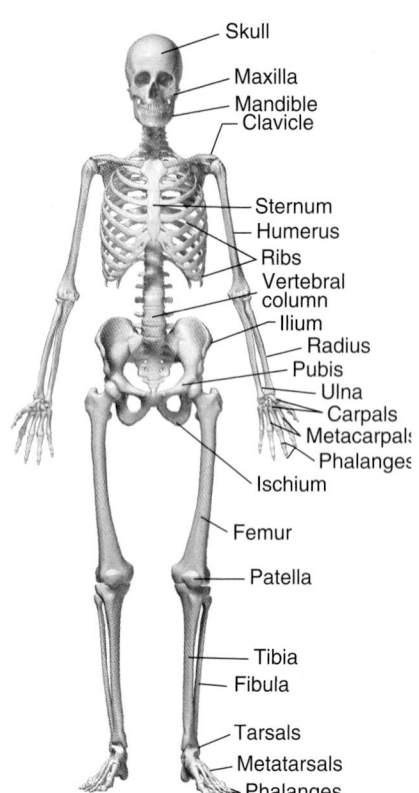

Appendicular skeleton (blue)
Axial skeleton (orange)

FIGURE 18-1 **Adult Skeleton:**
Anterior View

The musculoskeletal system provides the ability to maintain and change body position in response to both internal and external stimuli. Muscle tone and bone strength allow an individual to maintain an upright and erect posture position. Muscle contraction and joint movement allow an individual to move toward positive stimuli and away from noxious stimuli. Alterations in the musculoskeletal system will affect an individual's ability to complete activities of daily living, occupation, and recreation. The musculoskeletal system functions closely with the neurological system, such that a disturbance in the neurological system can grossly impact the musculoskeletal system.

ANATOMY AND PHYSIOLOGY

The musculoskeletal system consists of an intricate framework of bones, joints, skeletal muscles, and supportive connective tissue (cartilage, tendons, and ligaments). Although the primary purpose of the musculoskeletal system is to support body position and promote mobility, it also protects underlying soft organs and allows for mineral storage. In addition, it produces select blood components (platelets, red blood cells, and white blood cells). Only those aspects of the musculoskeletal system that are responsible for body position and mobility are discussed in this chapter.

BONES

The adult human skeleton is composed of 206 bones (Figure 18-1). Bone is ossified connective tissue. The skeleton is divided into the central **axial skeleton** (facial bones, skull, auditory ossicles, hyoid bone, ribs, sternum, and vertebrae) and the peripheral **appendicular skeleton** (limbs, pelvis, scapula, and clavicle). A bone's size and shape are directly related to the mobility and weight-bearing function of that bone. In some cases, bone size and shape are also related to the protection of underlying internal organs and tissues (e.g., the ribs in relation to the lungs, heart, and thoracic aorta).

Shape and Structure

Bones have long, short, flat, rounded, and irregular shapes. The long bone is a shaft (**diaphysis**) with two large ends (**epiphyses**). The two epiphyses each articulate with another bone to form a joint. A 1- to 4-cm layer of cartilage covers each epiphysis in order to minimize stress and friction on the bone ends during movement and weight bearing. The thickness of the cartilage layer varies, depending on the amount of stress placed on that joint. The interior of the diaphysis is the **medullary cavity**, which contains the bone marrow.

Short bones are found in the hands (carpals) and feet (tarsals). Flat bones, such as the skull and parts of the pelvic girdle, are associated with the protection of nearby soft body parts. Rounded, or sesamoid, bones are often encased in the fascia or in a tendon near a joint, such as is the patella. Irregular bones include the mandible, vertebrae, and the auditory ossicles of the inner ear.

MUSCLES

There are over 600 muscles in the human body, and they can be characterized as one of three types. Cardiac and smooth muscles are involuntary, meaning that the individual has no conscious control over the initiation and termination of the muscle contraction. The largest type of muscle, and the only type of voluntary muscle, is called skeletal muscle. Skeletal muscle provides for mobility by exerting a pull on the bones near a joint. In addition, skeletal muscle provides for body contour and contributes to overall body weight. Figure 18-2 illustrates the major

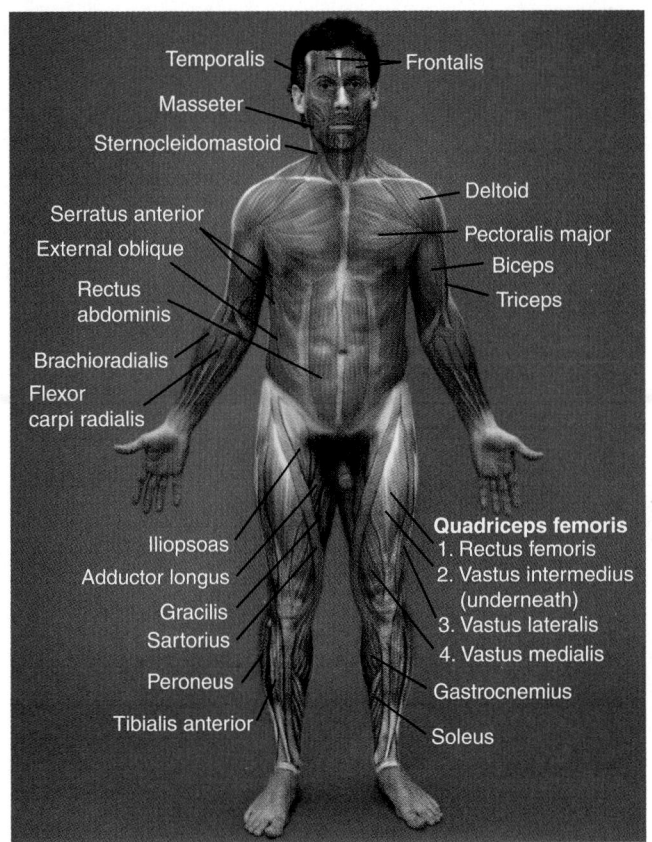

A. Anterior View

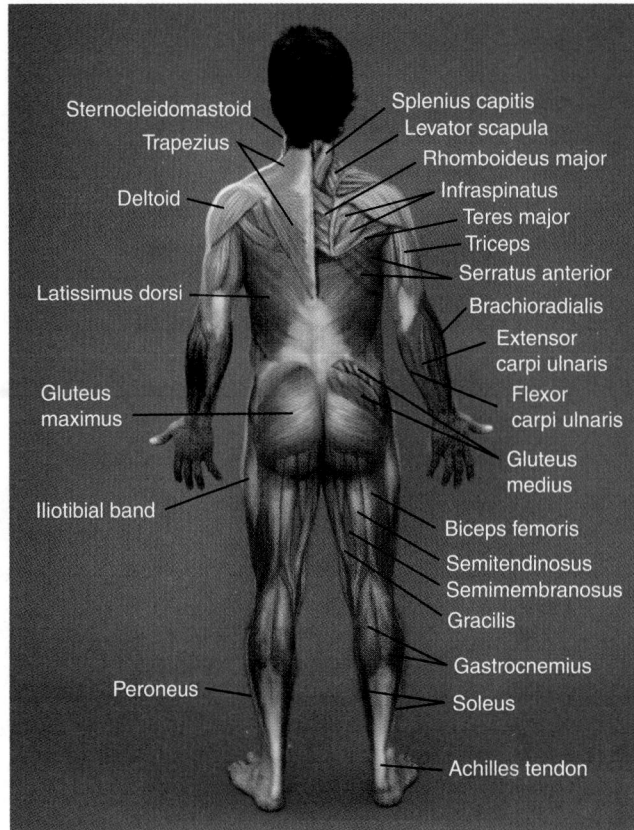

B. Posterior View

FIGURE 18-2 **Muscles of the Body**

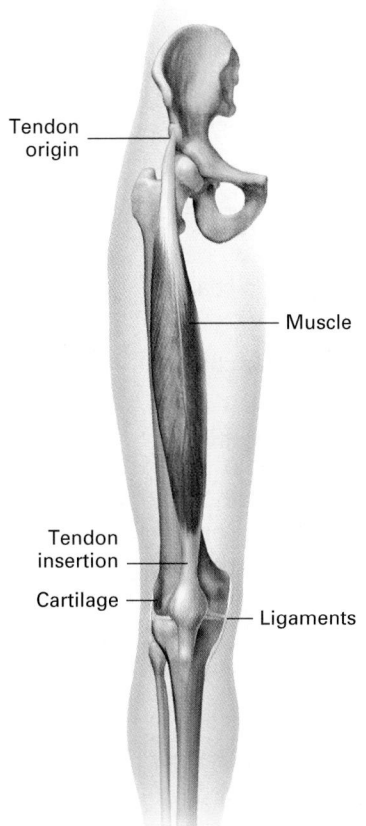

FIGURE 18-3 **Connective Tissue Structures of the Leg**

muscles. It is estimated that 40% to 50% of adult body weight is due to the weight of the skeletal muscles. Muscles vary in size and strength in every person and are affected by age, sex, exercise, and nutrition.

TENDONS

A strong connective tissue sheath (**epimysium**) acts as the outer covering of the muscle belly. The ends of the epimysium extend beyond the muscle belly to form the **tendons** of the muscle. The tendon attaches the muscle to a bone (Figure 18-3).

CARTILAGE

Cartilage is an avascular, dense, connective tissue that covers the ends of opposing bones. Its resilience allows it to withstand increased pressure and tension.

LIGAMENTS

Ligaments are composed of strong, fibrous, connective tissue. They connect bones to each other at the joint level and encase the joint capsule. Ligaments may be seen as oblique to or parallel to a joint (e.g., knee) or encircling the joint (e.g., hip). Ligaments support purposeful joint movement and prevent joint movement that is detrimental to that type of joint.

BURSAE

Bursae are sacs filled with fluid. Bursae act as cushions between two nearby surfaces (e.g., between tendon and bone or between tendon and ligament) to reduce friction. They can also develop in response to prolonged friction or pressure.

JOINTS

A **joint** is a union between two bones. Joints secure the bones firmly together but allow for some degree of movement between the two bones. Contraction of overlying skeletal muscle will act to alter the angle of the two bones by pulling the distal bone toward or away from the proximal bone. Terms used for joint range of motion are described in Table 18-1.

Of the three classifications of skeletal joints found in the adult human skeleton (synarthroses, amphiarthroses, and diarthroses), only the synovial joint (diarthroses) is considered freely movable. Examples of each joint are provided in Table 18-2. Table 18-3 shows categories of the major synovial joints. The synovial joint allows body movement.

TABLE 18-1 Descriptive Terms for Joint Range of Motion

TERM	DESCRIPTION	CHANGE IN JOINT ANGLE
Flexion	Bending of a joint so that the articulating bones on either side of the joints are moved closer together	Decreased
Extension	Bending the joint so that the articulating bones on either side of the joint are moved farther apart	Increased
Hyperextension	Extension beyond the neutral position	Increased beyond the angle of extension
Adduction	Moving the extremity medially and toward the midline of the body	Decreased
Abduction	Moving the extremity laterally and away from the midline of the body	Increased
Internal rotation	Rotating the extremity medially along its own axis	No change
External rotation	Rotating the extremity laterally along its own axis	No change
Circumduction	Moving the extremity in a conical fashion so that the distal aspect of the extremity moves in a circle	No change
Supination	Rotating the forearm laterally at the elbow so that the palm of the hand turns laterally to face upward	No change
Pronation	Rotating the forearm medially at the elbow so that the palm of the hand turns medially to face downward	No change
Opposition	Moving the thumb outward to touch the little finger of the same hand	No change
Eversion	Tilting the foot inward, with the medial side of the foot lowered	No change
Inversion	Tilting the foot outward, with the lateral side of the foot lowered	No change
Dorsiflexion	Flexing the foot at the ankle so that the toes move toward the chest	Decreased
Plantar flexion	Moving the foot at the ankle so that the toes move away from the chest	Increased
Elevation	Raising a body part in an upward direction	No change
Depression	Lowering a body part	No change
Protraction	Moving a body part anteriorly along its own axis (parallel to the ground)	No change
Retraction	Moving a body part posteriorly along its own axis (parallel to the ground)	No change
Gliding	One joint surface moves over another joint surface in a circular or angular nature	No change

A synovial membrane lines the interior of the joint space (Figure 18-4). The primary purpose of the synovial membrane is to secrete fluid for joint lubrication, nourishment, and waste removal. Normally, the joint space contains only 1 to 3 mL of synovial fluid. Excessive synovial joint fluid is called a **synovial effusion**.

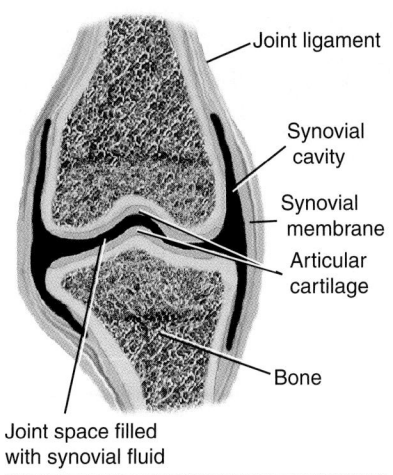

Joint ligament

Synovial cavity

Synovial membrane

Articular cartilage

Bone

Joint space filled with synovial fluid

FIGURE 18-4   Synovial Joint

TABLE 18-2   Categories of Skeletal Joints

CATEGORY	DEGREE OF MOVEMENT	EXAMPLES
Diarthroses (synovial)	Freely movable	Shoulder, elbow, wrist, thumb, hip, knee, ankle, and proximal cervical vertebrae
Amphiarthroses	Slightly movable	Vertebrae, manubriosternal joint, radioulnar joint, and symphysis pubis
Synarthroses	Immovable	Epiphyseal growth plate (adult), skull sutures (child), between the distal ends of the radius and ulna, between the distal ends of the tibia and fibula, and the attachment of the root of a tooth to the alveolar process of the maxilla or mandible

TABLE 18-3   Categories of Synovial Joints

CATEGORY	DESCRIPTION	EXAMPLES
Uniaxial Joints		
Hinge joint	Angular movement in one axis and in one plane	Elbow, fingers, knee
Pivot joint (trochoid)	Rotary movement in one axis; a ring rotates around a pivot, or a pivotlike process rotates within a ring	Radioulnar joint, atlantoodontal joint of the first and second cervical vertebrae
Biaxial Joints		
Saddle joint (sellar)	Articulating surface of one bone is convex and articulating surface of second bone is concave	Metacarpal bone of thumb, trapezium bone of carpus
Condyloid joint	Angular motion in two planes without axial rotation	Wrist between the distal radius and the carpals
Multiaxial Joints		
Ball and socket (spheroidal) joint	Round end of bone fits into cuplike cavity of another bone; provides movement around three or more axes, or in three or more planes	Shoulder, hip
Gliding joint	Gliding movement	Vertebrae, tarsal bones of ankle

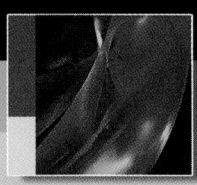

HEALTH HISTORY

The musculoskeletal health history provides insight into the link between a patient's life and lifestyle and musculoskeletal information and pathology.

PATIENT PROFILE

Diseases that are age-, gender-, and race-specific for the musculoskeletal system are listed.

Age

Osteosarcoma (10–20 and 50–60)
Ankylosing spondylitis (20–40)
Bursitis (20–40)
Rheumatoid arthritis (onset 20–40 unless juvenile form of the disease)
Systemic lupus erythematosus (SLE) (25–35)
Low back pain (30–50)
Gout (onset over 30, postmenopausal female)
Osteoporosis (menopausal female)
Carpal tunnel syndrome (pregnant or menopausal female)
Degenerative joint disease or osteoarthritis (onset after 55 in the female and before 45 in the male)
Multiple myeloma (50–70)
Paget's disease (50–70)
Fibromyalgia (40–75)

Gender

Female

Osteoporosis, rheumatoid arthritis, scoliosis, carpal tunnel syndrome, SLE, postmenopausal gout, polymyalgia rheumatica, scleroderma, myasthenia gravis, multiple sclerosis (MS), senile kyphosis, fibromyalgia

Male

Ankylosing spondylitis, gout, Paget's disease, Reiter's syndrome, Dupuytren's contracture, psoriatic arthritis, muscular dystrophy (MD), amyotrophic lateral sclerosis (ALS), low back pain

Race

Caucasian

Rheumatoid arthritis, primary osteoarthritis, polymyalgia rheumatica, osteoporosis, Paget's disease, Dupuytren's contracture, ALS, ankylosing spondylitis

African American

SLE, rheumatoid arthritis

CHIEF COMPLAINT

Common chief complaints for the musculoskeletal system are defined and information on the characteristics of each sign or symptom is provided.

1. Pain

The subjective sense of discomfort in the axial or appendicular skeleton

Location

Muscle, bone, tendon, ligament, or joint

Quantity

Degree of interruption in the patient's usual activities of daily living (ADL) (changes in ambulation, bathing, dressing, food preparation, working, sitting, transfer to a sitting or standing position, climbing stairs, lifting, pushing, and pulling)

Associated Manifestations

Inflammation, skin abrasion, laceration, bruising, hematoma, stiffness, deformity, muscle spasm, paresthesia, decreased joint mobility, restriction

continues

	of weight bearing and movement, excessive weakness or fatigue, mental depression, insomnia, guarding of the painful area, crying, moaning, facial grimacing, anxiety, social withdrawal, agitation, restlessness, diaphoresis, tachycardia, elevated blood pressure, tachypnea
Aggravating Factors	Muscle contraction, muscle spasm, joint movement, partial or full weight bearing, obesity, dependent position, cold and damp weather, noncompliance to physical or occupational therapy guidelines
Alleviating Factors	Restriction of movement, position change, nonweight bearing, limb elevation and rest, ice, heat, analgesics, anti-inflammatory agents, steroids, muscle relaxants, local anesthetic agents, whirlpool therapy, transcutaneous electrical nerve stimulation (TENS), acupuncture, acupressure, assistive devices for use during weight bearing and mobility, splints
Setting	Recent untreated streptococcal infection
Timing	Sudden, insidious, intermittent, continuous
2. Weakness	The subjective sense of an overall decrease in strength and endurance
Location	Local or diffuse, central or peripheral
Quantity	Effect on ADL
Associated Manifestations	Fatigue, muscle atrophy, decreased sensation, decreased joint mobility, decreased muscle strength, discomfort, decreased ability to do ADL
Aggravating Factors	Overexertion, fatigue, immobility, noncompliance to physical or occupational therapy guidelines, physical or emotional stress
Alleviating Factors	Rest, adequate nutrition and hydration, electrolyte replacement therapy, physical and occupational therapy geared toward muscle-strengthening exercises and adaptive techniques
3. Limited Movement	Decrease in mobility caused by a problem with impulse transmission to the muscle, stimulation of a muscle, the ability of that muscle to contract sufficiently to move the joint, or bone stability
Location	Diffuse, or localized to a specific joint
Quantity	Range of joint motion compared to maximum potential or previous measurement
Associated Manifestations	Pain, inflammation, stiffness, muscle atrophy, weakness, deformity, crepitus, joint effusion
Aggravating Factors	Overexertion, immobility, excessive weight gain, noncompliance to medication regime (e.g., anti-inflammatory agents), noncompliance to physical and occupational therapy guidelines
Alleviating Factors	Physical and occupational therapy, anti-inflammatory agents, analgesics, ice, heat, rest, reduction of fractures, correction of dislocation or subluxation
4. Stiffness	The subjective sense of inflexibility
Location	Diffuse, or localized to a specific joint

continues

Health History (continued)

Quantity	Effect on ADL
Associated Manifestations	Joint inflammation, muscle atrophy, deformity, contracture, immobility, pain, palpable joint crepitus, limited range of joint motion
Aggravating Factors	Immobility, aging, overexertion (especially without adequate warming-up and cooling-down sessions during exercise), noncompliance to medication regime (e.g., anti-inflammatory agents), noncompliance to physical and occupational therapy guidelines
Alleviating Factors	Physical and occupational therapy, exercise, anti-inflammatory agents, analgesics, heat, rest, massage, muscle relaxants
Setting	Cold and damp environment
Timing	Sudden or insidious, time of day (e.g., morning stiffness for more than 30 minutes is associated with rheumatoid arthritis), in relation to vigorous or excessive physical exercise
5. Deformity	The congenital or acquired alteration in the configuration of the axial or appendicular skeleton
Location	General (e.g., decreased overall body size) or localized (e.g., disruption in limb length and alignment due to a fracture)
Quality	Degree of cosmetic alteration, degree of musculoskeletal dysfunction (adverse changes in mobility, weight bearing, and the ability to maintain body posture and position)
Associated Manifestations	Enlarged skull, jaw protrusion, forehead protrusion, abnormal joint angle, limb malalignment, missing or extra digits, missing limb, discrepancy in limb length or width, abnormal posture, muscle atrophy, joint contractures
Aggravating Factors	Certain body positions or movements
Alleviating Factors	Surgery, skeletal or skin traction, manual reduction of a fracture or dislocation, limb elevation, ice, physical therapy, splint, cast, brace
Timing	Sudden or insidious, temporary or permanent
PAST HEALTH HISTORY	*The various components of the past health history are linked to musculoskeletal pathology and musculoskeletal-related information.*
Medical History	
Musculoskeletal Specific	Rheumatoid arthritis, osteoarthritis, osteoporosis, Paget's disease, gout, ankylosing spondylitis, osteogenesis imperfecta, loosening or malfunction of joint prosthesis, aseptic necrosis, chronic low back pain, herniated nucleus pulposus, chronic muscle spasms or cramps, scoliosis, poliomyelitis, polymyalgia rheumatica, osteomalacia, rickets, Marfan's syndrome, scleroderma, spina bifida, congenital deformity, MD, MS, myasthenia gravis, ALS, Guillain-Barré syndrome, Reiter's syndrome, carpal tunnel syndrome, paralysis

continues

Health History (continued)

Non-musculoskeletal Specific	Immunosuppression, necrotizing fasciitis, gas gangrene, tetanus, sickle cell anemia, SLE, Lyme disease, blood dyscrasias (including hemophilia), multiple myeloma, diabetes mellitus with or without peripheral neuropathy, hypo- or hypercalcemia, hypo- or hyperpituitarism, hyper- or hypoparathyroidism, hyper- or hypothyroidism, peripheral vascular disease with or without claudication, malnutrition, obesity, menopause
Surgical History	Joint aspiration, therapeutic joint arthroscopy, joint arthroplasty, joint replacement, synovectomy, meniscectomy, arthrodesis, open reduction and internal fixation (ORIF), discectomy, laminectomy, spinal fusion, Harrington rod placement or other spinal instrumentation, repair of torn rotator cuff, debridement, limb or digit amputation, reattachment of a limb or digit
Medications	Narcotic analgesics, nonnarcotic analgesics, anti-inflammatory agents, anti-gout agents, muscle relaxants, steroids, calcitonin, calcium and vitamin D supplements, intra-articular injections, bisphosphonates, selective estrogen receptor modulator, human parathyroid hormone
Communicable Diseases	Poliomyelitis
Injuries and Accidents	Fracture, dislocation, subluxation, tendon tear, tendonitis, muscle contusion, joint strain or sprain, spinal cord injury, torn rotator cuff, traumatic amputation of a digit or limb, crush injury, back injury (including herniated vertebral disc), sports-related injury (e.g., golf elbow, pitcher's shoulder), cartilage damage. See Table 18-4 for age-related trauma.
Special Needs	Amputation, hemiplegia, paraplegia, quadriplegia, need for brace or splint, limb in a cast, need for supportive devices, muscle atrophy
Childhood Illnesses	Poliomyelitis, juvenile arthritis
FAMILY HEALTH HISTORY	*Musculoskeletal diseases that are familial are listed.*
	Rheumatoid arthritis, osteoporosis, ankylosing spondylitis, gout, Paget's disease, Dupuytren's contracture, SLE, Marfan's syndrome, osteomalacia, congenital defect
SOCIAL HISTORY	*The components of the social history are linked to musculoskeletal factors and pathology.*
Alcohol Use	Increased use associated with increased risk of osteoporosis
Tobacco Use	Increased use associated with increased risk of osteoporosis
Work Environment	Manual movement of heavy objects (lifting, pushing, pulling), duties requiring repetitive motions (e.g., keyboard use), duties requiring prolonged standing or ambulation, use of hazardous equipment, availability and use of safety equipment (e.g., lifting equipment, availability of back support vest or brace)
Roles and Relationships	Decreased self-esteem, decreased independence, or isolation secondary to immobility or pain
Home Environment	Design of home (e.g., number of floors, width of doorways, stairs, location of bedroom and bathroom), elevated toilet seat, bar in bathtub or shower, access ramp

continues

Health History (continued)

Hobbies and Leisure Activities	Basketball, wrestling, gymnastics, hockey, ballet, aerobics, use of free weights and exercise machines, baseball, football, lacrosse, rugby, cycling, running, horseback riding, skiing, hiking, tennis, racquetball, swimming, camping, gardening, painting, needlepoint, carpentry, rollerblading, skateboarding
Stress	Stress can be deleterious to patients with autoimmune chronic diseases affecting the musculoskeletal system, such as multiple sclerosis, systemic lupus erythematosus, and rheumatoid arthritis. During times of stress, these patients may experience additional discomfort, stiffness, loss of mobility, and fatigue.
HEALTH MAINTENANCE ACTIVITIES	*This information provides a bridge between the health maintenance activities and musculoskeletal function.*
Sleep	Sleeping positions, need for pillow support, need for firm mattress
Diet	Intake of dairy products and protein, use of dietary supplements or vitamins (especially calcium and vitamin D)
Exercise	Prevents disuse atrophy, promotes bone growth (especially weight-bearing exercise), can aggravate existing musculoskeletal conditions and cause musculoskeletal trauma
Use of Safety Devices	Use of back support vest or lifting equipment for movement of heavy objects (e.g., Hoyer lift, forklift), safety shields when using hazardous equipment, protective padding (wrist or knee guards), helmet, use of gait belt for adult assistance/moving
Health Check-ups	Immunizations up-to-date, especially polio and tetanus, DEXA scan

TABLE 18-4 Common Age-Related Trauma

AGE RANGE	COMMON TRAUMA
10 to 20	Sports-related injuries, motorcycle accidents, high-energy falls (e.g., downhill skiing or cycling)
20 to 50	Sports-related injuries, stress or overuse injuries (e.g., stress fractures, tendonitis), pedestrian accidents
50 to 65+	Recreation-related injuries, falls, pathological fractures, pedestrian accidents

NURSING**TIP**

Weakness Rating Scale

A 0–10/10 scale can be used to obtain the patient's subjective rating of the intensity of the weakness. When a 0–10/10 scale is being utilized, 0 represents complete absence of weakness and 10 represents weakness necessitating complete bed rest.

NURSING**TIP**

Stiffness Rating Scale

When assessing a patient's ability to complete ADL, question the patient's family as well as the patient. The changes in activities of daily living over time may be too subtle to have been noticed by the patient, or the patient may have developed compensatory measures so that these activities can still be accomplished (although they may take longer to complete). A 0–10/10 scale can be used to obtain the patient's subjective rating of the intensity of the stiffness. When utilizing a 0–10/10 scale, 0 represents the complete absence of stiffness and 10 represents total inflexibility.

NURSING**ALERT**

Diet and Vitamin D

Calcium and phosphorous are the primary components of healthy bone. Vitamin D is essential for promoting the absorption of both of these elements from the gastrointestinal tract. Protein is essential for healthy muscle. A diet that is lacking in calcium, phosphorous, vitamin D, and/or protein can promote adverse changes in the musculoskeletal system, such as osteoporosis and osteomalacia. Exposure to sunlight helps to promote vitamin D production in the body. Supplemental vitamins and minerals may be necessary in the patient with lactose intolerance who cannot consume these essential elements easily through dietary intake of dairy products. Fortunately, calcium is also available in dark green, leafy vegetables.

NURSING**ALERT**

Risk Factors for Sports Injuries

Although exercise has been proven beneficial for good health and mobility, noncompliance to recommended guidelines can increase the risk of injury during exercise. Identification of risk factors for sports injury should be included in nursing assessment. These include, but are not limited to:
- The lack of medical clearance prior to the initiation of any aggressive exercise program following a period of prolonged sedentary activity.
- Aggressive cardiovascular activity not accompanied by adequate warm-up (before) or cool-down (after) periods.
- The lack of adequate and appropriate instruction on the use of all exercise equipment such as treadmill and weight machines.
- Not using a "spotter" assistant during gymnastic movements and heavy weightlifting.
- Improperly fitting and unsecured protective equipment such as bicycle helmets, equestrian helmets, a mouthpiece, eye goggles, and shin pads.
- Improperly fitting and unsupportive running shoes.
- The lack of "rest days" between long-distance runs (e.g., 20 miles during marathon training).

NURSING**TIP**

Obesity

Obesity adversely affects multiple body systems. In addition to the increased risk for cardiovascular disease and type 2 diabetes, excess body weight puts additional wear and tear on weight-bearing joints. Degenerative joint disease (also known as osteoarthritis) is associated with obesity. The stress of bearing excess body weight in the standing and ambulating positions can lead to loss of protective joint cartilage and joint pain in the hips and knees.

NURSING**TIP**

Assessing Musculoskeletal Pain

Musculoskeletal pain may be of an acute or a chronic nature. Acute pain is associated with a recent onset and a short duration. Chronic pain has a malignant or nonmalignant etiology and lasts longer than 6 months. Pain is the most common musculoskeletal complaint verbalized to health care providers.

LIFE ⊙ 360°

Assessing Home Safety

Examine the safety of your personal living quarters and the immediate outside environment. Next, reexamine your living quarters for safety as if you had an 85-year-old person living with you. Are there internal or external changes that would need to be made for the safety of the older adult?

EQUIPMENT

- **Measuring tape:** cloth tape measure that will not stretch
- **Goniometer:** protractor-type instrument with two movable arms to measure the angle of a skeletal joint during range of motion
- Sphygmomanometer and blood pressure cuff
- Felt-tip marker

NURSINGTIP

The Musculoskeletal Screening Assessment

The complete musculoskeletal assessment described in this chapter is designed for patients who have musculoskeletal complaints or disease or who have difficulty with ADL. The screening, or musculoskeletal mini-assessment, is conducted on all other patients and should include only general assessment: inspection and palpation of major muscles and joints, inspection of range of motion (ROM) as the patient moves through the examination, and muscle strength of the arms and legs.

NURSINGTIP

Ensuring Home Safety

To ensure a safe home environment, encourage patients (especially those who have an increased risk for injury in the home) to avoid:

- Loose or unsecured rugs (e.g., scatter rugs, rugs on stairways)
- Stairways without banisters or stairways with loose banisters
- Stairs with a slippery surface
- Dim lighting, especially near stairways or steps
- Ill-fitting shoes; loose, nonlaced shoes; shoes with high heels; or shoes with slippery soles
- Household clutter beneath waist level
- Electrical or phone cords that are too long and fall on the floor
- Only one phone or a phone that is not easily accessible during most of the day
- Wet or waxed floors
- Unrestrained small pets
- Bathtubs or shower stalls without a nonskid surface
- Lack of grab bars in the bathroom near the toilet and tub or shower stall
- Objects that are not within easy reach
- Wet or icy outdoor steps and sidewalks

ASSESSMENT OF THE MUSCULOSKELETAL SYSTEM

NURSINGCHECKLIST

General Approach to Musculoskeletal Assessment

1. Assist the patient to a comfortable position.
2. Offer pillows or folded blankets to support a painful body part.
3. If necessary because of a painful body part or limited mobility, provide the patient assistance in disrobing. Allow the patient extra time to remove clothing.
4. To maximize patient comfort during the physical assessment, maintain a warm temperature in the exam room.
5. Be clear in your instructions to the patient if you are asking the patient to perform a certain body movement or to assume a certain position. Demonstrate the desired movement if necessary.
6. Notify the patient before touching or manipulating a painful body part.
7. Inspection, palpation, range of motion, and muscle testing are performed on the major skeletal muscles and joints of the body in a cephalocaudal, proximal-to-distal manner. Always compare paired muscles and joints.
8. Examine nonaffected body parts before examining affected body parts.
9. Avoid unnecessary or excessive manipulation of a painful body part. If the patient complains of pain, stop the aggravating motion.
10. If necessary because of a painful body part or limited mobility, provide the patient assistance in dressing after the physical assessment. Allow the patient extra time to get dressed.
11. Some musculoskeletal disorders may affect the patient more during certain parts of the day. Arrange for the follow-up appointment to be during the patient's time of optimal function.

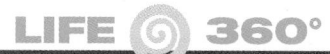

Dealing with Physical Anomaly

- Have you ever worked with a person who had a severe physical anomaly?
- Were you hesitant to start a relationship (personal or professional) with this person?
- Did you ever discuss the anomaly with the person?
- Were you comfortable discussing it? Was the other person comfortable with the discussion?
- What can you do to prepare yourself to communicate comfortably with a patient who has a physical anomaly?

GENERAL ASSESSMENT

Overall Appearance

E 1. Obtain height and weight. Refer to Chapter 7.

2. Observe the patient's ability to tolerate weight bearing on the lower limbs during standing and ambulation. Assess the amount of weight bearing placed on each of the lower limbs. Table 18-5 for a description of weight-bearing terms.

3. Identify obvious structural abnormalities (e.g., atrophy, scoliosis, kyphosis, amputated limbs, contractures). Figure 18-5.

4. Note indications of discomfort (e.g., restricted weight bearing or movement, frequent shifting of position, facial grimacing, excessive fatigue).

N Body height and weight should be appropriate for age and gender. See Chapter 7. The patient should be able to enter the assessment area via independent ambulation. Structural defects should be absent. There should be no outward indications of discomfort during rest, weight bearing, or joint movement. There should be a distinct and symmetrical relationship among the limbs, torso, and pelvis.

A An excessively tall or short, or overweight or underweight patient is abnormal.

P Marfan's syndrome affects multiple systems. The musculoskeletal changes are increased height for age due to an increased length of the distal limbs, extra digits, joint instability, pectus excavatum, and kyphosis.

P Dwarfism, a congenital disorder, is manifested by a decrease in body size. It is regarded as proportionate if both limb and trunk size are smaller than average. The decrease in size may affect only the limbs, which then appear out of proportion to the torso size.

P Severe osteoporosis and ankylosing spondylitis can result in height loss due to vertebral compression fractures and thoracic kyphosis.

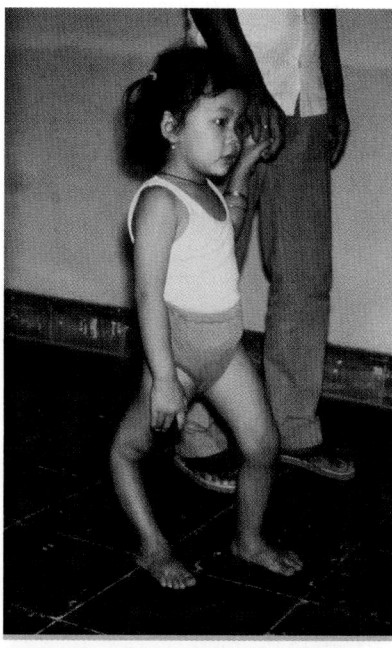

FIGURE 18-5 The musculoskeletal examination begins with assessing a patient's general appearance. The girl in this photo has an obvious deformity from polio. *Courtesy of the World Health Organization.*

TABLE 18-5 Weight-Bearing Status

DEGREE OF WEIGHT BEARING	DESCRIPTION
Nonweight bearing	Patient does not bear weight on the affected extremity. The affected extremity does not touch the floor.
Touchdown weight bearing	Patient's foot of the affected extremity may rest on the floor, but no weight is distributed through that extremity.
Partial weight bearing	Patient bears 30% to 50% of his or her weight on the affected extremity.
Weight bearing as tolerated	Patient bears as much weight as can be tolerated on the affected extremity without undue strain or pain.
Full weight bearing	Patient bears weight fully on the affected extremity.

Reprinted with permission from *Orthopedic Nursing* (3rd ed.), by A. Maher, S. Salmond, & T. Pellino, copyright 2002, Philadelphia: Elsevier.

| 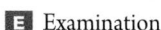 Examination | 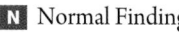 Normal Findings | 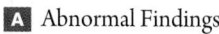 Abnormal Findings | 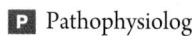 Pathophysiology |

Deviation of Normal Posture

Examine Figure 18-6. Describe the variations from normal that you observe in this man's posture. What additional observations can you make?

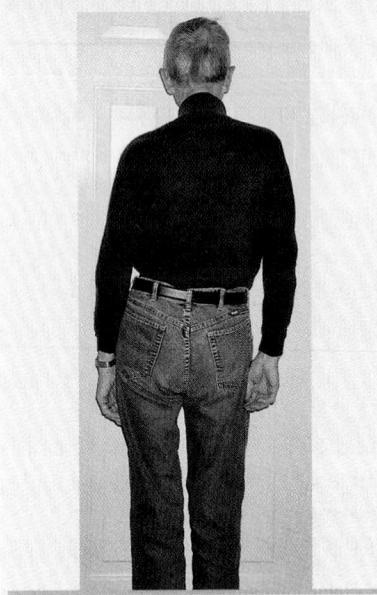

FIGURE 18-6 Deviation of Normal Posture

NURSINGALERT

Guarding Against Patient Falls

Use caution when assessing the patient with limited ability, poor coordination, poor balance, or a sensory deficit (e.g., visual loss, hearing loss, limb amputation, peripheral neuropathy, hemiplegia). Some of the positions and movements that are necessary may place the patient at increased risk for falling during the assessment. Be prepared to support the patient to prevent a fall. If necessary, omit those components of the musculoskeletal assessment that would place the patient at high risk for injury, or seek the assistance of a second nurse.

P Obesity is considered to be a factor in both degenerative joint disease and low back pain.

A Any weight-bearing status other than full weight bearing is abnormal.

P Low back pain may cause a patient to lean forward or toward the affected side.

A Structural defects are abnormal.

P **Acromegaly**, due to hyperpituitary function, may result in an enlarged skull with jaw protrusion, and an increase in the size of the hands, feet, and long bones. The increased length of the long bones can contribute to increased height.

P A missing limb can be due to a congenital defect, surgery, or trauma.

P Pectus excavatum and pectus carinatum are abnormal findings. See Chapter 15.

P Scoliosis and kyphosis are abnormal findings. They are discussed later in this chapter in the section entitled Spine.

Posture

P
1. Stand in front of the patient.
2. Instruct the patient to stand with the feet together.
3. Observe the structural and spatial relationship of the head, torso, pelvis, and limbs. Assess for symmetry of the shoulders, scapulae, and iliac crests.
4. Ask the patient to sit; observe posture.

N In the standing position, the torso and head are upright. The head is midline and perpendicular to the horizontal line of the shoulders and pelvis. The shoulders and hips are level, with symmetry of the scapulae and iliac crests. The arms hang freely from the shoulders. The feet are aligned and the toes point forward. The extremities are proportional to the overall body size and shape, and the limbs are also symmetrical with each other. The knees face forward, with symmetry of the level of the knees. There is usually less than a 2-inch interval between the knees when the patient stands with the feet together, facing forward. When full growth is reached, the arm span is equal to the height. In the sitting position, both feet should be placed firmly on the floor surface, with toes pointing forward.

A Forward slouching of the shoulders produces a false thoracic kyphosis.

P These findings can be caused by poor posture habits.

Gait and Mobility

E
1. Instruct the patient to walk normally across the room.
2. Ask the patient to walk on the toes and then on the heels of the feet.
3. Ask the patient to walk by placing one foot in front of the other, in a "heel-to-toe" fashion (tandem walking).
4. Instruct the patient to walk forward, then backward.
5. Ask the patient to sidestep to the left, then to the right.
6. Instruct the patient to ambulate forward a few steps with the eyes closed.
7. Observe the patient during transfer between the standing and sitting positions.

| **E** Examination | **N** Normal Findings | **A** Abnormal Findings | **P** Pathophysiology |

TABLE 18-6 Examples of Abnormal Gait Patterns

TYPE OF ABNORMAL GAIT	ETIOLOGY	DESCRIPTION
Antalgic	Degenerative joint disease of the hip or knee	Limited weight bearing is placed on an affected leg in an attempt to limit discomfort.
Short leg	Discrepancy in leg length, flexion contracture of the hip or knee, congenital hip dislocation	A limp is present during ambulation unless shoes have been adapted to compensate for length discrepancy.
Spastic hemiplegia	Cerebral palsy, unilateral upper motor neuron lesion (e.g., stroke)	Extension of one lower extremity with plantar flexion and foot inversion; arm is flexed at the elbow, wrist, and fingers. The patient walks by swinging the affected leg in a semicircle. The foot is not lifted off the floor. The affected arm does not swing with the gait.
Scissors	Multiple sclerosis, bilateral upper motor neuron disease	Adduction at the knee level produces short, slow steps. Gait is uncoordinated, stiff, and jerky. The foot is dragged across the floor in a semicircle.
Cerebellar ataxia	Cerebellar disease	Gait is broad based and uncoordinated, and the patient appears to stagger and sway during ambulation.
Sensory ataxia	Disorders of peripheral nerves, dorsal roots, and posterior column that interfere with proprioceptive input	Stance is broad based. Patient lifts feet up too high and abruptly slaps them on the floor, heel first. The patient watches the floor carefully to help ensure correct foot placement because the patient is unaware of position in space.
Festinating	Parkinson's disease	Decreased step height and length, but increased step speed, resulting in "shuffling" (feet barely clearing the floor). Patient's posture is stooped and patient appears to hesitate both in initiation and in termination of ambulation. Rigid body position, with flexion of the knees during standing and ambulation.
Steppage or footdrop	Peroneal nerve injury, paralysis of the dorsiflexor muscles, damage to spinal nerve roots L5 and S1 from poliomyelitis	Hip and knee flexion are needed for step height in order to lift the foot off the floor. Instead of placing the heel of the foot on the floor first, the whole sole of the foot is slapped on the floor at once. May be unilateral or bilateral.
Apraxic	Alzheimer's disease, frontal lobe tumors	Patient has difficulty with walking despite intact motor and sensory systems. The patient is unable to initiate walking, as if stuck to the floor. After walking is initiated, the gait is slow and shuffling.
Trendelenburg	Developmental dysplasia of hip, muscular dystrophy	During ambulation, pelvis of the unaffected side drops when weight bearing is performed on the affected side. When both hips are affected, a "waddling" gait may be evident.

Reprinted with permission from *Orthopedic Nursing* (3rd ed.), by A. Maher, S. Salmond, & T. Pellino, copyright 2002, Philadelphia: Elsevier.

N Walking is initiated in one smooth, rhythmic fashion. The foot is lifted 2.5 to 5 cm (1 to 2 inches) off the floor and then propelled 30–45 cm (12 to 18 inches) forward in a straight path. As the heel strikes the floor, body weight is then shifted onto the ball of that foot. The heel of the foot is then elevated off the floor before the next step forward. The patient remains erect and balanced during all stages of gait. Step height and length are symmetrical for each foot. The arms swing freely at the side of the torso but in opposite direction to the movement of the legs. The lower limbs are able to bear full body weight during standing and ambulation. Prior to turning, the head and neck turn toward the intended direction, followed by the rest of the body. The patient should be able to transfer easily to various positions.

A Indications of gait disturbance include hesitancy or multiple attempts to initiate ambulation, unsteadiness, staggering, grasping for external support, high stepping, foot scraping due to inability to raise the foot completely off the floor, persistent toe or heel walking, excessive pointing of the toes inward or outward, asymmetry of step height or length, limping, stooping during walking, wavering gait, shuffling gait, waddling gait, excessive swinging of the shoulders or pelvis, and slow or rapid step speed. See Table 18-6 provides examples of abnormal gait patterns.

P Causes of abnormal gait include muscle weakness, joint deterioration, malalignment of the lower limbs, paralysis, lack of coordination or balance, fatigue, and pain.

P Limited mobility due to stiffness is associated with degenerative joint disease, rheumatoid arthritis, Paget's disease, and Parkinson's disease.

P Severe thoracic kyphosis will alter the body's center of gravity and affect balance during both standing and ambulation.

P Pathological fracture of the femoral shaft during the stress of weight bearing may occur during standing or ambulation. Pathological fracture can occur if the bone has been significantly weakened by malignancy, osteoporosis, Paget's disease, or osteomalacia.

A When rising from or sitting in a chair, the patient may have to lean on the armrest for external support. The patient may also tend to rock forward and push off from the armrest for propulsion upward into the standing position. Discomfort felt while bearing the body's weight in the standing position may be reduced in the sitting position. In see Table 18-7, transfer techniques that will assist you in documenting the type of patient transfer are described.

P Because of stiffness and discomfort, the patient with degenerative joint disease of the hip joint often has difficulty rising from a sitting position without assistance.

INSPECTION

Muscle Size and Shape

E 1. Survey the overall appearance of the muscle mass.
2. Ask the patient to contract the muscle without inducing movement (isometric muscle contraction), relax the muscle, and then repeat the muscle contraction.
3. Look for any obvious muscle contraction.

N Muscle contour will be affected by the exercise and activity patterns of the individual. Muscle shape may be accentuated in certain body areas (e.g., the limbs and upper torso) but should be symmetrical. There may be hypertrophy in the dominant hand. During muscle contraction, you should be able to visualize sudden tautness of the muscle area. Muscle relaxation will be associated with termination of muscle tautness. There is no involuntary movement.

Hypertrophy refers to an increase in muscle size and shape due to an increase in the muscle fibers. Hypertrophy is detected as a unilateral

---

| **E** Examination | **N** Normal Findings | **A** Abnormal Findings | **P** Pathophysiology |

TABLE 18-7 Transfer Techniques

TECHNIQUE	DESCRIPTION
Independent	The patient is safe with transfers and requires no assistance.
Standby assist of 1	The patient is basically independent but may need verbal cues or observation.
Contact guard of 1	The patient transfers well with hands-on contact by a nurse. This method is used if the patient's judgment is questionable or for patients with slightly decreased balance.
Minimal assistance of 1	The patient requires minimal physical assistance from a nurse to stand or sit (e.g., for lower extremity placement on footrest of wheelchair).
Maximal assistance of 1	The patient requires maximal physical assistance and many verbal cues from a nurse to transfer (e.g., for extremity placement, trunk placement).
Maximal assistance of 2	Same as for the previous example but requires two nurses. This necessitates good body mechanics and often calls for assistive devices (e.g., Hoyer lift, total lift).

Reprinted with permission from *Orthopedic Nursing* (3rd ed.), by A. Maher, S. Salmond, & T. Pellino, copyright 2002, Philadelphia: Elsevier.

or bilateral increase in the contour of the muscle. During contraction, the borders of the muscle will become accentuated. An increase in muscle strength will accompany the increase in muscle size. Bilateral hypertrophy is common among athletes involved in weightlifting or other activities that require repetitive motion against opposing resistance. Hypertrophy of the proximal arms is often seen in patients who are dependent on a wheelchair for mobility yet are able to propel the wheelchair manually.

A **Atrophy** describes a reduction in muscle size and shape. Atrophy is evidenced by the appearance of thin, flabby muscles. The contour of the skeletal muscle is less distinct than usual. The muscle will appear relaxed, even during voluntary isometric contraction. Atrophy may be local or diffuse.

P Generalized atrophy is directly related to prolonged immobility of the body as a whole (disuse atrophy), unless isometric exercises were routinely performed during the period of immobility. It is accentuated by poor nutrition.

P Generalized atrophy may also be noted in grossly obese patients who lead sedentary lifestyles.

P Local atrophy is often detected in the limb or limbs affected by hemiparesis, paraplegia, or quadriplegia. It is also seen following the removal of a limb cast or splint.

A There is involuntary muscle movement.

P See Table 18-8.

Joint Contour and Periarticular Tissue

E 1. Observe the shape of the joint while the joint is in its neutral anatomic position.
2. Visually inspect the 5 to 7.5 cm (2 to 3 inches) of skin and subcutaneous tissue surrounding that joint. Assess the periarticular area for erythema, swelling, bruising, nodules, deformities, masses, skin atrophy, or skin breakdown.

TABLE 18-8 Involuntary Muscle Movements

TYPE	DESCRIPTION
Fasciculation	Visible twitching of a group of muscle fibers that may be stimulated by the tapping of a muscle.
Fibrillation	Ineffective, uncoordinated muscle contraction that resembles quivering.
Spasm	Sudden muscle contraction. A cramp is a muscle spasm that is strong and painful. Clonic muscle spasms are contractions that alternate with a period of muscle relaxation. A tonic muscle spasm is a sustained contraction with a period of relaxation.
Tetany	Paroxysmal tonic muscle spasms, usually of the extremities. The face and jaw may also be affected by spasm. Tetany may be associated with discomfort.
Chorea	Rapid, irregular, and jerky muscle contractions of random muscle groups. It is unpredictable and without purpose. It can involve the face, upper trunk, and limbs. Sometimes, the patient tries to incorporate the movement into voluntary movement, which may appear grotesque and exaggerated. The patient may have difficulty with chewing, speaking, and swallowing.
Tremors	A period of continuous shaking due to muscle contractions. Although the quality of the tremors will be influenced by the cause, the amplitude and the frequency should remain the same. Tremors may be fine or coarse, rapid or slow, continuous or intermittent. They may be exacerbated during rest and attempts at purposeful movements, or by certain body positions.
Tic	Sudden, rapid muscle spasms of the upper trunk, face, or shoulders. The action is often repetitive and may decrease during purposeful movement. It can be persistent or limited in nature.
Ballism	Jerky, twisting movements due to strong muscle contraction.
Athetosis	Slow, writhing, twisting type of movement. The patient is unable to sustain any part of the body in one position. The movements are most often in the fingers, hands, face, throat, and tongue, although any part of the body can be affected. The movements are generally slower than in chorea.
Dystonia	Similar to athetosis but differing in the duration of the postural abnormality, and involving large muscles such as the trunk. The patient may present with an overflexed or overextended posture of the hand, pulling of the head to one side, torsion of the spine, inversion of the foot, or closure of the eyes along with a fixed grimace.
Myoclonus	A rapid, irregular contraction of a muscle or group of muscles, such as the type of jerking movement that occurs when drifting off to sleep.
Tremors at rest	Asymmetrical and coarse movements that disappear or diminish with action. They tend to diminish or cease with purposeful movement.
Action tremors	Symmetrical or asymmetrical movements that increase in states of fatigue, weakness, drug withdrawal, hypocalcemia, uremia, or hepatic disease. This type of tremor may be induced in a normal individual when he or she is required to maintain a posture that demands extremes of power or precision. Action tremors are also called postural tremors.
Intention tremors	These tremors may appear only on voluntary movement of a limb and may intensify on termination of movement.
Asterixis	This is a variant of a tremor. The rate of limb flexion and extension is irregular, slow, and of wide amplitude. The outstretched limb temporarily loses muscle tone.

 Joint contour should be somewhat flat in extension, and smooth and rounded in flexion. You should be unable to detect any difference between periarticular tissue, the skin, and subcutaneous tissue. Bilateral joints should be symmetrical in position and appearance. There should be no observable erythema, swelling, bruising, nodules, deformities, masses, skin atrophy, or skin breakdown.

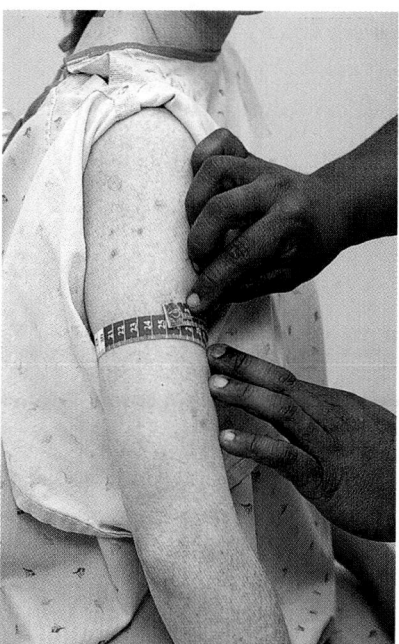

FIGURE 18-7 Measuring Limb Circumference

ADVANCED TECHNIQUE

Measuring Limb Circumference

Limb circumference is measured when a limb looks larger or smaller than its counterpart during inspection.

E During muscle relaxation or nonweight bearing, measure the limbs at exactly the same distance from a nearby joint (e.g., the knee or elbow) at the site of maximal limb diameter (Figure 18-7).

N Bilateral measurements should be within 1 to 3 cm of each other. A slight increase in the girth of the dominant arm is normal.

A A discrepancy in limb girth of 3 cm or more is abnormal.

P Atrophy results from disuse of a limb, as may occur in stroke.

P Swelling following trauma to soft tissue or bone (e.g., crush injury or fracture) results in an increased limb circumference.

P Unilateral hypertrophy can result from selected activities that use one side of the body more than the other (e.g., tennis arm).

P Unilateral hypertrophy may also be the result of compensating for a deficit in the corresponding limb. For example, a patient with hemiparesis of a limb will present with some degree of hypertrophy of the nonaffected arm muscles.

P A unilateral increase in calf girth may indicate a deep vein thrombosis. Calf girth alters prior to the development of a positive Homan's sign.

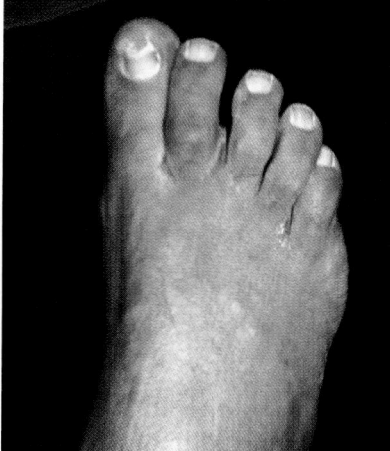

FIGURE 18-8 Joint Inflammation of Gout. Note the erythema and edema of the right 2nd metatarsal interphalangeal joint.

A Enlargement of the joint is an abnormal finding.

P Joint inflammation can result from inflammatory disorders such as rheumatoid arthritis and gout Figure 18-8.

P Trauma to the joint and its extra-articular structures will also result in joint inflammation.

A Deformity of the joint capsule is an abnormal finding.

P Immobility results in joint contractures, which cause the joint to be permanently fixated in one position. The acquired joint position may be one within its normal range of joint motion or an abnormal joint position.

P Joint destruction from rheumatoid arthritis may result in a joint becoming fixated in one position.

P Joint dislocation or subluxation will alter the normal contour of a joint. **Dislocation** refers to a complete dislodgment of one bone out of the joint cavity. **Subluxation** is a partial dislodgment of a bone from its place in the joint cavity.

A Alteration in periarticular skin and subcutaneous tissue is an abnormal finding.

P Trauma to the joint results in inflammation and bruising of the periarticular tissue. Joint trauma may include strain, sprain, contusion, dislocation, subluxation, or fracture within or near the joint capsule.

| **E** Examination | **N** Normal Findings | **A** Abnormal Findings | **P** Pathophysiology |

P The patient with rheumatoid arthritis often presents with periarticular skin atrophy and subcutaneous nodules near a joint (e.g., elbow).

P Synovial effusion within the joint capsule may cause a bulging appearance that extends into the periarticular area.

PALPATION

Muscle Tone

E 1. Palpate the muscle by applying light pressure with the finger pads of the dominant hand. Note any tenderness.

2. Note the change in muscle shape as the muscle belly (wide central aspect of the muscle) tapers off to become a tendon.

3. Ask the patient to alternately perform muscle relaxation and isometric muscle contraction. Note the change in palpable muscle tone between relaxation and isometric contraction.

4. Palpate the muscle belly during contraction induced by voluntary movement of a nearby joint.

5. Perform passive range of motion to all extremities and note whether these movements are smooth and sustained.

N Muscle tone refers to the partial muscle contraction state that is maintained in order for the muscle to respond quickly to the next stimulus. On palpation, the muscle should feel smooth and firm, even during the phase of muscle relaxation. There should be no pain. Normal muscle tone provides light resistance to passive stretch. During muscle contraction, especially against moderate external resistance to nearby joint movement, you will be able to palpate a significant overall increase in the firmness of the muscle belly. Muscle tone increases during anxiety or excitable states. Tone decreases during rest and sleep. You will be able to palpate the muscle belly and detect a change in its shape as it tapers down to become a tendon. The hypertrophied muscle will have a distinctive contour. You will detect muscle tautness even during the phase of relaxation.

A **Hypotonicity** (flaccidity) is a decrease in muscle tone. When the muscle is palpated, it feels flabby and soft to the touch. When a flaccid limb is held away from the body and then released, it falls quickly with gravity.

P Etiology of flaccidity may include diseases involving the muscles, anterior horn cells, or peripheral nerves.

A **Spasticity** refers to an increase in muscle tension on passive stretching (especially rapid or forced stretching of the muscle). It is often noted with extreme flexion or extension.

P Upper motor neuron dysfunction is associated with spasticity.

A The atrophied muscle will feel small and flabby, even during the phase of muscle contraction.

P Refer to the description of atrophy in the section Muscle Size and Shape.

A A muscle spasm represents persistent muscle contraction without relaxation. The muscle belly will feel taut and the patient may complain of discomfort over the muscle area. The spasm may also result in involuntary joint movement or a change in body position.

P Spasm follows fracture and may alter the distance between the bone fragments. Spasm is also common in the affected limbs of patients with paralysis, electrolyte imbalance, peripheral vascular disease, and cerebral palsy.

A Muscle pain may occur with or without palpation.

P Moderate to severe muscle pain of the neck, shoulders, or proximal thigh is associated with fibromyalgia. Palpation of certain trigger points located on the back of the neck, upper chest, trunk, low back, and lower extremities often result in burning and gnawing pain.

A Crepitus refers to a grating or crackling sensation caused by two rough musculoskeletal surfaces rubbing together. Crepitus is more commonly detected with joint movement than it is with muscle contraction.

P Crepitus detected during palpation of muscle contraction, especially in a nonarticulating area, may indicate shaft fracture due to trauma or loss of bone density. Muscle spasm following fracture may bring bone fragments in contact with each other, resulting in crepitus.

A Muscle masses detected on palpation are to be considered an abnormal finding.

P Muscle rupture (e.g., of the long head of the biceps muscle) will present as an inappropriate muscle mass above the joint. The muscle mass may be accentuated by muscle contraction.

P Tendon rupture may also result in an inappropriate muscle mass. An example is a complete rupture of the Achilles tendon, resulting in a mass noted in the calf area.

P Displaced fracture (e.g., of the femoral shaft near the hip joint) will often result in palpation of the displaced bone near a muscle.

P Complete dislocation (e.g., of the hip joint) will also result in palpation of the displaced bone near a muscle.

Joints

E 1. With the joint in its neutral anatomic position, begin palpating the joint by applying light pressure with the finger pads of the dominant hand 5 to 7 cm (2 to 3 inches) away from the center of the joint.

2. Palpate from the periphery inward to the center of the joint.

3. Note any swelling, pain, tenderness, warmth, or nodules.

N When the major skeletal joints are palpated in their neutral anatomic positions, the external joint contour will feel smooth, strong, and firm. The shape of the joint corresponds to that specific joint type. The area surrounding the joint (periarticular tissue) is free from swelling, pain, tenderness, warmth, and nodules. As the joint is moved through its normal range of motion, it should be able to articulate in proper alignment without any visible or palpable deformity. Palpation of joint movement produces a smooth sensation, without tactile detection of grating or popping. A synovial membrane is not palpable under normal circumstances.

A Bony enlargement or bony deformities of the joint are considered abnormal findings. See Table 18-9, which provides a tool for grading joint swelling, tenderness, and limitations.

P Urate deposits associated with gout will result in a reactive synovitis, producing joint enlargement. Urate crystals accumulate in the joint as a result of a prolonged elevation of serum uric acid. The affected joint will

| **E** Examination | **N** Normal Findings | **A** Abnormal Findings | **P** Pathophysiology |

TABLE 18-9 Grading of Joint Swelling, Tenderness, and Limitation

GRADE	SWELLING (S)	TENDERNESS (T)	LIMITATION (L)
0	None	None	None
1	Mild	Mild, but tolerable tenderness upon palpation	25% decrease in joint range of motion
2	Moderate	Moderate tenderness upon palpation (which the patient can tolerate but prefers not to)	50% decrease in joint range of motion
3	Marked	Light pressure or palpation induces an intolerable tenderness	75% decrease in joint range of motion
4	Maximum	Slight skin motion or sensation induces an intolerable tenderness	Complete loss of joint range of motion

0 = normal　　　　　　*2 = moderate abnormality*　　　*4 = maximum abnormality*
1 = mild abnormality　　*3 = marked abnormality*

Example: S3/T3/L4 = marked joint swelling with intolerable joint tenderness upon light pressure and with complete loss of joint range of motion.

be extremely warm and tender to the touch. Although the great toe is most commonly affected, gout can also affect other joints.

A Subcutaneous nodules detected in the periarticular area are abnormal.

P Rheumatoid arthritis is associated with subcutaneous nodules over the bony prominences and extensor joint surfaces (e.g., olecranon process of the elbow). These nodules are painless, firm but movable, and of normal skin color. They are more of a cosmetic concern than a threat to nearby joint function, although the overlying skin is at risk for breakdown due to irritation or pressure.

P Tophi nodules may be detected in the patient with chronic gout, and they represent soft tissue reaction to uric acid crystal deposition. They are often found on the great toes.

A Palpable, audible, severe crepitus that presents as more of a coarse than a fine sensation is abnormal.

P Crepitus is often palpated in joints affected by acute rheumatoid arthritis and degenerative joint disease due to the contact of bone surfaces.

P Bony overgrowth, muscle contracture, dislocation, and subluxation are associated with joint crepitus.

A Any tenderness felt on light touch or joint palpation is considered abnormal. You must differentiate between tenderness on palpation of the joint at rest versus palpation during joint movement.

P Joint pain due to septic arthritis can occur 10 to 14 days after an untreated streptococcal pharyngitis or tonsillitis.

P Increased joint capsule pressure with a significant joint effusion may induce discomfort with light touch or pressure to the joint in the neutral position.

P Localized joint tenderness may be detected in the presence of joint contusion, infection, or synovitis.

A Periarticular warmth, with temperature exceeding overall body temperature, indicates an underlying problem.

E Examination	**N** Normal Findings	**A** Abnormal Findings	**P** Pathophysiology

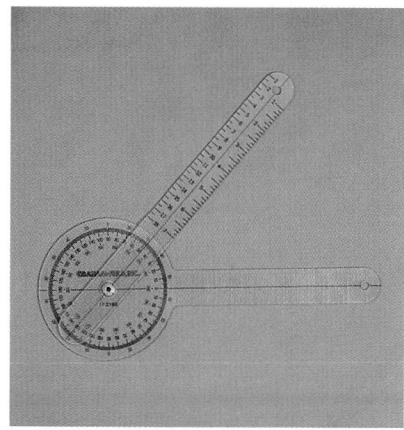

A. Goniometer

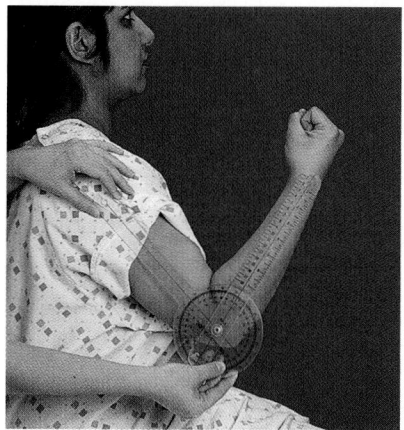

B. Use of Goniometer

FIGURE 18-9 Goniometer and Its Use

Assessing Joint ROM: Using a Goniometer

E 1. With the joint in its neutral position, place the center of the goniometer over the joint so that the two distal arms of the goniometer are in alignment with the proximal and distal bones adjacent to that joint.

2. Move the joint through its ROM and note the degree of the joint angle visible on the center of the goniometer (Figure 18-9).

N Refer to the specific sections on joints for the ROM for each joint movement.

A Abnormalities of joint function are indicated by the inability of the patient to voluntarily and comfortably move a joint in the directions and to the degrees that are considered the norms for that joint.

P Degenerative joint disease, rheumatoid arthritis, and joint trauma are some of the many musculoskeletal disorders that prevent the affected joint from moving through its normal ROM.

P Joint inflammation (e.g., due to acute rheumatoid arthritis or recent trauma) and gout produce significant joint warmth because of the increased localized perfusion associated with the inflammatory process.

RANGE OF MOTION (ROM)

E 1. Ask the patient to move the joint through each of its various ROM movements.

2. Note angle of each joint movement.

3. Note any pain, tenderness, or crepitus.

4. If the patient is unable to perform active ROM, then passively move each joint through its ROM.

5. Always stop if the patient complains of pain, and never push a joint beyond its anatomic angle.

6. Use a goniometer to determine exact ROM in joints with limited ROM. Refer to the Advanced Technique on Using a Goniometer.

MUSCLE STRENGTH

Each muscle group is assessed for strength via the same movements as are performed in range of motion.

E 1. Note whether muscle groups are strong and equal.

2. Always compare right and left sides of paired muscle groups.

3. Note involuntary movements.

N Normal muscle strength allows for complete voluntary range of joint motion against both gravity and moderate to full resistance. Muscle strength is equal bilaterally. There is no observed involuntary muscle movement.

A A decrease in skeletal muscle strength is significant if complete range of joint motion is either impossible or possible only without resistance or gravity.

TABLE 18-10 Muscle Strength Grading Scale

FUNCTIONAL ABILITY DESCRIPTION	SCALE (%)	0–5/5 SCALE
Complete range of joint motion against both gravity and full manual resistance from the nurse.	100%	5/5 Normal (N)
Complete range of joint motion against both gravity and moderate manual resistance from the nurse.	75%	4/5 Good (G)
Complete range of joint motion possible only without manual resistance from the nurse.	50%	3/5 Fair (F)
Complete range of joint motion possible only with the joint supported by the nurse to eliminate the force of gravity and without any manual resistance from the nurse.	25%	2/5 Poor (P)
Muscle contraction detectable but insufficient to move the joint even when the forces of both gravity and manual resistance have been eliminated.	10%	1/5 Trace (Tr)
Complete absence of visible and palpable muscle contraction.	0%	0/5 None (0)

P Local decrease in muscle strength will accompany muscle atrophy of the limbs secondary to disuse.

P Diffuse reduction in muscle strength is associated with general atrophy, severe fatigue, malnutrition, muscle relaxant medications, long-term steroid use, and deteriorating neuromuscular disorders. These deteriorating neuromuscular diseases include but are not limited to ALS, MD, MS, myasthenia gravis, and Guillain-Barré syndrome.

A One-sided muscle weakness or paralysis is considered abnormal.

P Unilateral weakness or paralysis is indicative of **hemiparesis** (**hemiplegia**) from a cerebrovascular accident, brain tumor, or head trauma.

EXAMINATION OF JOINTS
Temporomandibular Joint

E 1. Stand in front of the patient.
2. Inspect the right and left temporomandibular joints (see Figure 18-10).
3. Palpate the temporomandibular joints (see Figure 18-11).
   a. Place your index and middle fingers over the joint.
   b. Ask the patient to open and close the mouth.
   c. Feel the depression into which your fingers move with an open mouth.
   d. Note the smoothness with which the mandible moves.
   e. Note any audible or palpable click as the mouth opens.
4. Assess ROM (see Figure 18-12). Ask the patient to:
   a. Open the mouth as wide as possible.

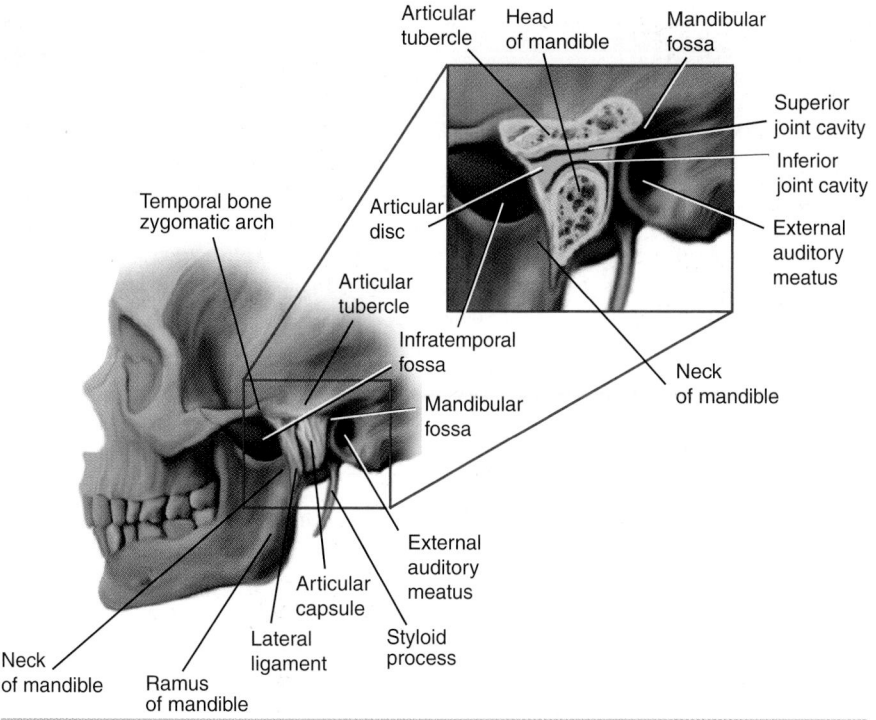

FIGURE 18-10   Anatomy of the Temporomandibular Joint (Sagittal Section)

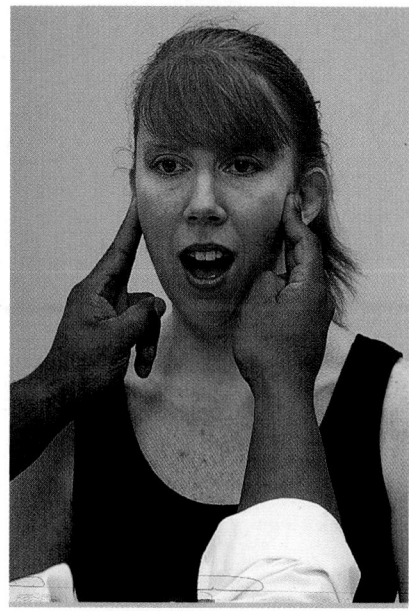

FIGURE 18-11   Palpation of the Temporomandibular Joint

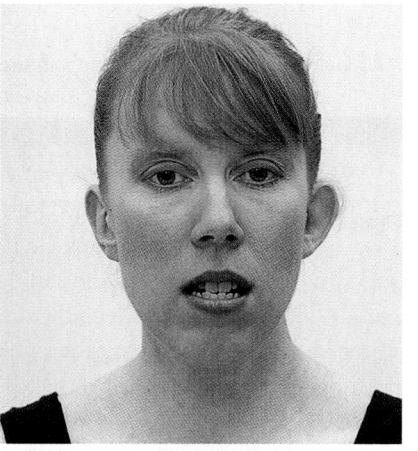

A. Pushing Out the Lower Jaw

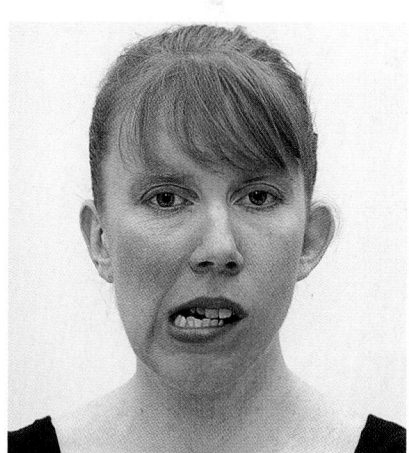

B. Moving the Jaw from Side to Side

FIGURE 18-12   Range of Motion of the Temporomandibular Joint

    b. Push out the lower jaw.

    c. Move the jaw from side to side.

5. Palpate the strength of the masseter and temporalis muscles as the patient clenches the teeth. This assesses cranial nerve V.

N It is normal to hear or palpate a click when the mouth opens. The mouth can normally open 3 to 6 cm with ease. The lower jaw protrudes without deviating to the side and moves 1 to 2 cm with lateral movement.

A Pain, limited ROM, and crepitus can occur in temporomandibular joint dysfunction.

P Temporomandibular joint dysfunction can occur secondary to malocclusion, arthritis, dislocation, poorly fitting dentures, myofacial dysfunction, and trauma.

| **E** Examination | **N** Normal Findings | **A** Abnormal Findings | **P** Pathophysiology |

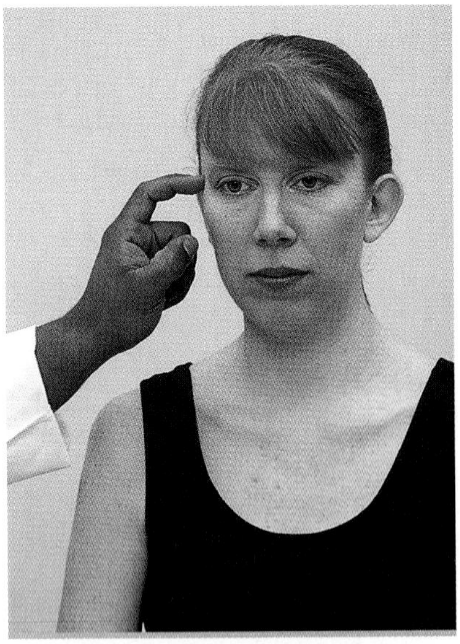

FIGURE 18-13 Assessing for Chvostek's Sign

Assessing for Neuroexcitability: Chvostek's Sign

E
1. The patient can be assessed in the standing, sitting, or supine position.
2. While the patient is facing forward, tap the side of the face just below the temple area, using the middle or index finger (Figure 18-13).
3. Observe for ipsilateral changes in facial expression immediately after tapping the face.
4. Repeat the procedure on the other side of the face.

N There will be no change in the patient's facial expression when the temple area is stimulated.

A A positive Chvostek's sign, indicated by ipsilateral muscle spasm of the mouth and cheek, is abnormal. The muscle spasm will occur in an upward direction, toward the temple.

P A positive Chvostek's sign is suggestive of neuroexcitability associated with hypocalcemia and tetanus infection.

Cervical Spine

E
1. Stand behind the patient.
2. Inspect the position of the cervical spine.
3. Palpate the spinous processes (see Figure 18-14) of the cervical spine and the muscles of the neck.
4. Stand in front of the patient.
5. Assess the ROM of the cervical spine (see Figure 18-15). Ask the patient to:
   a. Touch the chin to the chest (flexion).
   b. Look up at the ceiling (hyperextension).
   c. Move each ear to the shoulder on its respective side without elevating the shoulder (lateral bending).
   d. Turn the head to each side to look at the shoulder (rotation).
6. Assess strength of the cervical spine by repeating the movements in step 5d while applying opposing force. This also assesses the function of cranial nerve XI.

N The cervical spine's alignment is straight and the head is held erect. The normal ROM for the cervical spine is flexion—45°, hyperextension—55°, lateral bending—40° to each side, rotation—70° to each side. Hypertrophy of the neck muscles due to weight-lifting exercises will produce the appearance of a thick neck.

A A neck that is not erect and straight is abnormal.

P Degenerative joint disease of the cervical vertebrae may result in lateral tilting of the head and neck.

P Torticollis is discussed in Chapter 11.

A A change in the size of the neck is abnormal.

P Klippel-Feil syndrome is the congenital absence of one or more cervical vertebrae along with fusion of the upper cervical vertebrae and bilateral elevation of the scapulae, resulting in a shortened neck appearance. It may be accompanied by a low hairline, webbing of the neck, and decreased neck mobility.

E Examination		**N** Normal Findings		**A** Abnormal Findings		**P** Pathophysiology

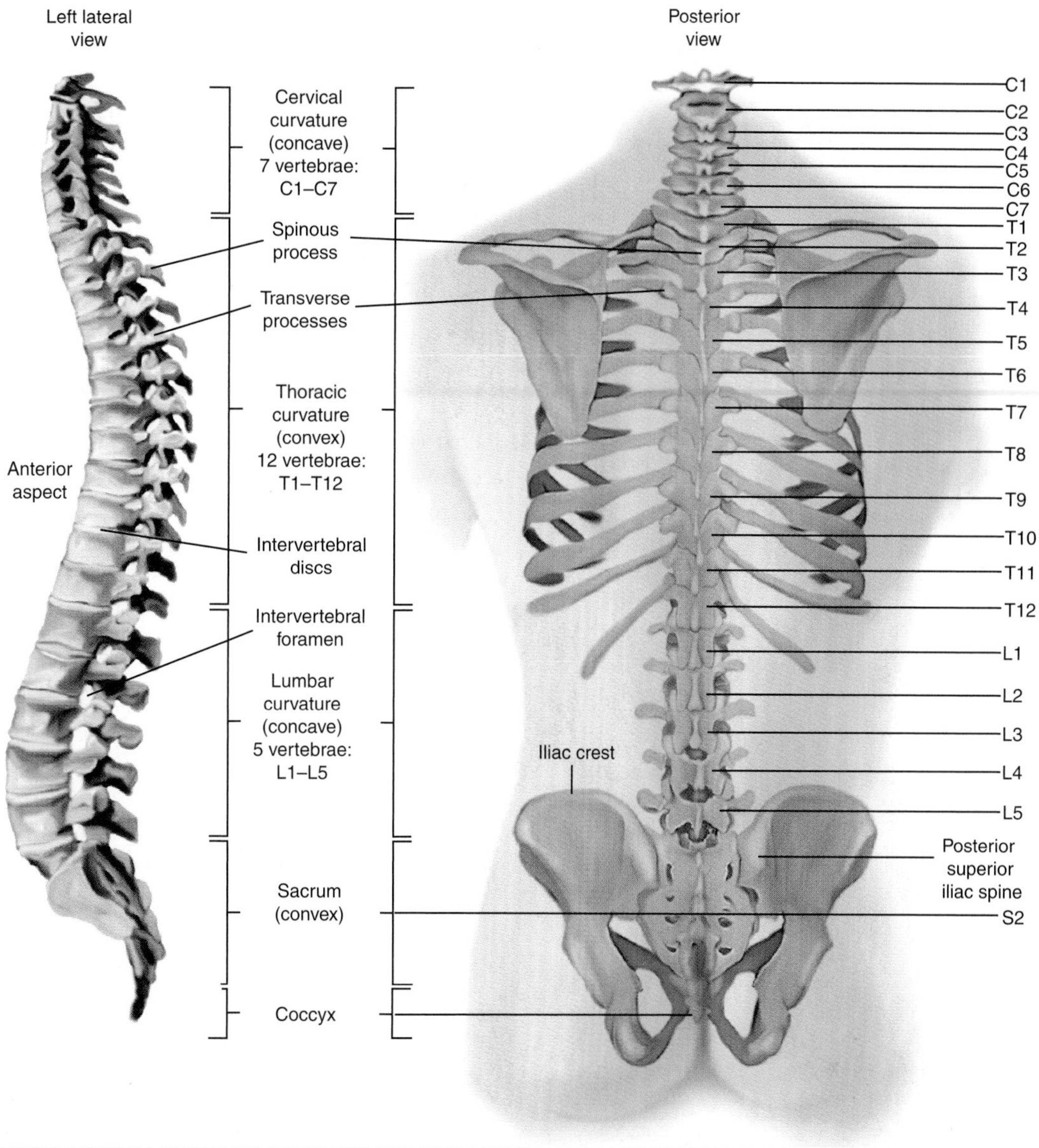

Left lateral view
Posterior view
Cervical curvature (concave) 7 vertebrae: C1–C7
Spinous process
Transverse processes
Thoracic curvature (convex) 12 vertebrae: T1–T12
Anterior aspect
Intervertebral discs
Intervertebral foramen
Lumbar curvature (concave) 5 vertebrae: L1–L5
Sacrum (convex)
Coccyx
Iliac crest
Posterior superior iliac spine
C1
C2
C3
C4
C5
C6
C7
T1
T2
T3
T4
T5
T6
T7
T8
T9
T10
T11
T12
L1
L2
L3
L4
L5
S2

FIGURE 18-14 Anatomy of the Spine

Hyperextension
Flexion
0
55
45
Right
Left
0
40
40
0
Left
Right
70
70

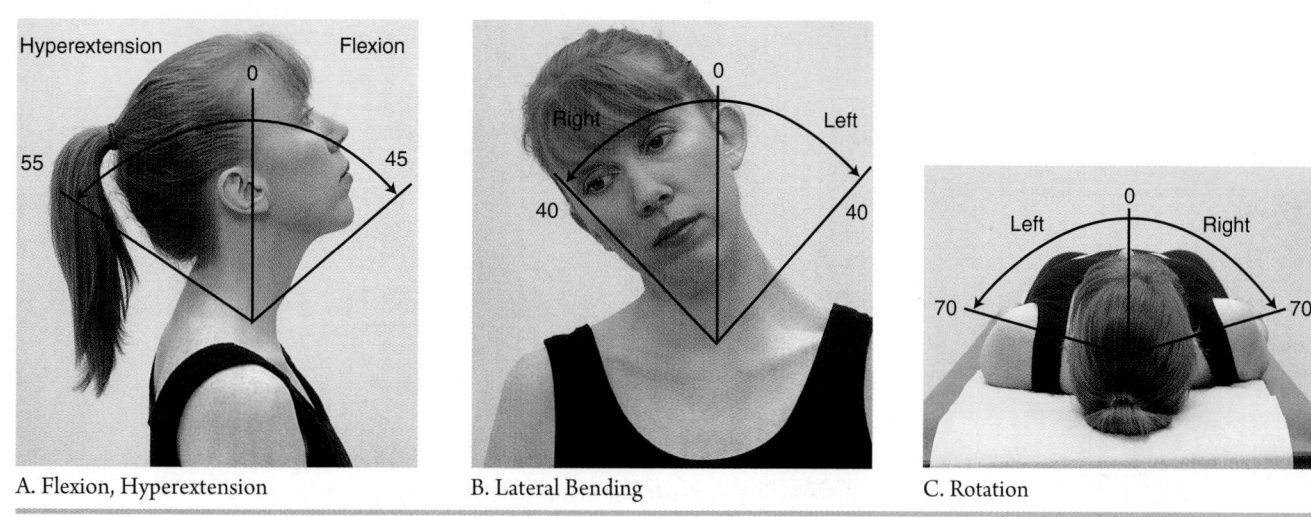

A. Flexion, Hyperextension B. Lateral Bending C. Rotation

FIGURE 18-15 Range of Motion of the Cervical Spine

A Inability of the patient to perform ROM, and pain and tenderness on palpation are abnormal.

P Osteoarthritis, neck injury, disc degeneration (among aging patients or from occupational stress), and spondylosis can cause these cervical spine signs or symptoms.

Shoulders

E 1. Stand in front of the patient.
2. Inspect the size, shape, and symmetry of the shoulders (Figure 18-16).
3. Move behind the patient and inspect the scapula for size, shape, and symmetry.
4. Palpate the shoulders and surrounding muscles.
   a. Move from the sternoclavicular joint along the clavicle to the acromioclavicular joint.
   b. Palpate the acromion process, subacromial area, greater tubercle of the humerus, the anterior aspect of the glenohumeral joint, and the biceps groove.
5. Assess ROM of the shoulders (see Figure 18-17). Ask the patient to:
   a. Place arms at the side, elbows extended, and move the arms forward in an arc (forward flexion).
   b. Move the arms backward in an arc as far as possible (hyperextension).
   c. Place arms at side, elbows extended, and move both arms out to the sides in an arc until the palms touch together overhead (abduction).
   d. Move one arm at a time in an arc toward the midline and cross it as far as possible (adduction).
   e. Place hands behind the back and reach up, trying to touch the scapula (internal rotation).

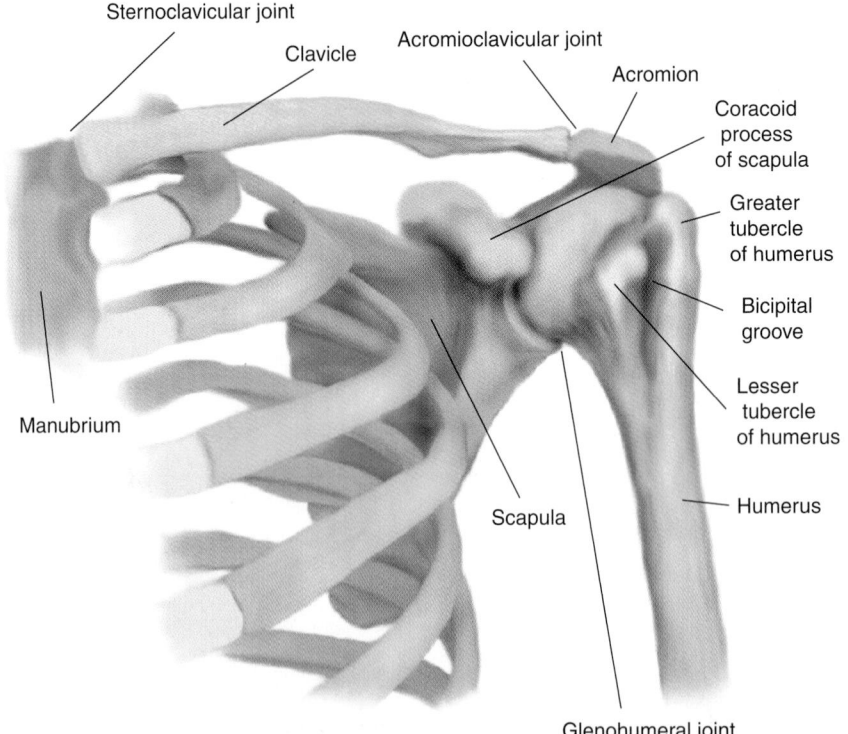

FIGURE 18-16 Anatomy of the Shoulder Joint

| **E** Examination | **N** Normal Findings | **A** Abnormal Findings | **P** Pathophysiology |

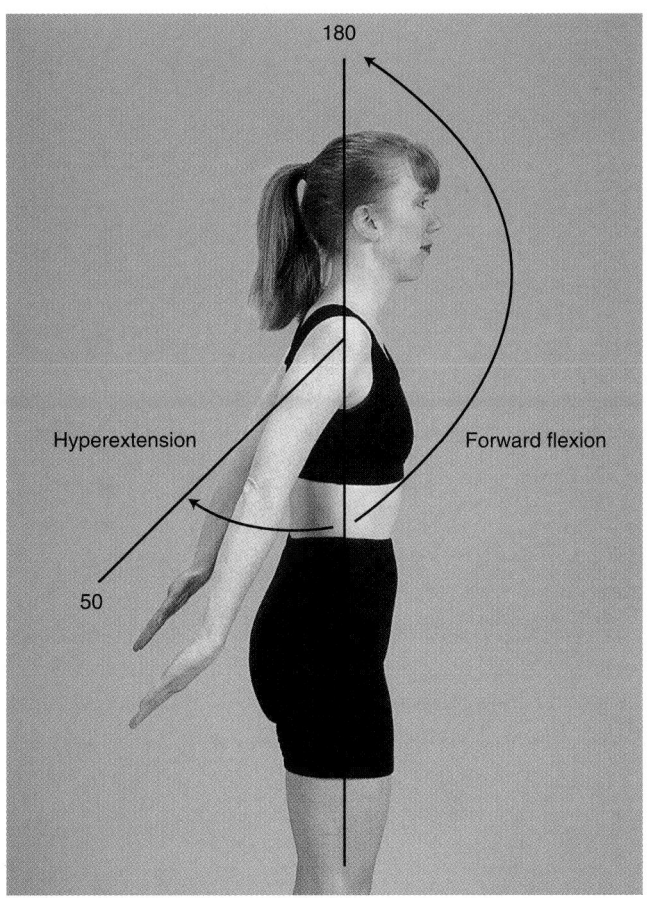

A. Forward Flexion, Hyperextension

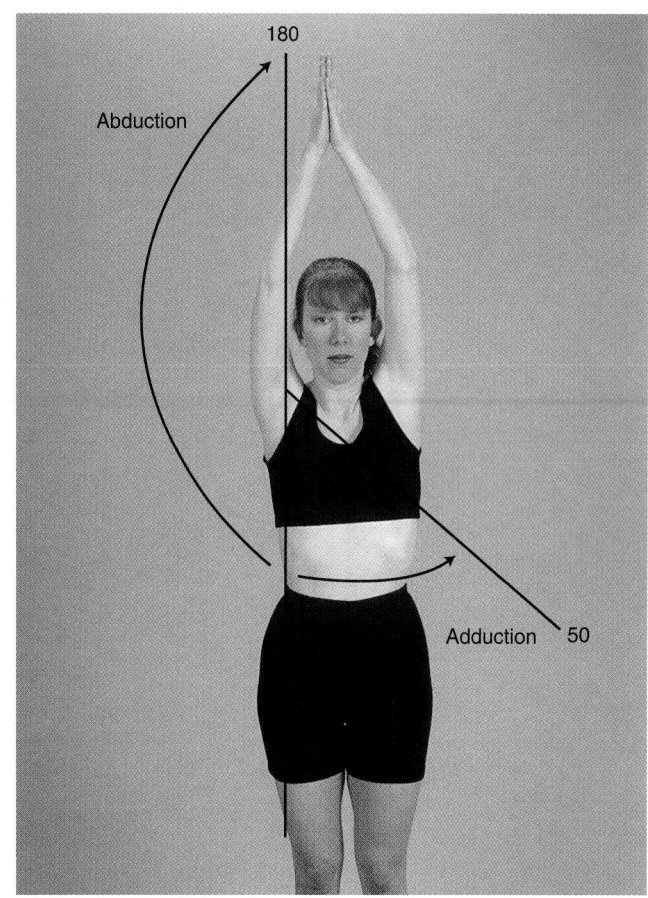

B. Abduction, Adduction

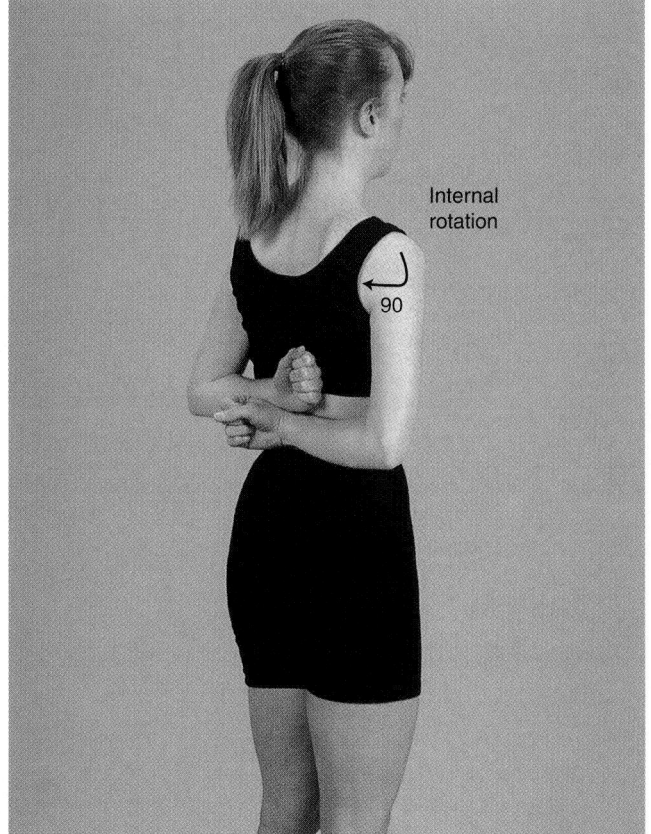

C. Internal Rotation

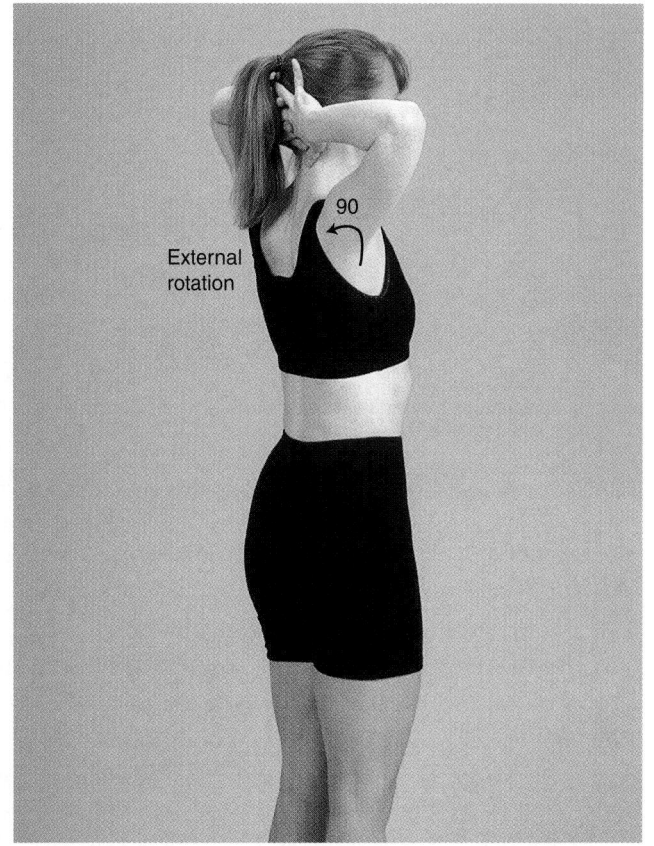

D. External Rotation

FIGURE 18-17   **Range of Motion of the Shoulder Joint**

f. Place both hands behind the head with elbows flexed (external rotation).

g. Shrug the shoulders. This assesses cranial nerve XI function.

6. Assess strength of the shoulders by applying opposing force to the ROM movement in step 5 g.

N The shoulders are equal in height. There is no fluid palpable in the shoulder area. Crepitus is absent. The normal ROM for the shoulder is forward flexion—180°, hyperextension—50°, abduction—180°, adduction—50°, internal rotation—90°, external rotation—90°.

A Increased outward prominence of the scapula (winging) is an abnormal finding.

P Scapular winging is indicative of serratus anterior muscle injury or weakness.

A Decreased movement, pain with movement, swelling from fluid, and asymmetry are abnormal.

P These findings are associated with immobility, osteoarthritis, and injury. Swelling from fluid is usually best seen anteriorly.

P A significant decrease in shoulder ROM is seen in frozen shoulder (adhesive capsulitis). In frozen shoulder, the glenohumeral joint gradually loses function, especially abduction and external rotation. Stroke with loss of shoulder movement and rotator cuff pathology are common etiologies.

P Bursitis of the shoulder can result from overuse of the shoulder in repetitive activity (either a new activity such as leaf raking and car polishing or a familiar activity such as swimming).

P An acromioclavicular joint separation (separated shoulder) causes pain in the acromioclavicular joint. Swelling frequently occurs at the distal end of the clavicle.

P Shoulder subluxation and dislocation are common athletic injuries. Patients with recurrent subluxations may feel the glenohumeral joint pop out of the socket and pop back in without medical intervention. The shoulder may lose its usual rounded contour. With an anterior dislocation, fluid is usually seen anteriorly, whereas with a posterior dislocation, fluid is usually best seen posteriorly.

P In biceps tendinitis, the patient is tender in the bicipital groove. Excessive straining, as with lifting heavy objects, can rupture an inflamed biceps tendon. This can lead to a bulge in the antecubital fossa.

ADVANCED TECHNIQUE

Assessing for Rotator Cuff Damage: Drop Arm Test

The rotator cuff is composed of four muscles (supraspinatus, infraspinatus, teres minor, and subscapularis) and their tendons. The tendons insert into the humeral tuberosities. The rotator cuff stabilizes the glenohumeral joint.

The drop arm test assesses for rotator cuff damage.

E 1. Manually abduct the patient's affected arm.

2. Ask the patient to slowly lower the raised arm to the side while maintaining extension of the arm.

3. Observe the speed at which the patient lowers the arm.

N The patient will be able to slowly lower the arm to the side while maintaining the arm in extension.

A An abnormal drop arm test is manifested by the inability of the patient to slowly lower the arm to the side (e.g., the arm quickly falls to the side of the torso), or by severe pain occurring in the shoulder while the arm is slowly lowered to the side.

P An abnormal drop arm test is indicative of a rotator cuff tear. It is caused by trauma to the shoulder.

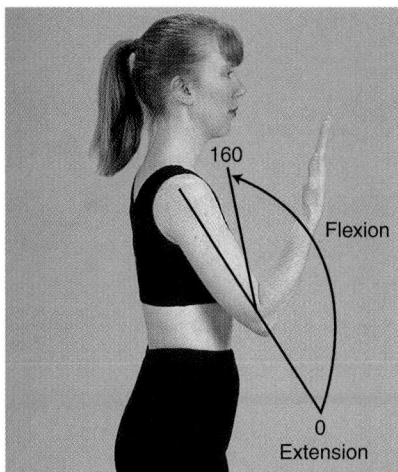

160

Flexion

0
Extension

A. Flexion, Extension

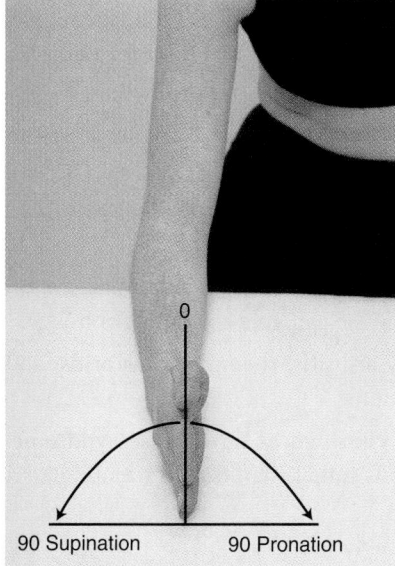

0

90 Supination   90 Pronation

B. Supination, Pronation

FIGURE 18-19 Range of Motion of the Elbow Joint

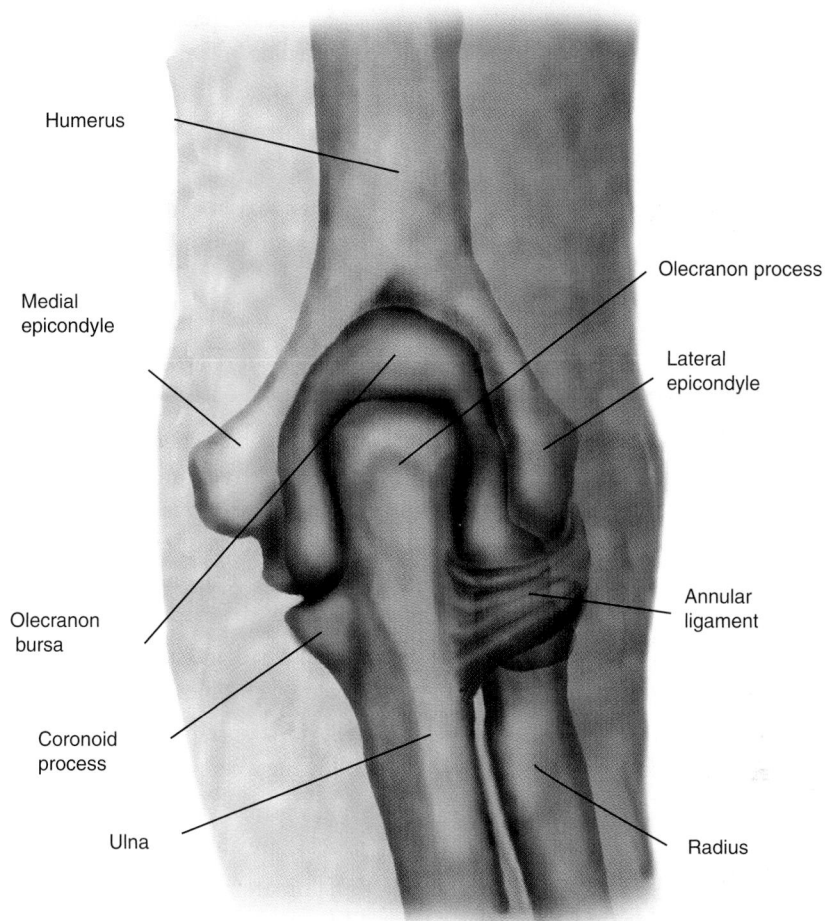

Humerus

Olecranon process

Medial epicondyle

Lateral epicondyle

Annular ligament

Olecranon bursa

Coronoid process

Ulna

Radius

FIGURE 18-18 Anatomy of the Elbow Joint (Posterior View, Right Elbow)

Elbows

E 1. Stand to the side of the elbow being examined.

2. Support the patient's forearm on the side that is being examined (approximately 70°).

3. Inspect the elbow in flexed and extended positions. Note the olecranon process and the grooves on each side of the olecranon process (Figure 18-18).

4. Using your thumb and middle fingers, palpate the elbow. Note the olecranon process, the olecranon bursa, the groove on each side of the olecranon process, and the medial and lateral epicondyles of the humerus.

5. Assess ROM of the elbows (Figure 18-19). Ask the patient to:
   a. Bend the elbow (flexion).
   b. Straighten the elbow (extension).
   c. Hold the arm straight out, bent at the elbow, and turn the palm upward toward the ceiling (supination).
   d. Turn the palm downward toward the floor (pronation).

6. Assess strength of the elbow:
   a. Stabilize the patient's arm at the elbow with your nondominant hand. With your dominant hand, grasp the patient's wrist.
   b. Ask the patient to flex the elbow (pulling it toward the chest) while you apply opposing resistance (see Figure 18-20).

E Examination   **N** Normal Findings   **A** Abnormal Findings   **P** Pathophysiology

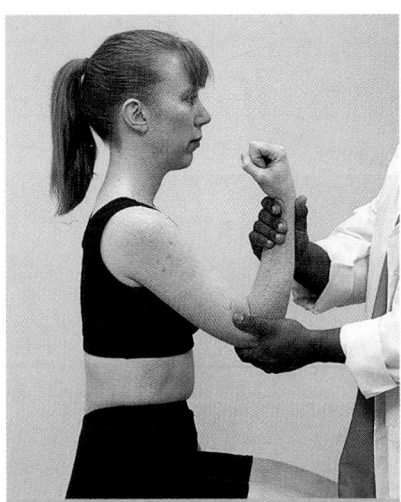

FIGURE 18-20 Muscle Strength of the Elbow

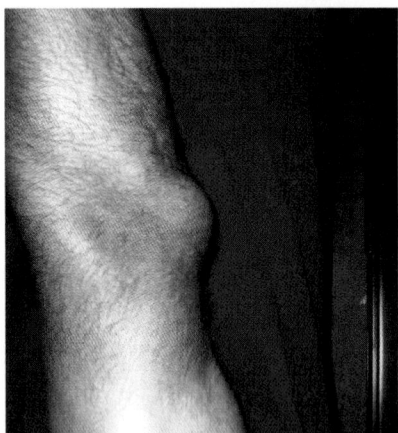

FIGURE 18-21 Olecranon Bursitis

c. Ask the patient to extend the elbow (pushing it away from the chest) while you apply opposing resistance.

N The elbows are at the same height and are symmetrical in appearance. The normal ROM for the elbow is flexion—160°, extension—0°, supination—90°, pronation—90°.

A Elbows that are not symmetrical are abnormal. The forearm is not in its usual alignment. Pain is present.

P These findings occur in a dislocation or a subluxation of the elbow. They usually occur from sports-related injuries, falls, or motor vehicle accidents.

A Localized tenderness and pain with elbow flexion, extension, or both are abnormal.

P Epicondylitis occurs from repetitive motions such as swinging a tennis racquet, hammering, using a screwdriver, tight gripping, and other activities involving repetitive movements of the forearm. Lateral epicondylitis (tennis elbow) is caused by injury to the extensor tendon at the lateral epicondyle, and medial epicondylitis (golfer's elbow) is caused by injury to the flexor tendon at the medial epicondyle.

P Radial head fractures usually result from falls. Frequently, the elbow is flexed in a 90° position.

P A flexion contracture of the elbow may be seen in a patient with hemiparesis following a cerebrovascular accident.

A Red, warm, swollen, and tender areas in the grooves beside the olecranon process are abnormal. Synovial fluid may be palpable and is soft or boggy.

P Inflammatory processes such as gouty arthritis, rheumatoid arthritis, and SLE can cause these clinical manifestations.

P Olecranon bursitis (Figure 18-21) is classified as an overuse syndrome. It usually results from repetitive motions rather than from an acute injury. ROM is usually not affected.

Wrists and Hands

E 1. Stand in front of the patient.
2. Inspect the wrists and the palmar and dorsal aspects of the hands. Note the shape, position, contour, and number of fingers (see Figure 18-22).

ADVANCED TECHNIQUE

Assessing for Neuroexcitability: Trousseau's Sign

E 1. Place the patient in a sitting or a supine position.
2. Apply a blood pressure cuff to the patient's upper arm.
3. Inflate the blood pressure cuff to 10mm Hg above the patient's systolic blood pressure for 1 to 3 minutes.
4. Observe for twitching of the hand and fingers on the side being tested.

N There will be no visible twitching of the hand and fingers during cuff inflation.

A A positive Trousseau's sign, indicated by visible ipsilateral twitching of the hand and fingers during cuff inflation, is abnormal.

P A positive Trousseau's sign is suggestive of neuroexcitability associated with hypocalcemia and tetanus infection.

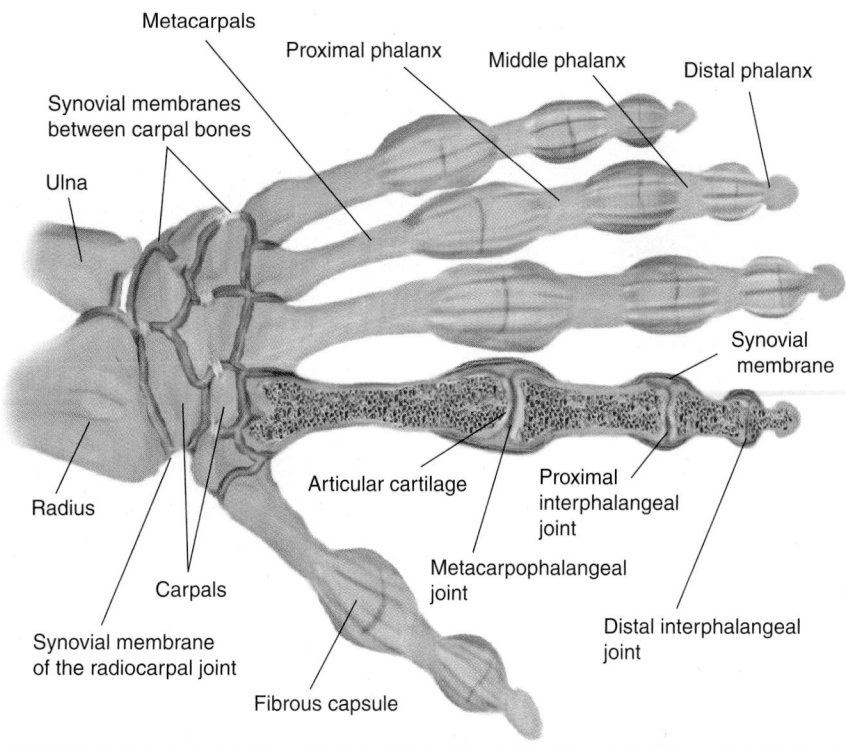

FIGURE 18-22 Anatomy of the Wrist and Hand

Labels on figure: Metacarpals; Proximal phalanx; Middle phalanx; Distal phalanx; Synovial membranes between carpal bones; Ulna; Synovial membrane; Radius; Articular cartilage; Proximal interphalangeal joint; Carpals; Metacarpophalangeal joint; Distal interphalangeal joint; Synovial membrane of the radiocarpal joint; Fibrous capsule

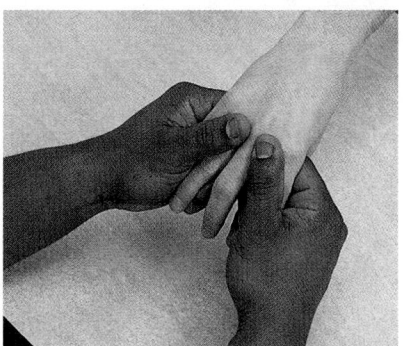

FIGURE 18-23 Palpating the Wrist Joint

A. Metacarpophalangeal Joint

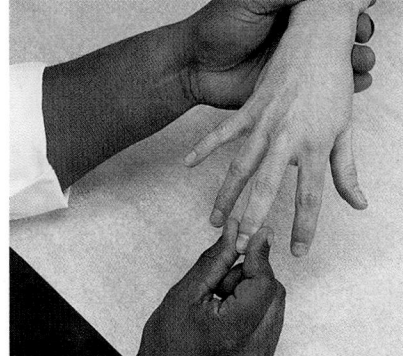

B. Interphalangeal Joint

FIGURE 18-24 Palpating the Hand Joints

3. Inspect the **thenar eminence** (the rounded prominence at the base of the thumb).

4. Support the patient's hand in your two hands, with your fingers underneath the patient's hands and your thumbs on the dorsum of the patient's hand.

5. Palpate the joints of the wrists by moving your thumbs from side to side. Feel the natural indentations (Figure 18-23).

6. Palpate the joints of the hand:
   a. Use your thumbs to palpate the metacarpophalangeal joints, which are immediately distal to and on each side of the knuckle (Figure 18-24A).
   b. Between your thumb and index finger, gently pinch the sides of the proximal and distal interphalangeal joints (Figure 18-24B).

7. Assess the ROM of the wrists and hands (Figure 18-25). Ask the patient to:
   a. Straighten the hand (extension) and bend it up at the wrist toward the ceiling (hyperextension).
   b. Bend the hand down at the wrist toward the floor (flexion).
   c. Bend the fingers up at the metacarpophalangeal joint toward the ceiling (hyperextension).
   d. Bend the fingers down at the metacarpophalangeal joint toward the floor (flexion).
   e. Place the hands on a flat surface and move them side to side (radial deviation is movement toward the thumb, and ulnar deviation is movement toward the little finger) without moving the elbow.
   f. Make a fist with the thumb on the outside of the clenched fingers.
   g. Spread the fingers apart.

| **E** Examination | **N** Normal Findings | **A** Abnormal Findings | **P** Pathophysiology |

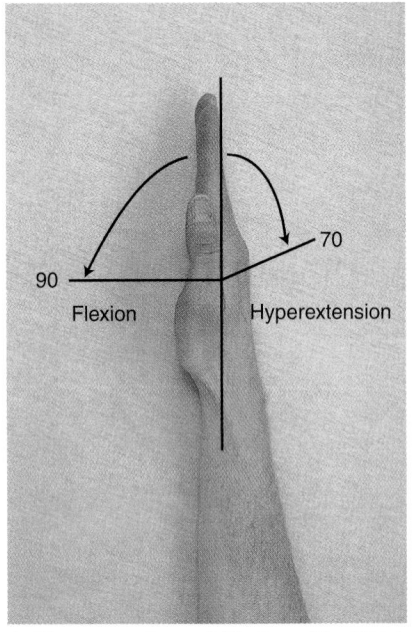

A. Hyperextension and Flexion of the Wrist

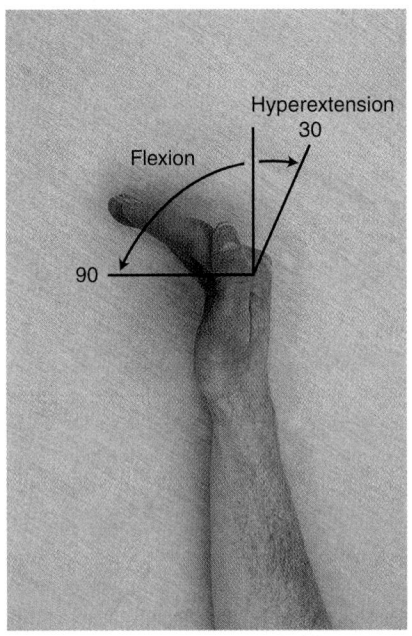

B. Flexion and Hyperextension of the Fingers

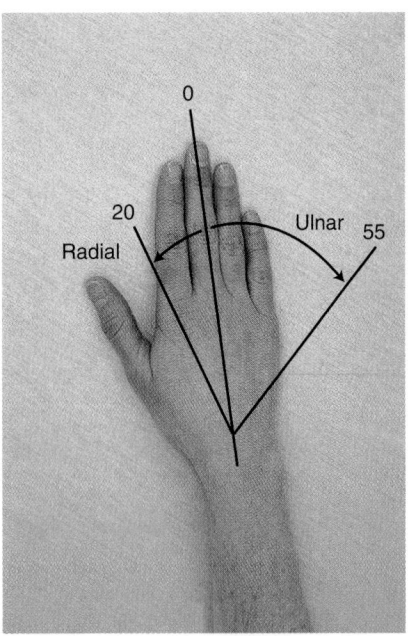

C. Radial and Ulnar Deviation of the Wrist

FIGURE 18-25 **Range of Motion of the Wrist and Hand Joints**

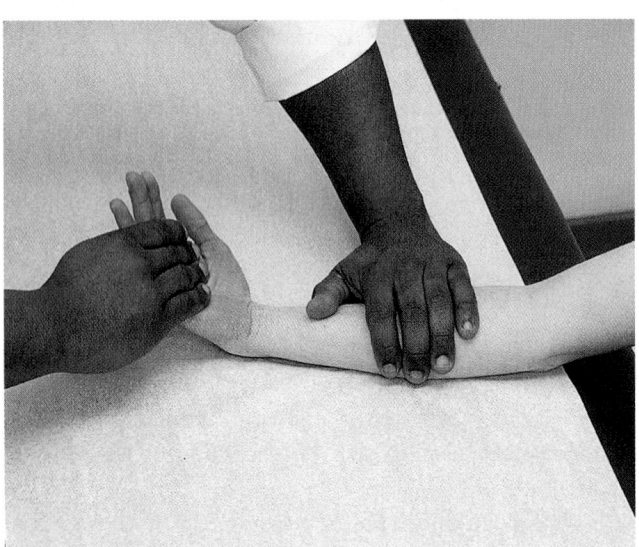

FIGURE 18-26 **Muscle Strength of the Wrist**

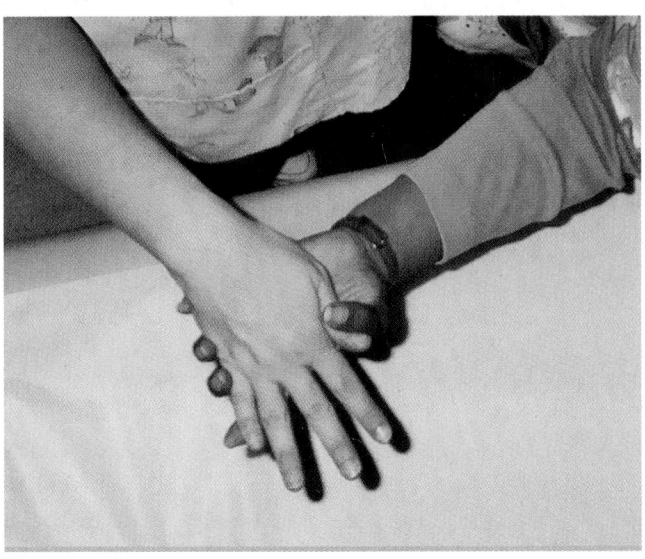

FIGURE 18-27 **Muscle Strength of the Fingers**

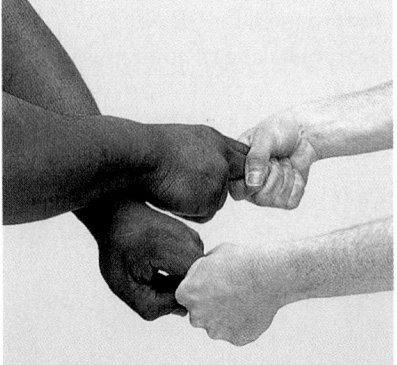

FIGURE 18-28 **Muscle Strength of the Hand Grasp**

    h. Touch the thumb to each fingertip. Touch the thumb to the base of the little finger.

8. Assess the strength of the wrists. Ask the patient to:

    a. Place the arm on a table with the forearm supinated. Stabilize the forearm by placing your nondominant hand on it.

    b. Flex the wrist while you apply resistance with your dominant hand (Figure 18-26).

    c. Extend the wrist while you apply resistance.

9. Assess the strength of the fingers. Ask the patient to:

    a. Spread the fingers apart while you apply resistance (Figure 18-27).

    b. Push the fingers together while you apply resistance.

10. Assess the strength of the hand grasp. Ask the patient to:

    a. Grasp your dominant index and middle fingers in the patient's dominant hand and your nondominant index and middle fingers in the patient's nondominant hand (Figure 18-28).

b. Squeeze your fingers as hard as possible.
c. Release the grasp.

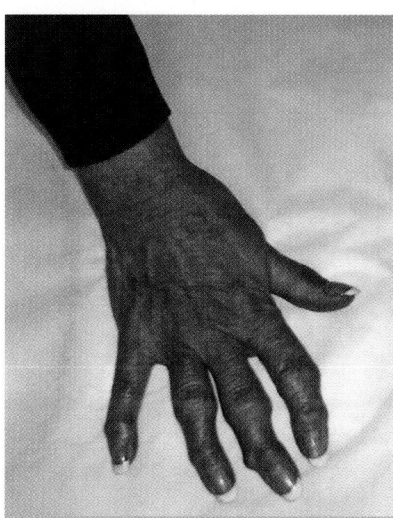

FIGURE 18-29 Bouchard's Nodes and Heberden's Nodes

N There are five fingers on each hand. The normal range of motion for the wrists is extension—0°, hyperextension—70°, flexion—90°, radial deviation—20°, ulnar deviation—55°. The normal range of motion for the metacarpophalangeal joints is: hyperextension—30° and flexion—90°.

A Extra fingers, loss of fingers, or webbing between fingers is abnormal.

P **Polydactyly** is the congenital presence of extra digits. **Syndactyly** is the congenital webbing or fusion of fingers or toes.

A Bony enlargement or bony deformities of the joints of the hand are abnormal.

P Osteoarthritis is associated with bony enlargement of the proximal interphalangeal joint (**Bouchard's node**) and the distal interphalangeal joint (**Heberden's node**) of the finger. These enlargements are hard and nontender. Bony enlargement may be masked by subcutaneous swelling. Bony enlargement is usually symmetrical (Figure 18-29).

P Rheumatoid arthritis results in ulnar deviation (Figure 18-30), swan-neck deformity, and boutonniere deformities of the fingers. In ulnar deviation, the fingers deviate to the ulnar side of the body. In swan-neck deformity, there is flexion of the metacarpophalangeal joint, hyperextension of the proximal interphalangeal joint, and flexion of the distal interphalangeal joint. In other words, the finger appears to go up, down, and up again. In boutonniere deformity, there is flexion of the proximal interphalangeal joint with hyperextension of the distal interphalangeal joint. The patient frequently complains of pain, especially early in the morning. The joints may feel boggy on palpation. ROM may be restricted.

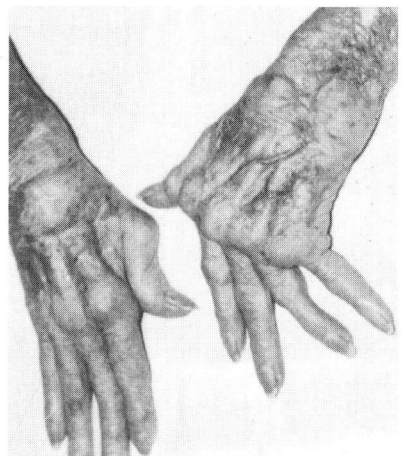

FIGURE 18-30 Ulnar Deviation

LIFE 360°

Living with Rheumatoid Arthritis

Look at the hand of the patient in Figure 18-29. How would you feel if you had a condition such as this? What would the impact be on your body image? Self-esteem? What environmental challenges might you encounter? What types of biases might you experience? What resources are available in the community to assist you?

NURSING**TIP**

Significance of Hand Grasp Strength

Although some nurses measure hand grasp strength as part of assessment, the true significance of this measurement may be in representing the patient's ability to respond to a command. A strong hand grasp around an object (e.g., the nurse's fingers or hand) as demonstrated by patients with brain disorders may actually represent a reflex action. When assessing muscle strength, arm muscle strength should thus always be considered more representative of muscle strength than is hand grasp strength.

E Examination   **N** Normal Findings   **A** Abnormal Findings   **P** Pathophysiology

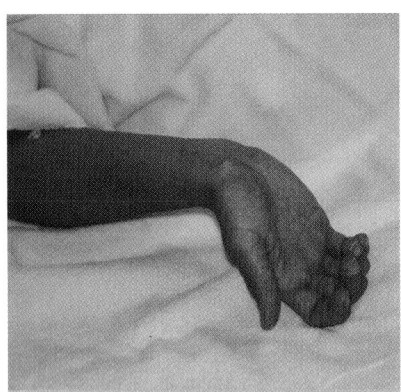

FIGURE 18-31 **Ganglion Cyst.**
Courtesy of Mary A. Hitcho.

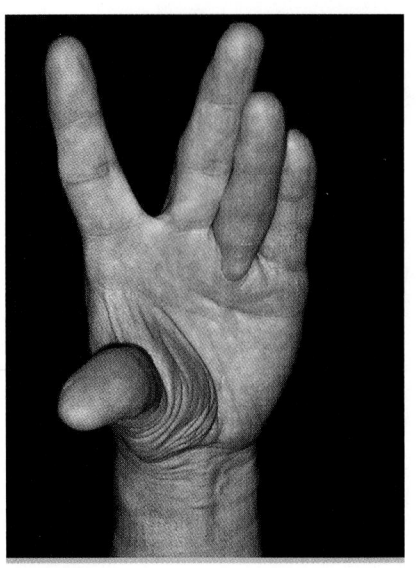

FIGURE 18-32 **Dupuytren's Contracture**

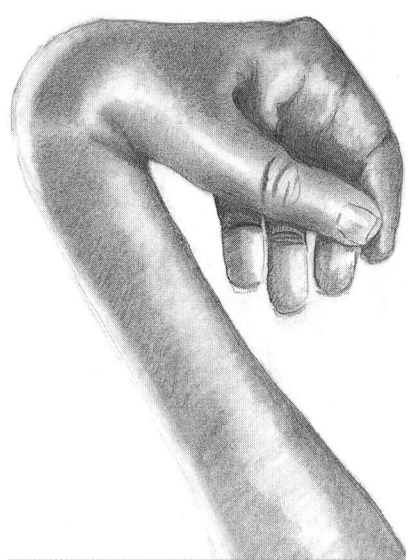

FIGURE 18-33 **Flexion Ankylosis**

A A round, cystic growth near the tendons of the wrist or joint capsule is abnormal.

P A **ganglion** is a benign growth that is usually nontender and more prominent on the dorsum of the hand and wrist (Figure 18-31). Its etiology is unknown.

A Flexion of the fingers is abnormal.

P Dupuytren's contracture is a flexion contracture that affects the little finger, ring finger, and middle finger. Pain does not normally accompany this disorder. It is caused by the progressive contracture of the palmar fascia from an unknown etiology (Figure 18-32).

A Muscular atrophy of the thenar eminence is abnormal.

P This disorder occurs in median nerve compression such as in carpal tunnel syndrome.

A Severe flexion ankylosis of the wrist is abnormal.

P Ankylosis can be caused by rheumatoid arthritis or severe disuse (Figure 18-33).

A Tenderness over the distal radius is abnormal.

P This can occur in Colles fracture or fracture of the distal radius. This is the most common type of wrist fracture.

A Wrist drop, demonstrated by the inability of the patient to flex the fisted hand downward at the wrist, is abnormal.

P Radial nerve injury may cause wrist drop.

A Inability of the patient to prevent moving of spread fingers together is abnormal.

P Ulnar nerve injury causes weakness of the fingers.

A Weakness of opposition of the thumb and ipsilateral finger against resistance is abnormal.

| **E** Examination | **N** Normal Findings | **A** Abnormal Findings | **P** Pathophysiology |

P Median nerve disorders, such as carpal tunnel syndrome, affect thumb opposition. Weak thumb opposition usually occurs from injuries where the hand is outstretched during a fall or from a twisting motion.

ADVANCED TECHNIQUE

Assessing Grip Strength Using a Blood Pressure Cuff

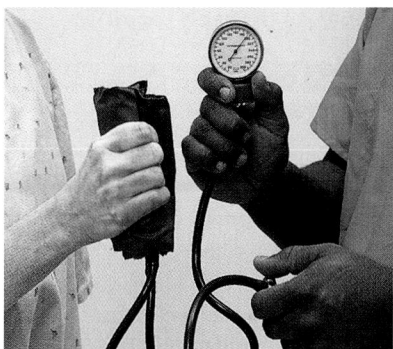

FIGURE 18-34 Assessing Grip Strength Using a Blood Pressure Cuff

E
1. Roll up a blood pressure cuff into a ball and inflate the cuff to 20 mm Hg.
2. Ask the patient to squeeze the inflated cuff (to determine the strength of the hand grasp action).
3. Note the increase in mm Hg during the grasp (Figure 18-34).
4. Assess the strength of the other hand.

N A healthy individual can usually achieve 150 mm Hg during a strong hand grasp action.

A A hand grasp that measures below 150 mm Hg is abnormal.

P Neurological pathology such as in stroke and myasthenia gravis, as well as musculoskeletal disease such as MS and rheumatoid arthritis can lead to decreased grip strength.

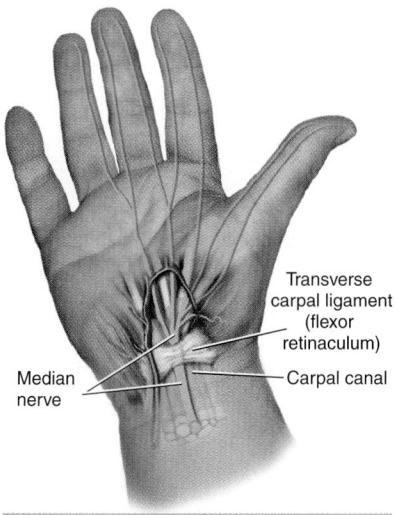

Transverse carpal ligament (flexor retinaculum)

Median nerve

Carpal canal

FIGURE 18-35 Anatomy of the Carpal Tunnel

ADVANCED TECHNIQUE

Assessing for Carpal Tunnel Syndrome: Tinel's Sign

The median nerve lies within the carpal tunnel of the wrist (Figure 18-35). Compression of the tunnel leads to median nerve neuropathy.
The patient may complain of paresthesias and burning, especially in the first three fingers, pain in the wrist and forearm, and a decreased ability to grasp objects due to a weak grip.

E
1. Place the patient in a sitting position with the arm flexed at the elbow and the palm facing up.
2. Using the index or middle finger of the dominant hand, briskly tap the center of the patient's wrist (median nerve) (Figure 18-36).
3. Ask the patient to describe the sensations that occur in the forearm, hands, thumb, or fingers.
4. Repeat the technique on the other wrist.

N There will be no tingling or burning noted in the hand, thumb, or fingers.

A A positive Tinel's test, indicated by a tingling or pricking sensation that occurs in the hand, thumb, and index and middle fingers when the median nerve is tapped, is abnormal.

P A positive Tinel's test is indicative of median nerve compression (carpal tunnel syndrome).

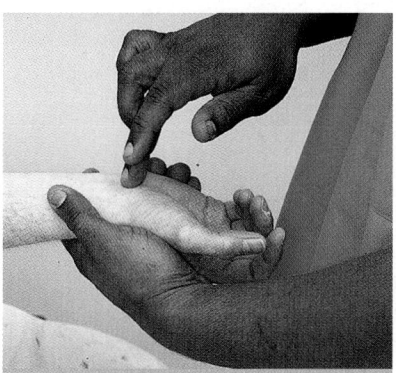

FIGURE 18-36 Assessing for Tinel's Sign

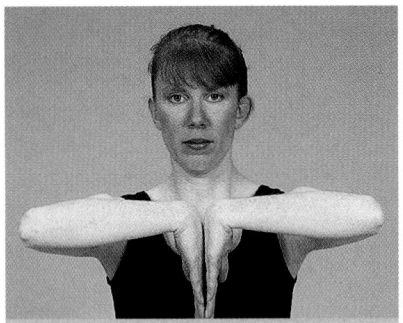

FIGURE 18-37 Assessing for Phalen's Sign

Assessing for Carpal Tunnel Syndrome: Phalen's Sign

E 1. Place the patient in a sitting position with the arms flexed at the elbow and the backs of the hands pressed together (Figure 18-37).

2. Ask the patient to maintain the wrist flexion of 90° for at least 1 minute.

3. Ask the patient to describe the sensations that occur in the hands and fingers.

N There will be no change in the sensation of the hands and fingers.

A A positive Phalen's test, indicated by sensations of numbness and paresthesia in the palmar aspect of the hand and in the fingers (especially the first three fingers), is abnormal. These sensations disappear when the wrist joint is returned to its neutral anatomic position.

P A positive Phalen's test is indicative of carpal tunnel syndrome.

Hips

Assessing for Hip Dislocation: Trendelenburg Test

E 1. Ask the patient to stand on one foot, with the knee of the non-weight-bearing leg flexed to raise the foot off the floor.

2. Assess the symmetry of the iliac crests while the patient is standing on one leg.

3. Repeat this technique on the other leg.

N The iliac crest on the side opposite the weight-bearing leg elevates slightly.

A It is abnormal for the iliac crest on the non-weight-bearing leg to drop.

P This finding is a positive Trendelenburg test and it is indicative of hip dislocation. The weakness of the gluteus medius muscle causes the hip on the unaffected side to drop.

NURSING**ALERT**

Osteoporosis Risk Factors

- Increased age (> 50), especially postmenopausal women
- Asian and Caucasian races
- Slender body build
- Smoking
- Family history
- Decreased physical activity
- Increased alcohol intake
- High caffeine intake
- Malabsorption syndromes
- Malnutrition, including decreased calcium and vitamin D intake
- Increased stress
- Diabetes mellitus
- Blood disorders
- Anorexia and bulimia
- Surgical removal of ovaries
- Hyperparathyroidism
- Medications (steroids, anticonvulsants, lithium, tamoxifen, thyroxine, thiazide diuretics)

NURSING**ALERT**

Hip Fracture

Hip fracture is the most serious fall-related fracture, often resulting in disability and death. This injury is often the pivotal event in an older adult's ability to remain independent in the home. Clinical manifestations of hip fracture include pain, inability to move the affected leg, inability to walk, and shortening of the affected leg with possible external rotation.

E Examination   **N** Normal Findings   **A** Abnormal Findings   **P** Pathophysiology

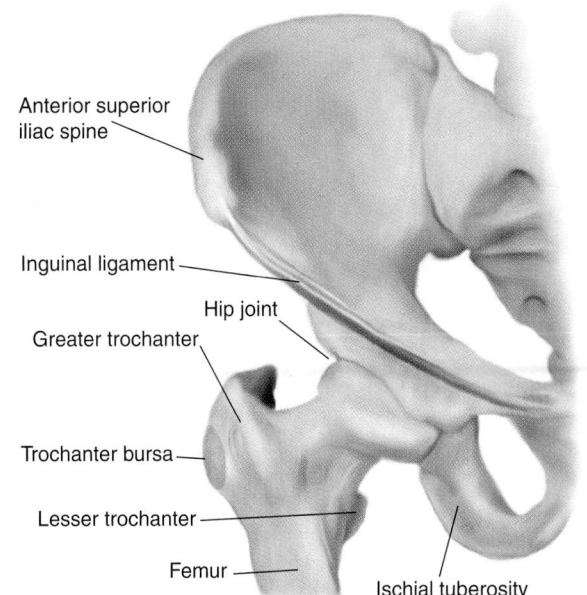

FIGURE 18-38   Anatomy of the Hip Joint

E 1. While the patient is standing, inspect the iliac crests (refer to the Advanced Technique for the Trendelenburg test), size and symmetry of the buttocks, and number of gluteal folds (Figure 18-38).

2. Observe the patient's gait, if not previously assessed (see General Assessment).

3. Assist the patient to a supine position on the examination table with the legs straight and the feet pointing toward the ceiling.

NURSING**ALERT**

DEXA Screening

Dual-energy X-ray absorptiometry (DEXA or DXA) screening is a painless procedure for measuring bone mineral density and for detecting bone density loss. Results can quantify bone as normal, osteopenic, or osteoporotic. Using a low level of radiation (or ultrasound waves in portable DEXA screening), the bones of the lower spine, hip, wrist, fingers, or heel can be scanned. The International Society for Clinical Densitometry recommends screening in the following individuals:

- Females 65 years old and older
- Females on HRT for extended periods of time
- Males 70 years old and older
- Individuals with fragility fractures
- Individuals with a disease associated with osteoporosis (e.g., eating disorder, hyperparathyroidism, celiac disease, chronic liver disease, irritable bowel disease, male hypogonadism)
- Individuals on medications associated with osteoporosis (e.g., steroids, anticonvulsants, androgen deprivation treatment such as leuprolide)
- Individuals with a condition associated with osteoporosis (e.g., menopause before age 45, X-ray findings of vertebral abnormality)
- Individuals being treated for osteoporosis to monitor the effects of treatment

DEXA scans are usually repeated no more than every 2 years, as treatment protocols do not have short-term results.

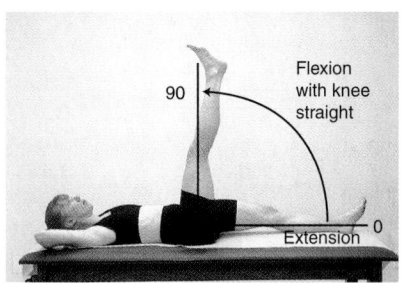

A. Flexion with Knee Straight

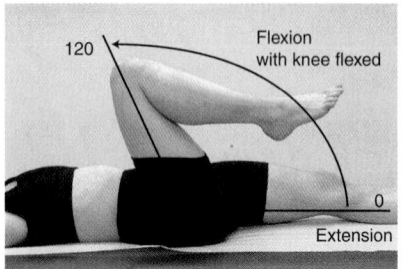

B. Flexion with Knee Flexed

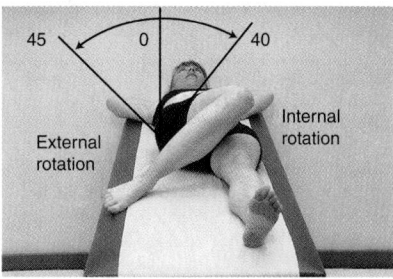

C. Internal and External Rotation

4. Palpate the hip joints.
5. Assess ROM of the hips (Figure 18-39). Ask the patient to:
   a. Raise the leg straight off the examination table with the knee extended (hip flexion with knee straight). The other leg should remain on the table.
   b. With the knee flexed, raise the leg off the examination table toward the chest as far as possible (hip flexion with knee flexed). The other leg should remain on the table. This is called the Thomas test.
   c. Flex the hip and knee. Move the flexed leg medially as the foot moves outward (internal rotation).
   d. Flex the hip and knee. Move the flexed leg laterally as the foot moves medially (external rotation).
   e. With the knee straight, swing the leg away from the midline (abduction).
   f. With the knee straight, swing the leg toward the midline (adduction).
   g. Roll over onto the abdomen and assume a prone position.
   h. From the hip, move the leg back as far as possible while maintaining the pelvis on the table (hyperextension). This can also be performed while the patient is standing.
6. Assist the patient to a supine position.
7. Assess strength of the hips.
   a. Place the palm of your hand on the anterior thigh, above the knee. Instruct the patient to raise the leg against your resistance (Figure 18-40A). Repeat on the other leg.
   b. Place the palm of your hand posteriorly above and behind the knee. Instruct the patient to lower the leg against your resistance. Repeat on the other leg.
   c. Place your hands on the lateral aspects of the patient's legs at the level of the knee. Instruct the patient to move the legs apart against your resistance (Figure 18-40B).

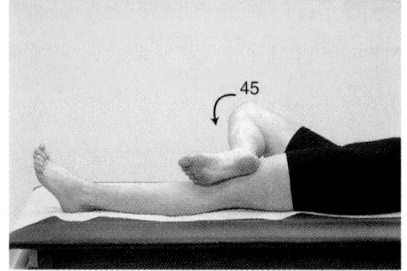

D. Position of the Leg for Full External Rotation

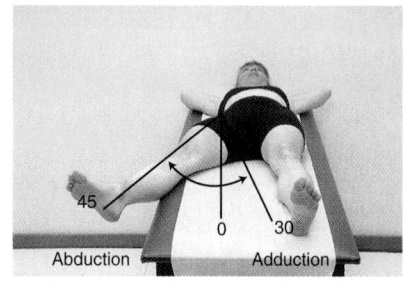

E. Abduction and Adduction

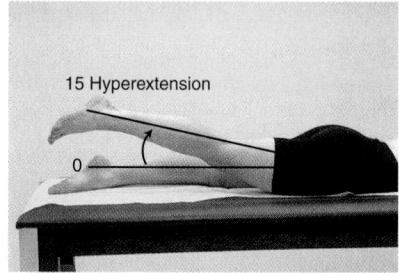

F. Hyperextension

FIGURE 18-39 **Range of Motion of the Hip Joint**

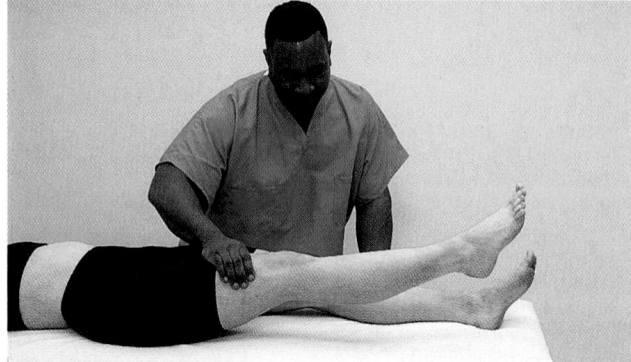

A. Flexion with Opposing Force

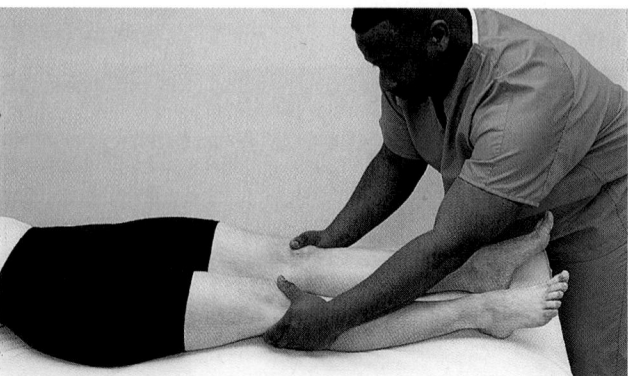

B. Abduction with Opposing Force

FIGURE 18-40 **Muscle Strength of the Hip**

Missed Diagnosis

A 45-year-old Asian woman is brought in by her son to be evaluated for her hip and leg pain. The son informs you that his mother was seen at another clinic 3 days ago for her leg pain after she fell down the steps. At that time she was told that she had pulled some muscles and to rest. Since then the woman has had increasingly severe leg and hip pain. After conducting the health history and physical examination you suspect that she has a hip fracture. What questions would you ask the patient and her son? What assessments would you perform? Why might a 45-year-old woman sustain a hip fracture? What explanation would you give to the family concerning the initial clinical evaluation?

d. Place your hands on the medial aspects of the patient's legs just above the knee. Instruct the patient to move the legs together against your resistance.

N The normal ROM for the hips is flexion with knee straight—90°, flexion with knee flexed—120°, internal rotation—40°, external rotation—45°, abduction—45°, adduction—30°, hyperextension—15°.

A A leg that is externally rotated and painful on movement is abnormal.

ADVANCED TECHNIQUE

Measuring Limb Length

E 1. Place the patient in a supine position on the examination table with the legs extended.
   2. Measure the leg from the anterior superior iliac spine to the medial malleolus (Figure 18-41).
   3. Repeat on the other limb.
   4. Compare measurements.

N Limb length measurements should be within 1 to 3 cm of each other.

A A more than 3 cm difference in the length of limbs is abnormal.

P Unilateral discrepancy in lower limb length may be a congenital defect.

P Sudden unilateral decrease in limb length occurs with fracture and dislocation of the hip and leg.

P A displaced proximal femoral shaft fracture (hip fracture) can result in limb shortening and internal or external rotation. Internal rotation is common if the patient fell forward during the fall, and external rotation is common if the patient fell onto the buttocks. The patient is unable to straighten the leg into its neutral anatomic position.

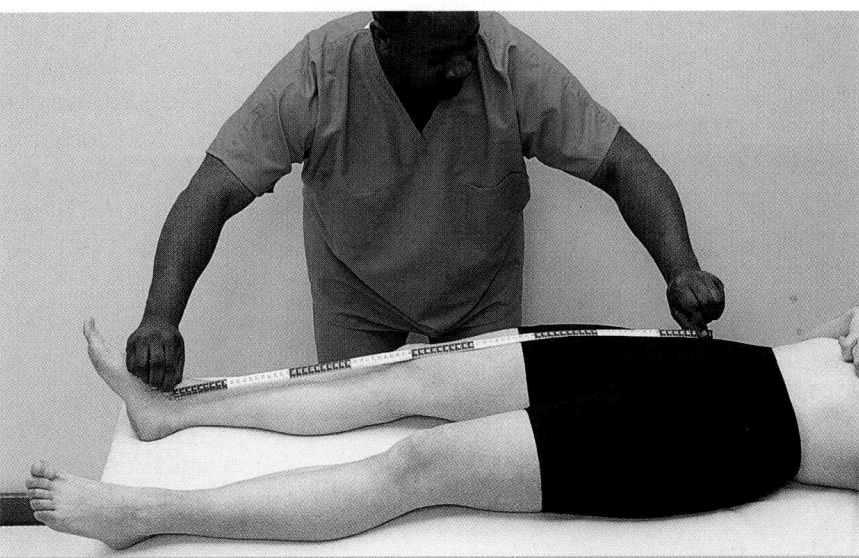

FIGURE 18-41 Measuring Limb Length

| **E** Examination | **N** Normal Findings | **A** Abnormal Findings | **P** Pathophysiology |

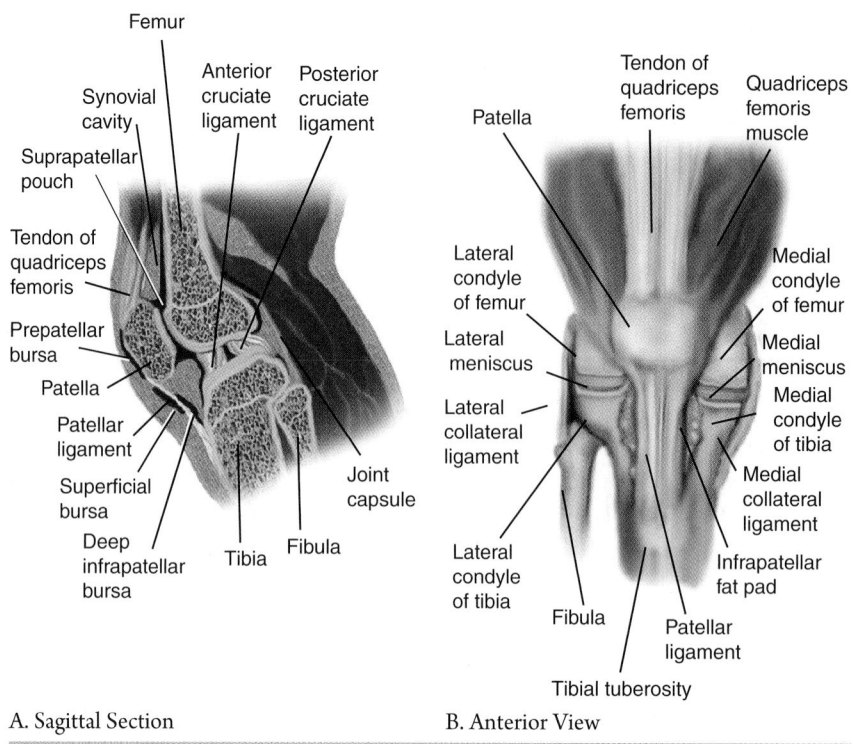

A. Sagittal Section

B. Anterior View

FIGURE 18-42 **Anatomy of the Right Knee Joint**

P These findings occur in hip fractures, which usually result from falls (especially in elderly persons). The affected leg may also be shorter. See the Advanced Technique for guidelines on measuring limb length.

A A positive Thomas test, when the patient is unable to flex one knee and hip while simultaneously maintaining the other leg in full extension, is abnormal. There may be slight to moderate hip and knee flexion of the extended leg.

P Flexion contractures of the hip joint, such as in long-term degenerative joint diseases, will result in a positive Thomas test. This test will identify hip flexion contractures that are masked by lumbar lordosis.

Knees

E 1. With the patient standing, note the position of the knees in relation to each other and in relation to the hips, thighs, ankles, and feet.

2. Ask the patient to sit on the examination table with the knees flexed and resting at the edge of the table.

3. Inspect the contour of the knees. Note the normal depressions around the patella (Figure 18-42).

4. Inspect the suprapatellar pouch and the prepatellar bursa.

5. Note the quadriceps muscle, located on the anterior thigh.

6. Palpate the knees. The patient may assume a supine position if this is more comfortable.

   a. Grasp the anterior thigh approximately 10 cm above the patella, with your thumb on one side of the knee and the other four fingers on the other side of the knee (Figure 18-43).

   b. As you palpate, gradually move your hand down the suprapatellar pouch.

7. Palpate the tibiofemoral joints. It is best to have the knee flexed to 90° when performing this assessment.

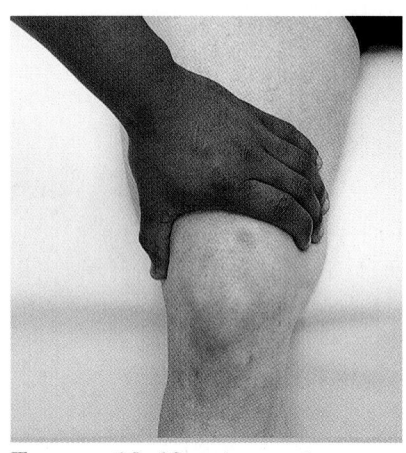

FIGURE 18-43 **Palpating the Knee**

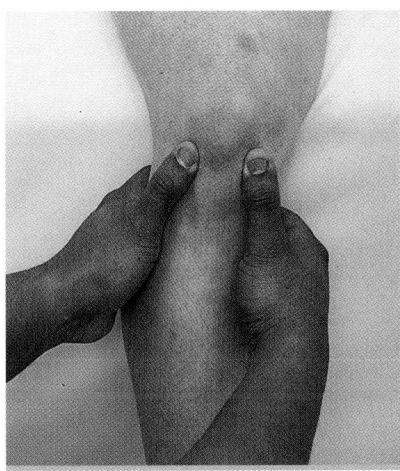

FIGURE 18-44 Palpating the Tibiofemoral Joint

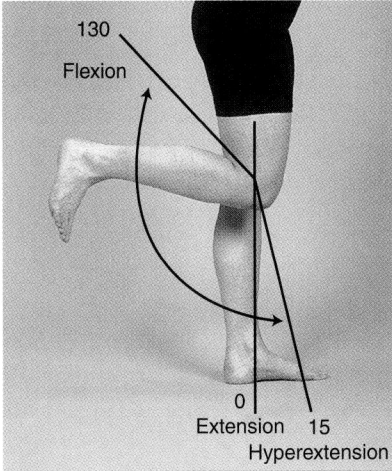

FIGURE 18-45 Range of Motion of the Knee Joint: Flexion, Extension, and Hyperextension

a. Place both thumbs on the knee, with the fingers wrapped around the knee posteriorly.

b. Press in with the thumbs as you palpate the tibial margins (Figure 18-44).

c. Palpate the lateral collateral ligament.

8. If knee fluid is suspected, test for the bulge sign and ballottement. See the Advanced Techniques on Bulge Sign and Patellar Ballottement.

9. Assess ROM of the knees (Figure 18-45). Ask the patient to stand and:

a. Bend the knee (flexion).

b. Straighten the knee (extension). The patient may also be able to hyperextend the knee during this movement.

10. Assess strength of the knees with the patient seated and the legs hanging off the table.

a. Ask the patient to bend the knee. Place your nondominant hand under the knee and place your other hand over the ankle.

b. Instruct the patient to straighten the leg against your resistance (Figure 18-46).

c. Ask the patient to place the foot on the bed and the knee at approximately 45° of flexion. Place one hand under the knee and place the other hand over the ankle.

d. Instruct the patient to maintain the foot on the table despite your attempts to straighten the leg.

N The knees are in alignment with each other and do not protrude medially or laterally. The normal ROM for the knees is flexion—130°, extension—0°; in some cases, hyperextension is possible up to 15°.

A Alteration in lower limb alignment is considered an abnormal finding.

P **Genu valgum** (knock knees) is inward deviation toward the midline at the level of the knees (Figure 18-47). Both legs are usually affected by the disorder. It is detected as an increased distance between the medial malleoli when the femoral condyles are close together and the patella are facing forward. The knees appear closer together than is normal. Genu valgum can be congenital or acquired (rickets).

P **Genu varum** (bow legs) is outward deviation away from the midline at the level of the knees (Figure 18-48). Both legs are usually affected by the disorder. It is detected as an increased distance between the femoral condyles

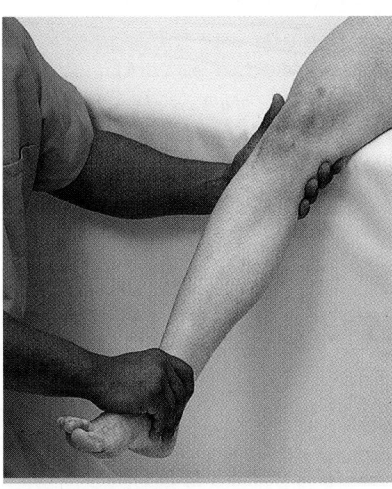

FIGURE 18-46 Strength of Knee Joint

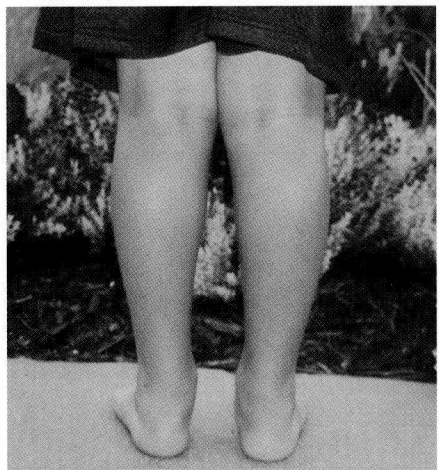

FIGURE 18-47 Genu Valgum

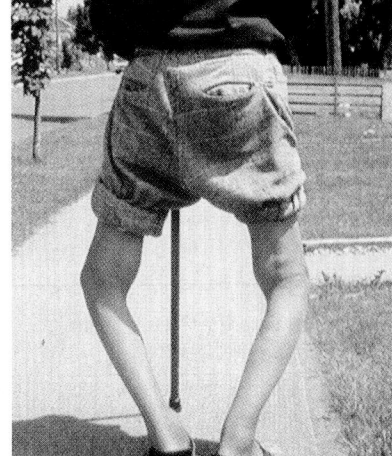

FIGURE 18-48 Genu Varum

| **E** Examination | **N** Normal Findings | **A** Abnormal Findings | **P** Pathophysiology |

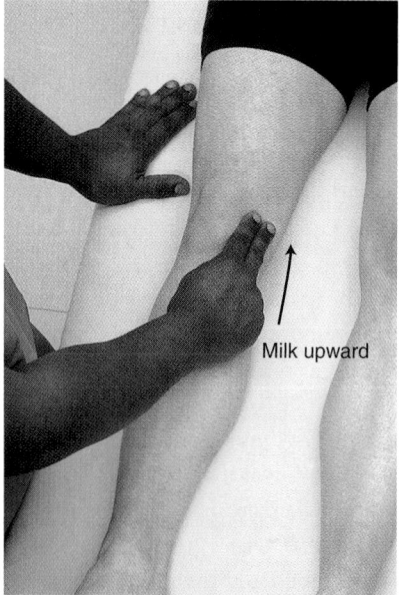

Milk upward

A. Milking the Patella

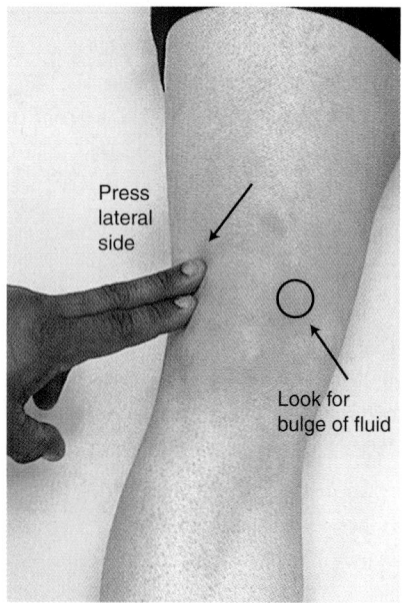

Press lateral side

Look for bulge of fluid

B. Observing for Fluid

FIGURE 18-49 Assessing for Bulge Sign

ADVANCED TECHNIQUE

Assessing for Small Effusions: Bulge Sign

The bulge sign tests for small effusions (4 to 8 mL) in the knee.

E 1. Place the patient in a supine position with the legs extended.

2. Firmly milk upward the medial aspect of the patella several times. This displaces any fluid (Figure 18-49A).

3. Press or tap the lateral aspect of the knee.

4. Observe the hollow on the medial aspect of the knee for a bulge of fluid (Figure 18-49B).

N Normally there is no fluid return to the knee. This is a negative bulge sign.

A The return of fluid to the medial aspect of the patella is abnormal.

P A positive bulge sign is present in joint effusion.

when the medial malleoli are close together and the patella are facing forward. The knees appear farther apart than is normal. Genu varum can be congenital or acquired. This syndrome is common in horse jockeys due to the stretching of the nearby ligaments. It may also be seen in rickets, rheumatoid arthritis, and osteomalacia due to the body's attempt to bend bone shape in order to tolerate the weight of the upper body.

A A knee effusion is present.

P A knee effusion can be associated with a Baker's cyst (see Figure 18-50). A Baker's cyst is a cystic mass in the medial popliteal fossa. If large enough, it can decrease the anatomic ROM of the knee. It is often detected in patients with rheumatoid arthritis.

ADVANCED TECHNIQUE

Assessing for Large Effusions: Patellar Ballottement

Ballottement is performed to detect large effusions in the knee.

E 1. Place the patient either in a supine position with the legs extended or sitting up with the knees flexed at 90° and hanging over the edge of the examination table.

2. Firmly grasp the thigh (with your thumb on one side and the four fingers on the other side) just above the patella. This compresses fluid out of the suprapatellar pouch.

3. With your other hand, push the patella back toward the femur (see Figure 18-51).

4. Feel for a click.

N There is no palpable click. Normally, the patella is close to the femur because there is no excess fluid.

A A palpable click is abnormal.

P When fluid is present between the femur and the patella, the patella "floats" on top of the femur. As the patella is pushed back, fluid is displaced and a palpable click is felt when the patella hits the femur.

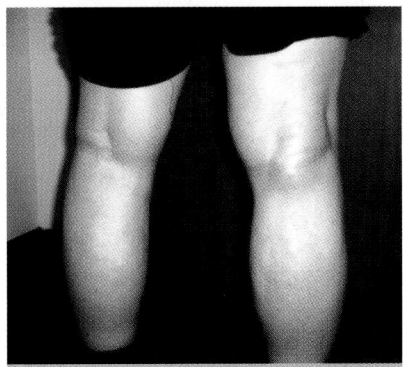

FIGURE 18-50 Baker's Cyst in the Right Popliteal Fossae

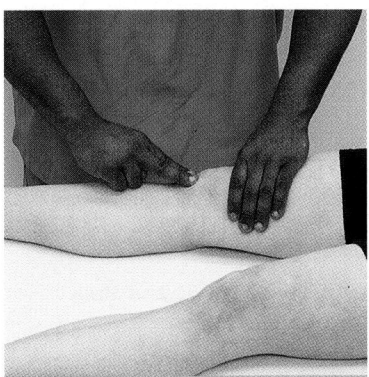

FIGURE 18-51 Patellar Ballottement

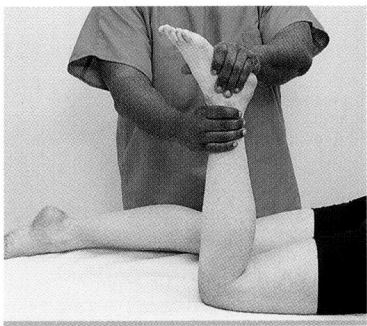

FIGURE 18-52 Assessing for Apley's Grinding Sign

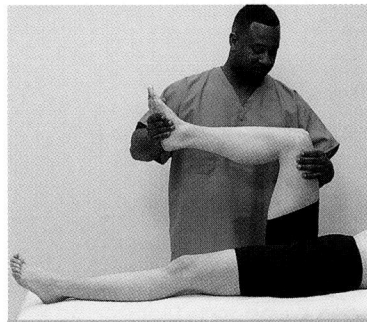

FIGURE 18-53 Assessing for McMurray's Sign

ADVANCED TECHNIQUE

Assessing for Meniscal Tears: Apley's Grinding Sign

This test is performed to identify meniscal tears.

E
1. Place the patient into a prone position on the examination table.
2. Manually flex the affected knee to a 90° angle so that the lower leg is perpendicular to the table.
3. With the dominant hand, apply firm downward pressure on the foot while simultaneously rotating the lower leg inward and then outward (Figure 18-52).
4. Assess for limited knee joint movement or audible clicks during knee joint movement.

N The patient will be able to flex the knee joint to a 90° angle, and no audible clicks will be heard during joint movement.

A A positive Apley's sign of the knee joint is indicated by limited movement of the knee joint (locking of the knee joint) or audible clicks.

P A positive Apley's sign is suggestive of torn meniscal cartilage within the knee joint.

ADVANCED TECHNIQUE

Assessing for Meniscal Tears: McMurray's Sign

This test is performed to assess the integrity of the meniscus of the knee.

E
1. Place the patient in a supine position on the examination table and stand on the affected side.
2. Manually flex the hip and knee. Hold the patient's heel with one hand and stabilize the knee with the other hand (Figure 18-53).
3. Using the hand that is holding the heel, internally rotate the leg while applying resistance to the medial aspect of the knee joint. This assesses the medial meniscus.
4. Move the knee to a position of full extension. Note if full extension of the knee joint can be achieved or tolerated by the patient.
5. Flex the hip and knee and externally rotate the leg. While stabilizing the knee joint, apply resistance to the lateral aspect of the knee joint. This assesses the lateral meniscus.
6. Assess for an audible or palpable click of the knee joint.

N The patient will be able to extend the leg at the knee joint and there will be no audible or palpable click detected.

A A positive McMurray's sign is indicated when the patient is unable to extend the leg at the knee joint or when an audible or palpable click is detected.

P A positive McMurray's sign is suggestive of torn meniscus cartilage of the knee. The patient may also state that full extension of the knee joint is impossible, that the knee joint "locks into place," or that "it feels like something is in the knee joint." If the torn meniscus cartilage is obstructing the articulating function of the joint, knee joint extension will be limited.

| **E** Examination | **N** Normal Findings | **A** Abnormal Findings | **P** Pathophysiology |

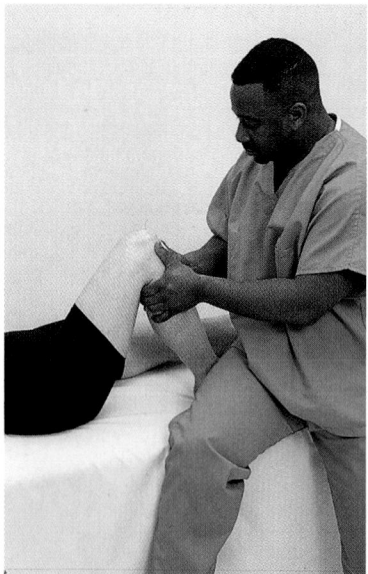

FIGURE 18-54 Drawer Test

ADVANCED TECHNIQUE

Assessing the Cruciate Ligaments: Drawer Test

This test is performed to assess the stability of the anterior and posterior cruciate ligaments of the knee.

E 1. Assist the patient to a supine position on the examination table.

2. Instruct the patient to flex the right knee to 90° and to flex the right hip joint to 45°, placing the right foot flat on the examination table.

3. Sit on the patient's right foot to stabilize it in place.

4. Observe for "sagging" of the tibia resulting in visible concavity below the patella (gravity drawer test, or "sag" sign).

5. Place both hands on the patient's right tibia, with the thumb of the right hand on the medial aspect of the knee, and the left thumb on the lateral aspect of the knee (Figure 18-54).

6. Attempt to move the tibia forward (anterior drawer test) and then backward (posterior drawer test).

7. Repeat on the left leg. Compare results.

N You will not be able to pull the tibia forward more than 6 mm or to move the tibia backward at all. Concavity should not be detected distal to the patella.

A An abnormal result is indicated by the ability to move the tibia forward more than 6 mm or to move the tibia backward.

P Forward movement of the tibia more than 6 mm indicates a tear in the anterior cruciate ligament of the knee. A false positive result may occur if the patient has instability of the posterior cruciate ligament of the knee.

P Sagging of the tibia or backward movement of the tibia indicates a tear in the posterior cruciate ligament of the knee.

ADVANCED TECHNIQUE

Assessing the Anterior Cruciate Ligament: Lachman's Test

This test is performed to assess for stability of the anterior cruciate ligament of the knee. It is considered the most reliable assessment technique for detecting instability of the anterior cruciate ligament.

E 1. Place the patient in a supine position on the examination table with the unaffected knee flexed to approximately 30°. The affected leg should be fully extended and in contact with the examination table.

2. Stabilize the femur of the affected leg by holding the leg above the knee joint with the right hand.

3. Grasp the affected lower leg beneath the knee with the left hand and move the tibia forward.

4. Note any changes in the infrapatellar slope.

N When the tibia is moved forward, the infrapatellar tendon slope should still be noticeable.

A It is abnormal for the infrapatellar tendon slope to no longer be noticeable when the tibia is moved forward.

P A positive Lachman's test is indicative of damage to the anterior cruciate ligament of the knee.

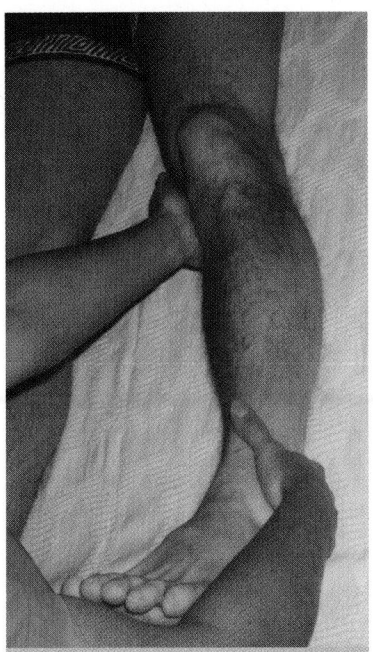

FIGURE 18-55 Varus Stress Test

ADVANCED TECHNIQUE

Assessing the Lateral Collateral Ligament: Varus Stress Test

E 1. Place the patient in a supine position on the examination table.
2. Slightly abduct the affected leg.
3. Place your left hand on the medial aspect of the affected knee.
4. Place your right hand on the lateral aspect of the same ankle.
5. Apply varus stress (lateral movement) to the knee and push the right hand at the ankle medially (Figure 18-55).
6. Note pain with movement.

N There should be no pain when varus stress is applied.

A Pain with varus stress is abnormal.

P Pain with varus stress may indicate a tear in the lateral collateral ligament.

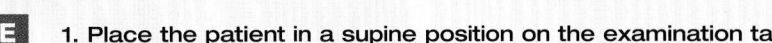

ADVANCED TECHNIQUE

Assessing the Medial Collateral Ligament: Valgus Stress Test

E 1. Place the patient in a supine position on the examination table.
2. Slightly abduct the affected leg.
3. Place your right hand on the lateral aspect of the affected knee.
4. Place your left hand on the medial aspect of the same ankle.
5. Apply valgus stress (medial movement) to the knee and push the left hand at the ankle laterally (Figure 18-56).
6. Note pain with movement.

N There should be no pain when valgus stress is applied.

A Pain with valgus stress is abnormal.

P Pain with valgus stress may indicate a tear in the medial collateral ligament.

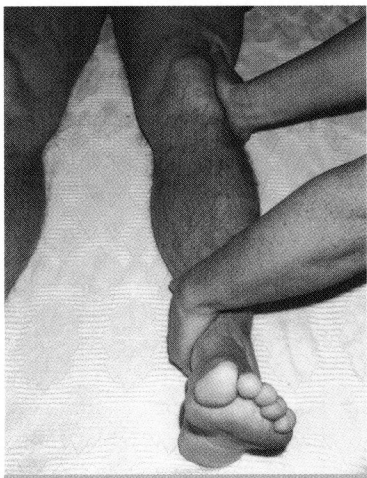

FIGURE 18-56 Valgus Stress Test

NURSING**TIP**

Assessing a Patient's Shoes

Examine the patient's shoes and observe for wear in unusual areas. This provides information on the patient's weight bearing. Keep this in mind as you watch the patient stand and walk.

Ankles and Feet

E 1. Inspect the ankles and feet (see Figure 18-57) as the patient stands, walks, and sits (bearing no weight).
2. Inspect the alignment of the feet and toes with the lower leg.
3. Inspect the shape and position of the toes.
4. Assist the patient to a supine position on the examination table.
5. Stand by the patient's feet.
6. Palpate the ankle and foot (see Figure 18-58).
   a. Grasp the heel with the fingers of both hands. Palpate the posterior aspect of the heel at the calcaneus.

E Examination 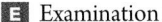 Normal Findings 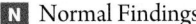 Abnormal Findings **P** Pathophysiology

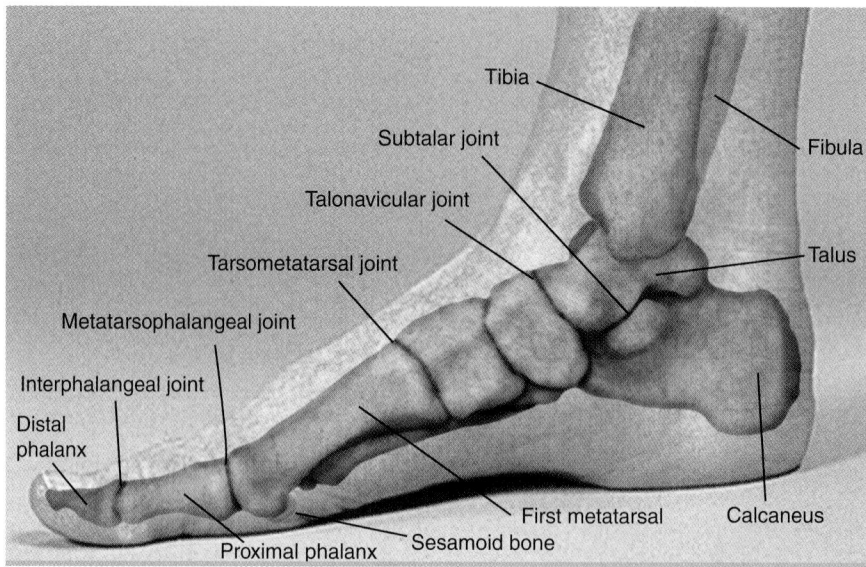

FIGURE 18-57 Anatomy of the Ankle and Foot

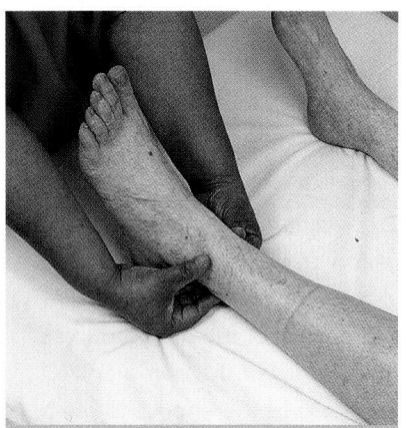

FIGURE 18-58 Palpation of the Ankle

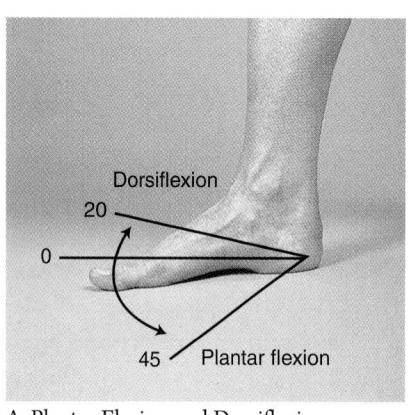

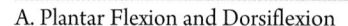

A. Plantar Flexion and Dorsiflexion

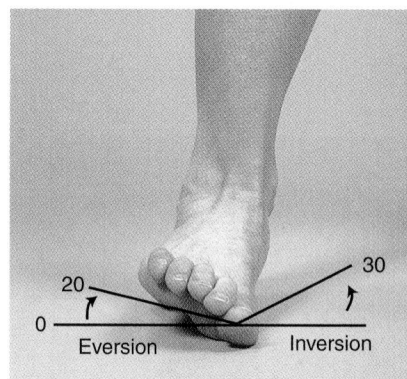

B. Eversion and Inversion

FIGURE 18-59 Range of Motion of the Ankle and Foot

    b. Use your thumbs to palpate the medial malleolus (bony prominence on the distal medial aspect of the tibia) and the lateral malleolus (bony prominence on the distal lateral aspect of the fibula).

    c. Move your hands forward and palpate the anterior aspects of the ankle and foot, particularly at the joints.

    d. Palpate the inferior aspect of the foot over the plantar fascia.

    e. Use your finger pads to palpate the Achilles tendon.

    f. Palpate with your thumb and index finger each metatarsophalangeal joint.

    g. Between your thumb and index finger, palpate the medial and lateral surfaces of each interphalangeal joint.

7. Assess ROM of the ankles and feet (Figure 18-59). Ask the patient to:

    a. Point the toes toward the chest by moving the ankle (dorsiflexion).

    b. Point the toes toward the floor by moving the ankle (plantar flexion).

    c. Turn the soles of the feet outward (eversion).

    d. Turn the soles of the feet inward (inversion).

    e. Curl the toes toward the floor (flexion).

    f. Spread the toes apart (abduction).

    g. Move the toes together (adduction).

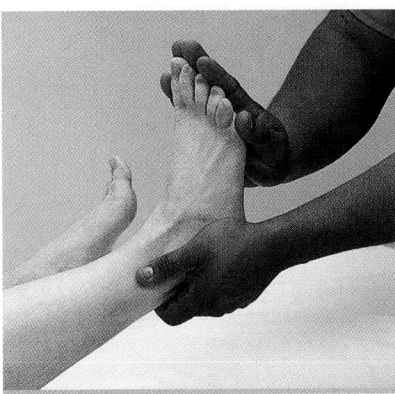

FIGURE 18-60   **Strength of the Ankle and Foot**

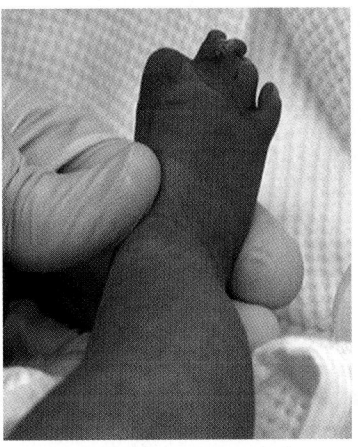

A. Congenital loss of the right big toe. Also note the syndactyly. *Courtesy of Mary Ellen Estes.*

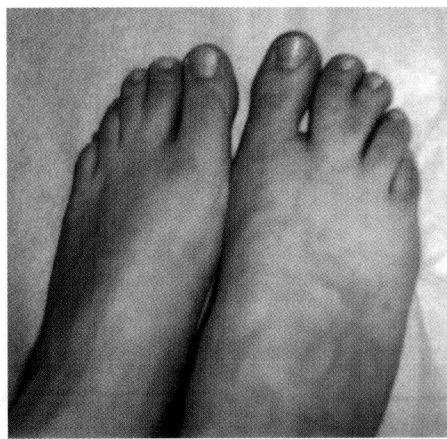

B. Syndactyly in the 2nd and 3rd metatarsals of the right foot.

FIGURE 18-61   **Toe Abnormalities**

8. Assess strength of the ankles and feet.
   a. Assist the patient to a supine position on the examination table with the legs extended and the feet slightly apart.
   b. Stand at the foot of the examination table.
   c. Place your left hand on top of the patient's right foot and place your right hand on top of the patient's left foot.
   d. Ask the patient to point the toes toward the chest (dorsiflexion) despite your resistance.
   e. Place your left hand on the sole of the patient's right foot and place your right hand on the sole of the patient's left foot.
   f. Ask the patient to point the toes down (plantar flexion) despite your resistance. This technique can also be performed one foot at a time as demonstrated in Figure 18-60.

N The foot is in alignment with the lower leg. The foot has a longitudinal arch. There is no pain over the plantar fascia. The normal ROM for the ankles and feet is dorsiflexion—20°, plantar flexion—45°, eversion—20°, inversion—30°, abduction—30°, and adduction—10°.

A Extra toes or webbing between the toes is congenital. Loss of toes can be congenital or acquired (Figure 18-61A).

P Polydactyly is the presence of extra digits. Syndactyly is the congenital webbing or fusion of toes (Figure 18-61B).

A An alteration in the shape and the position of the foot is considered abnormal.

P **Pes varus** describes a foot that is turned inward toward the midline.

P **Pes valgus** occurs when the foot is turned laterally away from the midline.

P **Pes planus** (flat foot) refers to a foot with a low longitudinal arch.

P **Pes cavus** refers to a foot with an exaggerated arch height.

P In **hallux valgus** (bunion), the big toe is deviated laterally while the first metatarsal is deviated medially (Figure 18-62). The metatarsophalangeal joint enlarges and becomes inflamed from the pressure. A bursa may form at this point. Hallux valgus can be congenital or caused by narrow shoes and arthritis.

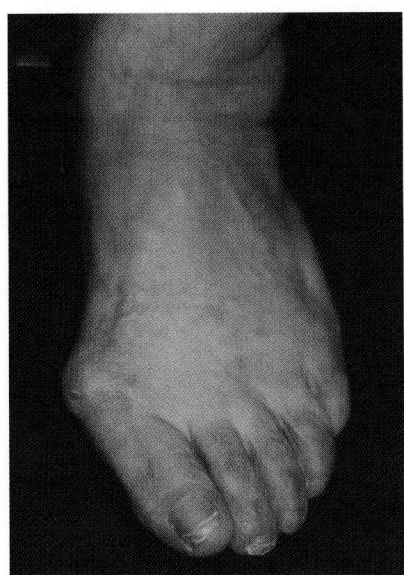

FIGURE 18-62   **Hallux Valgus.**
Courtesy of Mary A. Hitcho.

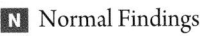 Examination   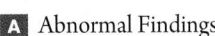 Normal Findings   **A** Abnormal Findings   **P** Pathophysiology

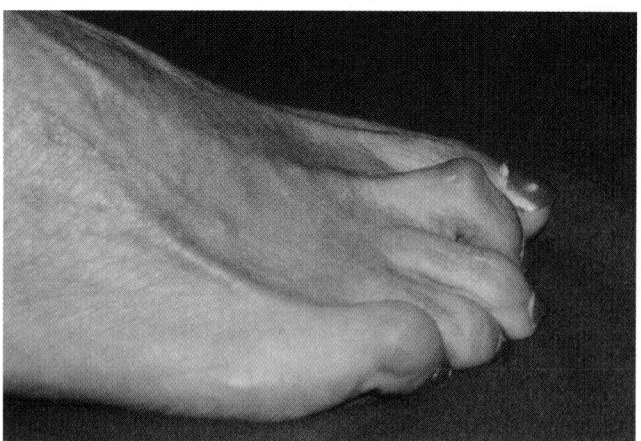

FIGURE 18-63 **Hammertoe with Corn**

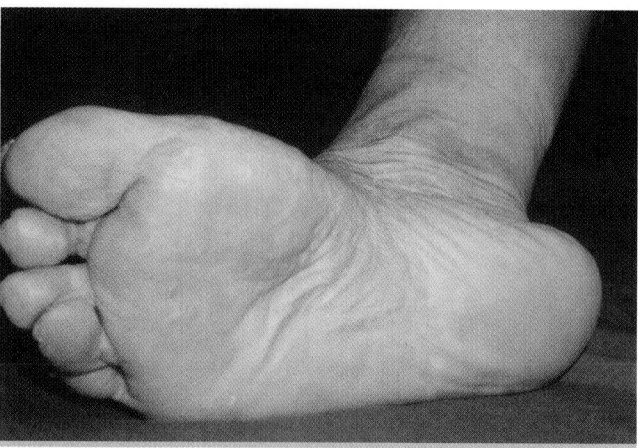

FIGURE 18-64 Callus

P Tight shoes can also cause **hammertoe**. In hammertoe, there is a flexion of the proximal interphalangeal joint and hyperextension of the distal metatarsophalangeal joint. A corn or callus can develop from undue pressure at the point of flexion (Figure 18-63).

P A **corn** is a conical area of thickened skin. It extends into the dermis and can be painful. Corns are caused by pressure on the affected area, particularly over bony prominences. Tight shoes and hammertoe can cause corns.

P A **callus** is a thickening of the skin due to prolonged pressure (Figure 18-64). It usually occurs on the sole of the foot and is not painful.

A Pain over the plantar fascia is abnormal.

P Plantar fasciitis (heel-spur syndrome) is an inflammation of the plantar fascia where it attaches to the calcaneus. The pain tends to be worse first thing in the morning, and with prolonged standing, sitting, or walking.

A A swollen, red, warm, and painful metatarsophalangeal joint is abnormal.

P The first metatarsophalangeal joint is usually affected in acute gouty arthritis.

A Decreased ROM of the ankle is abnormal.

ADVANCED TECHNIQUE

Assessing for Ankle Sprain: Anterior Drawer Test

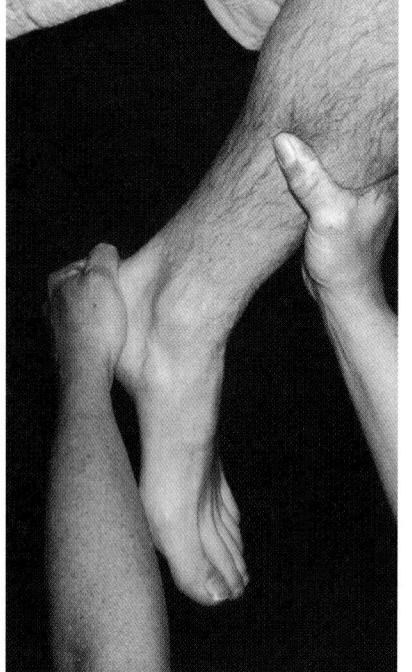

FIGURE 18-65 **Anterior Drawer Test of the Ankle**

E 1. Have the patient sit with the feet hanging freely.
   2. Grasp the heel of the foot with the injured ankle with the left hand.
   3. Place the right hand over the anterior aspect of the tibia on the affected side and firmly grasp the leg about 6 cm above the joint line (Figure 18-65).
   4. Firmly hold the tibia as you apply an anterior forward motion with your left hand.
   5. Note any movement of the ankle.

N There should be no forward movement of the ankle.

A It is abnormal to have anterior movement of the ankle.

P Anterior movement of the ankle indicates a possible tear in the anterior talofibular ligament (see Figure 18-66).

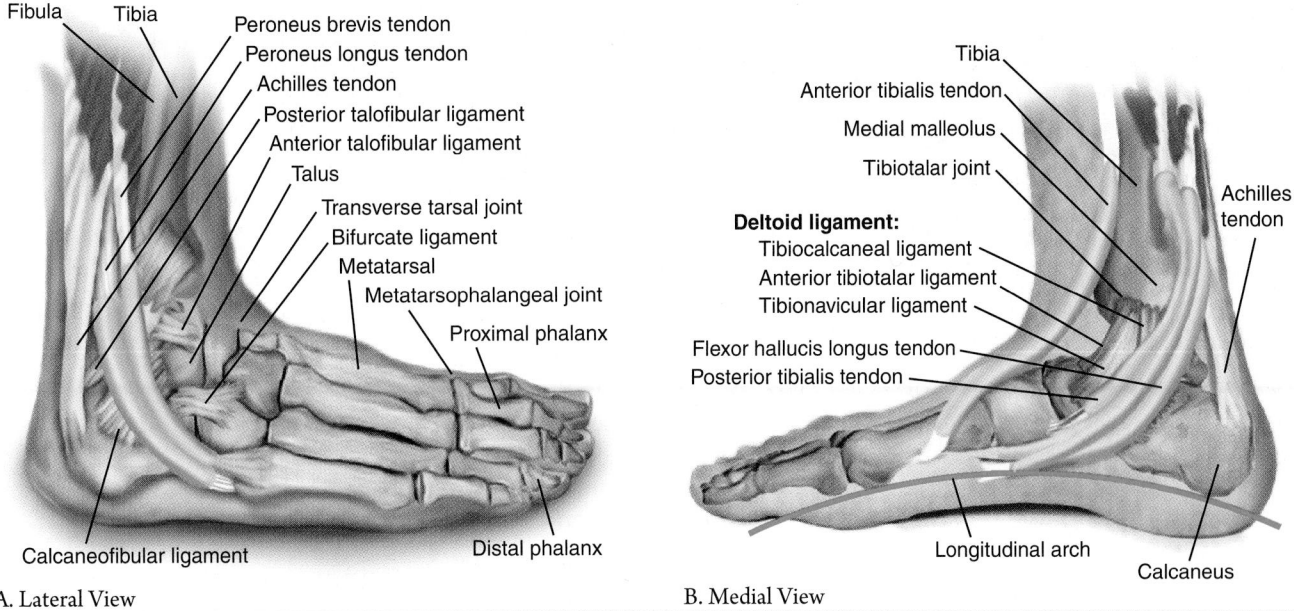

A. Lateral View

B. Medial View

FIGURE 18-66 **Ligaments of the Ankle**

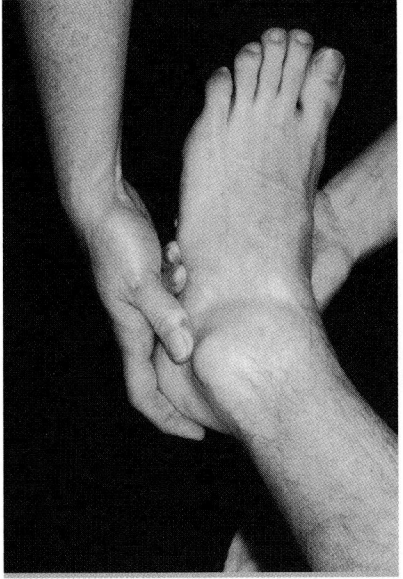

FIGURE 18-67 **Talar Tilt Test**

ADVANCED TECHNIQUE

Assessing for Ankle Sprain: Talar Tilt Test

E 1. Have the patient sit with the feet hanging freely.
2. Place your hands around the ankle of the affected leg so that the thumbs are inferior to the malleoli.
3. Passively invert and evert the ankle through range of motion (Figure 18-67).
4. Note the movement of the ankle.
5. Compare with the unaffected ankle.

N Normally, there should be an equal talar tilt, or range of motion, through inversion and eversion of both ankles.

A It is abnormal if the injured ankle has a talar tilt that is more than 5–10° than the unaffected ankle.

P A talar tilt greater than 5–10° may indicate a tear in the calcaneofibular ligament.

P The patient with an ankle sprain or fracture secondary to injury or trauma complains of pain on palpation and ROM. Crepitus may be present in an ankle fracture. Ankle sprain cannot always be differentiated from ankle fracture without the use of X-rays. Refer these patients to an orthopedist.

Spine

E 1. Ask the patient to stand and to leave the back of the gown open.
2. Stand behind the patient so that you can visualize the posterior anatomy.
3. Inspect the position and alignment of the spine from a posterior and a lateral position.

E Examination	**N** Normal Findings	**A** Abnormal Findings	**P** Pathophysiology

Compartment Syndrome

Acute compartment syndrome is a complication of limb injury with extensive soft tissue trauma. The lower leg and forearm are vulnerable to this complication. Increasing edema or hemorrhage within a muscle compartment reaches the point where it can no longer be accommodated by the elasticity of the fascia and skin. The continuing edema redirects itself inward, compressing muscle, nerves, and blood vessels. Muscular necrosis can result from lack of perfusion. Clinical manifestations include increased and uncontrolled pain despite narcotic analgesia, with pain aggravated by passive movement of the distal limb. Other manifestations include increased limb girth; shiny, tight skin; slow capillary refill; skin pallor; and decreased digit sensation and movement. Decreased peripheral pulse volume is a late indicator of compartment syndrome. The pressure within the muscle compartment can be measured using various invasive monitoring devices. A direct pressure reading of more than 20 mm Hg is indicative of compartment syndrome.

ADVANCED TECHNIQUE

Assessing Status of Distal Limbs and Digits

When you suspect distal limb or digit hypoperfusion due to trauma, injury, or pathology, conduct the following assessment:

E 1. Uncover the distal aspects of both limbs being assessed. A bilateral assessment allows for comparison of the affected and unaffected limbs. When assessing an injured limb, assess the limb areas proximal and distal to the site of injury.

2. Assess for swelling.

3. Assess the vascular status of the distal limb and its digits (peripheral pulses, skin color, skin temperature, and capillary refill).

4. Ask the patient to perform specific movements of the distal limb on command.

   a. To assess the ulnar nerve, ask the patient to perform abduction of the fingers.

   b. To assess the radial nerve, ask the patient to perform hyperextension of the thumb or wrist.

   c. To assess the median nerve, ask the patient to perform opposition of the thumb to the little finger of the same hand.

   d. To assess the peroneal nerve, ask the patient to perform dorsiflexion of the toes and ankle.

   e. To assess the tibial nerve, ask the patient to perform plantar flexion of the toes and ankle.

5. When assessing sensation, instruct the patient to close the eyes to prevent biased results. Use the thumb and index finger of the dominant hand to pinch certain areas of the distal limb.

   a. To assess the ulnar nerve, pinch the finger pad of the little finger.

   b. To assess the radial nerve, pinch the web space between the thumb and the index finger.

   c. To assess the median nerve, pinch the distal aspect of the index finger.

   d. To assess the peroneal nerve, pinch the lateral aspect of the great toe and the medial surface of the second toe.

   e. To assess the tibial nerve, pinch the medial and lateral surfaces of the sole of the foot.

N The individual with normal perfusion to the limbs and digits will appear comfortable during rest and muscle contraction. Pain will not occur with movement of the distal limb or digits. Limb perfusion will be manifested by strong peripheral pulses, warm skin temperature, and a brisk capillary refill. There will be complete motor and sensory function of the distal limb and digits. The patient will not experience any numbness or tingling.

A Neurovascular deterioration, manifested by the "5 P's" (pain, pallor, decreased perfusion, paresthesia, and paralysis) is abnormal.

P Neurovascular deterioration can occur in compartment syndrome. It is a severe complication of musculoskeletal trauma in which swelling is limited due to a confined space. Pain is the most significant and the earliest clinical manifestation of acute compartment syndrome. It occurs distal to the site of injury and is induced by the contraction of the muscle compartment being compressed. Pain results from stretching of a muscle that is experiencing vascular compromise.

continues

Assessing Status of Distal Limbs and Digits *continued*

P Inadequate arterial flow is a complication of digit or limb replantation following traumatic amputation.

P Arterial occlusion may also be detected as a complication of fracture or dislocation.

A Inadequate venous flow from the distal limb or digits, manifested by cyanosis, mottling, skin temperature that is warmer than usual, immediate capillary refill, and a distended or tense tissue turgor, is abnormal.

P Inadequate venous flow is a complication of digit or limb replantation following traumatic amputation.

ADVANCED TECHNIQUE

Assessing for Ruptured Achilles Tendon: Thompson Squeeze Test

E 1. Assist the patient to a prone position with the feet hanging over the edge of the examination table.
   2. Manually squeeze the calf muscles of the leg.
   3. Observe for plantar flexion of the foot being examined.

N When the calf muscles are squeezed, you should be able to visualize plantar flexion of the foot on the leg being examined.

P A positive Thompson test is manifested by the absence of plantar flexion when the calf muscles are squeezed.

P A positive Thompson test is suggestive of a ruptured Achilles tendon.

4. Draw an imaginary line:
   a. From the head down through the spinous processes (see Figure 18-68).
   b. Across the top of the scapula (see Figure 18-68).
   c. Across the top of the iliac crests.
   d. Across the bottom of the gluteal folds.
5. Palpate the spinous processes with your thumb.
6. Palpate the paravertebral muscles.
7. Assess ROM of the spine (see Figure 18-69). Ask the patient to bend forward from the waist and touch the toes (flexion).
8. If necessary, stabilize the patient's pelvis with your hands during the ROM assessment. Ask the patient to:
   a. Bend to each side (lateral bending).
   b. Bend backward (hyperextension).
   c. Twist the shoulders to each side (rotation).

N The normal spine has a cervical concavity, a thoracic convexity, and a lumbar concavity. An imaginary line can be drawn from the head straight down the spinous processes to the gluteal cleft. The imaginary lines drawn from the scapula, iliac crests, and gluteal folds are symmetrical

NURSING**TIP**

Differentiating Back Pain

Keep in mind that tenderness of the costovertebral angle can indicate a musculoskeletal problem or a kidney problem. Integrate the information obtained during the health history with clinical findings to guide your nursing interventions.

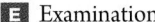 **E** Examination   **N** Normal Findings   **A** Abnormal Findings   **P** Pathophysiology

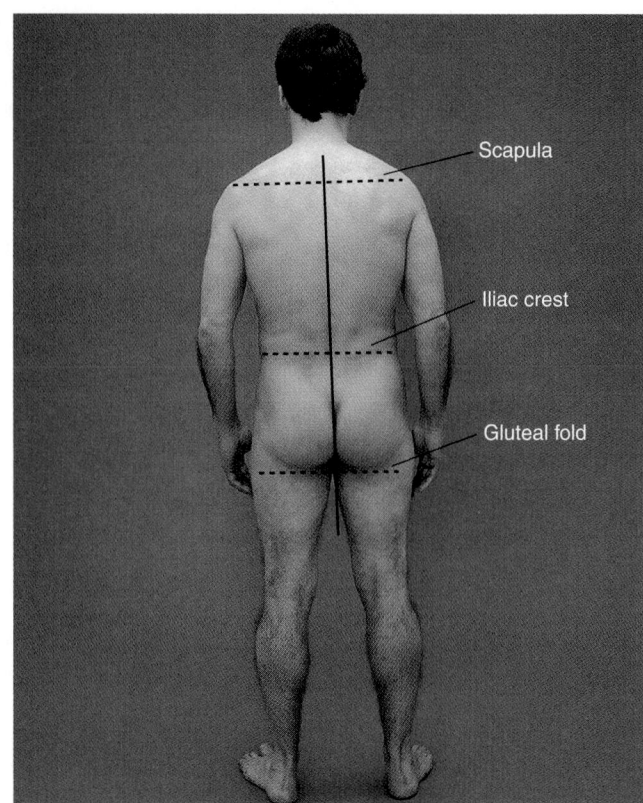

A. Lateral View

B. Posterior View

FIGURE 18-68 **Alignment of Spinal Landmarks**

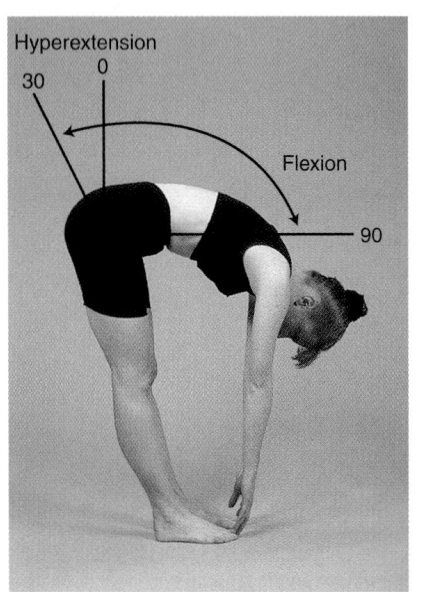

A. Flexion and Hyperextension

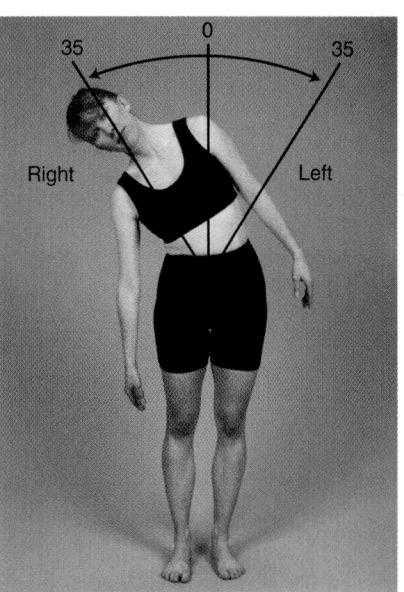

B. Lateral Bending

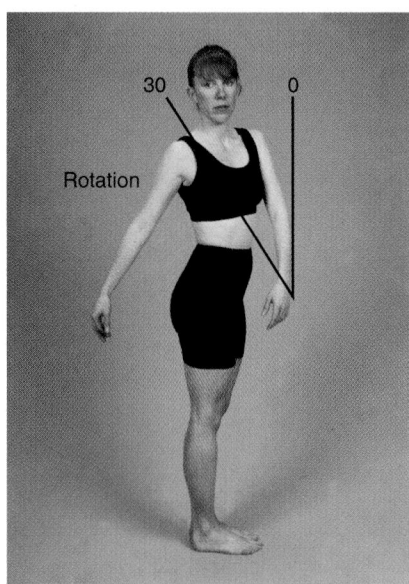

C. Rotation

FIGURE 18-69 **Range of Motion of the Spine**

with each other. The normal ROM of the spine is flexion—90°, hyperextension—30°, lateral bending—35°, and rotation—30°. As the patient flexes forward, the concavity of the lumbar spine disappears and the entire back assumes a convex C shape.

A From a posterior view, **scoliosis** (lateral curvature of the thoracic or lumbar vertebrae) may be detectable (Figure 18-70A, B) and is an abnormal finding.

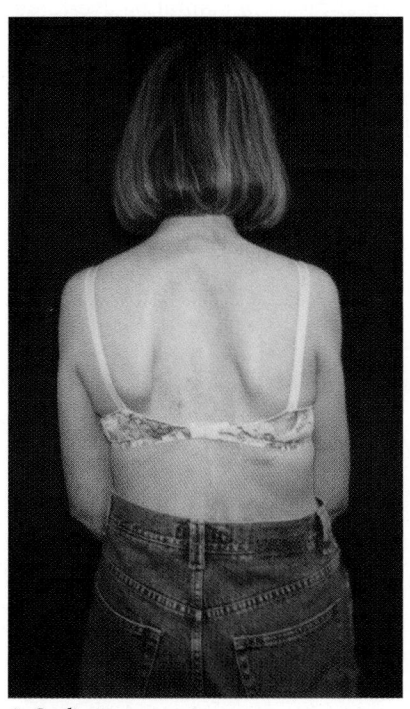

A. Scoliosis

The curvature is visible despite voluntary attempts at proper posture. This is structural scoliosis. The curvature becomes accentuated on forward flexion from the waist. Scoliosis may also be accompanied by asymmetry of the clavicles, uneven shoulder and iliac crest levels, and a visible prominence of a scapula. If the lateral curvature is allowed to progress beyond 55°, cardiopulmonary problems can occur. Surgery may be indicated if the curve exceeds 40°.

P Structural scoliosis occurs most frequently in adolescence, especially in females.

A Functional scoliosis, which manifests itself only in a standing position, is abnormal.

P Functional scoliosis is due to unequal leg length or poor posture. Limb length should be measured.

A **Kyphosis,** an excessive convexity of the thoracic spine (Figure 18-70C), is abnormal. The patient with kyphosis presents with the chin tilted downward onto the chest and with abdominal protrusion. There is also a decrease in the interval between the lower rib cage and the iliac crests. This appearance is due to forward and downward hunching of the head, neck, shoulders, and upper back.

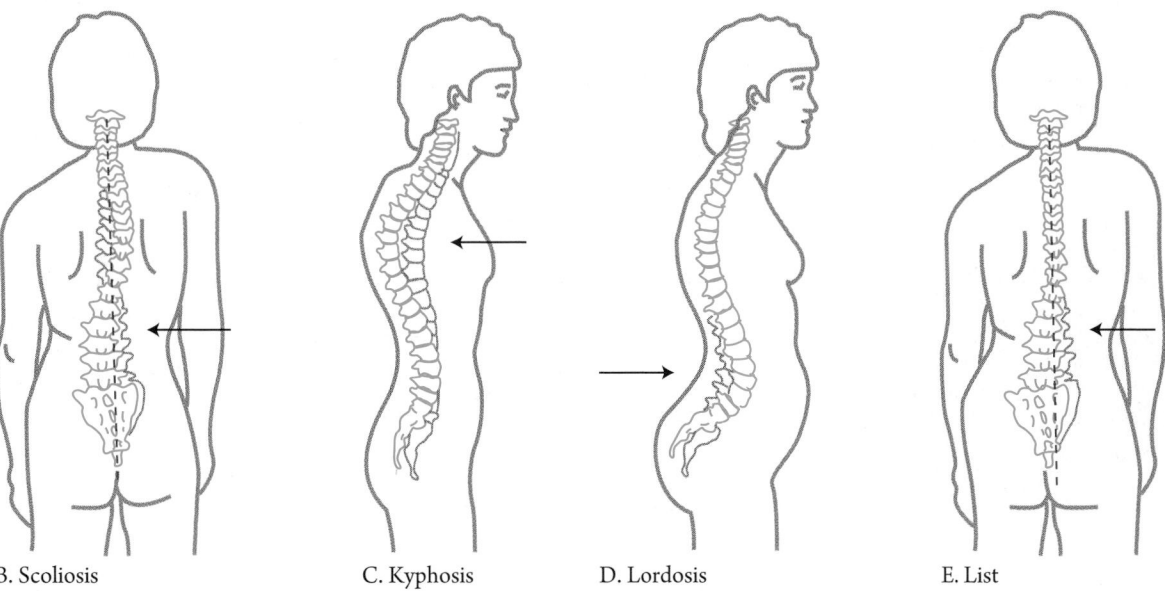

B. Scoliosis   C. Kyphosis   D. Lordosis   E. List

FIGURE 18-70 **Abnormalities of the Spine**

| **E** Examination | **N** Normal Findings | **A** Abnormal Findings | **P** Pathophysiology |

P Kyphosis is seen in elderly patients and in patients with osteoporosis, ankylosing spondylitis, and Paget's disease.

A **Lordosis**, an excessive concavity of the lumbar spine (see Figure 18-70D), is abnormal.

P Lordosis is accentuated in obesity and pregnancy due to the change in the center of gravity.

A A **list**, a leaning of the spine (see Figure 18-70E), is abnormal. If an imaginary line is drawn straight down from T1, the gluteal cleft is lateral to it. In scoliosis, the imaginary line rests in the gluteal cleft, and the spine deviates from this straight line.

P A list can result from a herniated vertebral disc and painful paravertebral muscle spasms.

A It is abnormal to have iliac crests that are unequal in height.

P Scoliosis and congenital or acquired limb length discrepancies lead to iliac crests that are not equal in height.

A Decreased ROM is abnormal. This is usually accompanied by pain.

P These clinical findings are found in back injury, osteoarthritis, and ankylosing spondylitis.

ADVANCED TECHNIQUE

Assessing for Scoliosis: Adams Forward Bend Test and Use of the Scoliometer

E 1. Instruct the patient to disrobe to the underclothing.

2. Have the patient stand upright with the feet together.

3. Stand behind the patient.

4. Ask the patient to bend forward from the waist with the hands held downward toward the feet and palms together (similar to a diving position). The head should be down, with the patient looking at the floor.

5. Inspect and palpate the progression of the spinous processes, starting at the cervical spine and progressing in an inferior direction to the sacral area.

6. Draw an imaginary line through the spinous processes (or use a felt-tip marker to connect the spinous processes).

7. Place the scoliometer (Figure 18-71A) on the thoracic vertebrae in the midspinal line. Measure the angle of trunk rotation on the scoliometer.

8. Place the scoliometer on the lumbar vertebrae (Figure 18-71B) in the midspinal line and measure the angle of trunk rotation.

N The imaginary (or real) line drawn through the spinous processes should be straight or with minimal deviation. The angle of trunk rotation reading on the scoliometer should be less than 7°.

A It is abnormal to have moderate to severe lateral deviation of the spine. An angle of trunk rotation reading greater than 7° indicates scoliosis.

P Structural scoliosis usually develops in adolescence.

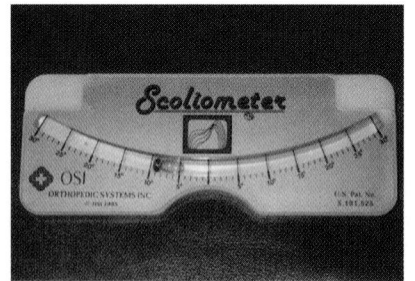

A. Scoliometer

B. Use of Scoliometer

FIGURE 18-71 Scoliometer and Its Use

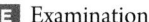

E Examination   **N** Normal Findings   **A** Abnormal Findings   **P** Pathophysiology

ADVANCED TECHNIQUE

Assessing for Herniated Disc: Straight Leg Raising Test (Lasègue's Test)

E 1. Assist the patient to a supine position on the examination table.

2. Place one hand on the heel of the right foot and place the other hand behind the upper calf area of the same leg.

3. Maintain the foot in its neutral anatomic position.

4. Raise the leg to the angle at which low back pain occurs.

5. With the extended leg still raised to its maximum height, manually dorsiflex the foot (Figure 18-72).

6. Repeat the technique on the left leg.

N The patient will be able to flex the hip joint and raise the straight leg to a hip flexion angle of 90°. There will be no low back pain with lifting of the extended leg or with dorsiflexion of the foot while the leg is raised.

A A positive straight leg raising test is abnormal. The patient will be unable to raise the extended leg to a 90° angle of hip joint flexion. Low back pain will occur with any lifting of the straight leg, and this discomfort will increase when the foot is dorsiflexed while the leg is in the raised position.

P Irritation of the nerve roots of the lumbosacral area causes pain in the sciatic nerve. Pain at less than 40° generally means an irritated nerve root caused by a herniated vertebral disc in the lumbosacral area. Pain may also occur in the other leg.

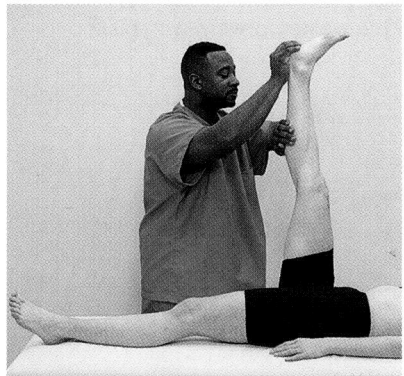

FIGURE 18-72 Straight Leg Raising Test

ADVANCED TECHNIQUE

Assessing for Herniated Disc: Milgram Test

E 1. Place the patient in a supine position on the examination table with both legs fully extended and resting on the table.

2. Instruct the patient to raise both legs at least 5 cm (2 inches) off the examination table while maintaining the legs in extension for at least 30 seconds.

N The patient will be able to hold the extended legs in the raised position for at least 30 seconds.

A The inability to maintain the straight legs in the raised position for at least 30 seconds is suggestive of pressure on the spinal nerves and is abnormal.

P A positive Milgram test is often indicative of a herniated intervertebral disc.

MUSCULOSKELETAL ASSISTIVE DEVICES
CHECKLIST

Assessing Patients with Musculoskeletal Assistive Devices

Assistive devices may be necessary to support musculoskeletal structure and function. The need for such devices automatically indicates an underlying musculoskeletal disorder. For each assistive device, determine the reason for its use.

Crutches
Determine the following:
  1. Amount of weight bearing allowed on affected lower limb
  2. Appropriate crutch height

continues

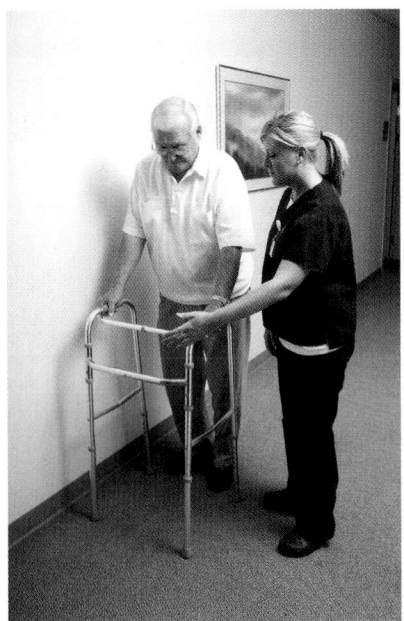

FIGURE 18-73 The nurse assesses the patient's ability to use the walker correctly.

Assessing Patients with Musculoskeletal Assistive Devices
continued

3. Type of crutch gait and appropriateness for the amount of weight bearing on affected leg: two-point crutch gait (partial weight-bearing); three-point crutch gait (partial or non-weight-bearing); four-point alternate crutch gait (partial or full weight-bearing); swing gait (non-weight-bearing)
4. Condition of crutches (padded handles, rubber tips)
5. Ease of transfer into and out of a chair
6. Ease of stair climbing with the crutches
7. Patient wearing flat, properly fitted shoes with nonskid surfaces
8. Signs or symptoms of skin breakdown or distal limb hypoperfusion

Cane
Determine the following:
1. Shape of handle (C or T)
2. Number of points on contact surface
3. Appropriateness for patient's height
4. Cane used on unaffected side
5. Refer to numbers 4–8 in the section on crutches

Walker
Determine the following:
1. Amount of weight bearing allowed on the lower limb
2. Type of walker (e.g., rolling or pickup walker)
3. Appropriateness for patient's height
4. Patient's ability to grip and propel the walker forward with rolling walker; patient's ability to grip, lift, and propel the walker forward with pickup walker (Figure 18-73)
5. Refer to numbers 4–8 in the section on crutches

Brace, Splint, Immobilizer
Determine the following:
1. Location of device (e.g., limb, neck, torso, lower back, or pelvis)
2. Joint position maintained by device (e.g., extension, flexion, or abduction)
3. Joint motion allowed by device
4. If a movable device is used, whether the hinge joint of the device is aligned with the skeletal joint
5. Padding under pressure points of device
6. Amount of weight bearing allowed on the affected leg (lower leg device)
7. Refer to numbers 7 and 8 in the section on crutches

Cast
Determine the following:
1. Plaster or nonplaster (e.g., synthetic, fiberglass)
2. Location of cast
3. Joint position maintained (e.g., extension, flexion, or abduction)
4. Joint motion allowed
5. Edges of the cast covered ("petaled") with tape to prevent skin irritation
6. Amount of weight bearing allowed (lower leg cast)
7. Damage to cast (e.g., cracked, flaking or crumbling, dented, wet, softening)
8. Visible discoloration on the cast (e.g., from underlying wound drainage or bleeding)
9. Significant odor around the cast (e.g., a musty or foul smell)
10. Refer to number 8 in the section on crutches

NURSINGALERT

Osteoarthritis Risk Factors

- Obesity
- Family history
- Age > 40–50
- Joint abnormality
- Overuse of joint
- History of joint trauma

The Patient with Musculoskeletal Trauma

This case study illustrates the application and objective documentation of the musculoskeletal assessment. Milton was hit by a car while crossing the street and presents to the Emergency Department for evaluation and treatment.

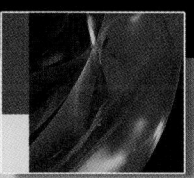

HEALTH HISTORY

PATIENT PROFILE	38 yo MBM
CHIEF COMPLAINT	"Everything hurts!"
HISTORY OF PRESENT ILLNESS	Patient transported to the ER 15 min ago following an MVA. While crossing a busy street against the cross signal, pt was hit by an SUV going approximately 35 mph. Upon impact, pt was thrown into the air, landing 20 ft away onto the street. Brief loss of consciousness at the scene as reported by EMS. EMS reports admission VS are HR 120 regular, BP 110/80 mm Hg from the Ⓛ thigh, RR 32 and labored, axillary temp 98.2 °F. 2+/3+ femoral pulses, EMS reports from transport: PERRLA, S1 and S2 present s̄ MGR; airway is patent s̄ tracheal deviation, breath sounds are ↓ over the Ⓛ lung fields. O2 saturation by pulse oximetry is 95% using a partial non-rebreather mask. No facial pallor or lip cyanosis. New ecchymosis is seen over most of the body, especially the Ⓛ side of the chest. Bleeding lacerations/abrasions are noted on the Ⓡ upper arm and over the Ⓡ thigh. 18-gauge IV in Ⓡ forearm and 18-gauge IV in Ⓡ dorsal foot vein, both inserted by EMS prior to ER transport. IV fluid of normal saline is infusing at wide-open rate via both IVs (total of 375 cc normal saline infused upon ER admission).
PAST HEALTH HISTORY	
Medical History	Seasonal allergic rhinitis during the summer mos, as manifested by nasal congestion and sneezing Nondisplaced complete fx of the Ⓡ humerus at age 14 due to a playground jungle gym fall. Treated by manual reduction under sedation/narcotic analgesia and casting. No complications or long-term adverse effects of injury
Surgical History	Dental removal of 4 impacted wisdom teeth under local anesthesia/conscious sedation at age 17. No complications or adverse effects of procedure Appendectomy under general anesthesia at age 22. No complications or adverse effects of procedure
Allergies	SAR as above requiring OTC medication. No comprehensive allergy testing or desensitizing tx performed Shellfish, had torso hives and facial angioedema following consumption of lobster at age 24; does not have Epi Pen

continues

CASE STUDY   (Continued)

The Patient with Musculoskeletal Trauma

	No medication allergies
	Denies bee sting/insect allergies
Medications	OTC allergy medication, either loratadine 10 mg po daily prn or cetirizine 10 mg po daily prn
	Occasional acetaminophen 325–650 mg po prn headache or other discomfort
	Daily MVI "when he remembers to take it" per spouse
	No daily prescription medication
Communicable Diseases	None. Annual PPD was negative last month.
Injuries and Accidents	Past humerus fracture as per PHH
Special Needs	Denies
Blood Transfusions	Denies
Childhood Illnesses	Healthy childhood c̄ an occasional otitis media and strep throat episode requiring antibiotic Rx. Pt received an annual physical exam during elementary, middle, and high school as a requirement for athletic activities. No other significant childhood health events.
Immunizations	Pt was fully immunized against childhood illnesses. Pt received his annual flu shot 4 weeks ago. Last tetanus shot was 2 yrs ago following a Ⓡ hand laceration that required suturing. Military reserve duty mandates compliance to recommended immunizations as well as to immunizations recommended for deployment to underdeveloped areas.

FAMILY HEALTH HISTORY

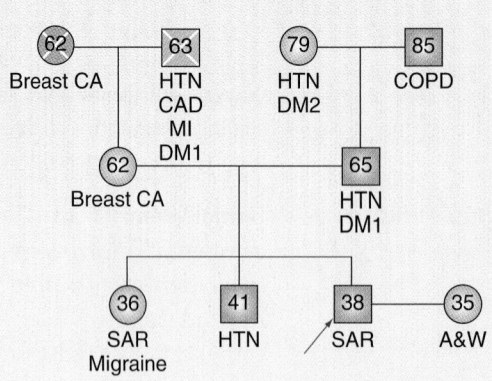

LEGEND

- ⬤ Living female
- ◼ Living male
- ⊗ Deceased female
- ⊠ Deceased male
- ↗ Points to patient

A&W = Alive & well
CA = Cancer
CAD = Coronary artery disease
COPD = Chronic obstructive pulmonary disease
DM = Diabetes mellitus
HTN = Hypertension
MI = Myocardial infarction
SAR = Seasonal allergic rhinitis

Denies FH of rheumatoid arthritis, osteoporosis, lupus, gout

continues

CASE STUDY   (Continued)

The Patient with Musculoskeletal Trauma

SOCIAL HISTORY	
Alcohol Use	2–3 beers (8 oz) per wk maximum. Occasional glass of red or white wine on wkend. Dislikes "hard liquor."
Tobacco Use	Never smoked, never used chewing tobacco or snuff
Drug Use	Occasional use of marijuana during college years, no recent use of such. No other illegal drug use. No reported abuse of OTC or prescription medication.
Domestic and Intimate Partner Violence	Denies
Sexual Practice	"Wild in college" per spouse. Multiple sexual partners in college but pt reports compliance c̄ recommended condom use c̄ each partner. No history of STD. Annual HIV testing for military reserve requirements has been negative (last done 6 mos ago). Monogamous for the last 12 yrs since meeting spouse.
Travel History	Various trips to Central/Western Europe, as well as to Hawaii. Last visit 11 mos ago to U.S. Virgin Islands. No major illness or injury during travel. Pt was preparing to go to Iraq c̄ his Army National Guard unit in the next year.
Work Environment	University security supervisor officer on a full-time basis. Pt has worked at his job for the last 8 years. Pt also holds the rank/rate of Captain/03 in the Army National Guard, with 12 yrs of military service (3 on active duty).
Home Environment	Married. Lives nearby c̄ wife in a 2-story townhouse. 10 steps needed to enter home, c̄ bedroom upstairs. Modern conveniences in the home. No children (wife recently had a miscarriage, pt and wife undergoing infertility treatments as well as considering adoption). Pets in the home environment include 2 domestic indoor kittens and an adult male German shepherd dog.
Hobbies and Leisure Activities	Travel, running, weightlifting
Stress	Couple currently undergoing expensive infertility treatments. Wife recently experienced a miscarriage. Pt was recently alerted of his pending military deployment to Iraq for 12–18 mos c̄ his military reserve unit.
Education	Bachelor's degree in criminal justice. Pt currently completing a part-time Master of Business Administration degree program by attending classes at night and on the weekend. Pt was hoping to complete graduate education prior to military deployment to Iraq.

continues

CASE STUDY (Continued)

The Patient with Musculoskeletal Trauma

Economic Status	"Stable without frills" per spouse. School loans have been paid off, leaving only car payment and mortgage. Both pt and spouse work full time and have comprehensive health and dental insurance, c̄ prescription coverage. Pt's military reserve pay provides extra income.
Military Service	As previously stated
Religion	Both pt and spouse are UUA (Unitarian-Universalist Association of Congregations) and attend Church every Sunday.
Ethnic Background	Both pt and spouse are Caribbean Americans from the island of St. Thomas.
Roles and Relationships	Both immediate and extended family are in the nearby area, c̄ frequent family gatherings. Family members and close friends are available and willing to help in times of need. Pt and spouse return to St. Thomas q yr to visit extended family.
Characteristic Patterns of Daily Living	Wakes at 6 AM to run 3–5 miles 3×per wk. Reports to work by 8:30 AM. Often brings lunch to work. "Tries to buy healthy lunches" at work per wife, but often eats fast food items for convenience and time limits. Home from work by 6 PM. Attends graduate night classes on Tuesdays and Thursdays from 7 PM to 9:30 PM. Usually in bed by 11:30 PM p̄ the nightly news.
HEALTH MAINTENANCE ACTIVITIES	
Sleep	7 to 7.5 hours per night. "Restless sleeper" per spouse due to caffeine intake during the day. No routine use of sedative/hypnotic agents to induce sleep. Occasional nap on the weekend.
Diet	Trying to avoid high-fat foods due to biannual military "weigh in" per spouse. Occasional fast food intake. Favorite food is hot and spicy meat chili. No lactose intolerance reported.
Exercise	Running and weightlifting as noted above. Pt needs to meet biannual military running time requirement for 1.5 miles.
Stress Management	Pt and spouse trying to deal c̄ the stress of infertility and pending military deployment to Iraq. Both are attending counseling as part of infertility therapy, as well as the nearby military family readiness program.
Use of Safety Devices	Pt routinely wears a seat belt while driving. Usually obeys pedestrian traffic guidelines per spouse, but was late for an appointment at the time of injury today.
Health Check-ups	Military reserve duty mandates an annual physical exam by a military hl care provider, including annual HIV and PPD testing.

continues

CASE STUDY (Continued)

The Patient with Musculoskeletal Trauma

PHYSICAL ASSESSMENT

General Assessment

Overall Appearance

Height: 6 feet 2 inches Weight: 185 lbs per spouse

Other than reported injuries, there are no obvious structural defects of the musculoskeletal system. All limbs and digits are present and in proportion to overall body size. No assistive devices. Pt is alert and fully oriented, but moaning in pain. There are visible lacerations and new ecchymosis of the face, forehead, and ℝ temporal area. There is no obvious clear or bloody drainage from the ears or the nose. Continuous bloody oozing from the mouth, and traumatic loss of several front teeth noted. There are bony deformities of the Ⓛ forearm, ℝ upper arm, and ℝ thigh. Bleeding wounds are noted on the ℝ upper arm and the ℝ thigh. No immobilizing splints were applied to the affected limbs by EMS prior to transport.

Posture

Pt is currently supine, secured to a backboard c̄ cervical collar in place by EMS pending vertebral integrity clearance. The ℝ leg measures 2 in. shorter than the Ⓛ leg. There is slight internal rotation of the ℝ leg. The Ⓛ leg remains in neutral position The wife reports no preinjury disturbance of pt posture, or of his ability to stand and sit. There is no preinjury reported discrepancy in limb length.

Gait and Mobility

Not observed, due to current injuries and vertebral immobilization. Spouse reports no problem with gait or mobility prior to today's MVA. Upon command, the patient is able to perform a hand grip, and wiggle all distal digits.

Inspection

Muscle Size and Shape

Well developed and contoured limb muscles.
Muscle hypertrophy of bilateral deltoid and bicep muscles.
No indication of muscle atrophy. No obvious involuntary muscle movement. Extensive swelling noted of both upper extremities and the ℝ upper leg.

Joint Contour and Periarticular Tissue

Joint contour WNL in the extension position. There is edema of the Ⓛ elbow and ℝ shoulder; ecchymosis extends to these areas.

Palpation

Muscle Tone

Nl tone associated c̄ muscle contraction over the noninjured muscles, c̄ hypertrophy. Muscle spasm is noted on the ℝ thigh muscles. Edema and tenderness over the muscles of the Ⓛ forearm and ℝ upper arm. Crepitus is palpated over the mid Ⓛ forearm in the extension position.

continues

CASE STUDY (Continued)

The Patient with Musculoskeletal Trauma

Joints	Pain over the Ⓛ elbow, Ⓡ shoulder, and posterior cervical joints. No crepitus over any body joint. There is no joint subluxation or joint dislocation. Pt is able to fully open and close his mouth.
Range of Motion	Not attempted upon ER admission due to pending radiological confirmation of vertebral stability and radiological assessment of possible multiple fx of the upper extremities and Ⓡ femur.
Muscle Strength	Limited assessment of muscle strength performed due to probable fractures of the upper extremities and the Ⓡ femur 4/5 muscle strength in the Ⓛ leg
Advanced Technique	Ⓡ thigh edematous, skin warm, dry Rapid capillary refill in all 4 limbs
Assessing Status of Distal Limbs and Digits	Ⓡ dorsalis pedis pulse is 1+/3+, Ⓛ dorsalis pedis is 2+/3+; all other pulses 2+/3+

ASSESSMENT IN BRIEF

Musculoskeletal Assessment

General Assessment
- Overall appearance
- Posture
- Gait and mobility

Inspection
- Muscle size and shape
- Joint contour and periarticular tissue

Palpation
- Muscle tone
- Joints

Range of Motion

Muscle Strength

Examination of Joints
- Temporomandibular joint
- Cervical spine
- Shoulders
- Elbows
- Wrists and hands
- Hips
- Knees
- Ankles and feet
- Spine

Advanced Techniques
- Measuring limb circumference
- Using a goniometer
- Chvostek's sign (assessing for neuroexcitability)
- Drop arm test (assessing for rotator cuff damage)
- Trousseau's sign (assessing for neuroexcitability)
- Assessing grip strength using a blood pressure cuff
- Tinel's sign (assessing for carpal tunnel syndrome)
- Phalen's sign (assessing for carpal tunnel syndrome)
- Trendelenburg test (assessing for hip dislocation)
- Measuring limb length
- Bulge sign (assessing for small effusions)
- Patellar ballottement (assessing for large effusions)
- Apley's grinding sign (assessing for meniscal tears)
- McMurray's sign (assessing for meniscal tears)
- Drawer test (assessing the cruciate ligaments)
- Lachman's test (assessing the anterior cruciate ligament)

continues

ASSESSMENT IN BRIEF *Continued*

- Varus stress test (assessing the lateral collateral ligament)
- Valgus stress test (assessing the medial collateral ligament)
- Anterior drawer test (assessing for ankle sprain)
- Talar tilt test (assessing for ankle sprain)
- Assessing status of distal limbs and digits
- Thompson squeeze test (assessing for ruptured Achilles tendon)
- Adams forward bend test (assessing for scoliosis) and use of the scoliometer

- Straight leg raising test (Lasègue's test) (assessing for herniated disc)
- Milgram test (assessing for herniated disc)

Assistive Devices
- Crutches
- Cane
- Walker
- Brace, splint, immobilizer
- Cast

REVIEW QUESTIONS

1. Following total hip joint replacement, the patient is instructed to avoid turning his affected leg and hip inward toward midline, or crossing the affected leg over the nonaffected leg. What are these movements called?
   a. External rotation, adduction
   b. Internal rotation, abduction
   c. Internal rotation, adduction
   d. External rotation, abduction
   The correct answer is (c).

2. What electrolyte imbalance is associated with a positive Trousseau's sign?
   a. Hypochloremia   c. Hypokalemia
   b. Hyponatremia   d. Hypocalcemia
   The correct answer is (d).

3. David is a 44-year-old male who enjoys long-distance running. He has been running 5 days a week for over 20 years. This year he has experienced increasing pain and stiffness in his knees, especially his right knee, which is his lead leg. David is most likely experiencing which musculoskeletal change?
   a. Rheumatoid arthritis   c. Osteomyelitis
   b. Osteoarthritis   d. Osteoporosis
   The correct answer is (b).

4. Painful involuntary muscle contraction near an area of acute bony deformity following trauma may represent which involuntary muscle movement?
   a. Asterixis   c. Fasciculation
   b. Tremor   d. Spasm
   The correct answer is (d).

5. Marion is a clerical worker who reports to the clinic complaining of painful tingling in the digits of her right hand, accompanied by wrist pain. With the patient positioned with the palmar surface of her right hand facing up, the examiner taps the median nerve over the center of the wrist. If Marion has carpal

tunnel syndrome, what would she now report to the examiner?
   a. Sudden onset of numbness in the thumb
   b. Burning wrist pain that radiates to the elbow
   c. Tingling sensation of the thumb, index, and middle fingers
   d. Sudden onset of numbness of the little finger
   The correct answer is (c).

6. Jimmy is a 22-year-old male who presents to ER triage complaining of severe pain in his left knee that suddenly occurred this afternoon while he was playing basketball. Which assessment technique would be used to assess the stability of the anterior cruciate ligament in his knee?
   a. Lachman's test   c. Straight-leg raising test
   b. Varus stress test   d. Valgus stress test
   The correct answer is (a).

7. What could be used as a quantitative technique for measuring grip strength in the conscious and cooperative patient?
   a. Instruct the patient to squeeze the examiner's hand.
   b. Instruct the patient to squeeze a caliper held in the examiner's hand.
   c. Instruct the patient to squeeze the examiner's finger.
   d. Instruct the patient to squeeze a rolled-up and slightly inflated blood pressure cuff.
   The correct answer is (d).

8. Sammy is a 10-year-old boy undergoing annual screening by the elementary school nurse. Following assessment of height, weight, visual acuity, and hearing, the nurse asks Sammy to bend forward from the waist and touch his toes. What disorder is characterized by lateral curvature of the spine in this position?
   a. Kyphosis   c. Lordosis
   b. Scoliosis   d. List
   The correct answer is (b).

9. Immediately following plaster cast application to a lower leg for immobilization of a reduced fracture, what assessment foci should the nurse monitor frequently?

a. Skin color, capillary refill, sensation, and movement of affected digits

b. Limb girth, limb length, and limb color

c. Cast odor, quantity of blood on the cast, and time until the plaster cast sets

d. Amount of weight bearing allowed on the cast

The correct answer is (a).

10. A 52-year-old right-handed woman who plays tennis every day comes to have her right shoulder evaluated for sudden pain and decreased mobility. You manually abduct the affected arm and ask the patient to slowly lower the arm while maintaining extension. You note that the patient's arm quickly falls to her side. What injury does this woman most likely have?

a. Adhesive capsulitis   c. Biceps tendonitis

b. Rotator cuff damage d. Shoulder subluxation

The correct answer is (b).

Visit the Estes online companion resource at
www.delmar.cengage.com
for additional content and study aids.
Click on Online Companions and then select
the Nursing discipline.

REFERENCE

Maher, A., Salmond, S., & Pellino, T. (2002). Orthopedic nursing (3rd ed.). Philadelpha: Elsevier.

BIBLIOGRAPHY

Best, J. T. (2005). Revision total hip and total knee arthroplasty. **Orthopedic Nursing, 24**(3), 174–179.

Brown, F. M. (2008). Nursing care after a shoulder arthroplasty. **Orthopedic Nursing, 27**(1), 3–9.

Diem, S. J., Blackwell, T. L., Stone, K. L., Yaffe, K., Haney, E. M., Bliziotes, M. M., & Ensrud, K. E. (2007). Use of antidepressants and rates of hip bone loss in older women. **Archives of Internal Medicine, 167**(12), 1240–1245.

DiFazio, D., & Atkinson, C. (2005). Extremity fracture in children: When is it an emergency? **Journal of Pediatric Care, 20**(4), 298–304.

Felson, D. (2006). Osteoarthritis of the knee. **New England Journal of Medicine, 354**(8), 841–848.

Folden, S., & Tappen, R. (2007). Factors influencing function and recovery following hip repair surgery. **Orthopedic Nursing, 26**(4), 234–241.

Hanna, J., & Letizia, M. J. (2007). A treatment for osteoporotic vertebral compression fracture. **Orthopedic Nursing, 26**(6), 342–346.

Ignatavicius, D., & Workman, M. L. (2006). **Medical-surgical nursing: Critical thinking for collaborative practice.** St. Louis: Elsevier-Saunders.

Lucas, B. (2006). Through the keyhole: An examination of minimally invasive hip surgery. **Orthopedic Nursing, 10**(1), 38–48.

Marter, A., & Agruss, J. C. (2008). Solving the riddle of fibromyalgia: An evidence-based practice protocol for the advanced practice nurse. **The Journal for Nurse Practitioners, 4**(6), 424–437.

McCaffrey, R., & Locsin, R. (2004). The effect of music listening on acute confusion and delirium in elders undergoing elective hip and knee surgery. **Orthopedic Nursing, 13**(6), 91–96.

Miller, N., & Askew, A. (2007). Tibia fractures: An overview of evaluation and treatment. **Orthopedic Nursing, 26**(4), 216–223.

Monahan, F., Sands, J., Neighbors, M., Marek, J., & Green, C. (2007). **Phipps' medical-surgical nursing: Health and illness perspectives.** St. Louis: Mosby.

Newman, A. M. (2007). Arthritis and sexuality. **Nursing Clinics of North America, 42**(4), 621–630.

Paice, J., Foog, L., Hollinger-Smith, L., Sikorski, K., & Stanaitis, H. (2008). Comparison of self-reported pain and the PAINAD scale in hospitalized cognitively impaired and intact older adults after hip fracture surgery. **Orthopedic Nursing, 27**(1), 21–28.

Richardson, R., & Engel, C. (2004). Evaluation and management of medically unexplained physical symptoms. **Neurologist, 10**(1), 18–30.

Shea, S. (2007). Emergency department evaluation of the knee. **Advanced Emergency Nursing, 29**(3), 241–248.

Wrotny, C. (2005). Osteoporosis: What women want to hear. **MEDSURG Nursing, 14**(6), 405–407, 415.

Zagaria, M. A. E. (2008). Relapsing-remitting multiple sclerosis: Primary and symptomatic management. **The American Journal for Nurse Practitioners, 12**(4), 22–26.

WEB SITES

American Academy of Orthopaedic Surgeons/American Association of Orthopaedic Surgeons:
http://www.aaos.org

Arthritis Foundation:
http://www.arthritis.org

Lupus Foundation of America:
http://www.lupus.org

National Association of Chronic Disease Directors:
http://www.chronicdisease.org

National Association of Orthopaedic Nurses:
http://www.orthonurse.org

National Osteoporosis Foundation:
http://www.nof.org

CHAPTER 19

Mental Status and Neurological Techniques

COMPETENCIES

1. Discuss the divisions of the nervous system and their functions.

2. Relate blood flow to the brain to the functional area supplied.

3. Describe the characteristics of the most common neurological complaints.

4. Perform a mental status assessment and document the results.

5. Assess the neurological system in a systematic manner and document the results.

6. Explain the pathophysiology of any abnormal results obtained.

7. Document a complete health history as it relates to the neurological system.

The nervous system controls all body functions and thought processes. The complex interrelationships among the various divisions of the nervous system permit the body to maintain homeostasis; to receive, interpret, and react to stimuli; and to control voluntary and involuntary processes, including cognition.

ANATOMY AND PHYSIOLOGY

The structure and function of the central nervous system and the peripheral nervous system are discussed.

MACROSTRUCTURE

The scalp and skull are two protective layers covering the brain. The scalp performs a unique function in that it moves freely, helping to protect and cushion the head from traumatic injury. The skull is a rigid, bony cavity that has a fixed volume of approximately 1,500 mL.

MENINGES

There are three layers of meninges (protective membranes), known as the dura mater, arachnoid mater, and pia mater, located between the brain and the skull (Figure 19-1). The dura mater is the thick, tough, outermost layer. Below the dura mater is a small serous space known as the subdural space.

The arachnoid mater lies between the dura mater and the pia mater. Below the arachnoid mater is the subarachnoid space, where cerebrospinal fluid (CSF) is circulated. Portions of the arachnoid mater, called arachnoid villi, project into the subarachnoid space (also shown in Figure 19-1). These serve to absorb CSF.

The pia mater is thin and vascular. It is the innermost layer of the meninges. The pia mater helps form the choroid plexuses, which are vascular structures located in the ventricles of the brain that form CSF.

CENTRAL NERVOUS SYSTEM

The brain and the spinal cord make up the central nervous system (CNS). The brain is divided into four main components: the cerebrum, the diencephalon, the cerebellum, and the brain stem. Each of these areas is subdivided into various anatomic areas.

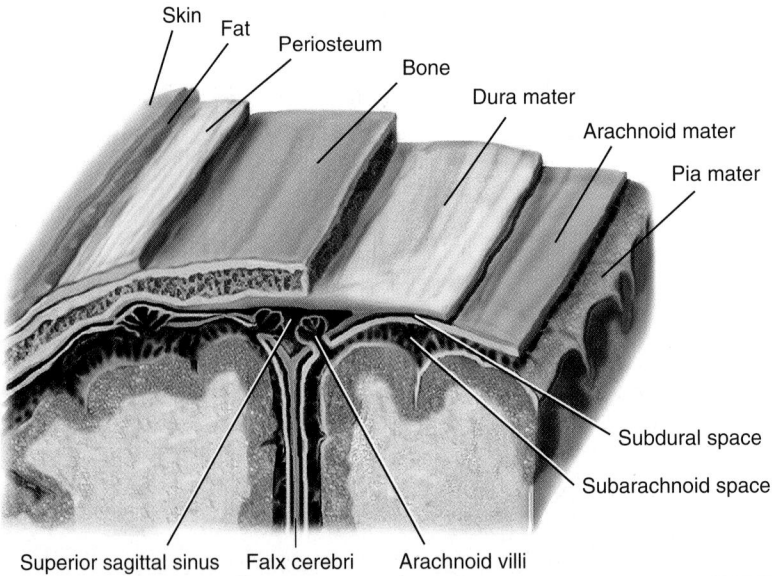

FIGURE 19-1 The Meninges

Cerebrum

The cerebrum is the largest portion of the brain. It is incompletely divided into right and left hemispheres by the longitudinal fissure. The two hemispheres are connected by the corpus callosum, which serves as a communication link between the left and right hemispheres.

The cerebral cortex, or the outermost layer of the cerebrum, contains gray matter. Higher cognitive functioning is dependent on the cerebral cortex and its interaction with other parts of the nervous system. The cerebral cortex is involved in memory storage and recall, conscious understanding of sensation, vision, hearing, and motor function. The basal ganglia are located deep within the cerebral hemispheres and function intricately with the cerebral cortex and the cerebellum in regulating motor activity.

Each cerebral hemisphere is divided into four lobes: the frontal, parietal, temporal, and occipital lobes. The locations and functions of each of the cerebral lobes are illustrated in Figure 19-2. A fifth lobe called the limbic lobe is anatomically part of the temporal lobe and is involved in emotional behavior and self-preservation.

Diencephalon

The diencephalon, a relay center for the brain, is composed of the thalamic structures: the thalamus, the epithalamus, and the hypothalamus. The hypothalamus is important in body temperature regulation, pituitary hormone control, and autonomic nervous system responses. It also plays a role in behavior via its connections with the limbic system.

Cerebellum

The cerebellum lies inferior to the occipital lobe and behind the brain stem. It is divided into two lateral lobes and a medial part called the vermis. The vermis is

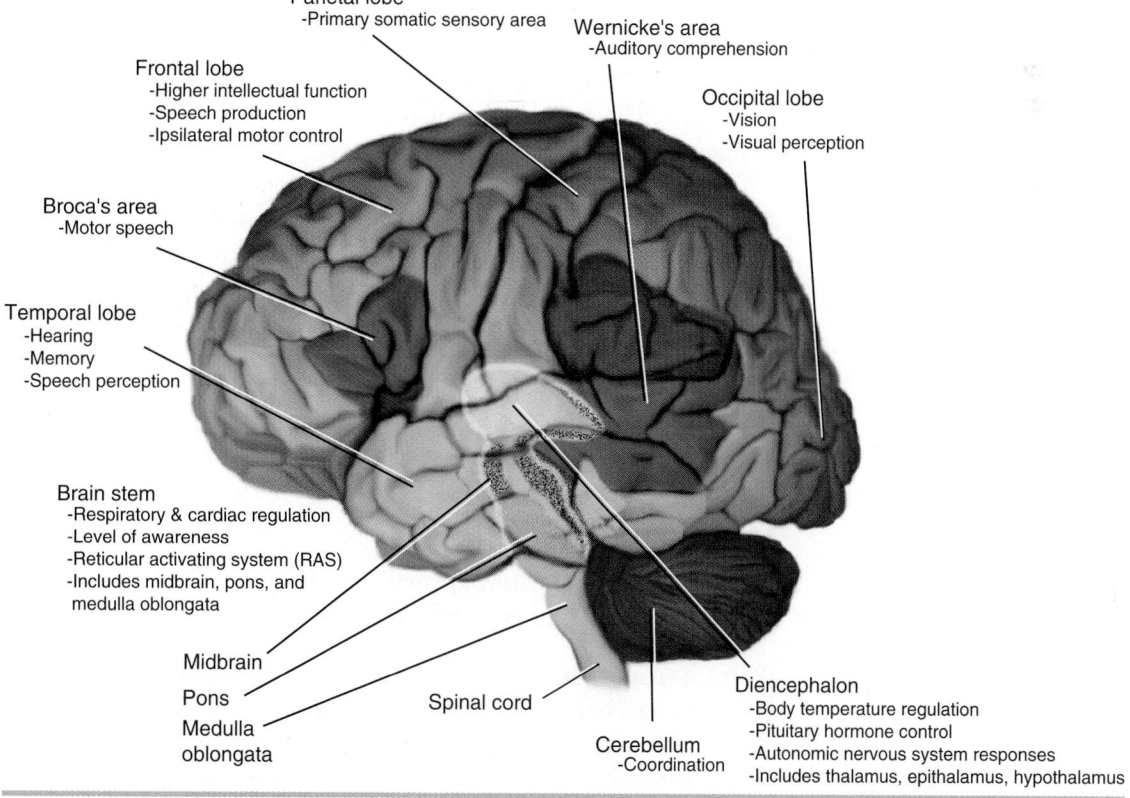

FIGURE 19-2 **The Locations and Functions of the Cerebral Lobes, Diencephalon, Cerebellum, and Brain Stem**

the part of the cerebellum concerned primarily with maintenance of posture and equilibrium. Each cerebellar hemisphere is responsible for coordination of movement of the ipsilateral (same) side of the body.

Brain Stem

The brain stem is located immediately below the diencephalon and is divided into the midbrain, the pons, and the medulla oblongata. The reticular formation, a complex network of sensory fibers in the brain stem, contains centers that control respiratory, cardiovascular, and vegetative functions. The ascending reticular activating system (RAS) is located in the brain stem and extends to the cerebral cortex. The RAS is mostly excitatory and is essential for arousal from sleep, maintaining attention, and perception of sensory input.

The midbrain contains the nuclei of cranial nerves III (oculomotor) and IV (trochlear), which are associated with control of eye movements. The pons is located between the midbrain and the medulla oblongata. Sensory and motor nuclei of cranial nerves V (trigeminal), VI (abducens), VII (facial), and VIII (acoustic) are located in the pons. The medulla oblongata is located between the pons and the spinal cord. It contains the nuclei of cranial nerves IX (glossopharyngeal), X (vagus), XI (spinal accessory), and XII (hypoglossal). Also located in the medulla oblongata are the centers for reflexes such as sneezing, swallowing, coughing, and vomiting, as well as the centers regulating the respiratory and cardiovascular systems.

Spinal Cord

The spinal cord is a continuation of the medulla oblongata. It exits the skull at the foramen magnum and begins at the upper border of the atlas (C1), continuing downward to the conus medullaris, a tapered ending of the cord at about the level of the first or second lumbar vertebrae (see Figure 19-3A). From the conus medullaris, a connective tissue filament called the filum terminale continues down to its attachment at the coccyx (see Figure 19-3B).

A cross section of the spinal cord will show that the central part of the cord is gray matter. The gray matter is in the shape of an H. White matter surrounds the gray matter.

The gray matter is made up of nerve cell bodies and short segments of unmyelinated fibers. The posterior portion of the H is called the dorsal horn, and the anterior portion is the ventral horn. Small lateral horns are also present in thoracic and upper lumbar sections of the spinal cord.

The dorsal horn contains cell bodies of sensory (afferent) neurons, which receive and transmit sensory messages from the afferent fibers in the spinal nerve. The ventral horn contains cell bodies of motor (efferent) neurons, which send axons into the spinal nerves and innervate skeletal muscles, carrying signals from the brain and the spinal cord.

Motor Pathways of the CNS

There are three motor pathways in the CNS: the corticospinal or pyramidal tract, the extrapyramidal tract, and the cerebellum.

PYRAMIDAL TRACT. The corticospinal pathway descends from the motor area of the cerebral cortex, through the midbrain, the pons, and the medulla. At the level of the medulla, 90% of the fibers of the corticospinal tract decussate (cross) to travel down the opposite side of the spinal cord, becoming the lateral corticospinal tract. The remaining fibers travel down the spinal cord in a tract

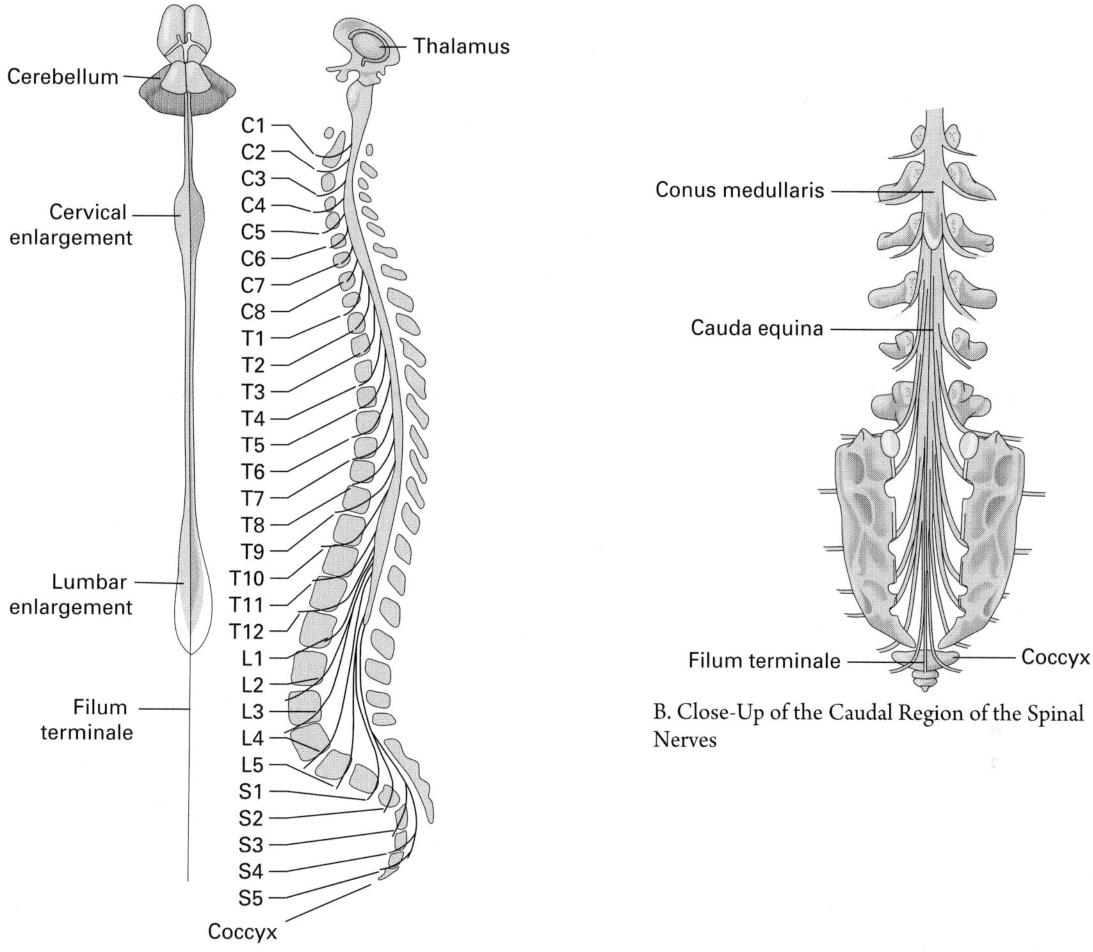

Cerebellum

Thalamus

Cervical enlargement

C1
C2
C3
C4
C5
C6
C7
C8
T1
T2
T3
T4
T5
T6
T7
T8
T9
T10
T11
T12
L1
L2
L3
L4
L5
S1
S2
S3
S4
S5

Lumbar enlargement

Filum terminale

Coccyx

A. The Spinal Cord and Spinal Nerves

Conus medullaris

Cauda equina

Filum terminale

Coccyx

B. Close-Up of the Caudal Region of the Spinal Nerves

FIGURE 19-3 **The Spinal Cord**

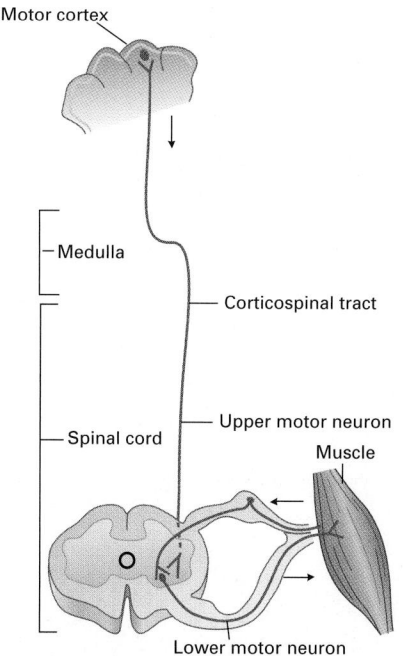

Motor cortex

Medulla

Corticospinal tract

Spinal cord

Upper motor neuron

Muscle

Lower motor neuron

FIGURE 19-4 **Motor Pathways of the CNS**

known as the anterior corticospinal tract. Fibers of the lateral corticospinal tract synapse in the anterior horn (gray matter) at all levels of the cord just before they leave the cord (Figure 19-4). The motor neurons above this synapse in the anterior horn are known as upper motor neurons. Upper motor neurons connect the cerebral cortex with the anterior horn and are entirely contained within the CNS. Lower motor neurons are motor neurons below the level of the upper motor neurons. Lower motor neuron cell bodies are located in the anterior horn, where they connect with the corticospinal tract. Lower motor neurons innervate skeletal muscle at the myoneural junction. They are responsible for purposeful, voluntary movement.

EXTRAPYRAMIDAL TRACT. This pathway includes all motor neurons in the motor cortex, basal ganglia, brain stem, and spinal cord that are outside the corticospinal, or pyramidal, tract (henceforth referred to as extrapyramidal). The extrapyramidal tract is responsible for controlling body movement, particularly gross automatic movements (e.g., walking), and for controlling muscle tone.

Sensory Pathways of the CNS

The sensory portion of the peripheral nervous system consists of afferent neurons divided into somatic afferent and visceral afferent neurons. Somatic afferent fibers

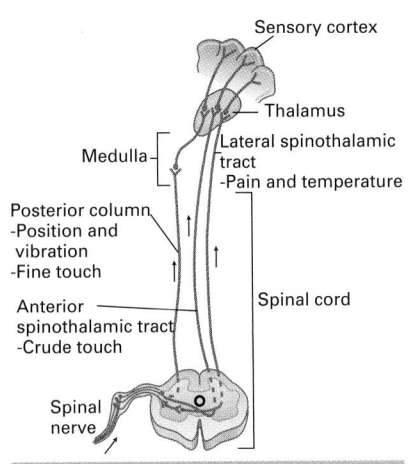

FIGURE 19-5 Sensory Pathways of the CNS

originate in skeletal muscles, joints, tendons, and skin. Visceral fibers originate in the viscera. Both types of afferent fibers carry impulses from both the external and the internal environments to the CNS.

Afferent fibers containing impulses, or messages, enter the spinal cord through the dorsal roots. From the spinal cord the message travels via the spinothalamic tracts or the posterior column to the thalamus and sensory cortex. The thalamus receives the message and interprets a general sensation. The impulse synapses with another sensory neuron to the sensory cortex, where the message is fully interpreted (Figure 19-5).

SPINOTHALAMIC TRACTS. In the spinal cord, the spinothalamic tracts synapse with a second sensory neuron and then decussate to the opposite side. The message is then carried up the tract. The lateral spinothalamic tract carries pain and temperature sensations, and the anterior spinothalamic tract carries the sensations of crude or light touch.

POSTERIOR COLUMN. The posterior column carries position, vibration, and fine-touch sensations. The nerve impulse enters the spinal cord and travels upward to the medulla, where a synapse with a second sensory neuron occurs. The neuron decussates to the opposite side of the medulla and continues on to the thalamus and sensory cortex.

BLOOD SUPPLY

Blood is supplied to the brain by two pairs of arteries, the internal carotid arteries (anterior circulation) and the vertebral arteries (posterior circulation). At the base of the brain lies the circle of Willis, an arterial anastomosis that links the anterior and posterior blood supplies (Figure 19-6). The functional areas supplied by each of the main cerebral arteries are listed in Table 19-1.

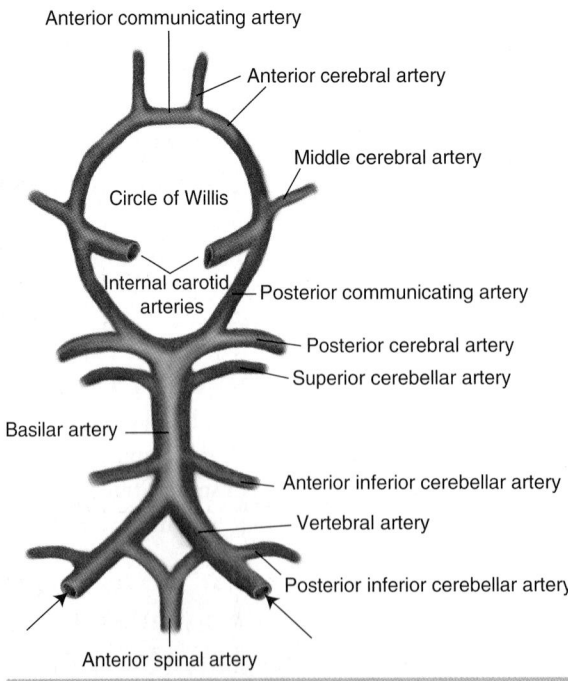

FIGURE 19-6 Major Arteries of the Brain

TABLE 19-1 Cerebral Blood Supply

ARTERY	FUNCTIONAL AREA
Anterior cerebral artery	Medial and inferior surfaces of each hemisphere: • Frontal lobe • Parietal lobe
Middle cerebral artery	Lateral surface of each hemisphere: • Frontal lobe • Temporal lobe • Parietal lobe • Occipital lobe
Posterior cerebral artery	Medial and inferior surfaces of each hemisphere: • Temporal lobe • Medial occipital lobe • Midbrain
Basilar artery	• Midbrain • Upper brain stem • Medulla oblongata
Cerebellar arteries	• Pons • Midbrain • Cerebellum

PERIPHERAL NERVOUS SYSTEM

The peripheral nervous system consists of nervous tissue found outside the CNS, including the spinal nerves, cranial nerves, and the autonomic nervous system.

Spinal Nerves

The 31 pairs of spinal nerves include 8 cervical, 12 thoracic, 5 lumbar, 5 sacral, and 1 coccygeal. Each spinal nerve is made up of a dorsal (afferent) root and a ventral (efferent) root. Each afferent spinal nerve root innervates a specific area of the skin, called a **dermatome**, for superficial cutaneous sensations. Figure 19-7 illustrates both the anterior and the posterior dermatomal distributions. Spinal nerves leaving the right side of the cord supply the right side of the body, and those leaving the left side supply the left side.

Each of the eight cervical nerves exits above its corresponding vertebra. Each of the spinal nerves below the cervical portion exits below its corresponding vertebra. The spinal cord is not as long as the vertebral column, so the lumbar and sacral nerves are comparatively long. These longer roots are called the cauda equina, meaning "horse's tail" (see Figure 19-3B).

Cranial Nerves

There are 12 pairs of cranial nerves. They are designated in order of their position with roman numerals I through XII. Some cranial nerves have purely motor functions and some have only sensory functions. Others have mixed sensory and motor functions. Table 19-2 summarizes the functions of the cranial nerves.

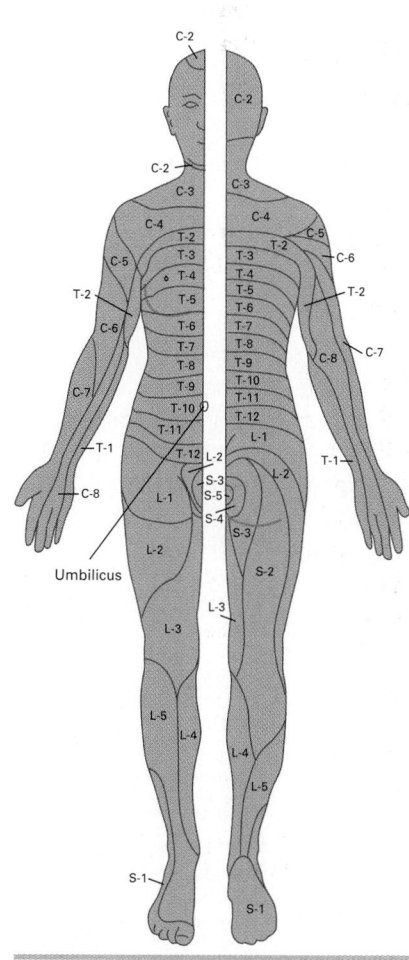

FIGURE 19-7 Anterior and Posterior Dermatomal Distributions

TABLE 19-2 The 12 Cranial Nerves and Their Functions

NAME AND NUMBER	FUNCTION
Olfactory (I)	Smell
Optic (II)	Visual acuity, visual fields, funduscopic examination
Oculomotor (III)	Cardinal fields of gaze (EOM movement), eyelid elevation, pupil reaction, doll's eyes phenomenon
Trochlear (IV)	EOM movement
Trigeminal (V)	Motor: strength of temporalis and masseter muscles Sensory: light touch, superficial pain and temperature to face, corneal reflex
Abducens (VI)	EOM movement
Facial (VII)	Motor: facial movements Sensory: taste anterior two-thirds of tongue Parasympathetic: tears and saliva secretion*
Acoustic (VIII)	Cochlear: gross hearing, Weber and Rinne tests Vestibular: vertigo, equilibrium, nystagmus
Glossopharyngeal (IX)	Motor: soft palate and uvula movement, gag reflex, swallowing, guttural and palatal sounds Sensory: taste posterior one-third of tongue Parasympathetic: carotid reflex, chemoreceptors*
Vagus (X)	Motor and Sensory: same as CN IX Parasympathetic: carotid reflex, stomach and intestinal secretions, peristalsis, involuntary control of bronchi, heart innervation*
Spinal Accessory (XI)	Sternocleidomastoid and trapezius muscle movements
Hypoglossal (XII)	Tongue movement, lingual sounds

Cannot be directly assessed.

EOM = extraocular muscle; CN = cranial nerve.

NURSING**TIP**

Cranial Nerve Mnemonics

Mnemonics can assist you in remembering the name of each cranial nerve and whether each nerve has a sensory function, a motor function, or both.

FIRST LETTER OF CRANIAL NERVE	NUMBER OF CRANIAL NERVE	FUNCTION OF CRANIAL NERVE
On (Olfactory)	I	**S**ome
Old (Optic)	II	**S**ay
Olympus's (Oculomotor)	III	**M**arry
Towering (Trochlear)	IV	**M**oney
Tops (Trigeminal)	V	**B**ut
A (Abducens)	VI	**M**y
Finn (Facial)	VII	**B**rother
And (Acoustic)	VIII	**S**ays
German (Glossopharyngeal)	IX	**B**ad
Viewed (Vagus)	X	**B**usiness
Some (Spinal Accessory)	XI	**M**arry
Hops (Hypoglossal)	XII	**M**oney

For cranial nerve function: **S** = sensory nerve, **M** = motor nerve, **B** = both sensory and motor nerves.

TABLE 19-3 Sympathetic versus Parasympathetic Response

SYSTEM	SYMPATHETIC RESPONSE	PARASYMPATHETIC RESPONSE
Neurological	Pupils dilated Heightened awareness	Pupils normal size
Cardiovascular	Increased heart rate Increased myocardial contractility Increased blood pressure	Decreased heart rate Decreased myocardial contractility
Respiratory	Increased respiratory rate Increased respiratory depth Bronchial dilation	Bronchial constriction
Gastrointestinal	Decreased gastric motility Decreased gastric secretions Increased glycogenolysis Decreased insulin production Sphincter contraction	Increased gastric motility Increased gastric secretions Sphincter dilatation
Genitourinary	Decreased urine output Decreased renal blood flow	Normal urine output

Autonomic Nervous System

The autonomic nervous system (ANS) is divided into two functionally different subdivisions: the sympathetic and the parasympathetic nervous systems. The ANS functions without voluntary control to maintain the body in a state of homeostasis. Most organs that are under the influence of the ANS have dual innervation of both sympathetic and parasympathetic systems.

The sympathetic nervous system, sometimes called the thoracolumbar system, controls "fight or flight" actions. The parasympathetic nervous system (craniosacral) is responsible for "general housekeeping" of the body. See Table 19-3 for specific system responses to autonomic stimulation.

REFLEXES

A reflex action, a specific response to an adequate stimulus, occurs without conscious control. The stimulus can occur in a joint, muscle, or the skin, and is transmitted to the CNS by one or more afferent, or sensory, neurons. The impulse enters the spinal cord through the dorsal root of a spinal nerve, where it synapses. Following synapse in the cord, the anterior motor neurons send an impulse via efferent neurons to the endplates of the skeletal muscle, causing the effector muscle to react (Figure 19-8).

A monosynaptic reflex, such as the patellar reflex, involves two neurons: one afferent and one efferent. Polysynaptic reflexes involve many neurons in addition to the afferent and efferent limbs of the reflex arc. Reflexes are classified into three main categories: muscle stretch, or deep tendon reflexes (DTR); superficial reflexes; and pathological reflexes.

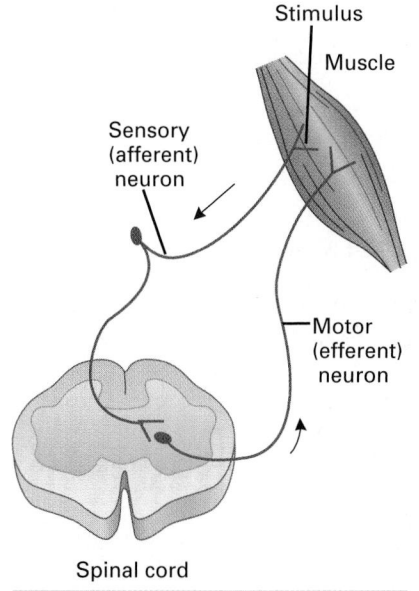

Stimulus

Muscle

Sensory (afferent) neuron

Motor (efferent) neuron

Spinal cord

FIGURE 19-8 Monosynaptic Reflex Arc

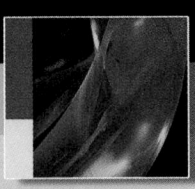

HEALTH HISTORY

The neurological health history provides insight into the link between a patient's life and lifestyle and neurological information and pathology.

PATIENT PROFILE	*Diseases that are age-, gender-, and race-specific for the neurological system are listed.*
Age	Multiple sclerosis (MS) (20–40)
	Myasthenia gravis (20–30)
	Fibromyalgia (25–50)
	Syringomyelia (30)
	Huntington's chorea (30–40)
	Parkinson's disease (>50)
	Alzheimer's disease (middle age–old age)
Gender	
Female	Myasthenia gravis, MS, meningiomas, pseudotumor cerebri, migraine headaches, fibromyalgia
Male	Cervical spine injuries, cluster headache, dyslexia (boys)
Race	
African American	Intracerebral hemorrhage (due to increased incidence of hypertension)
Asian or Pacific Islander	Intracranial hemorrhage
Hispanic	Intracranial hemorrhage
Caucasian	Multiple sclerosis
CHIEF COMPLAINT	*Common chief complaints for the neurological system are defined and information on the characteristics of each sign or symptom is provided.*
1. Headache	See Chapter 11
2. Seizure	A transient disturbance of cerebral function caused by an excessive discharge of neurons
Location	Body parts involved
Quality	General or localized
Quantity	Number of minutes or seconds, weekly, monthly, every few months
Associated Manifestations	Incontinence, injury (tongue, cheeks, limbs), memory loss, cyanosis, respiratory arrest; postictal headache, somnolence, or confusion
Aggravating Factors	Television viewing, bright lights, sleep deprivation, stress, flashing lights, hyperventilation, fever in children or infants, alcohol (use or withdrawal), hyperglycemia, hypoglycemia
Alleviating Factors	Medications
Setting	Sequence of events: warning (aura) such as headache, abdominal discomfort, euphoria or depression, visual hallucination; phases: tonic, clonic, postictal, fugue states

continues

Health History (continued)

Timing	First occurrence, age at onset of seizures, associated trauma or presumed cause, sleeping hours, first awakening, menses
3. Syncope	Abrupt loss of consciousness of brief duration due to decreased oxygen or glucose supply to the brain
Quality	Total versus partial loss of consciousness
Quantity	Duration of seconds, minutes, or hours; daily, monthly
Associated Manifestations	Nausea, diaphoresis, dimmed vision, increased salivation, gastrointestinal bleeding, dyspnea, chest pain, palpitations, hemiparesis, transient focal deficits, seizures, migraine headache, associated illness (myocardial infarction, diabetes mellitus type 1)
Aggravating Factors	Injury, intense emotion, carotid occlusion, cardiovascular disorders, exertion, anemia, hypoglycemia, insulin peak, crowded space, decreased atmospheric oxygen
Alleviating Factors	Cool air, change in position, oxygen, glucose, medication, volume infusions
Setting	Hot, stuffy room; standing still for long periods of time
4. Tremor	Repetitive, often regular, oscillatory movements of a body part caused by contraction of opposing muscle groups; usually voluntary
Location	Voice, face, arms, hands, trunk
Quality	Postural, intention/essential, rest
Aggravating Factors	Fatigue, anxiety, caffeine, movement; hyperthyroidism, cerebellar disease, MS, Parkinson's disease; lithium, tricyclic antidepressants
Alleviating Factors	Rest, propranolol, benzodiazepines, L-dopa, primidone, alcohol intake
Setting	Head or hands outstretched against gravity; with tasks requiring precision or fine motor grasp
Timing	Age of onset; intermittent, constant
5. Pain	A sensation of discomfort, distress, or suffering
Location	Anatomic location (e.g., lower back, head)
Quality	Aching, stabbing, throbbing, cramping
Associated Manifestations	Crying, hysteria, muscular tenseness, depression, shortness of breath, diaphoresis, splinting or protective behaviors, focal deficits, limited range of motion, sleep disturbance
Aggravating Factors	Stress, excessive exercise, lifting, coughing or sneezing, posture changes, trauma, illness, extreme temperatures, humidity
Alleviating Factors	Medications, heat, cold, distraction, physical therapy
Timing	Minutes to constant; early morning, late day; daily, monthly
6. Paresthesia	Abnormal sensations such as numbness, pricking, tingling
Location	Anatomic location (e.g., arms, hands, legs, feet)
Quality	Aching, stabbing, pins and needles, numbness

continues

Associated Manifestations	Pain, stiffness, changes in gait, pulseless extremities, pallor, injury, ulcers, muscle wasting, traumatic injury
Aggravating Factors	Activity, extreme cold, diabetes mellitus
Alleviating Factors	Medication, warmth, position changes
7. Disturbances in Gait	Abnormal way of moving on foot, walking, or running
Quality	Ataxic, spastic hemiplegia, hemiplegic, scissors, festinating, steppage, antalgic, apraxic, Trendelenburg
Associated Manifestations	Vertigo, visual impairments, blackouts, stroke, focal weakness, muscle wasting, abnormal movements or posture, spasticity, falling
Aggravating Factors	Fatigue, alcohol ingestion, vitamin D deficiency
Alleviating Factors	Rest, assistive devices
Setting	Level ground versus uneven terrain, CVA, neuromuscular pathology
8. Visual Changes	Changes in visual acuity, visual fields, color perception, depth perception
Quality	Blindness in particular field of vision; scotoma; perception of flashing, bright lights; blurriness
Associated Manifestations	Vertigo, dizziness, nausea, weakness, headache
Aggravating Factors	Darkness, fatigue, bright lights, reading, alcohol ingestion, medication
Alleviating Factors	Rest, medications, glasses
Timing	Abrupt, gradual, constant, intermittent, morning, evening
9. Vertigo	The sensation of moving in space or objects moving around the person; also may be referred to as dizziness, lightheadedness
Quality	Spinning sensations, dizziness, or lightheadedness
Associated Manifestations	Nausea, vomiting, headache, tinnitus, deafness, discharge from ear, cranial nerve palsies, hemiparesis, seizure, loss of consciousness, chest pain, palpitations, falling
Aggravating Factors	Motion, movement of head, changes in atmospheric pressure (weather), heights, amusement rides, anxiety, alcohol ingestion, pain, medications
Alleviating Factors	Medications, lying down, maintaining a still posture
Setting	Amusement rides, glassed-in elevators, rising from a seated or supine position
Timing	Sudden, gradual; seconds, minutes, days, months; constant, intermittent
10. Memory Disorders	Change in ability to remember events or facts
Quality	Recent or remote memory loss
Associated Manifestations	Irritability, anxiety, agitation, confabulation, associated trauma, depression, fearfulness
Aggravating Factors	Distraction, anxiety, medications, alcohol ingestion, drug abuse, unfamiliar environment, sleep deprivation, anesthesia, hypoxia, electrolyte imbalance, high altitude

continues

Health History (continued)	
Alleviating Factors	Visual or auditory cues, familiarity with environment, oxygen, electrolyte replacement, narcotic reversal, detoxification
Setting	Unfamiliar environment
Timing	Nighttime, upon awakening
11. Difficulty with Swallowing or Speech	Inability to swallow food or drink, choking, or aspiration; changes in enunciation of words, volume of speech, content of speech, or comprehension of written or verbal language
Associated Manifestations	Excessive drooling and saliva, paresis, dysarthria, weight loss, dehydration, irritability, depression, disease or damage to the CNS such as stroke or cerebral palsy
Aggravating Factors	Fatigue, position, prolonged tracheal intubation, alcohol intake
Alleviating Factors	Rest, quiet environment, thickened liquids, soft foods, varied communication tools
Setting	Loud, chaotic environment; after prolonged intubation
PAST HEALTH HISTORY	*The various components of the past health history are linked to neurological pathology and neurology-related information.*
Medical History	
Neurologic Specific	Amyotrophic lateral sclerosis (ALS), multiple sclerosis (MS), tumors, Guillain-Barré syndrome, cerebral aneurysm, arteriovenous malformations (AVM), cerebrovascular accident (CVA), migraines, Alzheimer's disease, myasthenia gravis, congenital defects, metabolic disorders, childhood seizures, head trauma, neuropathies, peripheral vascular disease, Parkinson's disease
Non-Neurologic Specific	Hypertension, heart disease, cardiac surgery, invasive procedures, diabetes mellitus, leukemia, hypoglycemia
Surgical History	Craniotomy, laminectomy, carotid endarterectomy, transsphenoidal hypophysectomy, cordotomy, aneurysmectomy or repair
Medications	Antidepressants, antiseizure medications, narcotics, antianxiety medications, antipsychotic medications
Communicable Diseases	Encephalitis, meningitis or poliomyelitis, AIDS dementia, botulism, syphilis, cat scratch disease, rickettsial infections, toxoplasmosis
Injuries and Accidents	Closed head injury, chronic subdural hematoma, spinal cord injury, peripheral nerve damage
FAMILY HEALTH HISTORY	*Neurological diseases that are familial are listed.*
	Congenital defects such as neural tube defects, hydrocephalus, AVM, headaches, epilepsy, Alzheimer's disease, Huntington's chorea, muscular dystrophies, lipid storage diseases, Gaucher's disease, Niemann-Pick's disease
SOCIAL HISTORY	*The components of the social history are linked to neurological factors and pathology.*

continues

Health History (continued)

Alcohol Use	Patients suffering from chronic alcoholism may exhibit the following abnormal findings: Korsakoff's psychosis, polyneuropathy, Wernicke's encephalopathy, tremor
Tobacco Use	Increased risk of stroke
Drug Use	Neurological signs of drug use are listed in Table 19-4.
Sexual Practice	Neurosyphilis; impotence secondary to neuropathies, MS, or lower motor neuron lesions
Travel History	Arthropod-borne encephalitis (Venezuelan equine, Japanese B, Murray-Valley, Russian spring-summer, Central European, Colorado tick), malaria
Work Environment	Exposure to continuous loud noise, performing repetitive-motion tasks, toxic chemical exposure (carbon dioxide, insecticides)
Home Environment	Exposure to toxic chemicals (carbon dioxide, insecticides), lead paint
Hobbies and Leisure Activities	Use of protective equipment; participation in contact sports or high-risk activities such as football, soccer, hockey, boxing, race car driving, motorcycling; hobbies involving repetitive motion (needlework)
Stress	Headaches; migraine H/A, fibromyalgia flares, or MS can be exacerbated by stress
Ethnic Background	
Jewish	Tay-Sachs disease
Northern European	MS
HEALTH MAINTENANCE ACTIVITIES	*This information provides a bridge between the health maintenance activities and neurological function.*
Sleep	Narcolepsy, insomnia
Diet	Beriberi (vitamin B_1), pellagra (niacin)
Exercise	Increased muscle strength, increased coordination
Use of Safety Devices	Helmet, seat belt, eye shields
Health Check-ups	Developmental milestones

NURSINGALERT

Risk Factors for Stroke

Significant risk factors for stroke include:

- Hypertension
- Diabetes mellitus
- Cocaine use
- Cigarette smoking
- Hyperlipidemia
- Atrial fibrillation and flutter
- History of cerebral aneurysm
- Sickle cell disease
- IV drug abuse
- Alcohol abuse
- Obesity
- Oral contraceptive use, especially in women over age 35 who smoke and have hypertension

TABLE 19-4 Neurological Signs of Drug Ingestion

ASSESSMENT PARAMETER	DRUG				
	HALLUCINOGENS	CANNABIS (MARIJUANA)	NARCOTICS	SEDATIVE-HYPNOTICS	CNS STIMULANTS
Pupils	Dilated React to light	Normal	Pinpoint Fixed	Normal	Dilated React to light
Deep tendon reflexes	Hyperactive	Normal	Normal	Hypoactive	Hyperactive
Speech	Normal	Often normal	Normal or dulled	Slurred	N/A
Coordination	Normal	Normal	Normal or unsteady	Ataxia	N/A
Sensorium	Often clear	Usually clear	Dulled	Confusion	May be confused
Sensory perception	Distorted	Distorted	Dulled	Dulled	Heightened
Memory	Unchanged	Transient loss	Unchanged	Impaired	Unchanged
Hallucinations	Any type	Rare	Rare	N/A	N/A
Delusions	Variable	Paranoid	N/A	N/A	Paranoid

N/A = not applicable.

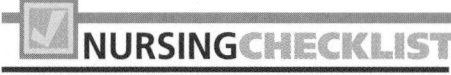

NURSINGCHECKLIST

General Approach to Neurological Assessment

1. Greet the patient and explain the assessment techniques that you will be using.
2. Maintain a quiet, unhurried, self-confident demeanor to help relieve any feelings of anxiety or discomfort and to help the patient relax during the assessment.
3. Provide a warm, quiet, and well-lit environment.
4. After the mental status examination, instruct the patient to remove all street clothes, and provide an examination gown for the patient to put on.
5. Begin the assessment with the patient in a comfortable, upright sitting position, or for the patient on bed rest, position the patient comfortably, preferably with the head of the bed elevated, or flat, whichever is tolerated best or is within activity orders for the patient.

EQUIPMENT

- Cotton wisp
- Cotton-tipped applicators
- Penlight
- Tongue blade
- Tuning fork: 128 Hz or 256 Hz
- Reflex hammer
- Sterile needle or a sterile safety pin
- Familiar small objects (coins, key, paper clip)
- Vials containing odorous materials (coffee, orange extract, vinegar)
- Vials containing hot and cold water
- Vials with solutions for tasting: quinine (bitter), glucose solution (sweet), lemon or vinegar (sour), saline (salty)
- Snellen chart or Rosenbaum pocket screener
- Pupil gauge in millimeters

ASSESSMENT OF THE NEUROLOGICAL SYSTEM

A complete neurological assessment includes an assessment of mental status, sensation, cranial nerves, motor function, cerebellar function, and reflexes. For patients with minor or intermittent symptoms, a rapid screening assessment may be used, as outlined in Table 19-5.

MENTAL STATUS

Much of the mental status assessment should be done during the interview, with the patient comfortably positioned facing you. Mental status may also be assessed throughout the neurological assessment. Assess physical appearance and behavior, communication, level of consciousness, cognitive abilities, and mentation while conversing with the patient.

TABLE 19-5 Neurological Screening Assessment

ASSESSMENT PARAMETER	ASSESSMENT SKILL	COMMENTS
Mental status	Note general appearance, affect, speech content, memory, logic, judgment, and speech patterns during the history.	If any abnormalities or inconsistencies are evident, perform full mental status assessment.
	Perform Glasgow Coma Scale (GCS) with motor assessment component and pupil assessment.	If GCS < 15, perform full assessment of mental status and consciousness. If motor assessment is abnormal or asymmetrical, perform complete motor and sensory assessment.
Sensation	Assess pain and vibration in the hands and feet, light touch on the limbs.	If deficits are identified, perform a complete sensory assessment.
Cranial nerves	Assess CN II, III, IV, VI: visual acuity, gross visual fields, funduscopic examination, pupillary reactions, and extraocular movements. Assess CN VII, VIII, IX, X, XII: facial expression, gross hearing, voice, and tongue.	If any abnormalities exist, perform complete assessment of all 12 cranial nerves.
Motor system	• Muscle tone and strength • Abnormal movements • Hand grasp	If deficits are noted, perform a complete motor system assessment.
Cerebellar function	Observe the patient's: 1. Gait on arrival 2. Ability to: • Walk heel-to-toe • Walk on toes • Walk on heels • Hop in place • Perform shallow knee bends 3. Check Rombergs' test. 4. Finger-to-nose test 5. Fine repetitive movements with hands	If any abnormalities exist, perform complete cerebellar assessment.
Reflexes	Assess the deep tendon reflexes and the plantar reflex.	If an abnormal response is elicited, perform a complete reflex assessment.

Physical Appearance and Behavior

POSTURE AND MOVEMENTS.

E 1. Observe the patient's ability to wait patiently.

2. Note if patient's posture is relaxed, slumped, or stiff.

3. Observe the patient's movements for control and symmetry.

4. Observe the patient's gait (see Chapter 18).

N The patient should appear relaxed with the appropriate amount of concern for the assessment. The patient should exhibit erect posture, a smooth gait, and symmetrical body movements.

A Restlessness, tenseness, and pacing can be abnormal.

P These may be signs of anxiety or metabolic disorders, which should alert you to further investigate these problems.

NURSINGTIP

Focusing the Mental Status Assessment

In most cases, the information obtained during the health history is sufficient to assess mental status. A more specific mental assessment should be performed if the following are noted:

- Known brain lesion (stroke, tumors, trauma)
- Suspected brain lesion (new seizures, headaches, behavioral changes)
- Memory deficits
- Confusion
- Vague behavioral complaints (by significant others if patient is unaware of or denies behavioral changes)
- Aphasia
- Irritability
- Emotional lability/depression

NURSINGTIP

Patient History and Mental Status Assessment

1. Begin your assessment as the patient approaches you. Observe gait, posture, mode of dress, involuntary movements, voice, and other features that will help guide and refine your assessment priorities.
2. The history should be holistic because neurological disorders can affect all body systems.
3. The history should be age-sensitive:
   - Utilize other family members when appropriate.
   - Acknowledge adolescents' ability to speak for themselves.
   - Do not make assumptions regarding elderly patients' ability to relate their own health histories.
4. Allow the patient to remain clothed during the history and mental status assessment.
5. Consider language and cultural norms when obtaining the history and performing the mental status assessment.

A Slumped posture, slow gait, poor eye contact, and slow responses can be abnormal findings.

P These may be signs of depression.

A Stooped, flexed, or rigid posture; drooping neck; deformities of the spine; and tics are abnormal findings.

P Patients with kyphosis, scoliosis, Parkinson's disease, cerebral palsy, osteoporosis, schizophrenia, muscular atrophy, myasthenia gravis, or stroke may exhibit these signs.

DRESS, GROOMING, AND PERSONAL HYGIENE.

E 1. Note the appearance of the patient's clothing, specifically:

   a Cleanliness

   b. Condition

   c. Age appropriateness

   d. Weather appropriateness

   e. Appropriateness for the patient's socioeconomic group

2. Observe the patient's personal grooming (hair, skin, nails, teeth) for:

   a. Adequacy

   b. Symmetry

   c. Odor

NURSINGTIP

Influences on Dress and Grooming

Dress and grooming are influenced by the patient's economic status, age, home situation, and ethnic background. Information obtained during the health history will assist you in determining appropriate dress and grooming for each patient. It is helpful to directly ask the patient about grooming routines and clothing choices when there is a question as to appropriateness.

N The patient should be clean and well groomed, and should wear appropriate clothing for age, weather, and socioeconomic status.

A Poor personal hygiene such as uncombed hair, body odor, or unkempt clothing is abnormal.

P These signs may be indications of depression, schizophrenia, or dementia.

A Excessive, meticulous care and attention to clothing and grooming are abnormal behaviors.

P These signs may indicate obsessive-compulsive behavior.

A Obvious one-sided differences in grooming and dressing or the use of only one side of the body is abnormal.

P Stroke in the parietal lobe may cause the patient to be aware of only one side of the body, which is termed one-sided neglect.

FACIAL EXPRESSION.

E Observe for appropriateness of, variations in, and symmetry of facial expressions.

N Facial expressions should be appropriate to the content of the conversation and should be symmetrical.

A Extreme, inappropriate, or unchanging facial expressions, or asymmetrical facial movements are abnormal.

P Abnormal facial expressions demonstrate anxiety, depression, or the unchanging facial expression of a patient with Parkinson's disease. They may also indicate a lesion in the facial nerve (CN VII).

AFFECT.

E 1. Observe the patient's interaction with you, paying particular attention to both verbal and nonverbal behaviors.

2. Note if the patient's affect appears labile, blunted, or flat.

3. Note the variations in the patient's affect with a variety of topics.

4. Note any extreme emotional responses during the interview.

N The appropriateness and degree of affect should vary with the topics and the patient's cultural norms, and be reasonable, or eurhythmic (normal).

A Blunted affect, manifested by the patient shuffling into the examination room, slumping into a chair, moving slowly, and not making eye contact, is abnormal.

P A blunted affect may indicate depression.

A Unresponsive, inappropriate affect is abnormal.

P A flat, unresponsive affect may indicate depression or schizophrenia.

A Anger, hostility, and paranoia are abnormal responses in most clinical situations.

P These may be the responses of a paranoid schizophrenic individual.

A Euphoric, dramatic, disruptive, irrational, or elated behaviors are abnormal in most clinical situations.

P A manic-depressive patient might display these responses during the manic phase.

COMMUNICATION.
Communication skills should be assessed throughout the entire interview and physical assessment.

E 1. Note voice quality, which includes voice volume and pitch.

2. Assess articulation, fluency, and rate of speech by engaging the patient in normal conversation. Ask the patient to repeat words and sentences after you or to name objects you point out.

3. Note the patient's ability to carry out requests during the assessment, such as pointing to objects within the room as requested. Ask questions that require "yes" and "no" responses.

Handedness

Note handedness prior to language testing. Handedness and cerebral dominance for language are closely allied. Patients with dominant hemisphere lesions will frequently show communication abnormalities; for example, aphasia in the right-handed individual almost always indicates left-hemisphere disease.

4. Write simple commands for the patient to read and perform, for example, "point to your nose" or "tap your right foot." Reading ability may be influenced by the patient's educational level or visual impairment.

5. Ask the patient to write his or her name, birthday, a sentence the patient composes, or a sentence that you dictate. Note the patient's spelling, grammatical accuracy, and logical thought process.

N The patient should be able to produce spontaneous, coherent speech. The speech should have an effortless flow with normal inflections, volume, pitch, articulation, rate, and rhythm. Content of the message should make sense. Comprehension of language should be intact. The patient's ability to read and write should match the patient's educational level. Non-native speakers may exhibit some hesitancy or inaccuracy in written and spoken language.

A Aphasia, an impairment of language functioning, is abnormal.

P Aphasias are classified by involved anatomy, behavioral speech manifestations, fluency of speech (fluent: rhythm, grammar, and articulation are normal; nonfluent: speech production is limited and speech is poorly articulated), and comprehension (receptive) versus expression (expressive) deficits. Other categories include amnesic, the inability to recall specific types of words, and central, a deficit in the coordination among the speech areas. Table 19-6 for a summary of the characteristics and pathophysiology

TABLE 19-6 Classification of Aphasias

APHASIA	PATHOPHYSIOLOGY	EXPRESSION	CHARACTERISTICS
Broca's aphasia	Motor cortex lesion, Broca's area	Expressive Nonfluent	Speech slow and hesitant, the patient has difficulty in selecting and organizing words. Naming, word and phrase repetition, and writing impaired. Subtle defects in comprehension.
Wernicke's aphasia	Left hemisphere lesion in Wernicke's area	Receptive Fluent	Auditory comprehension impaired, as is content of speech. Patient unaware of deficits. Naming severely impaired.
Anomic aphasia	Left hemisphere lesion in Wernicke's area	Amnesic Fluent	Patient unable to name objects or places. Comprehension and repetition of words and phrases intact.
Conduction aphasia	Lesion in the arcuate fasciculus, which connects and transports messages between Broca's and Wernicke's areas	Central Fluent	Patient has difficulty repeating words, substitutes incorrect sounds for another sound (e.g., *dork* for *fork*).
Global aphasia	Lesions in the frontal-temporal area	Mixed Fluent	Both oral and written comprehension severely impaired; naming, repetition of words and phrases, ability to write impaired.
Transcortical sensory aphasia	Lesion in the periphery of Broca's and Wernicke's areas (watershed zone)	Fluent	Impairment in comprehension, naming, and writing. Word and phrase repetition intact.
Transcortical motor aphasia	Lesion anterior, superior, or lateral to Broca's area	Nonfluent	Comprehension intact. Naming and ability to write impaired. Word and phrase repetition intact.

E Examination   **N** Normal Findings   **A** Abnormal Findings   **P** Pathophysiology

of specific aphasias. Most patients with an aphasia will have some components of several aphasia classifications (e.g., a patient with transcortical motor aphasia will usually have some degree of transcortical sensory aphasia).

A **Dysarthria**, a disturbance in muscular control of speech, is abnormal.

P Dysarthria is due to ischemia affecting motor nuclei of CN X and CN XII; defects in the premotor or motor cortex that provide motor input for the face, throat, and mouth; or cerebellar disease.

A **Dysphonia**, difficulty making laryngeal sounds, is abnormal and can progress to **aphonia** (total loss of voice).

P Dysphonia is usually caused by lesions of CN X or swelling and inflammation of the larynx.

A **Apraxia**, the inability to convert the intended speech into the motor act of speech, is abnormal.

P Apraxia is due to dysfunction in the precentral gyrus of the frontal lobe.

A **Agraphia**, the loss of the ability to write, is abnormal.

P Agraphia is caused by lesions of Broca's and Wernicke's areas in the dominant side of the brain.

A **Alexia**, the inability to grasp the meaning of written words and sentences (word blindness), is abnormal.

P Alexia is usually due to a lesion of the angular gyrus and the occipital lobe.

Level of Consciousness (LOC)

Consciousness is the level of awareness of the self and the environment. Conscious behavior requires arousal, or wakefulness, and awareness, or cognition and affect. Arousal is controlled by the reticular activating system (RAS). The RAS activates the cortex after receiving stimuli from the somatic and special sensory pathways. Awareness is a higher-level function of the cerebral cortex, which interprets incoming sensory stimuli. Aspects of awareness at a higher level include judgment and thinking, which are generally assessed as part of the cognitive assessment. Orientation is awareness of self and environment.

E **1.** Observe the patient's eyes when entering the room (environmental stimuli). Note whether the patient's eyes are open or whether they open when you enter the room (prior to any verbalization). Note the patient's response to any general environmental stimuli, such as noises or lights.

2. If the patient's eyes are closed, call out the patient's name (verbal stimuli). Observe whether the patient's eyes open, whether he or she responds verbally and appropriately, and whether he or she follows verbal commands.

3. If the patient does not respond to verbal stimuli, lightly touch the patient's hand or gently shake the patient awake.

4. If the patient is not responding to environmental or verbal stimuli, proceed to the application of a painful stimulus.

   a. Apply pressure with a pen to the nailbed of each extremity, or

   b. Firmly pinch the trapezius muscle, or

   c. Apply pressure to the supraorbital ridge or the manubrium.

5. Observe the patient's reaction to the painful stimulus. Note whether the patient's eyes open.

6. Observe whether the patient can localize the painful stimulus by reaching for the area being stimulated. Strength of the patient's extremities can be assessed by the strength and distance of movement during his or her attempt to reach the painful stimulus. Note any abnormal motor responses.

7. Compare the motor responses and strength of the responses of right versus left sides of the patient.

8. Note whether the patient responds verbally to the painful stimulus.

9. Assess orientation by asking questions related to person, place, and time:

   a. Person: name of the patient, name of spouse or significant other

   b. Place: where the patient is now (what town, what state), where the patient lives

   c. Time: the time of day, month, year, season

10. Determine the **Glasgow Coma Scale** (GCS) (see Figure 19-9) score, an international method for grading neurological responses of the injured or severely ill patient. It is monitored in patients who have the potential for rapid deterioration in level of consciousness. The GCS assesses three parameters of consciousness: eye opening, verbal response, and motor response.

N The patient's best response to each of these categories is what is recorded. The sum of the three categories is the total GCS score. The highest score of responsiveness is 15 and the lowest is 3. A score of 15 would indicate a fully alert, oriented individual.

A/P See Table 19-7.

E Examination   **N** Normal Findings   **A** Abnormal Findings   **P** Pathophysiology

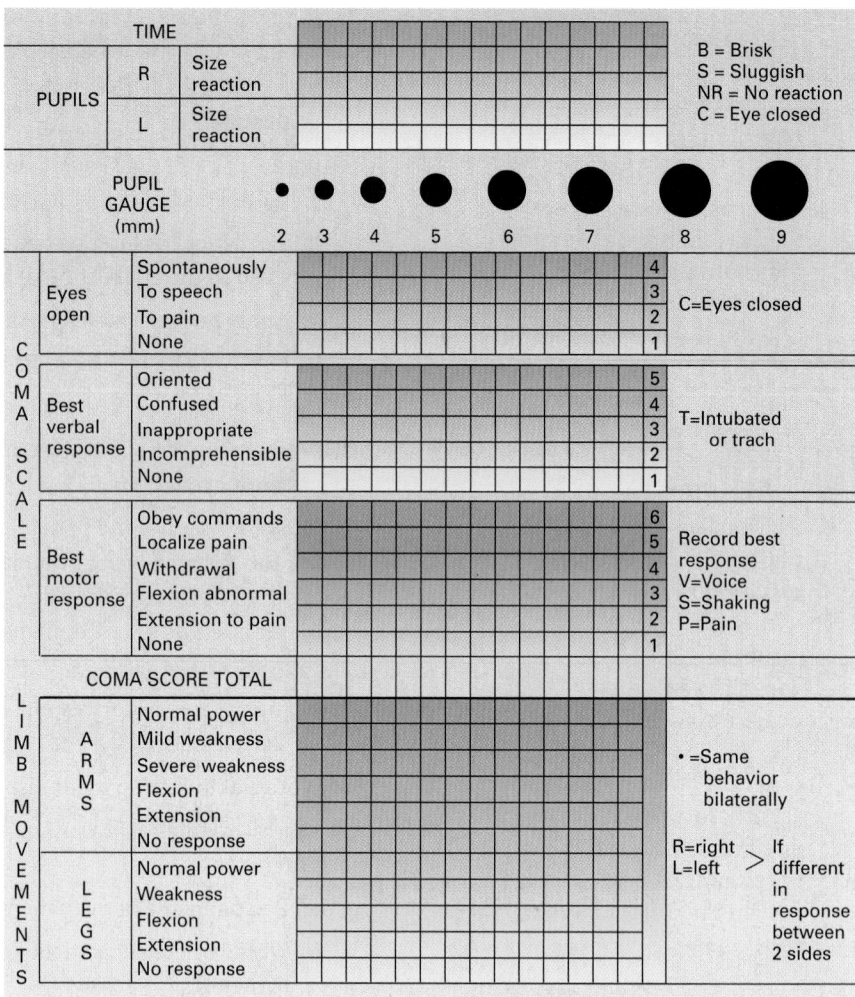

FIGURE 19-9 Neurological Flow Sheet, Including Glasgow Coma Scale

Cognitive Abilities and Mentation

Assessment of cognitive function includes testing for attention, memory, judgment, insight, spatial perception, calculation, abstraction, thought processes, and thought content.

ATTENTION.

 1. Pronounce a list of numbers slowly (approximately 1 second apart), starting with a list of two numbers and progressing to a series of five or six numbers. For example: 2, 5; 3, 7, 8; 1, 9, 4, 3; 1, 5, 4, 9, 0.

2. Ask the patient to repeat the numbers in correct order, both forward and backward.

3. Give the patient a different series of the same number of digits if the patient is unable to repeat the first series correctly. Stop after two misses of any length series.

TABLE 19-7 Levels of Consciousness: Abnormalities and Pathophysiology

LOC	GCS	RESPONSE TO STIMULI	PUPIL RESPONSE	PATHOPHYSIOLOGY	PROGNOSIS
Confusion	14	Spontaneous but may be inappropriate Memory faulty Reflexes intact	Normal	Metabolic derangements Diffuse brain dysfunction	Good chance of recovery Must treat primary cause
Lethargy	13–14	Requires stimulus to respond (verbal, touch) Reflexes intact	Normal to unequal	Metabolic derangements Medications Increased ICP	Good chance of recovery Must treat primary cause
Stupor	12–13	Requires vigorous, continuous stimuli to respond Reflexes intact	Normal, unequal, or sluggish	Metabolic derangements Medications Increased ICP	Good chance of recovery Must treat primary cause
Permanent vegetative state	8–10	Responds to pain No cognitive response Reflexes abnormal	Normal	Anoxic ischemic insults	Irreversible
Locked-in syndrome	6	Awake and aware	Normal	Lesion in ventral pons All four extremities and lower cranial nerves paralyzed Myasthenia gravis Acute polyneuritis	Poor prognosis
Coma	3–6	Abnormal Varied response to pain Reflexes abnormal or absent	Abnormal Dilated or pinpoint	Anoxia Traumatic injury Space-occupying lesion Cerebral edema	Prognosis dependent on length of time in coma
Brain death	3	No response Reflexes abnormal or absent	Abnormal Dilated or pinpoint	Anoxia Structural damage	Irreversible

LOC = level of consciousness; GCS = Glasgow Coma Scale; ICP = intracranial pressure

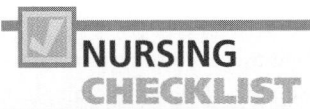

NURSING CHECKLIST

Assessment of Cognitive Function

You should have on hand:

- Preprinted lists of objects, phrases, and numbers for patient recall and explanation
- Answers to long-term memory questions to accurately assess recall
- Alternate tests prepared for patients with language barriers, aphasia, deafness, blindness, etc.
- Paper and pencils for patient to use to respond

NURSING**TIP**

Cognitive Mental Status Screening

The Mini Mental State Exam (MMSE) is a widely used tool for assessing cognitive mental status, detecting impairment following the course of an illness, and monitoring response to treatment. The MMSE is most useful in screening for the cognitive deficits seen in syndromes of dementia and delirium.

The MMSE contains 11 cognitive tasks and takes 5 to 10 minutes to administer. Time orientation, place orientation, immediate recall, short-term memory recall, serial 7's, reading, writing, drawing, and verbal/motor comprehension compose the bulk of the examination. The maximum score on the MMSE is 30, and scores greater than 24 are considered within the normal range. Patients who have scores lower than 24 need to have a more detailed neuropsychological evaluation.

The MMSE is a copyrighted screening tool that can be purchased from Psychological Assessment Resources, Inc. at: 16204 North Florida Avenue, Lutz, Florida 33549; phone: 1-800-331-8378; Fax: 1-800-727-9329; e-mail: copyright@parinc.com

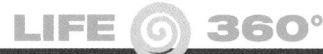

Serial 7's

Try beginning with the number 100 and counting backward by subtracting 7 each time.

- Were you able to successfully complete the serial 7's in 1 minute?
- Imagine how a patient feels when asked to perform this activity.
- How could you make the patient feel more comfortable when performing calculations?

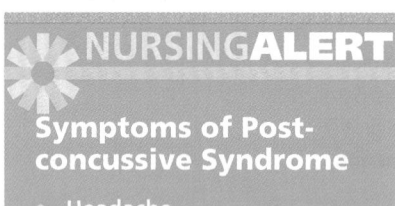

Symptoms of Post-concussive Syndrome

- Headache
- Subtle memory deficit
- Fatigue
- Dizziness
- Temporary inattention
- Impaired concentration
- Altered school or work performance
- Change in disposition

4. Serial 7's is another way of assessing attention and concentration. Instruct the patient to begin with the number 100 and to count backward by subtracting 7 each time: 100, 93, 86, 79, 72, 65, etc.

5. The patient may also try serial 3's (counting backward from 100 by threes) if unable to perform serial 7's.

N The patient should be able to correctly repeat the series of numbers up to a series of five numbers. The patient should be able to recite serial 7's or serial 3's accurately to at least the 40's or 50's from 100 within 1 minute.

A If the patient has a short attention span, the patient will not be able to repeat the numbers in sequence or perform serial 7's or 3's.

P Dementia, neurological injury or disease, and mental retardation may impair attention.

MEMORY.

E **1.** Assess immediate recall in conjunction with attention span as discussed previously.

2. Give a list of three items that the patient is to remember and repeat in 5 minutes. Have the patient repeat the items to check initial understanding. During the 5 minutes, carry on conversation as usual. Ask the patient to repeat the items again after the 5-minute time frame.

3. If the patient is unable to remember one or more of the objects, show a list containing the objects along with others, and check recognition.

4. Record the number of objects remembered over the number of objects given.

5. Long-term memory is memory that is retained for at least 24 hours. Commonly asked questions for testing long-term memory include: name of spouse, spouse's birthday, mother's maiden name, name of the president, or the patient's birthday.

N The patient should be able to correctly respond to questions and to identify all the objects as requested.

A Memory loss is abnormal.

P Memory loss may be caused by pathologies such as nervous system infection, trauma, stroke, tumors, Alzheimer's disease, seizure disorders, alcohol, and drug toxicity. Memory is located in the temporal lobe and the hippocampus. Damage to these areas, in the form of hemorrhage, ischemia, compression, or herniation, will cause memory impairment.

JUDGMENT.

E **1.** During the interview, assess whether the patient is responding appropriately to social, family, and work situations that are discussed.

2. Note whether the patient's decisions are based on sound reasoning and decision making.

3. Present hypothetical situations and ask the patient to make decisions as to what his or her responses would be. For example: "What would you do if followed by a police car with flashing lights?" or "What would you do if you saw a house burning?"

4. Interview the patient's family or directly observe the patient to assess judgment more carefully.

N The patient should be able to evaluate and act appropriately in situations requiring judgment.

A Impaired judgment, the inability to act appropriately in situations, is abnormal.

P Frontal lobe damage, dementia, psychotic states, and mental retardation may cause the patient to exhibit lack of appropriate judgment.

INSIGHT.   Insight is the ability to realistically understand oneself.

E 1. Ask the patient to describe personal health status, reason for seeking health care, symptoms, current life situation, and general coping behaviors.

2. If the patient describes symptoms, ask what life was like prior to the appearance of the symptoms, what life changes the illness has introduced, and whether the patient feels a need for help.

3. Ask the patient to draw a self-portrait; note the emphasis put on specific body parts, the patient's ability to reproduce figures on paper, and the representation of any part of the self-portrait. Note the facial features and the feelings portrayed by the picture.

N The patient should demonstrate a realistic awareness and understanding of self.

A Unrealistic perceptions of self are abnormal.

P Lack of insight may occur in the euphoric stages of bipolar affective disorders, endogenous anxiety states, or depressed states.

SPATIAL PERCEPTION.   Spatial perception is the ability to recognize the relationships of objects in space.

E 1. Ask the patient to copy figures that you have previously drawn, such as a circle, triangle, square, cross, and a three-dimensional cube.

2. Ask the patient to draw the face of a clock, including the numbers around the dial.

3. Ask the patient to identify a familiar sound while keeping the eyes closed, for example, a closing door, running water, or a finger snap.

4. Have the patient identify right from left body parts.

N The patient should be able to draw the objects without difficulty and as closely as possible to the original drawing, and to identify familiar sounds and left and right body parts.

A **Agnosia**, the inability to recognize the form and nature of objects or persons, is abnormal. It may be visual, auditory, or somatosensory. For example, the patient may be unable to name or recognize objects, faces, or familiar objects by touch, or to identify the meaning of nonverbal sounds.

P Lesions in the nondominant parietal lobe impair the patient's ability to appreciate self in relation to the environment and to conceive three-dimensional objects. Lesions in the occipital lobe will cause visual agnosia, and temporal lesions will cause auditory agnosia.

A Apraxia, the inability to perform purposeful movements despite the preservation of motor ability and sensation, is abnormal. **Constructional apraxia** is the inability to reproduce figures on paper (Figure 19-10).

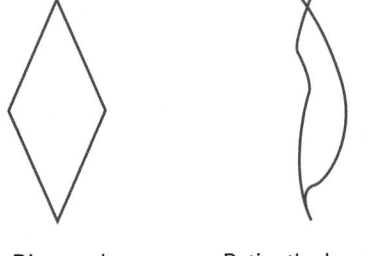

Diamond   Patient's drawing

FIGURE 19-10 Constructional Apraxia

| **E** Examination | **N** Normal Findings | **A** Abnormal Findings | **P** Pathophysiology |

P Apraxia is usually associated with lesions of the precentral gyrus of the frontal lobe.

CALCULATION.

The patient's ability to perform serial 7's was discussed in the section on attention and is also an assessment of calculation.

E 1. Ask the patient to add 3 to 100, then 3 to that number, until numbers greater than 150 are reached.

2. Note the amount of time and difficulty associated with the calculations.

N The patient should be able to calculate the correct numbers upon subtraction or addition within educational abilities and with fewer than four errors in less than 1½ minutes.

A **Dyscalculia**, the inability to perform calculations, is abnormal.

P Dyscalculia may be caused by depression or anxiety, dementia, or mental retardation. The most common cause of dyscalculia is focal lesions in the dominant parietal lobe; however, calculation deficits have also been ascribed to focal lesions in the frontal, temporal, and occipital lobes.

ABSTRACT REASONING.

E 1. Ask the patient to describe the meaning of a familiar fable, proverb, or metaphor. Use examples that are meaningful within the context of the patient's culture and language. Some examples from American culture are:
   - The squeaky wheel gets the grease.
   - A rolling stone gathers no moss.
   - A stitch in time saves nine.
   - People in glass houses should not throw stones.
   - Don't count your chickens before they hatch.

2. Note the degree of concreteness versus abstraction in the answers.

N Patients should be able to give the abstract meanings of proverbs, fables, or metaphors within their cultural understanding.

A Conceptual concreteness, the inability to describe in abstractions, to generalize from specifics, and to apply general principles, is abnormal.

P Alterations of cognitive processes causing concreteness in thought may occur in patients with dementia, frontal tumors, or schizophrenia. Concreteness in thought processes may also indicate low intelligence.

THOUGHT PROCESS AND CONTENT.

E 1. Observe the patient's pattern of thought for relevance, consistency, coherence, logic, and organization.

2. Listen throughout the interview for flaws in content of conversation.

N Thought processes should be logical, coherent, and goal oriented. Thought content should be based on reality.

A Unrealistic, illogical thought processes and interruptions of the thinking processes, such as blocking, are abnormal. Blocking is demonstrated when an extended pause occurs during a sentence due to a repressed or painful subject matter. Sometimes, the thoughts following are unrelated to what the patient was discussing.

E Examination **N** Normal Findings **A** Abnormal Findings **P** Pathophysiology

Risk Factors for Suicide

- Personal attempt history
- Mental illness
- Female (more suicide attempts)
- Male (more successful suicides)
- Prior suicide attempts
- Family member with attempt history
- Drug abuse
- Unwillingness to seek help because of stigma
- Barriers to accessing mental health treatment
- Stressful life events or loss
- Easy access to lethal methods such as guns
- Suicidal ideation with or without a plan
- Posttraumatic stress disorder

P Abnormal thought processes are often due to schizophrenia.

A Flight of ideas, demonstrated when the patient changes from subject to subject within a sentence, is abnormal. This is frequently due to distractions or word associations with a resultant lack of sense of purpose of the conversation.

P Patients suffering from manic episodes of bipolar affective disorder often demonstrate flight of ideas.

A **Confabulation**, the making up of answers unrelated to facts, is abnormal.

P Confabulation is often related to aging, memory loss, disorientation, Korsakoff's psychosis, and psychopathic disorders.

A **Echolalia**, the involuntary repetition of a word or sentence that was uttered by another person, is abnormal.

P Schizophrenics and patients suffering from dementia often demonstrate echolalia.

A **Neologism**, a word coined by the patient that is meaningful only to the patient, is an abnormal finding.

P Patients who are delirious or schizophrenic may exhibit neologism.

A Delusions of persecution, grandiose delusions, hallucinations, illusions, obsessive-compulsiveness, and paranoia are examples of abnormal thoughts.

P Abnormal thought content is demonstrated in patients suffering from schizophrenia or dementia and in patients who use illegal drugs.

Table 19-8 compares and contrasts the various clinical parameters that distinguish dementia, depression, delirium, and acute confusion.

SUICIDAL IDEATION. If the patient has expressed feelings of sadness, hopelessness, despair, worthlessness, or grief, explore his or her feelings further with more specific questions such as:

E 1. Have you ever felt so bad that you wanted to hurt yourself?

2. Do you feel like hurting yourself now?

N The patient should provide a negative response and be able to verbalize his or her self-worth.

A An affirmative response is abnormal and requires probing such as:

Do you have a plan to hurt yourself?
What would happen if you were dead?

Depression Acronym

An easy way to remember the symptoms of clinical depression is to use the acronym "IN SAD CAGES."

IN   Interest (loss of pleasure)

S   Sleep disturbance

A   Appetite change (increases or decreases)

D   Depressed mood

C   Concentration difficulties

A   Activity level (retardation or agitation)

G   Guilt feelings (low self-esteem)

E   Energy loss (fatigue)

S   Suicidal ideation

The Elderly Depressed Patient

It is often difficult to differentiate between depression and early dementia in the elderly. The clinical presentation of apathy, difficulty concentrating, memory loss, and general inability to keep up with the demands of everyday life is common to both depression and early dementia. It is imperative to also remember that the elderly may have other etiologies that may account for their behavior, such as thyroid disease, altered glucose metabolism, electrolyte imbalance, and polypharmacy. A complete health history and physical examination are warranted.

TABLE 19-8 Distinguishing Dementia, Depression, Delirium, and Acute Confusion

PARAMETER	DEMENTIA	DEPRESSION	DELIRIUM	ACUTE CONFUSION
Definition	Deterioration of all cognitive function with little or no disturbance of consciousness or perception Onset: gradual	An abnormal emotional state characterized by feelings of sadness, despair, and discouragement Onset: variable	A disorder of perception with heightened awareness, hallucinations, vivid dreams, and intense emotional disturbances Onset: sudden	An inability to think with customary speed, clarity, and coherence Onset: variable
Pathophysiology	Alzheimer's disease Metabolic disorders Stroke Head injury	Inherited: neurochemical abnormalities Situational: acute loss of significant person CVA Parkinson's disease Alzheimer's disease Medications (e.g., steroids)	Withdrawal from alcohol and other drugs Drug intoxication Encephalitis Traumatic injury Febrile states Hypoxia Fluid and electrolyte imbalance	Metabolic disorders Drug intoxication Traumatic injury Febrile states
Attention	Impaired	Intact	Impaired: heightened or dulled	Impaired: dulled
Memory	Short term: impaired first Long term: intact for a while	Intact	Short term: impaired Long term: intact	Short term: impaired Long term: may be intact
Judgment	Impaired	Intact	Grossly impaired Impulsive Volatile	Impaired
Insight	Impaired	Impaired if in manic phase	Impaired	Impaired
Spatial perception	Impaired	Intact	Intact	May be impaired
Calculation	Impaired	May be intact	May be intact	Impaired
Abstract reasoning	Impaired	Intact	Impaired	Impaired
Thought process and content	Impaired	Intact but may demonstrate flight of ideas	Impaired, hallucinations present	Impaired, incoherent

CVA = cerebrovascular accident.

Continued affirmative responses and expressions of worthlessness and hopelessness should be interpreted as suicidal ideation, a psychiatric emergency that requires immediate referral to a specialist.

P Suicidal ideation is associated with mental disorders, particularly depression, substance abuse, and schizophrenia.

Mental Health

Findings during the cognitive functioning examination may indicate the need for further mental health screening. Table 19-9 summarizes findings common to mental illness that may lead the practitioner to refer the patient for further diagnostic study.

SENSORY ASSESSMENT

Sensation should be tested early in the neurological assessment because of the detail involved and because the cooperation of the patient is required. The conclusions of the assessment may be unreliable if the patient becomes fatigued.

The sensory assessment is divided into three sections. First, the exteroceptive sensations (superficial sensations that originate in the sensory receptors in the skin and mucous membranes) are tested. These are the sensations of light touch, superficial pain, and temperature.

Next, the proprioceptive sensations (deep sensations, with sensory receptors in the muscles, joints, tendons, and ligaments) are assessed. **Proprioception** is tested with the modalities of motion and position, and vibration sense.

Finally, the cortical sensations (those that require cerebral integrative and discriminative abilities) are assessed. Stereognosis, graphesthesia, two-point discrimination, and extinction are tested.

Exteroceptive Sensation

For the entire exteroceptive sensation assessment, expose the patient's legs, arms, and abdomen.

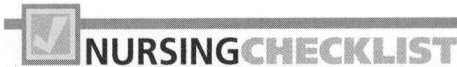

✓ NURSING CHECKLIST

Assessing Sensation

1. Explain the procedure to the patient before starting the assessment.
2. The sensory assessment is carried out with the patient's eyes closed.
3. For a thorough sensory examination, the patient should be in a supine position.
4. The patient should be cooperative and reliable, although the pain assessment may be performed on comatose patients.
5. Note the patient's ability to perceive the sensation.
6. Much of the sensory component of the neurological assessment is subjective; observe the reactions of the patient by watching the face for grimacing, or withdrawal of the stimulated extremity.
7. Compare the patient's sensation on the corresponding areas bilaterally.
8. Note whether any sensory deficits follow a dermatome distribution.
9. The borders of any area exhibiting changes in sensation should be mapped by dermatomes (see Figure 19-7).

TABLE 19-9 Mental Illnesses

DISORDER	DEFINING CHARACTERISTICS	POPULATION CHARACTERISTICS
Anxiety Disorders • Panic • Phobias • Generalized anxiety disorder • Obsessive-compulsive disorder • Acute and posttraumatic stress disorders	A group of conditions that share extreme or pathological anxiety as the principal disturbance of mood or emotional tone	• Common across cultures • Early age onset • Relapsing or recurrent episodes • Periods of disability • Significant overlap with mood and substance abuse disorders
Panic Disorder • Panic attack • Panic disorder	The patient has experienced at least two unexpected panic attacks and develops persistent concern over having recurring attacks or changes behavior to avoid or minimize such attacks.	• Twice as common in women as men • Onset most common between adolescence and midadult life • Significant overlap with mood, substance abuse, and panic disorders
Phobias • Agoraphobia • Social phobia • Specific phobias	Marked fear of specific objects or situations	• Experienced by approximately 8% of the population • Typically begin in childhood • There is a second peak in the middle 20s of adulthood
Generalized anxiety disorder	Protracted period of anxiety and worry accompanied by multiple associated physical and cognitive symptoms.	• Twice as common in women as men • Half of cases begin in childhood or adolescence • Symptoms increase with life stress or difficulties
Obsessive-compulsive disorder	Obsessions are recurrent, intrusive thoughts, impulses, or images that are perceived as inappropriate, grotesque, or forbidden. Compulsions are repetitive behaviors or mental acts that reduce the anxiety that accompanies an obsession.	• Equally common among the sexes • Begins in adolescence to young adult life in males • Female onset typically is young adult life • Familial pattern • Strongly associated with Tourette's disorder • Significant overlap with other anxiety disorders and major depressive disorder
Acute and posttraumatic stress disorders	Acute: The anxiety and behavioral disturbances that develop within the first month after exposure to an extreme trauma. If the symptoms persist for more than 1 month and are associated with functional impairment, the diagnosis is changed to posttraumatic stress disorder.	• Twice as prevalent in females as males • Develop in approximately 9% of those exposed to extreme trauma • Rape • Physical assault • Near-death experience • Witnessing murder and combat

Mood Disorders
 	
• Major depressive disorder
• Dysthymia
• Bipolar disorder
• Cyclothymia
	A cluster of mental disorders best recognized by depression or mania.	• Rank among the top 10 causes of worldwide disability
		• More prevalent in women
		• Leading cause of absenteeism and diminished productivity at work
		• Common comorbidities include anxiety disorder, personality disorders, and chronic medical conditions
		• May be caused by:
		  – Dominant hemispheric strokes
		  – Hyperthyroidism – Antihypertensives

continues

TABLE 19-9 (Continued)

DISORDER	DEFINING CHARACTERISTICS	POPULATION CHARACTERISTICS
		– Cushing's disease – Oral contraceptives – Pancreatic cancer – Alcohol withdrawal
Major depressive disorder	Five or more of the following symptoms have been present for the same 2-week period and represent a change from previous functioning; at least one symptom is either depressed mood or loss of interest or pleasure: • Depressed mood • Loss of interest or pleasure • Significant weight loss when not dieting • Insomnia or hypersomnia • Psychomotor agitation or retardation • Fatigue or loss of energy • Feeling of worthlessness • Diminished ability to think or concentrate; indecisiveness • Recurrent thoughts of death or suicidal ideation	• More common among women • Most severe depressions more common among the elderly • At least 50% will recur
Dysthymia	A chronic form of depression, symptoms are constant for a 2-year period (1 year for children)	• Twice as many women as men are diagnosed • Affects about 2% of adults each year • If onset in childhood, associated strongly with subsequent substance abuse • Susceptible to major depression episode superimposed on dysthymia
Bipolar disorder • Type I (prior mania) • Type II (prior hypomanic episodes only)	Recurrent mood disorder featuring one or more episodes of mania or mixed episodes of mania and depression	• Equally common in men and women • Affects about 2% of adult population
Cyclothymia	Manic and depressive states of insufficient intensity or duration to merit a diagnosis of bipolar disorder or major depressive disorder	• 33% higher risk than general population to develop bipolar disorder
Schizophrenia	Profound disruption in cognition and emotion. Two or more of the following symptoms persist for a significant portion of time during a 1-month period: — Delusions — Hallucinations — Disorganized speech — Grossly disorganized or catatonic behavior — Negative symptoms: affective flattening, alogia (inability to express oneself through speech), or avolition (lack of motivation for work or other goal-directed activity)	• Onset during young adulthood • Women experience later onset than men • One-year prevalence in adults is estimated to be 1.3% • Associated with significantly higher mortality rate than the general population • Suicide • Comorbid medical illness: visual and dental problems, hypertension, diabetes, and sexually transmitted diseases

Information condensed from *Mental Health: A Report of the Surgeon General,* 1999, by U.S. Department of Health and Human Services, Substance Abuse and Mental Health Services Administration, Center for Mental Health Services, National Institutes of Health, National Institute of Mental Health, Rockville, MD: Author.

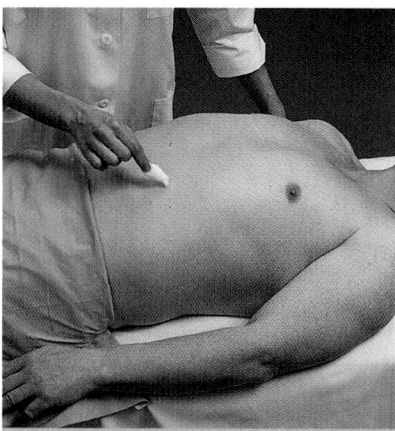

FIGURE 19-11 **Assessment of Light Touch**

LIGHT TOUCH.

E 1. Use a wisp of cotton and apply the stimulus with very light strokes (Figure 19-11). If the skin is calloused, or for thicker skin on the hands and soles, the stimulus may need to be intensified, although care must be taken not to stimulate subcutaneous tissues.

2. Begin with distal areas of the patient's limbs and move proximally.

3. Test the hand, lower arm, abdomen, foot, and leg. Assessment of sensation of the face is discussed in the Cranial Nerve section.

4. To prevent the patient from being able to predict the next touch, alter the rate and rhythm of stimulation. Also, vary the sites of stimulation, keeping in mind that the right and left sides must be compared.

5. Instruct the patient to respond by saying "now" or "yes" when the stimulus is felt, and to identify the area that was stimulated either verbally or by pointing to it.

N/A/P Refer to Temperature, following.

SUPERFICIAL PAIN.

E 1. Use a sharp object: sterile needle or sterile safety pin.

2. Establish that the patient can identify sharp and dull sensations by touching the patient with each stimulus and asking the patient to describe what is felt. This will help alleviate some of the fears the patient may have about being touched with a sharp object.

3. Hold the object loosely between the thumb and first finger to allow the sharp point to slide if too much pressure is applied.

4. Begin peripherally, moving in a distal to proximal direction and following the dermatomal distribution. If impaired sensation is identified, move from impaired sensation to normal sensation for comparison. Attempt to define the area of impaired sensation (mapping) by proceeding from the analgesic area to the normal area.

5. Alternate the sharp point with the dull end to test the patient's accuracy of shear sensation.

6. Instruct the patient to reply "sharp," "dull," or "I don't know" as quickly as the stimulus is felt and to indicate areas of the skin that perceive differences in pain sensation.

7. Again, compare the two sides, taking care not to proceed too fast or to cue the patient with regularity in the stimulus presentation.

N/A/P Refer to Temperature on the following page.

TEMPERATURE. Assess temperature sensation only if abnormalities in superficial pain sensation are noted.

E 1. Use glass vials containing warm water (40° to 45°C or 104° to 113°F) and cold water (5° to 10°C or 41° to 50°F). Hotter or colder temperatures will stimulate pain receptors.

2. Touch the warm or cold test tubes on the skin, distal to proximal and following dermatome distribution.

3. Instruct the patient to respond "hot," "cold," or "I can't tell" and to indicate where the sensation is felt.

E Examination   **N** Normal Findings   **A** Abnormal Findings   **P** Pathophysiology

N The patient should be able to perceive light touch, superficial pain, and temperature accurately, and be able to correctly perceive the location of the stimulus.

A Anesthesia refers to an absence of touch sensation. **Hypesthesia** is a diminished sense of touch; this may also be called hypoesthesia. **Hyperesthesia** is marked acuteness to the sensitivity of touch. **Paresthesia** is numbness, tingling, or a pricking sensation. **Dysesthesia** is an abnormal interpretation of a stimulus such as burning or tingling from a stimulus such as touch or superficial pain. All of these findings are abnormal.

P Peripheral nerve lesions may cause anesthesia, hypesthesia, or hyperesthesia, which may be mapped out in the specific sensory distribution of the affected nerve. Lesions of the nerve roots produce areas of anesthesia and hypesthesia limited to the segmental distribution of the roots involved. Lesions in the brain stem or spinal cord can cause anesthesia, paresthesia, or dysesthesia.

A Analgesia refers to insensitivity to pain. **Hypalgesia** refers to diminished sensitivity to pain. **Hyperalgesia** is increased sensitivity to pain. These findings are abnormal.

P Lesions of the thalamus and the peripheral nerves and nerve roots can cause analgesia, hypalgesia, and hyperalgesia.

A Total unilateral loss of all forms of sensation is an abnormal finding.

P This is due to an extensive lesion of the thalamus and results in gross disability.

A A "saddle" pattern of sensation loss is abnormal.

P A lesion of the cauda equina produces the "saddle" pattern of sensation loss, the loss of leg reflexes, and the loss of sphincter control. If touch is preserved, the lesion is in or near the conus medullaris.

A The loss of touch sensation in the hands and lower legs (glove and stocking anesthesia) is abnormal.

P Glove and stocking anesthesia is common in polyneuritis of any cause.

A Unilateral loss of all exteroceptive sensation is abnormal.

P This is caused by a partial lesion of the thalamus or a lesion laterally situated in the upper brain stem. It may also be caused by hysteria.

Proprioceptive Sensation

MOTION AND POSITION.

E 1. Grasp the patient's index finger with your thumb and index finger. Hold the finger at the sides (parallel to the plane of movement) in order not to exert upward or downward pressure with your fingers and thus give the patient any clues as to which direction the finger is moving. The patient's fingers should be relaxed.

2. Have the patient shut the eyes, and show the patient what "up" and "down" feel like by moving the finger in those directions.

3. Use gentle, slow, and deliberate movements. Begin with larger movements that become smaller and less perceptible.

4. Instruct the patient to respond "up," "down," or "I can't tell" after each time you raise or lower the finger.

5. Repeat this several times. Vary the motion in order not to establish a predictable pattern.

6. Repeat steps 2 through 5 with the finger of the patient's opposite hand, and then with the great toes.

7. If there appears to be a deficit in motion sense, proceed to the proximal joints such as wrists or ankles, and repeat the test.

N The patient should be able to correctly identify the changes of position of the body.

A Inability to perceive direction of movement is abnormal.

P Peripheral neuropathies will interfere with position sense. A lesion of the posterior column will cause an ipsilateral loss of position sense. Lesions of the sensory cortex, the thalamus, or the connections between them (thalamocortical connections) may also disrupt position sense.

VIBRATION SENSE.

E 1. Strike the prongs of a low-pitch tuning fork (128 or 256 Hz) against the ulnar surface of your hand or your knuckles, and place the base of the fork firmly on the patient's skin over bony prominences (Figure 19-12). Be sure that your fingers touch only the stem of the fork, not the tines.

2. Begin with distal prominences such as a toe or finger, testing each extremity.

3. Instruct the patient to say "now" when the buzzing, vibrating tuning fork is felt, and to report immediately when the vibrations are no longer felt.

4. Be sure that the patient is reporting the vibration sense rather than hearing a humming sound or just feeling pressure from the tuning fork.

5. After the patient can no longer feel the vibrations, determine whether the vibrations can, in fact, still be felt by holding the prongs while the tuning fork is left on the patient.

6. If you detect a deficit in vibratory sense in the peripheral bony prominences, progress toward the trunk by testing ankles, knees, wrists, elbows, anterior superior iliac crests, ribs, sternum, and spinous processes of the vertebrae.

N Normally, the patient should be able to perceive vibration over all bony prominences.

A The inability to perceive vibration sense is abnormal.

P Vibratory sense may be lost as a result of polyneuropathies (e.g., diabetic) or spinal cord lesions involving the posterior columns. Vibratory sensation is normally lower in patients over age 65.

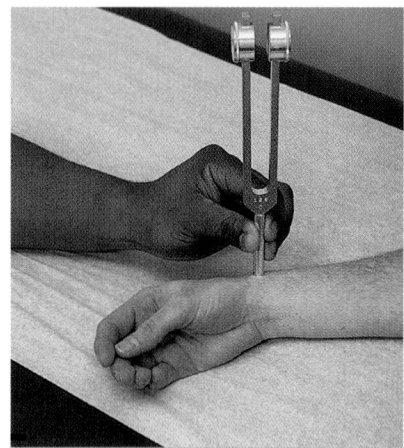

FIGURE 19-12 Assessment of Vibration

Cortical Sensation

STEREOGNOSIS.

STEREOGNOSIS. Stereognosis is the ability to identify objects by manipulating and touching them.

E 1. Place a familiar object (coin, button, closed safety pin, key) into the patient's hand (Figure 19-13).

2. Ask the patient to manipulate the object, appreciating size and form.

3. Ask the patient to name the object.

4. Repeat in the opposite hand with a different object.

N The patient should be able to identify the objects by holding them.

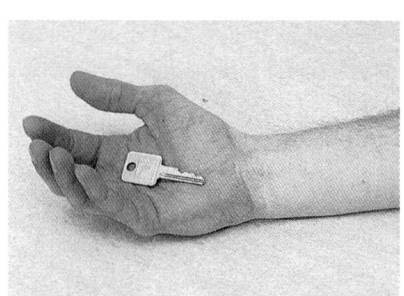

FIGURE 19-13 Assessment of Stereognosis

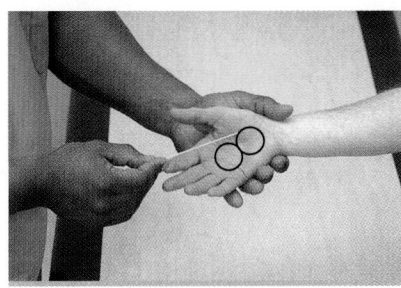

FIGURE 19-14 Assessment of Graphesthesia

A The inability to recognize the nature of objects by touch manipulation, termed **astereognosis**, is abnormal.

P Astereognosis is related to dysfunction of the parietal lobe, where the sensory cortex is located.

GRAPHESTHESIA.

The ability to identify numbers, letters, or shapes drawn on the skin is termed **graphesthesia**.

E 1. Draw a number or letter with a blunt object (such as a closed pen or the stick of a cotton-tipped applicator) on the patient's outstretched palm. Make sure the number or letter is facing the patient's direction (Figure 19-14).

2. Ask the patient to identify what has been written.

3. Repeat on the opposite side.

N The patient should be able to identify what number or letter has been written on the palm or other skin surface.

A **Graphanesthesia** is the inability to recognize a number or letter drawn on the skin and is abnormal.

P Graphanesthesia, in the presence of intact peripheral sensation, indicates parietal lobe dysfunction.

TWO-POINT DISCRIMINATION.

Two-point discrimination is tested by simultaneously and closely touching various parts of the body with two identical, sharp objects.

E 1. With two sterile pins or broken cotton-tipped applicators, simultaneously touch the tip of one of the patient's fingers, starting with the objects far apart.

2. Ask the patient whether one or two points are felt.

3. Continue to move the two points closer together until the patient is unable to distinguish two points. Note the minimum distance between the two points at which the patient reports feeling the objects separately.

4. Irregularly alternate, using one or two pins throughout the test, to verify that the patient is feeling two points.

5. Repeats steps 1–4 with the fingers of the opposite hand.

6. Other areas of the body that may be tested include the dorsum of the hand, the tongue, the lips, the feet, or the trunk.

N The patient should be able to identify two points at 5 mm apart on the fingertips. Other parts of the body vary widely in normal distance of discrimination, such as the dorsum of the hand or feet, where a separation of as much as 20 mm may be necessary for discrimination. The patient may be able to detect two points as close as 2 to 3 mm ($^1/_{16}$ to $^1/_8$ inch) on the tip of the tongue.

A Distances greater than those described previously that are required to identify two points are abnormal.

P Lesions in the parietal lobe impair two-point discrimination (with intact tactile sensation).

EXTINCTION.

Extinction (sensory inattention) is tested by simultaneously touching opposite sides of the body at the identical site. Use cotton-tipped applicators or your fingers.

E 1. Ask the patient if one or two points are felt and where they are felt.

2. Remove the stimulus from one side while maintaining the stimulus on the opposite side.

3. Ask the patient if one or two points are felt and where the sensations are felt.

N The patient should be able to feel both stimuli.

A The inability to feel the two points simultaneously and to discriminate that one point has been removed is abnormal.

P A lesion in one parietal lobe may prevent the patient from feeling the stimulus on the opposite side of the body even if sensation is intact on that side during routine assessment.

CRANIAL NERVES

A complete assessment of the 12 cranial nerves is necessary when a baseline assessment is desired, if a tumor of a specific cranial nerve is suspected, or if periodic assessment is needed after surgery or radiation treatments. An abbreviated cranial nerve assessment is an integral part of a neurological screening examination. The screening examination would include cranial nerves II, III, IV, and VI: visual acuity and gross visual fields, funduscopic examination, pupillary reactions, and extraocular movements; cranial nerves VII, VIII, IX, X, and XII: facial musculature and expression, gross hearing, voice, and inspection of the tongue.

Olfactory Nerve (CN I)

E 1. Ask the patient to close the eyes.

2. Test each side separately by asking the patient to occlude one nostril by pressing against it with a finger.

3. Ask the patient to inhale deeply in order to cause the odor to surround the mucous membranes and adequately stimulate the olfactory nerve (Figure 19-15).

4. Ask the patient to identify the contents of each vial.

5. Present one odor at a time and alternate them from nostril to nostril.

6. Allow enough time to pass between presentation of vials to prevent confusion of the olfactory system.

7. Record the number of substances tested and the number of times the patient was able to correctly identify the contents.

8. Note whether a difference between the right and the left sides was apparent.

N The patient should be able to distinguish and identify the odors with each nostril.

A Anosmia, the loss of the sense of smell, is abnormal.

P Total loss of the sense of smell may be caused by trauma to the cribriform plate, sinusitis, colds, or heavy smoking. Unilateral anosmia may be the result of an intracranial neoplasm, such as a meningioma of the sphenoid ridge compressing the olfactory tract or bulb.

Optic Nerve (CN II)

VISUAL ACUITY. (ENAP: See Chapter 12.)

VISUAL FIELDS. (ENAP: See Chapter 12.)

FUNDUSCOPIC EXAMINATION. (ENAP: See Chapter 12.)

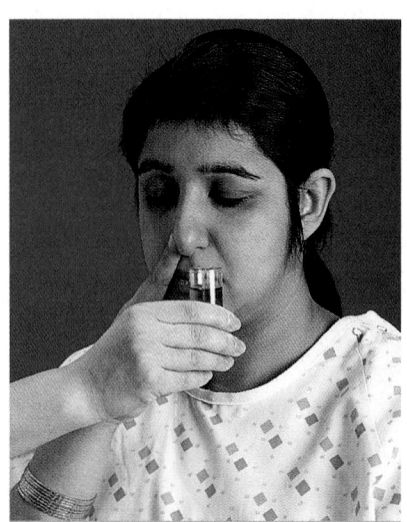

FIGURE 19-15 **Assessment of CN I**

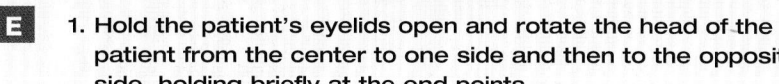

Doll's Eyes Phenomenon

Assess doll's eyes phenomenon (oculocephalic reflex) (CN III) in the unconscious patient. This tests the intactness of the vestibular and oculomotor pathways. Doll's eyes phenomenon should not be tested in the patient with suspected neck injury.

E
1. Hold the patient's eyelids open and rotate the head of the patient from the center to one side and then to the opposite side, holding briefly at the end points.
2. Watch for eye movement.
3. Further evaluate the oculocephalic reflex by alternately flexing and extending the head with the eyelids held as before.

N Normally, the eyes should deviate in the direction opposite the head (e.g., head up, eyes look down; head turned to the right, eyes look left) (Figure 19-16).

A The patient with an abnormal response will have eyes that appear to be painted onto a doll's head, hence the term *doll's eyes phenomenon*. Loss of doll's eyes phenomenon is abnormal and is demonstrated when the eyes remain fixed with neither lateral nor vertical deviation in response to head movement (Figure 19-16).

P Patients with low brain stem lesions will exhibit abnormal doll's eyes phenomenon.

Normal (reflex present)

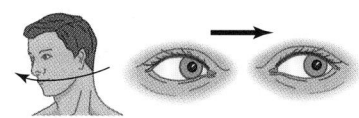

Head rotated to the right   Eyes move to the left

Abnormal (reflex absent)

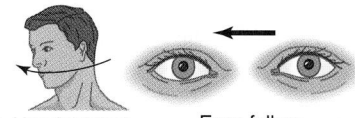

Head rotated to the right   Eyes follow

FIGURE 19-16 Assessing the Oculocephalic Reflex

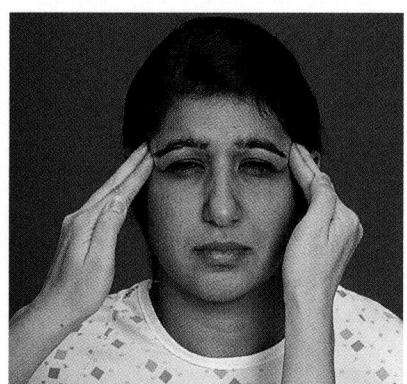

A. Temporalis Muscles

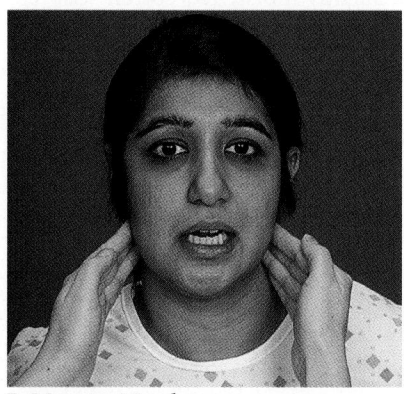

B. Masseter Muscles

FIGURE 19-17 Assessment of the Motor Component of CN V

Oculomotor Nerve (CN III)

CARDINAL FIELDS OF GAZE. (ENAP: See Chapter 12.)

EYELID ELEVATION. (ENAP: See Chapter 12.)

PUPIL REACTIONS (DIRECT, CONSENSUAL, ACCOMMODATION). (ENAP: See Chapter 12.)

Trochlear Nerve (CN IV)

CARDINAL FIELDS OF GAZE. (ENAP: See Chapter 12.)

Trigeminal Nerve (CN V)

MOTOR COMPONENT.

E
1. Instruct the patient to clench the jaw.
2. Palpate the contraction of the temporalis (Figure 19-17A) and masseter (Figure 19-17B) muscles on each side of the face by feeling for contraction of the muscles with the finger pads of the first three fingers.
3. Ask the patient to move the jaw from side to side against resistance from your hand. Feel for weakness on one side or the other as the patient pushes against resistance.
4. Test the muscles of mastication by having the patient bite down with the molars on each side of a tongue blade and comparing the depth

---

E Examination   **N** Normal Findings   **A** Abnormal Findings   **P** Pathophysiology

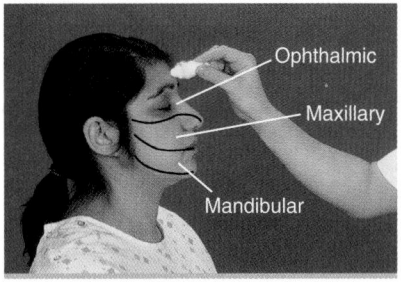

FIGURE 19-18 Assessment of the Sensory Component of CN V: Light Touch

of the impressions made by the teeth. If you can pull the tongue blade out while the patient is biting on it, there is weakness of the muscles of mastication.

5. Observe for fasciculation and note the bulk, contour, and tone of the muscles of mastication.

SENSORY COMPONENT.

E 1. Instruct the patient to close the eyes.

2. Test light touch by using a cotton wisp to lightly stroke the patient's face in each area of the sensory distribution of the trigeminal nerve (Figure 19-18).

3. Instruct the patient to respond by saying "now" each time the touch of the cotton wisp is felt.

4. Test and compare both sides of the face.

5. To assess superficial pain sensation, use a sterile needle. Before testing, show the patient how the sharpness of the needle feels compared to the dullness of the opposite, blunt end. Testing with the blunt end will give some reliability to the assessment.

   a. Instruct the patient to respond by saying "sharp" or "dull" when each sensation is felt.

   b. Irregularly alternate the sharp and dull ends, and again test each distribution area of the trigeminal nerve on both sides of the face.

6. Test temperature sensation if other abnormalities have been detected. Use vials of hot and cold water.

   a. Touch the vials to each dermatomal distribution area, alternating hot and cold.

   b. The patient should respond by saying "hot" or "cold."

7. Because sensation to the cornea is supplied by the trigeminal nerve, test the corneal reflex (the motor component is CN VII). The corneal reflex should not be routinely assessed in conscious patients, unless there is a clinical suspicion of trauma to CN V or CN VII.

   a. Ask the patient to open the eyes and look away from you.

   b. Approach the patient out of the line of vision to eliminate the blink reflex. You can stabilize the patient's chin with your hand if it is moving.

   c. Lightly stroke the cornea with a slightly moistened cotton wisp (to avoid irritating the cornea) (Figure 19-19). Avoid stroking just the sclera or the lashes of the eye. An alternative technique is to instill normal saline eye drops instead of a light stroke of a cotton wisp.

   d. Observe for bilateral blinking of the eyes.

   e. Repeat on the opposite eye.

N The temporalis and masseter muscles should be equally strong on palpation. The jaw should not deviate and should be equally strong during side-to-side movement against resistance. The volume and bulk of the muscles should be bilaterally equal. Sensation to light touch, superficial pain, and temperature should be present on the sensory distribution areas of the trigeminal nerve. The corneal reflex should cause bilateral blinking of eyes.

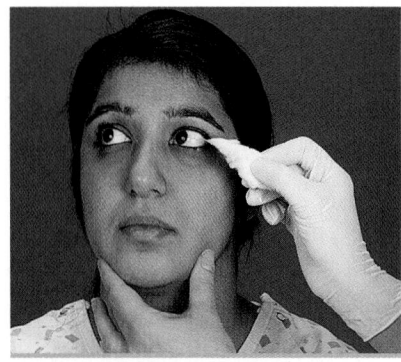

FIGURE 19-19 Assessment of the Sensory Component of CN V and Motor Component of CN VII: Corneal Reflex

A Lesions of the trigeminal nerve may give rise to either reduced sensory perception or to facial pain, both of which are abnormal.

P Aneurysms of the internal carotid artery next to the cavernous sinus may give rise to severe pain in the ophthalmic or mandibular distribution of the trigeminal nerve due to the pressure of the aneurysm on the nerve. Neoplasms that compress the gasserian ganglion or root, such as meningiomas, pituitary adenomas, and malignant tumors of the nasopharynx, may cause facial pain and impairment of sensation. Head injuries, especially basilar skull fractures, may give rise to facial anesthesia and paralysis of the muscles of mastication.

A Trigeminal neuralgia (tic douloureux), characterized by brief, paroxysmal, unilateral facial pain along the distribution of the trigeminal nerve, is abnormal. The pain can be provoked by touch or movement of the face, such as in tooth brushing, yawning, chewing, or talking. There is no associated motor weakness.

P Trigeminal neuralgia may occur in patients with multiple sclerosis due to demyelinization of the root of CN V. The patient with a posterior fossa tumor may have trigeminal neuralgia. In most cases, there is no etiology found.

A Postherpetic neuralgia is found most often in the elderly. The pain is continuous and is described as a constant, burning ache with occasional stabbing pains. The stabbing pain may begin spontaneously or may be provoked by touch. The pain is unilateral and tends to follow the distribution of the ophthalmic distribution of the trigeminal nerve. It is abnormal.

P Herpes zoster involvement of the trigeminal nerve causes postherpetic neuralgia. Inflammatory lesions are found throughout the trigeminal pathways.

A Tetanus is characterized by tonic spasms interfering with the muscles that open the jaw (trismus). Dysphagia and spasms of the pharyngeal muscles are also observed in tetanus. Tetanus is abnormal.

P Motor root involvement of the trigeminal nerve causes the spasm of the masseter muscles.

Abducens Nerve (CN VI)

CARDINAL FIELDS OF GAZE. (ENAP: See Chapter 12.)

Facial Nerve (CN VII)

MOTOR COMPONENT.

E 1. Observe the patient's facial expressions for symmetry and mobility throughout the assessment.

2. Note any asymmetry of the face, such as wrinkles or lack of wrinkles on one side of the face or one-sided blinking.

3. Test muscle contraction by asking the patient to:

   a. Frown

   b. Raise the eyebrows

   c. Wrinkle the forehead while looking up

   d. Close the eyes lightly and then keep them closed against your resistance (Figure 19-20).

   e. Smile, show teeth, purse lips, and whistle

   f. Puff out the cheeks against the resistance of your hands

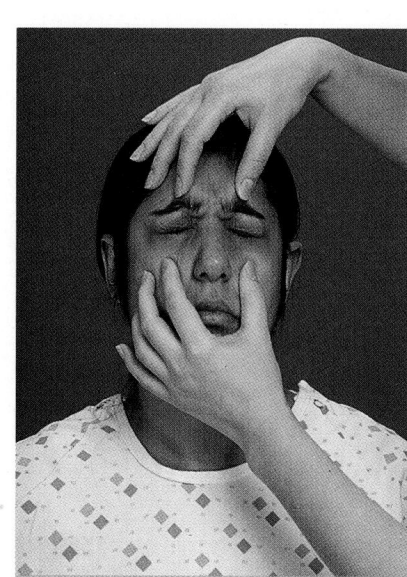

FIGURE 19-20 **Assessment of the Motor Component of CN VII: Opening the Patient's Eyes Against Resistance**

E Examination   **N** Normal Findings   **A** Abnormal Findings   **P** Pathophysiology

4. Observe for symmetry of facial muscles and for weakness during the above maneuvers.

5. Note any abnormal movements such as tremors, tics, grimaces, or immobility.

N Normal findings of the motor portion of the facial nerve include symmetry between the right and the left sides of the face as well as between the upper and lower portions of the face at rest and while executing facial movements. There should be an absence of abnormal muscle movement.

A **Bell's palsy** (idiopathic facial palsy), characterized by complete flaccid paralysis of the facial muscles on the involved side, is abnormal. The affected side of the face is smooth, the eye cannot close, the eyebrow droops, the labiofacial fold is gone, and the mouth may droop. Loss of the sensation of taste in the anterior two-thirds of the tongue may occur.

P Bell's palsy is caused by damage to the facial nerve. It is a lower motor neuron paralysis because the damage occurs along the facial nerve from its origin to its periphery.

A Supranuclear facial palsy is characterized by paralysis in the lower one-third to two-thirds of the face; the upper portion of the face is spared. The nasolabial fold is flat, and the eye on the affected side can close, although more weakly. The patient may be unable to keep the eye closed against resistance applied by the nurse. The muscles of the upper portion of the face remain intact. Supranuclear facial palsy is abnormal.

P Supranuclear facial palsy is due to an upper motor neuron lesion of the facial nerve.

SENSORY COMPONENT.

E **1.** Sensory assessment of the facial nerve is limited to testing taste. The portions of the tongue that are tested are:

    a. The tip of the tongue for sweet and salty tastes

    b. Along the borders and at the tip for sour taste

    c. The back of the tongue and the soft palate for bitter taste

2. Test both sides of the tongue with each solution.

3. The patient's tongue should protrude during the entire assessment of taste, and talking is not allowed. In order for the patient to identify the substance, the words sweet, salty, bitter, and sour should be written on a card so that the patient can point to what is tasted. Be sure the patient does not see which solution is being tested.

4. Cotton swabs may be used as applicators, using a different one for each solution.

5. Dip the cotton swab into the solution being tested and place it on the appropriate part of the tongue.

6. Instruct the patient to point to the word that best describes the taste perception.

7. Instruct the patient to rinse the mouth with water before the next solution is tested.

8. Repeat steps 5, 6, and 7 until each solution has been tested on both sides of the tongue.

N Normal sensation would be accurate perceptions of sweet, sour, salty, and bitter tastes.

E Examination   **N** Normal Findings   **A** Abnormal Findings   **P** Pathophysiology

A Ageusia (loss of taste) and **hypogeusia** (diminution of taste) are abnormal.

P Age, excessive smoking, extreme dryness of the oral mucosa, colds, medications, lesions of the medulla oblongata, and lesions of the parietal lobe may cause alterations in the sense of taste.

Acoustic Nerve (CN VIII)

COCHLEAR DIVISION.

Hearing. (ENAP: See Chapter 13.)
Weber and Rinne Tests. (ENAP: See Chapter 13.)

VESTIBULAR DIVISION.
The vestibular division of CN VIII assesses for vertigo.

E 1. During the history, ask the patient if vertigo is experienced.

2. Note any evidence of equilibrium disturbances. Refer to the section on cerebellar assessment.

3. Note the presence of nystagmus.

N Vertigo is not normally present.

A Vertigo describes an uncomfortable sensation of movement of the environment or the movement of self within a stationary environment; it is often accompanied by nausea, vomiting, and nystagmus.

P Vertigo is caused by a disorder of the labyrinth or the vestibular nerve. Causative factors may include migraine headache, which causes a disruption in the supply of the internal auditory artery. Tumors of the cerebellopontine angle may cause vertigo by compressing the vestibular nerve. Head injuries that involve the labyrinth may cause vertigo. Blockage of the eustachian tube during ascent in an airplane may lead to vertigo.

A Ménière's disease, characterized by vertigo that lasts for minutes or hours, low-pitched roaring tinnitus, progressive hearing loss, nausea, and vomiting, is abnormal. The patient also experiences pressure in the ear.

P The main pathological finding is distension of the endolymphatic system, with degenerative changes in the organ of Corti.

Glossopharyngeal and Vagus Nerves (CN IX and CN X)

The glossopharyngeal and vagus nerves are tested together because of their overlap in function.

E 1. Examine soft palate and uvula movement and gag reflex as described in Chapter 13.

2. Assess the patient's quality of speech for a nasal quality or hoarseness. Ask the patient to produce guttural and palatal sounds, such as *k, q, ch, b,* and *d*.

3. Assess the patient's ability to swallow a small amount of water. Observe for regurgitation of fluids through the nose. If the patient is unable to swallow, observe how oral secretions are handled.

4. The sensory assessment of the glossopharyngeal and vagus nerves is limited to taste on the posterior one-third of the tongue. This assessment was previously discussed in the section on CN VII.

N Refer to Chapter 13 for normal soft palate and uvula movement and gag reflex findings. The speech is clear, without hoarseness or a nasal quality. The patient is able to swallow water or oral secretions easily.

Taste (sweet, salty, sour, and bitter) is intact in the posterior one-third of the tongue.

A Unilateral lowering and flattening of the palatine arch; weakness of the soft palate; deviation of the uvula to the normal side; mild dysphagia, regurgitation of fluids, and nasal quality of the voice; loss of taste in the posterior one-third of the tongue; and hemianesthesia of the palate and pharynx are abnormal.

P Unilateral glossopharyngeal and vagal paralysis, such as with trauma or skull fractures at the base of the skull, will cause these symptoms.

A Marked nasal quality of the voice, difficulty with guttural and palatal sounds, severe dysphagia with liquids, and inability of the palate to elevate on phonation are abnormal.

P Bilateral vagus nerve paralysis will cause these more marked symptoms, and often occurs simultaneously with signs and symptoms of other lower brain stem cranial nerve dysfunctions such as in progressive bulbar palsy in amyotrophic lateral sclerosis (ALS).

Spinal Accessory Nerve (CN XI)

E 1. Place the patient in a seated or a supine position. Inspect the sternocleidomastoid muscles for contour, volume, and fasciculation.

2. Place your right hand on the left side of the patient's face. Instruct the patient to turn the head sideways against the resistance of your hand (Figure 19-21A).

3. Use the other hand to palpate the sternocleidomastoid muscle for strength of contraction. Inspect the muscle for contraction.

4. Repeat steps 2 and 3 in the opposite direction. Compare the strength of the two sides.

5. To assess the function of the trapezius muscle, stand behind the patient and inspect the shoulders and scapula for symmetry of contour. Note any atrophy or fasciculation.

6. Place your hands on top of the patient's shoulders and instruct the patient to raise the shoulders against the downward resistance of your hands (Figure 19-21B). This can be performed in front of or behind the patient.

7. Observe the movements and palpate the contraction of the trapezius muscles. Compare the strength of the two sides.

N The patient should be able to turn the head against resistance with a smooth, strong, and symmetrical motion. The patient should also demonstrate the ability to shrug the shoulders against resistance with strong, symmetrical movement of the trapezius muscles.

A Inability to turn the head toward the paralyzed side, and a flat, noncontracting muscle on that side are abnormal findings. The contralateral sternocleidomastoid muscle may be contracted.

P These findings are the result of unilateral paralysis of the sternocleidomastoid muscle due to trauma, tumors, or infection affecting the spinal accessory nerve.

A The inability of the patient to elevate one shoulder, asymmetrical drooping of the shoulder and scapula, and a depressed outline of the neck are abnormal findings. The involved shoulder may also show atrophy and fasciculation of the muscles.

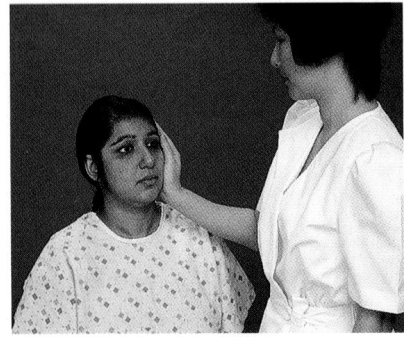

A. Strength of Sternocleidomastoid Muscle

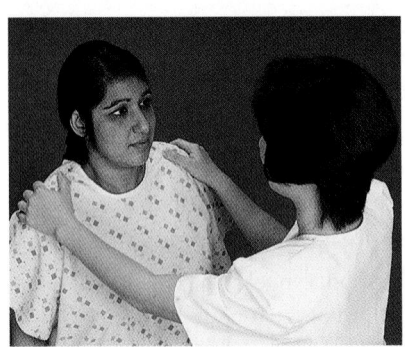

B. Strength of Trapezius Muscle

FIGURE 19-21 Assessment of CN XI

E Examination	**N** Normal Findings	**A** Abnormal Findings	**P** Pathophysiology

P   Unilateral paralysis of the trapezius muscle may be suspected, usually due to trauma, tumors, or infection.

A/P   For information on torticollis, see Chapter 11.

Hypoglossal Nerve (CN XII)

E   **1.** See Chapter 13 for assessment of tongue movement.

   2. Assess lingual sounds by asking the patient to say "la la la."

N   See Chapter 13 for normal tongue movements. Lingual speech is clear.

A   Inability or difficulty in producing lingual sounds is abnormal. The speech sounds lispy and clumsy.

P   Lesions of the hypoglossal nerve will cause difficulty in pronunciation of lingual sounds.

MOTOR SYSTEM

For ENAP on muscle size, tone, and strength, and involuntary movements, see Chapter 18. See the following for additional abnormal findings and pathophysiology.

A   Extrapyramidal rigidity is evident when resistance is present during passive movement of the muscles in all directions and lasts throughout the entire range of motion. It may involve both flexor and extensor muscles and is abnormal.

P   Extrapyramidal rigidity is due to lesions located in the basal ganglia.

A   **Decerebrate rigidity** (decerebration) is characterized by rigidity and sustained contraction of the extensor muscles and is abnormal. The arms are adducted, extended, and hyperpronated. The legs are stiffly extended and the feet are plantar flexed (Figure 19-22A). The back and neck may be arched and the teeth clenched (opisthotonos).

P   Decerebration may be found in unconscious patients with deep, bilateral diencephalic injury that progresses to midbrain dysfunction. Decerebrate rigidity may also occur due to midbrain and pontine damage, which occurs with compression of these structures due to expanding cerebellar or posterior fossa lesions. Severe metabolic disorders that depress diencephalic and forebrain function may also cause decerebration.

A   **Decorticate rigidity** (decortication) is characterized by hyperflexion of the arms (flexion of the arm, wrist, and fingers, adduction of the arms), hyperextension and internal rotation of the legs, and plantar flexion (Figure 19-22B). It is abnormal.

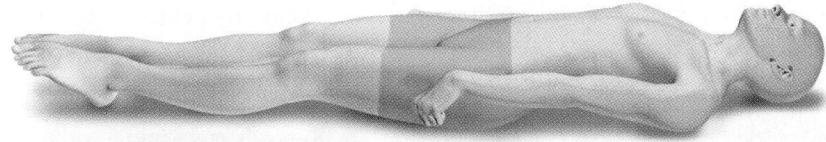

A. Decerebrate Rigidity (Abnormal Extension)

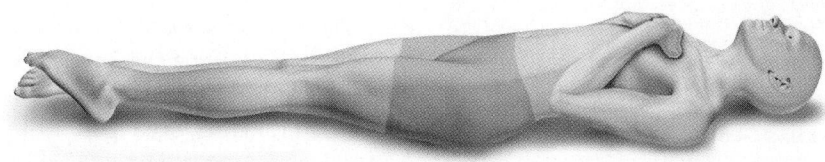

B. Decorticate Rigidity (Abnormal Flexion)

FIGURE 19-22   **Motor System Dysfunction**

P Decorticate rigidity is found in unconscious patients with cerebral hemisphere lesions that interfere with the corticospinal tract.

Pronator Drift

E 1. Have the patient extend the arms out in front with palms up for 20 seconds.

2. Observe for downward drifting of an arm.

N There should be no downward drifting of an arm.

A Downward drifting of an arm is abnormal.

P Downward drifting of an arm may indicate hemiparesis, such as in stroke.

CEREBELLAR FUNCTION (COORDINATION, STATION, AND GAIT)

Motor coordination refers to smooth, precise, and harmonious muscular activity. Movement requires the coordination of many muscle groups. Coordination is an integrated process involving complicated neural integration of the motor and premotor cortex, basal ganglia, cerebellum, vestibular system, posterior columns, and peripheral nerves.

Equilibratory coordination refers to maintenance of an upright stance and depends on the vestibular, cerebellar, and proprioceptive systems. Nonequilibratory coordination refers to smaller movements of the extremities and involves the cerebellar and proprioceptive mechanisms.

Incoordination is categorized into three different types of syndromes: cerebellar, vestibular, and posterior column syndromes. Incoordination is not considered to be secondary to involuntary movements, paresis, or alterations of muscle tone.

Station refers to the patient's posture, and gait refers to the patient's manner of walking.

Coordination

E 1. Instruct the patient to sit comfortably facing you, with eyes open and arms outstretched.

2. Ask the patient to first touch the index finger to the nose, then to alternate rapidly with the index finger of the opposite hand.

3. With the patient's eyes closed, have the patient continue to rapidly touch the nose with alternate index fingers (Figure 19-23).

4. With the patient's eyes open, ask the patient to again touch finger to nose. Next, ask the patient to touch your index finger, which is held about 45 cm (18 inches) away from the patient.

5. Change the position of your finger as the patient rapidly repeats the maneuver with one finger.

6. Repeat steps 4 and 5 with the other hand.

7. Observe for intention tremor or overshoot or undershoot of the patient's finger.

8. To assess rapid alternating movements, ask the patient to rapidly alternate patting the knees, first with the palms and then alternating palms with the backs of the hands (rapid supinating [see Figure 19-24A] and pronating [see Figure 19-24B] of the hands).

9. Ask the patient to repeatedly touch the thumb to each of the fingers of the hand in rapid succession from index to the fifth finger, and back.

NURSINGTIP

Patients Who Require Corrective Lenses for Coordination

Ensure that patients who wear corrective lenses (eyeglasses or contacts) are wearing them prior to assessing their coordination.

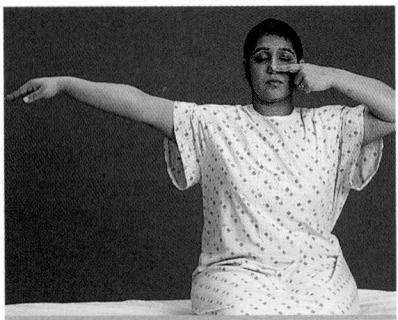

FIGURE 19-23 Assessment of Coordination: Fingertip-to-Nose Touch

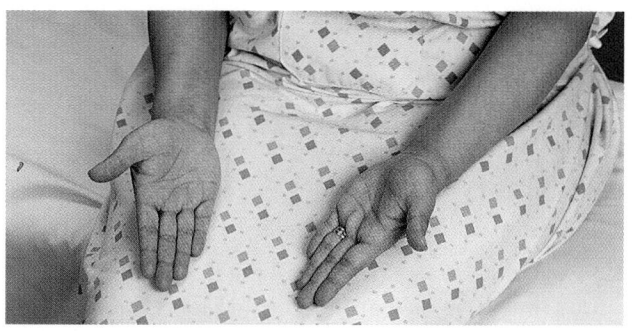

A. Supination

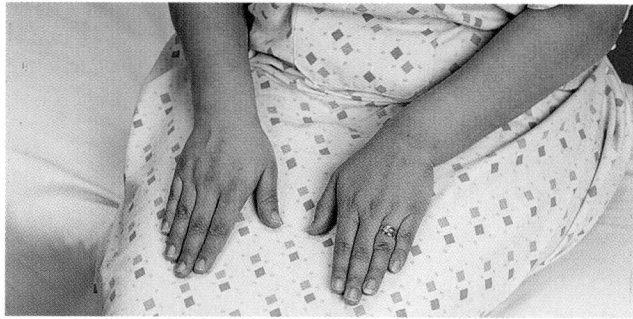

B. Pronation

FIGURE 19-24 **Assessment of Coordination: Rapid Alternating Hand Movements**

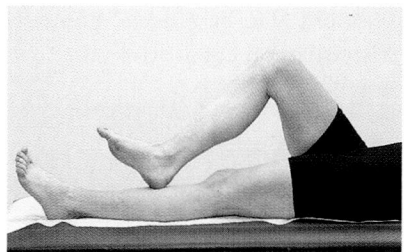

FIGURE 19-25 **Assessment of Coordination: Heel Slide**

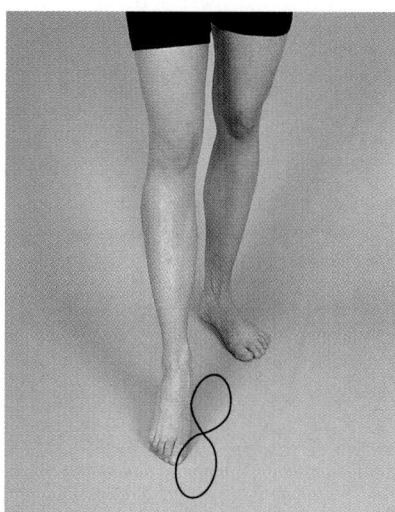

FIGURE 19-26 **Assessment of Coordination: Figure 8**

10. Repeat step 9 with the other hand.

11. Observe coordination and the ability of the patient to perform these in rapid sequence.

12. With the patient in a seated or supine position, ask the patient to place the heel just below the knee on the shin of the opposite leg and to slide it down to the foot (Figure 19-25).

13. Repeat with the opposite foot.

14. Observe coordination of the two legs.

15. Ask the patient to draw a circle or a figure 8 with a foot either on the ground or in the air (Figure 19-26).

16. Repeat with the other foot.

17. Observe for coordination and regularity of the figure.

18. Test the lower extremities for rapid alternating movement by asking the patient to rapidly extend the ankle ("tap your foot") or to rapidly flex and extend the toes of one foot.

19. Repeat with the opposite foot.

20. Note rate, rhythm, smoothness, and accuracy of the movements.

N The patient is able to rapidly alternate touching finger to nose and moving finger from nose to your finger in a coordinated fashion. The patient is able to perform alternating movements in a purposeful, rapid, coordinated manner. The patient demonstrates the ability to purposefully and smoothly run heel down shin with equal coordination in both feet and to draw a figure 8 or circles with the foot.

A **Dyssynergy**, the lack of coordinated action of the muscle groups, is abnormal. The patient is unable to carry out smooth, coordinated movements. The patient's movements appear jerky, irregular, and uncoordinated.

A **Dysmetria**, impaired judgment of distance, range, speed, and force of movement, is abnormal. The patient misjudges distance and overshoots.

A **Dysdiadochokinesia**, the inability to perform rapid alternating movements, is abnormal. The patient is unable to abruptly stop one movement and begin another opposite movement.

P Cerebellar disease causes all of these abnormal findings.

| **E** Examination | **N** Normal Findings | **A** Abnormal Findings | **P** Pathophysiology |

Station

(ENAP: See Chapter 18.)

Gait

E 1. See Chapter 18 for gait assessment technique.

2. Ask the patient to walk on tiptoes, then on heels.

3. Ask the patient to walk in a straight line, touching heel to toe (tandem walking). The arms should be held at the side and the eyes should be open.

4. Note the patient's ability to maintain balance.

5. Ask the patient to hop in place, first on one foot and then on the other.

N See Chapter 18 for normal gait findings. The patient should be able to walk unaided on tiptoes and heels, and walk heel to toe in a straight line without losing balance. The patient should also be able to maintain balance while hopping on one foot, with bilateral equal strength.

A/P See Chapter 18.

NURSING**ALERT**

Romberg Test

Stand close to the patient during this test in order to catch the patient if she or he begins to fall.

NURSING**TIP**

Deep Tendon Reflex Reinforcement

Even when the deep tendon reflex (DTR) is stimulated correctly, the patient may not exhibit a DTR because of conscious thought. If this occurs, reinforcement may be necessary. Reinforcement is a technique used to distract conscious thought of the DTR by concentrating on another action. Examples include the patient clenching the teeth, grasping the thigh with the hand not being assessed, and grasping and pulling the wrists with the contralateral hand.

ADVANCED TECHNIQUE

Romberg Test

E 1. Ask the patient to stand erect, feet together and arms at side, first with eyes open, then closed.

2. Note the patient's ability to maintain balance with eyes first open, then closed.

N The patient should be able to maintain balance with eyes open or closed for 20 seconds and with minimal swaying.

A The Romberg test is positive if the patient becomes unsteady and tends to fall when the eyes are closed.

P In cerebellar disease, the patient remains unsteady with the eyes open and closed. In posterior column disease with proprioceptive loss, the patient becomes appreciably more unsteady with eye closure.

☑ REFLEX ASSESSMENT CHECKLIST

Assessing Reflexes

1. When testing reflexes, the patient should be relaxed and comfortable.
2. Position the patient so the extremities are symmetrical.
3. To elicit true reflexes, distract the patient by talking about another topic.
4. Hold the reflex hammer loosely between the thumb and index finger and strike the tendon with a brisk motion from the wrist. The reflex hammer should make contact with the correct point on the tendon in a quick, direct manner.
5. Observe the degree and speed of response of the muscles after the reflex hammer makes contact. Grading of DTR is as follows:
   0: absent
   + (1+): present but diminished

continues

| **E** Examination | **N** Normal Findings | **A** Abnormal Findings | **P** Pathophysiology |

REFLEX ASSESSMENT CHECKLIST *Continued*

++ (2+): normal

+++ (3+): mildly increased but not pathological

++++ (4+): markedly hyperactive, clonus may be present

6. Compare reflex responses of the right and the left sides. The normal response to taps in the correct area should elicit a brisk (++ or +++) contraction of the muscles involved.

7. When documenting the DTRs, you can use a stick figure.

REFLEXES

Deep Tendon Reflexes

BRACHIORADIALIS.

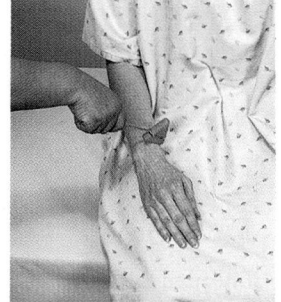

A. Brachioradialis

E **1.** Flex the patient's arm to 45°.

2. Support the patient's relaxed arm either on the lap or semipronated on your forearm.

3. With the blunt end of the reflex hammer, strike the tendon of the brachioradialis above the styloid process of the radius (a few centimeters above the wrist on the thumb side) (Figure 19-27A).

N Observe for flexion and supination of the forearm. An exaggerated reflex may also show flexion of the wrist and fingers and adduction of the forearm. Innervation of this reflex is through the radial nerve, with segmental innervation of C5, C6.

A/P See Achilles on following page.

BICEPS.

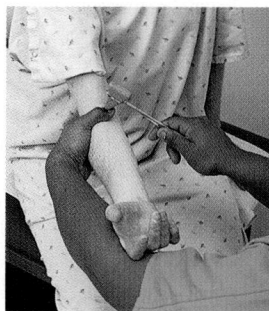

B. Biceps

E **1.** Flex the patient's arm to between 45° and 90°.

2. Support the patient's forearm on your forearm.

3. Place your thumb firmly on the biceps tendon just above the crease of the antecubital fossa (Figure 19-27B).

4. Wrap your fingers around the patient's arm and rest them on the biceps muscle to feel it contract.

5. Tap the thumb briskly with the pointed end of the reflex hammer.

N Observe for contraction of the biceps muscle and flexion of the elbow. Innervation of the biceps reflex is through the musculocutaneous nerve with segmental innervation of C5, C6.

A/P See Achilles, on following page.

TRICEPS.

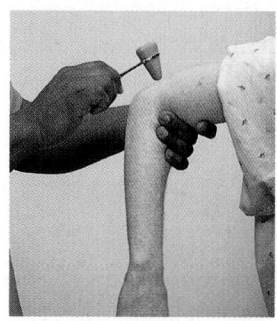

C. Triceps

FIGURE 19-27 **Assessment of Deep Tendon Reflexes** *continues*

E **1.** Flex the patient's arm to between 45° and 90°.

2. Support the patient's arm either on the lap or on your hand as shown in Figure 19-27C.

3. With the pointed end of the reflex hammer, tap the triceps tendon just above its insertion above the olecranon process (elbow).

N Observe for contraction of the triceps muscle and extension of the arm. Innervation of the triceps reflex is through the radial nerve, with segmental innervation of C7, C8.

A/P See Achilles on following page.

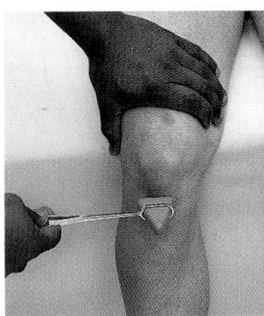

D. Patellar

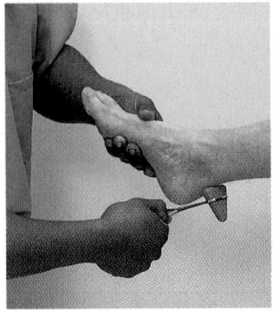

E. Achilles

FIGURE 19-27   **Assessment of Deep Tendon Reflexes** *continued*

PATELLAR.

E   **1.** Ask the patient to sit in a chair or at the edge of the examination table.

2. Place your hand over the quadriceps femoris muscle to feel contraction.

3. With the other hand, tap the patellar tendon just below the patella with the blunt end of the reflex hammer (Figure 19-27D).

4. If the patient cannot tolerate a sitting position, support the flexed knee with your hand under it so the foot is hanging freely.

N   There should be contraction of the quadriceps muscle and extension of the leg. Innervation of the patellar reflex is through the femoral nerve, with segmental innervation of L2, L3, L4.

A/P   See Achilles, below.

ACHILLES.

E   **1.** Ask the patient to sit with the feet dangling.

2. Slightly dorsiflex the patient's foot.

3. With the blunt end of the reflex hammer, tap the Achilles tendon just above its insertion in the heel.

4. If the patient is lying down, flex the leg at the knee and externally rotate the thigh. Place your nondominant hand under the foot to produce dorsiflexion (Figure 19-27E). Apply the stimulus as described in step 3.

N   The normal response is contraction of the muscles of the calf (gastrocnemius, soleus, and plantaris) and plantar flexion of the foot. Innervation of the Achilles reflex is through the tibial nerve, with segmental innervation of L5, S1, S2.

A   Absent or decreased deep tendon reflexes are abnormal.

P   Diminished deep tendon reflexes usually result from interference in the reflex arc, and an absence may indicate a break in the reflex arc. Deep tendon reflexes are lost in deep coma, narcosis, or deep sedation. Hypothyroidism, sedative or hypnotic drugs, and infectious diseases may also diminish reflexes. Patients with increased intracranial pressure frequently show decreased or absent deep tendon reflexes. Spinal shock also causes loss of these reflexes.

A   Hyperactive deep tendon reflexes are abnormal. Hyperactive deep tendon reflexes are characterized by an increase in speed of response and enhancement of the vigor of movement. The muscle contraction is sustained, with a minimal stimulus needed to elicit the response. Sometimes the adjacent muscles may also contract. Clonus may be present.

P   Hyperactivity is associated with a loss of inhibition of the higher centers in the cortex and reticular formation and in lesions of the pyramidal system. Muscle stretch reflexes are also exaggerated in light coma, tetany, and tetanus.

Superficial Reflexes

ABDOMINAL.

E   **1.** Drape and place the patient in a recumbent position, arms at sides and knees slightly flexed. Stand to the right of the patient.

2. Use a moderately sharp object to stroke the skin, such as the wooden tip of a cotton-tipped applicator or a split tongue blade.

3. To elicit the upper abdominal reflex, stimulate the skin of the upper abdominal quadrants. From the tip of the sternum, stroke in a diagonal (downward and inward) fashion (Figure 19-28).

4. Repeat step 3 on the opposite side.

5. To elicit the lower abdominal reflex, stimulate the skin of the lower abdominal quadrants. From the area below the umbilicus, stroke in a diagonal (downward and inward) fashion to the symphysis pubis.

6. Repeat step 5 on the opposite side.

N Observe for contraction of the upper abdominal muscles upward and outward with a deviation of the umbilicus toward the stimulus. The upper abdominal reflex is innervated by the intercostal nerves through T7, T8, T9. Observe for contraction of the lower abdominal muscles and contraction of the umbilicus toward the stimulus. The lower abdominal reflex is innervated by the lower intercostal, iliohypogastric, and ilioinguinal nerves through segments T10, T11, T12.

A/P See Bulbocavernosus, below.

PLANTAR.

E 1. With the handle of the reflex hammer, stroke the outer aspect of the sole of the foot from the heel across the ball of the foot to just below the great toe (Figure 19-29).

2. Repeat on the opposite foot.

N Observe for plantar flexion of the toes. The plantar reflex is innervated by the tibial nerve with segmental innervation of L5, S1, S2.

A/P See Bulbocavernosus, below.

CREMASTERIC.

E 1. The male patient should be lying down with the thighs exposed and the testicles visible.

2. Stroke the skin of the inner aspect of the thigh near the groin from above downward (Figure 19-30).

3. Repeat step 2 on the opposite side.

N Observe contraction of the cremasteric muscle with corresponding elevation of the ipsilateral testicle. Innervation of the cremasteric reflex is through the ilioinguinal and genitofemoral nerves with segmental innervation of T12, L1, L2.

A/P See Bulbocavernosus, next.

BULBOCAVERNOSUS.

E 1. Pinch the skin of the foreskin or the glans penis.

2. Observe for a contraction of the bulbocavernosus muscle in the perineum at the base of the penis.

N Contraction of the bulbocavernosus muscle occurs. The presence of this reflex in a paraplegic patient after acute spinal cord injury indicates that the initial stage of spinal shock is past. The bulbocavernosus reflex is innervated by segments S3 and S4.

A Decreased or absent superficial reflexes are abnormal.

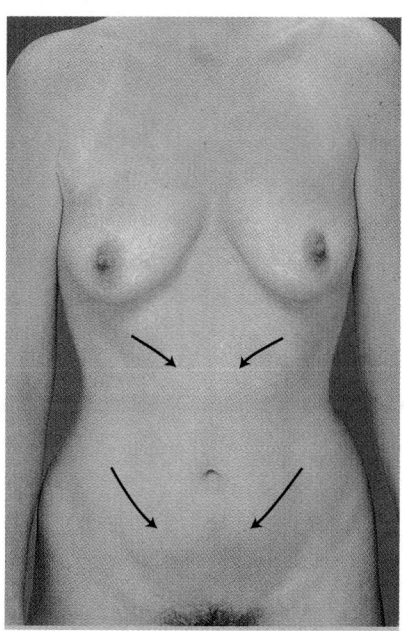

FIGURE 19-28 Assessment of Superficial Reflexes: Direction of Stimulus for Abdominal Reflexes

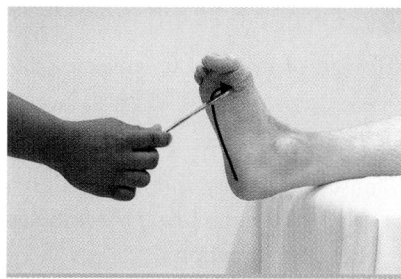

FIGURE 19-29 Assessment of Superficial Reflex: Plantar

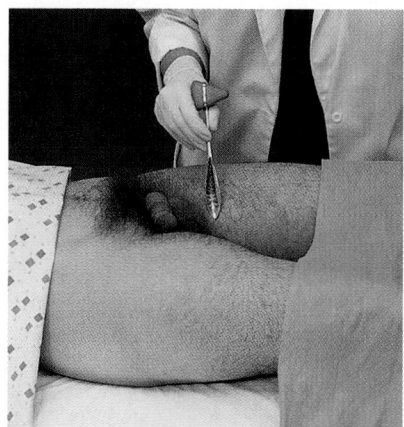

FIGURE 19-30 Assessment of Superficial Reflex: Cremasteric

| **E** Examination | **N** Normal Findings | **A** Abnormal Findings | **P** Pathophysiology |

P Superficial reflexes are diminished or absent with dysfunction of the reflex arc as in the muscle stretch reflexes. Superficial reflexes are complex because they involve the parietal areas and the motor centers of the premotor area and the pyramidal system. Lesions in the pyramidal tracts will cause decrease or absence of superficial reflexes. These reflexes may also be lost in deep sleep and coma.

Pathological Reflexes

All the following reflexes described are abnormal findings in adults and are not usually assessed unless the patient's clinical presentation warrants it.

GLABELLAR.

E 1. With your finger, tap the patient on the forehead between the eyebrows.

2. Observe for a hyperactive blinking response.

A The presence of this reflex is abnormal.

P Patients with lesions of the corticobulbar pathways from the cortex to the pons, patients with Parkinson's disease, and patients with glioblastoma of the corpus callosum will have this reflex.

CLONUS.

E 1. Have the patient assume a recumbent position. Stand to the side.

2. Support the patient's knee in a slightly flexed position.

3. Quickly dorsiflex the foot and maintain it in that position.

4. Assess for **clonus** (a rhythmic oscillation of involuntary muscle contraction).

A Sustained clonus is an abnormal finding.

P Sustained clonus, in combination with muscle spasticity and hyperreflexia, indicates upper motor neuron disease. Table 19-10 summarizes the findings associated with upper and lower motor neuron dysfunction.

P Women with preeclampsia and eclampsia can also demonstrate clonus.

BABINSKI.

E With the handle of the reflex hammer, stroke the patient's sole as you did for the plantar reflex. Use a slow and deliberate motion.

TABLE 19-10 Comparison of Upper Motor Neuron and Lower Motor Neuron Lesions

PARAMETER	UPPER MOTOR NEURON	LOWER MOTOR NEURON
Muscle tone	Spasticity	Flaccidity
Muscle bulk	Late atrophy from disease; no fasciculations	Atrophy; fasciculations
Pronator drift	Positive	Absent
Deep tendon reflexes	Hyperreflexia	Hyporeflexia or absent
Babinski reflex	Positive	Absent
Clonus	Present	Absent

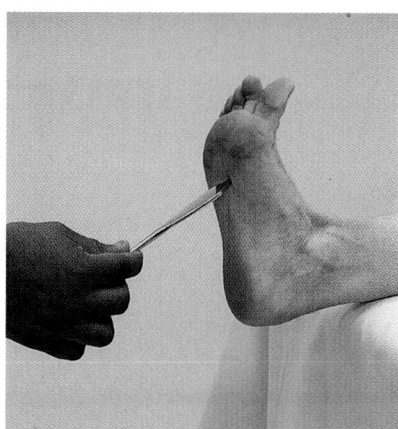

FIGURE 19-31 Assessment of Pathological Reflex: Babinski

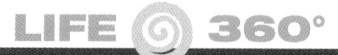

Meningococcal Meningitis

The meningococcal meningitis vaccine is widely recommended for college students. Meningitis is rapidly spread in crowded living quarters and through exposure to respiratory tract infections among close contacts.

* What measures could limit the risks of acquiring meningitis?
* Should the meningitis vaccine be required or recommended?
* What other populations share similar risks for contracting meningitis?

NURSING**ALERT**

Signs/Symptoms of Lyme Disease

* Erythema migrans (EM) lesion
* Secondary additional EM lesions
* Headache
* Fever/chills
* Lymphadenopathy
* Neck stiffness or painful neck flexion
* Malaise, fatigue, lethargy
* Arthralgias, myalgias

N A Babinski reflex is normal in infants and toddlers until 15–18 months of age.

A A positive Babinskis' reflex is noted when the patient's toes abduct (fan) and the great toe dorsiflexes (Figure 19-31).

P Patients with lesions in the pyramidal system, such as in stroke or trauma, display a positive Babinskis' reflex.

ADVANCED TECHNIQUE

Meningeal Irritation

To assess the patient for signs of meningeal irritation, look for nuchal rigidity, Kernig's sign, and Brudzinski's sign, all abnormal findings. Other signs and symptoms include violent headache, photophobia, fever, nausea and vomiting, decreasing level of consciousness, and seizures. Definitive diagnosis is obtained through cultures of cerebrospinal fluid.

NUCHAL RIGIDITY. Nuchal rigidity is the tendency of the patient to maintain the head in an immobile, extended position. The patient resists movement of the neck. Severe pain and spasms occur with movement.

E 1. Place the patient in a supine position.

   2. Flex the patient's neck.

A The patient resists the movement.

P Nuchal rigidity can be caused by meningeal irritation such as in meningitis. Meningitis is an infectious process of the meninges caused by bacteria, viruses, mycobacteria, fungi, or spirochetes. The organisms enter the subarachnoid space, causing an acute inflammatory response.

P Irritation of the subarachnoid space due to subarachnoid hemorrhage may cause meningeal irritation.

KERNIG'S SIGN.

E 1. Place the patient in a recumbent position.

   2. Lift the patient's leg and flex the knee at a right angle.

   3. Attempt to extend the patient's knee by pushing down on it.

A A positive Kernig's sign is a resistance to extension and pain (due to spasm of the hamstring), preventing extension of the leg.

P Kernig's sign is caused by stretching of irritated nerve roots and meninges.

BRUDZINSKI'S SIGN.

E 1. Place one hand under the patient's neck and the other hand on top of the patient's chest to prevent elevation of the body.

   2. Flex the patient's neck with a deliberate motion.

A Brudzinski's sign is positive if the patient responds with flexion of one or both legs up to the pelvis. The arms may also flex.

P Refer to Nuchal Rigidity.

E Examination   **N** Normal Findings   **A** Abnormal Findings   **P** Pathophysiology

CASE STUDY

The Patient with a Potential Stroke

This case study illustrates the application and objective documentation of the neurological assessment.
Mr. Lewis is a 24-year-old ex-military enlistee in a large East Coast city.

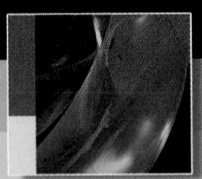

HEALTH HISTORY

PATIENT PROFILE	24 yo, Ⓡ handed, SWM
CHIEF COMPLAINT	"I had numbness and tingling in my Ⓛ hand and lower arm for a few seconds after bending forward. My speech was slurred, I had difficulty swallowing, and then I got a right sided H/A."
HISTORY OF PRESENT ILLNESS	Patient bent down to tie his boot this morning and felt momentary Ⓛ-arm numbness and "shooting, shocking" pain in his Ⓛ hand. Temporary Ⓡ frontal, then diffuse H/A, which resolved s̄ intervention. He then experienced dysphagia for liquids, Ⓛ-sided apraxia, and slurred speech for less than 5 minutes. He did not lose consciousness. All symptoms abated spontaneously within 5 minutes.
PAST HEALTH HISTORY	
Medical History	Migraine H/A without aura, triggered by stress and hunger Epididymitis at 21 yo; resolved c̄ Atb therapy, no sequelae Premature birth at 33-wks gestation; no mechanical ventilation, no intracranial bleed, no respiratory/motor/cognitive sequelae
Surgical History	Denies
Allergies	Penicillin—rash
Medications	Ibuprofen prn for H/A
Communicable Diseases	Mononucleosis at 15 yo, no sequeale
Injuries and Accidents	Denies
Special Needs	Denies
Blood Transfusions	Denies
Childhood Illnesses	Chickenpox at 5 yo
Immunizations	Hepatitis A, hepatitis B, malaria, typhoid, tetanus, yellow fever for military duty in Iraq, 2006; dates of childhood immunizations unknown

continues

CASE STUDY (Continued)

The Patient with a Potential Stroke

FAMILY HEALTH HISTORY

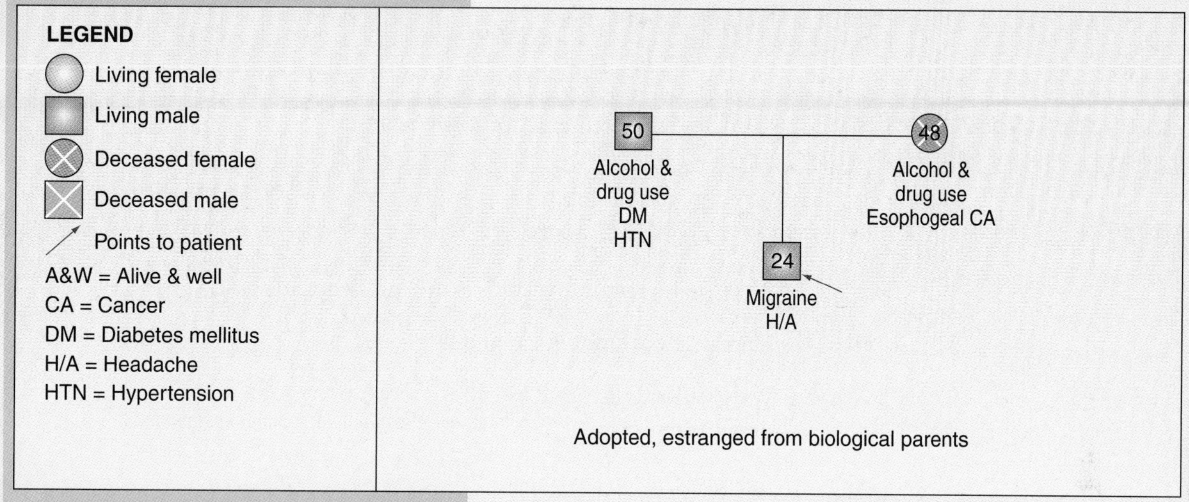

LEGEND

- ⬤ Living female
- ◻ Living male
- ⊗ Deceased female
- ⊠ Deceased male
- ╱ Points to patient

A&W = Alive & well
CA = Cancer
DM = Diabetes mellitus
H/A = Headache
HTN = Hypertension

50 — Alcohol & drug use DM HTN

48 — Alcohol & drug use Esophogeal CA

24 — Migraine H/A

Adopted, estranged from biological parents

SOCIAL HISTORY

Alcohol Use	6–12 servings/wk. Drinks only on weekends. No drinking and driving, no passing out
Tobacco Use	Denies
Drug Use	Denies
Sexual Practice	Heterosexual, monogamous re/ship $\bar{c}$ girlfriend
Domestic and Intimate Partner Violence	Denies
Travel History	Domestic travel $\bar{x}$ military duty in Iraq
Work Environment	Security guard at defense contractor; has security clearance; feels safe even though he is required to carry a firearm
Home Environment	Lives with adoptive mother and stepfather, foster sister also lives in the home; comfortable house $\bar{c}$ all modern appliances
Hobbies and Leisure Activities	Weightlifting 3 days/wk for 1 hr
Stress	Minimal, works 40 hrs/week
Education	High school and 1 yr of college
Economic Status	Middle class
Military Status	2 yrs active duty $\bar{c}$ 7 mos active duty deployment in Iraq—2006

continues

CASE STUDY (Continued)

The Patient with a Potential Stroke

Religion	Baptist; aspires to be a minister or military chaplain
Ethnic Background	No specific affiliation
Roles and Relationships	Son, stepbrother, nephew, boyfriend, military veteran
Characteristic Patterns of Daily Living	Work and social interaction with peers
HEALTH MAINTENANCE ACTIVITIES	
Sleep	8 hrs/night, restorative and restful; no sleep aids used
Diet	Unrestricted, limits sugar and fats
Exercise	Weightlifts 3 days/wk for 60 minutes; no aerobic exercise or organized sports
Stress Management	Exercises, listens to music
Use of Safety Devices	Wears seat belts; helmet when cycling; used appropriate safety devices when in military, no hazmat exposure
Health Check-ups	Only when ill or per military requirements
PHYSICAL ASSESSMENT	

Mental Status	1. Physical appearance and behavior:
	  a. Posture and movements: sitting on exam table c̄ no demonstrated deficits
	  b. Dress, grooming, and personal hygiene: work uniform, neatly groomed and clean
	  c. Facial expression: calm and relaxed
	  d. Affect: appropriate
	2. Communication: Clear, fluent speech
	3. Level of consciousness: Awake, alert, and oriented; GCS = 15
	4. Cognitive abilities and mentation:
	  a. Attention: focused, on-task
	  b. Memory: intact short and long term
	  c. Judgment: intact
	  d. Insight: appropriate
	  e. Spatial perception: intact
	  f. Calculation: intact
	  g. Abstract reasoning: intact
	  h. Thought process and content: consistent
	  i. Suicidal ideation: denies

continues

CASE STUDY (Continued)

The Patient with a Potential Stroke

Sensory
1. Exteroceptive sensation:
   a. Light touch: = & intact bilaterally
   b. Superficial pain: = & intact bilaterally
   c. Temperature: = & intact bilaterally
2. Proprioceptive sensation:
   a. Motion and position: = & intact bilaterally
   b. Vibration sense: = & intact bilaterally
3. Cortical sensation:
   a. Stereognosis, graphesthesia, two-point discrimination, extinction: intact bilaterally

Cranial Nerves

I: Smells lemon bilaterally

II: Visual acuity 20/20 c̄ glasses; visual fields by confrontation intact; no papilledema

III, IV, and VI: EOM intact, PERRLA

V: Temporalis and masseter muscles strong; corneal reflex intact; superficial pain and light touch present in all areas of face

VII: Intact s̄ facial palsy, ptosis, or asymmetry; taste deferred

VIII: Gross hearing intact; Weber: no lateralization; Rinne: AC > BC; no nystagmus

IX and X: Intact gag reflex, uvula midline; taste deferred

XI: Sternocleidomastoid and trapezius muscles strong and = bilaterally

XII: Tongue midline, speech clear

Motor
1. Size: = bilaterally
2. Tone: firm and supple bilaterally
3. Strength: RUE 5/5, LUE 5/5, RLE 5/5, LLE 5/5
4. Involuntary movements: none
5. Pronator drift: none

Cerebellar Function
1. Coordination
   a. Finger to nose: intact bilaterally c̄ eyes open and closed
   b. Rapid alternating movements: rapid supination and pronation of the hands: intact bilaterally; heel slide: intact bilaterally
2. Station: posture erect
3. Gait: steady
   a. Tiptoes and heel walking: intact
   b. Heel to toe in a straight line: intact
   c. Hopping on one leg: intact bilaterally

continues

CASE STUDY (Continued)

The Patient with a Potential Stroke

Reflexes

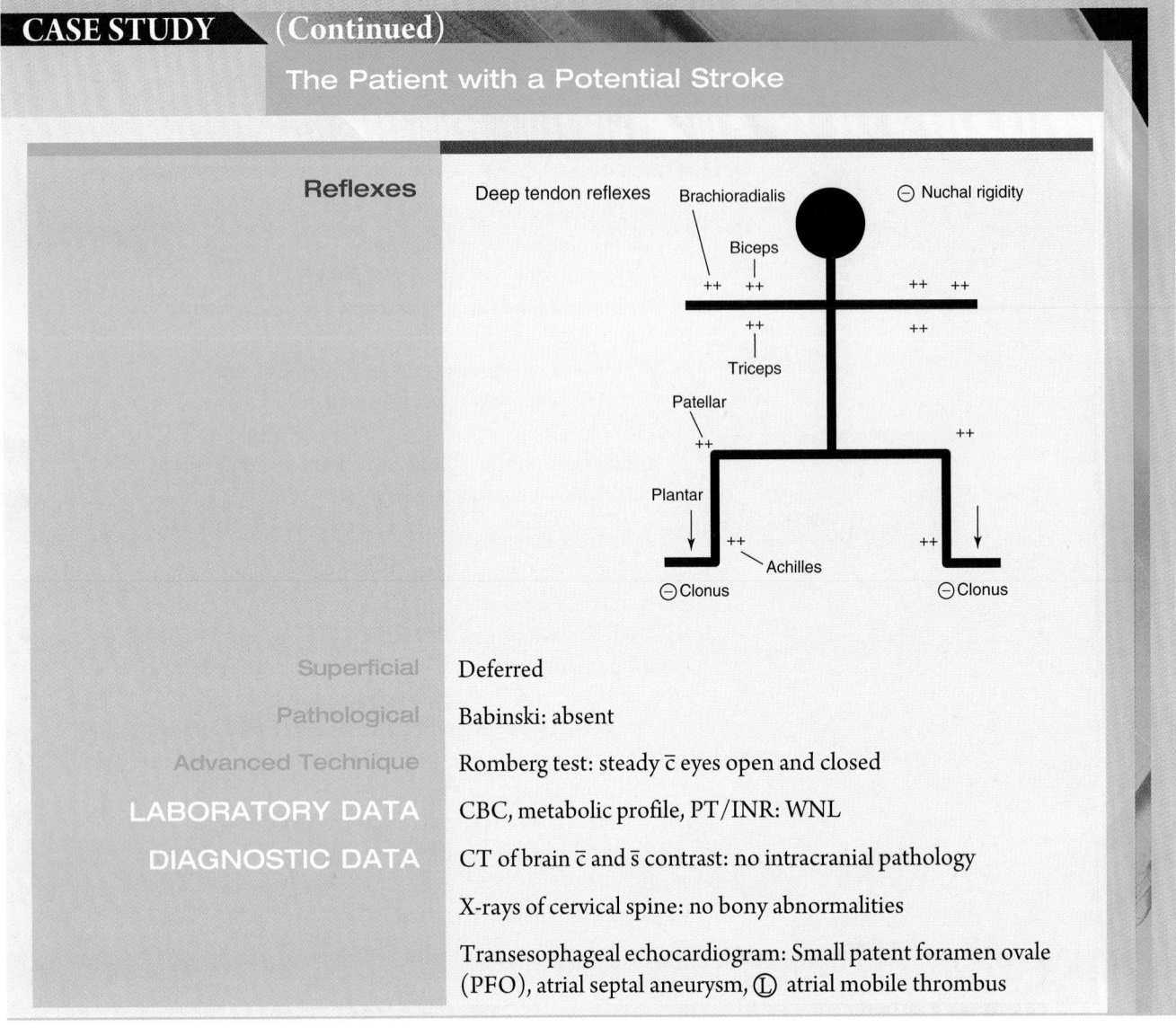

Deep tendon reflexes

Superficial	Deferred
Pathological	Babinski: absent
Advanced Technique	Romberg test: steady c̄ eyes open and closed
LABORATORY DATA	CBC, metabolic profile, PT/INR: WNL
DIAGNOSTIC DATA	CT of brain c̄ and s̄ contrast: no intracranial pathology
	X-rays of cervical spine: no bony abnormalities
	Transesophageal echocardiogram: Small patent foramen ovale (PFO), atrial septal aneurysm, Ⓛ atrial mobile thrombus

ASSESSMENT IN BRIEF

Mental Status Assessment and Neurological Techniques

Mental Status Assessment

- Physical appearance and behavior
  - Posture and movements
  - Dress, grooming, and personal hygiene
  - Facial expression
  - Affect
- Communication
- Level of consciousness
- Cognitive abilities and mentation
  - Attention
  - Memory

- Judgment
- Insight
- Spatial perception
- Calculation
- Abstract reasoning
- Thought process and content
- Suicidal ideation

Sensory Assessment

- Exteroceptive sensation
  - Light touch

continues

ASSESSMENT IN BRIEF *Continued*

- – Superficial pain
- – Temperature
- Proprioceptive sensation
  - – Motion and position
  - – Vibration sense
- Cortical sensation
  - – Stereognosis
  - – Graphesthesia
  - – Two-point discrimination
  - – Extinction

Cranial Nerves Assessment
- Olfactory nerve (CN I)
- Optic nerve (CN II)
  - – Visual acuity
  - – Visual fields
  - – Funduscopic examination
- Oculomotor nerve (CN III)
  - – Cardinal fields of gaze
  - – Eyelid elevation
  - – Pupil reactions
- Trochlear nerve (CN IV)
  - – Cardinal fields of gaze
- Trigeminal nerve (CN V)
  - – Motor component
  - – Sensory component
- Abducens nerve (CN VI)
  - – Cardinal fields of gaze
- Facial nerve (CN VII)
  - – Motor component
  - – Sensory component
- Acoustic nerve (CN VIII)
  - – Cochlear division
    - Hearing
    - Weber test
    - Rinne test
  - – Vestibular division
- Glossopharyngeal nerve (CN IX)
- Vagus nerve (CN X)

- Spinal accessory nerve (CN XI)
- Hypoglossal nerve (CN XII)

Motor System Assessment
- Muscle size
- Muscle tone
- Muscle strength
- Involuntary movements
- Pronator drift

Cerebellar Function
- Coordination
- Station
- Gait

Reflexes
- Deep tendon reflexes
  - – Brachioradialis
  - – Biceps
  - – Triceps
  - – Patellar
  - – Achilles
- Superficial reflexes
  - – Abdominal
  - – Plantar
  - – Cremasteric
  - – Bulbocavernosus
- Pathological reflexes
  - – Glabellar
  - – Clonus
  - – Babinski

Advanced Techniques
- Doll's eyes phenomenon
- Romberg test
- Meningeal irritation
  - – Nuchal rigidity
  - – Kernig's sign
  - – Brudzinski's sign

REVIEW QUESTIONS

1. Reflexes are conducted in the nervous system by:
   a. Motor efferent neurons
   b. Sensory afferent neurons
   c. Pyramidal tract
   d. Extrapyramidal tract
   The correct answer is (b).

2. When assessing your patient's mental status, you note that she is alert but cannot identify where she is. This indicates:
   a. Flat affect
   b. Aphasia
   c. Altered level of consciousness
   d. Acute confusion
   The correct answer is (d).

3. You are conducting a cranial nerve assessment on a new patient. She cannot feel vibration of the tuning fork when the Weber test is performed. She exhibits a deficit of which cranial nerve?
   a. II   c. VI
   b. III   d. VIII
   The correct answer is (d).

4. The unit admits a 20-year-old male who fell off his bike, hitting his head on the sidewalk. His neurological assessment reveals opening his eyes to speech, inaccurate perception of time and place, and localization of pain. With these findings, this patient's Glasgow Coma Scale score would be:
   a. 15   c. 10
   b. 12   d. 11
   The correct answer is (b).

5. The son of your 80-year-old female patient expresses concern about his mother's cognitive mental status. You tell the patient a list of three items and have the patient repeat them to check initial understanding. By having the patient repeat the three items after 5 minutes pass, you are assessing what cognitive function?
   a. Judgment   c. Memory
   b. Attention   d. Abstract reasoning
   The correct answer is (c).

6. Your 30-year-old male patient reports difficulty maintaining balance and coordination for the past 3 weeks. He denies headache, blurred vision, or change in level of consciousness. You perform a Romberg Test to assess cerebellar function. Your patient should:
   a. Maintain balance if standing with feet together with eyes open and closed
   b. Maintain balance if sitting with eyes closed
   c. Maintain balance if standing with feet separated and eyes closed

   d. Maintain balance if sitting with eyes open
   The correct answer is (a).

7. You are assessing exteroceptive sensation in your patient. When the patient's hand is stroked with a wisp of cotton, the patient reports a burning sensation in the area tested. This is an example of:
   a. Hypesthesia   c. Paresthesia
   b. Hyperalgesia   d. Dysesthesia
   The correct answer is (d).

8. CN III is assessed to verify intact function of the vestibular and oculomotor pathways. You are asked to check your ICU patient for doll's eyes phenomenon. Normal findings reveal:
   a. Eyes deviate in the opposite direction of lateral or vertical head rotation
   b. Pupils are fixed and dilated
   c. Eyes appear painted on, and remain midline with head rotation
   d. Nystagmus develops with repeated testing
   The correct answer is (a).

9. Sitting relaxed and facing you, have your patient perform the following sequence of activities: With arms outstretched, alternately bring in each hand and touch the tip of each index finger to his nose. Next, have the patient rapidly alternate patting his knees with the palmar, then the dorsal aspects of his hands. Finally, have the patient rapidly extend and tap his foot. Which component of the neurological exam are you assessing?
   a. Sensory function   c. Cranial nerves
   b. Cerebellar function   d. Mental status
   The correct answer is (b).

10. Patients with Parkinson's disease will often exhibit a positive glabellar reflex. This is characterized by:
    a. Flexion and supination of the forearm when the brachioradialis tendon is struck with a reflex hammer
    b. Ataxia/unsteadiness when feet are together, arms down at the side, eyes closed
    c. Hyperactive blinking reflex when tapped between the eyebrows
    d. Plantar flexion of toes with stimulation to the lateral dorsal foot
    The correct answer is (c).

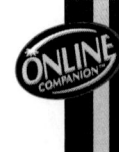

BIBLIOGRAPHY

American Psychiatric Association. (2000). *Diagnostic and statistical manual of mental disorders (4th ed.). Text Revision*. Washington, DC: Author.

Dodick, D. W., & Gladstone, J. P. (2005). An evidence-based and experience-based approach to acute migraine treatment. *Excellence in Migraine Management, 1*(2), 4–10, 15.

French, M. (2006). Assessing pain from diabetic neuropathy. *The Clinical Advisor, 9*(4), 51.

Goldberg, R. J. (2007). *Practical guide to the psychiatric patient* (33rd ed.). St. Louis: Mosby.

Goroll, A. H., & Mulley, A. G. (2006). *Primary care medicine* (5th ed.). Philadelphia: Lippincott Williams, & Wilkins.

Henry, G. L., Little, N., Jagoda, A., & Pelligrino, T. R. (2003). *Neurological emergencies: A symptom-oriented approach*. New York: McGraw-Hill.

Hickey, J. V. (Ed.). (2008). *The clinical practice of neurological and neurosurgical nursing* (6th ed.). Philadelphia: Lippincott Williams, & Wilkins.

Kasper, D. L., Braunwald, E., Hauser, S. L., Longo, D. L., Jameson, J. L., & Fauci, A. S. (2008). *Harrison's principles of internal medicine* (17th ed.). New York: McGraw-Hill.

Lehman, C. A., Hayes, J. M., LaCroix, M., Owen, S. V., & Nauta, H. J. (2003). Development and implementation of a problem-focused neurological assessment system. *Journal of Neuroscience Nursing, 35*(4), 185–192.

Martins, D. A. (2007). Burning pain that's too heavy for a weight lifter. *Consultant, 47*(11), 965.

McPhee, S. J., Papadakis, M. A., & Tierney, L. M. (2006). *Current medical diagnosis and treatment* (46th ed.). New York: McGraw-Hill.

Poss, J. P. (2005). Mindfulness-based stress reduction. *Applications for Nurse Practitioners, 9*(7/8), 9–18.

Rauen, C. A., Vollman, K., Arbour, R. B., & Chulay, M. (2008). Challenging nursing's sacred cows. *American Nurse Today, 3*(4), 24–26.

Romanoff, M. R. (2006). Assessing military veterans for post-traumatic stress disorder: A guide for primary care clinicians. *Journal of the American Academy of Nurse Practitioners, 18*(9), 409–413.

Ropper, A. H., Gress, D. R., Diringer, M. N., Green, D. M., Mayer, S. A., & Bleck, T. P. (2004). *Neurological and neurosurgical intensive care* (4th ed.). Philadelphia: Lippincott Williams, & Wilkins.

Roth, B. (2006). Meningococcal meningitis. *Advance for Nurse Practitioners, 14*(10), 88–89.

Sultan, L. L. (2007). Brain injury: A primary-care perspective. *The Clinical Advisor, 10*(7), 84–88.

Wijdicks, E. F. M. (2004). *Catastrophic neurological disorders in the emergency department* (2nd ed.). Washington, DC: American Psychiatric Association.

Wright, W. L. (2008). Assessing functional impairment during and between migraine attacks. *The Journal for Nurse Practitioners, 4*(3), 201–207.

Zagaria, M. A. E. (2008). Relapsing-remitting multiple sclerosis: Primary and symptomatic management. *The American Journal for Nurse Practitioners, 12*(4), 22–26.

WEB SITES

Alzheimer's Association:
http://www.alz.org

Alzheimer's Foundation of America:
http://www.alzfdn.org

American Stroke Foundation:
http://www.americanstroke.org

Brain Trauma Foundation:
http://www.braintrauma.org

The Internet Stroke Center at Washington University in St. Louis [Missouri]:
http://www.strokecenter.org

Mayo Clinic:
http://www.mayoclinic.com

MS ActiveSource:
http://www.msactivesource.com

National Multiple Sclerosis Society:
http://www.nationalmssociety.org

National Stroke Association:
http://www.stroke.org

Psychiatry 24 × 7.com:
http://www.dementia.com

CHAPTER 20
Female Genitalia

COMPETENCIES

1. Describe the anatomy and physiology of the female genitalia, including age-relevant transformations.

2. Demonstrate the techniques necessary for assessment of the female genitalia, including patient positioning, external and internal inspection, speculum procedures, and palpation methods.

3. Identify anatomic landmarks during bimanual vaginal, uterine, and rectovaginal examinations.

4. Identify normal findings as well as atypical findings of the vulva, vagina, cervix, uterus, and adnexa.

5. Describe procedures for genital and anal smears and cultures.

Assessment of the genitalia is often the last phase of a woman's physical assessment. Deaths attributed to uterine and cervical cancers have declined by more than 50% since the 1960s. This decline in morbidity and mortality rates can be attributed to early detection by physical assessment and Papanicolaou Test (Pap smears) and, to a lesser extent, increased patient knowledge of routine screening techniques. However, previous experiences of painful or embarrassing examinations may contribute to a patient's apprehension of the assessment process. By using a few commonsense techniques to diminish patient discomfort and by empowering the patient through education and participation in the assessment process, you can encourage the patient in the management of her own health care. The female reproductive system is an area in which you can have a major impact on patient health through routine screening, education, and integrating the patient in the process of self-care.

ANATOMY AND PHYSIOLOGY

EXTERNAL FEMALE GENITALIA

The components of the external female genitalia are collectively referred to as the vulva. They consist of the mons pubis, labia majora, labia minora, clitoris, vulval vestibule and its glands, urethral meatus, and vaginal introitus (Figure 20-1).

The **mons pubis** is a pad of subcutaneous fatty tissue lying over the anterior symphysis pubis. At puberty, a characteristic triangular pattern of coarse, curly hair known as **escutcheon** develops over the mons pubis. The function of the mons pubis is to protect the pelvic bones, especially during coitus.

The **labia majora** are two longitudinal folds of adipose and connective tissue. They extend from the clitoris anteriorly and gradually narrow to merge and form the posterior commissure of the perineum. The outer surface of the labia

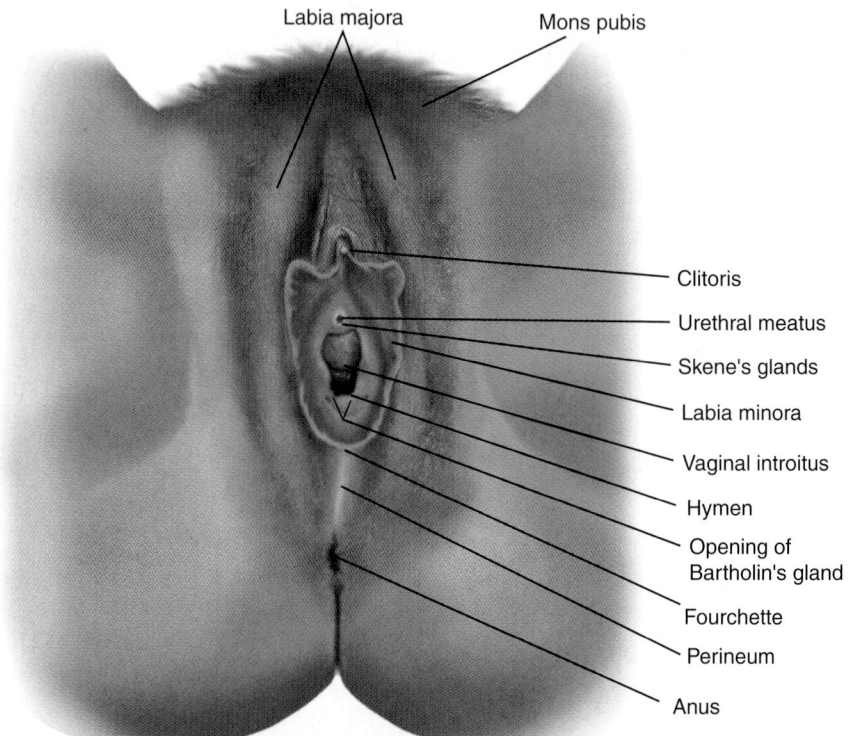

FIGURE 20-1 External Female Genitalia

majora becomes pigmented, wrinkled, and hairy at puberty. The inner surface is smoother, softer, and contains sebaceous glands. The function of the labia majora is to protect the vulva components that it surrounds.

Tucked within the labia majora are the **labia minora**, which enclose the vestibule. They are two thin folds of skin that extend to form the prepuce, or hood, of the clitoris anteriorly and a transverse fold of skin forming the **fourchette**, or frenulum, posteriorly. The labia minora contain sebaceous glands, erectile tissue, blood vessels, and involuntary muscle tissue but no adipose tissue or hair follicles. The secretions of the sebaceous glands are bactericidal and aid in lubricating the vulval skin and protecting the skin from urine. Both the labia majora and the labia minora contain genital corpuscles that transmit erotic sensation.

The **clitoris** is a cylinder-shaped erectile body approximately 2.5 cm (1 inch) in length and 0.5 cm (¼ inch) in diameter, but normally less than 2.0 (¾ inch) cm of the body is visible on inspection. It is located at the superior aspect of the vulva and between the labia minora. The clitoris contains erectile tissue and has a significant supply of nerve endings.

The **vestibule** is the area between the two skin folds of the labia minora. The vestibule is a boat-shaped area that contains the urethral meatus, openings of the Skene's glands, hymen, openings of the Bartholin's glands, and vaginal introitus.

The external urethral meatus is located in the superior aspect of the vestibule, approximately 2.5 cm (1 inch) inferior to the clitoris. It is characterized as an elongated dimple or slit. Surrounding the urethral meatus are **Skene's glands**, also known as paraurethral glands, which provide lubrication to protect the skin. These tiny glands open in a posterolateral position to the urethral meatus, but they are not readily visible.

The **vaginal introitus** or orifice is situated at the inferior aspect of the vulval vestibule and is the entrance to the vagina. The size and shape of the vaginal introitus may vary. Surrounding the vaginal introitus is the **hymen**, an avascular, thin fold of connective tissue. It may be annular or crescentic in shape. The hymen may be broken by first-time sexual intercourse, strenuous physical activity, the use of tampons, masturbation, or menstruation, or it may be congenitally absent. Once the hymenal ring is perforated, small, irregular tags of tissue may be visible at the vaginal opening.

In the cleft between the labia minora and the hymenal ring lie the **Bartholin's glands**, also known as the greater vestibular glands. Bartholin's glands are small, pea-shaped glands located deep in the perineal structures. The ductal openings are not usually visible. The glands secrete a clear, viscid, odorless, alkaline mucus that improves the viability and motility of sperm along the female reproductive tract.

The **perineum** is located between the fourchette and the anus. Its composition of muscle, elastic fibers, fascia, and connective tissue gives it an exceptional capacity for stretching during childbirth. The **anal orifice** is located at the seam of the gluteal folds, and it serves as the exit to the gastrointestinal tract.

INTERNAL FEMALE GENITALIA

The components of the internal female genitalia are the vagina, uterus, fallopian tubes, and ovaries (see Figure 20-2).

The **vagina** is a pink, hollow, muscular tube extending from the cervix to the vulva. It is located posterior to the bladder and anterior to the rectum, and it slopes backward at an angle of approximately 45° with the vertical plane of the body. The cervix projects into the vagina. This projection creates pouch-like recesses around the cervix. These recesses are divided into anterior, posterior, and lateral **fornices**. Abdominal organs such as the uterus, ovaries, appendix, cecum, colon, ureters, and distended bladder can be palpated through the thin walls of these fornices.

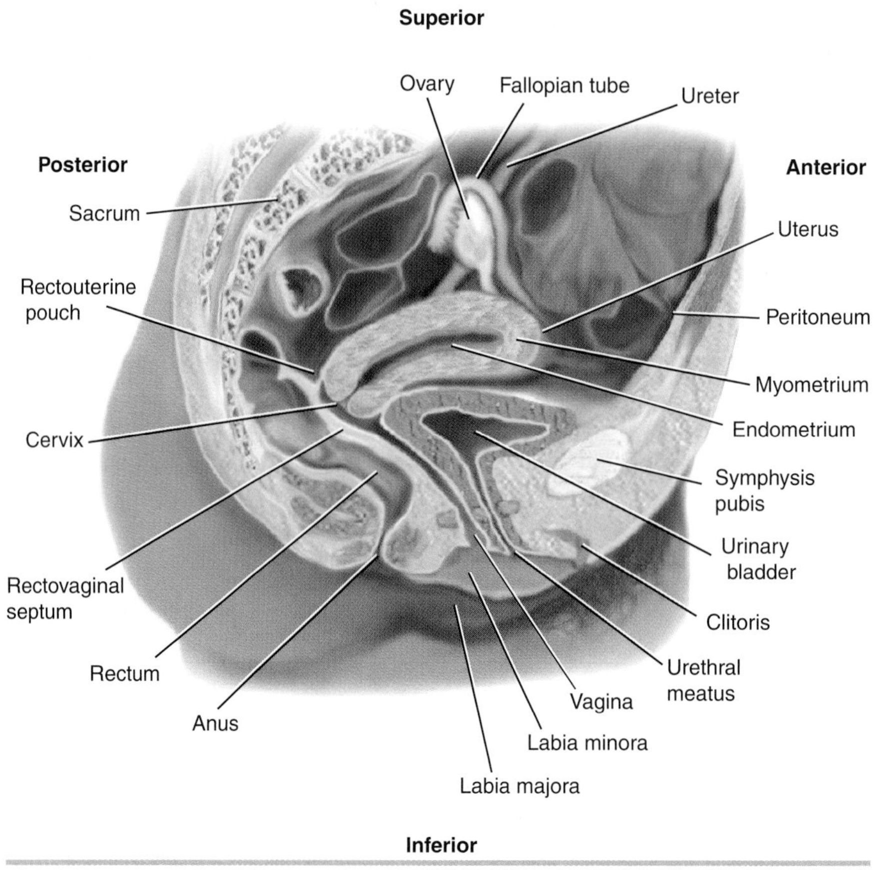

FIGURE 20-2 Left-Sided Sagittal Section at Midline of Internal Pelvic Organs

The vaginal walls consist of an outer layer of longitudinal and circular muscle fibers and a stratified squamous epithelium arranged in folds called rugae. Lactic acid is formed by the normal vaginal flora in conjunction with glycogen, which is contained in the superficial cells of the vagina. This maintains the vaginal pH and assists in the prevention of vaginal infections.

The **uterus** is an inverted, pear-shaped, hollow, muscular organ in which an impregnated ovum develops into a fetus. The inferior aspect is the **cervix**; the superior aspect is the **fundus**. The most common position of the uterus is anteverted, but it may also be anteflexed, retroverted, retroflexed, or in midplane position (see Figure 20-3). The mature, nonpregnant uterus weighs about 60 gm and is approximately 5.5 to 8.0 cm (2¼ –3¼ inches) long, 3.5 to 4.0 cm (1⅜–1⅝ inches) wide, and 2.0 to 2.5 cm (¾–1 inch) thick. The uterus of a parous patient, or one who has given birth, may be enlarged by 2 to 3 cm (¾–1¼ inches) in any of the above dimensions.

Anatomically, the uterus can be divided into three parts: the body, the isthmus, and the cervix (see Figure 20-4). The body consists of the fundus, a raised, dome-shaped area on the superior portion of the uterus, and the cornu, the points of insertion of the fallopian tubes. The uterine body has three layers: an outer layer of peritoneum; a middle layer of muscle, called the myometrium; and an inner layer of columnar epithelium, mucous glands, and stroma, called the endometrium. It is this innermost layer that is shed and regenerated under normal hormonal influence during the menstrual cycle. The outer layer of the peritoneum forms a deep recess called the **rectouterine pouch**, or pouch of Douglas. It is the lowest point in the pelvic cavity and encompasses the lower posterior wall of the uterus, the upper portion of the vagina, and the intestinal surface of the rectum.

The **isthmus** is a constricted area between the body of the uterus and the cervix. The cervix is an open-ended canal approximately 2 to 3 cm (¾ –1¼ inches) in length and diameter. Its internal os (opening) is at the isthmus and its external os extends into the vagina. The os of the **nulliparous** woman, one who has not given birth, will be closed and tight. The os of a **parous** woman, one who has given birth to one or more neonates, may be open by 1 cm (⅜ inch) and the orifice may be elongated and irregular. The endocervical canal is lined with mucus-secreting columnar epithelium. The ectocervix, which protrudes into the vagina, is covered with the same squamous epithelial cells that line the vagina. The point at which the two types of cells merge is the **squamocolumnar junction**. Its exact location varies with age but is clinically important because it is the point at which most cervical cancer originates.

The **adnexa** of the uterus consists of the fallopian tubes, the ovaries, and their supporting ligaments. The **fallopian tubes** extend from the cornu of the uterus to the ovaries and are supported by the broad ligaments. The tubes are approximately 8 to 14 cm (3¼–5½ inches) long. The distal, funnel-shaped end of the fallopian tube is called the infundibulum. It has moving, fingerlike projections called fimbriae, which help direct ova from the ovary into the tube, where fertilization takes place. The fallopian tubes are lined with ciliated squamous epithelium. The movement of the cilia and the peristaltic waves of the muscular layer of the tube propel the ovum toward the uterus, where implantation occurs.

The **ovaries** are a pair of almond-shaped glands, approximately 3 to 4 cm (1¼ –1⅝ inches) in length, in the upper pelvic cavity. **Oogenesis**, the development and formation of an ovum, and hormonal production are the ovaries' principal functions. The rectovaginal septum separates the rectum from the posterior aspect of the vagina.

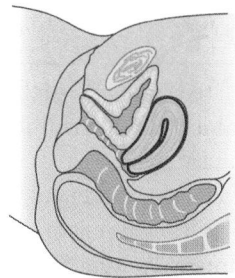

Anteverted
(most common)

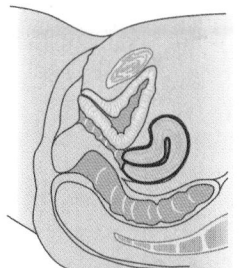

Anteflexed

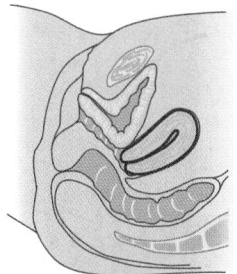

Midposition
(midplane)

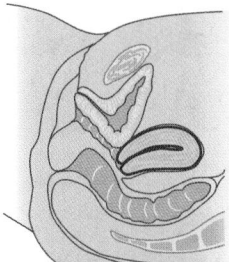

Retroverted
(palpable only during
rectovaginal exam)

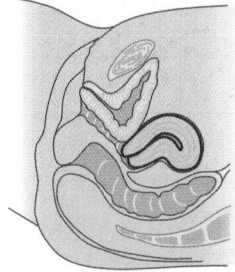

Retroflexed
(palpable only during
rectovaginal exam)

FIGURE 20-3 Positions of the Uterus

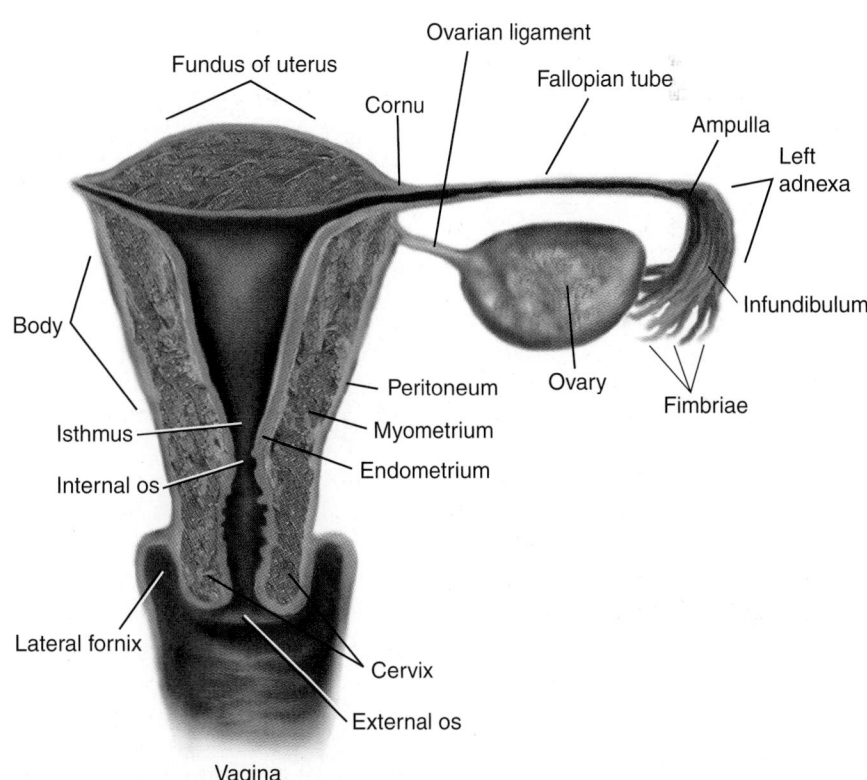

FIGURE 20-4 Coronal Section of Uterus and Adnexal Structures

THE FEMALE REPRODUCTIVE CYCLE

The female reproductive cycle consists of two interrelated cycles called the ovarian and the menstrual cycles. These cycles occur synchronously under neurohormonal control from the hypothalamus and the anterior pituitary gland.

The ovarian cycle consists of two phases: the follicular phase and the luteal phase. During the follicular phase, the actions of the follicle-stimulating hormone (FSH) and the luteinizing hormone (LH) from the anterior pituitary gland stimulate the ripening of one ovarian follicle called the graafian follicle. The remaining follicles are suppressed by LH. Ovulation occurs when high levels of LH cause the release of the ovum from the graafian follicle. During the luteal phase, LH stimulates the development of the corpus luteum. This yellow pigment that fills the

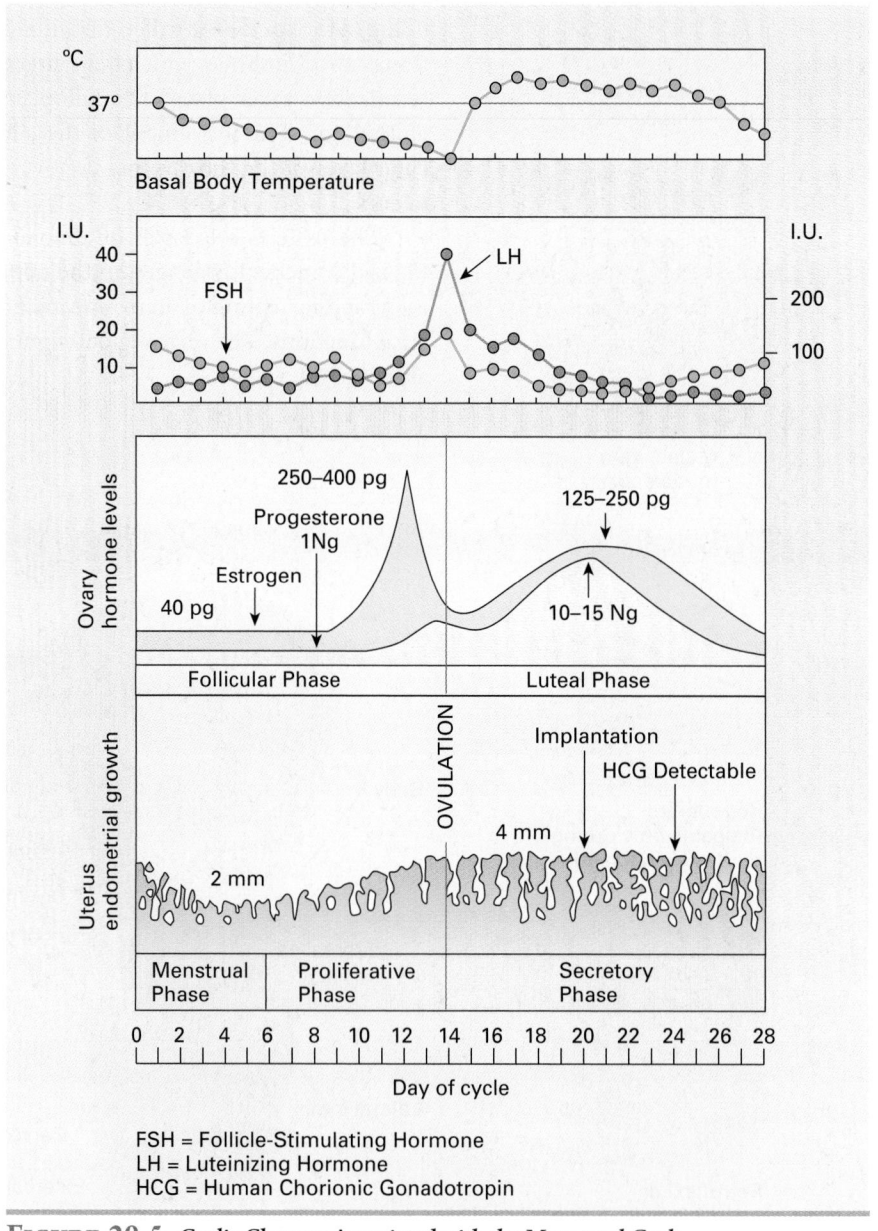

FSH = Follicle-Stimulating Hormone
LH = Luteinizing Hormone
HCG = Human Chorionic Gonadotropin

FIGURE 20-5 **Cyclic Changes Associated with the Menstrual Cycle**

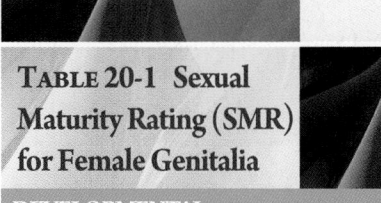

TABLE 20-1 Sexual Maturity Rating (SMR) for Female Genitalia

DEVELOPMENTAL STAGE	DESCRIPTION
Stage 1 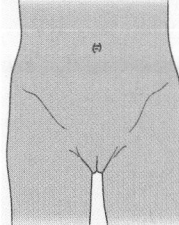	**Preadolescent Stage** (before age 8) No pubic hair, only body hair (vellus hair)
Stage 2 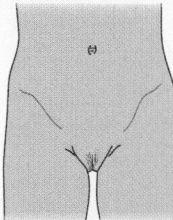	**Early Adolescent Stage** (ages 8 to 12) Sparse growth of long, slightly dark, fine pubic hair, slightly curly and located along the labia
Stage 3 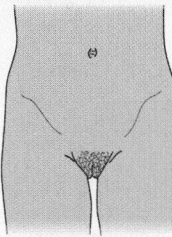	**Adolescent Stage** (ages 12 to 13) Pubic hair becomes darker, curlier, and spreads over the symphysis
Stage 4 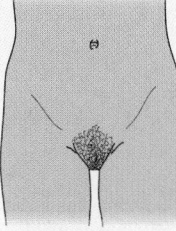	**Late Adolescent Stage** (ages 13 to 15) Texture and curl of pubic hair is similar to that of an adult but not spread to thighs
Stage 5 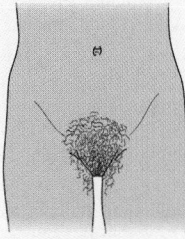	**Adult Stage** Adult appearance in quality and quantity of pubic hair; growth is spread to inner aspect of thighs and abdomen

graafian follicle produces high levels of progesterone and low levels of estrogen. The basal body temperature rises, indicating that ovulation has occurred.

The menstrual cycle begins if implantation does not occur. The corpus luteum degenerates and the levels of progesterone and estrogen decrease, causing the endometrium to degenerate and shed. The menstrual flow lasts from 2 to 7 days and the cycles continue every 25 to 34 days, with the average being 28 days. The first day of the cycle is the first day of menstruation. The menstrual flow consists of blood and mucus and normally does not exceed 150 mL. Menstrual blood lacks fibrin; therefore, it does not clot. If clots do occur, they usually form in the vagina and are a combination of red blood cells, glycoproteins, and mucus. Cyclic changes associated with the menstrual cycle are shown in Figure 20-5.

The proliferative phase of the menstrual cycle occurs when the endometrial lining begins to regenerate under the influence of estrogen. Changes in the cervical mucosa also occur during this phase. The cervical mucus becomes clearer, thinner, and threadlike.

If conception and implantation of the fertilized ovum occur, the corpus luteum is maintained by the presence of human chorionic gonadotropin (HCG), which is secreted by the implanting blastocyst. HCG is the hormone tested in at-home pregnancy kits.

The female reproductive cycle begins at **menarche**, the onset of menstruation, which occurs between 9 and 16 years of age, and ends at menopause, which occurs between 45 and 55 years of age. The onset of puberty, which occurs between the ages of 8 and 9, is marked by significant increases in estrogen production and the development of secondary sex characteristics such as breast enlargement, hair distribution on the mons pubis, and contour changes of the hips and abdomen. Tanner's stages of pubic hair development provide objective criteria for the evaluation of developmental changes in the appearance of female genitalia (Table 20-1).

NURSING**TIP**

Patient Education on the Reproductive Cycle

Educating the patient about the reproductive cycle and its effects on the body will help the patient to better understand her own body's functioning and will assist her in planning for gynecological examinations and birth control measures. The cervical mucus becomes clearer, thinner, and threadlike, indicating the onset of ovulation. The patient can perform her own **spinnbarkeit** test, the point at which the mucus can be drawn to a maximal length, by stretching vaginal mucus between her thumb and index finger. Tell the patient it is normal to feel low abdominal or flank pain when the ovum is released during ovulation. Rise in basal body temperature indicates that ovulation has occurred. Spotting may also be present after ovulation.

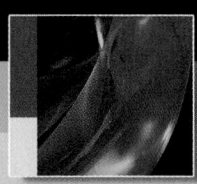

HEALTH HISTORY

The female genitalia health history provides insight into the link between a patient's life and lifestyle and female genitalia information and pathology.

PATIENT PROFILE

Diseases that are age- and race-specific for the female genitalia are listed.

Age

Sexually transmitted diseases (STDs), also referred to as sexually transmitted infections (STIs) (increased incidence 15–25)

Uterine myomas (30–50)

Cervical cancer (40–60)

Vulval cancer (postmenopause)

Uterine prolapse (postmenopause)

Cystocele (postmenopause)

Rectocele (postmenopause)

Atrophic vaginitis (postmenopause)

Endometrial cancer (diagnosis is usually made between 55 and 69)

Vaginal cancer (over 60)

Ovarian cancer (risk increases with age; highest rates are between 65 and 84)

Race

Fibroids are more common in African Americans.

Ethnicity (Female genital mutilation, or cutting, is still practiced in some African nations.)

CHIEF COMPLAINT

Common chief complaints for the female genitalia are defined and information on the characteristics of each sign or symptom is provided.

1. Uterine Bleeding

The presence of bleeding from the endometrium

Quality

Odor, consistency, color, clotting

Quantity

Amount (number and size of tampons or pads used in 24 hours), duration and frequency of flow

Associated Manifestations

Abdominal pain or cramping, passage of clots or tissue

Aggravating Factors

Stress, anxiety, medications (aspirin, NSAIDs), rapid weight loss or gain, obesity, sexual intercourse

Alleviating Factors

Medication, dilatation and curettage, surgery

Setting

Traumatic abortion or dilatation and curettage

Timing

Relationship to menses (intermenstrual, oligomenorrhea, polymenorrhea, menometrorrhagia, metrorrhagia); use of intrauterine device (IUD); perimenopausal

2. Vaginal Discharge

The presence of a leaky discharge of fluid from the vagina

Quality

Color, consistency, odor

Quantity

Number and size of tampons or pads used in 24 hours

Associated Manifestations

Itching, presence of discharge in sexual partner, **dyspareunia** (painful sexual intercourse), dysuria, abdominal pain or cramping, spotting

Aggravating Factors

Tight pants, wet bathing suits, antibiotics, birth control pills, diet, pregnancy, deodorant tampons, bubble bath, chemical douches, lubricated condoms, contraceptive creams, preexisting disease such as diabetes mellitus, increased number of sexual partners, semen, vaginal films, latex products

continues

Health History (continued)	
Alleviating Factors	Position, loose-fitting pants, cotton underpants and pantyhose with cotton crotch, medication
Timing	Postcoitus, while taking antibiotics
3. Urinary Symptoms	Changes in the normal voiding pattern and in characteristics of the urine
Quality	Color: straw, amber; microscopic or macroscopic hematuria; consistency: clear, cloudy; presence of particles; odor
Quantity	Polyuria, oliguria or anuria
Associated Manifestations	Flank pain, abdominal pain or cramping, dysuria, abdominal distention, vaginal discharge, urgency and frequency in voiding, stress incontinence, pneumaturia, fever
Aggravating Factors	Douches, intravaginal devices, traumatic coitus, alcohol, caffeine, spices, delaying urination
Alleviating Factors	Medication, warm baths, hydration
Setting	Postcoitus, nocturia
Timing	At beginning, throughout, or end of stream
4. Pelvic Pain	The subjective sense of discomfort in the pelvis
Quality	Stabbing, burning, cramping, aching, throbbing, drawing, pulling
Associated Manifestations	Abdominal distension, pelvic fullness, vaginal discharge or bleeding, gastrointestinal symptoms, menstruation, fever, ectopic pregnancy, pelvic inflammatory disease (PID)
Aggravating Factors	Exercise, sexual activity, cultural perception
Alleviating Factors	Rest, medication, surgery, heating pad, NSAIDs
Setting	During coitus, ovulation
Timing	Sudden or gradual onset, association with activity, duration, recurrence, relation to menstrual cycle
PAST HEALTH HISTORY	*The various components of the past health history are linked to female genitalia pathology and female genitalia-related information.*
Medical History	
Female Genitalia Specific	See Table 20-2.
Nonfemale Genitalia Specific	Diabetes mellitus, thyroid disease, incontinence, constipation, urinary tract infections
Surgical History	Hysterectomy, myomectomy, salpingectomy, oophorectomy, dilatation and curettage, laparoscopy, vulvectomy, tubal ligation, colpotomy, cesarean section, colposcopy, cryotherapy, uterine cryoablation, hysteroscopy
Allergies	Numerous feminine hygiene products may cause allergic reactions or increase the incidence of *Candida* vaginosis. Be aware of any latex allergies; condoms and diaphragms are usually made of latex. The spermicide nonoxynol 9 may also cause allergic reactions.
Medications	Antibiotics may increase incidence of *Candida* vaginosis and lessen the effectiveness of oral contraceptives

continues

Health History (continued)

Communicable Diseases	STD: gonorrhea, syphilis, herpes, HIV/AIDS, hepatitis, *Chlamydia*, human papillomavirus, hepatitis B and C, trichomoniasis, chancroid, molluscum contagiosum
Injuries and Accidents	Abdominal trauma, rape, sexual abuse, vaginal trauma or injuries, pelvic fractures, lumbar spine, sacrococcygeal injuries
Special Needs	Paraplegic and quadriplegic patients are at increased obstetric risk depending on level of injury, tone of uterus, and competency of cervix.
Childhood Illnesses	Fetal diethylstilbestrol (DES) exposure
Immunizations	Gardasil
FAMILY HEALTH HISTORY	*Female genitalia diseases that are familial are listed.* Cancers of the reproductive organs, mother received DES while pregnant with patient, transfer of STDs during delivery, placental transfer of hepatitis B and hepatitis C, HIV/AIDS, multiple pregnancies, congenital anomalies
SOCIAL HISTORY	*The components of the social history are linked to female genitalia factors and pathology.*
Alcohol Use	There is a significant positive correlation between alcohol use and date rape in the college-aged population.
Tobacco Use	There is an increased incidence of strokes and thrombotic events in women who concurrently smoke and use hormonal therapy. Smoking is a risk factor for cervical cancer.
Sexual Practice	Often, sexual favors are exchanged for narcotics, leading to increased rates of STDs. Prostitution increases the risk of STDs, HIV/AIDS, hepatitis, and cervical carcinoma (an increase in the number of partners increases the risk of human papillomavirus, which can lead to dysplasia and possible cervical cancer).
Home Environment	Poor sanitation may lead to numerous forms of vaginitis and infections; overcrowding is an ideal condition for mite infestation.
Hobbies and Leisure Activities	Wearing wet bathing suits for extended periods of time may increase the likelihood of *Candida* vaginosis. Strenuous equestrian sports and off-road cycling increase the likelihood of external genitalia trauma from saddle injuries. Female athletes may suffer from **amenorrhea** (absent menses).
Stress	Stress can have significant effects on menstruation, causing amenorrhea and exacerbating genital herpes simplex.
HEALTH MAINTENANCE ACTIVITIES	*This information provides a bridge between the health maintenance activities and female genitalia function.*
Sleep	Lack of sleep or extreme fatigue can lead to amenorrhea.
Diet	Increased levels of refined sugars, salt, and caffeine enhance PMS symptomology. Extreme dieting can affect menstruation and lead to amenorrhea. Elevated sugar and lactose can lead to vaginal candidiasis.
Exercise	Exercise may diminish **dysmenorrhea** (pain or cramping during menses) and **menorrhagia** (heavy menses).
Use of Safety Devices	Condom use
Health Check-ups	Date of last Pap smear and results, HPV status, and last STD screen

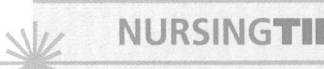

NURSING**TIP**

Late Onset of Menarche

Late onset of menarche can result from a multiplicity of pathologies. If you encounter a patient who has not experienced the onset of menstruation by 16 years of age or 14 years of age when secondary sex characteristics are present, this is called primary amenorrhea. Evaluate the patient for the following:

1. Pregnancy
2. Inadequate nutrition or eating disorders
3. Chronic diseases such as Crohn's disease, thyroid disease
4. Environmental stressors
5. Intensive athletic training
6. Use of opiates or steroids
7. Polycystic ovary syndrome
8. Autoimmune diseases
9. Anatomic obstruction to menstrual flow
10. Genetic or chromosomal syndromes
11. Hypothalamic-pituitary-ovarian axis disorders

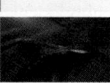

TABLE 20-2 Female Reproductive Health History

MENSTRUAL HISTORY

Age of menarche, last menstrual period (LMP), length of cycle, regularity of cycle, duration of menses, amenorrhea, menorrhagia, presence of clots or vaginal pooling, number and type of tampons or pads used during menses, dysmenorrhea, spotting between menses, missed menses.

REPRODUCTIVE MEDICAL HISTORY

Vaginal infections, yeast infections, salpingitis, endometritis, endometriosis, cervicitis, fibroids, ovarian cysts, cancer of the reproductive organs, infertility, Pap smear records.

OBSTETRIC HISTORY

See Chapter 23.

PREMENSTRUAL SYNDROME (PMS)

Symptoms occur from 3 to 7 days before the onset of menses, with cessation of symptoms after second day of cycle. Symptoms include: breast tenderness; bloating; moodiness; cravings for salt, sugar, or chocolate; fatigue; weight gain; headaches; joint pain; nausea and vomiting.

MENOPAUSE HISTORY

Menopause (cessation of menstruation), spotting, associated symptoms of menopause (such as hot flashes, palpitations, numbness, tingling, drenching sweats, mood swings, vaginal dryness, itching), treatment for symptoms (including estrogen replacement therapy), feelings about menopause.

VAGINAL DISCHARGE

See Chief Complaint section.

HISTORY OF UTERINE BLEEDING

See Chief Complaint section.

SEXUAL FUNCTIONING

Sexual preference, number of partners, interest, satisfaction, dyspareunia, inorgasmia.

METHOD OF BIRTH CONTROL

Type, frequency of use, methods to prevent STDs, any associated problems with birth control or STD-prevention methods, such as a reaction to the spermicides used with the vaginal sponges, diaphragms, and condoms.

NURSING**TIP**

Maintaining Gynecological Health

Encourage patients to adopt healthy gynecological practices:

1. Avoid douches and feminine hygiene sprays or films, or use sparingly because both products disrupt the natural vaginal flora and increase the vaginal pH.
2. Do not leave tampons in the vagina for longer than 8 hours at a time because of the increased risk of toxic shock syndrome.
3. Always wash and wipe the vaginal area from front to back to prevent contamination of the vagina and urethra with fecal material.
4. Thoroughly wash diaphragms, pessaries (device used to maintain the position of the uterus/bladder), and sexual aid devices before and after each use.
5. Void immediately after coitus.

EQUIPMENT

Assemble items before placing the patient on the examination table; materials should be arranged in order of use and within easy reach.

- Examination table with stirrups
- Stool, preferably mounted on wheels
- Large hand mirror
- Gooseneck lamp
- Clean gloves
- Linens for draping
- Vaginal specula (Figure 20-6):
  - Graves' bivalve specula, sizes medium and large, useful for most adult sexually active women
  - Pederson bivalve specula, sizes small and medium, useful for nonsexually active women, children, menopausal women
- Cytological materials (Figure 20-7):
  - Ayre spatulas
  - Cervical broom
  - Cytobrushes
  - Cotton-tipped applicators
  - Liquid-based preparation vials
  - Microscope slides, cover slips, culture probes labeled with the patient's name, identification number, and date specimen was collected
  - Cytology fixative spray
  - Reagents: normal saline solution, potassium hydroxide (KOH), acetic acid (white vinegar)
  - Thayer-Martin plate
- Warm water
- Water-soluble lubricant

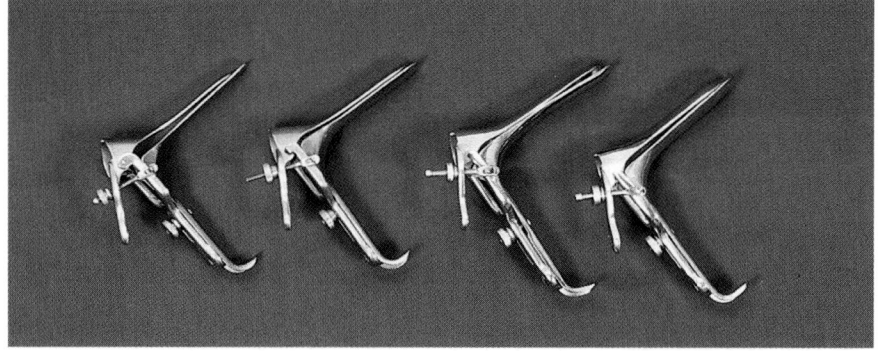

A. Lateral View

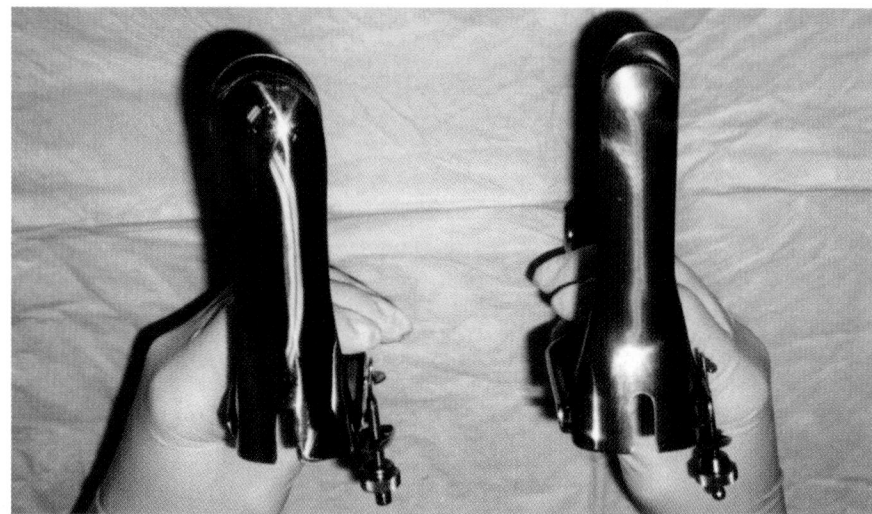

B. Superior View. Graves' Speculum (left), Pederson Speculum (right)

FIGURE 20-6 Vaginal Specula

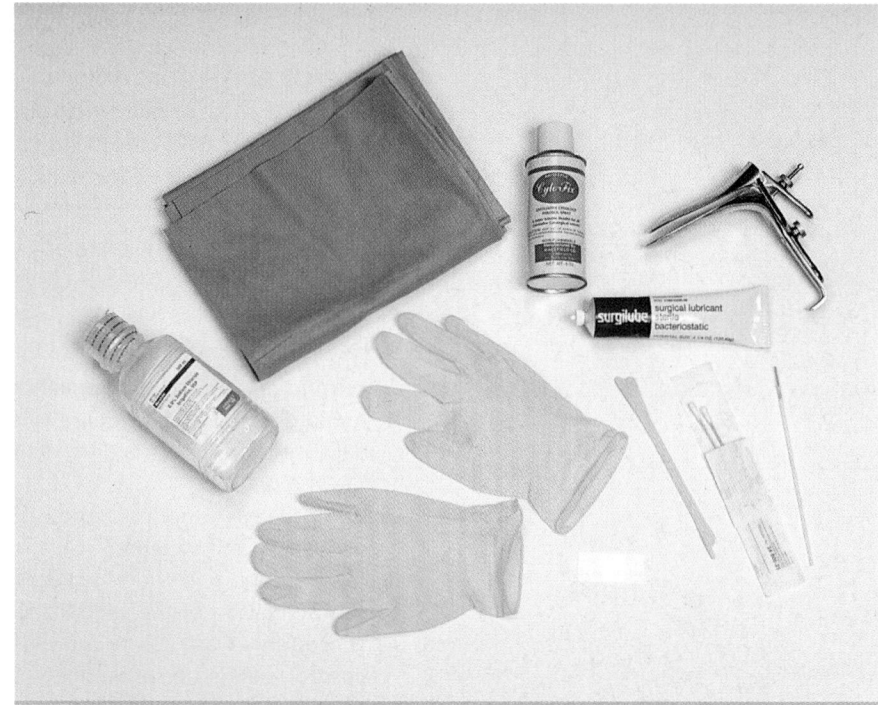

FIGURE 20-7 Cytological Materials Needed for Gynecological Examination

ASSESSMENT OF THE FEMALE GENITALIA

Assessment of the female reproductive system consists of inspection and palpation only, and includes assessment of the abdomen (see Chapter 17), inspection of the external genitalia, palpation of the external genitalia, speculum assessment of the internal genitalia, collection of specimens for laboratory analysis, inspection of the vaginal walls, bimanual examination, and rectovaginal assessment (see Chapter 22 for the complete rectal examination). The assessment process requires somewhat uncomfortable positioning for the patient; therefore, it should be completed as quickly and as efficiently as possible.

NURSING TIP

Preparing for a Gynecological Examination

If you are a beginning nurse or if you have not performed a gynecological examination:

- Ask another nurse to assist you with the first few examinations.
- Familiarize yourself with the equipment. Practice opening and closing the speculum. Plastic specula make significant audible clicking sounds when opening and closing, so you should prepare the patient for this event.
- Review the anatomy and physiology of the female genitalia; visualize the underlying structures of the anatomic landmarks.
- Review and practice any procedures to be done. Some nurses find it difficult to prepare slides and cultures without assistance if they are novices to these procedures.
- Know your institution's policies regarding the option of having a female nurse present if a male nurse is performing the gynecological exam.

NURSING TIP

Liquid-Based Cervical Cytology

Two methods of liquid-based cervical cytology are available: AutoCyte Prep system (Shure-Path system) and the ThinPrep system for the detection of squamous epithelial abnormalities (Figure 20-8). These methods clean the specimens for Pap smears by removing blood and mucus prior to mounting the cells on the slide. The cell sample is placed in a preservative vial, and the specimen is centrifuged, filtered, or both at the laboratory.

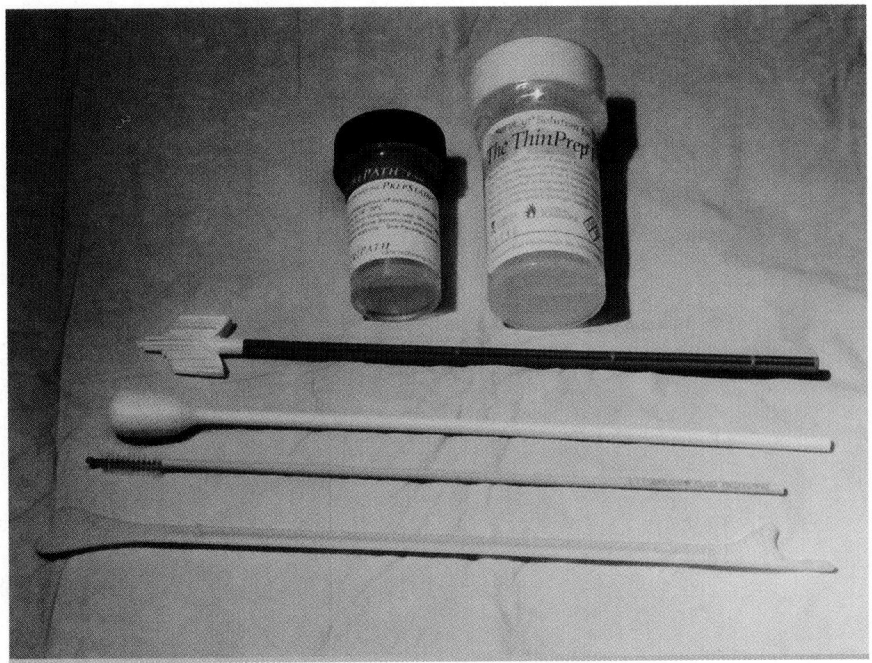

FIGURE 20-8 Liquid-Based Cervical Cytology Preparations

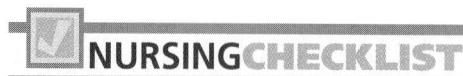

General Approach to Female Genitalia Assessment

Prior to the assessment

1. Ensure that the patient will not be menstruating at the time of the examination for optimal cytological specimen collection.
2. Instruct the patient not to use vaginal sprays, to douche, or to have coitus 24 to 48 hours before the scheduled physical assessment. The products of coitus and commercial sprays and douches may affect the Pap smear and other vaginal cultures.
3. Encourage the patient to express any anxieties and concerns about the physical assessment. Reassure the patient by acknowledging anxieties and validating concerns. Virgins need reassurance that the pelvic assessment should not affect the hymen.
4. Show the speculum and other equipment to the patient and allow her to touch and explore any items that do not have to remain sterile.
5. Inform the patient that the assessment should not be painful but may be uncomfortable at times, and tell her to inform you if she is experiencing any pain.
6. Instruct the patient to empty her bladder and then to undress from the waist to the ankles.
7. Ensure that the room is warm enough to prevent chilling, and provide additional draping material as necessary.
8. Place drapes or sheep skin over the stirrups to increase patient comfort.
9. Warm your hands with warm water prior to gloving.
10. Ensure that privacy will be maintained during the assessment. Provide screens and a closed door.
11. Warm the speculum with warm water or a warming device before insertion.

During the assessment

1. Inform the patient of what you are going to do before you do it. Tell her she may feel pressure when the speculum is opened and a pinching sensation when the Pap smear is done.
2. Adopt a nonjudgmental and supportive attitude.
3. Maintain eye contact with the patient as much as possible to reinforce a caring relationship.
4. Use a mirror to show the patient what you are doing and to educate her about her body. Help her with positioning the mirror during the examination so she will feel comfortable using this technique at home to assess her genitalia.
5. Offer the patient the opportunity to ask questions about her body and sexuality.
6. Encourage the patient to use relaxation techniques such as deep breathing or guided imagery to prevent muscle tension during the assessment.

After the assessment

1. Assess whether the patient needs assistance in dressing.
2. Offer tissues with which to wipe excess lubrication.
3. After the patient is dressed, discuss the experience with her, invite questions and comments, listen carefully, and provide her with information regarding the assessment and any laboratory information that is available.
4. Tell the patient she may experience a small amount of spotting following the Pap smear.

E Examination   **N** Normal Findings   **A** Abnormal Findings   **P** Pathophysiology

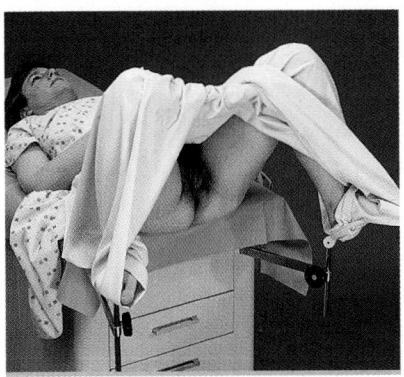

FIGURE 20-9 Patient Positioning and Draping for Gynecological Examination

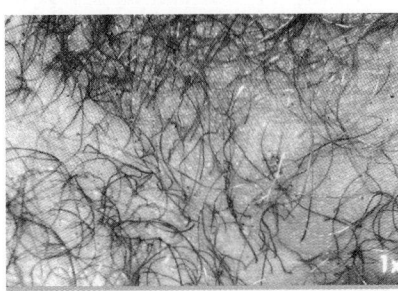

FIGURE 20-10 Pubic Lice, or *Phthirus pubis.* Note the reddish-brown crab lice feces. *Courtesy of the Centers for Disease Control and Prevention (CDC) and Joe Miller.*

INSPECTION OF THE EXTERNAL GENITALIA

1. With the patient seated, place a drape over the patient's torso and thighs until positioning is completed.
2. Instruct the patient to first sit on the examination table between the stirrups, facing away from the head of the table.
3. Assist the patient in assuming a dorsal recumbent or lithotomy position on the examination table. Assist the patient in placing her heels in the stirrups, thus abducting her legs and flexing her hips.
4. Don clean gloves.
5. Assist the patient as she moves her buttocks down to the lower end of the examination table so that the buttocks are flush with the edge of the table. If the patient desires, raise the head of the examination table slightly to elevate her head and shoulders. This position allows you to maintain eye contact with the patient and prevents abdominal muscle tension (Figure 20-9).
6. Readjust the drape to cover the abdomen, thighs, and knees; adjust the stirrups as necessary for patient comfort. Push the drape down between the patient's knees so you can see the patient's face.
7. Sit on a stool at the foot of the examination table facing the patient's external genitalia.
8. Adjust your lighting source and provide the patient with a mirror. Instruct her on how to hold the mirror in order to view the examination prior to your touching her genitalia.
9. Finally, remember to inform the patient of each step of the assessment process before it is performed, and be gentle.

Pubic Hair

E 1. Observe the pattern of pubic hair distribution.

 2. Note the presence of nits or lice.

N The distribution of the female pubic hair should be shaped like an inverse triangle. There may be some growth on the abdomen and upper inner thighs. A diamond-shaped pattern from the umbilicus may be due to cultural or familial differences. There are no nits or lice.

A A diamond-shaped pattern from the umbilicus, not associated with cultural or familial differences, is abnormal.

P This distribution pattern may occur with hirsutism, which is indicative of an endocrine disorder.

A Hair distribution is sparse or hair is absent at the genitalia area. This is called **alopecia** and it is abnormal.

A Alopecia in the genital area may result from genetic factors, aging, or local or systemic disease. These include developmental defects and hereditary disorders, infection, neoplasms, physical or chemical agents, endocrine diseases, deficiency states (nutritional or metabolic), destruction, damage to the follicles, and obesity. Note: This variant may be expected if the patient shaves or waxes this region.

A The presence of nits or lice is abnormal.

P Pubic lice (pediculosis pubis) is the infestation of the hairy regions of the body, usually the pubic area (Figure 20-10), but it sometimes involves the hairy aspects of the abdomen, chest, and axillae.

Skin Color and Condition

Mons Pubis and Vulva.

E 1. Observe the skin coloration and condition of the mons pubis and vulva.

2. Inform the patient that you will touch the inside of her thigh before you touch her genitals.

3. With gloved hands, separate the labia majora using the thumb and index finger of the dominant hand.

4. Observe both the labia majora and the labia minora for coloration, lesions, or trauma.

N The skin over the mons pubis should be clear except for nevi and normal hair distribution. The labia majora and minora should appear symmetrical with a smooth to somewhat wrinkled, unbroken, slightly pigmented skin surface. There should be no ecchymosis, excoriation, nodules, swelling, rash, or lesions. An occasional sebaceous cyst is within normal limits. These cysts are nontender, yellow nodules that are less than 1 cm in diameter.

A Ecchymosis over the mons pubis or labia is abnormal.

P This may be due to blunt trauma that may have resulted from an accident or intentional abuse.

A Edema or swelling of the labia is an abnormal finding.

P This may be due to hematoma formation, Bartholin's cyst, or obstruction of the lymphatic system.

A Broken areas on the skin surface are abnormal.

P These may be due to ulcerations or abrasions secondary to infection or trauma.

A Rash over the mons pubis and labia is abnormal.

P Rashes have multiple etiologies including contact dermatitis and infestations.

A A nontender, reddish, round ulcer with a depressed center, and raised, indurated edges (**chancre**) is an abnormal finding (Figure 20-11).

P A chancre appears during the primary stages of syphilis at the site where the *Treponema* enters the body. The chancre lasts for 4 weeks and then disappears.

A Flat or raised, round, wartlike papules that have moist surfaces covered by gray exudate (condyloma latum) are abnormal (Figure 20-12).

P These lesions occur during the secondary stage of syphilis.

A White, dry, cauliflower-like growths that have narrow bases are suggestive of condyloma acuminatum (see Figure 20-13) and are abnormal.

P These warts are caused by the human papillomavirus and may be dysplastic.

A Small, swollen, red vesicles that fuse together to form a large, burning ulcer that may be painful and itch (see Figure 20-14) are abnormal.

P These ulcers are indicative of herpes simplex virus (HSV). Primary HSV (or genital herpes) outbreaks can last up to 21 days. Recurrent HSV outbreaks are usually shorter in duration and last about 2 weeks. Serologic testing must be performed to determine if an outbreak is HSV-1 or HSV-2.

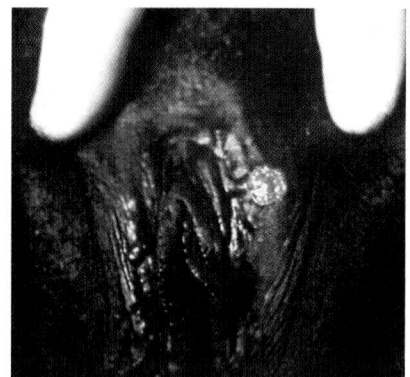

FIGURE 20-11 **Syphilitic Chancre.**
Courtesy of the Centers for Disease Control and Prevention (CDC).

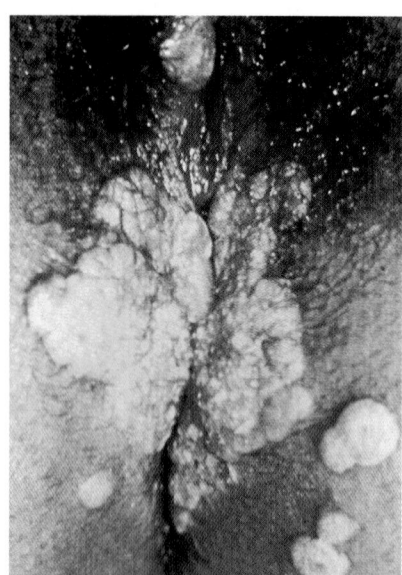

FIGURE 20-12 **Secondary Syphilis (Condyloma Latum).** *Courtesy of the Centers for Disease Control and Prevention (CDC).*

| **E** Examination | **N** Normal Findings | **A** Abnormal Findings | **P** Pathophysiology |

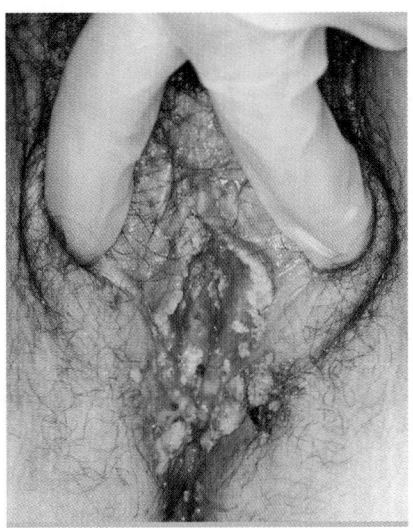

FIGURE 20-13 Genital Warts (Condyloma Acuminatum). *Courtesy of the Centers for Disease Control and Prevention (CDC).*

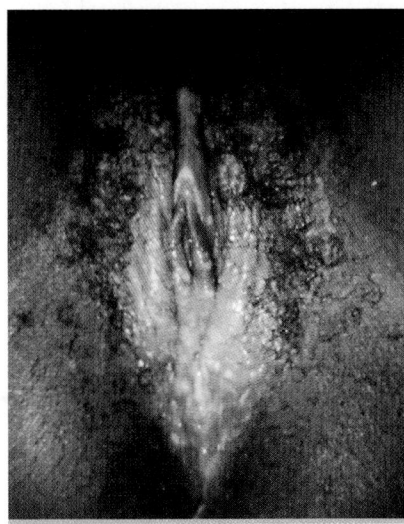

FIGURE 20-14A Genital Herpes Simplex Virus. *Courtesy of the Centers for Disease Control and Prevention (CDC).*

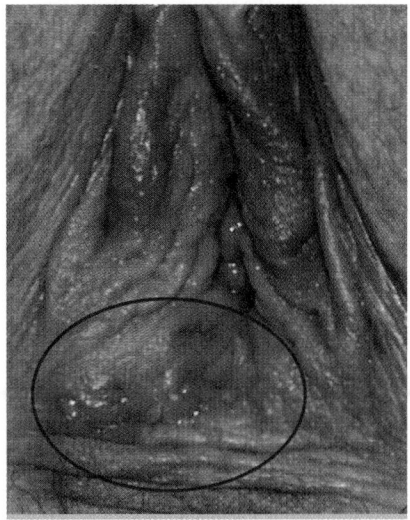

FIGURE 20-14B Primary Herpes Simplex Virus, First Episode. Serology tests are negative for HSV. *Copyright GlaxoSmithKline. Used with permission.*

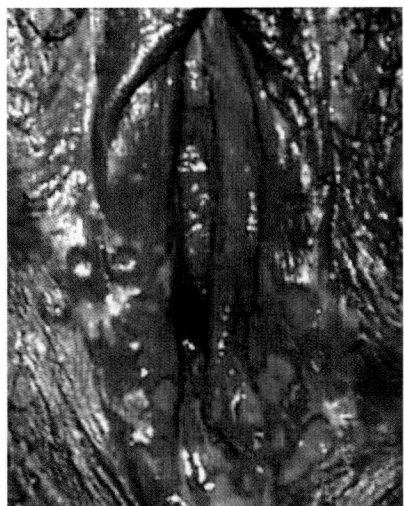

FIGURE 20-14C Nonprimary Herpes Simplex Virus, First Episode. Serology tests are positive for HSV (type 1 or type 2), meaning the patient has had previous exposure to the virus at another body site. *Copyright GlaxoSmithKline. Used with permission.*

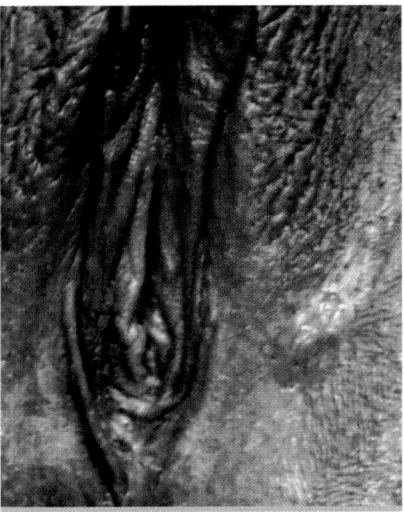

FIGURE 20-14D Recurrent HSV. After the initial primary outbreak, frequent recurrences (four to eight episodes per year) can occur at the primary outbreak site. *Copyright GlaxoSmithKline. Used with permission.*

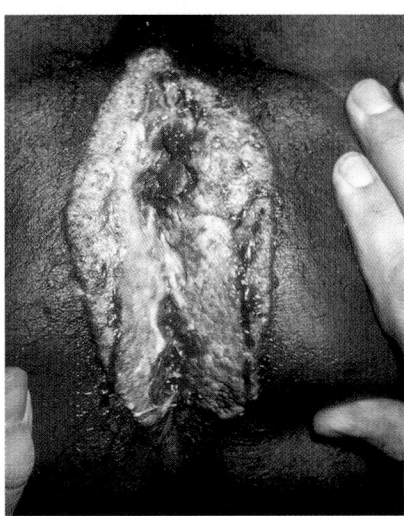

FIGURE 20-15 Granuloma Inguinale. *Courtesy of the Centers for Disease Control and Prevention (CDC).*

A Firm, painless, papular, granular lesions that are beefy red are abnormal (Figure 20-15).

P Granuloma inguinale is caused by the bacteria *Calymmatobacterium granulomatis*. It is also referred to as donovanosis and granuloma venereum. This STD tends to occur on the external genitalia, inguinal region, and the anus.

A A painless mass that may be accompanied by pruritus or a mass that develops into a cauliflower-like growth is an abnormal finding.

P This type of mass is highly suggestive of malignancy.

A Venous prominences of the labia may be abnormal.

P Varicose veins may develop due to a congenital predisposition, prolonged standing, pregnancy, or aging.

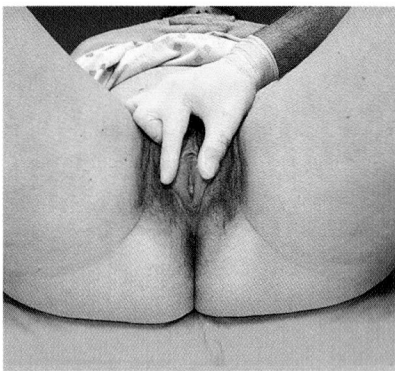

FIGURE 20-16 Inspection of the Clitoris

CLITORIS.

E **1.** Using the dominant thumb and index finger, separate the labia minora laterally to expose the prepuce of the clitoris (Figure 20-16).

2. Observe the clitoris for size and condition.

N The clitoris is approximately 2.0 cm ($\frac{3}{4}$ inch) in length and 0.5 cm ($\frac{1}{4}$ inch) in diameter and without lesions.

A Hypertrophy of the clitoris is an abnormal finding.

P This may indicate female pseudohermaphroditism due to androgen excess.

A A reddish, round ulcer with a depressed center and raised, indurated edges (chancre) is an abnormal finding.

P Refer to the chancre discussion (see Figure 20-11)

A Excision of the clitoris is a post-surgical finding

P Female genital mutilation (clitoridectomy), a practice in some cultures, can result in this finding.

URETHRAL MEATUS.

E **1.** Using the dominant thumb and index finger, separate the labia minora laterally to expose the urethral meatus. Do not touch the urethral meatus; this may cause pain and urethral spasm.

2. Observe the shape, color, and size of the urethral meatus.

N The urethral opening is slitlike in appearance and midline; it is free of discharge, swelling, or redness and is about the size of a pea.

A Discharge of any color from the meatus is an abnormal finding.

P Discharge indicates possible urinary tract infection.

A Swelling or redness around the urethral meatus is an abnormal finding.

P Swelling indicates possible infection of the Skene's glands, urethral caruncle (small, red growth that protrudes from the meatus, shown in Figure 20-17), urethral carcinoma, or prolapse of the urethral mucosa (Figure 20-18).

VAGINAL INTROITUS.

E **1.** Keep the labia minora retracted laterally to inspect the vaginal introitus.

2. Ask the patient to bear down.

3. Observe for patency and bulging.

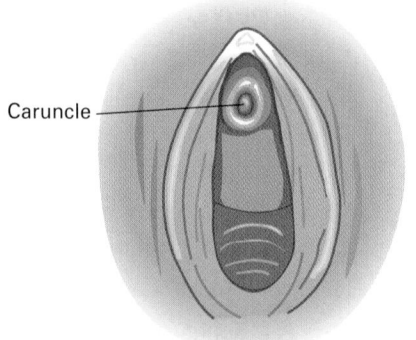

FIGURE 20-17 Urethral Caruncle

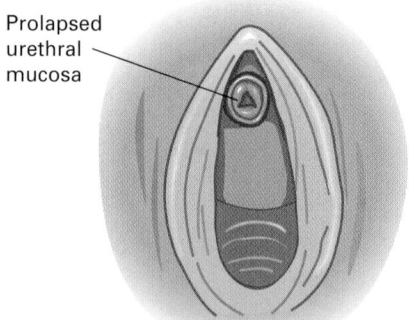

FIGURE 20-18 Prolapse of the Urethral Meatus

TABLE 20-3 Description of Vaginal Discharges

DISCHARGE	NORMAL PHYSIOLOGICAL DISCHARGE	BACTERIAL VAGINOSIS (BV)	TRICHOMONAS	CANDIDA	GONOCOCCAL
Color	White	Gray	Grayish yellow	White	Greenish yellow
Odor	Absent	Fishy	Fishy	Absent	Absent
Consistency	Nonhomogenous	Homogenous	Purulent, often with bubbles	Cottage cheeselike	Mucopurulent
Location	Dependent	Adherent to walls	Often pooled in fornix	Adherent to walls	Adherent to walls
Vaginal pH	4	5–6	5–6	4–4.5	—
Anatomic Appearance					
Vulva	Normal	Normal	Edematous	Erythematous	Erythematous
Vaginal Mucosa	Normal	Normal	Usually normal	Erythematous	Normal
Cervix	Normal	Normal	May show red spots	Patches of discharge	Pus in os

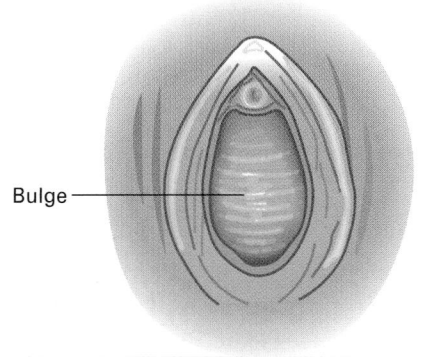

Bulge

FIGURE 20-19 Cystocele

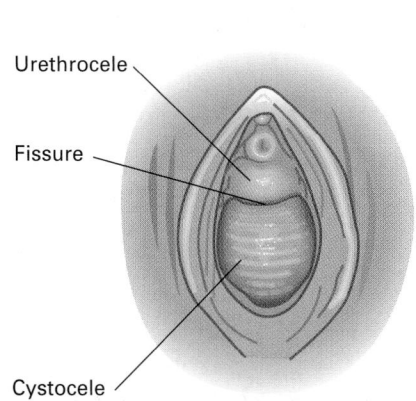

Urethrocele

Fissure

Cystocele

FIGURE 20-20 Cystourethrocele

N The introitus mucosa should be pink and moist. Normal vaginal discharge is clear to white and free of foul odor; some white clumps may be seen that are mass numbers of epithelial cells. The introitus should be patent and without bulging.

A Pale color and dryness of the introitus are abnormal.

P Possible etiologies include atrophy from topical steroids, the aging process, and estrogen deficiency.

A Foul-smelling discharge that is any color other than clear to slightly pale white is abnormal. Malodorous white, yellow, green, or gray discharge that may be purulent are some possible findings.

P Gonorrhea, *Chlamydia*, *Candida* vaginosis, *Trichomonas* vaginitis, bacterial vaginosis, atrophic vaginitis, or cervicitis are possible infectious processes or vectors (Table 20-3).

A An external tear or impatency of the vaginal introitus is abnormal.

P Possible causes include trauma and fissure of the introitus. An external tear may indicate trauma from sexual activity or abuse, and a fissure may indicate a congenital malformation or childbirth trauma.

A Bulging of the anterior vaginal wall indicates a **cystocele** (Figure 20-19) and is abnormal.

P The upper two-thirds of anterior vaginal wall along with the bladder push forward into the introitus due to weakened supporting tissues and ligaments.

A Closure of the vaginal introitus is abnormal.

P Trauma to the area and possible female gential mutilation are potential etiologies.

A Bulging of the anterior vaginal wall, bladder, and urethra into the vaginal introitus indicates a **cystourethrocele** (Figure 20-20) and is abnormal.

| **E** Examination | **N** Normal Findings | **A** Abnormal Findings | **P** Pathophysiology |

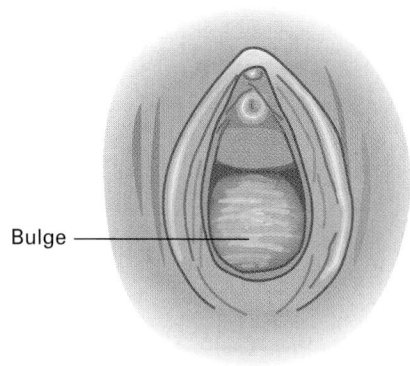

Bulge

FIGURE 20-21 Rectocele

P The etiology is usually a weakening of the entire anterior vaginal wall. A fissure may define the urethrocele and cystocele.

A Bulging of the posterior vaginal wall with a portion of the rectum indicates a **rectocele** (Figure 20-21) and is abnormal.

P This is caused by a weakening of the entire posterior vaginal wall.

PERINEUM AND ANUS.

E 1. Observe for color and shape of the anus.

2. Observe texture and color of the perineum.

N The perineum should be smooth and slightly darkened. A well-healed episiotomy scar is normal after vaginal delivery. The anus should be dark pink to brown and puckered. Skin tags are not uncommon around the anal area.

A A fissure or tear of the perineum is an abnormal finding.

P Possible causes include trauma, abscess, or unhealed episiotomy.

A Venous prominences of the anal area indicate external hemorrhoids and are abnormal.

P An external hemorrhoid is the varicose dilatation of a vein of the inferior hemorrhoidal plexus and is covered with modified anal skin.

PALPATION OF THE EXTERNAL GENITALIA

Labia

E 1. Palpate each labium between the thumb and the index finger of your dominant hand.

2. Observe for swelling, induration, pain, or discharge from a Bartholin's gland duct.

N The labium should feel soft and uniform in structure with no swelling, pain, induration, or purulent discharge.

A Swelling, redness, induration, or purulent discharge from the labial folds with hot, tender areas are abnormal findings (see Figure 20-22).

P These findings indicate a probable Bartholin's gland infection. Causative organisms include gonococci, *Chlamydia trachomatis*, and syphilis.

A A firm mass that is possibly painful in the labia majora is abnormal.

P This might indicate an inguinal hernia. If this is suspected, repalpate the mass with the patient in a standing position. See Chapter 21 for a more thorough explanation of hernias.

Urethral Meatus and Skene's Glands

E 1. Insert your dominant index finger into the vagina.

2. Apply pressure to the anterior aspect of the vaginal wall and milk the urethra (see Figure 20-23).

3. Observe for discharge and patient discomfort.

N Milking the urethra should not cause pain or result in any urethral discharge.

A Pain on contact and discharge from the urethra are abnormal findings.

P These findings indicate a Skene's gland infection or urinary tract infection.

E Examination **N** Normal Findings **A** Abnormal Findings **P** Pathophysiology

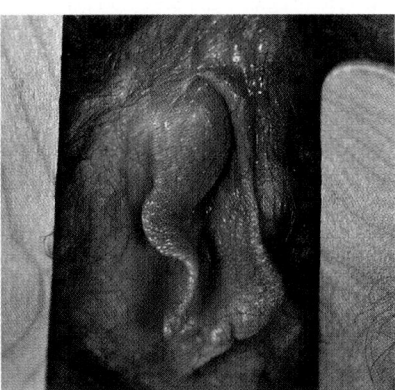

FIGURE 20-22 **Bartholinitis.** *Courtesy of the Centers for Disease Control and Prevention (CDC).*

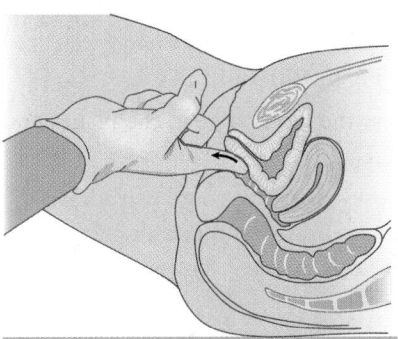

FIGURE 20-23 **Milking the Urethra**

Vaginal Introitus

E **1.** While your finger remains in the vagina, ask the patient to squeeze the vaginal muscles around your finger.

2. Evaluate muscle strength and tone.

N Vaginal muscle tone in a nulliparous woman should be tight and strong; in a parous woman, it will be diminished.

A Significantly diminished or absent vaginal muscle tone and bulging of vaginal or pelvic contents are abnormal findings.

P Weakened muscle tone may result from injury, age, childbirth, or medication. Bulging results from cystocele, rectocele, or uterine prolapse (Figure 20-24).

Perineum

E **1.** Withdraw your finger from the introitus until you can place only your dominant index finger posterior to the perineum and place the dominant thumb anterior to the perineum.

2. Assess the perineum between the dominant thumb and index finger for muscular tone and texture.

N The perineum should be smooth, firm, and homogenous in the nulliparous woman, and thinner in the parous woman. A well-healed episiotomy scar is also within normal limits for a parous woman.

A A thin, tissuelike perineum, fissures, or tears are abnormal.

P A thin perineum is indicative of atrophy, and fissures and tears may indicate trauma or an unhealed episiotomy.

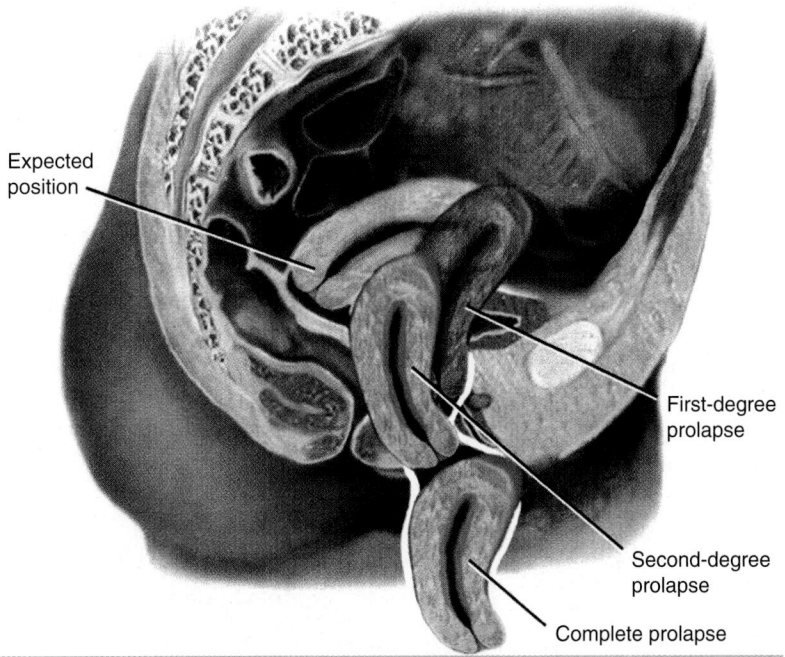

Expected position

First-degree prolapse

Second-degree prolapse

Complete prolapse

FIGURE 20-24 **Uterine Prolapse. In first-degree prolapse, the cervix is contained within the vagina with straining. In second-degree prolapse, the cervix is at the introitus with straining, and in third-degree prolapse, complete prolapse, the cervix, uterus, and vagina are outside the introitus, even without straining.**

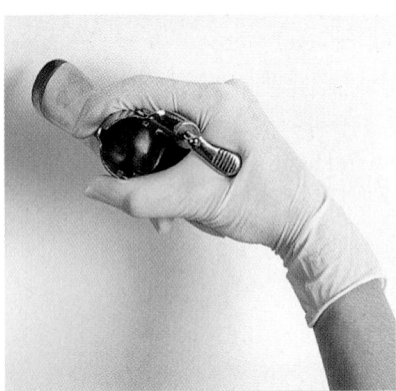

FIGURE 20-25 Holding the Speculum

SPECULUM EXAMINATION OF THE INTERNAL GENITALIA

Cervix

E 1. Select the appropriate-sized speculum. This selection should be based on the patient's history, size of vaginal introitus, and vaginal muscle tone.

2. Lubricate and warm the speculum by rinsing it under warm water. Do not use other lubricants because they may interfere with the accuracy of cytological samples and cultures.

3. Hold the speculum in your dominant hand with the closed blades between the index and middle fingers. The index finger should rest at the proximal end of the superior blade. Wrap the other fingers around the handle, with the thumbscrew over the thumb (Figure 20-25).

4. Insert your nondominant index and middle fingers, ventral sides down, just inside the vagina and apply pressure to the posterior vaginal wall. Encourage the patient to bear down. This will help to relax the perineal muscles.

5. Encourage the patient to relax by taking deep breaths. Be careful not to pull on pubic hair or pinch the labia.

6. When you feel the muscles relax, insert the speculum at an oblique angle on a plane parallel to the examination table until the speculum reaches the end of the fingers that are in the vagina (see Figure 20-26A).

7. Withdraw the fingers of your nondominant hand.

8. Gently rotate the speculum blades to a horizontal angle and advance the speculum at a 45° downward angle against the posterior vaginal wall until it reaches the end of the vagina (see Figures 20-26B and C).

9. Using your dominant thumb, depress the lever to open the blades and visualize the cervix (see Figure 20-26D).

10. If the cervix is not visualized, close the blades and withdraw the speculum 2 to 3 cm (¾–1¼ inches) and reinsert it at a slightly different angle to ensure that the speculum is inserted far enough into the vagina.

11. Once the cervix is fully visualized, lock the speculum blades into place. This procedure varies based on the type of speculum being used.

12. Adjust your light source so that it shines through the speculum.

13. If any discharge obstructs the visualization of the cervix, clean it away with a cotton-tipped applicator.

14. Inspect the cervix and the os for color, position, size, surface characteristics such as polyps or lesions, discharge, and shape.

COLOR.

N The normal cervix is a glistening pink; it may be pale after menopause or blue (**Chadwick's sign**) during pregnancy.

A Cyanosis not associated with pregnancy is abnormal.

P Possible causes include venous congestion of the area or systemic hypoxia as in congestive heart failure.

A Redness or a friable appearance is an abnormal finding.

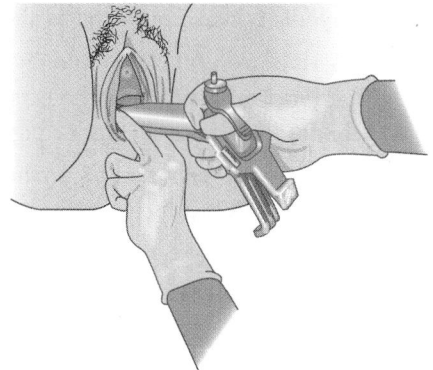
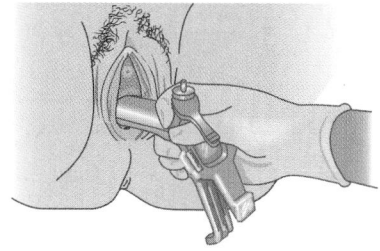

A. Opening of the Vaginal Introitus   B. Oblique Insertion of the Speculum

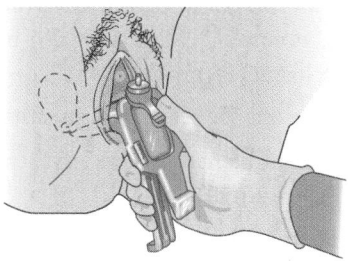
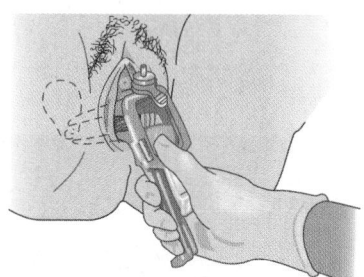

C. Final Advancement of the Speculum   D. Opening the Speculum Blades

FIGURE 20-26 Speculum Examination

P   Possible causes include infection and inflammation, such as *Chlamydia* or gonorrhea.

POSITION.

N   The cervix is located midline in the vagina with an anterior or posterior position relative to the vaginal vault and projecting approximately 2.5 cm (1 inch) into the vagina.

A   Lateral positioning of the cervix may present as an abnormal finding.

P   Possible causes include tumor or adhesions that would displace the cervix.

A   Projection of the cervix into the vaginal vault greater than normal limits is suspect.

P   Uterine prolapse is caused by weakened vaginal wall muscles and pelvic ligaments, and may push the cervix into the vaginal vault.

SIZE.

N   Normal size is 2.5 cm (1 inch).

A   Cervical size greater than 4 cm (1⅝ inches) is indicative of hypertrophy and is abnormal.

P   Inflammation or tumor could result in the morbid enlargement of the cervix.

SURFACE CHARACTERISTICS.

N   The cervix is covered by the glistening pink squamous epithelium, which is similar to the vaginal epithelium, and the deep pink to red columnar epithelium, which is a continuation of the endocervical lining.

E Examination   **N** Normal Findings   **A** Abnormal Findings   **P** Pathophysiology

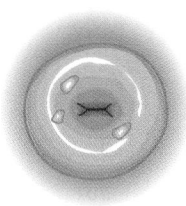

FIGURE 20-27 Nabothian Cysts

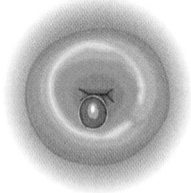

FIGURE 20-28 Cervical Polyp

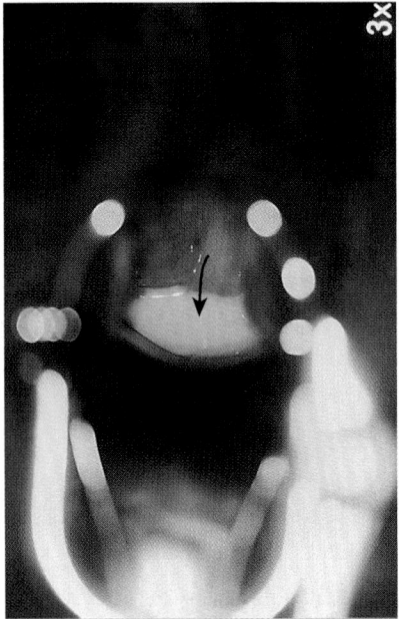

FIGURE 20-29 *Trichomonas vaginalis* is the cause of the purulent cervical discharge. *Courtesy of the Centers for Disease Control and Prevention (CDC).*

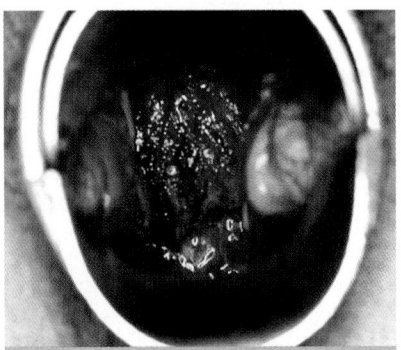

FIGURE 20-30 This woman's cervix is erythematous with erosions due to ***Chlamydia.*** *Courtesy of the Centers for Disease Control and Prevention (CDC).*

A A reddish circle around the os may be abnormal.

P This is known as **ectropion** or **eversion**. It occurs when the squamocolumnar junction appears on the ectocervix. It results from lacerations during childbirth or, possibly, from congenital variation.

A Small, cystic, yellow lesions on the cervical surface indicate **nabothian cysts** (Figure 20-27), which are abnormal.

P These benign cysts result from the obstruction of cervical glands.

A A bright red, soft protrusion through the cervical os indicates a cervical polyp (Figure 20-28) and is abnormal.

P Polyps originate from the endocervical canal; they are usually benign but tend to bleed if abraded.

A Hemorrhages dispersed over the surface and known as strawberry spots are abnormal. There may also be a foul-smelling, frothy, green or yellow discharge (Figure 20-29).

P These may be seen in conjunction with trichomonal infections.

A Mucopurulent discharge, erythema, and friability of the cervix are abnormal (Figure 20-30).

P Many women with *Chlamydia trachomatis* are asymptomatic; others can have pelvic pain, fever, and dysuria. Chlamydia is the most common STD in the United States. Patients infected with this STD frequently have gonorrhea.

A Irregularities of the cervical surface that may look cauliflower-like are an abnormal finding.

P Carcinoma of the cervix may manifest as a cauliflower-like overgrowth (see Figure 20-31).

A Columnar epithelium covering most of the cervix and extending to the vaginal wall (vaginal adenosis), and a collar-type ridge between the cervix and the vagina are abnormal (see Figure 20-32).

P This denotes fetal exposure to DES.

DISCHARGE.

E Note characteristics of any discharge.

N/A/P See Table 20-3.

SHAPE OF THE CERVICAL OS.

N In the nulliparous woman, the os is small and either round or oval. In the parous woman who has had a vaginal delivery, the os is a horizontal slit.

A A unilateral transverse, bilateral transverse, stellate, or irregular cervical os is abnormal (Figure 20-33).

P Possible causes include cervical tears that have occurred during rapid second-stage childbirth delivery, forceps delivery, and trauma.

COLLECTING SPECIMENS FOR CYTOLOGICAL SMEARS AND CULTURES

After inspection of the cervix and the cervical os, obtain any laboratory specimens that are indicated.

E Examination **N** Normal Findings **A** Abnormal Findings **P** Pathophysiology

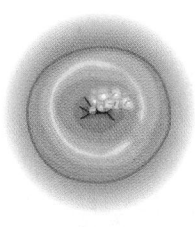

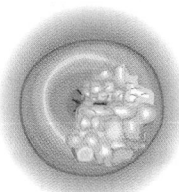

FIGURE 20-31 Carcinoma of the Cervix

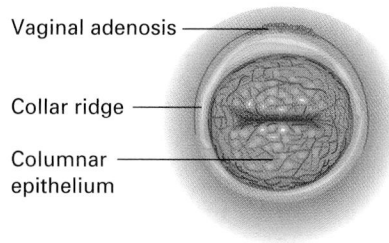

Vaginal adenosis —

Collar ridge —

Columnar epithelium —

FIGURE 20-32 Fetal Exposure to DES

NURSING**ALERT**

DES Exposure

Most patients with DES exposure were born prior to 1971. These patients are at greater risk for carcinoma of the upper vagina.

Normal

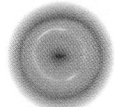 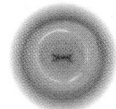

Nulliparous   Parous

Lacerations

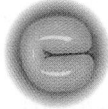 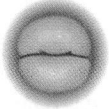 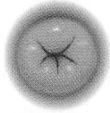

Unilateral transverse   Bilateral transverse   Stellate

FIGURE 20-33 Shapes of the Cervical Os

NURSING**ALERT**

Risk Factors for Female Genitalia Cancer

Evaluate each patient for risk factors, and counsel the patient regarding diminishing risk factors that are behavior dependent. Suspected carcinoma of the female genitalia requires an immediate referral.

Cervical Cancer
- Early age at first intercourse
- Multiple sex partners or male partners who have had multiple partners
- Prior history of herpes simplex virus
- Current or prior history of human papillomavirus or condylomata, or both
- Family history
- Tobacco use
- Drug use
- HIV
- Immunosuppressed
- History of STDs, cervical dysplasia or cervical cancer, endometrial, vaginal, or vulvar cancer
- Women of lower socioeconomic status

Endometrial Cancer
- Early or late menarche (before age 11 or after age 16)
- History of infertility
- Failure to ovulate
- Unopposed estrogen therapy
- Use of tamoxifen
- Obesity
- Family history
- Family history of nonpolyposis colon cancer

Ovarian Cancer
- Advancing age
- Nulliparity
- History of breast cancer
- Family history of ovarian cancer
- Infertility treatment

Vaginal Cancer
- Daughters of women who ingested DES during pregnancy
- Prior human papillomavirus

Collect the Pap smear first, followed by the gonococcal and any other vaginal smears. There are many accepted variations among laboratories regarding the collection and fixing of vaginal specimens. It is prudent to identify the procedure recommended by the laboratory testing the specimens.

Pap Smear

The Pap smear is actually a collection of specimens that are obtained from two sites: the endocervix and the cervix. If the patient has had a hysterectomy, the specimen is obtained from the vaginal cuff. The purpose of the Pap smear is to evaluate cervicovaginal cells for pathology that may indicate carcinoma. See Table 20-4 for guidelines.

Most providers use liquid-based cytology systems, such as ThinPrep and AutoLyte Prep.

TABLE 20-4 Cervical Cancer Screening Guidelines

SCREENING TEST	AMERICAN CANCER SOCIETY	U.S. PREVENTATIVE SERVICES TASK FORCE	AMERICAN COLLEGE OF OBSTETRICIANS AND GYNECOLOGISTS
When to start	Within 3 years of engaging in vaginal intercourse, but no later than 21 years old	Within 3 years of engaging in intercourse, or age 21, whichever occurs first	Within 3 years of engaging in vaginal intercourse, but no later than 21 years old
Conventional Pap test	Perform yearly	At least every 3 years	Perform yearly
	If over 30, with three normal serial Pap tests, the interval may be 2 to 3 years*		If over 30, with three normal serial Pap tests, the interval may be 2 to 3 years*
Liquid-based cytology Pap test	Perform every 2 years If over 30, with three normal serial Pap tests, the interval may be 2 to 3 years*	Inadequate evidence	Perform yearly If over 30, with three normal serial Pap tests, the interval may be 2 to 3 years*
If HPV testing used	Pap smear every 3 years for women over 30 years of age when combined with HPV-DNA testing*	Inadequate evidence	Pap smear every 3 years for women over 30 years of age when combined with HPV-DNA testing*
When to stop	70 years of age or older when there are three or more normal Pap smears within the past 10 years*	Optimal age for cessation is unclear; however, 65 years of age is adequate when there are three or more normal Pap smears within the past 10 years*	Upper age limit not established
Post-total hysterectomy	Discontinue if for benign reasons and no prior history of high-grade CIN*	Discontinue if for benign reasons and no prior history of high-grade CIN*	Continuation of screening if history of high-grade CIN or DES exposure

*Exceptions that apply are women who are immunocompromised such as those with HIV infection, organ transplant, chemotherapy, chronic steroid use, prenatal exposure to DES, or history of high-grade CIN.

ENDOCERVICAL SMEAR.

 1. Using your dominant hand, insert the Cytobrush or cervical broom through the speculum into the cervical os approximately 1 cm. Many patients find that this procedure causes a cramping sensation, so forewarn your patient that she may feel discomfort during this element of the assessment.

2. Rotate the Cytobrush between your index finger and thumb 360° clockwise, then counterclockwise. Keep the Cytobrush in contact with the cervical tissue (Figure 20-34). Note: If you have to use a cotton-tipped applicator instead of a Cytobrush, leave the applicator in the cervical os for 30 seconds to ensure saturation. If you use the cervical broom, rotate the broom 6 times clockwise and place the broom in the liquid-based preparation container.

3. Remove the Cytobrush and, using a rolling motion, spread the cells on the section of the slide marked *E,* if a sectional slide is being used. Do not press down hard or wipe the Cytobrush back and forth because doing so will destroy the cells.

4. Discard the brush.

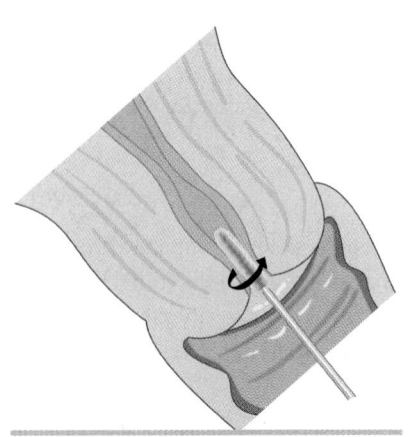

FIGURE 20-34 Endocervical Smear

N Normal classifications for all cervicovaginal cytology should read "Specimen Adequacy—adequate for evaluation" and "General Categorization—negative for intraepithelial lesion or malignancy," using the Bethesda System 2001, which denotes a lack of pathogenesis (Table 20-5).

A A report finding of benign cellular changes is abnormal.

P Benign cellular changes have a multiplicity of causes including fungal, bacterial, protozoan, or viral infections.

A A report finding of "atypical squamous cells of undetermined significance" is abnormal.

P Causes of this finding include inflammatory or infectious processes, a preliminary lesion, or an unknown phenomenon.

A A report finding of epithelial cell abnormalities is aberrant.

TABLE 20-5 The 2001 Bethesda System for Reporting Cervical Cytological Diagnoses

SPECIMEN ADEQUACY
Adequate for evaluation
Presence or absence of endocervical or transformation zone components
Unsatisfactory for evaluation
Specimen rejected or not processed (specify reason)
Specimen processed but unsatisfactory for evaluation

GENERAL CATEGORIZATION
Negative for intraepithelial lesion or malignancy
Organisms (*Trichomonas vaginalis, Candida* species)
Shift in flora suggestive of bacterial vaginosis
Cellular changes consistent with herpes simplex virus
Reactive cellular changes associated with inflammation, radiation, IUD
Glandular cells posthysterectomy
Atrophy

EPITHELIAL CELL ABNORMALITIES

Squamous Cell
Atypical squamous cells (ASC)
ASC of undetermined significance (ASC-US)
ASC, cannot exclude high-grade squamous intraepithelial lesion (ASC-H)
Low-grade squamous intraepithelial lesion (LSIL) encompassing human papillomavirus, mild dysplasia, and cervical intraepithelial neoplasm (CIN 1)
High-grade squamous intraepithelial lesion (HSIL) encompassing moderate and severe dysplasia, carcinoma in situ, CIN 2, and CIN 3
Squamous cell carcinoma

Glandular Cell
Atypical glandular cells (AGC), specify endocervical, endometrial, or glandular cells not otherwise specified
Atypical glandular cells, favor neoplastic
Endocervical adenocarcinoma in situ (AIS)
Adenocarcinoma
Endometrial cells in a woman 40 years or older

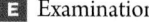 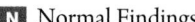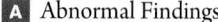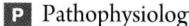

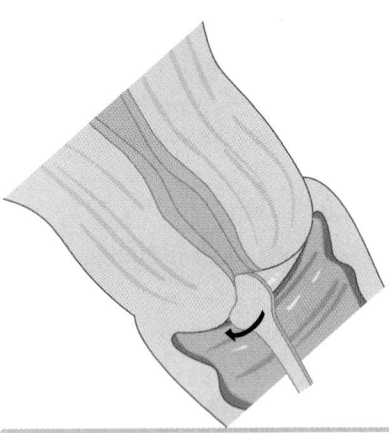

FIGURE 20-35 **Cervical Smear**

P This finding is indicative of squamous intraepithelial lesion, which may or may not be transient; squamous cell carcinoma; or glandular cell abnormalities that are seen in postmenopausal women who are not on hormone replacement therapy.

CERVICAL SMEAR.

E 1. Insert the bifurcated end of the Ayre spatula through the speculum base. Place the longer projection of the bifurcation into the cervical os. The shorter projection should be snug against the ectocervix.

2. Rotate the spatula 360° one time only (Figure 20-35). Make sure the transformation zone is well sampled.

3. Remove the spatula and gently spread the specimen on the section of the slide labeled *C*, if a sectional slide is being used.

N/A/P Refer to Endocervical Smear.

Chlamydia Culture Specimen

E 1. Insert a sterile cotton swab applicator 1 cm (⅜ inch) into the cervical os.

2. Hold the applicator in place for 20 seconds.

3. Remove the swab.

4. Place the swab in a viral, *Chlamydia*, or mycoplasma culture transport tube.

5. Dispose of the cotton swab applicator.

6. Submit the specimens to the appropriate laboratory per your institution's guidelines for culture specimens.

N Cervicovaginal tissues are normally free of *Chlamydia trachomatis.*

A It is abnormal to find *trachomatis*, serotypes D through K, or obligate, intracellular bacteria in cervicovaginal secretions.

P *Trachomatis* may invade the cervix or fallopian tubes, but it is often asymptomatic in women.

Note: Nonculture laboratory test methods include direct fluorescent antibody (DFA), enzyme immunoassay (EIA), DNA probes, or polymerase chain reaction (PCR).

Gonococcal Culture Specimen

E 1. Insert a sterile cotton swab applicator 1 cm (⅜ inch) into the cervical os.

2. Hold the applicator in place for 20 to 30 seconds.

3. Remove the swab.

4. Place the swab in a Gonoccal or culture transport tube.

5. Submit the specimens to the appropriate laboratory per your institution's guidelines for culture specimens.

N Cervicovaginal tissues are normally free of *Neisseria gonorrhoeae.*

A It is abnormal to find a large number of gram-negative diplococci present in cervicovaginal secretions.

P *N. gonorrhoeae* are gram-negative diplococci organisms that prefer to invade columnar and stratified epithelium.

Saline Mount or "Wet Prep"

This test is performed for the rapid evaluation of white blood cells and protozoa.

E 1. Spread a sample of the cervical specimen onto a microscope slide, add one drop of normal saline solution, and apply a cover slip.

2. Examine under a microscope.

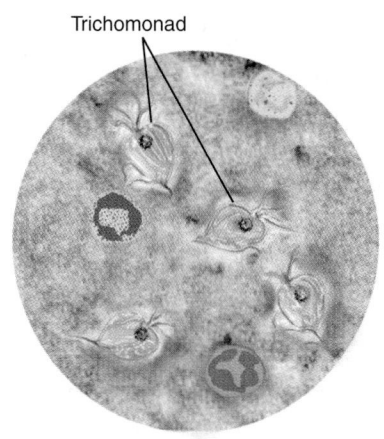

FIGURE 20-36 Microscopic View of *Trichomonas*

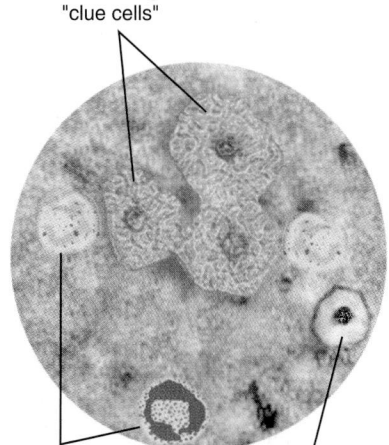

FIGURE 20-37 Microscopic View of Clue Cells

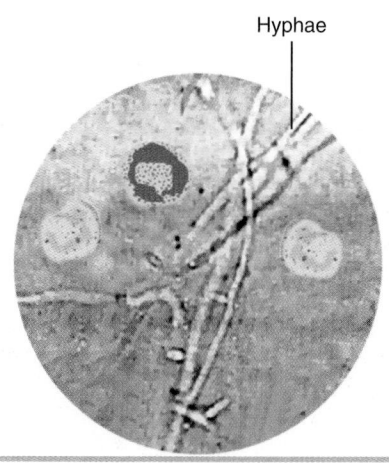

FIGURE 20-38 Microscopic View of Hyphae

N The sample should have fewer than 10 white blood cells (WBCs) per field.

A A sample with more than 10 WBCs per field, protozoa (Figure 20-36), bacteria-filled epithelial cells (clue cells) (Figure 20-37), or other organisms is abnormal.

P A large number of WBCs can be indicative of an inflammatory response, *Chlamydia trachomatis*, or a bacterial infection. Protozoa are indicative of trichomoniasis.

KOH Prep

This test is performed for the rapid evaluation of *Candida*.

E 1. Spread a sample of the cervical specimen onto a microscope slide, add one drop of potassium hydroxide (KOH), and apply a cover slip.

2. Note any odor.

3. Examine under a microscope.

N Cervicovaginal tissues are normally free of *Candida albicans* except in a small percentage of women. There should be no odor.

A The presence of yeast and pseudohyphae forms (chains of budding yeast) (Figure 20-38) is abnormal.

P The presence of budding yeast is indicative of an overgrowth of *Candida*.

A An odor is abnormal.

P A fishy odor ("the whiff test") indicates bacterial vaginosis.

Five Percent Acetic Acid Wash

E After completing all other vaginal specimens, swab the cervix with a cotton-tipped applicator that has been soaked in 5% acetic acid.

N The normal response is no change in the appearance of the cervix.

A A rapid acetowhitening or blanching with jagged borders is an abnormal finding.

P The cause may be the human papillomavirus, which is the causative agent of genital warts.

Anal Culture

E 1. Insert a sterile cotton swab applicator 1 cm (⅜ inch) into the anal canal.

2. Hold the applicator in place for 20 to 30 seconds.

3. Remove the swab. If fecal material is collected, discard the applicator and start again.

4. Roll and rotate the swab in a large "Z" pattern over a Thayer-Martin culture plate.

5. Dispose of the swab.

N Anal tissues are normally free of *Neisseria gonorrhoeae*.

A The presence of a large number of gram-negative diplococci is abnormal.

P This is indicative of *N. gonorrhoeae*.

E Examination   **N** Normal Findings   **A** Abnormal Findings   **P** Pathophysiology

INSPECTION OF THE VAGINAL WALL

E 1. Disengage the locking device of the speculum.

2. Slowly withdraw the speculum but do not close the blades.

3. Rotate the speculum into an oblique position as you retract it to allow full inspection of the vaginal walls. Observe vaginal wall color and texture.

N The vaginal walls should be pink, moist, deeply rugated, and without lesions or redness.

A Spots that appear as white paint on the walls are abnormal.

P A possible cause is leukoplakia from *Candida albicans.* Repeated occurrences even after treatment may indicate HIV infection.

A Pallor of the vaginal walls is abnormal.

P Possible causes include anemia and menopause.

A Redness of the vaginal walls is abnormal.

P Possible causes include inflammation, hyperemia, and trauma from tampon insertion or removal.

A Vaginal lesions or masses are abnormal findings.

P Possible causes include carcinoma, tumors, and DES exposure.

BIMANUAL EXAMINATION

E 1. Observe the patient's face for signs of discomfort during the assessment process.

2. Inform the patient of the steps of the bimanual assessment, and warn her that the lubricant gel may be cold.

3. Squeeze water-soluble lubricant onto the fingertips of your dominant hand.

4. Stand between the legs of the patient as she remains in the lithotomy position, and place your nondominant hand on her abdomen and below the umbilicus.

5. Insert your dominant index and middle fingers 1 cm into the vagina. The fingers should be extended with the palmar side up. Exert gentle posterior pressure.

6. Inform the patient that pressure from palpation may be uncomfortable. Instruct the patient to relax the abdominal muscles by taking deep breaths.

7. When you feel the patient's muscles relax, insert your fingers to their full length into the vagina. Insert your fingers slowly so that you can simultaneously palpate the vaginal walls.

8. Remember to keep your thumb widely abducted and away from the urethral meatus and clitoris throughout the palpation in order to prevent pain or spasm.

Vagina

E Complete steps 1–8 from bimanual examination. Rotate the wrist so that the fingers are able to palpate all surface aspects of the vagina.

N The vaginal wall is nontender and has a smooth or rugated surface with no lesions, masses, or cysts.

A The presence of lesions, masses, scarring, or cysts is abnormal.

P These findings may be indicative of benign lesions such as inclusion cysts, myomas, or fibromas. The most common site for malignant lesions of the vagina is the upper one-third of the posterior vaginal wall.

Cervix

E 1. Position the dominant hand so that the palmar surface faces upward.

2. Place the nondominant hand on the abdomen approximately one-third of the way down between the umbilicus and the symphysis pubis.

3. Use the palmar surfaces of the dominant hand's finger pads, which are in the vagina, to assess the cervix for consistency, position, shape, and tenderness.

4. Grasp the cervix between the fingertips and move the cervix from side to side to assess mobility (Figure 20-39).

N The normal cervix is mobile without pain, smooth and firm, symmetrically rounded, and midline.

A The presence of pain on palpation or the assessment of mobility is a positive **Chandelier's sign** and is abnormal.

P This is indicative of possible pelvic inflammatory disease or ectopic pregnancy.

A Softening of the cervix (Goodell's sign) is a significant finding.

P This sign is seen at the fifth to sixth week of pregnancy.

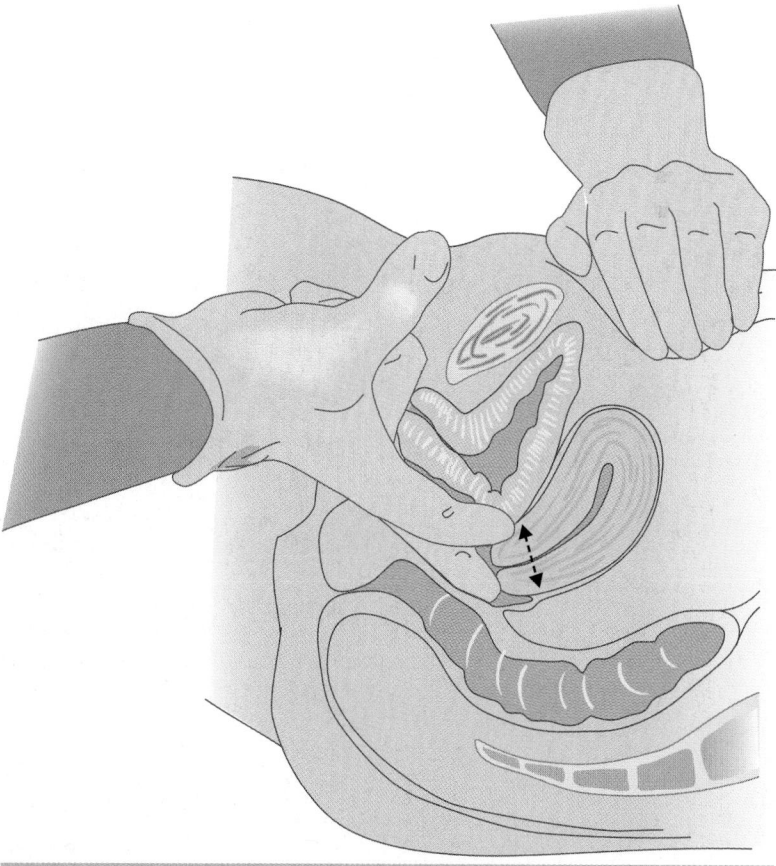

FIGURE 20-39 **Assessment of Cervical Mobility**

E Examination   **N** Normal Findings   **A** Abnormal Findings   **P** Pathophysiology

A Irregular surface, immobility, or nodular surface structure of the cervix indicates abnormality.

P Possible causes include malignancy, fibroids, nabothian cysts, and polyps.

Fornices

E 1. With the fingertips and palmar surfaces of the fingers, palpate around the fornices.

2. Note nodules or irregularities.

N The walls should be smooth and without nodules.

A The presence of nodules or irregularities is abnormal.

P Possible causes include malignancy, polyps, and herniations if the walls of the fornices are impatent.

Uterus

E 1. With the dominant hand, which is in the vagina, push the pelvic organs out of the pelvic cavity and provide stabilization while the nondominant hand, which is on the abdomen, performs the palpation (Figure 20-40).

2. Press the hand that is on the abdomen inward and downward toward the vagina, and try to grasp the uterus between your hands.

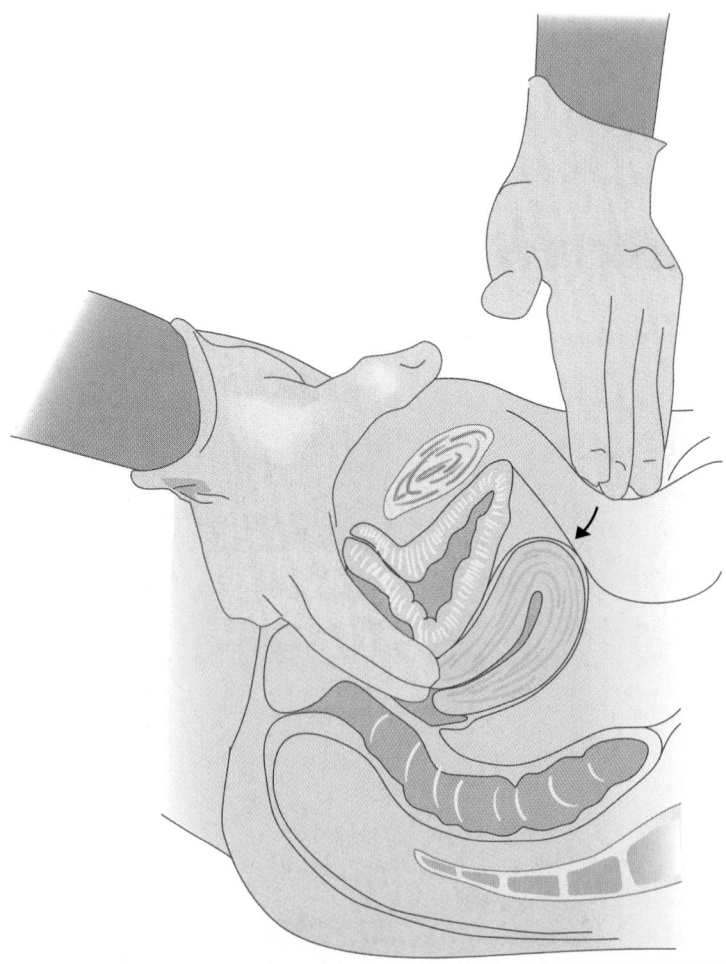

FIGURE 20-40 Uterine Palpation

3. Evaluate the uterus for size, shape, consistency, mobility, tenderness, masses, and position.

4. Place the fingers of the intravaginal hand into the anterior fornix and palpate the uterine surface.

N The size of the uterus varies based on parity; it should be pear-shaped in the nongravid patient and more rounded in the parous patient. The uterus should be smooth, firm, mobile, nontender, and without masses. For uterine positions, see Figure 20-3. A uterus may be nonpalpable if it is retroverted or retroflexed. The uterus in these positions can be assessed only via rectovaginal examination. A nonpalpable uterus in the older woman may be a normal finding secondary to uterine atrophy.

A Significant exterior enlargement and changes in the shape of the uterus are abnormal.

P Uterine enlargement indicates possible intrauterine pregnancy or tumor.

A Presence of nodules or irregularities indicates leiomyomas.

P Leiomyomas are tumors containing muscle tissue.

A Inability to assess the uterus may be abnormal.

P A hysterectomy may account for a nonpalpable uterus.

Adnexa

Fallopian tubes are rarely palpable, and palpation of the ovaries depends on patient age and size. Many times, the ovaries are not palpable, and this procedure can be painful to the patient during the luteal phase of the menstrual cycle (postovulation) or due to normal visceral tenderness.

E 1. Move the intravaginal hand to the right lateral fornix, and the hand on the abdomen to the right lower quadrant just inside the anterior iliac spine. Press deeply inward and upward toward the abdominal hand.

2. Push inward and downward with the abdominal hand and try to catch the ovary between your fingertips.

3. Palpate for size, shape, consistency, and mobility of the adnexa.

4. Repeat the above maneuvers on the left side (see Figure 20-41).

N The ovaries are normally almond shaped, firm, smooth, and mobile without tenderness.

A Presence of enlarged ovaries that are irregular, nodular, painful, with decreased mobility, or pulsatile indicate pathology.

P Abnormal adnexal presentation may indicate ectopic pregnancy, ovarian cyst, pelvic inflammatory disease, or malignancy.

RECTOVAGINAL EXAMINATION

E 1. Withdraw your dominant hand from the vagina and change gloves. Apply additional lubricant to the fingertips of your dominant hand.

2. Tell the patient you will be inserting one finger into her vagina and one finger into her rectum. Remind her that the lubricant jelly will feel cold and that the rectal examination will be uncomfortable.

3. Insert the dominant index finger back into the vagina.

4. Ask the patient to strain down as if she is having a bowel movement, in order to relax the anal sphincter. Assess anal sphincter tone.

| **E** Examination | **N** Normal Findings | **A** Abnormal Findings | **P** Pathophysiology |

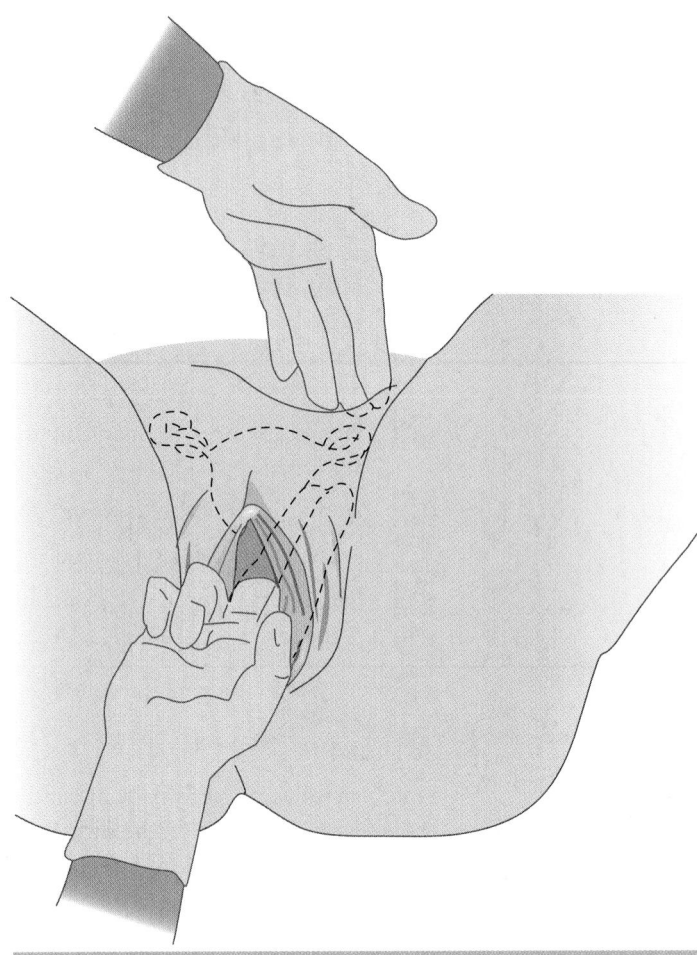

FIGURE 20-41 Palpation of the Left Adnexa

5. Insert the middle finger of the dominant hand into the patient's rectum as she strains down (see Figure 20-42). If the rectum is full of stool, carefully remove the stool digitally from the rectum.

6. Advance the rectal finger forward while using the nondominant hand to depress the abdomen. Assess the rectovaginal septum for patency, the cervix and uterus for anomalies such as posterior lesions, and the rectouterine pouch for contour lesions.

7. On completion of the assessment, withdraw the fingers from the vagina and rectum, and if any stool is present on the glove, test for occult blood.

8. Clean the patient's genitalia and anal area with a tissue and assist her back to a sitting position.

N The rectal walls are normally smooth and free of lesions. The rectal pouch is rugated and free of masses. Anal sphincter tone is strong. The cervix and uterus, if palpable, are smooth. The rectovaginal septum is smooth and intact. Refer to Chapter 22 for further information on the complete rectal examination.

A The presence of masses or lesions indicates pathology.

P Possible causes include malignancy and internal hemorrhoids.

A Lax sphincter tone is an abnormal finding.

P Possible causes include perineal trauma from childbirth or anal intercourse and neurological disorders.

| **E** Examination | **N** Normal Findings | **A** Abnormal Findings | **P** Pathophysiology |

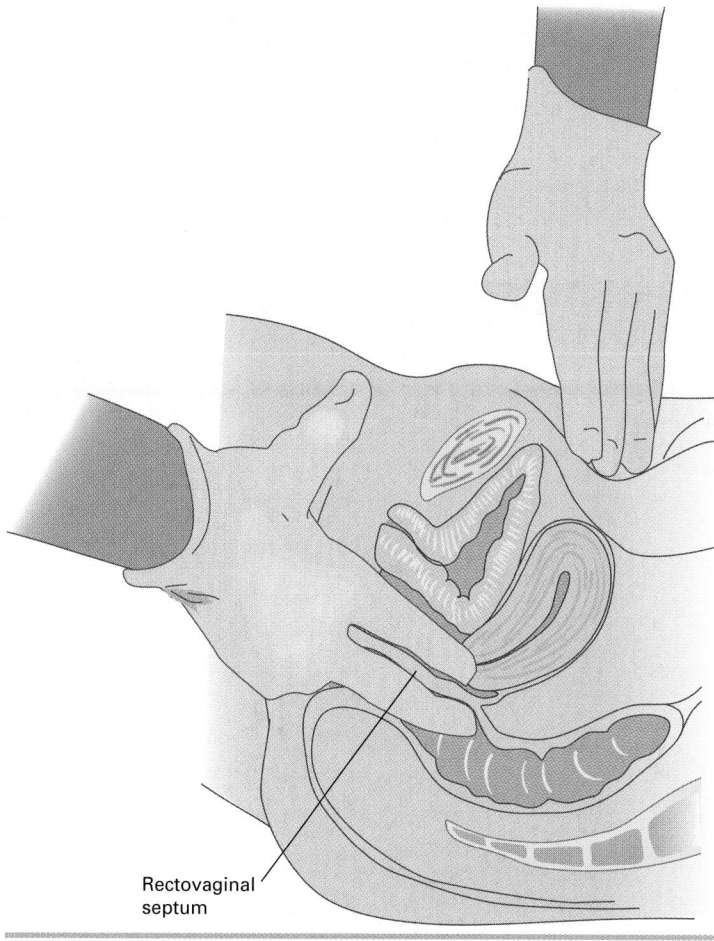

Rectovaginal
septum

FIGURE 20-42 Rectovaginal Examination

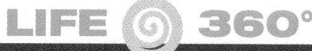

Gynecological Assessments for Women after Hysterectomies

Some women feel that it is unnecessary to have gynecological examinations after hysterectomies. Many of these women had surgery because of malignancy and therefore are at risk for recurrence. All women who have had this type of surgery must be encouraged to continue seeking annual gynecological examinations. Yearly monitoring helps to determine if malignancy has returned or if other pathologies have developed; for instance, women whose ovaries were not removed in the hysterectomy are still at risk for ovarian cancer.

How can you get this topic out into the public arena? How can you increase women's awareness of the need for annual gynecological check-ups even if they have had hysterectomies?

NURSING**TIP**

Maintaining Sexual Function in the Menopausal Woman

Sexually active older women may benefit from:

- Water-soluble lubricant if vaginal secretions are decreased
- Extended foreplay in order to attain orgasm
- A reminder that there is no risk of pregnancy

NURSING**TIP**

Examining the Patient with a Hysterectomy

If the patient has had a hysterectomy, follow the same assessment sequence but omit the following items: cervical palpation, uterine inspection and palpation, endocervical smear, and cervical smear. The vaginal walls and adnexa are evaluated if they were not surgically removed during the hysterectomy.

The Patient with Uterine Fibroids

This case study illustrates the application and objective documentation of the female genitalia assessment.
Joyce is a 42-year-old married mother with uterine fibroids.

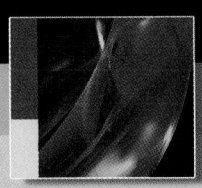

HEALTH HISTORY

PATIENT PROFILE	42-year-old MBF
CHIEF COMPLAINT	"My periods are heavier and painful, and I'm passing clots."
HISTORY OF PRESENT ILLNESS	Pt states that she has noted heavier menstrual cycles for the past 6 mos c̄ ↑ use of 10–14 maxi pads per day and cycles lasting up to 10 days. She notes quarter-size clots on many pads and severe cramping, which keeps her from going to work. She has noted ↑ lower abdominal girth in the past 2 mos and ↑ urinary urgency and some constipation. OTC NSAIDs ↓ the pain.

PAST HEALTH HISTORY

Medical History

Female Reproductive Health History
Menstrual history: menarche age 12, 28–30 d cycle c̄ heavy flow lasting up to 10 days; LMP 2 wks ago
Reproductive medical history: no sexually transmitted infections, endometriosis, cancer of the reproductive organs, or abnormal Pap smears
Obstetric history: G: 2; P: 2; T: 2; P: 0; A: 0; E: 0; LC: 2; SVD for first child and C-section for breech presentation of second child
Premenstrual syndrome: denies
Menopause history: N/A
Vaginal discharge: clear
History of uterine bleeding: describes heavier menstrual bleeding c̄ longer cycles; denies midcycle bleeding
Sexual functioning: heterosexual, sexually active for 22 years, 2 lifetime partners; c̄ husband for past 18 yrs, has some dyspareunia, denies inorgasmia
Method of birth control: bilateral tubal ligation in 1994

Surgical History
C-section '94 c̄ bilateral tubal ligation s̄ sequelae

Allergies
Denies food or drug allergies

Medications
Ibuprofen 400–1,000 mg every 4–6 hrs prn for menstrual pain

Communicable Diseases
Denies, has not been tested x̄ for HPV in the past 13 yrs

Injuries and Accidents
MVA in 2002 whiplash-type cervical injury c̄ no residual problems

Special Needs
Denies

continues

CASE STUDY (Continued)

The Patient with Uterine Fibroids

Blood Transfusions	Denies
Childhood Illnesses	Chickenpox
Immunizations	Adacel last year

FAMILY HEALTH HISTORY

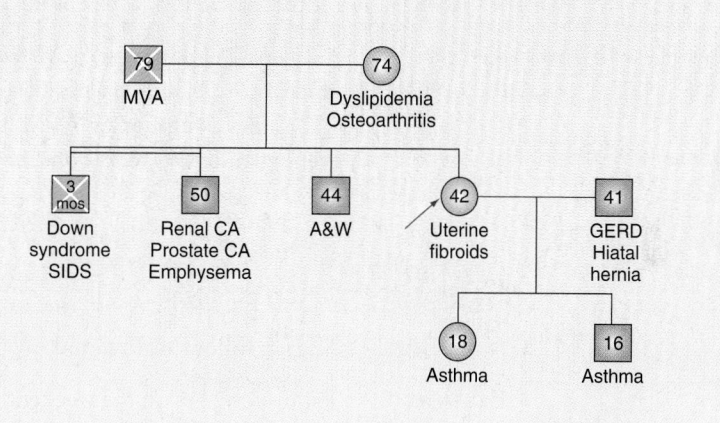

LEGEND

○ Living female

□ Living male

⊗ Deceased female

⊠ Deceased male

⟋ Points to patient

⊓ Twin males

A&W = Alive & well

CA = Cancer

GERD = Gastroesophageal reflux disease

MVA = Motor vehicle accident

SIDS = Sudden infant death syndrome

Denies family hx of CA of the female reproductive organs, DES exposure, congenital anomalies

SOCIAL HISTORY

Alcohol Use	2 glasses of wine on the weekends
Tobacco Use	Denies
Drug Use	Denies
Domestic and Intimate Partner Violence	Denies
Sexual Practice	Monogamous for 18 yrs
Travel History	Mission trip c̄ church group every spring to Haiti; likes to vacation in Florida
Work Environment	CPA for health insurance company for 12 yrs
Home Environment	2-story colonial in suburbs, lives c̄ spouse and 2 children; house well maintained
Hobbies and Leisure Activities	Sewing and tennis
Stress	Children are teenagers and are causing stress
Education	Master's degree in accounting

continues

CASE STUDY (Continued)

The Patient with Uterine Fibroids

Economic Status	Middle-upper income
Military Status	None
Religion	Southern Baptist; active member of congregation; attends wkly worship services and serves on a few committees
Ethnic Background	African American
Roles and Relationships	Mother, daughter, wife, employee. Spouse is supportive.
Characteristic Patterns of Daily Living	Awakens c̄ children at 7 AM. Oatmeal for breakfast or fruit; in office by 9 AM, lunch at 12:00 noon usually fast food; home by 6 PM, makes dinner by 7 PM, bedtime at 10 PM. Sews in the evening and plays tennis on the weekend.
HEALTH MAINTENANCE ACTIVITIES	
Sleep	7–8 hrs per night
Diet	Tries to follow MyPyramid
Exercise	Tennis for 2 hrs on the weekends
Stress Management	Talking to spouse, talks to friends from her church
Use of Safety Devices	Wears seat belt in the car
Health Check-ups	Last Pap smear 2 mos ago WNL; vision and dental exams last yr WNL
PHYSICAL ASSESSMENT	
Inspection of the External Genitalia	
Pubic Hair	Inverse triangle formation, no nits or lice
Skin Color and Condition	Mons pubis and vulva: well-healed low abdominal transverse scar; labia majora and labia minora are s̄ lesions, brown skin color, moist s̄ external discharge, no sign of mutilation Clitoris: no lesions Urethral meatus: midline s̄ swelling or discharge Vaginal introitus: pink s̄ lesion, no discharge Perineum and anus: pink-brown perineum, old episiotomy scar well healed; anus dark brown
Palpation of the External Genitalia	
Labia	No tenderness
Urethral Meatus and Skene's Glands	No pain or discharge

continues

CASE STUDY (Continued)

The Patient with Uterine Fibroids

Vaginal Introitus	Tone strong s̄ bulging of pelvic contents
Perineum	Palpable episiotomy scar, nontender
Speculum Examination of the Internal Genitalia	
Cervix	Color: pink Position: slightly Ⓛ of midline Size: 4 cm Surface characteristics: laceration at 3:00 position Discharge: none Shape of the cervical os: parous
Inspection of the Vaginal Wall	Pink c̄ rugae
Bimanual Examination	
Vagina	No masses, nontender
Cervix	Mobile, nontender, firm
Fornices	No polyp or mass
Uterus	Palpable 2 cm mass on anterior fundus, nontender; uterus is anteverted and parous
Adnexa	Mobile, round s̄ masses or tenderness
Rectovaginal Examination	Septum intact, no masses or fissures; cervix and uterus WNL, strong anal sphincter tone, no occult blood
LABORATORY DATA	Pap smear negative of intraepithelial lesion or malignancy HPV Hybrid Capture 2, negative
DIAGNOSTIC DATA	Transabdominal and transvaginal sonogram confirm 2 cm anterior uterine fibroid

ASSESSMENT IN BRIEF

Female Genitalia Assessment

Inspection of the External Genitalia

- Pubic hair
- Skin color and condition
  - Mons pubis and vulva
  - Clitoris
  - Urethral meatus
  - Vaginal introitus
  - Perineum and anus

Palpation of the External Genitalia

- Labia
- Urethral meatus and Skene's glands
- Vaginal introitus
- Perineum

Speculum Examination of the Internal Genitalia

- Cervix
  - Color

continues

ASSESSMENT IN BRIEF *Continued*

– Position
– Size
– Surface characteristics
– Discharge
– Shape of the cervical os

Collecting Specimens for Cytological Smears and Cultures

• Pap smear
   – Endocervical smear
   – Cervical smear
• Chlamydia culture specimen
• Gonococcal culture specimen
• Saline mount or "wet prep"

• KOH prep
• Five percent acetic acid wash
• Anal culture

Inspection of the Vaginal Wall

Bimanual Examination

• Vagina
• Cervix
• Fornices
• Uterus
• Adnexa

Rectovaginal Examination

REVIEW QUESTIONS

1. During the examination of the external genitalia, you notice a bulging area between the labia minora and the hymenal ring. These greater vestibular glands are also known as the:
   a. Skene's glands
   b. Parathyroid glands
   c. Bartholin's glands
   d. Adrenal glands
   The correct answer is (c).

2. The endometrium of the uterus is composed of all of the following structures except:
   a. Stroma
   b. Columnar epithelium layer
   c. Myometrium
   d. Mucous glands
   The correct answer is (c).

3. Menarche represents:
   a. Stage 1 of the Sexual Maturity Rating Scale
   b. Presence of human chorionic gonadotropin
   c. An increase in estrogen production
   d. A decrease in basal body temperature
   The correct answer is (c).

4. A cause of primary amenorrhea is:
   a. Parathyroid disease
   b. Intensive athletic training
   c. Ovarian cysts
   d. Obesity
   The correct answer is (b).

5. When advising a patient regarding maintaining gynecological health, which statement is incorrect?
   a. Void after coitus to prevent UTIs
   b. Do not leave tampons in place for more than 8 hours at a time due to risk of toxic shock syndrome

   c. Wipe from front to back to prevent contamination of the vagina with fecal material
   d. Douches may be used routinely to make the patient feel refreshed
   The correct answer is (d).

6. Normal vaginal discharge has which of the following properties?
   a. pH of 5–6
   b. Fishy odor
   c. Nonhomogenous
   d. Gray in color
   The correct answer is (c).

7. A second-degree uterine prolapse is marked by which physical assessment finding?
   a. The cervix is at the introitus with straining
   b. The uterus is at the introitus with straining
   c. The cervix is in the vagina with straining
   d. The uterus is outside of the vagina
   The correct answer is (a).

8. A 29-year-old who has had two normal Pap smears in the last decade would need a Pap smear how often, according to the American Cancer Society?
   a. Yearly
   b. Every 2 years
   c. Every 3 years
   d. No longer needs Pap smears
   The correct answer is (a).

9. The KOH Prep is a rapid evaluation for:
   a. HPV
   b. *Candida*
   c. *Neisseria gonorrhoeae*
   d. *Gardnerella vaginalis*
   The correct answer is (b).

10. Vaccination for prevention of HPV is indicated for:
    a. Girls and women ages 13 to 26
    b. Girls and women ages 15 to 25
    c. Girls and women ages 9 to 26
    d. Girls and women ages 6 to 25
    The correct answer is (c).

Visit the Estes online companion resource at
www.delmar.cengage.com
for additional content and study aids.
Click on Online Companions and then select
the Nursing discipline.

BIBLIOGRAPHY

Albers, J. R., Hull, S. K., & Wesley, R. M. (2004). Abnormal uterine bleeding. *American Family Physician, 69*(8), 1915–1926, 1931–1932.

Bogart, L. M., Berry, S. H., & Clemens, J. Q. (2007). Symptoms of interstitial cystitis, painful bladder syndrome and similar diseases in women: A systematic review. *The Journal of Urology, 177*(2), 450–456.

Centers for Disease Control and Prevention. (2007). Update to CDC's Sexually Transmitted Treatment Guidelines, 2006: Fluoroquinolones no longer recommended for treatment of Gonococcal infections. *MMWR, 56*(14), 332–336.

DuRant, E., & Leslie, N. S. (2007). Polycystic ovary syndrome: A review of current knowledge. *The Journal for Nurse Practitioners, 3*(3), 180–185.

Gregory, D. S. (2006). *Case studies in maternity & women's health.* Clifton Park, NY: Delmar Cengage Learning.

Haggerty, C. L., Totten, P. A., Astete, S. G., & Ness, R. B. (2006). Mycoplasma genitalium among women with nongonococcal, nonchlamydial pelvic inflammatory disease. *Infectious Diseases in Obstetrics and Gynecology, 2006*, article ID 30184, 5 pages, doi: 10.1155/ IDOG/2006/30184.

Karan, A., DeVuyst, H., Luchters, S., Othigo, J., Mandaliya, K., Chersich, M. F., & Temmerman, M. (2007). The pap smear for detection of bacterial vaginosis. *International Journal of Gynecology and Obstetrics, 98*(1), 20–23.

Kurman, R. J., Visvanathan, K., Roden, R., Wu, T. C., & Shih, Ie-M. (2008). Early detection and treatment of ovarian cancer: Shifting from early stage to minimal volume of disease based on a new model of carcinogenesis. *American Journal of Obstetrics and Gynecology, 198*(4), 351–356.

Leung-Chen, P. (2008). Syphilis makes another comeback. *American Journal of Nursing, 108*(2), 28–31.

Lobo, R. (2007). *Treatment of the postmenopausal women: Basic and clinical aspects* (3rd ed.). London: Academic Press.

Mahoney, M. C., Cox, J. T., & Kimmel, S. R. (2006). New options in HPV prevention. *Journal of Family Practice, 55*(Suppl.), S2–S22.

Mobley, A. M. (2008). A trichomoniasis primer. *The Journal for Nurse Practitioners, 4*(6), 455–458.

Novi, J. M., Jeronis, S., Morgan, M. A., & Arya, L. A. (2005). Sexual function in women with pelvic organ prolapse compared to women without pelvic organ prolapse. *The Journal of Urology, 173*(5), 1669–1672.

Nucci, M., & Oliva, E. (2008). *Gynecologic pathology.* Oxford: Churchill Livingstone.

Oyelowo, T. (2007). *Mosby's guide to women's health.* St. Louis: Mosby.

Saraiya, M., Ahmed, F., Krishnan, S., Richards, T. B., Unger, E. R., & Lawson, H. W. (2007). Cervical cancer incidence in a prevaccine era in the United States, 1998–2002. *Obstetrics & Gynecology, 109*(2), 360–370.

Schorges, O., Cunningham, G., Hoffman, B., Halvorson, L. M., Bradshaw, K. D., & Schaffer, J. (2008). *Williams' gynecology.* New York: McGraw Hill.

Siddiqui, M. A., & Perry, C. M. (2006). Human papillomavirus quadrivalent (types 6, 11, 16, 18) recombinant vaccine (Gardasil). *Drugs, 66*(9), 1263–1271.

Sobel, J. D. (2005). What's new in bacterial vaginosis and trichomonas? *Infectious Disease Clinics of North America, 19*(2), 387–406.

Sperloff, L., & Fritz, M. (2005). *Clinical gynecologic endocrinology and infertility* (7th ed.). Baltimore: Lippincott, Williams & Wilkins.

Varela, J. A., Otero, L., Espinosa, E., Sanchez, C., Luisa Junquera, M., & Vazquez, F. (2003). Phthirus pubis in a sexually transmitted disease unit: A study of 14 years. *Sexually Transmitted Diseases, 30*(4), 292–296.

World Health Organization. Female genital mutilation. Retrieved May 14, 2009, from http://www.who.int/topics/female_genital_mutilation/en/

Xu, F., Sternberg, M. R., Kottiri, B. J., McQuillan, G. M., Lee, F. K., Nahmias, A. J., Berman, S. M., & Markowitz, L. E. (2006). Trends in herpes simplex virus type 1 and type 2 seroprevalence in the United States. *JAMA, 296*(8), 964–973.

Zimmerman, R. K. (2006). Ethical analysis of HPV vaccine policy options. *Vaccine, 24*(22), 4812–4820.

WEB SITES

Bethesda 2001 Workshop:
    http://www.bethesda2001.cancer.gov

Centers for Disease Control and Prevention:
    http://www.cdc.gov

National Cancer Institute:
    http://www.cancer.org

UNICEF:
    http://www.unicef.org

U.S. National Library of Medicine:
    http://www.nlm.nih.gov

World Health Organization:
    http://www.who.int

CHAPTER 21

Male Genitalia

COMPETENCIES

1. Identify the anatomic landmarks of the male genitalia.

2. Describe the characteristics of the most common male reproductive chief complaints.

3. Perform inspection, palpation, and auscultation on an adult male.

4. Explain the pathophysiological rationale for abnormal findings.

5. Document male reproductive assessment findings.

The male reproductive system includes essential and accessory organs, ducts, and supporting structures (see Figure 21-1). The essential organs are the testes, or male gonads. The accessory organs include the seminal vesicles and bulbourethral glands. There are also several ducts, including the epididymis, ductus (vas) deferens, ejaculatory ducts, and urethra. The supporting structures include the scrotum, penis, and spermatic cords. The prostate is discussed in Chapter 22.

ANATOMY AND PHYSIOLOGY

Organs, ducts, supporting structures, and sexual development are discussed.

ESSENTIAL ORGANS

The **testes**, or testicles, are two oval glands located in the scrotum. Each measures about 5 cm (2 inches) in length and 2.5 cm (1 inch) in width. The testes are partially covered by a serous membrane called the tunica vaginalis (see Figure 21-2). This membrane separates the testes from the scrotal wall. Interior to the tunica vaginalis is a dense, whitish membrane covering each testicle called the tunica albuginea. This membrane enters the testes and divides each testis into sections called lobules, which contain tightly coiled tubules called the seminiferous tubules. These coiled structures are the main component of testicular mass, and they produce sperm by spermatogenesis.

ACCESSORY ORGANS

The **seminal vesicles** are two pouches located posteriorly to and at the base of the bladder. They contribute about 60% of the volume of semen. The fluid secreted by the seminal vesicles is rich in fructose and helps provide a source of energy for sperm metabolism. Prostaglandins, which contribute to sperm motility and viability, are also produced by the seminal vesicles.

The **bulbourethral glands**, or Cowper's glands, are pea-sized glands located just below the prostate. Secretions are emptied from the bulbourethral glands at the time of ejaculation. The bulbourethral glands secrete an alkaline substance that protects sperm by neutralizing the acidic environment of the vagina. These glands also provide lubrication at the end of the penis during sexual intercourse.

DUCTS

The **epididymis** is a comma-shaped, tightly coiled tube that is located on the top and behind the testis and inside the scrotum. Each epididymis is composed of three parts: the head, which is connected to the testis; the body; and the tail, which is continuous with the vas deferens. Sperm mature and develop the power of motility as they pass through the epididymis.

The **ductus (vas) deferens** is an extension of the tail of the epididymis. Each duct ascends from the scrotum and permits sperm to exit from the scrotal sac upward into the abdominal cavity. The ductus deferens loops over the side and down the posterior surface of the bladder. This is where the duct enlarges into the ampulla of the vas deferens and joins the duct from the seminal vesicles to form the ejaculatory ducts.

The **ejaculatory ducts** are two short tubes posterior to the bladder. They descend through the prostate gland and terminate in the urethra. The ducts eject spermatozoa into the prostatic urethra just prior to ejaculation.

The **urethra** is the terminal duct of the seminal fluid passageway. It measures about 20 cm (8 inches) in length, passes through the prostate gland and penis, and terminates at the external urethral orifice.

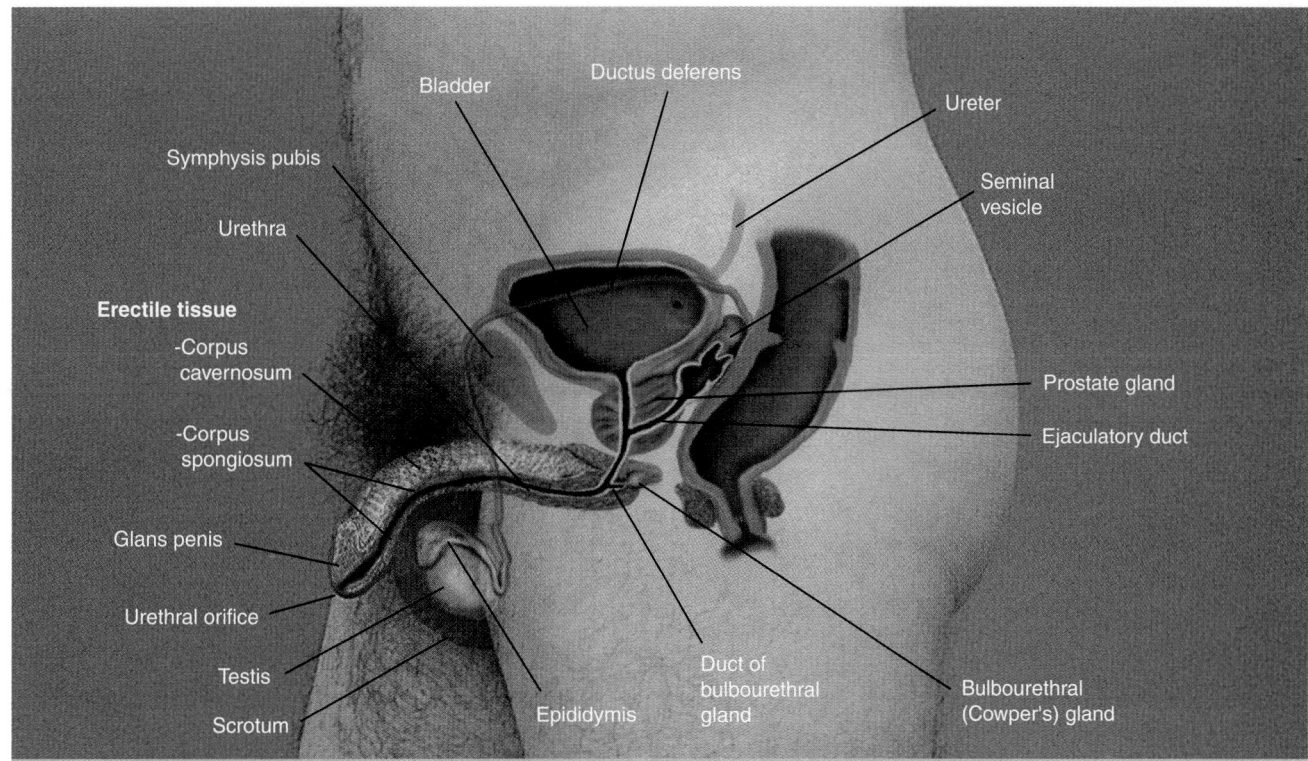

FIGURE 21-1 Male Genitalia

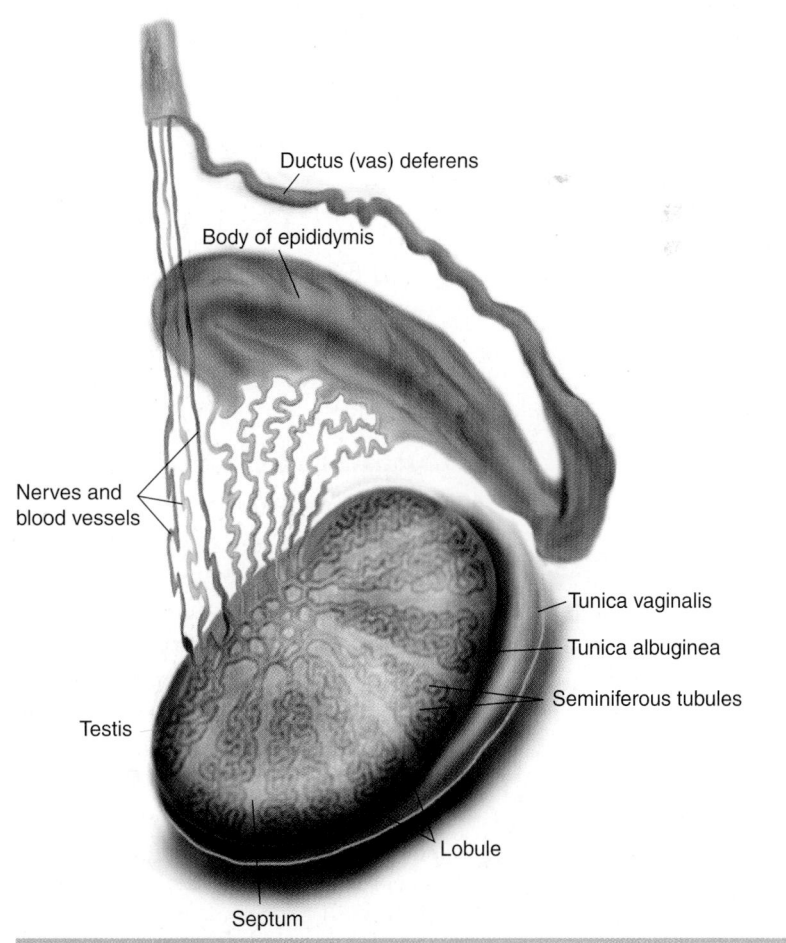

FIGURE 21-2 Testicle

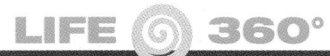

Supporting Structures

The **scrotum** is a pouchlike supporting structure for the testes and consists of rugated, deeply pigmented, loose skin. Inside, the scrotum is divided by a single septum into two sacs, each containing a single testis. The production and survival of sperm requires a temperature that is 1°C cooler than normal body temperature (37°C). This is achieved by the scrotum's exposed location.

The **penis**, or male organ of copulation and urination, is hairless, slightly pigmented, and cylindrical in shape. It consists of three compartments of erectile tissue. The corpus spongiosum surrounds the urethra and is located ventromedially. The two corpora cavernosa are located on the dorsolateral sides of the corpus spongiosum. Distally, the corpus spongiosum expands to form the **glans penis**, or the bulbous end of the penis. In the uncircumcised male, a fold of loose skin, the **prepuce** (foreskin), covers the glans penis. The corona forms the border between the glans penis and the penile shaft. The penis contains the urethra, a slitlike opening on the tip of the glans. The urethra terminates at the urethral meatus and is the passageway for urine.

The **spermatic cord** is made up of testicular arteries, autonomic nerves, veins that drain the testicles, lymphatic vessels, and the cremaster muscle. The testicles are suspended by the spermatic cord. The left side of the spermatic cord is longer than the right side, causing the left testicle to be lower in the scrotal sac. The cremaster muscle elevates the testes during sexual stimulation and exposure to cold. It also surrounds the testicles. The spermatic cord and ilioinguinal nerves pass through the inguinal canal into the abdomen. The inguinal canal is an oblique passageway in the anterior abdominal wall. The canal is about 4 to 5 cm (1.5 to 2 inches) long. It originates at the deep inguinal ring. The distal opening of the inguinal canal is called the external inguinal ring and is accessible to palpation. Superior to the inguinal canal lies the inguinal ligament, or Poupart's ligament. The inguinal ligament extends from the anterior iliac spine to the pubic tubercle.

Sexual Development

Sexual development can be assessed according to the five stages described by Tanner (see Table 21-1). Most of the changes in the male genitalia occur during puberty, starting between ages 9½ and 13½. The development of male genitalia to adult size and shape can take 2 to 5 years, with 3 years being the average.

Spermatogenesis

The primary function of the male reproductive system is to produce sperm to fertilize eggs. In order for this to be achieved, there are several essential features of male reproduction that must take place. These are the manufacture of sperm and the deposition of sperm into the female genital tract.

The testes produce sperm by a process called **spermatogenesis**. Specialized cells found between the seminiferous tubules, called the interstitial cells of Leydig, secrete the male hormone testosterone. Testosterone is sometimes called an androgen and is responsible for the development of secondary sexual characteristics and the attainment of reproductive capacity. Testosterone is responsible for male sexual feelings and performance as well as muscle development. The testes prepare for sperm production at approximately 13 years of age.

TABLE 21-1 Sexual Maturity Rating (SMR) for Male Genitalia

DEVELOPMENTAL STAGE	PUBIC HAIR	PENIS	SCROTUM
1.	No pubic hair, only fine body hair (vellus hair)	Preadolescent; childhood size and proportion	Preadolescent; childhood size and proportion
2.	Sparse growth of long, slightly dark, straight hair	Slight or no growth	Growth in testes and scrotum; scrotum reddens and changes texture
3.	Becomes darker and coarser; slightly curled and spreads over symphysis	Growth, especially in length	Further growth
4.	Texture and curl of pubic hair is similar to that of an adult but not spread to thighs	Further growth in length; diameter increases; development of glans	Further growth; scrotum darkens
5.	Adult appearance in quality and quantity of pubic hair; growth is spread to medial surface of thighs	Adult size and shape	Adult size and shape

MALE SEXUAL FUNCTION

The male sexual act consists of four stages: erection, lubrication, emission, and ejaculation. Erection of the penis is the first stage and is achieved through either physical or psychogenic stimulation of sensory nerves in the genital area. Parasympathetic impulses from the sacral portion of the spinal cord cause a vascular effect. The arterioles dilate and blood fills the corpora cavernosa, causing the penis to expand and become rigid. The corpora cavernosa can hold from 20 to 50 mL of blood. The veins from the tissue are compressed to occlude venous outflow.

Parasympathetic impulses at the same time cause the bulbourethral glands to secrete mucus, which provides lubrication during intercourse. When the sexual stimulus reaches a critical intensity, the reflex centers of the spinal cord send sympathetic impulses to the genital organs, and an orgasm occurs. Emission begins with contraction of the epididymis and the vas deferens, causing expulsion of sperm into the internal urethra. Ejaculation follows with contractions of the penile urethra.

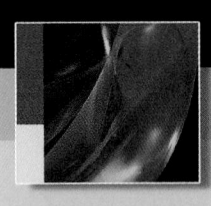

HEALTH HISTORY

The male genitalia health history provides insight into the link between a patient's life and lifestyle and male genitalia information and pathology.

PATIENT PROFILE   *Diseases that are age- and race-specific for the male genitalia are listed.*

Age
Chlamydia trachomatis (14–35)
Testicular torsion (12–25)
Varicocele (15–35)
Testicular cancer (16–35)
Gonococcal urethritis (< 35)
Epididymitis, sexually associated (< 35)
Epididymitis, urinary pathogens (> 35)
Hydrocele (> 30)
Spermatocele (> 30)
Testicular lymphoma (50+)
Erectile dysfunction (50+)
Bacteriuria (> 65)

Race

Caucasians   Testicular cancer

CHIEF COMPLAINT   *Common chief complaints for the male genitalia are defined and information on the characteristics of each sign or symptom is provided.*

1. Urethral Discharge   Excretion of substance from the urethra

Quality   Color: clear, white, purulent, blood-tinged, green, yellow, pink; consistency: thin, moderate, thick, mucoid; foul odor

Quantity   Absent, scant, mild, moderate, copious

continues

Health History (continued)

Associated Manifestations	Dysuria, painful ejaculation, fever, urethral meatal discharge, change in frequency of urination, pruritus, conjunctivitis, arthritis, dermatological rash, STD
Aggravating Factors	Urethral trauma
Alleviating Factors	Medications (antibiotics, analgesics)
Setting	A new sexual partner in the last 6 months, multiple partners, a partner known to have other partners, unprotected intercourse
Timing	More prominent in the morning before urinating
2. Palpable Mass	A lump in the male genitalia
Quality	Firm, smooth, stellate, soft, mobile, nonmobile, well circumscribed, poorly circumscribed, "bag of worms," hard, heavy, transilluminating, nontransilluminating, fluctuant, separate from testes
Associated Manifestations	Pain, scrotal enlargement, absence of pain, vague back or abdominal pain, gynecomastia (if mass produces estrogen or human chorionic gonadotropin), nausea, vomiting, generalized edema
Aggravating Factors	Positioning, palpation or pressure, obesity, lifting, edema
Alleviating Factors	Medications, surgical removal or repair, positioning
Setting	Post-trauma, recurrent testicular pain
Timing	Mumps orchitis present 7–10 days following parotitis
3. Scrotal Pain	Discomfort in the scrotal sac
Quality	Dull, sharp, heavy
Associated Manifestations	Scrotal swelling, groin pain, lower abdominal pain, flank pain, dysuria, urinary frequency, fever, nausea, vomiting, pyuria, urethral discharge, scrotal edema, erythema, infertility
Aggravating Factors	Sexual encounter, urinary tract infection, scrotal trauma
Alleviating Factors	Medications (antibiotics, analgesics), bed rest, scrotal elevation, surgery
Setting	New sexual partner months prior, unprotected intercourse, recent urinary instrumentation
Timing	Epididymitis may present months following a new or unprotected sexual encounter; it may also present shortly after a urinary tract infection.
4. Erectile Dysfunction	The inability or decrease in ability to achieve and maintain a penile erection or to ejaculate seminal fluid
Quality	Inability to achieve erection (failed nocturnal tumescence test), ability to achieve with failure to maintain erection, inability to achieve complete erection, inability to ejaculate
Associated Manifestations	Anxiety, systemic disease (diabetes mellitus, hypertension, coronary artery disease), decreased libido, phimosis, decreased or absent cremasteric reflex, decreased femoral pulses, trauma, recent transurethral resection of the prostate or prostatectomy surgery, testicular atrophy

continues

Health History (continued)

Aggravating Factors	Medications (beta blockers, diuretics, reserpine, monoamine oxidase inhibitors, selective serotonin reuptake inhibitors, diazepam, alprazolam, chemotherapeutic agents, codeine, Darvon, Percocet), anxiety, unsupportive partner, alcohol, smoking, elevated blood sugar, hyperthyroidism, hypothyroidism
Alleviating Factors	Medications (hormone therapy, yohimbine, anxiolytics, sildenafil, alprostadil), injections, implants, vascular surgery, sex counseling, avoiding alcohol, smoking cessation, change in diet (avoiding foods high in saturated fat or cholesterol), maintaining ideal body weight, reducing tension and stress, vacuum erectile device
Setting	Uncomfortable physical environment, stress
Timing	Nocturnal tumescence
5. Penile Lesion	A growth on the penis
Quality	Color: erythematous, hyperpigmented, hypopigmented, pink, brown, black; presentation: flat, raised, indurated, papular, macular, multiple, isolated, ulcerated, warty, exudative (clear, purulent, bloody drainage)
Associated Manifestations	Fever, malaise, inguinal lymphadenopathy, pain, prodromal numbness and tingling at lesion site, myalgias, headache, pruritus, immunosuppression, systemic illness, recurrent herpes simplex virus (HSV), human papillomavirus (HPV)
Aggravating Factors	Stress, systemic illness, immunosuppression
Alleviating Factors	Medications (antivirals, antibiotics), surgical removal, lifestyle changes
Setting	Unprotected intercourse, multiple sexual partners
Timing	Lymphogranuloma venereum: papule appears 1–3 weeks after inoculation; primary HSV: lesions appear 2–7 days after inoculation, vesicles ulcerate in 3–4 days; recurrent HSV: lesions appear a few hours to days after prodromal symptoms, lesions last approximately 10 days
PAST HEALTH HISTORY	*The various components of the past health history are linked to male genitalia pathology and male genitalia-related information.*
Medical History	
Male Genitalia Specific	Prior history of sexually transmitted disease (STD), prostatitis, urinary tract infection, nephrolithiasis, cryptorchidism, trauma, cancer, benign prostatic hypertrophy (BPH), congenital or acquired deformity (epispadias, hypospadias), premature ejaculation, impotence, infertility
Nonmale Genitalia Specific	Mumps, rashes, joint pain, conjunctivitis, viral illness, renal disease, congestive heart failure, spinal cord injury, pelvic fracture, diabetes mellitus, hypertension, tuberculosis, multiple sclerosis, depression, anxiety
Surgical History	Prostatectomy, transurethral prostatectomy, circumcision, orchiectomy, correction of malposition of testes, vasectomy, lesion or nodule removal, epispadias repair, hypospadias repair, hernia repair
Allergies	Contact dermatitis from topical preparations, condoms, nonoxynol 9 or other spermicides

continues

Health History (continued)

Medications	Antibiotics, hormone replacements, 5-alpha-reductase inhibitors, antihypertensives, psychotropic agents
Communicable Diseases	HSV, HPV, molluscum contagiosum, condyloma acuminata, syphilis, penile lesion, chlamydia, gonorrhea, ureaplasma
Injuries and Accidents	Trauma, testicular torsion
Special Needs	Urinary incontinence, indwelling or intermittent urinary catheter, penile prosthesis, suprapubic urinary catheter
Childhood Illnesses	Mumps: orchitis, infertility
FAMILY HEALTH HISTORY	*Male genitalia diseases that are familial are listed.*
	Varicocele, testicular cancer, hypospadias, infertility, mother's use of hormones (diethylstilbestrol [DES]) during pregnancy
SOCIAL HISTORY	*The components of the social history are linked to male genitalia factors and pathology.*
Alcohol Use	Impairs gonadotropin release and accelerates testosterone metabolism, causing impotence and loss of libido; large doses can acutely depress the sexual reflexes; chronic alcoholism causes high levels of circulating estrogens, which decrease libido; alcohol intoxication may impair judgment, decreasing incidence of safe-sex practices and increasing risk of exposure to STDs.
Tobacco Use	Cigarette smoking increases risk of atherosclerotic disease, which may decrease penile blood flow; it is also associated with an increased risk of bladder cancer.
Drug Use	May impair judgment, increasing the risk for unsafe sex practices and STD exposure Cocaine: priapism with chronic abuse, impotence, increased sexual excitability Barbiturates: impotence Amphetamines: increased libido and delayed orgasm in moderate users, impotence in chronic users
Sexual Practice	Multiple partners, partner with multiple partners, new sexual partner, condom use (frequency and accuracy of use), sexual orientation, anal or oral intercourse
Work Environment	Radiation exposure has been linked to cancer of the male genitalia.
HEALTH MAINTENANCE ACTIVITIES	*This information provides a bridge between the health maintenance activities and male genitalia function.*
Sleep	Nocturia secondary to urethritis
Diet	Erectile dysfunction: foods high in saturated fat or cholesterol
Exercise	Trauma to the testicle may cause a hydrocele
Use of Safety Devices	Condoms used for vaginal and anal intercourse; supportive device worn while participating in sports
Health Check-ups	Testicular exam

EQUIPMENT

- Nonsterile gloves
- Penlight
- Stethoscope
- Culturette tube
- Sterile cotton swabs
- Chux
- 1½ "–2" gauze wrap
- Five percent acetic acid solution in spray bottle
- Thayer-Martin plate
- Gen probe
- 10× power magnifying lens

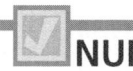

Sensitivity during the Male Genitalia Examination

Before beginning the genitalia examination, consider your patient's cultural background and what beliefs or attitudes he may have about having the examination. Does the patient's culture prohibit a female nurse from examining a male patient? Does the patient's culture prohibit a male nurse from examining a male patient?

ASSESSMENT OF THE MALE GENITALIA

✅ NURSINGCHECKLIST

General Approach to Male Genitalia Assessment

1. Greet the patient and explain the assessment techniques that you will be using.
2. Ensure that the examination room is at a warm, comfortable temperature to prevent patient chilling and shivering.
3. Use a quiet room that will be free from interruptions.
4. Ensure that the light in the room provides sufficient brightness to adequately observe the patient.
5. Assess the patient's apprehension level about the assessment and address this with him, reassuring him that this is normal.
6. Instruct the patient to remove his pants and underpants.
7. Place the patient on the examination table in the supine position with the legs spread slightly, and cover with a drape sheet. Stand to the patient's right side or have the patient stand in front of you while you are sitting.
8. Don clean gloves.
9. Expose the entire genital and groin area.

INSPECTION

Sexual Maturity Rating

E 1. Using the Tanner stages in Table 21-1, assess the developmental stage of the pubic hair, penis, and scrotum.

2. Determine the Sexual Maturity Rating.

N Males usually begin puberty between the ages of 9½ and 13½ . The average male proceeds through puberty in about 3 years, with a possible range of 2 to 5 years.

A An SMR that is less than expected for a male's age is abnormal.

P Delayed puberty may be familial or caused by chronic illnesses.

A A normally formed but diminutive penis is abnormal. There is a discrepancy between the penile size and the age of the individual.

P A **microphallus** can result from a disorder in the hypothalamus or pituitary gland. It may be secondary to primary testicular failure due to partial androgen insensitivity. Maternal DES exposure has teratogenic effects caused by defects in nonandrogen-dependent regulatory agents. Microphallus can also be idiopathic in nature.

A It is abnormal when the penis appears larger than what is generally expected for the stated age. This condition is usually evident only before the age of normal puberty.

P Hormonal influence of tumors of the pineal gland or hypothalamus, tumors of the Leydig cells of the testes, tumors of the adrenal gland, or precocious genital maturity may cause penile hyperplasia.

A A testicle that is smaller and softer than normal (less than 5 cm × 2.5 cm [2 in. × 1 in.]) is abnormal.

P An atrophic testicle may be the result of Klinefelter's syndrome (hypogonadism), hypopituitarism, estrogen therapy, or orchitis.

| **E** Examination | **N** Normal Findings | **A** Abnormal Findings | **P** Pathophysiology |

NURSING**TIP**

Hygiene for the Uncircumcised Male

During the penis examination, it is important to review proper hygiene. Instruct the patient to retract the foreskin daily so that the underlying skin can be washed with soap and warm water. The skin should also be dried thoroughly and the foreskin returned to its original position.

NURSING**ALERT**

Risk Factors for Penile Cancer

- 50–70 years of age
- Intact foreskin
- Poor hygiene
- History of HPV types 16 and 18

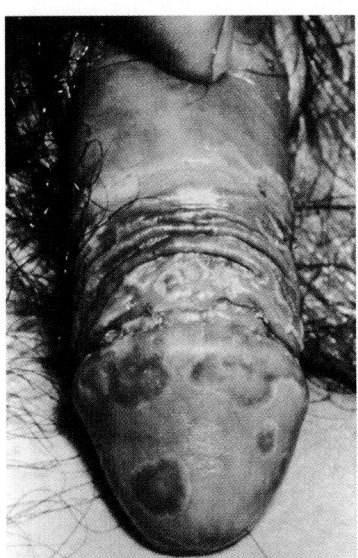

FIGURE 21-3 Balanitis of the Glans Penis. *Courtesy of the Centers for Disease Control and Prevention (CDC).*

Hair Distribution

E **1.** Note hair distribution pattern.

2. Note the presence of nits or lice.

N Pubic hair is distributed in a triangular form. It is sparsely distributed on the scrotum and inner thigh and absent on the penis. Genital hair is more coarse than scalp hair. There are no nits or lice.

A Hair distribution is sparse or hair is absent at the genitalia area. This is called **alopecia** and it is abnormal.

P Alopecia in the genital area may result from genetic factors, aging, or local or systemic disease. These include developmental defects and hereditary disorders, infection, neoplasms, physical or chemical agents, endocrine diseases, deficiency states (nutritional or metabolic), destruction, or damage to the follicles.

A The presence of nits or lice is abnormal.

P See Chapter 10.

Penis

E **1.** Inspect the glans, foreskin, and shaft for lesions, swelling, and inflammation. If the patient is uncircumcised, ask him to retract the foreskin so that the underlying area can be inspected. After the assessment, replace the foreskin.

2. Inspect the anterior surface of the penis first. Then lift the penis to check the posterior surface.

3. Note the shape of the penis.

N Skin is free of lesions and inflammation. The shaft skin appears loose and wrinkled in the male without an erection. The glans is smooth and without lesions, swelling, and inflammation. The foreskin retracts easily and there is no discharge. There may be a small amount of **smegma**, a white, cottage cheeselike substance, present. The dorsal vein is sometimes visible. The penis is cylindrical in shape. The glans penis varies in size and shape and may appear rounded or broad.

A Inflammation of the glans penis is abnormal.

P This inflammation is called balanitis. The prepuce may also be affected. This is a bacterial infection that is associated with phimosis and is seen in diabetic men.

P Balanitis can occur with sexually transmitted diseases. The patient in Figure 21-3 had balanitis of the glans penis from a chlamydial infection (nongonococcal urethritis) caused by *C. trachomatis*.

LIFE 360°

Gaining Confidence with the Male Genitalia Examination

Female nurses may feel anxious about examining male genitalia. Before you can help your patient talk comfortably about his concerns, you need to work through your own feelings to reach a level of comfort about sexuality and reproduction. Work through any reluctance you may have about discussing sexual situations by:

- Practicing phrasing questions
- Practicing interviewing a male friend or fellow student
- Practicing using correct terminology
- Familiarizing yourself with lay and slang terms

REFLECTIVE THINKING

Embarrassing Situations Encountered during the Male Genitalia Assessment

The genitalia examination may cause the patient to feel uncomfortable or embarrassed. How would you handle the following situations if they were to occur during the genitalia assessment?

- The patient has an erection during the examination.
- The patient asks you if you would like to go out with him for dinner.

A A small papular lesion that enlarges and undergoes superficial necrosis to produce a sharply marginated ulcer on a clean base is abnormal (Figure 21-4).

P The **chancre** is the lesion of primary syphilis. It contains a multitude of *Treponema pallidum* spirochetes and is highly infectious. The tissue reacts to the organism with infiltration of lymphocytes, fibroblasts, and plasma cells that cause swelling and proliferation of the endothelial tissue, manifesting as a chancre.

A A tender, painful, ulcerated, exudative, papular lesion with an erythematous halo, surrounding edema, and a friable base is abnormal (Figure 21-5).

P **Chancroid** is caused by inoculation of *Haemophilus ducreyi* through small breaks in epidermal tissue. Acute inflammatory response causes bubo formation. This is usually accompanied by inguinal adenopathy.

A Penile lesion that ranges from a relatively subtle induration to a small papule, pustule, warty growth, or exophytic lesion is abnormal. The distribution of lesions is most commonly on the glans and prepuce.

P Penile carcinoma usually begins with a small lesion that gradually extends to involve the entire glans, shaft, and corpora. Circumcision has been well established as a prophylactic measure that will eliminate the occurrence of penile carcinoma.

A Pinhead papules to cauliflower-like groupings of filiform, skin-colored, pink, or red lesions are abnormal (Figure 21-6).

P **Condyloma acuminatum** (genital warts) are caused by HPV infection of the epithelial cells. HPV may remain dormant for months to years after infection. There is a high incidence of recurrence of condyloma following appropriate treatment because of the persistence of latent HPV in normal-appearing skin. Lesions may be visualized by using acetowhitening. Refer to the Advanced Technique on Acetowhitening.

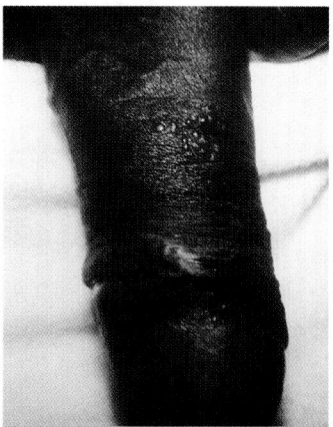

FIGURE 21-4 Syphilitic Chancre. *Courtesy of the Centers for Disease Control and Prevention (CDC).*

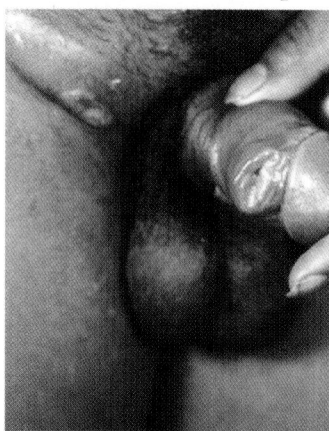

FIGURE 21-5 Chancroid of the Penis with Right Inguinal Lymphadenopathy. *Courtesy of the Centers for Disease Control and Prevention (CDC).*

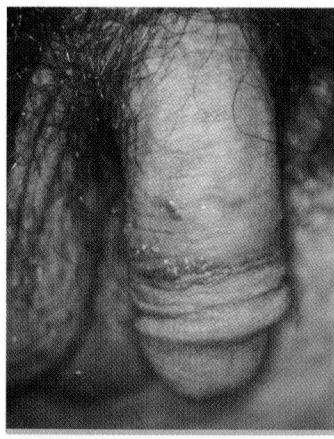

FIGURE 21-6 Genital Warts. *Courtesy of the Centers for Disease Control and Prevention (CDC).*

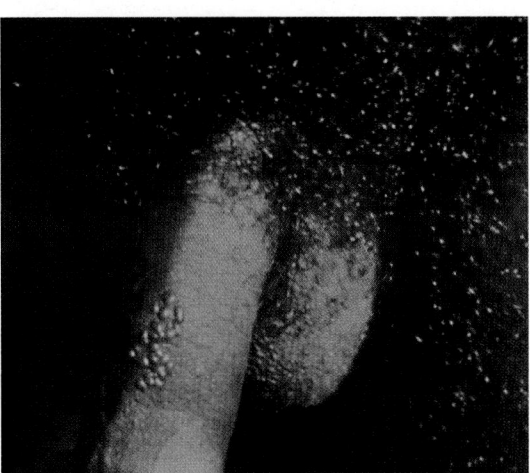

FIGURE 21-7A Herpes Simplex Virus of the Penis. *Courtesy of the Centers for Disease Control and Prevention (CDC).*

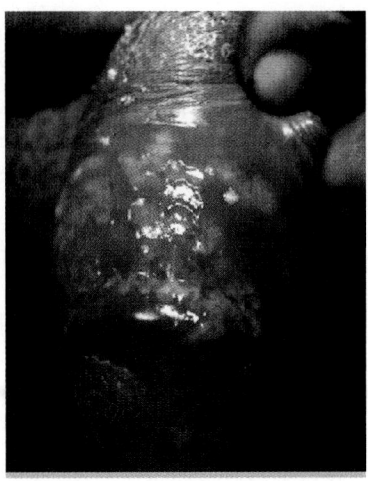

FIGURE 21-7B Primary Herpes Simplex Virus, First Episode. Serology test are negative for HSV. *Copyright GlaxoSmithKline. Used with permission.*

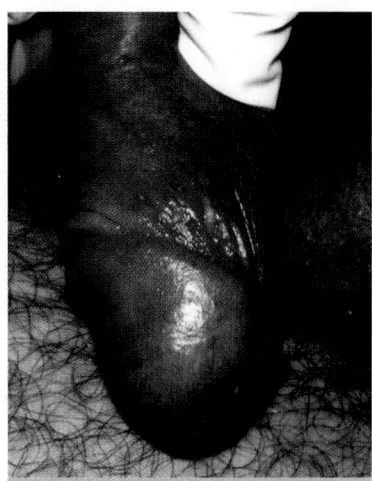

FIGURE 21-7C Nonprimary Herpes Simplex Virus, First Episode. Serology tests are positive for HSV (type 1 or type 2), meaning the patient has had a previous exposure to the virus at another body site. This patient had a cold sore (herpes labialis) **2 years ago.** *Copyright GlaxoSmithKline. Used with permission.*

A Multifocal maculopapular lesions that are tan, brown, pink, violet, or white are abnormal.

P This describes intraepithelial neoplasia. HPV oncogenic types 16, 18, 31, and 33 infection causes epidermal proliferation and koilocytotic, dyskeratotic cells. Female partners may have a history of cervical intraepithelial neoplasm (CIN). The majority of lesions are distributed on the glans penis and prepuce. Changes of squamous cell carcinoma in situ are seen on histological examination.

A Erythematous, painful ulcers developing into vesicular lesions that may become pustular, are abnormal (Figure 21-7).

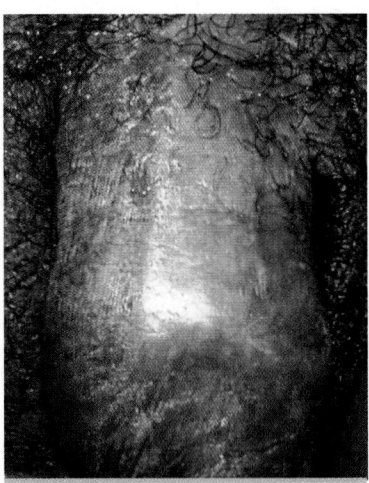

FIGURE 21-7D Recurrent HSV. After the initial, primary outbreak, frequent recurrences (four to eight episodes per year) can occur at the primary outbreak site. This outbreak was the second episode in 4 months for this patient. *Copyright GlaxoSmithKline. Used with permission.*

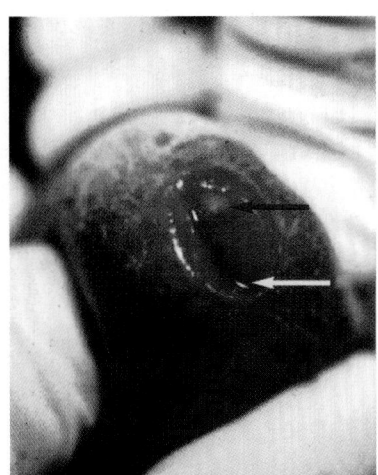

FIGURE 21-7E Atypical Recurrent HSV Presentation. The black arrow points to the Herpetic urethritis, and the yellow arrow points to the urethral discharge. *Copyright GlaxoSmithKline. Used with permission.*

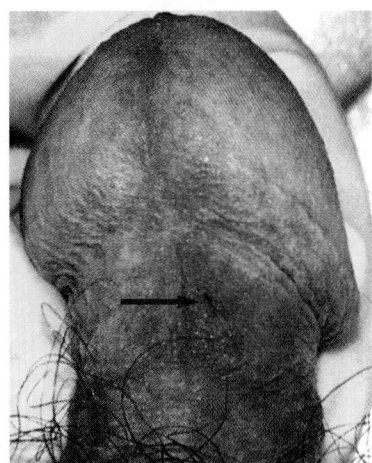

FIGURE 21-7F Atypical Recurrent HSV Presentation. The arrow points to a healed crusted lesion surrounded by erythema. *Copyright GlaxoSmithKline. Used with permission.*

| **E** Examination | **N** Normal Findings | **A** Abnormal Findings | **P** Pathophysiology |

LIFE ⊚ 360°

Male Sexual Assault

You need to be aware of the possibility that your male patients have experienced male sexual assault (MSA). MSA is forced intercourse or sexual contact that occurs without consent by another person. MSA includes fondling, forced anal sex, forced oral sex, stimulation of an erection, stimulation of ejaculation, and oral-to-anal contact. Patients may present with genital injuries, lacerations to the anal sphincter, rectal tears, fissures, or hematomas. Nongenital injuries may include a black eye, fractured jaw, cerebral concussion, or facial contusions/lacerations. MSA victims may experience confusion about their sexual orientation, nightmares, suicidal ideation, and self-blame. You may need to offer the patient referral to a therapist or counselor.

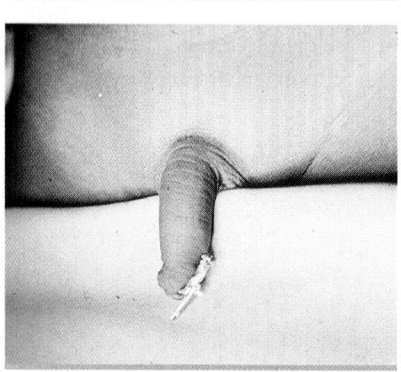

FIGURE 21-8 **Phimosis.** *Courtesy of Dr. James Mandell, Children's Hospital, Boston, MA.*

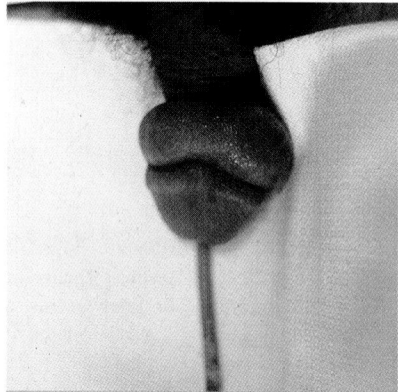

FIGURE 21-9 **Paraphimosis.** *Courtesy of Dr. James Mandell, Children's Hospital, Boston, MA.*

P This describes genital herpes simplex virus infection. Skin-to-skin contact infection of HSV 1 and 2 causes epidermal degeneration, acanthosis, and intraepidermal vesicles. Lesions become ulcerated and eroded and are moist or crusted. Epithelial changes resolve in 2 to 4 weeks and hyper- or hypopigmentation of these areas is common. Postinflammatory scarring is rare. Recurrent herpes lesions are smaller. Diagnosis may be confirmed by Tzanck test for microscopic acanthocytes, viral culture, or serology for HSV antibodies.

A Multiple, discrete, flat pustules with slight scaling and surrounding edema are abnormal.

P *Candida* is a superficial mycotic infection of moist cutaneous sites. Predisposing factors include moisture, diabetes mellitus, antibiotic therapy, and deficiencies in systemic immunity.

A Erythematous plaques with scaling; papular lesions with sharp margins, and occasionally clear centers; and pustules are abnormal.

P Tinea cruris is a fungal infection of the groin, usually caused by *Epidermophyton floccosum* or *Trichophyton rubrum*. Predisposing factors are a warm, humid environment, tight clothing, and obesity.

A An unusually long foreskin or one that cannot be retracted over the glans penis is abnormal.

P **Phimosis** occurs in uncircumcised males (Figure 21-8). Inability to retract the foreskin is normal in infancy. In later years, an acquired constricting circumferential scar may follow healing of a split foreskin.

A It is abnormal when the retracted foreskin develops a fixed constriction proximal to the glans (Figure 21-9). The penis distal to the foreskin may become swollen and gangrenous.

P This is called **paraphimosis**. If the foreskin is retracted and not returned to its original position, paraphimosis can ensue (e.g., a patient's penis is cleansed for indwelling catheter insertion and the foreskin remains retracted). The foreskin acts as a circulatory constrictor, causing decreased blood flow, edema, and potential tissue necrosis.

A A continuous and pathological erection of the penis is abnormal.

P The cause of **priapism** is unclear in most patients; however, it does not occur as the result of sexual desire. Some of the cases are associated with leukemia, metastatic carcinoma, sickle cell anemia, intracavernous injection, alcohol abuse, genital trauma, and neurologic disorders. Some drugs, such as antihypertensives, antipsychotics, and antidepressants, have also been associated with prolonged erections. The patient may also present after having used a medication for erectile dysfunction. Priapism is created by the positive imbalance between the arterial blood supply and its return, created by venous drainage.

A Penile curvature, or chordee, is either a ventral or a dorsal curvature of the penis and is abnormal.

P Curvature is usually congenitally caused by a fibrous band along the usual course of the corpus spongiosum. Ventral chordee is seen mostly with **epispadias** (see Figure 21-10), when the urethral meatus opens dorsally on the glans. In cases of congenital penile curvature without epispadias

---

E Examination   **N** Normal Findings   **A** Abnormal Findings   **P** Pathophysiology

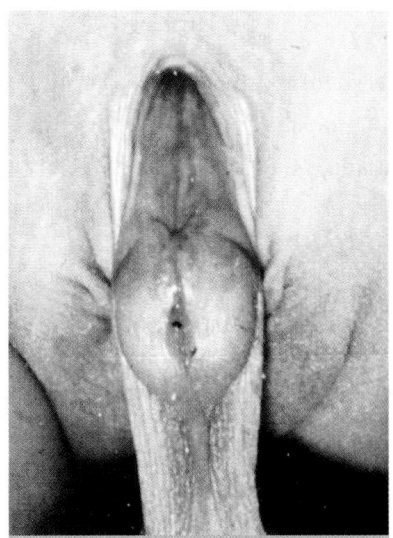

FIGURE 21-10 **Epispadias.** *Courtesy of Dr. James Mandell, Children's Hospital, Boston, MA.*

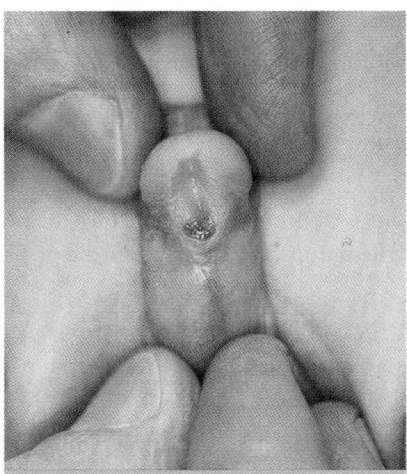

FIGURE 21-11 **Hypospadias.** *Courtesy of Dr. James Mandell, Children's Hospital, Boston, MA.*

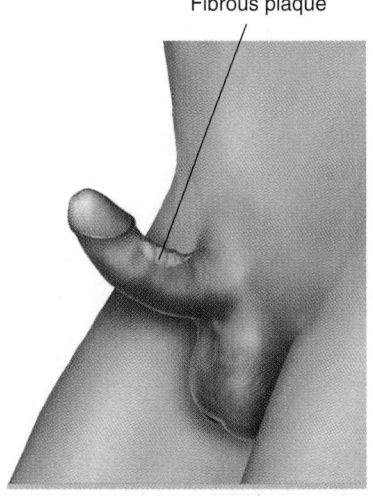

Fibrous plaque

FIGURE 21-12 **Dorsal Curvature of the Penis in Peyronie's Disease**

NURSING**ALERT**

Warning Signs of STDs in the Male Patient

- Urethral discharge, bloody or purulent
- Scrotal or testicular pain
- Burning or pain during urination
- Penile lesion

or **hypospadias** (when the urethral meatus opens ventrally on the glans), there is no additional tissue on or in any portion of the corpora cavernosa (Figure 21-11). This is caused by congenital maldevelopment of the tunica albuginea of the corpora.

P Peyronie's disease is a condition of penile curvature that occurs with erection (Figure 21-12). The dorsal surface of the corpora cavernosa becomes hardened with palpable, nontender plaques. Its cause is unknown.

ADVANCED TECHNIQUE

Acetowhitening: Assessing for HPV

The purpose of acetowhitening is to identify warty skin lesions that are not easily seen by the naked eye. It is indicated with a history of warts or HPV, of sexual contact with partner with warts or HPV, of high-risk sexual behavior, or of STD. The goal of treatment is the removal of exophytic warts and the elimination of signs and symptoms, not the eradication of HPV.

Equipment: clean gloves, 10× power magnifying lens, Chux, 1½"–2" gauze wrap, scissors, and 5% acetic acid solution (white vinegar) in spray bottle

E 1. Explain the procedure to the patient.

2. Have the patient undress from the waist down and sit on Chux at the edge of the examination table.

3. Wash hands. Don gloves.

4. Have the patient lie supine.

5. Wrap the penis and the scrotal area with gauze wrap that has been impregnated with 5% acetic acid solution.

6. Allow the area to soak in the saturated gauze for 5 minutes.

7. Remove the gauze from the penis and scrotal areas.

8. Examine the penis and scrotum with a magnifying lens.

N The penis and scrotal area should be free of any whitish-appearing areas.

A Condyloma acuminatum (HPV) appears as tiny white papules identified with a 10× hand lens.

P The "acetowhite" lesions are not always due to HPV, and the patient should be referred for a biopsy to confirm the diagnosis.

P Refer to the prior discussion on HPV infection.

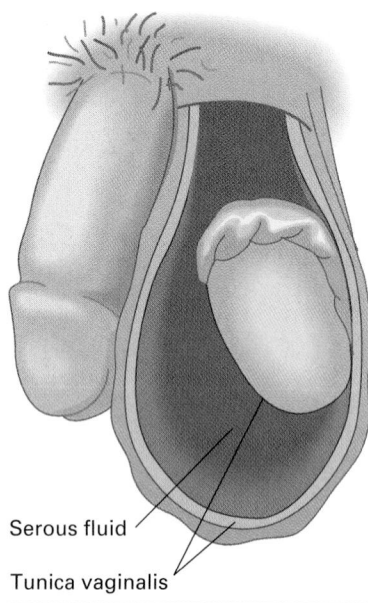

Serous fluid

Tunica vaginalis

FIGURE 21-13 **Hydrocele**

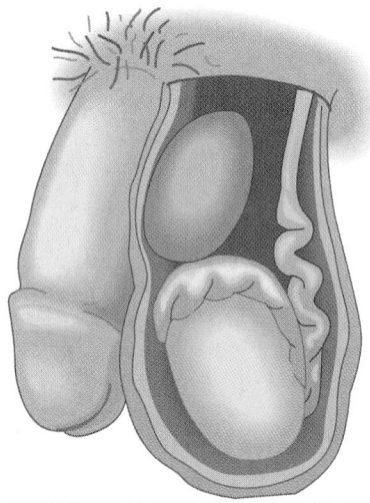

FIGURE 21-14 **Spermatocle**

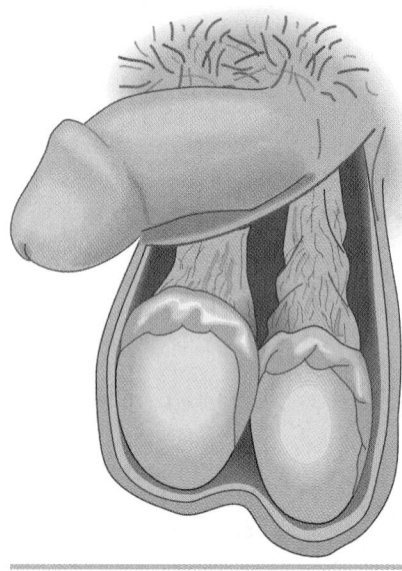

FIGURE 21-15 **Varicocele**

Scrotum

E 1. Displace the penis to one side in order to inspect the scrotal skin.

2. Lift up the scrotum to inspect the posterior side.

3. Observe for lesions, inflammation, swelling, and nodules.

4. Note size and shape.

5. The patient should then stand with legs slightly spread apart.

6. Have the patient perform the Valsalva maneuver.

7. Observe for a mass of dilated testicular veins in the spermatic cord above and behind the testes.

N Scrotal skin appears rugated and thin and more deeply pigmented than body color. The skin should hug the testicles firmly in the young male and become elongated and flaccid in the elderly male. All skin areas should be free of any lesions, nodules, swelling, or inflammation. Scrotal size and shape vary greatly from one individual to another. The left scrotal sac is lower than the right. There should be no dilated testicular veins.

A/P Condyloma acuminatum, tinea cruris, and *Candida* are abnormal findings. See prior discussion.

A Enlargement of or masses within the scrotum are abnormal.

P Scrotal masses can arise from benign or malignant conditions. Scrotal swelling is seen with inguinal hernia, hydrocele, varicocele, spermatocele, tumor, and edema.

A A large, pear-sized mass in the scrotum is abnormal (Figure 21-13). The scrotal skin is stretched, shiny, and erythematous, which may give the penis a shortened appearance.

P A **hydrocele** is created by the accumulation of fluid between the two layers of the tunica vaginalis. Hydroceles may be idiopathic or due to trauma, inguinal surgery, epididymitis, or testicular tumor.

A A well-defined cystic mass on the superior testis or in the epididymis is abnormal. It is usually < 2 cm (¾ inch) in diameter (Figure 21-14). Multiple masses may be present.

P This is called **spermatocele**. Blockage of the efferent ductules of the rete testis causes formation of sperm-filled cysts at the top of the testis or in the epididymis.

A In light-skinned individuals, a scrotal mass with a bluish discoloration is abnormal (Figure 21-15).

P Dilated veins in the pampiniform plexus of the spermatic cord cause **varicocele** formation and are usually accompanied by a decreased sperm count. Most appear in the left hemiscrotum; the remainder are bilateral. A right-sided varicocele may be indicative of an obstruction at the vena cava. Acute onset of a right-sided varicocele may be pathognomonic for a renal tumor extending into the renal vein or compression of the renal vein. It may increase in size with the Valsalva maneuver and decrease or disappear with supine positioning.

A Round, firm, cystic nodules confined within the scrotal skin are abnormal.

P A sebaceous cyst contains sebum, an oily, fatty matter secreted by the sebaceous glands. The cyst may result from a decrease in localized circulation and closure of sebaceous glands or ducts.

Urethral Meatus

E 1. Note the location of the urethral meatus.

2. Observe for discharge.

3. Obtain a culture of any discharge (see Advanced Technique on Urethral Culture).

4. If the patient complains of penile discharge but none is present, ask the patient to milk the penis from the shaft to the glans. This maneuver may express a discharge that can then be cultured.

N The urethral meatus is located centrally. It is pink and without discharge.

A Erythema and swelling at the urethral meatus are abnormal.

P Urethritis is a localized tissue inflammation resulting from bacterial, viral, or fungal infection as well as from urethral trauma.

A It is abnormal for the urethral meatus to be displaced dorsally (see Figure 21-10).

P Epispadias is a congenital abnormality caused by a complete or partial dorsal fusion defect of the urethra.

A It is abnormal for the urethral meatus to open on the ventral aspect of the glans penis (see Figure 21-11). The urethral meatus may also open at the perineum.

P Hypospadias is a congenital abnormality, usually associated with chordee. Complications of this defect include urethral meatal stenosis, inability to direct the urine stream, and sexual dysfunction.

Inguinal Area

E 1. If the patient is supine, ask the patient to stand.

2. Stand facing the patient.

3. Observe for swelling or bulges.

4. Ask the patient to bear down.

5. Observe for swelling or bulges.

N The inguinal area is free of any swelling or bulges.

A A bulge in the inguinal area is abnormal.

P Hernia pathology is discussed further in the section on palpation.

PALPATION
Penis

E 1. Stand in front of the patient's genital area.

2. Don clean gloves.

3. Between the thumb and the first two fingers, palpate the entire length of the penis (Figure 21-16).

4. Note any pulsations, tenderness, masses, or plaques.

N Pulsations are present on the dorsal sides of the penis. The penis is nontender. No masses or firm plaques are palpated.

A It is abnormal to palpate fibrotic plaques or ridges along the dorsal shaft.

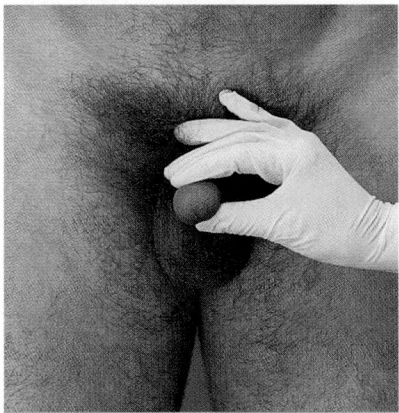

FIGURE 21-16 Palpation of the Penis

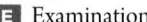 Examination   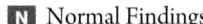 Normal Findings   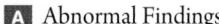 Abnormal Findings   **P** Pathophysiology

P Plaques develop from perivascular inflammation between the tunica albuginea and the underlying spongy erectile tissue.

A Vascular insufficiency is evidenced by diminished or absent palpable pulse or pulsations and is abnormal.

P Systemic disease, localized trauma, and localized disease may adversely affect normal blood flow in the penis.

A It is abnormal for the penis to be enlarged in a nonerect state. Generalized penile swelling may be present.

P Fluid accumulation in the loose tissue of the penile integument results from anasarcic states. Obstruction of the penile veins or inflammation of the penis results in local edema. Trauma to the penis may cause swelling secondary to penile contusion and extravasation of blood. Gentle finger pressure may cause pitting.

Urethral Meatus

E 1. Stand in front of the patient's genital area.

2. Between the thumb and forefinger, grasp the glans and gently squeeze to expose the meatus (Figure 21-17).

3. If discharge is seen, or if the patient complains of a urethral discharge, a culture should be taken.

N The urethral meatus is free of discharge and drainage.

A A urethral discharge of pus and mucus shreds is abnormal (Figure 21-18). The discharge may vary in color, consistency, and amount.

P Bacterial infection of the genitourinary tract causes inflammation and formation of a liquid composed of albuminous substances, leukocytes, shedding tissue cells, and bacteria.

Scrotum

E 1. Between the thumb and the first two fingers, gently palpate the left testicle (Figure 21-19).

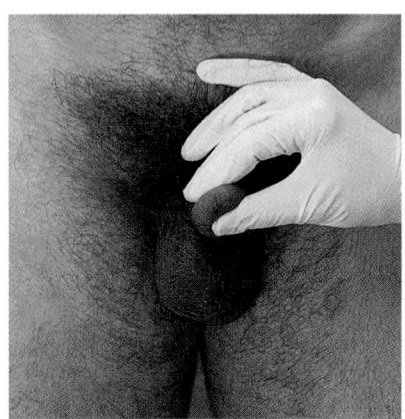

FIGURE 21-17 Palpation of the Urethral Meatus

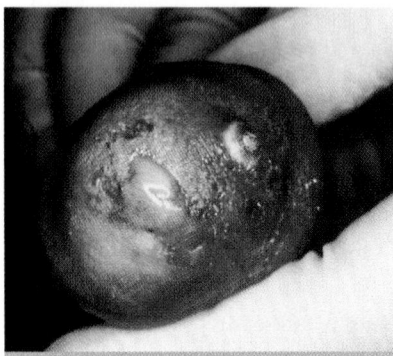

FIGURE 21-18 Purulent Penile Discharge from Gonorrhea. *Courtesy of the Centers for Disease Control and Prevention (CDC).*

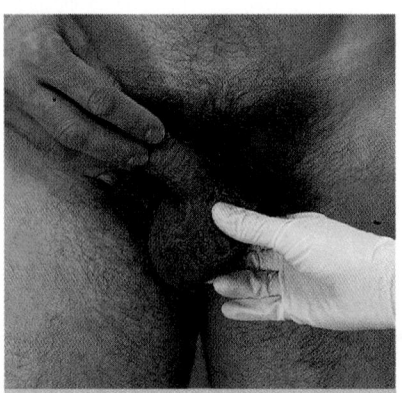

FIGURE 21-19 Palpation of the Testicle

ADVANCED TECHNIQUE

Urethral Culture: Identifying Penile Pathogens

Equipment: sterile cotton swabs, Culturette tube, Thayer-Martin plate.

E 1. Explain to the patient what you are going to do and that some discomfort may be involved.

2. Place the patient in the supine position.

3. Note the color, consistency, and odor of the discharge.

4. With the nondominant hand, hold the penis. With the dominant hand, roll a sterile cotton swab in the discharge.

5. Place the swab in a Culturette tube.

6. With a second sterile cotton swab, obtain another specimen for a gonorrheal culture.

7. Roll the swab over a Thayer-Martin plate in a "Z" pattern.

8. Label both cultures and send them to the laboratory for analysis.

E Examination   **N** Normal Findings   **A** Abnormal Findings   **P** Pathophysiology

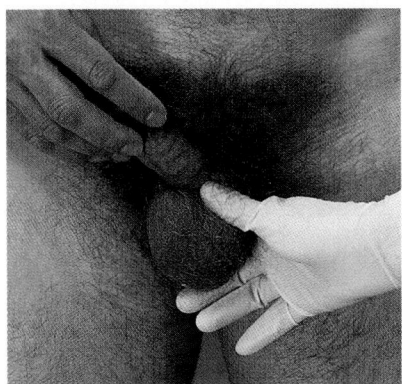

FIGURE 21-20 **Palpation of the Epididymis**

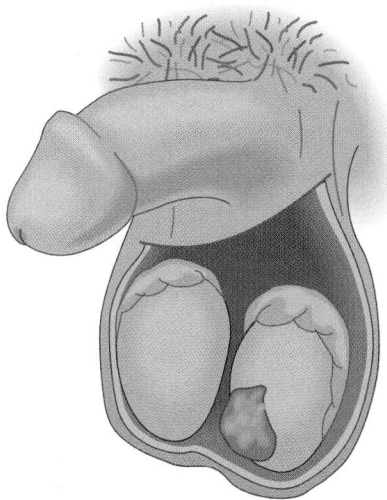

FIGURE 21-21 **Testicular Tumor**

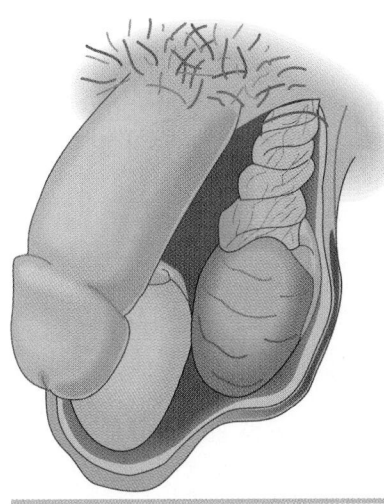

FIGURE 21-22 **Testicular Torsion**

2. Note the size, shape, consistency, and presence of masses.

3. Palpate the epididymis (Figure 21-20).

4. Note the consistency and presence of tenderness or masses.

5. Between the thumb and the first two fingers, palpate the spermatic cord from the epididymis to the external ring.

6. Note the consistency and presence of tenderness or masses.

7. Repeat on the left side.

N The scrotum contains on each side a testicle and an epididymis. The testicles should be firm but not hard, ovoid, smooth, and equal in size bilaterally. They should be sensitive to pressure but not tender. The epididymis is comma-shaped and should be distinguishable from the testicle. The epididymis should be insensitive to pressure. The spermatic cord should feel smooth and round.

A A unilateral mass palpated within or about the testicle is abnormal (Figure 21-21).

P Intratesticular masses should be considered malignant until proven otherwise. They are nodular and associated with painless swelling. The majority of intratesticular masses arise from germinal elements. Extratesticular tumors are uncommon and usually are benign. They can arise from any of the surrounding structures, including the epididymis, the testicular tunica vaginalis, or the spermatic cord. Testicular cancer should be suspected if a hard, fixed nodule is palpated.

P Inguinal hernia is discussed in the section entitled Inguinal Area.

P Refer to the section on scrotal inspection for a description of spermatocele.

A A large, pear-shaped mass that has a smooth wall is abnormal.

P Refer to the section on scrotal inspection for a description of hydrocele. The entire testicle must be palpated because underlying malignancies cause a small percentage of all hydroceles. Sonography must be performed if the entire testicle is not palpable.

A A soft testis is abnormal.

P This might indicate hypogonadism.

A Palpation of a scrotal mass superior to the testis that reveals a "bag of worms" is abnormal.

P Refer to the section on scrotal inspection for a description of varicocele.

A It is abnormal for the testicle to be enlarged, retracted, in a lateral position, and extremely sensitive (Figure 21-22). Sometimes it is difficult to distinguish between testicular torsion and epididymitis. Refer to the Advanced Technique on Prehn's Sign on the next page.

P Testicular torsion is a surgical emergency. Twisting or torsion of the testis causes venous obstruction, secondary edema, and eventual arterial obstruction. Doppler ultrasonography reveals absence of perfusion to the testicle.

A Palpation reveals an indurated, swollen, tender epididymis (see Figure 21-23).

P Epididymitis results from the retrograde spreading of pathogenic organisms from the urethra to the epididymis. The majority of infections are caused by bacterial pathogens such as *Chlamydia trachomatis* and *Neisseria gonorrhoeae*. An associated hydrocele may be present. The testis may also be enlarged and tender.

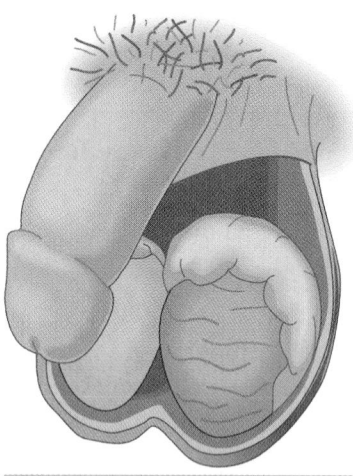

FIGURE 21-23 Epididymitis

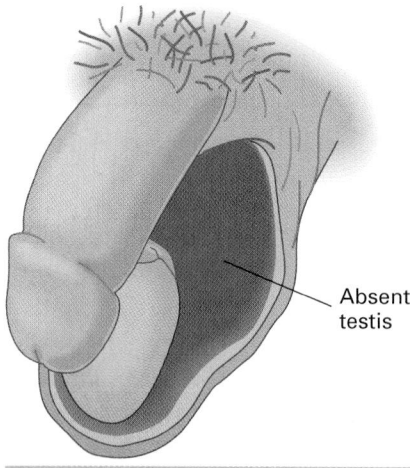

FIGURE 21-24 Cryptorchidism

Absent testis

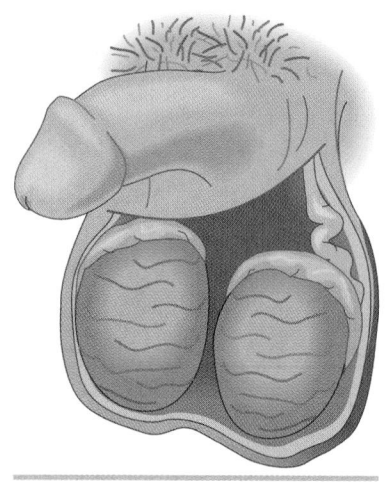

FIGURE 21-25 Orchitis

A It is abnormal for one or both testes to be undescended (Figure 21-24).

P The causes of **cryptorchidism** are not established but may be multiple and related to testicular failure, deficient gonadotrophic stimulation, mechanical obstruction, or gubernacular defects. The undescended testis is usually smaller than its normally descended mate. Unilateral cryptorchidism is more common than is bilateral. The undescended testicle is usually located in the inguinal canal or, less commonly, intra-abdominally. Spontaneous descent is unusual after 1 year of age.

A An acute, painful onset of swelling of the testicle along with warm scrotal skin is abnormal (Figure 21-25). The patient may complain of heaviness in the scrotum.

P **Orchitis** can be caused by mumps, coxsackievirus B, infectious mononucleosis, and varicella. Involvement of the testes is via the hematogenous route. Orchitis is unilateral in the majority of cases, but onset in the second testicle may occur up to 1 week after that in the first.

A In light-skinned individuals, it is abnormal for the scrotum to be enlarged, taut with pitting edema, and reddened (Figure 21-26).

P Scrotal edema accompanies edema associated with the lower half of the body, such as in congestive heart failure (CHF), renal failure, and portal vein obstruction. Scrotal edema may also be the result of local inflammation. Scrotal contents are usually nonpalpable.

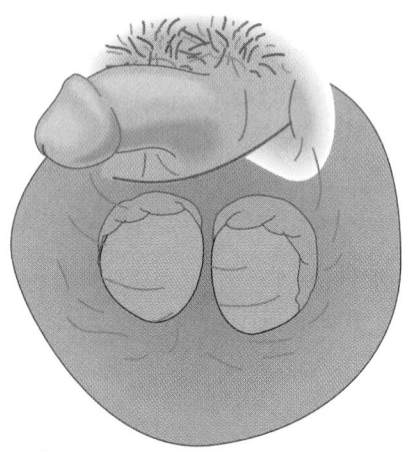

FIGURE 21-26 Scrotal Edema

NURSING**ALERT**

Risk Factors for Testicular Cancer

- Caucasian race, especially Scandinavian background
- Higher socioeconomic status
- Unmarried
- Rural resident
- History of cryptorchidism (even if previously repaired)

ADVANCED TECHNIQUE

Prehn's Sign: Assessing for Testicular Torsion

E 1. Elevate the scrotum with towels until it is fully supported.

2. Observe the patient's pain response.

N The patient with epididymitis will have decreased scrotal pain with scrotal elevation.

A/P The patient with testicular torsion will not have any change in his scrotal pain with this maneuver.

| **E** Examination | **N** Normal Findings | **A** Abnormal Findings | **P** Pathophysiology |

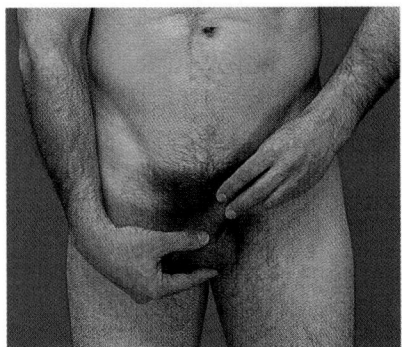

A. Palpating the Testis

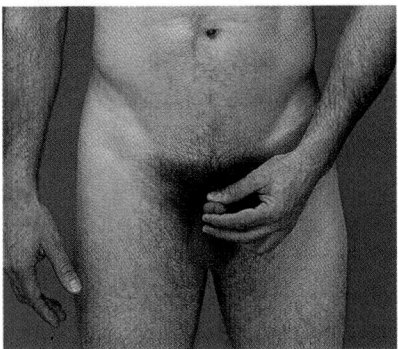

B. Assessing for Penile Discharge

FIGURE 21-27 Testicular
Self-Examination

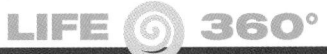

Teaching Testicular Self-Examination

You, a high school nurse, teach a group of male junior students the importance of performing a testicular self-examination. You proceed to demonstrate the technique on a mannequin. After the class is over, one student shyly approaches you and tells you that he is not sure he can perform testicular self-examination because "it is masturbation." How could you respond to the student?

NURSING**TIP**

Teaching Testicular Self-Examination

Testicular self-examination (TSE) should be taught to the patient during the scrotal examination.

- Ask the patient if monthly testicular self-examination is performed.
- Explain the rationale for the examination. Monthly testicular examination will allow for earlier detection of testicular cancer, which occurs most often in 16- to 35-year-old males.
- Tell the patient to pick a date to perform the exam every month. The best time to perform the examination is after a warm shower when both hands and the scrotum are warm.
- Instruct the patient to gently feel each testicle using the thumb and first two fingers (Figure 21-27A).
- Remind the patient that the testicles are ovoid and movable, and that they feel firm and rubbery. The epididymis is located on top and behind the testis, is softer, and feels ropelike.
- Instruct the patient to report any changes from these findings, including any lumps and nodules, especially if they are nonmobile.
- Instruct the patient to squeeze the tip of the penis and observe for any discharge (Figure 21-27B).

A Acute, painful, scrotal swelling may occur with a history of trauma. This is abnormal.

P Trauma is a major cause of acute scrotal swelling. Scrotal or testicular hematoma formation as well as testicular rupture may be present. A small percentage of all diagnosed testicular tumors are diagnosed through medical attention for trauma; therefore, any intratesticular hematoma must be followed to rule out neoplasm.

ADVANCED TECHNIQUE

Transillumination of the Scrotum: Assessing for a Scrotal Mass

If a scrotal mass or enlargement is detected, the scrotum should be transilluminated.

E 1. Tell the patient what you are going to do and that it should not be painful.
   2. Darken the room.
   3. Using a penlight, apply the light source to the unaffected side behind the scrotum and direct it forward.
   4. Apply the light source to the side of the scrotal enlargement or mass.
   5. Note whether there is transmission of a red glow (see Figure 21-28).

N A normal testicle does not transilluminate (i.e., there is no red glow).

A The transmission of a red glow indicates a serous fluid within the scrotal sac (see Figure 21-29). This can occur in hydrocele and spermatocele and is abnormal. Vascular structures such as a hernia and a tumor do not transilluminate.

P Refer to previous discussions of these conditions.

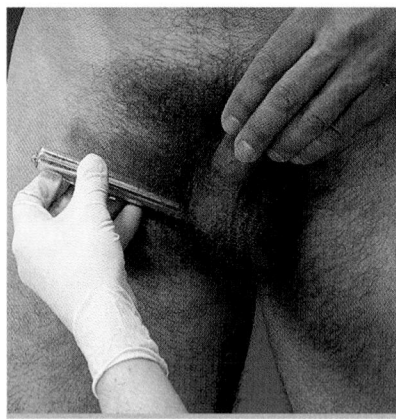

FIGURE 21-28 **Transillumination of the Scrotum**

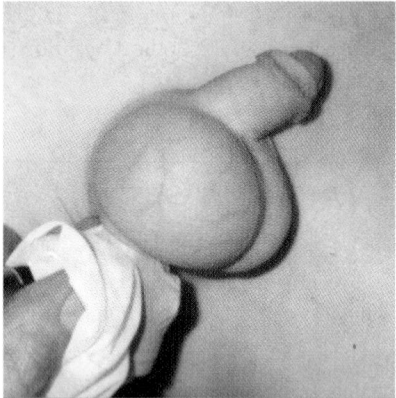

FIGURE 21-29 **Transillumination of a Hydrocele.** In this case a transilluminator was not available. The examiner used a penlight with a rubber glove on top of it to illuminate the scrotal mass, which was a hydrocele.

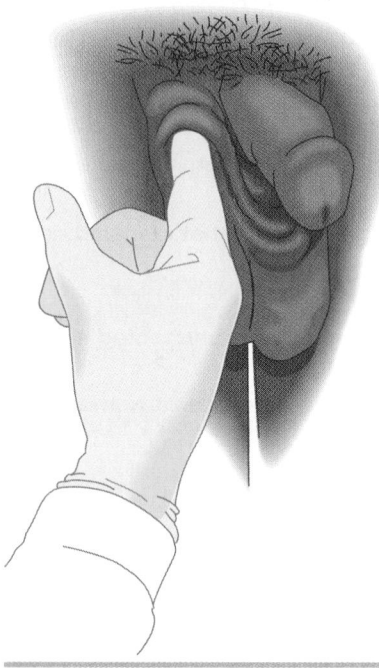

FIGURE 21-30 **Palpation for an Inguinal Hernia**

Inguinal Area

E 1. With the index and middle fingers of the right hand, palpate the skin overlying the inguinal and femoral areas for lymph nodes.

2. Note size, consistency, tenderness, and mobility.

3. Ask the patient to bear down while you palpate the inguinal area.

4. Place the right index finger in the patient's right scrotal sac above the right testicle and invaginate the scrotal skin. Follow the spermatic cord until you reach a triangular, slitlike opening (the external inguinal ring).

5. The finger is placed with the nail facing inward and the finger pad outward (Figure 21-30).

6. If the inguinal ring is large enough, continue to advance the finger along the inguinal canal and ask the patient to turn his head and cough.

7. Note any masses felt against the finger.

8. Repeat on the left side using the left hand to perform the palpation.

9. Palpate the femoral canal. Ask the patient to bear down.

N It is normal for there to be small (1 cm), freely mobile lymph nodes present in the inguinal area. There should not be any bulges present in the inguinal area. There should not be any palpable masses in the inguinal canal. No portions of the bowel should enter the scrotum. There should be no palpable mass at the femoral canal.

A Unilateral enlargement of the lymph nodes along with erythematous overlying skin that may contain adhesions is abnormal.

P Three of the 15 strains of *Chlamydia trachomatis*, specifically L1, L2, and L3, cause lymphogranuloma venereum (LV). These serovars are more invasive and virulent and selectively infect lymphoid tissue rather than columnar epithelial cells. Firm inguinal masses result when buboes involute.

A Unilateral or bilateral enlargement of the inguinal lymph nodes is abnormal. The nodes may be tender or painless.

P Lymphadenopathy occurs when the immune system responds to bacterial infections, trauma, or carcinoma. Bacterial infections commonly associated with inguinal lymphadenopathy include syphilis, chancroid, and gonorrhea.

A An **indirect inguinal hernia** palpated at the inguinal ring is abnormal (see Figure 21-31). An impulse may be felt on the fingertip when the patient is asked to cough. A larger indirect inguinal hernia may feel like a mass at the inguinal canal.

P Portions of the bowel or omentum enter the inguinal canal through the internal ring and exit at the external inguinal ring. All indirect hernias are congenitally related to a patent processus vaginalis. The severity of a combination of the congenital abnormality and a condition that increases abdominal pressure (e.g., obesity, chronic obstructive pulmonary disease [COPD], hard physical labor, coughing, ascites) determines the onset and degree of the hernia.

A Oval swelling found at the pubis on inspection represents a **direct inguinal hernia** and is abnormal (see Figure 21-32). Coughing causes enlargement on palpation of the mass.

| **E** Examination | **N** Normal Findings | **A** Abnormal Findings | **P** Pathophysiology |

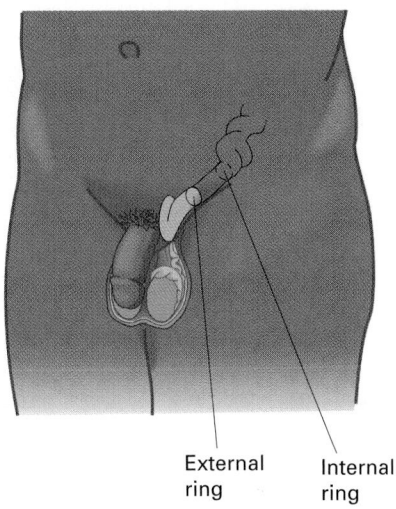

FIGURE 21-31 **Indirect Inguinal Hernia**

External ring   Internal ring

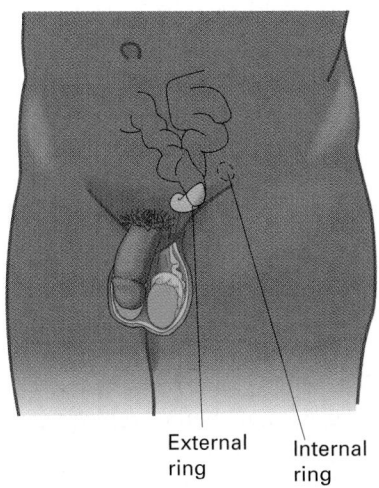

FIGURE 21-32 **Direct Inguinal Hernia**

External ring   Internal ring

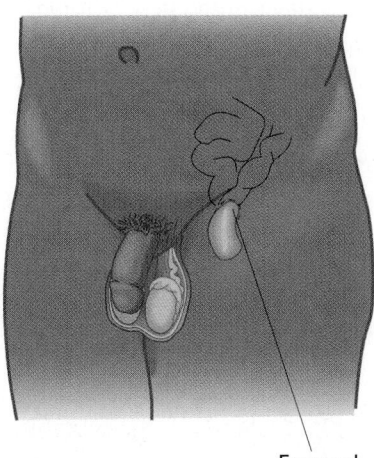

FIGURE 21-33 **Femoral Hernia**

Femoral canal

P In direct hernias, portions of the bowel or omentum protrude directly through the external inguinal ring. Direct hernias are acquired masses that are influenced by increases in intra-abdominal pressure and weakening of the inguinal structures as part of the normal aging process. Other related factors include heavy lifting, obesity, and COPD.

A Palpation of a mass medial to the femoral vessels and inferior to the inguinal ligament is indicative of a **femoral hernia** and is abnormal (Figure 21-33).

P A femoral hernia is caused by protrusion of the omentum or bowel through the femoral wall. Onset and size of the hernia may be affected by a congenitally large femoral ring, degradation of collagen and tissue attenuation associated with aging, increased intra-abdominal pressure, and presence of preperitoneal fat.

Table 21-2 compares the different types of hernias.

AUSCULTATION

Auscultation is performed if a scrotal mass is found on inspection or palpation.

Scrotum

E 1. Place the patient in a supine position.

2. Stand at the patient's right side at the genitalia area.

3. Place your stethoscope over the scrotal mass.

4. Listen for the presence of bowel sounds.

N No bowel sounds are present in the scrotum.

A An indirect inguinal hernia is present if bowel sounds are present in the enlarged scrotum.

P Loops of bowel extending into the scrotum via an indirect hernia continue to produce bowel sounds unless the hernia is strangulated (lack of blood flow to bowel tissue) and bowel tissue becomes ischemic or necrotic.

NURSING**TIP**

Reducing a Direct Inguinal Hernia

An attempt should be made by a qualified practitioner to reduce the hernia (to return the bowel to the abdominal cavity) if nausea, vomiting, and tenderness are absent. Have the patient lie down and gently push the hernia back into the abdominal cavity. An incarcerated hernia cannot be pushed back into the abdominal cavity. If nausea, vomiting, and tenderness are present, they may indicate a strangulated hernia (no blood supply to the affected bowel), which should be referred to a physician.

NURSING**TIP**

Hernias in Females

Be alert to females who experience lower quadrant pain; one of the differential diagnoses can be hernia. Hernias can occur in females as well as males, though they are more prevalent in males. When they occur in females, they are frequently femoral hernias. Assess for hernias in females in the inguinal area by palpating the femoral area while the patient bears down. A bulge or palpable mass would confirm the finding.

TABLE 21-2 Comparison of Inguinal and Femoral Hernias

FEATURE	INDIRECT INGUINAL HERNIA	DIRECT INGUINAL HERNIA	FEMORAL HERNIA
Occurrence	More common in infants < 1 year and males 16 to 25 years of age	Middle-aged and elderly men	More frequent in women
Origin of Swelling	Above inguinal ligament. Hernia sac enters canal at internal ring and exits at external ring. Can be found in the scrotum	Above inguinal ligament Directly behind and through external ring	Below inguinal ligament
Cause	Congenital or acquired	Acquired weakness brought on by heavy lifting, obesity, COPD	Acquired, due to increased abdominal pressure and muscle weakness
Signs and Symptoms	Lump or fullness in the groin that may be associated with a cough or crying	Lump or fullness in the groin area. It may cause an aching or dragging sensation.	Firm or rubbery lump in the groin. Pain may be severe.

NURSING**TIP**

Erectile Function

Treatment for impotence varies greatly depending on the cause and may include any of the following:
- Patience and a relaxed atmosphere
- Oral medication: Halotestin, yohimbine HCl, phosphodiesterase type 5 inhibitors
- Penile prosthesis
- Intracavernosal injections
- Vacuum erection device
- Transurethral suppositories

NURSING**TIP**

Sildenafil (Viagra), Vardenafil (Levitra), and Tadalafil (Cialis)

There are three phosphodiesterase type 5 inhibitors (PDE 5) now available for erectile dysfunction. All three are available only by prescription. PDE 5 inhibitors improve vasodilation and smooth muscle relaxation. Libido is not affected by PDE 5 inhibitors. All three have a contraindication in men using organic nitrates.

Sildenafil citrate was approved by the FDA in 1998. The recommended starting dose is a 50 mg tablet taken 30 to 60 minutes before initiating sexual activity, and it has a half-life of 4 to 5 hours. A 100 mg dose is recommended for patients who do not respond to the 50 mg dose. Sildenafil citrate should be taken on an empty stomach or after a low-fat meal. Ingesting a high-fat meal within 1 to 2 hours can reduce the onset of action by up to 70%. A blue discoloration of vision may be experienced.

Vardenafil received clearance from the FDA in 2003. Vardenafil is supplied in 2.5 mg, 5 mg, 10 mg, and 20 mg tablets. Initial starting dose is 10 mg taken 1 hour before sexual activity, and it usually lasts 4 to 5 hours. All alpha blockers are contraindicated in patients taking vardenafil due to potential orthostatic hypotension. Vardenafil can be taken without regard to food.

Tadalafil also became available in 2003. It is marketed in 5 mg, 10 mg, and 20 mg tablets. Patients should start with a 10 mg dose and increase to 20 mg if needed. It is taken 30 to 60 minutes before sexual activity. Tadalafil has a half-life of 17.5 hours. All alpha blockers except tamsulosin (Flomax) are contraindicated in patients taking tadalafil. Tadalafil can be taken without regard to food.

Side effects of all three drugs may include headache, nasal congestion, and flushing. Only rarely do these side effects cause men to stop using the drug.

The Patient with Epididymitis Caused by *Chlamydia Trachomatis*

This case study illustrates the application and objective documentation of the male genitalia assessment. Ho is a 46-year-old accountant who is experiencing testicular pain.

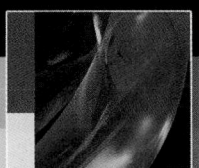

HEALTH HISTORY

PATIENT PROFILE	46 yo single Asian male
CHIEF COMPLAINT	"My left testicle hurts."
HISTORY OF PRESENT ILLNESS	Pt c/o of pain (5/10) and swelling in the left testicle over the past 4 days; he found a hard lump on the left testicle which is tender to touch; onset of chills/fever this morning; temp to 100.6°F; increase in urinary frequency for the past 3 days; divorced for 4 years; sexual relationships with new partner for 2 months; denies ever using any condoms; denies urethral discharge, denies any traumatic injury to the genital area. During the past 6 months has noticed nocturia × 3 most nights.
PAST HEALTH HISTORY	
Medical History	Negative
Surgical History	Ⓡ knee sgy age 24 s̄ sequelae
Allergies	Lactose intolerance since childhood
Medications	Denies
Communicable Diseases	Herpes simplex type 2 diagnosed age 26; denies medication use, rare outbreaks; denies past gonorrhea/chlamydia or other STD infections
Injuries and Accidents	Torn Ⓡ meniscus, age 24, surgically repaired; physical therapy twice wkly for 4 wks after sgy
Special Needs	Denies
Blood Transfusions	Denies
Childhood Illnesses	Chickenpox (age 5), mumps (age 6)
Immunizations	"Up to date," last tetanus unknown

continues

CASE STUDY (Continued)

The Patient with Epididymitis Caused by *Chlamydia Trachomatis*

FAMILY HEALTH HISTORY

LEGEND

 Living female

 Living male

 Deceased female

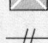 Deceased male

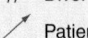 Divorced

Patient

A&W = Alive & well
dz = disease
HTN = Hypertension
CA = Cancer
CVA = Cerebrovascular accident
MI = Myocardial infarction

```
  50          81      71         70
  MI       Unknown  Prostate    CVA
                      CA        HTN

        73                68
       A&W               HTN

     44          46  //    42
    A&W         A&W      Crohn's dz

                 19
                A&W
```

Denies family hx of varicocele, testicular CA, hypospadias, infertility

SOCIAL HISTORY

Alcohol Use	Drinks 2–3 beers at Friday "happy hours"
Tobacco Use	Cigarettes 1½ PPD for 26 yrs (39 pack/yr history); chewing tobacco in high school and college, chews with recreational baseball team on wkends
Drug Use	Marijuana use in high school/college
Domestic and Intimate Partner Violence	Denies
Sexual Practice	Heterosexual; sexual contacts have involved women he meets through friends and work; 5 partners in life, denies condom use
Travel History	Germany 3× in the last 5 yrs to visit his sister
Work Environment	Accountant with a tax firm; at current job for 2 yrs
Home Environment	Rents luxury apt in the suburbs that was built 3 yrs ago; "I don't need to fool with a yard or house maintenance."
Hobbies and Leisure Activities	Listening to music; watching sporting events; recreational baseball league since college
Stress	Not seeing his 19 yo daughter as often as he would like; college tuition for her
Education	MBA, CPA
Economic Status	"I'm OK."

continues

CASE STUDY (Continued)

The Patient with Epididymitis Caused by *Chlamydia Trachomatis*

Military Service	None
Religion	Nonpracticing Presbyterian
Ethnic Background	3rd generation Asian American (family emigrated from Taiwan)
Roles and Relationships	Lives alone for the last yr; girlfriend moved out 1 yr ago, lived together 18 months; married 18 yrs; divorced 4 yrs ago, does not communicate with ex-wife; currently involved with new girlfriend for 2 mos; 1 daughter, whom he talks to q wk
Characteristic Patterns of Daily Living	Wakes up at 6:30 AM. Leaves for work at 7:30 AM. Has a ½ to 1 h commute, depending on traffic. Has lunch at his desk. Arrives back home between 6 PM and 6:30 PM. 2 nights a wk he plays basketball at the local rec center, baseball on the wkends; goes to bed around 11 PM
HEALTH MAINTENANCE ACTIVITIES	
Sleep	7½ hrs/night s̄ need for sleep medication
Diet	Breakfast: cereal/toast; lunch: sandwich from the local deli; dinner: picks up fast food 2–3 × wk; fixes meals other nights
Exercise	Basketball and baseball
Stress Management	Exercise
Use of Safety Devices	Wears seat belt while driving
Health Check-ups	Goes to his primary care provider for yearly BP checks/physicals
PHYSICAL ASSESSMENT	
Inspection	
Sexual Maturity Rating	Tanner stage 5
Hair Distribution	Triangular distribution of pubic hair
Penis	Circumcised, no erythema at meatus, skin free of lesions and inflammation, rounded glans penis, size equated c̄ developmental stage, no penile curvature
Scrotum	Skin rugated, erythematous c̄ Ⓛ sided edema
Urethral Meatus	Centrally located, no erythema
Inguinal Area	No swelling or bulges
Palpation	
Penis	Pulsations present on dorsal aspect, no masses or firm plaques

continues

CASE STUDY (Continued)
The Patient with Epididymitis Caused by *Chlamydia Trachomatis*

Urethral Meatus	Light yellow discharge expressed
Scrotum	Ⓛ testis tender, palpable swelling Ⓛ epididymis c̄ ↑ temperature Ⓡ testis soft, no masses or tenderness
Inguinal Area	No inguinal nodes, no hernia masses
Ascultation	
Scrotum	No bowel sounds
Advanced Technique	Transillumination of the scrotum: no red glow

LABORATORY DATA

		PT'S VALUES	NORMAL RANGE
CBC	RBC	4.8 M/mm^3	4.0–5.2 M/mm^3
	WBC	12.5 k/mm^3	4.0–11 k/mm^3
	PLT	400 k/mm^3	140–440 k/mm^3
	Hgb	15.6 g/dL	13.0–17 g/dL
	Hct	50%	39–51%
Urinalysis	WBCs	20–30/hpf	0–3/hpf
	RBCs	3–5/hpf	0–3/hpf
PSA		10.0 ng/mL	0–4.0 ng/mL
Urethral Discharge Culture		*Chlamydia trachomatis*	No bacteria

ASSESSMENT IN BRIEF

Male Genitalia Assessment

Inspection
- Sexual maturity rating
- Hair distribution
- Penis
- Scrotum
- Urethral meatus
- Inguinal area
- Scrotum
- Inguinal area

Palpation
- Penis
- Urethral meatus

Auscultation
- Scrotum

Advanced Techniques
- Acetowhitening: Assessing for HPV
- Urethral culture: Identifying penile pathogens
- Prehn's sign: Assessing for testicular torsion
- Transillumination of the scrotum: Assessing for a scrotal mass

REVIEW QUESTIONS

1. A 30-year-old man has had a painless swelling in his left testis for the past 6 months. Physical examination reveals enlargement of the left testis. The right testis appears normal. Which of the following would you be most suspicious of?
   a. Hydrocele
   b. Varicocele
   c. Tumor
   d. Epididymitis
   The correct answer is (c).

2. A 23-year-old healthy man has been unable to father a child. On physical examination both his testes are palpable in the scrotum. The testes and scrotum are normal in size, with no masses palpable. However, the spermatic cord on the left has the feel of a "bag of worms." Which of the following does the man most likely have?
   a. Hydrocele
   b. Varicocele
   c. Tumor
   d. Epididymitis
   The correct answer is (b).

3. On physical examination, a newborn has an abnormal opening of the urethra on the ventral surface of the penis. Which of the following is the most likely diagnosis?
   a. Hypospadias
   b. Phimosis
   c. Epispadias
   d. Cryptorchidism
   The correct answer is (a).

4. A 35-year-old man has a routine check of his health status. On physical examination, the prepuce cannot be fully retracted from the glans of his penis. No other abnormalities are noted. What condition does this man most likely have?
   a. Epispadias
   b. Hypospadias
   c. Phimosis
   d. Paraphimosis
   The correct answer is (c).

5. Which of the following statements describes the appearance of genital herpes?
   a. Inflammation of the glans penis with penile discharge
   b. Multifocal maculopapular lesions that are tan, brown, pink, violet, and white
   c. Papular lesion with erythematous halo and surrounding edema
   d. Superficial vesicles grouped on an erythematous base
   The correct answer is (d).

6. An indirect inguinal hernia can be differentiated from other causes of scrotal swelling by which of the following?
   a. Transillumination of the scrotum
   b. Palpating the inguinal canal and having the patient cough
   c. Scrotal X-ray
   d. Prehn's sign
   The correct answer is (b).

7. Which of the following are side effects of PDE 5 inhibitors?
   a. Nasal congestion, headache
   b. Stomach upset, flushing
   c. Elevated blood sugar, chest pain
   d. Ringing in the ears, priapism
   The correct answer is (a).

Questions 8 and 9 refer to the following situation:

Mr. Whitfield is a 60-year-old man who is in your office for his yearly physical. He reports that he is sexually active and denies any medical conditions. He is currently on no prescription medication.

8. While performing the genitalia examination on Mr. Whitfield, you observe that he is uncircumcised. You ask him to retract the foreskin and notice that the glans appears inflamed. This inflammation is called which of the following?
   a. Phimosis
   b. Balanitis
   c. Smegma
   d. Paraphimosis
   The correct answer is (b).

9. What laboratory test would you order because of the inflammation of the glans penis?
   a. Liver function tests
   b. Complete blood cell count
   c. Fasting blood sugar
   d. Thyroid stimulating hormone
   The correct answer is (c).

10. Which patient would be at the highest risk for developing penile cancer?
    a. 30-year-old sexually active, circumcised male with a history of HPV type 11
    b. 40-year-old uncircumcised male who is not sexually active
    c. 55-year-old sexually active, uncircumcised male
    d. 75-year-old sexually active, circumcised male
    The correct answer is (c).

BIBLIOGRAPHY

Blackwell, C. W. (2008). Anorectal carcinoma screening in gay men: Implications for nurse practitioners. *The American Journal for Nurse Practitioners, 12*(1), 60–63.

Ceo, P. (2006). Assessment of the male reproductive system. *Urologic Nursing, 26*(4), 290–296.

Chaney, S., & Esparza Fuentes, E. (2006). Genitourinary tract infections in men. *Advance for Nurse Practitioners, 14*(6), 47–49.

Diamond, D. A. (2007). Adolescent varicocele. *Current Opinions in Urology, 17*(4), 263–267.

Ellsworth, P., & Caldamone, A. A. (2006). *The little black book of urology* (2nd ed.). Boston: Jones and Bartlett.

Gee, R. (2006). Primary care health issues among men who have sex with men. *Journal of the American Academy of Nurse Practitioners, 18*(1), 144–153.

Goh, B. T. (2005). Syphilis in adults. *Sexually Transmitted Infections, 81*(6), 448–452.

Hellstrom, W. J. (2007). Current safety and tolerability issues in men with erectile dysfunction receiving PDE5 inhibitors. *International Journal of Clinical Practice, 61*(9), 1547–1554.

Johnson-Mallard, V., Lengacher, C., Kromrey, J., Campbell, D., Jevitt, C., Daley, E., & Schmitt, K. (2007). Increasing knowledge of sexually transmitted infection risk. *Nurse Practitioner, 32*(2), 26–32.

McVary, K. T. (2007). Clinical practice. Erectile dysfunction. *New England Journal of Medicine, 357*(24), 2472–2481.

Miller, K. E. (2006). Diagnosis and treatment of Neisseria gonorrhoeae infections. *American Family Physician, 73*(10), 1779–1784.

Mullen, B. A. (2004). Testicular complaints and the young man. *Journal of the American Academy of Nurse Practitioners, 16*(11), 490–495.

Parsons, J. K., & Wright, E. J. (2006). *Brady urology manual.* Westborough, MA: Informa.

Peate, I. (2005). Examining adult male genitalia: Providing a guide for the nurse. *British Journal of Nursing, 14*(1), 36–40.

Porche, D. J. (2005). Male sexual assault. *The Journal for Nurse Practitioners, 6*(4), 196–197.

Porche, D. J. (2007). Genital human papillomavirus infection in men. *The Journal for Nurse Practitioners, 3*(10), 684–685.

Porche, D. J. (2007). Male contraception. *The Journal for Nurse Practitioners, 3*(9), 595–597.

Raphaelidis, L. (2006). Making sense of HPV. *The Journal for Nurse Practitioners, 2*(5), 329–332.

Roehrborn, C. G. (2007). *Contemporary diagnosis and management of benign prostatic hypertrophy.* Newtown, PA: Handbooks in Health Care Co.

Sark, M., & Hilinski, A. (2008). Treating genital warts. *Advance for Nurse Practitioners, 16*(1), 24–28.

Tanagho, E. A., & McAninch, J. W. (2007). *Smith's general urology* (17th ed.). New York: McGraw Hill.

Tracy, C. R., Steers, W. D., & Constabile, R. (2008). Diagnosis and management of epididymitis. *Urology Clinics of North America, 35*(1), 101–108.

U.S. Preventive Services Task Force. (2007). Screening for chlamydial infection: U.S. Preventive Services Task Force recommendation statement. *Annals of Internal Medicine, 142*(11), 914–925.

Wein, A. J., Kavoussi, L. R., Novick, A. C., Partin, A. W., & Peters, C. A. (2007). *Campbell-Walsh urology review manual.* Philadelphia: Saunders.

Workowski, K. A., & Berman, S. M. (2006). Sexually transmitted diseases treatment guidelines. *MMWR Recommendations Report, 55*(RR-11), 1–94.

Wren, T. (2004). Penile and testicular disorders. *Nursing Clinics of North America, 39*(2), 319–326.

WEB SITES

American Urological Association:
http://www.auanet.org

Centers for Disease Control and Prevention:
http://www.cdc.gov

Digital Urology Journal:
http://www.duj.com

The Journal of Urology:
http://www.jurology.com

Society of Urologic Nurses and Associates:
http://www.suna.org

Urology Health.org:
http://www.urologyhealth.org

CHAPTER 22

Anus, Rectum, and Prostate

COMPETENCIES

1. Identify anatomic landmarks of the rectum and the prostate gland.

2. Describe the characteristics of the most common rectal and prostatic chief complaints.

3. Perform inspection and palpation of the anus, rectum, and prostate on an adult.

4. Explain the pathophysiological rationale for abnormal findings.

5. Document assessment findings.

The anorectal examination is an important part of the physical examination. In the male patient, this includes assessment of the anus, rectum, and prostate gland. In the female patient, assessment of the anus and rectum is performed. These assessments are usually performed last and should be performed on a regular basis because they provide vital screening for anorectal and prostate cancers.

ANATOMY AND PHYSIOLOGY

RECTUM

The large intestine is composed of the cecum, colon, rectum, and anal canal. The cecum and colon are discussed in Chapter 17. The sigmoid colon begins at the pelvic brim. Beyond the sigmoid colon, the large intestine passes downward in front of the sacrum. This portion is called the **rectum** (Figure 22-1). The rectum contains three transverse folds, or valves of Houston. These valves work to retain fecal material so it is not passed along with flatus.

ANUS

The terminal 3 to 4 cm (1¼ –1⅝ inches) of the large intestine is called the **anal canal**. The anal canal fuses with the rectum at the anorectal junction, or the dentate line, and together these structures form the **anorectum**. The anal orifice is located at the seam of the gluteal folds; it serves as the exit to the gastrointestinal tract and it is marked by corrugated skin. The anal orifice lies 2 cm (¾ inch) below the dentate line. The lower 2 cm of the anal canal is lined by **anoderm**, a thin, pale, stratified squamous epithelium that contains no hair follicles, sweat glands, or sebaceous glands.

In the superior half of the anal canal are **anal columns**, which are longitudinal folds of mucosa (also called columns of Morgagni). The **anal valves** are formed by

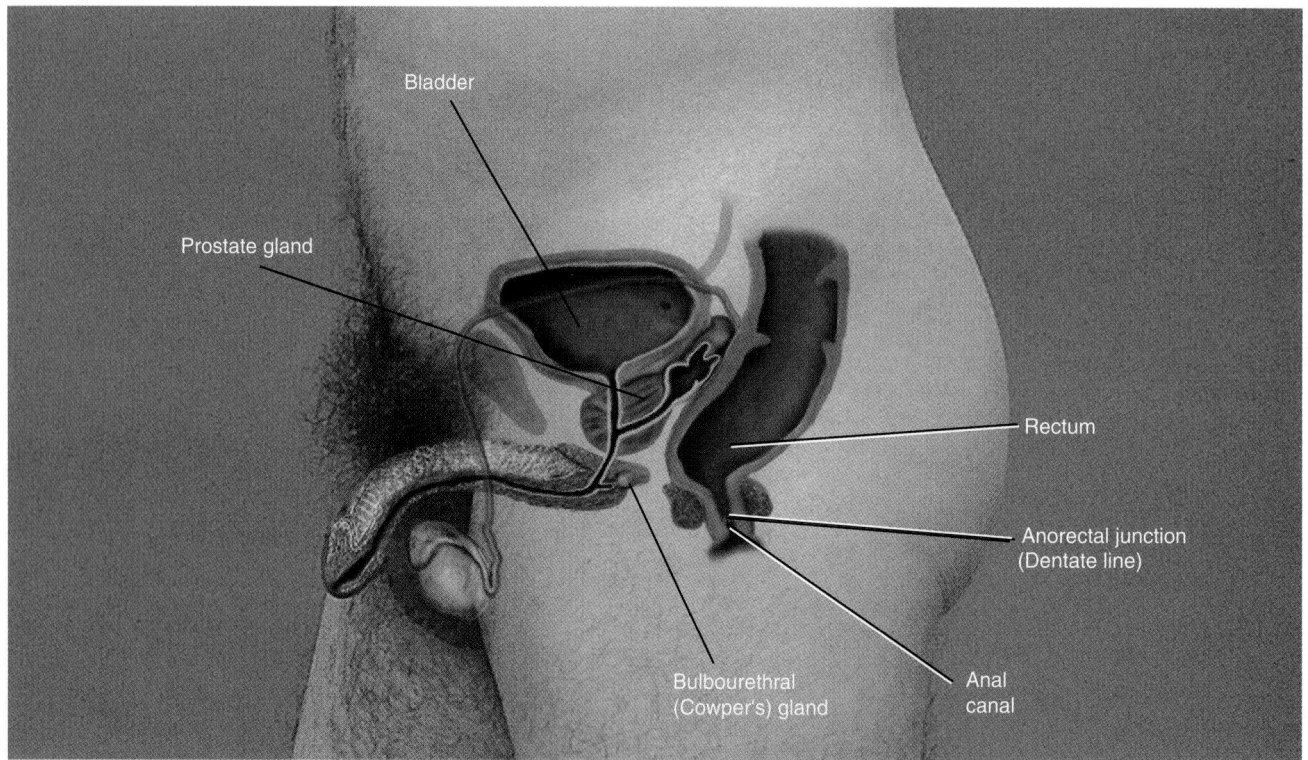

FIGURE 22-1 The Anorectum and Prostate

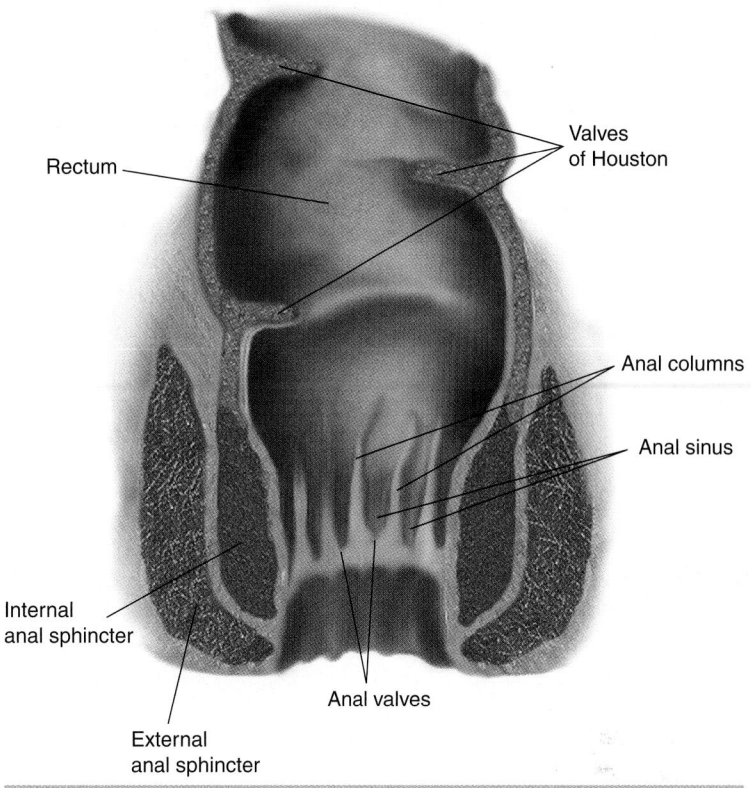

FIGURE 22-2 Anal Canal

inferior joining anal columns. There are pockets located superior to the valves called the **anal sinuses**. These sinuses secrete mucus when they are compressed by feces, providing lubrication that eases fecal passage during **defecation** (Figure 22-2).

The anal canal opens to the exterior through the anus. Internal and external anal sphincter muscles surround the anus. Smooth muscle, which is under involuntary control, forms the internal sphincter. Skeletal muscle forms the external sphincter and is under voluntary control, allowing a person to control bowel movements.

The motility of the large intestine is controlled mainly by its nerves. There are two types of nerves: those that lie within the large intestine (the intrinsic nerves) and those that lie outside it (the extrinsic nerves). The rectum has more segmental contractions than does the sigmoid colon. These contractions keep the rectum empty by retrograde movement of contents into the sigmoid colon. As fecal material is forced into the rectum by mass peristaltic movements, the stretching of the rectal wall initiates the defecation reflex. A parasympathetic reflex signals the walls of the sigmoid colon and rectum to contract and the internal anal sphincter to relax. During defecation, the musculature of the rectum contracts to expel the feces.

PROSTATE

Contiguous with part of the anterior rectal wall in the male is the **prostate** gland. The prostate is an accessory male sex organ the size and shape of a chestnut, approximately 3.5 cm (1⅜ inches) long by 3 cm (1¼ inches) wide. It consists of glandular tissue and muscle, and its small ducts drain into the urethra. The prostate lies just below the bladder and encircles the urethra like a doughnut.

The prostate has five lobes: anterior, posterior, median, and two lateral. The median sulcus is the groove between the lateral lobes. The right and left lateral lobes are accessible to examination.

Prostatic secretions are thin, milky, and alkaline. The secretions are made up of many different components. Citrate, a major component of prostatic fluid, provides a good transport medium for spermatozoa by maintaining the osmotic equilibrium of the seminal fluid. Prostatic fluid composes 15% to 30% of the ejaculate. Prostatic secretions have high levels of prostatic acid phosphatase (PAP) and prostate-specific antigen (PSA).

The prostate is primarily involved in reproduction, but it also provides a certain measure of protection against urinary tract infections. Semen contains high levels of zinc, which is derived from the prostate. Zinc is what provides the antibacterial properties to the prostate.

Within the prostatic cells, testosterone is converted to an androgen called dihydrotestosterone (DHT). DHT is the major androgen responsible for the benign enlargement of the prostate gland.

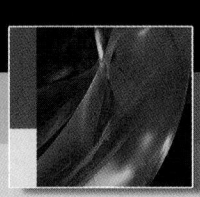

HEALTH HISTORY

The anus, rectum, and prostate health history provides insight into the link between a patient's life and lifestyle and anal, rectal, and prostatic information and pathology.

PATIENT PROFILE

Diseases that are age-, gender-, and race-specific for the anus, rectum, and prostate are listed.

Age

Pilonidal cyst or sinus (20–35)
Crohn's disease of the anorectum (20–40)
Anal fissure (20–45)
Rectal condyloma acuminatum (20–50)
Ulcerative colitis (20–50)
Gonococcal proctitis (20–50)
Herpes proctitis (20–50)
Prostatitis (20–60)
Anal stenosis (> 25)
Pruritus ani (> 25)
Anal skin tags (< 30)
Acute bacterial prostatitis (> 30)
Anorectal abscess (30–40)
Anorectal fistula (30–40)
Hemorrhoids (40–65)
Prostatic abscess (> 40)
Fecal incontinence (> 40)
Benign prostatic hypertrophy (> 40)
Rectal cancer (> 55)
Prostate cancer (> 50)
Fecal impaction (> 60)
Rectal prolapse (60–80)

Gender

Female

Rectal prolapse, fecal incontinence

continues

Male	Anorectal abscess, anorectal fistula, pruritus ani, rectal cancer, pilonidal cyst or sinus, hemorrhoids, gonococcal proctitis, herpes proctitis, benign prostatic hypertrophy, prostatitis, prostate abscess, prostate cancer
Race	
African American	Prostate cancer
Caucasian	Rectal cancer, Crohn's disease of the anorectum, pilonidal cyst or sinus, benign prostatic hypertrophy
CHIEF COMPLAINT	*Common chief complaints for the anus, rectum, and prostate are defined and information on the characteristics of each sign or symptom is provided.*
1. Rectal Bleeding	Discharge of blood from the rectum
Quality	Occult, melena, hematochezia, massive hemorrhage
Quantity	Scant, spotty, dripping, massive
Associated Manifestations	Pain, absence of pain, malaise, fever, mass at anus
Aggravating Factors	Defecation, constipation, diarrhea, minor trauma, pelvic irradiation
Alleviating Factors	Increased fiber diet, bulk agents, exercise, increased fluid intake, hemorrhoidectomy
Timing	Constant, intermittent
2. Rectal Pain	The subjective phenomenon of a sensation indicating real or potential tissue damage in the rectum
Quality	Acute, sharp, tearing, burning, throbbing
Associated Manifestations	Swelling, fever, blood, abdominal pain
Aggravating Factors	Defecation, sitting, movement, foreign bodies, pregnancy, anal sex
Alleviating Factors	High-fiber diet, bulk agents, exercise, increased fluid intake, warm sitz bath, topical emollients, surgery, removal of foreign body, lying down
Timing	More prominent with defecation; constant or episodic
3. Anal Incontinence	The involuntary passage of stool
Associated Manifestations	Diarrhea, urgency, rectal prolapse, prolapsed hemorrhoids, gaping anus
Aggravating Factors	Diarrhea, impaction, cognitive impairment, anxiety, physical handicaps, neurological disorders, trauma
Alleviating Factors	Bulk fiber, constipating agents, laxatives, enemas, biofeedback, anal continence plugs
4. Constipation	The infrequent, difficult passage of stool
Quantity	Fewer than three bowel movements per week
Associated Manifestations	Pain, blood, mucus, hard stool, straining with defecation, flatulence, decreased appetite
Aggravating Factors	Low-fiber diet, lack of exercise, drugs (e.g., narcotics, calcium channel blockers), chronic use of laxatives, ignoring urge to defecate, weak abdominal muscles, inadequate fluid intake, rectocele, rectal prolapse, anal stenosis

continues

Alleviating Factors	High-fiber diet, bulking agents, increased fluid intake, defecation schedule, exercise, laxatives, digital removal, suppositories
5. Diarrhea	Increased volume, fluidity, or frequency of bowel movements relative to the person's usual pattern
Associated Manifestations	Abdominal pain, blood, steatorrhea, weight changes, appetite changes
Aggravating Factors	Viral infection, bacterial infection, antibiotics, laxatives, fecal impaction, Crohn's disease, ulcerative colitis, lactose intolerance, specific foods (very indivualized), irritable bowel syndrome, caffeine, alcohol
Alleviating Factors	Constipating agents, anticholinergics, fluid replacement, certain foods (bananas, rice, apples, toast), antibiotics
Setting	Stressful situations, recent ingestion of improperly stored or prepared food, recent travel abroad
6. Pruritus	Itching of the anal and perianal skin
Associated Manifestations	Erythema, edema, psoriasis, candidiasis, contact dermatitis, hemorrhoids, anal fissures, rectal carcinoma
Aggravating Factors	Psoriasis, eczema, contact dermatitis, infections, parasites, oral antibiotics, diabetes mellitus, liver disease, obesity, poor hygiene, tight underclothes, wet clothing
Alleviating Factors	Discontinuing current antibiotics and topical agents; eliminating coffee, tea, cola, milk, beer, and wine; discontinuing laxatives; good rectal hygiene; loose clothing; nonmedicated talcum powder; topical fungicides
7. Palpable Mass	A mass at the anus, in the anal canal, or on the prostate
Quality	Firm, smooth, soft, mobile, nonmobile, nodular, fibrotic
Associated Manifestations	Pain, absence of pain, blood, pus, mucus, fever, hemorrhoids, rectal prolapse
Alleviating Factors	Warm sitz baths, high-fiber diet, bulk agents, surgery
PAST HEALTH HISTORY	*The various components of the past health history are linked to anal, rectal, and prostatic pathology and anal-, rectal-, and prostatic-related information.*
Medical History	
Anorectal Specific	Trauma, inflammatory bowel disease, prior history of STDs, polyps, rectal cancer, hemorrhoids, pruritus ani, constipation, diarrhea, incontinence
Nonanorectal Specific	Radiation, lymphogranuloma venereum, childbirth, arthritis, endocarditis, high serum testosterone, endometrial cancer, ovarian cancer, breast cancer, cervical cancer, HIV infection, penile or vaginal STDs
Prostate Specific	Prostate cancer, prostatitis, benign prostatic hypertrophy
Surgical History	
Anorectal	Sigmoidoscopy, colonoscopy, rubber band ligation, injection sclerotherapy, hemorrhoidectomy, drainage of fistula or abscess
Prostate	Prostatectomy, transurethral resection of the prostate (TURP)

continues

Allergies	Contact dermatitis of perianal area
Medications	Laxatives, constipating agents, alpha blockers, 5-alpha-reductase inhibitors, antifungals, astringent ointments, suppositories
Communicable Diseases	HIV, *Neisseria gonorrhoeae*, *Treponema pallidum*, *Chlamydia trachomatis*, HPV, HSV
Injuries and Accidents	Rectal trauma, foreign body in rectum
Childhood Illnesses	Anal stenosis, Hirschsprung's disease (with rectal pull through)
FAMILY HEALTH HISTORY	*Anal, rectal, and prostatic diseases that are familial are listed.* Rectal polyps, rectal cancer, pilonidal cyst, prostate cancer
SOCIAL HISTORY	*The components of the social history are linked to anal, rectal, and prostatic factors and pathology.*
Alcohol Use	Excess intake of alcohol associated with pruritus ani; increased amount of alcohol associated with rectal and prostate cancers
Tobacco Use	Cigarette smoking increases the risk for anal carcinoma and exacerbates Crohn's disease.
Drug Use	Illicit drug use may distort the user's perception, increasing the risk for unsafe sexual practices and STD exposure.
Sexual Practice	Rectal penetration increases the risk for anal carcinoma and anorectal STDs. Use of foreign objects in the rectum can lead to anal valve incompetence.
Work Environment	Excessive sitting causes direct pressure and increases venous pooling, which can lead to hemorrhoids.
Hobbies and Leisure Activities	Weightlifting (hemorrhoids, rectal prolapse)
Stress	Pruritus ani can be exacerbated by stress; diarrhea can be caused by stress; constipation can be caused by depression.
HEALTH MAINTENANCE ACTIVITIES	*This information provides a bridge between the health maintenance activities and anal, rectal, and prostatic function.*
Sleep	Nocturia secondary to an enlarged prostate
Diet	Increased amounts of dietary fats, cured and smoked meats, and charcoal-broiled foods, and decreased amounts of fiber, fruits, and vegetables are associated with prostate and rectal cancers; excessive intake of milk, coffee, tea, cola, and spices is associated with pruritus ani. Vitamins A, C, E, and folate may protect against developing rectal cancer.
Exercise	Exercise promotes regular bowel evacuation.
Use of Safety Devices	Condoms used with vaginal and anal intercourse
Health Check-ups	Hemoccult cards, digital rectal exam, flexible sigmoidoscopy, colonoscopy

EQUIPMENT

- Nonsterile gloves
- Water-soluble lubricant
- Hemoccult cards
- Gooseneck lamp

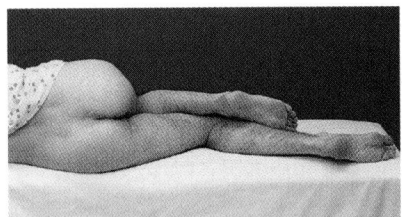

A. Left Lateral Decubitus

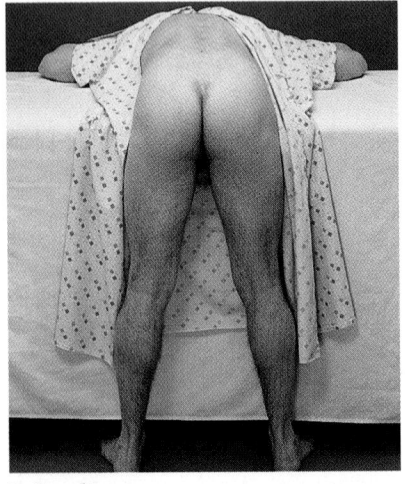

B. Standing

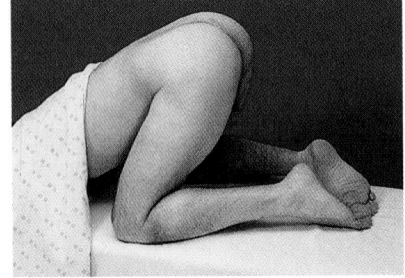

C. Knee-Chest

FIGURE 22-3A **Patient Positions for the Anus, Rectum, and Prostate Examination**

ASSESSMENT OF THE ANUS, RECTUM, AND PROSTATE

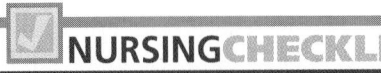

NURSING CHECKLIST

General Approach to Anus, Rectum, and Prostate Assessment

1. Greet the patient and explain the assessment techniques that you will be using.
2. Ensure that the examination room is at a warm, comfortable temperature to prevent patient chilling and shivering.
3. Use a quiet room that will be free from interruptions.
4. Ensure that the light in the room provides sufficient brightness to adequately observe the patient. It may be helpful to have a gooseneck lamp available for additional lighting when lesions are observed.
5. Instruct the patient to void prior to the assessment.
6. Instruct the patient to remove pants and underpants and to cover up with a drape sheet.
7. Assess the patient's apprehension level about the assessment and reassure the patient that apprehension is normal.
8. For inspection, place the patient in the left lateral decubitus position and visualize the perianal skin (Figure 22-3A). This position can also be used for palpation.
9. For palpation, have the patient stand at the side or end of the examination table, bending over the table, resting the elbows on the table, and spreading the legs slightly apart (Figure 22-3B). For the patient who cannot stand, have the patient assume the knee-chest position (Figure 22-3C). For the female who is undergoing a rectovaginal examination, have her assume the lithotomy position. See Chapter 20.
10. Don nonsterile gloves.
11. Use a systematic approach every time the assessment is performed. Proceed from the anus to the rectum in the female patient. Proceed from the anus to the prostate in the male patient.

NURSING**TIP**

Rectal Examination of the Female Patient

If a woman is to undergo a rectal examination without a vaginal exam, then the left lateral decubitus, standing, or knee-chest position can be used for the assessment.

LIFE 360°

Conversations during the Rectal Examination

You have your patient assume the standing position for the anorectal examination. Think how you would respond if your patient asked you one of the following:

- If you are free later that evening to catch dinner and a movie
- What you thought of the football game that was on TV last night
- If you enjoy this part of the examination

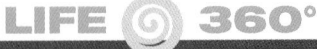

INSPECTION

Perineum and Sacrococcygeal Area

E Inspect the buttocks and sacral region for lesions, swelling, inflammation, and tenderness.

N This area should be smooth and free of lesions, swelling, inflammation, and tenderness. There should be no evidence of feces or mucus on the perianal skin.

A It is abnormal for one or several tiny openings to be seen in the midline over the sacral region, often with hair protruding from them (Figure 22-4).

P Pilonidal disease is an acquired condition of the midline coccygeal skin region induced by local stretching forces. There can be a cyst, an acute abscess, or chronic draining sinuses in the sacrococcygeal area. Small skin pits representing enlarged hair follicles precede development of the draining sinus or abscess. Lesions are often secondarily invaded by hair.

A Areas of hyperpigmentation, coupled with excoriation and thickened skin in the perianal area, are abnormal. The area may be intensely pruritic.

P Pruritis ani is caused by pinworms in children and by fungal infections in adults. The lesions are dull, grayish pink.

A Well-demarcated, erythematous, sometimes itchy exudative patches of varying size and shape rimmed with small, red-based pustules are abnormal.

P *Candida albicans* occurs in sites where heat and maceration provide a fertile environment. Systemic antibacterial, corticosteroid, or antimetabolic therapy; pregnancy; obesity; diabetes mellitus; blood dyscrasias; and immunologic defects increase susceptibility to candidiasis.

Anal Mucosa

E **1.** Spread the patient's buttocks apart with both hands, exposing the anus.

2. Instruct the patient to bear down as though moving the bowels.

3. Examine the anus for color, appearance, lesions, inflammation, rash, and masses.

N The anal mucosa is deeply pigmented, coarse, moist, and hairless. It should be free of lesions, inflammation, rash, masses, or additional openings. The anal opening should be closed. There should not be any leakage of feces or mucus from the anus with straining and there should not be any tissue protrusion.

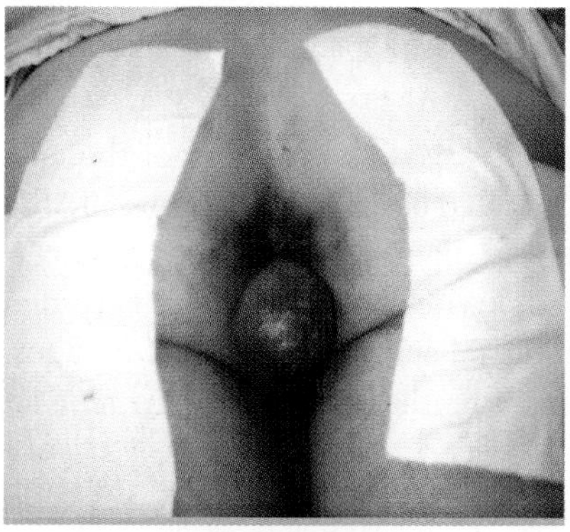

A A spherical, bluish lump that appears suddenly at the anus, and that ranges in size from a few millimeters to several centimeters in diameter, (Figure 22-5) is abnormal. The overlying anal skin may be tense and edematous. Pain and pruritus may be present in the perianal region.

P **Hemorrhoids** result from dilatation of the superior and inferior hemorrhoidal veins. These hemorrhoidal veins form a hemorrhoidal plexus, or cushion, in the submucosal layer of the anorectum. An external hemorrhoid is located below the dentate line. Thrombosed external hemorrhoids (blood clots within subcutaneous hemorrhoidal veins) occur as a

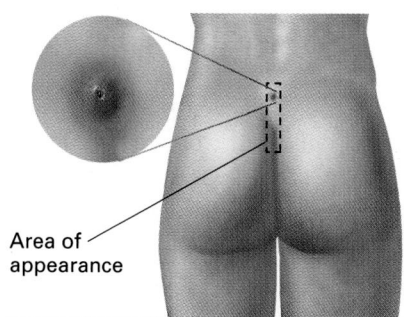

Area of appearance

FIGURE 22-4 Pilonidal Cyst

FIGURE 22-5 Thrombosed **Hemorrhoid.** *Courtesy of Dr. Haider Goussous, Albany, NY.*

E Examination   **N** Normal Findings   **A** Abnormal Findings   **P** Pathophysiology

result of heavy lifting, childbirth, straining to defecate (which may be due to a low-fiber diet), or other vigorous activity. Bleeding may occur with defecation.

A Excess anal or perianal tissue of varying sizes that is soft, pliable, and covered by normal skin is abnormal.

P Anal skin tags are the result of residual resolved thrombosed external hemorrhoids, pregnancy, or anal operations. In some cases, there is no known cause.

A Fecal incontinence is abnormal.

P Fecal incontinence is usually a sign of an underlying acute medical problem. Some causes of fecal incontinence include fecal impaction, diarrhea, irritable bowel syndrome, stroke, dementia, multiple sclerosis, rectal prolapse, rectal trauma, and anorectal carcinoma.

A The perianal area may have erythema, excoriations, cracking, and bleeding. In chronic cases the anal ring may have a shiny appearance.

P Pruritus ani is a condition in which itching around the rectum occurs. There are multiple causes of pruritus ani; however, excessive cleaning of the anal area is the most common cause. Moisture around the anus, associated with sweating or from passage of abnormal feces, can also exacerbate or induce this problem. Other possible causes of pruritus ani include pinworms, psoriasis, eczema, dermatitis, hemorrhoids, anal fissures, and sexually transmitted diseases.

A Linear tears in the epidermis of the anal canal beginning below the dentate line and extending distally to the anal orifice are abnormal (Figure 22-6). Extreme pain, pruritus, and bleeding may accompany these findings.

P **Anal fissures** are the result of trauma, such as the forced passage of a large, hard stool, and anal intercourse, especially forced intercourse. Fissures occur most often in the area of the posterior coccygeal midline and less frequently in the anterior midline. This is because of weakness in the superficial external sphincter in these sectors. Predisposition to fissure is increased by perianal inflammation, which causes the anoderm to lose its normal elasticity. A sentinel skin tag may be visible inferior to the anal fissure and at the anal margin. Sphincter spasms may occur during the examination. The use of a local anesthetic may be necessary to thoroughly examine the area.

A Undrained collections of perianal pus of the tissue spaces in and adjacent to the anorectum are abnormal.

P The most common cause of **anorectal abscesses** is infection of the anal glands, usually located posteriorly and situated between the internal and the external sphincters. These glands normally drain via the internal sphincter through small ducts and into anal crypts. When these ducts are occluded by impacted fecal material or trauma, ductal stasis and abscess formation results. An indurated mass with overlying erythema displaces the anus in cases of superficial abscess.

A An inflamed, red, raised area with purulent or serosanguineous discharge on the perianal skin is abnormal (Figure 22-7).

P An **anorectal fistula** is a hollow, fibrous tract lined by granulation tissue and having an opening inside the anal canal or rectum and one or more orifices

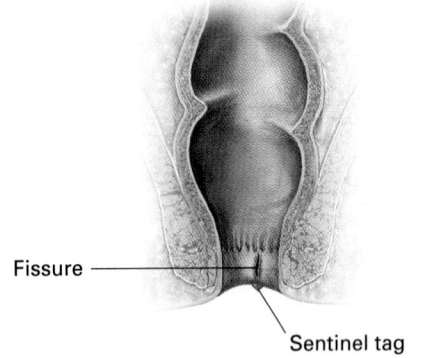

Fissure
Sentinel tag

FIGURE 22-6 Anal Fissure

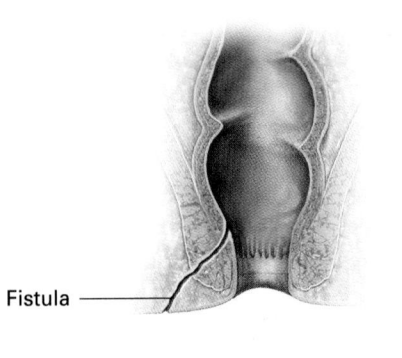

Fistula

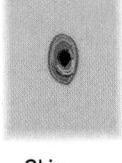

Skin surface opening

FIGURE 22-7 Anorectal Fistula

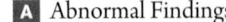

| **E** Examination | **N** Normal Findings | **A** Abnormal Findings | **P** Pathophysiology |

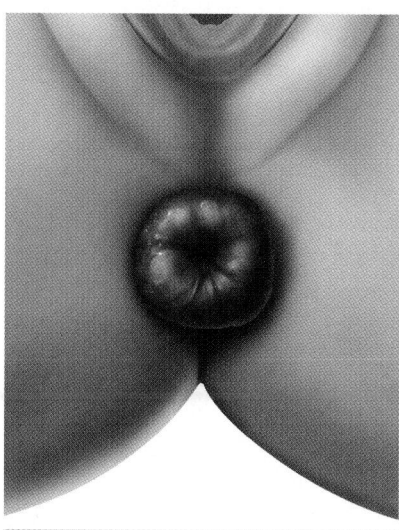

FIGURE 22-8 Rectal Prolapse

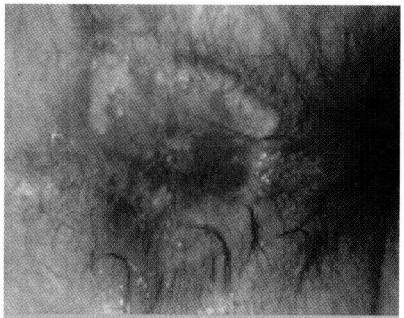

FIGURE 22-9 Perianal Herpes Simplex Virus. *Courtesy of Centers for Disease Control and Prevention (CDC).*

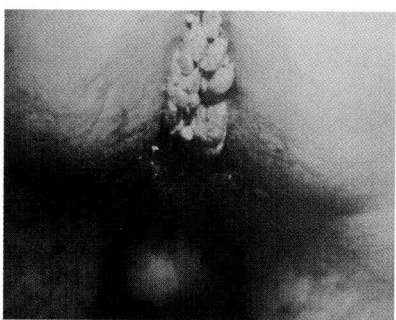

FIGURE 22-10 Human Papillomavirus in the Anal Region. *Courtesy of the Centers for Disease Control and Prevention (CDC).*

NURSING**TIP**

Documenting Abnormalities of the Anus

When documenting any abnormalities found in the anus, describe them with regard to anatomic location—e.g., posterior toward the patient's back; anterior toward the patient's abdomen; right and left, respectively. Be sure to note patient position and orientation.

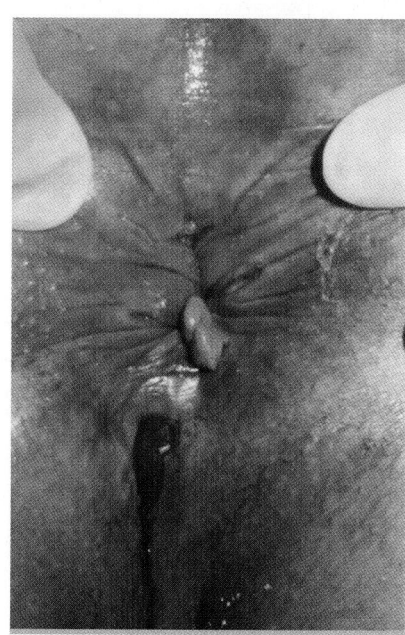

FIGURE 22-11 Perineal Chancroid. *Courtesy of Centers for Disease Control and Prevention (CDC).*

---

in the perianal skin. Fistulas are usually the result of incomplete healing of drained anorectal abscesses. However, they may occur in the absence of an abscess history. If this is the case, other causes for the fistula must be explored. Additional predisposing factors are inflammatory bowel disease, infectious disease, malignancy, Crohn's disease, radiation therapy, chemotherapy, chlamydial infections, and trauma.

A Soiling of the skin with stool and gaping of the anus are abnormal.

P **Anal incontinence** may be caused by neurological diseases, traumatic injuries, or surgical damage to the puborectalis or sphincter muscles. Perineal or intestinal disorders, diarrhea, fecal impaction, and constipating agents may also cause anal incontinence.

A The protrusion of the rectal mucosa (pinkish-red doughnut with radiating folds) through the anal orifice is abnormal (Figure 22-8).

P **Rectal prolapse** is associated with poor tone of the pelvic musculature, chronic straining at stool, fecal incontinence, and, sometimes, neurological disease or traumatic damage to the pelvis. A complete rectal prolapse involves the entire bowel wall. It is larger, red, and moist looking and has circular folds.

A Erythematous plaques that develop into vesicular lesions that may become pustules and ulcerate are abnormal (Figure 22-9).

P These lesions are suggestive of HSV. Most anorectal herpes is due to HSV-2, and infections are related to anal intercourse.

A Warts or lesions that are beefy red, flesh colored, irregular, and pedunculated are abnormal findings (Figure 22-10). The lesions may involve the anoderm but may also extend deep into the anal canal and involve the rectal mucosa. There may be a few scattered lesions or extensive involvement of the entire anus.

P Condylomata acuminatum are caused by HPV. Coital trauma allows entry into the anal epidermis in those in whom wart virus is latent in the anorectum. Anal warts may also develop in women via extension of genital warts along the perineum. Of the 50 strains of HPV, types 16, 18, and 31 have been associated with malignant lesions.

P Perineal chancroids (Figure 22-11) are caused by *Haemophilus ducreyi*. Chancroids can be seen on the genitalia as well as the perineal and perianal regions.

A Mucoid or creamy exudate, possibly blood, from the rectum is abnormal.

Rectal Assessment

A wide range of situations may be encountered during the rectal assessment. Consider how you would react in each of the following situations:

- Mr. DiCicco presents to you complaining of rectal bleeding and pain. While preparing him for examination, you notice the tip of a thermometer protruding from the rectum.

- Mrs. Kelly visits the office today for her annual Pap smear and pelvic examination. She states, "I am embarrassed to talk about this, but my husband would like me to participate in anal intercourse and I feel the need to discuss this with someone."

P Gonococcal proctitis is most often seen in homosexual men as a result of direct inoculation, but it also occurs in women through contamination by vaginal discharge.

A Multiple perianal fissures and edematous skin tags of varying degrees are abnormal.

P Anorectal involvement occurs in the majority of patients with Crohn's disease. Perianal disease may precede the onset of intestinal Crohn's disease by several years. Perianal disease may proceed to anal stricture and incontinence. The development of perianal Crohn's disease has no relation to other extraintestinal manifestations of the disease.

NURSING TIP

Assessing Risk through Anal Pap

The anal Pap is a screening tool used to identify premalignant cytologic changes in the anal epithelium in at-risk populations. There are currently no national guidelines available that specify when the anal Pap should be performed. Complete a comprehensive medical history with a focused anal cancer risk interview that facilitates the screening for risk factors. The interview should focus on the following areas:

- Sexual history, asking about anal intercourse and the number of sexual partners
- History of anal warts, genital warts, anal pain, anal discharge, anal dysplasia, or anal cancer
- Past history of an anal Pap; if yes, why, when, and the results

At-risk groups that may benefit from the anal Pap include:

- HIV-infected men with any history of receptive anal intercourse
- HIV-infected men with a history of injected drug use who might benefit from aggressive treatment
- Non-HIV-infected men who participate in receptive anal intercourse or who have a history of perianal or intra-anal condylomas
- Any recipient of allograft transplantation

ADVANCED TECHNIQUE

Anal Pap Collection

E
1. Inform the patient to avoid enemas and receptive anal intercourse for 24 hours prior to specimen collection.
2. Colonic preparation is not required, but the rectum should be emptied before obtaining the sample.
3. Moisten a Dacron-tipped swab with tap water and insert the swab about 2 inches into the anal canal.
4. Perform 10 to 12 spiral rotation movements of the swab against the walls of the rectum and anus as the swab encircles the anal canal during slow withdrawal of the swab.
5. Remove the swab and swirl it for 15 seconds in a container of liquid cytology fluid.
6. Perform a digital rectal examination after the anal Pap to rule out any masses.

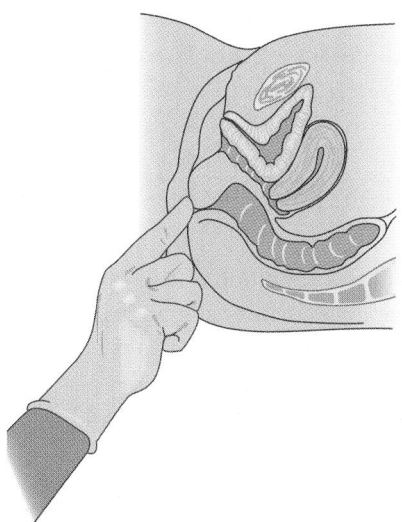

FIGURE 22-12 Position of the Index Finger for Anorectal Palpation

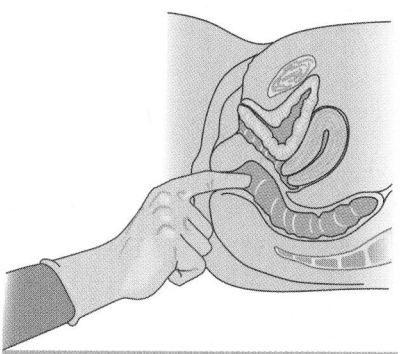

FIGURE 22-13 Position of the Index Finger in the Anorectum

PALPATION

Anus and Rectum

E To perform anal and rectal wall palpation:

1. Have the patient assume the most comfortable examination position.

2. Reassure the patient that sensations of urination and defecation are common during the rectal assessment.

3. Lubricate a gloved index finger.

4. Place your finger by the anal orifice and instruct the patient to bear down (Valsalva maneuver) as you gently insert the flexed tip of your gloved finger into the anal sphincter, with the tip of the finger toward the anterior rectal wall (pointed toward the umbilicus) (Figure 22-12). The anus should never be approached at a right angle (with the index finger extended).

4A. If the patient tightens the sphincter, remove your finger, reassure the patient, and try again, instructing the patient to use a relaxation technique such as deep breathing.

5. Feel the sphincter relax. Insert finger as far as it will go (Figure 22-13). Note anal sphincter tone.

6. Palpate the lateral, posterior, and anterior walls of the rectum in a sequenced manner. The lateral walls are felt by rotating the finger along the sides of the rectum. Palpate for nodules, irregularity, masses, and tenderness. Ask the patient to bear down again (which may help to palpate masses).

NURSING**ALERT**

Spotting Rectal Abuse

Suspect rectal abuse if you encounter any of the following in the assessment: bruises around the buttocks and hip area; cuts, tears, or bleeding around the anal mucosa; or refusal by the patient to undergo the rectal examination. Tell the patient about your concern and consult your institution's policy regarding suspected abuse.

LIFE ◎ 360°

Situations Encountered during the Rectal Assessment

The rectal examination may cause the patient to feel uncomfortable or embarrassed. How would you handle the following situations if they were to occur during the rectal assessment?

- Prior to the rectal examination, the patient is unable to sit still on the examination table.
- The patient develops an erection during the examination.
- The patient loses bowel control.
- The patient passes flatus during the examination.

TABLE 22-1 Common Causes of Rectal Bleeding

- Cancer of the colon
- Benign polyps of the colon
- Hemorrhoids
- Anal fissure
- Inflammatory bowel disease
- Forced or vigorous anal intercourse
- Traumatic sexual practices

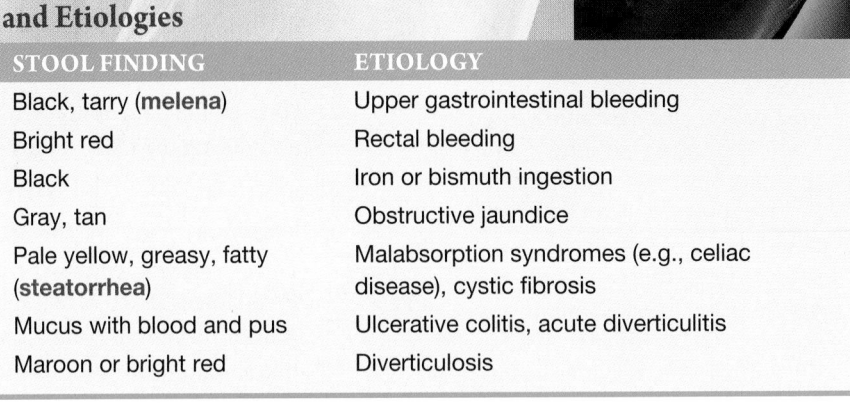

TABLE 22-2 Common Stool Findings and Etiologies

STOOL FINDING	ETIOLOGY
Black, tarry (**melena**)	Upper gastrointestinal bleeding
Bright red	Rectal bleeding
Black	Iron or bismuth ingestion
Gray, tan	Obstructive jaundice
Pale yellow, greasy, fatty (**steatorrhea**)	Malabsorption syndromes (e.g., celiac disease), cystic fibrosis
Mucus with blood and pus	Ulcerative colitis, acute diverticulitis
Maroon or bright red	Diverticulosis

7. Slowly withdraw the finger; inspect any fecal matter on your glove and test it for occult blood. Table 22-1 lists the common causes of rectal bleeding. Table 22-2 lists common stool findings and etiologies.

8. Offer the patient tissues to wipe off any remaining lubricant.

N The rectum should accommodate the index finger. There should be good sphincter tone at rest and with bearing down. There should be no excessive pain, tenderness, induration, irregularities, or nodules in the rectum or rectal wall.

A It is abnormal for the anal canal to be tight (making insertion of the index finger very difficult and painful or impossible).

P Anal stenosis can occur congenitally, but this condition usually is acquired. Anorectal operations, diarrheal disease, inflammatory conditions, and the habitual use of laxatives may cause anal stenosis. Chlamydial infections and malignancy must be excluded.

A Internal masses of vascular tissue in the anal canal are abnormal (Figure 22-14).

P Internal hemorrhoids arise from the superior (internal) hemorrhoidal vascular plexuses above the dentate line; they are covered by mucosa. Internal hemorrhoids are usually painless unless they are thrombosed or prolapsed through the anal orifice.

A A soft nodule or nodules in the rectum are abnormal (Figure 22-15).

P Rectal polyps occur frequently in the general population of the United States. Occasionally, they can be palpated, but more often they are diagnosed by proctoscopy. They vary in size and may be accompanied by rectal bleeding. Rectal polyps are of two types: pedunculated (attached to a stalk) or sessile (adhering to the rectal mucosal wall). A biopsy of the tissue is required to determine whether the polyp is benign or malignant.

A A tender, indurated mass in the anorectum is abnormal.

P This may be an anorectal abscess. Refer to the prior discussion on anorectal abscesses.

A An indurated cord palpated in the anorectum is abnormal.

P Anorectal fistula tracts may be palpated from the secondary orifice toward the anus. Digital rectal examination helps to determine the course of the tract. A drop of purulent drainage can be expressed from the opening if the opening is patent.

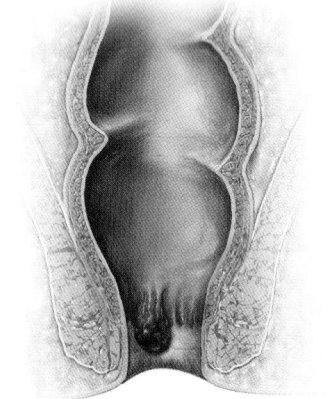

FIGURE 22-14 **Internal Hemorrhoid**

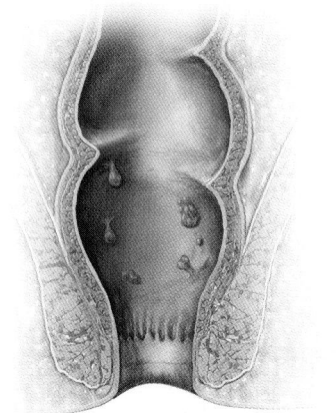

FIGURE 22-15 **Rectal Polyps**

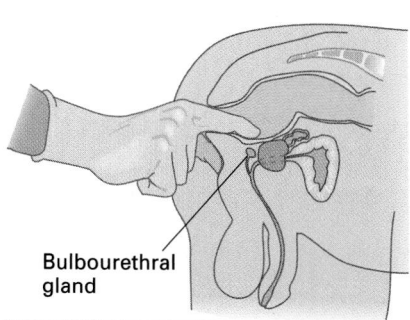

Bulbourethral gland

FIGURE 22-16 Bidigital Palpation of the Bulbourethral Gland

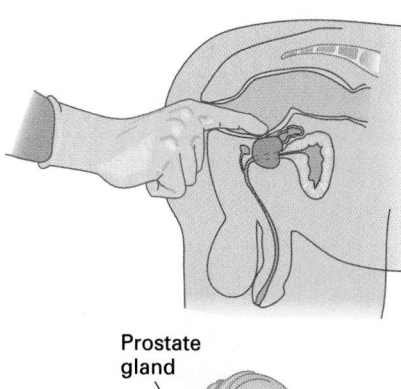

Prostate gland

Seminal vesicle

Bladder

FIGURE 22-17 Prostatic Palpation

A A small, symmetrical projection 2 to 4 cm long is abnormal.

P Rectal prolapse is best assessed with the patient in a squatting position. The anal sphincter is lax, and palpation between the finger and thumb reveals only two layers of mucosa. Refer to page 827 for additional information.

A Foreign bodies palpated in the rectum are abnormal.

P Thermometers, enema catheters, vibrators, bottles, and phallic objects may be introduced into the anus by accident, for erotic purposes, for concealment, for self-treatment, or by assault. Complications may include perforation of the rectum, obstruction, and pararectal infections.

A A hard mass in the anal canal is abnormal.

P This finding usually indicates anal carcinoma. There is a strong association between anal carcinoma (squamous cell) and HPV types 16 and 18.

A A firm, sometimes rocklike but often rubbery, puttylike mass is abnormal.

P In fecal impaction, the feces accumulates in the rectum because the colon does not respond to the usual stimuli promoting evacuation, or because accessory stimuli normally provided by eating and physical activity are lacking. Drugs, such as opiates, may compound the problem. Rectal sensitivity may be dulled by habitual disregard of the urge to defecate. The prolonged use of laxatives or enemas may also decrease rectal sensitivity.

Prostate

E To perform prostatic palpation:

1. Position the patient as tolerated (the standing position is preferred).

2. Reassure the patient that sensations of urination and defecation are common during the prostatic assessment.

3. Use a well-lubricated, gloved index finger.

4. Insert the gloved index finger and proceed as described in steps 4 and 5 on page 829.

5. Perform bidigital examination of the bulbourethral gland by pressing your gloved thumb into the perianal tissue while pressing your gloved index finger toward it (Figure 22-16). Assess for tenderness, masses, or swelling.

6. Release pressure of the thumb and index finger. Remove thumb from the perianal tissue and advance your index finger.

7. Palpate the posterior surface of the prostate gland (Figure 22-17). Note the size, shape, consistency, sensitivity, and mobility of the prostate. Note whether the median sulcus is palpable.

8. Attempt to palpate the seminal vesicles by extending your index finger above the prostate gland. Assess for tenderness and masses.

9. Slowly withdraw the finger; inspect any fecal matter on your glove and test it for occult blood (if not previously performed).

N The prostate gland should be small, smooth, mobile, and nontender. The median sulcus should be palpable.

| **E** Examination | **N** Normal Findings | **A** Abnormal Findings | **P** Pathophysiology |

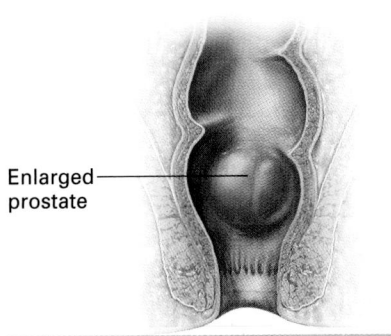

FIGURE 22-18 **Benign Prostatic Hypertrophy**

Enlarged prostate

A A soft, nontender, enlarged prostate gland is abnormal (Figure 22-18).

P The development of benign prostatic hypertrophy (BPH) is related to aging and the presence of testosterone, which converts to dihydrotestosterone and leads to prostatic cell growth. The size of the prostate gland on rectal assessment is not always indicative of the degree of symptoms because the lobes may not be palpable or they may be causing obstruction. In BPH, the median sulcus may not be palpable.

A A firm, tender, or fluctuant mass on the prostate is abnormal.

P A high percentage of patients with prostatic abscess have diabetes mellitus. An abscess is suspected in the patient with acute bacterial prostatitis or urinary tract infection who develops a spiked fever along with rectal pain. Prostatic abscesses are caused mainly by *Escherichia coli.*

A Firm, hard, or indurated nodules on the prostate are abnormal (Figure 22-19).

P The nodules of prostate cancer may be single or multiple. Early in the disease the nodules may be small, but late in the disease the entire prostate may seem irregular, hard, immobile, and quite large.

A An exquisitely tender and warm prostate is abnormal.

P Bacterial prostatitis is usually caused by *Escherichia coli.* When patients present with a sudden onset of high fever, chills, malaise, myalgias, and arthralgias, acute bacterial prostatitis is suspected.

NURSING**ALERT**

Guidelines for Early Detection of Prostate Cancer

Men who have reached 50 years of age need to be offered annual digital rectal examinations and PSA blood testing. More specific guidelines for the early detection of prostate cancer include:

• Age 50 for men who have at least a 10-year life expectancy
• Age 45 for African American men
• Age 45 for men who have a first-degree relative (father, brother) diagnosed with prostate cancer at an early age (younger than 65)
• Age 40 for men with several first-degree relatives diagnosed with prostate cancer at an early age

Source: www.cancer.org/docroot/PED/content/PED_2_3X_ACS_Cancer_Detection_Guidelines_36.asp. Accessed June 24, 2008.

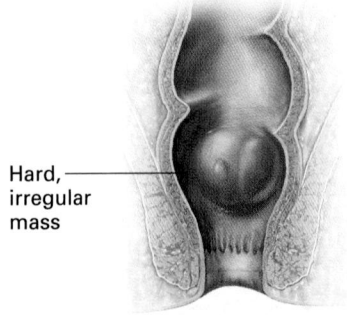

Hard, irregular mass

A. Single nodule

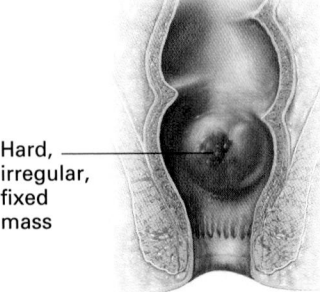

Hard, irregular, fixed mass

B. Multiple nodules

FIGURE 22-19 **Cancer of the Prostate**

E Examination | **N** Normal Findings | **A** Abnormal Findings | **P** Pathophysiology

NURSING**ALERT**

Risk Factors for Prostate Cancer

- Over 50 years of age
- Family history of prostate cancer
- African American race
- High intake of dietary fat, oil, and sugar
- High levels of serum testosterone

NURSING**TIP**

Prostate-Specific Antigen

The normal value for a serum PSA (prostate-specific antigen) is 0–4 ng/mL. Serum PSA elevations occur as a result of disruption of the normal prostatic architecture, which allows PSA to diffuse into the prostatic tissue and gain access to the circulation. This can occur with prostate disease such as prostate cancer, benign prostatic hypertrophy (BPH), and prostatitis. Prostate manipulation with prostate massage and prostate biopsy may also cause increases in the PSA level. There is no significant change, however, in PSA with a digital rectal exam.

Patients can have prostatic carcinoma with a normal PSA. Any time an abnormality (nodule, firmness, irregularity) is palpated during the prostate exam, a prostate biopsy needs to be performed to rule out carcinoma.

NURSING**TIP**

Acute Bacterial Prostatitis

Bacterial prostatitis is associated with a bladder infection caused by the same organism. Obtaining a urine culture will identify the pathogen. Rectal examination should be avoided in known cases of acute bacterial prostatitis because of the possibility of bacteremia.

CASE STUDY

An HIV-Positive Patient with Rectal Bleeding

This case study illustrates the application and objective documentation of the anal, rectal, and prostatic assessment. Spyridon is a 17-year-old male high school student who presents with rectal bleeding.

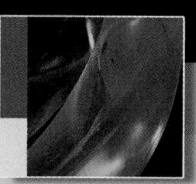

HEALTH HISTORY

PATIENT PROFILE	17 yo SWM
CHIEF COMPLAINT	"I have blood from my bottom and it hurts when I go to the bathroom."
HISTORY OF PRESENT ILLNESS	Pt reports that 3 days ago he started to experience some pain with defecation. The next day he noticed increased pain with defecation and blood on the surface of his stool. Yesterday the pain and bleeding worsened and they occurred without defecation. Pt also noted some mucopurulent anal discharge yesterday. Denies any previous history of rectal bleeding or pain. Pt denies any previous history of sexually transmitted diseases. He reports that he was screened for HIV infection 10 mos ago and was positive. He reports feeling "feverish" for the past 3 mos. Pt thinks he may have lost a few pounds but has not weighed himself. Has had some nausea and intermittent diarrhea.

continues

CASE STUDY (Continued)

An HIV-Positive Patient with Rectal Bleeding

PAST HEALTH HISTORY

Medical History

Celiac dz diagnosed last yr after 9–12 mos of abd pain, diarrhea, and 15 lb weight loss; follows gluten-free diet some days

Surgical History

Negative

Allergies

Wheat and wheat by-products (celiac dz)

Medications

None

Communicable Diseases

States that he has been tested for STDs and tests were always negative

Injuries and Accidents

MVA at 16 yo—hit another car at 40 mph (driving friend's car without a license), minor neck pain for 2 days, no long-term sequelae

Special Needs

Denies

Blood Transfusions

Denies

Childhood Illnesses

Chickenpox at a young age

Immunizations

Not sure

FAMILY HEALTH HISTORY

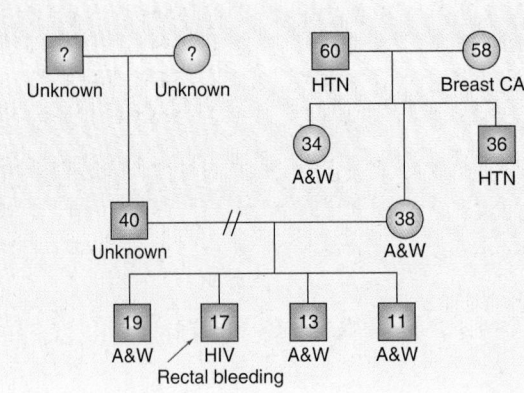

LEGEND

- ○ Living female
- □ Living male
- ⊗ Deceased female
- ⊠ Deceased male
- —//— Divorced
- ╱ Points to Patient
- A&W = Alive and well
- CA = Cancer
- HTN = Hypertension
- HIV = Human Immunodeficiency Virus

Denies FH of pilonidal cyst, colorectal CA, rectal polyps, prostate CA

SOCIAL HISTORY

Alcohol Use

Drinks beer with friends on weekends, 3–6 beers per night; usually drives home after partying

Tobacco Use

Cigarettes 1 PPD × 2 years

continues

Drug Use	Marijuana use every weekend, snorted cocaine once last year
Domestic and Intimate Partner Violence	One episode of sexual abuse at the age of 9 by a friend of the family. "I try to forget that night." Denies counseling. Mother is unaware of episode.
Sexual Practice	Sexually active at the age of 14 with 7 previous partners; "usually" uses condoms. 3 partners were female and 4 were male. His current sexual partner is a 30-yo man whom he has been with for the past 8 mos. Both anal receptive and nonanal receptive sexual practices.
Travel History	Travels to Greece every other summer to visit relatives; last summer he had 1 male and 1 female sexual partner in Greece
Work Environment	Store clerk for 1 yr; works 20 hrs/wk
Home Environment	Lives with his mother, 3 brothers, aunt, and uncle in a downtown apt complex; pt wants to move out as soon as he finishes high school; his aunt and uncle have "lots of money" and pay for his trips back to Greece
Hobbies and Leisure Activities	Riding around in his car and friends' cars, partying
Stress	Home situation is stressful. His mother works 2 jobs to support him and his brothers. Younger brother was recently expelled from school for carrying a knife. No contact with his father.
Education	Attends local high school, where he is a senior. Not sure what he is going to do after high school. GPA 2.5
Economic Status	"It's a struggle."
Military Service	Denies
Religion	Greek Orthodox; his aunt and uncle "demand" that he accompany them to Christmas and Easter services since they pay for his trips back to the "homeland"; describes self as "totally" nonreligious
Ethnic Background	Greek American, brings his friends to apt for dinner when his family is celebrating some Greek holidays
Roles and Relationships	Monogamous homosexual relationship for the last 8 months with male partner who is 13 years older. Poor relationship with teachers and classmates. Past month has spent less time with his friends for fear of them finding out about his homosexual relationship. Dislikes his aunt and uncle.
Characteristic Patterns of Daily Living	Wakes at 7:00 AM 5 days a week for school. Goes to class only when he "feels like it." No extracurricular activities at school or in the community. Works after school 3 days/wk and 1 shift on the weekend. Goes to bed at 12:00 AM.

continues

CASE STUDY (Continued)

An HIV-Positive Patient with Rectal Bleeding

HEALTH MAINTENANCE ACTIVITIES	
Sleep	7 hr every night, nonrestful, wakes feeling tired
Diet	Tries to stay away from gluten products but usually ends up eating whatever is in the pantry. Mother is not home to fix any meals, except on major holidays. Aunt will sometimes cook. Eats a lot of canned and frozen foods.
Exercise	Denies
Stress Management	Being with male partner
Use of Safety Devices	Denies using seat belt
Health Check-ups	Goes to ED or Health Clinic when he has a problem

PHYSICAL ASSESSMENT	
Inspection	
General	Thin young male in clear discomfort
Perineum and Sacrococcygeal Area	1 cm fissure at posterior coccygeal midline
Anal Mucosa	Deeply pigmented, coarse, moist and hairless, ⊕ mucous discharge, anal opening closed
Palpation	
Inguinal Area	Multiple 1–2 cm inguinal nodes in both groins
Anus and Rectum	Pain and tenderness with rectal exam; ⊕ gross blood and mucus; ⊕ sphincter tone; Ø nodules in the rectum or rectal wall
Prostate	Small, soft, smooth, mobile; extreme pain with rectal exam
Advanced Technique	
Anal Pap	Pt refused

LABORATORY DATA		PT'S VALUES	NORMAL RANGE
CBC	RBC	3.0 M/mm³	4–5.2 M/mm³
	WBC	3.2 k/mm³	4–11 k/mm³
	PLT	120 k/mm³	140–440 k/mm³
	Hgb	9.9 g/dL	12–16 g/dL
	Hct	32%	39–51%

continues

		PT'S VALUES	NORMAL RANGE
Chemistry Panel	ALT	82 units/L	5–60 units/L
	AST	90 units/L	5–43 units/L
	Sedimentation Rate (Westergren method)	90 mm/hr	0 to 15 mm/hr
Stool Hemoccult		Positive	Negative
HIV ELISA		Positive	Negative

ASSESSMENT IN BRIEF

Anus, Rectum, and Prostate Assessment

Inspection

- Perineum and sacrococcygeal area
- Anal mucosa

Palpation

- Anus and rectum
- Prostate

Advanced Technique

- Anal Pap collection

REVIEW QUESTIONS

1. Pruritus ani is a condition caused by which of the following?
   a. Constipation
   b. Excessive anal cleansing
   c. Use of cotton underwear
   d. Vigorous exercise
   The correct answer is (b).

2. Mr. Smith presents to your office and you obtain his sexual history. Which of the following causes you to consider performing an anal Pap?
   a. Mr. Smith is single and heterosexual
   b. Mr. Smith uses condoms intermittently
   c. Mr. Smith has a history of perianal condylomas
   d. Mr. Smith has had 8 sexual partners in the last 2 years
   The correct answer is (c).

3. On which of the following patients should you order a PSA?

   a. A 48-year-old Caucasian male with prostatitis
   b. A 42-year-old Hispanic male with hemorrhoids
   c. A 40-year-old Asian male whose uncle has prostate cancer
   d. A 47-year-old African American male with no complaints
   The correct answer is (d).

4. Which of the following instructions should a patient receive prior to having the anal Pap performed?
   a. Use a cleansing enema the evening before the procedure
   b. Eat clear liquids the entire day before the procedure
   c. Avoid receptive anal intercourse for 24 hours before the procedure
   d. Use a rectal suppository 12 hours before the procedure
   The correct answer is (c).

5. Which etiology would you suspect if, while performing the inspection portion of the rectal examination, you noted vesicular lesions?
   a. Condyloma acuminatum
   b. Crohn's disease
   c. Gonococcal prostatitis
   d. Herpes simplex virus
   The correct answer is (d).

6. Which statement is correct in regard to performing a successful rectal examination?
   a. Provide a step-by-step explanation about the examination
   b. Tell the patient that you are just as nervous about this as he is
   c. Perform the rectal examination at the beginning of the physical examination to decrease patient anxiety
   d. While performing the rectal examination, ask the patient about what he enjoys doing in his spare time, to try to get his mind off of the examination
   The correct answer is (a).

   Questions 7, 8, and 9 refer to the following situation:

   Mrs. Skiados, a 48-year-old heterosexual female, presents to you with the complaint of hematochezia.

7. Which etiology would you suspect from the patient's complaint of bright red stools?
   a. Upper gastrointestinal bleeding
   b. Iron ingestion
   c. Rectal bleeding
   d. Malabsorption syndrome
   The correct answer is (c).

8. After explaining to Mrs. Skiados that you would like her to roll over on her left side so that you can examine the rectal area, she seems reluctant. Upon inspection of the rectal area, you observe a linear tear in the anal canal and some scattered lesions that are pedunculated, beefy red and irregular. Which of the following would you suspect?
   a. Rectal prolapse
   b. Rectal abuse
   c. Anorectal abscess
   d. Ulcerative colitis
   The correct answer is (b).

9. Which of the following conditions is the probable etiology of Mrs. Skiados's rectal lesions?
   a. Condyloma acuminatum
   b. Pilonidal cyst
   c. Herpes simplex virus
   d. Pruritus ani
   The correct answer is (a).

10. During Mr. Goldman's rectal examination, you palpate a firm, tender, and fluctuant mass on the prostate. What etiology do these findings suggest?
    a. Prostate cancer
    b. Prostate abscess
    c. Benign prostatic enlargement
    d. Thrombosed internal hemorrhoid
    The correct answer is (b).

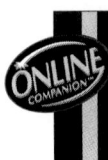

Visit the Estes online companion resource at
www.delmar.cengage.com
for additional content and study aids.
Click on Online Companions and then select
the Nursing discipline.

REFERENCE

www.cancer.org/docroot/PED/content/PED_2_3X_ACS_Cancer_Detection_Guidelines_36.asp. Accessed June 24, 2008.

BIBLIOGRAPHY

American Cancer Society. (2007). What are the risk factors for colorectal cancer? Retrieved February 22, 2007, from http://www.cancer.org/docroot/CRI/content/CRI_2_4_2X_What_are_the_risk_factors_for_colon_and_rectum_cancer.asp?sitearea=

Atiemo, H. O., Moy, L., Vasavada, S., & Rackley, R. (2007). Evaluating and managing urinary incontinence after prostatectomy: Beyond pads and diapers. *Cleveland Clinic Journal of Medicine, 74*(1), 57–63.

Benway B. M., & Moon T. D. (2008). Bacterial prostatitis. *Urology Clinics of North America, 35*(1), 23–32.

Blackwell, C. W. (2008). Anorectal carcinoma screening in gay men: Implications for nurse practitioners. *The American Journal for Nurse Practitioners, 12*(1), 60–63.

Carter, H. B., Ferrucci, L., Kettermann, A., Landis, P., Wright, E. J., Epstein, J. I., Trock, B. J., & Matter, E. J. (2006). Detection of life-threatening prostate cancer with prostate-specific antigen velocity during a window of curability. *Journal of the National Cancer Institute, 98*(21), 1521–1527.

Ficorelli, C. T., & Weeks, B. (2006). Facing up to prostate cancer. *Nursing 2006, 36*(5), 66–68.

Gee, R. (2006). Primary care health issues among men who have sex with men. *Journal of the American Academy of Nurse Practitioners, 18*(1), 144–153.

Gordon, P. H., & Nivatvongs, S. (2002). *Principles and practices of surgery for the colon, rectum and anus* (2nd ed.). New York: Informa Healthcare.

Holcomb, S. S. (2007). Prostate cancer screening: An individual decision. *Nurse Practitioner, 32*(8), 6–8.

Matthiesen, V., & DeWolff, D. (2006). Constipation and fecal incontinence. *Advance for Nurse Practitioners, 14*(10), 41–45.

Nickel, J. C. (2008). Inflammation and benign prostatic hypertrophy. *Urology Clinics of North America, 35*(1), 109–115.

Porche, D. J. (2006). Anal pap in men: A screening tool. *The Journal for Nurse Practitioners, 2*(9), 580–581.

Raper, J. L. (2006). Anal pap screening in men with HIV. *Advance for Nurse Practitioners, 14*(6), 30–36.

Smith R. A., Cokkinides, V., & Eyre H. J. (2006). American Cancer Society guidelines for the early detection of cancer. *CA: A Cancer Journal for Clinicans, 56*(1),11–25.

Tariman, J. D. (2006). Prostate cancer: Screening and early detection. *Advance for Nurse Practitioners, 14*(9), 20–24.

Warren, T., & Warren, R. (2005). *The updated herpes handbook.* Portland, OR: The Portland Press.

Wein, A. J., Kavoussi, L. R., Novick, A. C., Partin, A. W., & Peters, C. A. (2007). *Campbell-Walsh urology review manual.* Philadelphia: Saunders.

WEB SITES

The American College of Gastroenterology:
http://www.acg.gi.org

American Gastroenterological Association:
http://www.gastro.org

Digital Urology Journal:
http://www.duj.com

Gastrointestinal Nursing:
http://www.gastrointestinalnursing.com

National Cancer Institute:
http://www.cancer.org

National Comprehensive Cancer Network:
http://www.nccn.org

Prostate Cancer Foundation:
http://www.prostatecancerfoundation.org

Society of Urologic Nurses and Associates:
http://www.suna.org

Urology Health.org:
http://www.urologyhealth.org

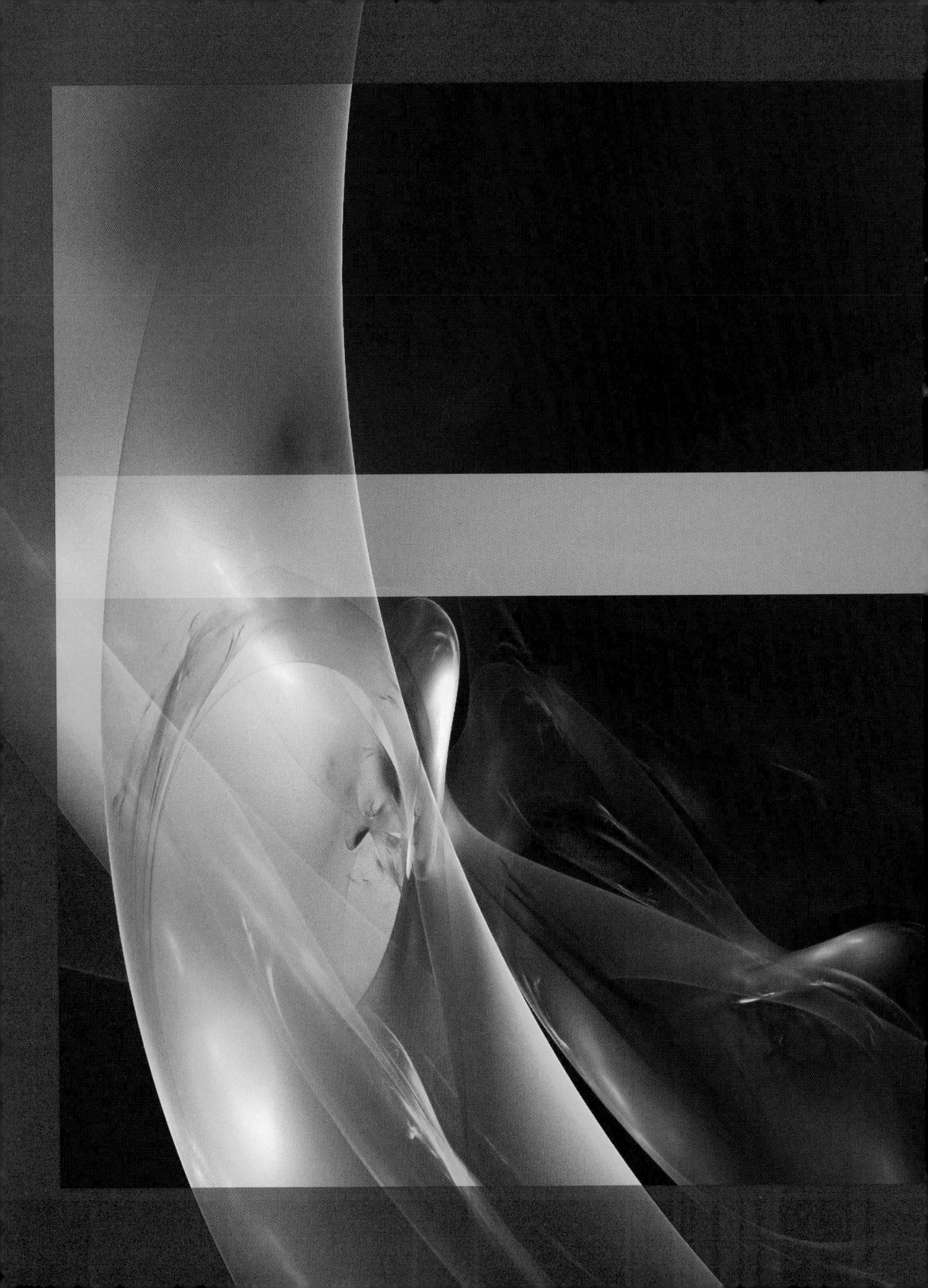

UNIT 4 | Special Populations

Conciseness and decision are, above all things, necessary with the sick. Let your thought expressed to them be concisely and decidedly expressed.

—Florence Nightingale

CHAPTER 23

The Pregnant Patient

COMPETENCIES

1. Describe the characteristics of the most common pregnancy-related complaints.

2. Assess the psychosocial status of a pregnant woman.

3. Differentiate the normal changes of pregnancy from pathological changes.

4. Perform a physical assessment on a pregnant woman.

5. Assess the learning needs of a pregnant woman.

Pregnancy imposes many physiological, hormonal, and psychological changes on a woman during the 280 days, or approximately 40 (normal range 37 to 40) weeks, of gestation. The pregnancy is subdivided into trimesters of a little more than 13 weeks each, and various symptoms and problems can be specific to certain trimesters. You are encouraged to review Chapters 14 and 20 before beginning this chapter.

The focus when assessing a pregnant patient is the wellness of the mother and the fetus. Much of prenatal care centers around educating and reassuring the pregnant patient and her family regarding physical changes that result from pregnancy. With the availability of accurate home pregnancy tests, a woman may know she's pregnant within 2 weeks of conception, affording an opportunity for early health care interaction. As a nurse, you will often be the primary contact during the pregnancy, and you can play a critical role in helping to ensure a healthy pregnancy. With active listening and a supportive attitude, you can also play an important role in educating the family on what to expect during the next 9 months, as well as educating them about warning signs of possible complications of pregnancy.

ANATOMY AND PHYSIOLOGY

Physiological changes during pregnancy affect every system in the body. These changes occur to maintain maternal health and accommodate the growth of a healthy fetus. This chapter provides an overview of these changes and is not all-inclusive.

SKIN AND HAIR

The skin is subjected to the influence of hormones during pregnancy. There is an increased subdermal fat deposit, along with thickening of the skin. Acne may develop or improve during pregnancy. Other changes include an increase in sweat and sebaceous gland production, which, along with the increase in superficial capillaries and peripheral vasodilation, serves to dissipate heat. Existing pigmentation increases in the nipples, areolae, external genitalia, and the anal region. The face may develop **melasma** (Figure 23-1), known as the mask of pregnancy, which manifests as blotchy, irregular pigmentation. Linea nigra, or darkening of the linea alba, may present on the abdomen as a darkened vertical midline between the fundus and the symphysis pubis (Figure 23-2). **Linea nigra** regresses, or fades, after delivery, but does not totally disappear. Nevi, circumscribed, pigmented areas of skin, may be stimulated to grow; and skin tags, molluscum fibrosum gravidarum, may develop from epithelial hyperplasia, especially on the upper body. With connective tissue changes of pregnancy, **striae gravidarum** (stretch marks) often develop on the abdomen, breasts, and upper thighs; after delivery, they regress or fade but do not totally disappear.

Vascular changes reflected in the skin can include the development or enlargement of spider angiomas, hemangiomas, varicosities, and palmar erythema, which may become more pronounced as pregnancy progresses.

Facial hair may increase, but the scalp hair may shed and thin, especially in the postpartum period. The scalp hair may become oily.

HEAD AND NECK

The thyroid gland may increase in size after approximately 12 weeks of gestation (although studies are conflicting as to whether or not there is an increase), related to the increase in vascularity. This may result in a shift in thyroid tests.

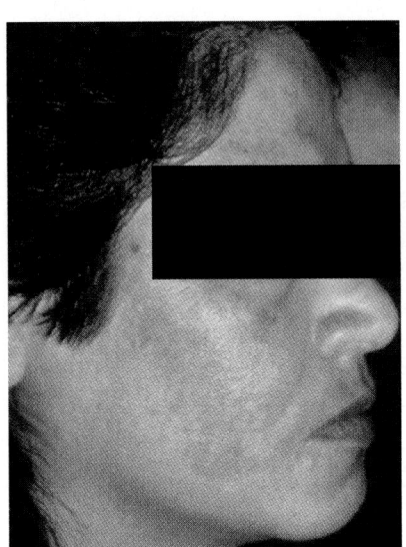

FIGURE 23-1 **Melasma.** *Courtesy of Timothy Berger, MD, Chief, Department of Dermatology at San Francisco General Hospital, San Francisco, CA.*

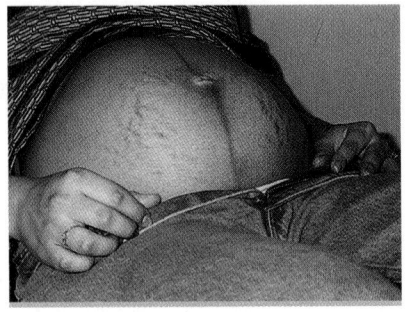

FIGURE 23-2 Linea Nigra with Striae Gravidarum

NURSING**TIP**

Chemical Hair Treatments

Chemical hair treatments such as color and permanents should be avoided during pregnancy, especially in the first trimester, because these chemicals are absorbed into the scalp and ultimately into the maternal circulation.

Eyes, Ears, Nose, Mouth, and Throat

Corneal thickening and edema (especially in the third trimester) may occur and the pregnant woman may experience visual changes. These changes may be discussed with the patient's ophthalmologist or optometrist, but pregnancy changes in vision are typically not treated because they may resolve shortly after delivery. Contact lens wearers may also experience blurry vision secondary to increased lysozyme in tears, which may lead to an oily sensation.

Increased vascularity and increased mucus production often lead to nasal stuffiness, snoring, congestion and epistaxis, impaired hearing or fullness in the ears, and a decreased sense of smell. The pregnant woman should be reassured that these are normal experiences that usually resolve after delivery.

Increased vascularity and hormonal changes often lead to soft, edematous, and bleeding gums, commonly noticed when brushing teeth. Epulis, or erythematous gingival nodules that bleed easily, can be present. **Ptyalism**, excessive secretion of saliva, may be an annoying symptom and, if marked, may require evaluation for other causes such as goiter. Vocal changes or cough may be noted due to hormonally induced changes in the larynx.

Breasts

Early breast changes may include enlargement, tingling, and tenderness secondary to hormonal changes. As the pregnancy progresses, the breasts continue to enlarge and the mammary glands prepare for lactation after delivery (alveoli increase in both number and size, Montgomery's tubercles enlarge, and lactiferous ducts proliferate). This may cause the breasts to feel more nodular on palpation than in the nonpregnant state. The areolae may darken. The nipples may become darker and more erect. **Colostrum**, a thick, yellow discharge known as early breast milk, may be secreted as early as the second trimester. Veins in the breasts may become more apparent and blue as they become engorged from increased vascularization.

Thorax and Lungs

The demands of the physiological changes of pregnancy and of the fetus lead to increased oxygen consumption and carbon dioxide excretion. This helps to increase oxygen use by the fetus and facilitate the transfer of carbon dioxide from the fetus to the maternal circulation for elimination. With advancing pregnancy, the diaphragm elevates approximately 4 cm and the movement of the diaphragm increases, so that most respiratory effort is diaphragmatic. Stimulated by progesterone, the thoracic cage relaxes and expands by 5 to 7 cm in circumference to accommodate these increased respiratory demands, which may cause discomfort or pain as the intercostal muscles stretch. The tidal volume increases by 30% to 40% during pregnancy, probably due to the stimulatory effects of increased levels of progesterone. These physiological changes often lead to an increased respiratory rate, hyperventilation, or shortness of breath, especially on exertion such as climbing stairs.

Heart and Peripheral Vasculature

Largely as an increase in plasma, blood volume increases by 30% to 50% (more with multiple births), thus increasing the cardiac output. This process begins at 12 weeks of gestation and peaks at 28 to 34 weeks. This increase protects the mother from hemorrhage at delivery, increases oxygen transport, increases renal filtration, and dissipates fetal heat production. With cardiac dilatation (maximal

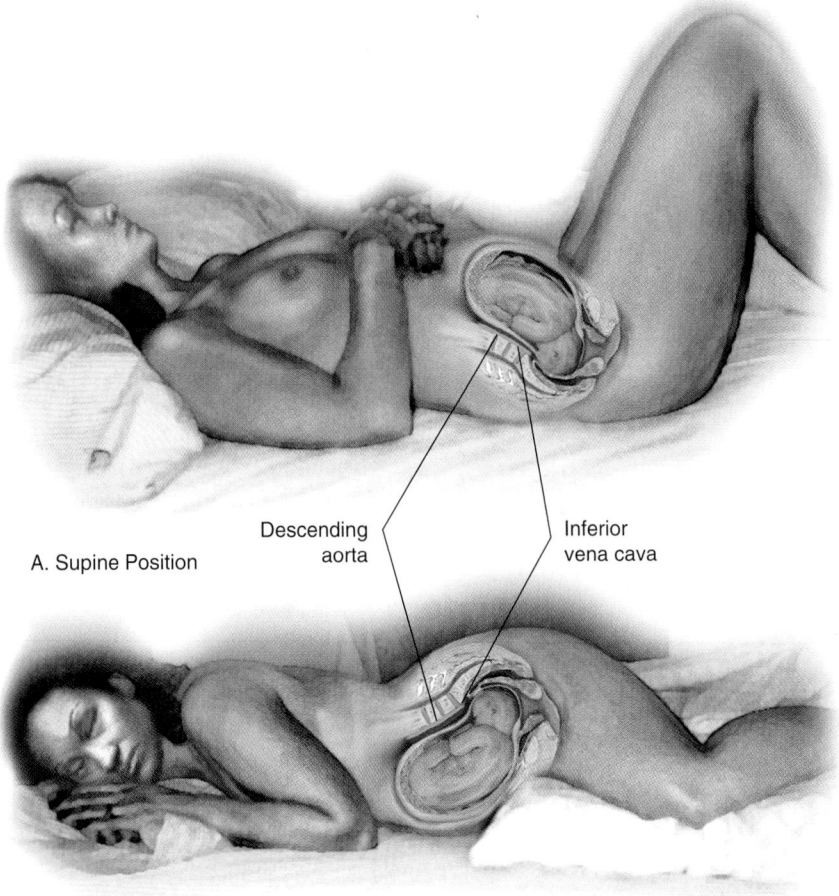

Descending aorta

Inferior vena cava

A. Supine Position

B. Right Lateral Position

FIGURE 23-3 **A. Supine hypotension can occur when the woman is in the supine position. The weight of the gravid uterus may partially occlude the descending aorta and vena cava. B. Maintaining a lateral position alleviates the compression.**

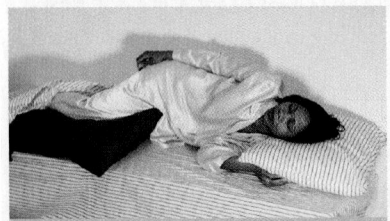

FIGURE 23-4 **Resting in the lateral position helps to alleviate pooling of blood in the lower extremities.**

by 10 weeks), the mother's heart lies more horizontally and shifts upward and to the left along with the apical impulse. Heart rate increases by 10 to 20 beats per minute, a split first heart and S_3 sound may be heard, physiological systolic murmurs of grade 2/6 may be heard, and blood pressure varies according to position and trimester. In addition, the increased breast vascularization may lead to a continuous murmur, especially near the end of the pregnancy, known as the "mammary souffle." Supine hypotension, resulting from the weight of the uterus on the inferior vena cava, is common; it is recommended that pregnant women avoid a supine position starting at 20 weeks, unless there is a uterine tilt to the side.

Systolic pressure is not significantly different throughout pregnancy, whereas the diastolic pressure may lower by 5 mm Hg in the second trimester and then rise to first-trimester levels after midpregnancy. The lower blood pressure in the second trimester occurs as the body adjusts to the changes in the intravascular volume and to the hormonal effects on the vascular walls. Monitoring of blood pressure during pregnancy is an important factor in determining complications such as preeclampsia. Many pregnant women also experience dependent edema partially due to peripheral vasodilation and decreased vascular resistance. This swelling is most commonly seen in the feet but can also occur in the hands and face.

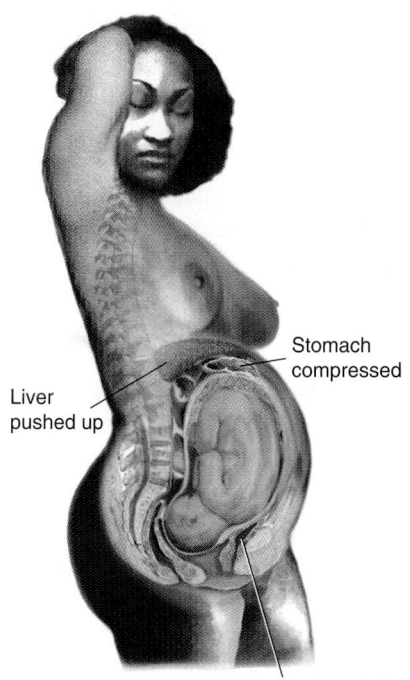

Liver pushed up

Stomach compressed

Bladder largely in pelvis therefore frequent urination

FIGURE 23-5 Crowding of Abdominal Contents by Gravid Uterus

ABDOMEN

The growing uterus gradually displaces the abdominal contents, leading to decreased tone and motility, decreased bowel sounds, and an increased emptying time for the stomach and intestines (Figure 23-5). These changes often bring about increased flatulence and constipation and can contribute to the development of hemorrhoids.

Indigestion (heartburn) is often experienced by the pregnant woman due to the relaxation of the esophageal sphincter, subsequent reflux, and slowed gastric emptying. Nausea and vomiting are common early in pregnancy and may even lead to a weight loss in the first trimester.

Increased emptying time and chemical changes in bile composition can put the pregnant woman at increased risk for cholelithiasis, the presence or formation of bilestones or calculi in the gallbladder or duct, and estrogen may augment any tendency to develop cholestasis (arrest of bile excretion).

Some women will also experience a separation of the rectus muscle of the abdominal wall, known as **diastasis recti**, which may be asymptomatic and noticed only as a vertical protrusion midline. Diastasis requires no medical intervention.

URINARY SYSTEM

Secondary to the increased intravascular volume, the glomerular filtration rate (GFR) increases by approximately 50% and the reabsorption rate of various chemicals, especially sodium and water, changes. Urinary frequency usually increases in the first trimester. **Glycosuria**, glucose in the urine, is common in pregnancy. There is also an increased loss of amino acids that may show as **proteinuria** on a urine dipstick. Dilation of the ureters and renal pelvises, a decrease in bladder tone, and the short female urethra place the pregnant woman at risk for urinary tract infections. In both early and late pregnancy, the bladder is encroached upon by the enlarging uterus and fetal presenting parts. **Nocturia**, or excessive nighttime urination, may disrupt the pregnant woman's sleep pattern.

MUSCULOSKELETAL SYSTEM

The hormones relaxin and progesterone affect all joints in the pregnant woman's body. This leads to a widening (and, occasionally, a separation) of the symphysis pubis at approximately 28 to 32 weeks, increased pelvic mobility to accommodate vaginal delivery, and an unsteady gait known as the "waddle of pregnancy." These hormones also allow the thoracic cage to change shape, which can lead to complaints of upper back or rib pain.

Developing lordosis of the lumbar spine keeps the center of gravity over the legs and is often associated with lower back pain. Sciatic nerve pain may also present as lower back pain, a shooting pain down the leg, or leg weakness. For unknown reasons, muscle cramps, particularly in the calves, thighs, and buttocks, may develop, especially at night.

Shoe size may increase by as much as one full size as pregnancy progresses, due to edema and relaxation of foot joints. Fat deposits increase throughout the body and are most noticeable on the hips and buttocks.

NEUROLOGICAL SYSTEM

The most commonly experienced neurological changes of pregnancy include headaches, numbness, and tingling. The more bothersome neuropathies include carpal tunnel syndrome, footdrop, facial palsy, fatigue, and difficulty remaining asleep at night. After ruling out any underlying disorder, reassure the patient that these are temporary symptoms. Headaches may be relieved by small, frequent meals; adequate rest; and posture and work environment adjustments. Seizure activity with no prior history may indicate the development of **eclampsia**, or seizures associated with hypertensive disorders of pregnancy (HDP), also called pregnancy-induced hypertension (PIH). Dizziness and lightheadedness may be due to the fetus' pressure on the vena cava. Lapses of memory are common but the etiology is poorly understood.

FEMALE GENITALIA

The pelvic organs experience vascular, hormonal, and structural changes during pregnancy. Uterine vessels dilate and at term can hold one-sixth of the maternal circulation, with a blood flow of 500 mL/min. With the increased blood flow, the pregnant woman may note a feeling of pelvic congestion as well as vulvar edema. Amenorrhea, secondary to the hormonal changes of pregnancy, is generally the first noticeable sign.

The pregnant woman's enlarging uterus begins as a pelvic organ, becoming, with bimanual examination, palpably enlarged at 6 to 7 weeks (Figures 23-6 and 23-7), and progresses to an abdominal organ at approximately 12 weeks of gestation.

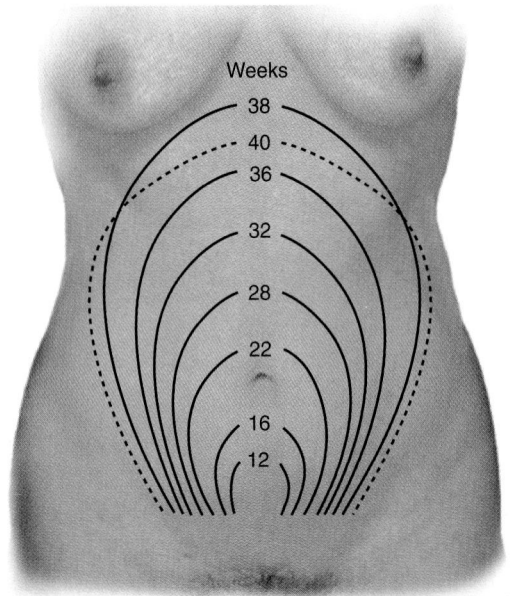

FIGURE 23-6 Uterine and Abdominal Enlargement of Pregnancy

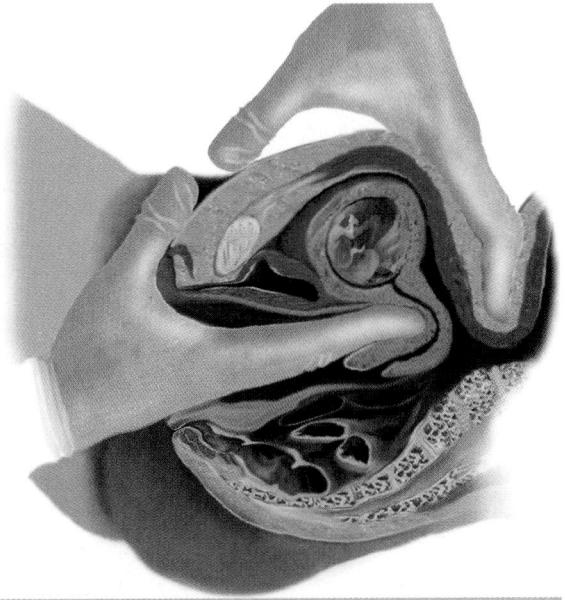

FIGURE 23-7 Bimanual Examination and Hegar's Sign

At 16 weeks the fundus of the uterus is midway between the symphysis pubis and the umbilicus, and at 20 weeks the fundus is typically at the umbilicus.

Between weeks 18 and 32 of gestation, the height of the uterine fundus above the symphysis pubis is measured in centimeters and is used to confirm the gestational age in weeks. After 32 weeks, although still used, this measurement is less accurate.

The round and broad ligaments elongate to accommodate the growing fetus, and may cause the patient lower quadrant pain. **Lightening**, also called dropping, is a decrease in fundal height due to the descent of the presenting fetal part into the pelvis. This typically occurs approximately 3 weeks prior to the onset of labor in a nulliparous woman, and is often indicated by increased pressure in the pelvis and increased frequency of urination. In a multiparous woman, lightening may not occur until after active labor begins. **Braxton Hicks contractions**, which are irregular and usually painless, begin as early as the first trimester.

The cervix experiences increased vascularity and increased **friability**, or susceptibility to bleeding, especially following a Pap smear or intercourse. Table 23-1 lists additional changes in the cervix and uterus in pregnancy. The endocervical glands increase in number and size. This causes a softening of the cervix. Mucus production occurs to form an endocervical protective plug, and the vaginal mucosa thickens secondary to hormonal changes. Throughout pregnancy, the vaginal discharge increases and is typically of a white, milky consistency. From 36 weeks on, vaginal discharge may become noticeably thicker and clumps may be present when the mucus plug is expelled. The hormonally induced changes in the vaginal environment lead to an increased risk of yeast infection.

NURSING**TIP**

Avoiding Vaginal Yeast Infections during Pregnancy

Teach your patients good perineal care during pregnancy:

- Avoid clothing that fits tightly in the crotch.
- Choose underwear with a cotton rather than a nylon crotch.
- Remove a wet bathing suit promptly.
- Monitor sugar and simple carbohydrates in the diet, if prone to yeast infection.
- Report recurrent yeast infections, which suggest the possibility of glucose intolerance.

NURSING**ALERT**

Physiological Anemia and Hypertensive Disorders of Pregnancy (HDP)

Failure of the normal physiological anemia of pregnancy to occur in the third trimester may be associated with HDP. HDP is commonly known as toxemia of pregnancy. Complications associated with HDP can include **HELLP syndrome** (hemolysis, elevated liver enzymes, and low platelets), which may lead to significant blood loss. Immediately refer patients with these symptoms for further evaluation.

TABLE 23-1 Changes in Pelvic Organs in Pregnancy

NAME	GESTATIONAL AGE	DESCRIPTION
Ladin's sign	5–6 weeks	Softening of cervical-uterine junction
Goodell's sign	6 weeks	Cervical softening
McDonald's sign	7–8 weeks	Easy flexion of fundus on cervix
Chadwick's sign	8 weeks	Cervical bluish hue
Hegar's sign	8 weeks	Softening of uterine isthmus

Providing Care to the Abused Pregnant Patient

The abused woman is often reluctant to seek help, sometimes out of fear (of retaliation from her partner, or of inability to survive on her own) and sometimes out of the hope that the partner will change and the abuse will end. The often-described "cycle of violence" (a period of tension-building followed by battery followed by remorse, calm, and even kindness on the part of the abuser) may keep the woman feeling trapped. What are some supportive nursing strategies you can provide to the abused pregnant woman that will respect her dignity and help allay her fears?

NURSING ALERT

Identifying Abuse in Pregnant Women

Abusive relationships are much more common in our society, across all socioeconomic groups, than is generally believed, and abusive situations often intensify when a woman announces her pregnancy. Suspect abuse if the pregnant patient:

- **Has a pattern of frequent visits, especially with vague complaints**
- **Presents with complaints inconsistent with a known injury (any unusual pattern of bruises on the head, neck, breasts, chest, abdomen, and genitalia)**
- **Frequently misses appointments**
- **Fails to plan appropriately for the baby's arrival**
- **Is always accompanied by an overly solicitous partner**

ANUS AND RECTUM

Decreased gastrointestinal tract tone and motility produce a sense of fullness, indigestion, constipation, bloating, and flatulence. Development of hemorrhoids is common and can become very problematic. As pregnancy progresses and the uterus enlarges, mechanical pressure may aggravate constipation and hemorrhoids. Vitamin and iron supplementation may increase the above symptoms and commonly darken the stool.

HEMATOLOGICAL SYSTEM

Common hematological changes include increased white blood cell (WBC) count, increased total red blood cell (RBC) volume, increased plasma volume, decreased number and increased size of platelets, and increased fibrinogen and clotting factors VII through X. The relatively larger increase in plasma volume compared to RBC volume leads to physiological anemia of pregnancy. The coagulation changes protect against hemorrhage at birth but may also put the pregnant woman at increased risk for thromboembolic disease, for example, deep vein thrombosis (DVT).

ENDOCRINE SYSTEM

The basal metabolic rate (BMR) increases by 15% to 25% due to the increased oxygen consumption and to fetal metabolic demands. This can often lead to feelings of warmth and heat intolerance.

As pregnancy progresses, an increasing resistance to insulin develops, causing pregnancy to be called a "diabetogenic state." Causes for this phenomenon are incompletely understood but are partially related to placental manufacture of the enzyme insulinase. This process occurs to ensure adequate amounts of glucose for fetal demands. Glycosuria may be noted because the distant renal tubules cannot respond to the increased amounts and duration of glucose in the circulatory system. Pregnancy-induced glucose intolerance can be a risk factor for future development of insulin-dependent diabetes mellitus. The maternal immunological system is also less resistant to infection due to a decreased cellular immune response.

The Battered Pregnant Woman

Because of a history of missed appointments, bruises on her chest and neck, a history of a broken arm, and a partner who is always with her and answers all questions for her, you want to investigate the possibility of abuse with your pregnant patient.

1. Does your office flow and physical layout allow you to see the patient by herself so she may talk freely?
2. Will you feel comfortable asking her directly whether she is being hurt or abused in any way or whether anyone has caused her injuries?
3. Do you know what resources and services are available to her, e.g., a residence home for battered women and their children?
4. If the woman does not respond to your questions or declines help now, do you have small, inconspicuous (so the partner cannot easily find them) cards with the names and numbers of agencies that can help?
5. Can you comfortably let the patient know you are available to help her if she decides she wants help?
6. Do you know the laws for reporting abuse in your state?

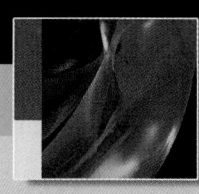

HEALTH HISTORY

The pregnant patient health history provides insight into the link between a patient's life and lifestyle and pregnancy-related information and pathology.

The health history for the pregnant woman is generally taken on a form designed specifically for pregnancy. It may be one of several nationally recognized forms or one created by the individual health care provider. These forms contain information on the patient, from a preconception visit through delivery, as well as on the newborn. They cover the standard health history questions, any prior obstetric history, genetic predispositions, current signs and symptoms including those of pregnancy, any change in normal routine, initial prenatal visit physical assessment, subsequent visits, and laboratory data. This comprehensive approach is essential for directing risk factor assessment and developing a plan of management. Table 23-2 illustrates a typical obstetric history.

PATIENT PROFILE

Diseases that are age- and race-specific for pregnancy are listed.

Age

Being under 17 or over 35 puts women at risk for various pregnancy complications such as HDP, gestational diabetes, genetic disorders, twins, miscarriage, operative delivery, and preterm labor and/or delivery.

Race

African Americans: sickle cell trait or disease, increased risk for hypertension and preterm delivery

CHIEF COMPLAINT

The pregnant patient may have a myriad of complaints as discussed throughout the chapter. The most common chief complaints have been discussed in previous chapters.

PAST HEALTH HISTORY

The various components of the past health history are linked to pregnancy pathology and pregnancy-related information.

Medical History

Asthma, diabetes mellitus, cardiac disease, renal disease, seizure disorder, autoimmune disorders

Surgical History

Uterine surgery, cone or excisional biopsy of the cervix, abdominal surgery leading to internal or external scarring or adhesions

Allergies

Symptoms may change with pregnancy; it is best to review all current allergy medications to ensure compatibility with pregnancy.

Medications

Certain medications for chronic conditions may be continued during pregnancy, such as methyldopa and hydralazine for hypertension. Other medications may be changed due to the teratogenic effect on the fetus; for example, coumadin would be changed to heparin, and an oral diabetic agent would be changed to insulin. Medications for seizure disorders or psychiatric conditions should be discussed with the health care provider in terms of risk-benefit ratio for both the mother and the fetus, as well as any possible alternate medications for use preconceptually and during pregnancy. Some OTC medications such as acetaminophen are considered safe during pregnancy, but any pregnant (or possibly pregnant) woman should consult her health care provider before taking any medications or therapies.

continues

Health History (continued)

Communicable Diseases	TORCH diseases (toxoplasmosis, rubella, cytomegalovirus, herpes), measles, varicella, mumps, human parvovirus B19, HIV, hepatitis B. A rubella titer, RPR or VDRL, and hepatitis B surface antigen are routinely drawn on pregnant patients. HIV testing is recommended, if the patient allows it. Rubella (German measles), especially in the first trimester, and syphilis during pregnancy can cause anomalies and complications. Other infectious diseases may affect the pregnancy, depending on their severity and the gestational age at which the disease is contracted—e.g., varicella may present a problem to the fetus if active at the time of delivery. Other infectious diseases to review include tuberculosis and sexually transmitted diseases (STDs).
Injuries and Accidents	Any trauma that leads to abdominal scarring or injury to the pelvic organs themselves may affect the pregnancy; injuries to the back may also be of concern.
Special Needs	Disabilities and handicaps do not generally interfere with pregnancy. Some neuromuscular disorders such as myasthenia gravis may affect muscle response as pregnancy progresses and during labor. Paralysis does not interfere with pregnancy other than with regard to the patient's decreased ability to note significant changes in her physical status, e.g., change in vaginal discharge or increase in uterine contractions.
Childhood Illnesses	Rheumatic heart disease, if mitral valve prolapse (MVP) developed, may put the patient at risk for endocarditis with an extremely long or complicated labor or delivery and could require prophylactic antibiotics with delivery. Knowledge of childhood diseases leading to immunity may decrease anxiety if exposure to those illnesses occurs during pregnancy.
Immunizations	Typically, immunizations, especially those containing live viruses, should be avoided during pregnancy. The hepatitis B series and tetanus toxoid are not contraindicated during pregnancy. Any unavoidable travel to an area with known infectious disease risk requires a discussion of the risk-benefit ratio of immunization. Immune status testing should be encouraged at any preconceptual visit. If immune status is unknown or immune status testing reveals a lack of adequate titers, rubella and varicella immunizations should be given, along with instructions to avoid pregnancy for 3 months. Flu vaccine is recommended.
FAMILY HEALTH HISTORY	*Pregnancy-related conditions and diseases that are familial are listed.*
	Preterm labor or delivery; hypertensive disorders of pregnancy; diethylstilbestrol (DES) exposure; multiple births in female relatives of patient's mother; chromosome abnormalities such as Down syndrome; genetic disorders such as Tay-Sachs or Gaucher's diseases or sickle cell disease; inheritable diseases such as Huntington's chorea; congenital anomalies such as cleft lip or palate; neural tube defects; cardiac deformities; blood disorders; diabetes (gestational, non-insulin dependent, insulin dependent); neuromuscular diseases; psychiatric disorders; any history of abuse, neglect, or substance abuse Family history of baby's father: genetic, hereditary, or chromosomal disorders, abuse or neglect, substance abuse
SOCIAL HISTORY	*The components of the social history are linked to pregnancy factors and pathology.*

continues

Health History (continued)

Alcohol Use	Can lead to fetal alcohol syndrome (FAS). The absolute safe level of alcohol consumption is unknown. Problems have been documented with >2 oz of alcohol per day and with binge drinking.
Tobacco Use	Smoking can lead to a small-for-gestational-age (SGA) infant, preterm labor, spontaneous abortions, and lower Apgar scores (refer to Chapter 24). The effects are dose related, and tobacco use during pregnancy should be discontinued. Referral to a smoking cessation program may be beneficial. With a history of smoking or secondary smoke exposure, status should be checked frequently throughout pregnancy.
Drug Use	Drug effects on the fetus vary according to the drug(s) used and the gestational age at time of use. The most common complications are spontaneous abortion, preterm delivery, congenital anomalies, and stillbirth. Some drugs, such as crack cocaine and heroin, lead to an addicted newborn, who must then go through withdrawal after birth. Cocaine use is associated with a high incidence of abruptio placenta and preterm delivery.
Sexual Practice	Sexual expression or practice throughout pregnancy is not contraindicated unless there are high-risk restrictions. Sexual intercourse should be avoided after the membranes have ruptured.
Travel History	Ask about travel outside the United States or to regions at risk for infectious diseases. Travel more than 1½ hours from home during the last month of pregnancy should be avoided. Air travel should be taken only in pressurized cabins. Pregnant women should move about every hour, drink plenty of liquids, and travel with enough food for small, frequent meals or snacks.
Work Environment	Prolonged sitting or standing; heavy lifting; an extremely loud, cold, or wet environment; work with chemicals, lead, or mercury; or a one-way commute greater than 1 hour may put the pregnant woman at risk for preterm labor or congenital anomalies in the newborn.
Home Environment	Stairs may make domestic chores even more difficult for the pregnant woman and may be a significant factor for a high-risk patient who needs to maintain bed rest. The pregnant woman should avoid toxic chemicals; exposure to toxoplasmosis should be avoided by not cleaning cat litter boxes and by wearing gloves and washing hands after gardening. Household chores should be avoided if they either lead to excessive contractions or aggravate pregnancy discomforts.
Hobbies and Leisure Activities	May be continued during the pregnancy unless they present a physical risk such as certain high-risk sports, including skiing and horseback riding.
Stress	The patient's perception that she has more stress in her life than she can cope comfortably with should be addressed by practicing relaxation techniques, seeking counseling if needed, and using family and social support systems. Excessive stress may be a risk factor for preterm labor.
Ethnic Background	People of Asian, Asian Indian, or Mediterranean origin (Greece, Italy, Cyprus, Middle East): thalassemia Ashkenazi Jews: Tay-Sachs and Gaucher's diseases French Canadians (and possibly Cajuns): Tay-Sachs disease African American: Sickle cell disease/trait

continues

Health History (continued)

HEALTH MAINTENANCE ACTIVITIES	*This information provides a bridge between the health maintenance activities and pregnancy.*
Sleep	Increased demand, complicated frequently by nocturia or difficulty in finding and maintaining a comfortable position
Diet	All meats should be well cooked and all dairy products should be pasteurized to prevent infections such as toxoplasmosis and listeria.
Exercise	Normal activities may be continued and exercise may help with some of the common complaints such as constipation. Exercise done in moderation is beneficial, but any exercise should be discontinued or modified if pain occurs; intensity and duration may need to be decreased from prepregnant exercise levels (e.g., heart rate should not exceed 150 beats per minute or moderate levels of perceived exertion). Care should be taken to avoid overheating, especially in humid weather, and water intake should be increased as needed. Physically dangerous exercise, such as waterskiing, downhill skiing, and horseback riding, should be discontinued. Some providers recommend discontinuing exercise in the first trimester due to the possibility of increased risk of miscarriage.
Use of Safety Devices	Seat belts are recommended, with the lap portion worn below the pregnant abdomen.
Health Check-ups	Gynecological evaluations; avoid X-rays

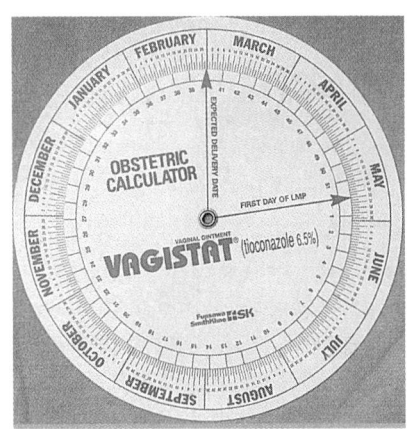

FIGURE 23-8 Gestation Calculation Wheel Used to Determine EDD. "First day of LMP" arrow is placed on that date. The other arrow, labeled "expected delivery date," shows the expected date of delivery.

NURSING**TIP**

Obstetric Abbreviations

You can classify pregnant patients according to their prior obstetric outcomes by using the following abbreviations. During the initial visit it is important to note all of the categories. In subsequent visits, every category may not be documented, just the number of pregnancies (gravida) and deliveries (para).

G = gravida

P = para

T = term

P = preterm

A = abortion (either therapeutic or spontaneous; may be listed separately)

E = ectopic pregnancy

LC = living children

Examples:

G 4, P 2, T 2, P 0, A 1, E 1, LC 2 = 4 pregnancies, 2 births, 2 term births, 0 preterm births, 1 abortion, 1 ectopic pregnancy, 2 living children

G 3, P 3, T 2, P 1, A 0, E 0, LC 4 = 3 pregnancies, 3 births, 2 term births, 1 preterm birth, 0 abortions, 0 ectopic pregnancies, 4 living children (preterm birth = 1 set of twins)

G 3, P 3 = 3 pregnancies, 3 births

G 4, P 3, A 1 = 4 pregnancies, 3 births, 1 abortion

G 4, P 3, T 2, P 1, A 1, E 0, LC 2 = 4 pregnancies, 3 births, 2 term births, 1 preterm birth, 1 abortion, 0 ectopic pregnancies, 2 living children

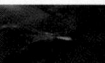

NURSING**TIP**

Drug Safety Categories in Pregnancy

The Food and Drug Administration has established drug safety categories that describe the potential risk of a drug during pregnancy. Only medications that have been developed since 1983 are required to assign a pregnancy-risk category.

Risk Categories of Medicine

Category A: Safety established using human studies

Category B: Presumed safety based on animal studies

Category C: Uncertain safety, no human studies, and animal studies show an adverse effect

Category D: Unsafe, with evidence of risk that may in certain clinical circumstances be justifiable

Category X: Highly unsafe—risk of use outweighs any possible benefits

Some drugs have not been assigned a category but may be described as:

+ Generally accepted as safe

? Safety unknown or controversial

− Generally regarded as unsafe

The use of selective serotonin reuptake inhibitor (SSRI) medications should be evaluated for benefit versus risk in each trimester and postpartum. The use or discontinuation of these medications should be done in conjunction with the patient's mental health provider.

TABLE 23-2 Obstetric History

PRESENT OBSTETRIC HISTORY

Last menstrual period (LMP)

Menstrual cycles (Menarche, frequency, duration)

History since LMP (e.g., fever, rashes, disease exposures, abnormal bleeding, nausea and vomiting, medication use, toxic exposures)

Signs and symptoms of pregnancy

Use of fertility drugs

Contraception

Estimated date of delivery (EDD) or estimated date of confinement (EDC)*

Genetic predispositions

Gynecology history

PAST OBSTETRIC HISTORY

Gravidity/gravida (number of pregnancies)

Parity/para (number of births 20 weeks or greater) usually listed as term (37–42 weeks gestational age), preterm (20–37 weeks gestational age), or postterm (> 42 weeks gestational age)

Spontaneous abortion

Therapeutic abortion

Ectopic pregnancy

Multiples or multiple births (more than one fetus or baby)

Number of living children

Pregnancy history (see Table 23-3 for high-risk factors):

- Complications during pregnancy
- Duration of gestation
- Date of delivery
- Type of delivery
  (vaginal versus cesarean)
  (if cesarean, reason)
  (forceps or vacuum extraction)
  (episiotomy or laceration, and degree)
- Length of labor
- Medications and anesthesia used
- Complications during labor and delivery
- Postpartum complications, including depression

Infant weight and sex, Apgar score

Type of feeding (breastfeeding versus bottle feeding)

Breastfeeding: difficulties

*Use Naegele's rule to determine EDD: subtract 3 months from the first day of the LMP, then add 7 days. This is based on a 28-day cycle and may have to be adjusted for shorter or longer cycles. For example, if the LMP is September 1,   9/1 − 3 months = 6/1
6/1 + 7 days = 6/8*

The EDD for this patient is June 8.
A pregnancy wheel may also be used (see Figure 23-8).

TABLE 23-3 Risk Factors for Pregnancy

There are many risk factor tools and scoring systems available with varying degress of sensitivity and specificity. Some prenatal forms include a risk screen in the history.

MATERNAL FACTORS

Age less than 17 or older than 35	Stress or unusual anxiety, or both, per patient perception
Single	Unplanned pregnancy or conflict about pregnancy, or both
Abusive relationship and other violence or family relationship stresses	Height less than 5 ft
	Weight less than 100 lbs
Low socioeconomic status, poverty, or low educational level	Inadequate diet
Long work hours, long commute, or long, tiring trip; excessive fatigue	Habits: smoking, excessive caffeine (greater than six cups of coffee per day), alcohol consumption, drug addiction

REPRODUCTIVE HISTORY

More than one prior abortion (some risk tools differentiate first and second trimester)	Delivery of infant less than 2500 g
	Delivery of infant greater than 4000 g
Uterine anomaly	Delivery of infant with congenital or perinatal disease
Molar pregnancy/hydatidiform mole	Delivery of infant with isoimmunization or ABO incompatibility
Myomas (leiomyomas)	Gestational diabetes
Sexually transmitted infections or diseases	Operative delivery
Perinatal death	Cervical incompetence
Preterm delivery or premature labor, or both	Prior cerclage

MEDICAL PROBLEMS

Hypertension	Pulmonary disease
Renal disease, pyelonephritis, asymptomatic bacteriuria	Endocrine disorder
Diabetes mellitus	Neurological disorder
Heart disease	Autoimmune disorder
Sickle cell disease	Hematological disorder
Anemia	

PRESENT PREGNANCY

Late, inadequate, or no prenatal care	Low or excessive weight gain
Abdominal surgery	Rh-negative sensitization
Bleeding	Teratogenic exposure
Placenta previa	Viral infections (especially fever-rash with first trimester)
Premature rupture of membranes	Sexually transmitted infection(s) or disease(s)
Anemia	Bacterial infections (bacterial vaginosis and group B streptococcus, in particular)
Hypertension	
Preeclampsia or eclampsia	Protozoal infections
Hydramnios	Abnormal presentation (i.e., breech, transverse) at approximately 36 weeks
Multiple pregnancy	
Abnormal glucose screen	Postdates

EQUIPMENT

- Stethoscope
- Doppler or **fetoscope**
- Centimeter tape measure
- Watch with a second hand
- Nonsterile gloves
- Speculum
- Genital culture supplies
- Pap smear supplies (see Chapter 20)
- Sphygmomanometer
- Urine cup
- Urine dipsticks

ASSESSMENT OF THE PREGNANT PATIENT

Assessment of the pregnant patient includes a complete initial assessment as well as subsequent specific follow-up prenatal visits. The initial assessment is done when the pregnant patient first seeks care. Encourage patients to seek prenatal care in the first trimester or as soon as pregnancy is suspected. Optimally, this should be preceded by a visit with the health care provider to assess health status prior to conception. This is especially important for women with preexisting medical problems such as diabetes mellitus, cardiac disease, or seizure disorders. The American College of Obstetricians and Gynecologists (ACOG) recommends the following schedule for prenatal visits: every 4 weeks for weeks 6–28 of gestation, every 2 weeks for weeks 28–36 of gestation, and weekly from 36 weeks until delivery. Patients going beyond the 40th week of gestation (postdates) require additional evaluations. The following examination guidelines discuss how each system examination is different for the pregnant patient than for the nonpregnant patient. See the previous chapters for the specific assessment of each system. The goal of the assessment is not only to confirm pregnancy and gestational age but also to evaluate general health so you can provide any needed intervention and educate the patient to maintain and promote her health as well as that of the fetus. See Table 23-4 for signs and symptoms of pregnancy.

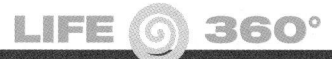

A Pregnant Woman Consuming Alcohol

You are a nurse in the OB/GYN clinic and obtain vital signs and a brief health history from a pregnant woman on her first prenatal visit. You smell alcohol on the patient's breath and ask her about it. The patient replies that she gargled with an alcohol-based mouthwash a few minutes ago. One month later, on a subsequent visit, you again smell alcohol on the pregnant woman's breath. The patient states that she was baking cookies and tasted the vanilla. You note that the pregnant woman is slurring her words, laughing loudly and inappropriately, and has an unsteady gait. What course of action should you take?

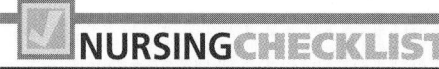

NURSING CHECKLIST

General Approach to Assessment of the Pregnant Patient

1. Greet the patient and explain how the assessment will proceed.
2. Ensure that the examination room is ready and supplies are at hand.
3. Use a quiet room that will be free from interruptions.
4. Ensure that there is adequate lighting, including a light that is appropriate for the pelvic assessment.
5. Prior to the physical assessment, complete the health history and the nutritional and psychosocial assessments. (This is usually done in an office before proceeding to the examination room.)
6. Ask the patient to void prior to the examination, both for patient comfort and to facilitate uterine and adnexal evaluation (which can be impeded by a full bladder). The urine should be saved and checked for sugar and acetone.
7. For the physical assessment, instruct the patient to remove all street clothes, don an examination gown, and cover her lap with a sheet.
8. Perform the initial assessment in a head-to-toe manner. Try to minimize the patient's time in the supine position—i.e., ask questions later. Assist the patient in assuming the lithotomy position via verbal guidance and by assisting in placing her feet in the foot or leg stirrups. Always inform the patient before touching her of what you will be doing and what to expect ("this may pinch," "you may feel some pressure," and so on). Special sensitivity should be given to adolescents and the patient who is having her first pelvic examination. The patient may be dizzy upon sitting up or upon standing. It may be beneficial to assist her to a sitting position or to brace her arm. She should be cautioned not to stand or sit up abruptly.

Signs of Pregnancy

Azaree, a 43-year-old female, visits you for the first time. You ask why she has made this appointment. She tells you that she is pregnant and that she wants to take good care of her baby. She informs you that she has had at least five miscarriages in the past 9 months, but these were never documented by any provider. She states, "A woman just knows when she is pregnant." She denies performing a home pregnancy test. The initial serum HCG report is negative for pregnancy. Azaree cries when you inform her of the lab results and states, "I'm getting so old, I will never have children!" How would you respond to Azaree? What information is vital for her to know? How would you proceed?

TABLE 23-4 Signs and Symptoms of Pregnancy

PRESUMPTIVE*	PROBABLE†	POSITIVE‡
Amenorrhea	Abdominal enlargement	Fetal heart beats
Breast tenderness and enlargement	Uterine changes	Fetal movement
Fatigue	Cervical changes	Fetal outline
Changes in skin pigmentation	Braxton Hicks contractions	
Nausea, vomiting, or both	Ballottement	Ultrasound
Urinary frequency	Quickening	
	Hegar's sign	
	Chadwick's sign	
	Goodell's sign	
	Positive pregnancy test— HCG in blood or urine	

*Presumptive: Signs or symptoms that are associated with pregnancy but are not conclusive.
†Probable: Signs or symptoms that are more indicative of pregnancy, including physical assessment changes.
‡Positive: Signs or symptoms that confirm a definite pregnancy.

GENERAL ASSESSMENT, VITAL SIGNS, AND WEIGHT

E **1.** Conduct a general assessment, including obtaining vital signs.

2. Obtain the patient's weight (Figure 23-9).

N See Chapter 9 for normal general assessment and the Anatomy and Physiology section of this chapter for blood pressure changes that occur in pregnancy. See Chapter 7 for the recommended weight gain in pregnancy. See Table 23-5 for common complaints of pregnancy.

A Hypertension at any time in pregnancy is considered abnormal. In pregnancy, hypertension is defined as a systolic pressure greater than 140 and a diastolic pressure greater than 90. This is assessed by taking the blood pressure twice, at least 6 hours apart. If a prepregnancy blood pressure is unknown, the greater than 140/90 criterion is used. Hypertension noted prior to 20 weeks is most likely chronic hypertension. After 20 weeks, hypertension is related to hypertensive disorders of pregnancy (HDP). See Table 23-6 for additional information on hypertensive disorders during pregnancy.

P The pathophysiology of HDP is still being researched. It is widely thought that vasospasms occurring throughout the vasculature contribute to HDP.

A A weight gain that is more than the recommended amount is abnormal.

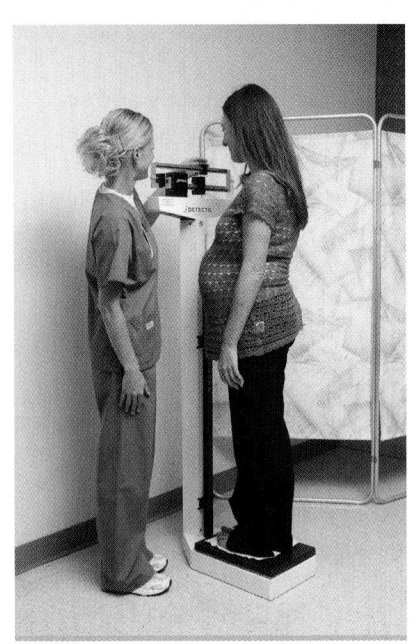

FIGURE 23-9 The patient's weight is determined at each prenatal visit.

E Examination	**N** Normal Findings	**A** Abnormal Findings	**P** Pathophysiology

TABLE 23-5 Common Complaints in Pregnancy

COMPLAINT	RELIEF MEASURES
Backache, sciatic pain, femoral nerve pain	For posture, stand with abdomen pulled in and buttocks tucked in. Do cat-arch exercises and stretching exercises for legs, gluteal muscles, and back. Avoid bending at waist—bend at knees to pick up objects from floor. If available, attend pregnancy exercise class or program. Wear flat, comfortable shoes. A maternity girdle or support can be helpful, as can local heat and massage.
Bleeding gums	Maintain good dental hygiene. Use a soft toothbrush.
Breast soreness, tenderness, or tingling	A well-fitting, supportive brassiere, worn as much as 24 hours a day.
Constipation	High-fiber diet and 8–10 glasses of water a day plus exercise.
Difficulty sleeping	Pillows for support, between legs, under abdomen, and shoulders. Exercise, a warm bath before bed. Avoid caffeine. Go to bed at the same time every night.
Dizziness	Avoid sudden position changes or prolonged standing, especially in heat or a closed room. Eat and drink frequently.
Edema	Left lateral position for rest. Plenty of fluids.
Fatigue	Increased rest and relaxation, which may necessitate a different division of duties at home or work and prioritization of projects and chores.
Headache	Frequent meals and increased rest. If severe, discuss with health care provider.
Heartburn	Small, frequent meals; avoid foods that aggravate heartburn, for example, spicy or fatty foods, carbonated drinks. If severe, discuss medication with provider.
Hemorrhoids	Avoid constipation. Local treatment with a witch hazel-type product may reduce burning and itching, at least temporarily. Rest in left lateral position.
Increased vaginal discharge	It is acceptable to wash more often with plain tepid water, or a mild, nonirritating soap and water. Avoid douching when pregnant. Panty liners may be necessary. Tell your provider if you notice an odor, itching, or unusual color. Report any episode of bleeding.
Leg cramps	Make sure dietary calcium is sufficient (dairy products, dark, leafy vegetables); there can even be an excess of milk intake (calcium in the form of phosphate); calcium carbonate supplement may be indicated (as well as for cases of lactose intolerance). Stretching exercises, flexing calf muscle; avoid hyperextending calf muscle.
Lapses or changes in memory	Lists! A sense of humor. Explain to family, friends, and coworkers that short-term memory is frequently affected by pregnancy. Store items like keys in the same place. Develop the habit of mentally checking for needed items (checkbook, wallet, address, and grocery lists) before leaving the house.
Loss of balance	Flat shoes. Avoid activities where loss of balance could present a serious problem (e.g., bicycle riding). Use caution when changing position.
Pelvic or abdominal discomfort or pressure	After ruling out a complication, increased rest, leg elevation, and maternity support devices may be beneficial.
Nausea or vomiting, or both	Small, frequent meals. Avoid foods that trigger nausea and avoid smoking and alcohol. A protein snack at bedtime or crackers before getting up in the morning can help. If severe, associated with weight loss, or if nausea or vomiting persist past the first trimester, be sure to consult your provider.
Shortness of breath	Extra pillows under head, shoulders, or upper back may help relieve pressure on the diaphragm, especially late in pregnancy.
Sweating/acne/melasma/ptyalism	Dress in layers. Fans may help at home or desk. Maintain hygiene, but avoid overcleaning, especially face so as not to irritate skin. Avoid prolonged sun exposure. Wear sunscreen when outside.

continues

TABLE 23-5 (Continued)

COMPLAINT	RELIEF MEASURES
Urinary changes (increased frequency, urinary incontinence)	Maintain fluid intake. Arrange work and errands to allow for restroom breaks or stops. Consult provider if dysuria or discharge is present.
Stuffy nose	Avoid allergens (cats, sleeping with window open) when possible. Saline nasal products may be helpful.
Varicose veins	Left lateral position for rest. Frequent movement of legs if work requires prolonged standing or sitting. Support hose or even antiembolism-type hose may be necessary.

TABLE 23-6 Hypertensive Disorders of Pregnancy

GESTATIONAL HYPERTENSION

Blood pressure elevation during the second half of pregnancy or in the first 24 hours postpartum without other symptoms

Blood pressure returns to normal usually within 10 days postpartum.

Gestational hypertension generally does not require treatment.

PREECLAMPSIA

Hypertension: Systolic blood pressure of 140 mm Hg or greater or a diastolic blood pressure of 90 mm Hg or greater

Proteinuria: 0.1 g/L or > in at least 2 urine samples 6 hours apart, or > 0.3 g/L in 24-hour urine sample

Severe preeclampsia:

- BP of at least 160/110 2 times at least 6 hours apart
- 5 g protein in 24-hour urine sample or persistent 3–4+ proteinuria on dipstick
- Oliguria: < 500 mL for 24 hours
- Neurological symptoms: altered LOC, headache, blurred vision, or scotomata
- Pulmonary edema
- Epigastric or RUQ pain
- Impaired liver function
- Thrombocytopenia—platelet count ≤ 100,000 mm^3
- Elevated serum creatinine > 1.2 g/dL
- Intrauterine growth restriction (IUGR)

ECLAMPSIA

Above signs or symptoms

Development of seizures

CHRONIC HYPERTENSION

Present prior to pregnancy or diagnosed < 20 weeks

BP > 140/90

Hypertension persists > 42 days postpartum

CHRONIC HYPERTENSION WITH SUPERIMPOSED PREECLAMPSIA

Chronic hypertension and showing signs of developing preeclampsia

Appearan ce of edema or proteinuria

P Excessive weight gain may be due to increased caloric intake, multiple pregnancies, polyhydramnios, and edema secondary to HDP.

A A weight gain that is less than the recommended amount is abnormal.

P Weight loss or insufficient weight gain in pregnancy can be due to hyperemesis gravidarum, decreased caloric intake, and malabsorption syndromes.

SKIN AND HAIR

E Examine the skin and hair.

N See Chapter 10 and the Anatomy and Physiology section of this chapter.

A **Prurigo** of pregnancy presents as excoriated papules, which are highly pruritic and usually distributed on the hands and feet but in more severe cases may be noted on the upper trunk. They are most commonly found in mid- to late pregnancy and are abnormal.

P Etiology is poorly understood, but there is no increase in fetal mortality, and the eruptions fade after delivery.

A Papular dermatitis of pregnancy may manifest at any time during pregnancy as erythematous, pruritic, widespread, soft papules. These papules are typically 3 to 5 mm in size and are surmounted by smaller, firmer papules or small crusts. There tend to be several new eruptions daily, and those already present heal in 7 to 10 days, possibly with hyperpigmentation. Papular dermatitis is abnormal.

P The pathophysiology of these lesions is poorly understood. Papular dermatitis is associated with an increased risk for fetal loss, which may be significantly reduced by the use of oral prednisone.

A Erythematous plaques that develop into vesicular lesions that may become pustular are abnormal.

P Primary herpes (see Chapter 10) contracted in the first trimester places the fetus at risk for abnormalities. It is more virulent and likely to cross the placental barrier, leading to fetal abnormalities. Recurrent genital herpes lesions contain fewer viral particles and carry a less severe outcome throughout the pregnancy, most often leading to a cesarean delivery when lesions are noted in and around the vagina.

A Rashes are generally abnormal and should be further investigated.

P These should be evaluated for infectious, collagen, or other disease etiology as described in Chapter 10.

HEAD AND NECK

E/N See Chapter 11 and the Anatomy and Physiology section of this chapter.

A The appearance of hyperthyroidism and hypothyroidism is abnormal in pregnancy.

P Neoplastic disorders such as choriocarcinoma, ovarian teratoma, and hydatidiform mole, as well as a single active thyroid nodule or multinodular goiter, should be considered with the diagnosis of hyperthyroidism in the pregnant patient.

| **E** Examination | **N** Normal Findings | **A** Abnormal Findings | **P** Pathophysiology |

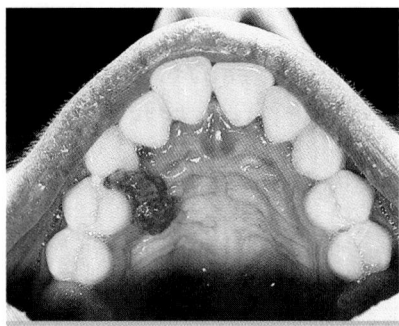

FIGURE 23-10 **Pregnancy Tumor.**
Courtesy of Dr. Joseph L. Konzelman, School of Dentistry, Medical College of Georgia.

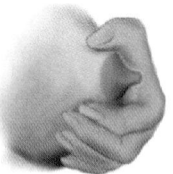
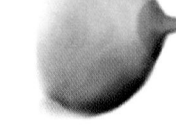

Press just behind areola

Normal nipple protraction

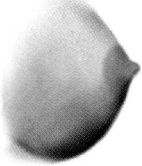
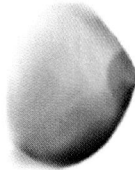

Pseudo-inverted

Inverted

FIGURE 23-11 **Assessing for Protractivity of the Nipple**

EYES, EARS, NOSE, MOUTH, AND THROAT

E/N See Chapters 12 and 13 and the Anatomy and Physiology section of this chapter.

A Arterial constriction of retinal vessels is abnormal. This may lead to blurred vision, scotomata, and, rarely, a retinal detachment.

P This can occur in HDP.

A Any growth in the mouth is abnormal.

P Some women develop pregnancy tumors in their mouths (Figure 23-10). These growths are usually benign. The vascular proliferation occurs secondary to hormonal changes. They may not resolve at the end of pregnancy.

BREASTS

E 1. Examine the breasts as described in Chapter 14.

2. Don gloves.

3. Assess the shape of each nipple by putting your thumb and index finger on the areola and pressing inward to express any discharge. Note whether the nipple protracts (becomes erect) or retracts (inverts) (Figure 23-11).

N Refer to Chapter 14 and the Anatomy and Physiology section of this chapter. Nipples normally protract when stimulated.

A Accessory breast tissue (supernumerary nipple), most commonly in the axilla, and secondary nipples on the nipple line are abnormal.

P This finding is a result of abnormal embryologic development, but does not present a problem in pregnancy. These areas may develop during the pregnancy along with the normal breast tissue.

THORAX AND LUNGS

E See Chapter 15.

N See Chapter 15 and the Anatomy and Physiology section of this chapter.

A/P Pathology noted in Chapter 15 would also be considered abnormal for the pregnant patient.

HEART AND PERIPHERAL VASCULATURE

E Assess the patient as described in Chapter 16.

N See Chapter 16 and the Anatomy and Physiology section of this chapter.

A Generalized edema, in contrast to the dependent edema of pregnancy, is abnormal.

P The most common causes for this are standing or sitting too long and HDP. This disease decreases the colloid osmotic pressure within the vasculature, therefore allowing fluid to leak into the tissues. Other potential causes to be considered are kidney disease and cardiovascular disease such as cardiomyopathy.

ABDOMEN

E Assess the patient as described in Chapter 17.

N See Chapter 17 and the Anatomy and Physiology section of this chapter.

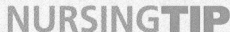
A Severe nausea and vomiting (**hyperemesis gravidarum**) leading to a significant weight loss in pregnancy is abnormal.

P Hyperemesis gravidarum is a disease of unknown etiology. It usually presents in the first trimester and may continue throughout the pregnancy. This is more severe than morning sickness and may persist throughout the day, leading to nutritional deficiencies. There often is associated hyperthyroidism. Other less common causes may include cholestasis, acute fatty liver disease, hepatitis, cirrhosis, appendicitis, and ulcers.

A Epigastric pain is abnormal.

P This is usually a result of liver inflammation or necrosis from HDP. It must be differentiated from cholecystitis or other liver disorders. It may be confused with commonly experienced pregnancy heartburn, but epigastric pain resulting from liver pathology is over the liver itself, whereas heartburn is felt more midline.

URINARY SYSTEM

E 1. Obtain a complete urinalysis at the initial prenatal visit.

2. Obtain a urine culture if indicated by urinalysis or patient history.

3. It is common (but not proven to affect outcome) to assess urine for protein, glucose, leukocytes, and nitrates at each subsequent prenatal visit.

N The urine may turn a brighter yellow as a result of prenatal vitamins. Trace amounts of protein may be noted. Glycosuria may be noted without pathology, but concern for diabetes mellitus cannot be ignored. Leukocytes and nitrates are normally absent.

A Nitrates or large amounts of leukocytes are abnormal.

P Nitrates, a breakdown product of bacteria, and large amounts of white blood cells (leukocytes) may indicate a urinary tract infection.

A Dysuria that presents as any of the following is abnormal: difficulty in initiating urinary flow, increased urinary frequency, a feeling of being unable to empty the bladder.

P Dysuria results most commonly from a bacterial infection, inflammation of the bladder (cystitis), or urinary tract infection.

A Pain in the flank area (costovertebral angle tenderness) is abnormal.

P The pregnant patient is more prone than the nonpregnant patient to develop pyelonephritis from a lower urinary tract infection secondary to the dilation of the ureters and renal pelvises, along with decreased tone and peristalsis, which lead to stasis. This results from the physiological changes that occur during pregnancy.

A Asymptomatic bacteriuria is abnormal.

P A clean-voided urine specimen containing more than 100,000 organisms of the same species per milliliter of urine is consistent with infection. Asymptomatic bacteriuria sometimes progresses to acute symptomatic infection unless treated. Through poorly understood mechanisms, bacteriuria is associated with an increased rate of preterm labor and birth.

A Proteinuria greater than trace as shown on a urine dipstick is abnormal.

E Examination   **N** Normal Findings   **A** Abnormal Findings   **P** Pathophysiology

P The most common cause is HDP. The vasospasms that occur also affect the kidneys and their ability to filter substances. Other possible causes are collagen disorders or kidney diseases.

Musculoskeletal System

E Assess the patient as described in Chapter 18.

N See Chapter 18 and the Anatomy and Physiology section of this chapter.

A Abnormalities and pathology described in Chapter 18 are also considered abnormal for the pregnant patient.

Neurological System

E Assess the patient as described in Chapter 19.

N See Chapter 19 and the Anatomy and Physiology section of this chapter.

A Seizures are abnormal.

P Eclampsia is the most common cause of seizures in the pregnant patient. Other less common causes are stroke, tumors, or epilepsy. The coagulation and vascular changes associated with pregnancy may exacerbate preexisting conditions.

A Hyperreflexia and clonus are abnormal.

P HDP can cause these findings.

Female Genitalia

E 1. For the initial prenatal visit, perform the assessment as described in Chapter 20.

2. Perform cultures as indicated in Table 23-7.

3. Postdate pregnancies and pregnancies complicated by preterm labor symptoms or preterm labor risk factors may require a cervical assessment at each visit.

N See Chapter 20 for normal findings of the female genitalia assessment. The multiparous vulva and vagina may appear more relaxed in tone, with a shorter perineum. There is often a visible, white, milky discharge during pregnancy, and the cervix may show more **ectropion** (also called eversion and friability). Ectropion is the condition in which the columnar epithelium extends from the os past the normal squamocolumnar junction, often producing a red, possibly inflamed appearance. See Table 23-1 for additional changes in pelvic organs.

Manual assessment should show uterine size appropriate for gestational age, and the uterus may be slightly more tender than in a nonpregnant woman. The retroverted and retroflexed uterus may be more difficult to assess. Palpation of the adnexa may demonstrate a slight tenderness and enlargement of the ovulatory ovary secondary to the corpus luteum of pregnancy.

A Persistent abdominal pain or tenderness is abnormal and should be evaluated.

P Either finding may indicate many underlying disorders related or unrelated to pregnancy. HDP and abruptio placenta are the most common causes of pain related to pregnancy. HDP pain is secondary to the hepatic involvement. Abruptio pain is from the retroplacental bleeding of the placental

| **E** Examination | **N** Normal Findings | **A** Abnormal Findings | **P** Pathophysiology |

TABLE 23-7 Laboratory Tests and Values in Pregnancy

TEST	REFERENCE RANGE—UNITS*	TIMING
Prenatal Panel includes		
Blood type	A, B, O, AB	Initial visit
Rh	Positive or negative	Initial visit
Antibody screen	Negative	Initial visit; as needed at 28 weeks
RPR (rapid plasma reagent) or VDRL (venereal disease research laboratory)	Nonreactive or negative. A positive result requires the more specific MHA-TP (microhemagglutination assay for *Treponema* pallidum antibodies) or FTA-ABS (fluorescent treponemal antibody absorbed).	Initial visit; may repeat at 36 weeks
Rubella	Immune (nonimmune patients should be cautioned to avoid contact with any possible exposure during the first trimester and will require a postpartum immunization)	Initial visit
Hepatitis B surface antigen	Negative	Initial visit; may repeat at 36 weeks
HIV (many states are mandating this test or that it at least be offered)	Negative	Initial visit; repeat based on history or exposure
Varicella	Immune	Initial visit if uncertain history
Human parvovirus B19 (fifth disease)	Negative	May be done on initial visit or as indicated by exposure
Hepatitis C antibody	Negative	Initial visit if indicated by history
CBC to include:		Initial visit; repeat at 26–28 weeks and 36 weeks
HGB	10.0–14.0 g/dL	
HCT	32.0–42.0%	
MCV	80.0–100.0 fL µL	
Platelets	50,000–400,000 mm^3	
Hemoglobin electrophoresis	Normal AA hemoglobin pattern	As indicated by race, ethnic background, or demonstrated anemia
Maternal serum alpha fetal protein (MSAFP) or triple marker screen	Both are maternal blood screening tests. MSAFP screens for neural tube defects and ventral wall defects, an elevation being a positive screen. As a screening test, there are false negatives (misses 20% of actual defects) and false positives, which may result from inaccurate dates, multiple fetus pregnancy, or bleeding with pregnancy. The MSAFP incidentally picks up 20% of Down-affected infants, as the alpha fetal protein will be diminished. Poorly understood is the association of an increased MSAFP with a normal fetus but increased pregnancy complications such as preterm labor or delivery or HDP. The triple screen adds estradiol and HCG to the test and thus increases the detection of Down to approximately 60%.	15–20 weeks; 16–18 weeks is optimal

continues

TABLE 23-7 (Continued)

TEST	REFERENCE RANGE—UNITS*	TIMING
Cystic fibrosis screening	Noncarrier This disease is inherited in an autosomal recessive pattern and may not manifest with symptoms until later in childhood. Caucasians (non-Jewish) carry at a rate of 1 in 25, while Ashkenazi Jews carry at a rate of 1 in 29; Hispanics are 1 in 46; African Americans are 1 in 65; and Asian Americans are 1 in 90.	Ideally, prior to pregnancy; if not, at initial prenatal visit
Genital Cultures or Probes		
Chlamydia by DNA probe or culture	Negative	Initial visit; may repeat at 36 weeks
Gonorrhea by DNA probe or culture	Negative	Initial visit; may repeat at 36 weeks
Genital bacterial/group β Streptococcus (GBBS)	Normal flora or negative for gonorrhea, bacterial vaginosis, GBBS and other pathogens	Initial visit; may repeat at 36 weeks
Urinalysis	Same as nonpregnant; glycosuria is a normal variant	Initial visit; as needed per symptoms and history
Urine culture	No notable pathogens	Initial visit; as needed per symptoms and history
Toxoplasma IgG	0–5 International Units/mL	As indicated by any history of exposures and symptoms
Glucose screen: 1 hour post 50 gram glucola glucose tolerance test	1 hour: 140 mg/dL or less (ACOG standard); may vary depending on regional variations, 130–135 mg/dL most common	26–30 weeks for all pregnant women and an early test, preferably with initial prenatal panel, for a woman with a family history of diabetes, a prior macrosomic baby, or who is 34 years or older or obese
3-hour glucose tolerance test		If indicated by elevated screening glucose or with history of failure in screening in prior pregnancies
Fasting blood sugar	95 or less mg/dL	
1 hour post 100 grams glucola	180 or less mg/dL	
2 hour post 100 grams glucola	155 or less mg/dL	
3 hour post 100 grams glucola	140 or less mg/dL	

*Reference range values may vary to some degree between laboratories

separation. Disorders unrelated to pregnancy include ulcers, cholecystitis, appendicitis, and pancreatitis.

A Painful adnexal masses are abnormal.

P In early pregnancy, these may indicate an **ectopic pregnancy** (pregnancy other than intrauterine, such as in the abdomen or fallopian tube), infection, or cancerous growth. Pain associated with an adnexal mass may be elicited via cervical motion during bimanual assessment.

UTERINE SIZE

Uterine size is determined by internal pelvic exam on the initial prenatal visit, by palpation if less than 18 weeks, and by fundal height in centimeters for subsequent visits. If the initial visit is late in pregnancy, it will include the internal pelvic exam and fundal height.

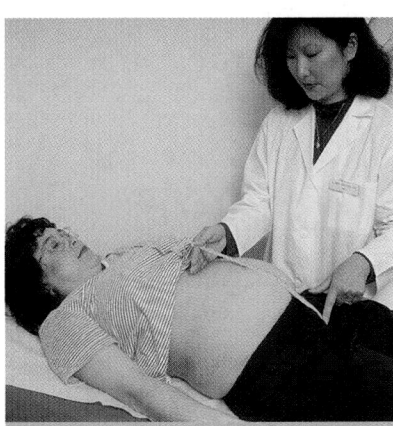

FIGURE 23-12 Measuring Fundal Height

Fundal Height by Centimeters

E
1. Place the patient in a supine position.
2. Place the zero centimeter mark of the tape measure at the symphysis pubis in the midline of the abdomen.
3. Palpate the top of the fundus and pull tape measure to the top (Figure 23-12).
4. Note the centimeter mark.

N A 16-week uterus is between the symphysis pubis and umbilicus, a 20-week uterus is at the umbilicus (20 cm), and from 18 to 32 weeks the size is equal to the centimeter height of the uterine fundus. After 32 weeks, although still used, this measurement is less accurate.

A Uterine size larger than expected given LMP is abnormal.

P This may indicate hydatidiform mole or molar pregnancy (especially in the absence of fetal heart tones), multiple gestation, inaccurate dating, uterine pathology (fibroid), polyhydramnios, or, later in pregnancy, **macrosomia** (newborn weighing greater than 4,000 gm).

A Uterine size smaller than expected given LMP is abnormal.

P This may indicate a nonviable pregnancy, inaccurate dating, or, later in pregnancy, intrauterine growth restriction (IUGR) or transverse lie of the fetus.

FETAL HEART RATE

E
1. Place the patient in the supine position.
2. Place Doppler or fetoscope (see Figure 23-13) on abdomen and move it around until FHTs are heard. Refer to Figure 23-14 to see the best location for auscultation based on fetal position.
3. Count the FHR for sufficient time to determine rate and absence of an irregularity (optimally 1 minute).

☀ NURSING**TIP**

FHR AKA FHT

The term *fetal heart tone* (FHT), described in beats per minute, is commonly used in antepartum assessment, whereas in much of the literature, especially intrapartum discussions, the term *fetal heart rate* (FHR) is used.

| **E** Examination | **N** Normal Findings | **A** Abnormal Findings | **P** Pathophysiology |

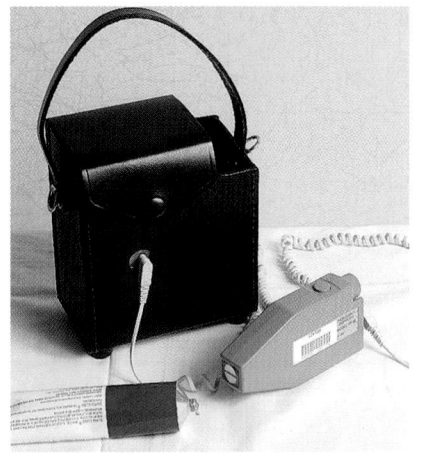

A. Doppler

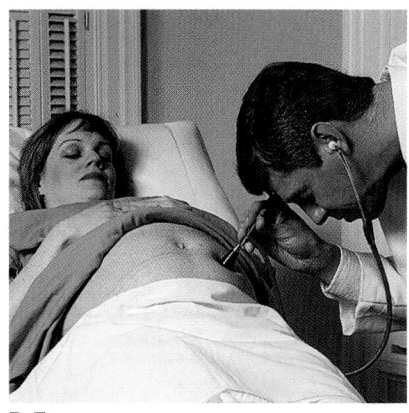

B. Fetoscope

FIGURE 23-13 Equipment Used for Fetal Heart Rate Determination

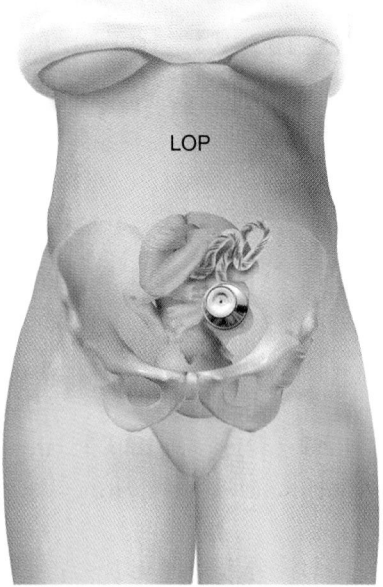

LOP

LOP = Left occiput posterior

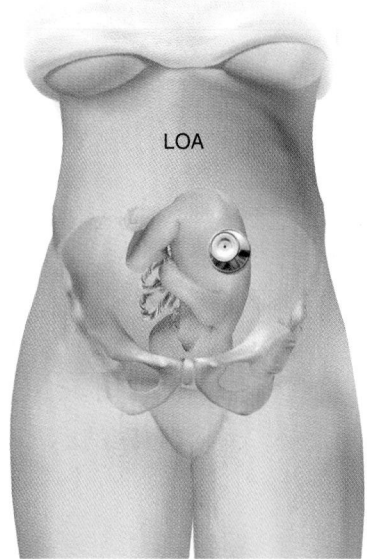

LOA

LOA = Left occiput anterior

FIGURE 23-14 Auscultating Fetal Heart Rate

N During early gestation, the fetal heart is generally heard in the midline area between the symphysis pubis and the umbilicus. It can be heard via Doppler by approximately 12 weeks (and maybe as early as 9 weeks). Use Doppler to auscultate FHT prior to 20 weeks; a fetoscope can be used after 20 weeks. Doppler is commonly used throughout pregnancy, as it is more convenient and also allows the patient to hear FHTs. The normal rate is 110 to 160 bpm. If the FHT seems low, check the mother's pulse rate to verify it is the FHT that you are listening to and not the mother's heart rate. Near-term FHTs are generally heard at maximum intensity in the left or right lower quadrant. If FHTs are best heard above the umbilicus, one should suspect a breech presentation or placenta previa. The fetal heart is best heard through the fetal back, which can be located by performing Leopold's maneuver as described on the following page.

A FHR below 110 bpm indicates bradycardia, which is abnormal.

P Bradycardia may be a sign of fetal distress or drug use. An FHR of 60 bpm or below may be indicative of a heart block. These conditions may be benign and convert to normal after delivery, but a consultation with a perinatologist is advised for consideration of intervention with the newborn.

A Absence of fetal heart activity is abnormal.

P Absence of fetal heart tones may indicate an ectopic pregnancy, a blighted ovum, fetal demise, or a molar pregnancy.

A FHR above 160 bpm indicates tachycardia, which is abnormal.

P Tachycardia may indicate a cardiac dysrhythmia, maternal fever, or drug use. Prior to approximately 28 weeks of gestation, tachycardia is a natural consequence of the immaturity of the fetal nervous system. In early gestation, the parasympathetic system exerts a greater influence. As the fetus matures, the sympathetic and parasympathetic systems mature and the FHR should remain within the normal range of 110 to 160 bpm.

LEOPOLD'S MANEUVER

Beginning at 36 weeks, determine fetal presentation using Leopold's maneuver (Figure 23-15).

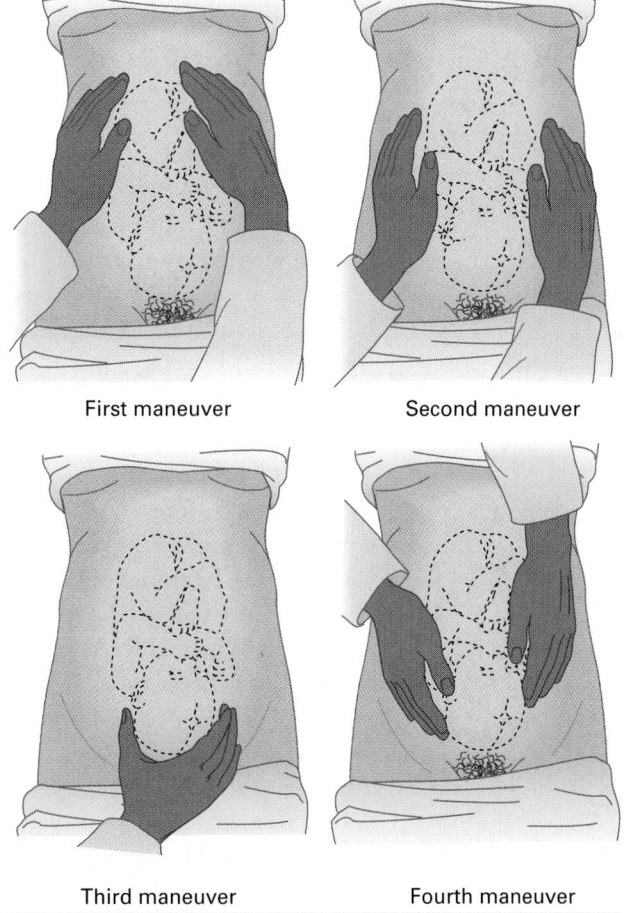

First maneuver | Second maneuver

Third maneuver | Fourth maneuver

FIGURE 23-15 Leopold's Maneuver

E Examination   **N** Normal Findings   **A** Abnormal Findings   **P** Pathophysiology

First Maneuver

E 1. Place the patient in a supine position with the knees bent.

2. Stand to the patient's right side facing her head.

3. Keeping the fingers of your hand together, palpate the uterine fundus.

4. Determine which fetal part presents at the fundus.

Second Maneuver

E 1. Move both hands to the sides of the uterus.

2. Keep your left hand steady and palpate the patient's abdomen with your right hand.

3. Determine the positions of the fetus' back and small parts.

4. Keep your right hand steady and palpate the patient's abdomen with your left hand.

Third Maneuver

E 1. Place your right hand above the symphysis pubis with your thumb on one side of the fetus' presenting part and your fingers on the other side.

2. Gently palpate the fetus' presenting part.

3. Determine whether the buttocks or the head is the presenting part in the pelvis. (This should confirm the findings of the first maneuver.)

Fourth Maneuver

E 1. Change your position so you are facing the patient's feet.

2. Place your hands on each side of the uterus above the symphysis pubis and attempt to palpate the cephalic prominence (forehead). This will assist you in determining the fetal lie (long axis of fetus in relationship to long axis of mother) and attitude (head flexed or extended).

N The fetus' head is usually the presenting part. It feels firm, round, and smooth. The head can move freely when palpated. If the baby is in a breech position, the buttocks feel soft and irregular. With palpation, the fetus' whole body seems to move but not with as much facility as the head. The fetus' back is firm, smooth, and continuous. The limbs are bumpy and irregular. The long axis is vertical, and the fetal head is flexed. A fetus not in a vertex presentation can affect the type of delivery; for example, a fetus in a persistent transverse or oblique lie will need to be delivered by cesarean. A breech fetus may be delivered vaginally or by cesarean, depending on the health care provider's comfort and experience in doing a vaginal breech delivery. Breech presentation, if uncorrected (i.e., by external version [the manual turning of the fetus by the health care provider]), is associated with an increased rate of perinatal morbidity and mortality, prolapsed umbilical cord, placenta previa, fetal anomalies and abnormalities (which may not manifest immediately after birth), and uterine anomalies.

A Inability to determine fetal outline is abnormal.

P   Polyhydramnios and maternal obesity can lead to an inability to outline the fetus.

Refer to a textbook on obstetrics for more specific information.

ANUS, PERINEUM, AND RECTUM

Inspection and Palpation

E   1. Observe for color and shape of anus.

      2. Observe texture and color of perineum.

      3. Palpate the rectum as described in Chapter 22. A digital rectal examination may be part of the bimanual examination in pregnancy.

N   The anus should be dark pink to brown and puckered. Skin tags are a normal variant and hemorrhoids may be seen with pregnancy, especially as the fetus enlarges. The perineum should be smooth and slightly darkened. A prior episiotomy scar may be visible. The perineum may vary significantly in length. The rectum should be free of masses and blood; however, constipation is common in early pregnancy. Discomfort is common with this examination.

A   Warty growths or abnormal lesions, fissures, or tears are not normally found.

P   Possible causes of fissures and tears are trauma, abscess, or unhealed episiotomy. Warty growths can represent HPV. Abnormal lesions can represent a malignancy.

HEMATOLOGICAL SYSTEM

E/N   See Table 23-7.

ENDOCRINE SYSTEM

E   See Table 23-7 for information on the glucose screen.

N   See Table 23-7.

A   Glucose screen greater than 130–140 mg/dL post glucola is abnormal.

P   Normal physiological changes that occur during pregnancy affect glucose metabolism. In some pregnant women, these changes accentuate and lead to gestational diabetes. These changes affect the known diabetic by altering her need for insulin throughout the pregnancy. The diabetic patient is at an increased risk for HDP, infection, macrosomia or intrauterine growth restriction (IUGR), fetal demise, polyhydramnios, and postpartum hemorrhage.

NUTRITIONAL ASSESSMENT

See Chapter 7.

SPECIAL ANTEPARTUM TESTS AND EVALUATIONS

Table 23-8 lists special antepartum tests and evaluations that can be performed in pregnant women.

NURSING**TIP**

Perinatal Depression

Depression can have a negative effect on pregnancy and on newborn care and development. It is important at prenatal visits to screen and postpartum to monitor for symptoms of depression. Screening questions may include: personal or family history of depression or anxiety, prior or current use of antidepressants, difficulty dealing with life stress, lack of support, relationship problems, equivocal feelings about pregnancy, and/or significant premenstrual moodiness.

E Examination   **N** Normal Findings   **A** Abnormal Findings   **P** Pathophysiology

TABLE 23-8 Special Antepartum Tests and Evaluations

TEST	DESCRIPTION
Ultrasound	At any time for pregnancy dating, although more accurate for dates early in prenancy. Confirm or rule out placenta previa, multiple pregnancy; confirm presenting fetal part. Evaluate amniotic fluid volume or fetal growth (especially to rule out intrauterine growth restriction or discordant growth with a multiple pregnancy). Evaluate for ectopic pregnancy or fetal demise.
Genetic testing: chorionic villi sampling (CVS), early amniocentesis, amniocentesis, chromosome studies	CVS for chromosome studies is best done at approximately 9-week gestational age, while early amniocentesis is done at approximately 13–16 weeks and traditional amniocentesis between 16–20 weeks, timing being the only difference between the two techniques. Early amniocentesis may carry a higher incidence of abortion. There may be an approximately 1% increased risk of limb deformities associated with CVS, as well as a 1% increased risk of spontaneous abortion. Blood or tissue chromosome studies can be done at any time but are best done with a known family history prior to conception.
Nonstress test (NST) or contraction stress test (CST) for fetal well-being, e.g., with decreased fetal movement, known decreased fluid volume, history of certain maternal diseases (insulin-dependent diabetes, collagen vascular disease), or obstetric complications such as IUGR, postdates, preeclampsia, discordant twin, or multiples	For a nonstress test, an electrical fetal monitor is applied to the woman's abdomen, with a tocodynamometer to monitor and record uterine activity and fetal movement and a Doppler to monitor and record FHR, looking at fetal heart response to fetal movement (and any spontaneous uterine contractions). Timing is typically 1 or 2 times per week, and may start as early as 32 weeks depending on the risk factor. With a contraction stress test, uterine activity is induced by timed breast nipple stimulation (which induces uterine contractions), and failing adequate uterine stimulation from nipple stimulation, pitocin intravenously via a pump is used to induce uterine activity. (Relative contraindications for a contraction stress test include any risk for uterine rupture, e.g., previous vertical cesarean section; premature delivery risk; any bleeding risk such as known placenta previa; or any unexplained vaginal bleeding.) Timing is typically once per week after 36 weeks.
Amniotic fluid volume (AFV), which may be described as amniotic fluid index (AFI), most commonly ordered with postdates pregnancies	Ultrasound measurement of AFV using an index to determine normal, increased, or decreased fluid levels.
Biophysical profile	A composite test that includes amniotic fluid volume, nonstress test, fetal breathing movements, fetal limb movements, and fetal tone; each rated on 0–2 score. This study is done most commonly for the same reasons as an NST or CST.
Fetal movement count	Can be done by all pregnant women, requires no equipment, and incurs no direct cost. There are many methods of doing fetal movement or kick counts, e.g., number of movements during the day or at certain times of the day, or noting the amount of time to discern 10 separate fetal movements after dinner.

PSYCHOSOCIAL ASSESSMENT AND LEARNING NEEDS

The diagnosis of pregnancy can normally lead to very mixed feelings. These feelings can range from ambivalence to anger, fear, or excitement. Crying for no apparent reason and mood swings are common in pregnant patients. Feelings of dependency may also present. Early physical changes such as nausea and fatigue may accentuate these feelings. Among the changes confronting the pregnant patient and her significant others are: role expectations (e.g., lifestyle and career); relationship expectations, definitions, and requirements (e.g., parent versus lover); and physiological changes.

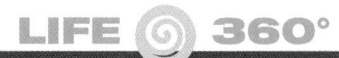

Assessing a Pregnant Woman's Learning Needs

You are teaching a childbirth preparation class and learn that you have 10 pregnant women in the class. Seven women are married with husbands. One woman is accompanied by her female companion. One woman is a single mother with no companion, and one woman has her three sisters with her (her husband is overseas with the military). Discuss how you would assess the learning needs of such a diverse group. Would this dictate a change in your lesson plan for the class?

Feelings may fluctuate throughout the pregnancy depending on the trimester and can be predicated on a change in medical status, such as the development of a high-risk condition. Early in pregnancy the patient often focuses on herself and on how these changes are affecting her physical state and her lifestyle. As pregnancy progresses, the patient usually shifts her focus from herself to the fetus as an individual and to the fetus' well-being. The patient's age, prior history, family history, prior pregnancy experience; whether the pregnancy was planned or accidental; and any known risk factors all serve to affect her state of mind. Social support systems, socioeconomic status, environmental hazards, and culture are also influencing factors.

The learning needs of the pregnant patient also change throughout pregnancy, and your assessments and teaching must change accordingly. Many communities offer pregnancy-related classes that start with early pregnancy and progress through the childbirth process, breastfeeding, infant care, and sibling involvement. The first-trimester classes typically focus on the physiological changes occurring during pregnancy and what the patient must do to develop a healthy infant, for example, nutrition, rest, exercise, and behaviors to avoid. During the second trimester, emphasis shifts to information on danger signs and symptoms (Table 23-9). At 24 to 26 weeks, the patient should be provided verbal and written information on signs and symptoms of preterm labor.

TABLE 23-9 Danger Signs of Pregnancy

SIGN OR SYMPTOM	ACTION
Vaginal bleeding*	Call health care provider immediately. Small amounts of bleeding may require only rest and observation at home. More significant bleeding or significant cramping, pain, or fever may require intervention at a hospital. Concerns would be for miscarriage, preterm labor, and placenta previa.
Leaking or gush of watery fluid*	Call health care provider immediately. Nothing should be put in the vagina unless the provider inserts a sterile speculum to evaluate for rupture of membranes. A sample of the fluid can be evaluated with the nitrazine test to evaluate if it is amniotic fluid.
Abdominal or pelvic pain or cramping*	Call health care provider immediately after consideration of the normal discomforts of pregnancy (e.g., round or broad ligament pain). It is important for the patient to describe the quality of the pain, duration, and location. Concerns would be for premature labor, ectopic pregnancy, placenta abruptio, or urinary tract infection.
Severe headache or blurring of vision	Call health care provider immediately because of the concern for HDP. Evaluation would include BP and labs (blood chemistries, liver function tests, and platelet count).
Persistent chills or fever greater than 102°F	Call health care provider. Associated symptoms may be helpful in determining underlying cause and its significance (e.g., infection, dehydration). Tylenol may be used to decrease the actual fever.
Persistent vomiting	Call health care provider immediately. Need is to determine underlying cause (e.g., gastritis, food poisoning) and treat symptoms before dehydration.
Decreased fetal movement or lack of fetal movement	Call health care provider immediately. At 20–24 weeks, lack of fetal movement could require an ultrasound to confirm dates and fetal viability. Decreased fetal movement or lack of movement later in pregnancy would require evaluation for fetal well-being.
Change in vaginal discharge or pelvic pressure before 36 to 37 weeks*	Call health care provider to evaluate for preterm labor.
Frequent (more than four per hour) uterine contractions or painless tightenings between 20 and 37 weeks*	Call health care provider. Rest, fluids, or snack may be recommended if uterine activity is not excessive or for prolonged period of time. If either is true, evaluation for preterm labor is required.

*Associated with preterm labor.

Third-trimester classes focus on the preparation for childbirth and the care of a newborn infant. The topic of breastfeeding should be introduced in the first trimester and discussed throughout the pregnancy. The patient should be informed of available childbirth education classes.

Adolescents may need additional support and educational reinforcement. Many school districts offer special programs for pregnant teens in addition to their normal school courses. Such programs typically encompass childbirth preparation and infant care assistance while the teen finishes school.

Learning needs must be assessed on an ongoing basis so that interventions can occur at the appropriate times. A social services consultation may be indicated for certain patients, such as those with a history of physical, emotional, or sexual abuse; those experiencing current drug and/or alcohol abuse; and those requiring help with basic housing and food needs. Learning may require reinforcement, and educational needs should be reviewed and documented throughout the pregnancy. Appropriate written or visual information should be used to reinforce verbal discussions.

Any couple who suffers fetal loss, whether intrauterine, stillborn, or newborn demise, should be offered supportive follow-up. Many communities have support groups, or couples may seek help from a counselor or religious leader. Couples who experience early miscarriages often find that they are not allowed by society to grieve their losses; supportive follow-up should thus be offered to these couples.

Sexual relations during pregnancy is often viewed as a taboo subject. Intercourse, unless specifically proscribed, is considered safe during pregnancy, although it may not always be easy or comfortable. During the first trimester, there may be no changes in libido for the woman, unless nausea and other physical changes leave her feeling excessively miserable. During the second trimester, the pregnant woman may even experience increased libido, whereas the physical and psychological changes of the third trimester may decrease the woman's interest in sexual relations. As pregnancy advances, the woman may find that she is

---

NURSING**TIP**

Pregnancy, Childbirth, Breastfeeding, and Sibling Education

Early in the pregnancy, encourage relevant preparation classes. These are offered by most health care systems and hospitals. The fees, if charged, vary widely. Give the pregnant woman a packet of information at the first visit and include information on the classes available and contact numbers to register for them. Some facilities offer a special class on pain relief and anesthesia. This initial packet may also include information on optimal nutrition, importance of normal weight gain, avoidance of excessive weight gain, safe activities during pregnancy, and warning signs of complications and preterm labor. Patients often enjoy pamphlets or books that show fetal development and pregnancy symptoms at various stages of the pregnancy.

Each laboratory, ultrasound, and/or genetic test may require specific explanation or education. At approximately 20 weeks, in addition to advising the pregnant woman to avoid sleeping on her back, you can again stress the importance of registering for preparation classes.

Some facilities also offer a class for siblings. These classes provide an opportunity for siblings to explore their feelings about changes in their mother's behavior and the possibility of a new person intruding into their world. The classes often offer tips to help the siblings adjust. Expectant parents may not have explored this issue and how to best parent the newborn and siblings.

Some women may need encouragement to take breastfeeding classes because they perceive that it is a natural process and therefore should require no teaching. If a pregnant woman is planning to breastfeed, classes should be highly encouraged because they can be very beneficial to helping her understand the physical and hormonal changes she is experiencing, not to mention the benefits of breastfeeding to the newborn.

At about 26 (24–28) weeks, in addition to appropriate laboratory studies, is the best time to review the signs and symptoms of preterm labor and appropriate action. There are generally handouts available. You can also teach the pregnant woman the fetal movement (kick) counting technique.

Prior Pregnancy Loss, Miscarriage, Fetal Demise, Stillborn, Genetic or Chromosomal Abnormality in Current or Prior Pregnancy

Prior pregnancy loss, miscarriage, fetal demise, stillborn, genetic or chromosomal abnormality in the current or prior pregnancy often requires professional counseling with grief counselors, religious leaders, support groups, therapists, and genetic counselors. A woman with a history of miscarriages may also benefit from referral to a reproductive specialist.

Each woman and family will bring to this event their own cultural beliefs and their own feelings. It is important to try to determine each woman's particular needs. What actions have already been taken? What support does the woman and her family have? Is there discord or blaming, acceptance or apathy?

When seeing the woman following a loss, try to schedule her and any family members to be seen when there are not pregnant women in the waiting room. Allow plenty of time and privacy for emotions and questions. Talk with the patient and have her health care provider talk with her and her family in a private office before performing any necessary physical examination.

Listen, offer empathy, and, when appropriate, arrange referrals.

most comfortable on her side, perhaps with a pillow under the abdomen, facing away from her partner. This position may decrease the depth of penetration of the penis. Male partners may express concern about injuring the fetus or the perceived discomfort of the pregnant woman.

SUBSEQUENT OR RETURN PRENATAL VISITS

Return prenatal visits include vital signs, FHR, fundal height, documentation of fetal movement appropriate for gestational age, weight, urine dipstick, assessment of any edema, assessment of uterine activity, assessment of any vaginal discharge or pelvic pain or pressure, and cervical exam, if done. Other issues discussed at return visits include concerns of the mother, weight gain, diet, childbirth preparation, breastfeeding, family planning, preparedness of the home, any family issues, and blood and other tests as appropriate to the gestational age.

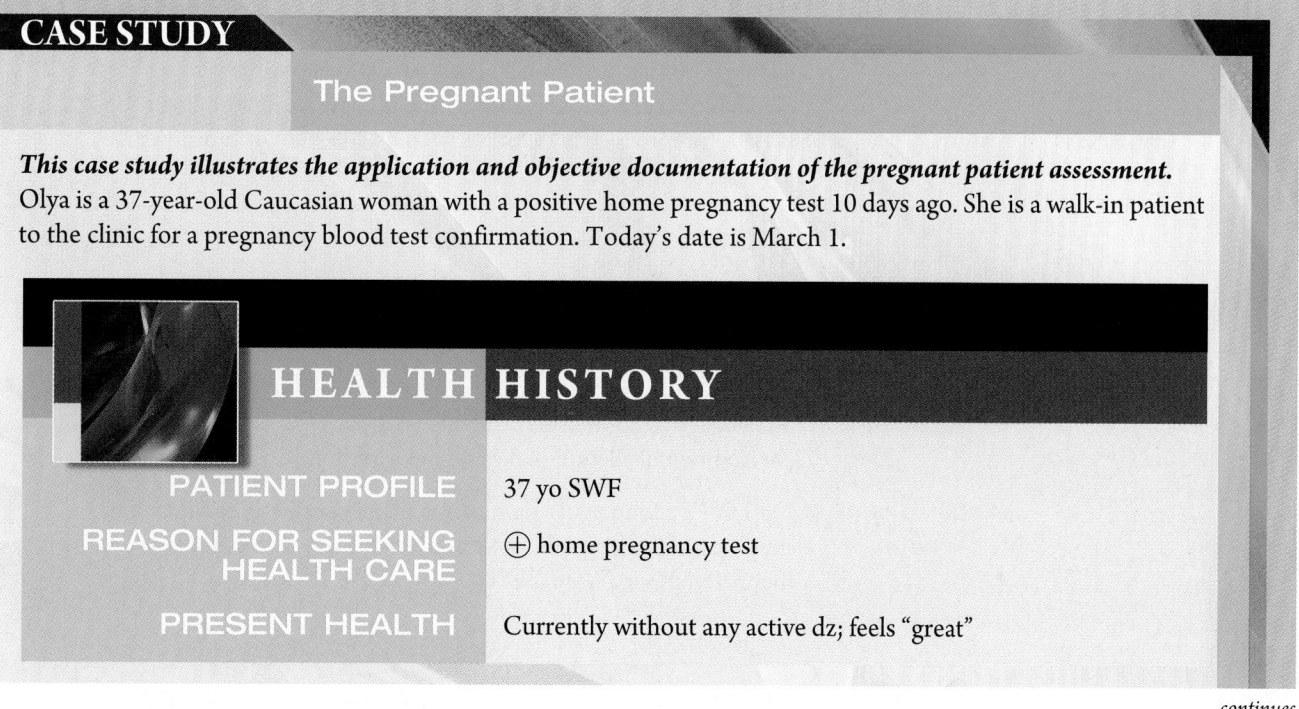

CASE STUDY

The Pregnant Patient

This case study illustrates the application and objective documentation of the pregnant patient assessment.
Olya is a 37-year-old Caucasian woman with a positive home pregnancy test 10 days ago. She is a walk-in patient to the clinic for a pregnancy blood test confirmation. Today's date is March 1.

HEALTH HISTORY

PATIENT PROFILE	37 yo SWF
REASON FOR SEEKING HEALTH CARE	⊕ home pregnancy test
PRESENT HEALTH	Currently without any active dz; feels "great"

continues

OBSTETRIC HISTORY	G 2, P 0, T 0, P 1, A 1, E 0, LC 0

G 2, P 0, T 0, P 1, A 1, E 0, LC 0
LMP: 12/9 (pt is sure of date)
Menstrual Cycles: Every 28–60 days, lasting 5–7 days, with menarche at age 14
History since LMP: No bleeding or cramping since LMP

Exposures since LMP: Denies fevers, rashes, or communicable diseases such as varicella, Fifth's disease, or exposure to dangerous chemicals, heavy metals, or radiation. She has a cat and sometimes changes the litter box, a task she shares with her partner. No history of toxemia or hypertensive disorders of pregnancy, glucose intolerance, bleeding or postpartum hemorrhage, isoimmunization, or postpartum depression. She did suffer hyperemesis requiring medications during her 1st trimester last pregnancy (age 29). Delivery at 28 weeks, after preterm labor arrested for 48 hours to allow steroids for fetal lung development, infant did not survive. No cause determined. She was under a lot of stress, completing law school at the time. Therapeutic abortion at age 20; was 14 weeks pregnant.

S/S of Pregnancy: Amenorrhea, breast tenderness, and nausea
Use of Fertility Drugs: None
Contraception: Condoms, unplanned pregnancy
EDD: 9/16 by dates
Genetic Predisposition: No family history; advanced maternal age

Gynecology History: History of one Pap smear with atypical squamous cells of undetermined significance (ASCUS) at age 27; no tx; all Pap smears since then have been WNL; no prior HPV testing with Pap smears. She has had 5 sexual partners in her life. She denies recurrent UTIs or genital infections, including Group B Beta Streptococcus (GBBS). Denies any known reproductive organ abnormality.

PAST HEALTH HISTORY

Medical History	Denies any medical problems
Surgical History	Wisdom teeth extraction under general anesthesia age 21 without complications
Allergies	Sulfa drugs (lead to rash); codeine (nausea). Occasional seasonal environmental allergies, takes no meds for this
Medications	No MVI or folic acid (pt was not planning this pregnancy and thus was not taking folic acid or prenatal vitamins beforehand); ibuprofen prn for headaches

continues

CASE STUDY (Continued)

The Pregnant Patient

Communicable Diseases	Positive history of Fifth's disease age 7; denies hx of TB, measles, mumps, or exposure to ill children or viral illnesses. Denies history of hepatitis, cytomegalovirus, and toxoplasmosis. Denies risk factors for HIV.
Injuries and Accidents	Denies
Blood Transfusion	Denies
Special Needs	Denies
Childhood Illnesses	Positive for varicella and Fifth's disease at age 7
Immunizations	Up-to-date, including all 3 shots in the hepatitis B vaccine series; last tetanus more than 10 years ago. Had influenza vaccine in November. Is out of recommended age range to have HPV vaccine series

FAMILY HEALTH HISTORY

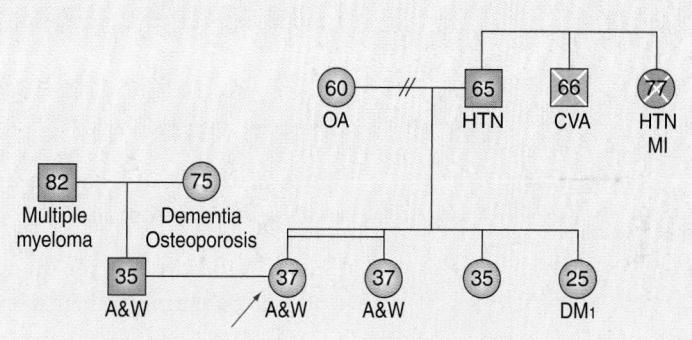

LEGEND

- ◯ Living female
- ◻ Living male
- ⊗ Deceased female
- ⊠ Deceased male
- ◯ ◯ Twin girls
- —//— Divorced
- ↗ Points to patient

A&W = Alive & well
CVA = Cerebrovascular accident
DM = Diabetes mellitus
HTN = Hypertension
MI = Myocardial infarction
OA = Osteoarthritis

Denies mother or sisters had any problems with pregnancies.
Denies mother took DES while pregnant with her.

Genetics: Denies family history of cerebral palsy, congenital anomalies, cystic fibrosis, Down syndrome, hemophilia, Huntington's chorea, mental retardation, muscular dystrophy, neural tube defects, thalassemia A or B

SOCIAL HISTORY

Alcohol Use	Occasional beer with friends or wine with dinner; none since pregnancy discovered; no binge or heavy drinking
Tobacco Use	Denies ever using. FOB does not smoke. Denies secondary smoke exposure.
Drug Use	She and FOB deny use and addictions in the family
Domestic and Intimate Partner Violence	Denies history of abuse and neglect

continues

Sexual Practice	Monogamous relationship for the past 10 years; 4 prior relationships
Travel History	Eastern Europe last year; denies infectious diseases
Work Environment	Long hours mostly sitting; feels safe at work; has building security guard walk her to her car after dark.
Home Environment	Secure and safe, comfortable. She has a dog and a cat and sometimes changes the litter box, last performed 1 week ago.
Hobbies and Leisure Activities	Cooking, movies, kayaking, skiing
Stress	She works long hours at a private law firm with lots of pressure; partner is an engineer working for the state government.
Education	JD
Economic Status	Pt and partner share all expenses, and they have a comfortable lifestyle with adequate savings for her postpartum absence. Her firm allows 1-month unpaid leave in addition to the regular maternity leave.
Military Service	Denies
Religion	Christian, nonpracticing
Ethnic Background	She is Caucasian of Ukranian descent; FOB is Caucasian Italian and Northern European.
Roles and Relationships	Pt and FOB have not yet thought about how they will manage work and parenting or their role expectations of each other.
Characteristic Patterns of Daily Living	Rises at 6:30 AM, showers, feeds cat and dog, has juice and one cup of coffee, drives to work; arrives 8 AM; often goes out for food and/or eats at desk and will sometimes have a deli sandwich or salad with chicken for lunch; finishes work 7 PM; sometimes attends exercise class; pt and partner take turns cooking dinner and cleaning up; may watch TV, do some chores; goes to bed about 11:30 PM
HEALTH MAINTENANCE ACTIVITIES	
Sleep	6–8 hrs every night
Diet	She has increased her dairy and vitamin C- and A-rich vegetables and fruits, as well as adding 1 serving daily from bread group. Has some protein with breakfast. Vegetables are well washed, and all meats are cooked to at least medium doneness to avoid toxoplasmosis. All dairy products are pasteurized.
Exercise	Attends an exercise class a few times a week

continues

CASE STUDY   (Continued)

The Pregnant Patient

Stress Management	Exercise, partner, friends, family support
Use of Safety Devices	Wears seat belt always; her car has front and side air bags
Health Check-ups	GYN check with Pap smear, most years, since age 20; dental visits annually; no hx of periodontal dz
PHYSICAL EXAMINATION	
General Assessment, Vital Signs, Height, and Weight	WDWN female in NAD T: 98.3°F P: 88 R: 18 BP: 102/75 LA sitting WT: 165 lbs (usual weight) HT: 68 inches
Skin and Hair	Intact without lesions, rashes, bruises
Head and Neck	Thyroid without enlargement, no lymphadenopathy
Eyes, Ears, Nose, Mouth, and Throat	WNL
Breasts	Tender with everted nipples
Thorax and Lungs	Breath sounds clear, no wheezing or crackles
Heart and Peripheral Vasculature	Heart: regular rhythm, no murmurs, no peripheral edema
Abdomen	Positive bowel sounds, no masses; no HSM
Urinary System	Clean catch urinalysis and urine culture sent to lab; negative glycosuria, negative proteinuria in dipstick
Musculoskeletal System	No limitations in ROM
Neurological System	CN II–XII grossly intact, mental status intact, DTRs 2+/4+ bilaterally
Female Genitalia	External genitalia: Without lesions, abnormalities or tenderness
	Internal genitalia: Vagina and cervix without lesions or abnormalities, with normal softening of the cervix and cervical/ uterine junction, the uterus is 8 weeks post LMP size. DNA probe for chlamydia and gonorrhea sent. Informed of Group Beta Strep culture at 36 weeks.
Anus, Perineum, and Rectum	WNL
Hematological System	Prenatal panel requisition given
Endocrine	Early glucose tolerance test ordered with prenatal lab panel
Nutrition	Reports now eating several small meals; fairly balanced diet; without physical s/s of malnutrition; not obese, BMI 27.3

continues

CASE STUDY (Continued)

The Pregnant Patient

Psychosocial Assessment/ Learning Needs	Unplanned pregnancy; encouraged to seek childbirth, infant care, and breastfeeding classes. Encouraged to discuss finances with partner. Had grief counseling after demise of preterm infant. No personal history or family history of depression. History of significant premenstrual moodiness. Pt and FOB desire 1st-trimester screening and cystic fibrosis testing. Referral given for prenatal diagnosis with appropriate time intervals noted.

ASSESSMENT IN BRIEF

Assessment of the Pregnant Patient*

Fundal Height

Fetal Heart Rate

Leopold's Maneuvers

- First maneuver
- Second maneuver
- Third maneuver
- Fourth maneuver

Only pregnancy-specific assessments are listed.

REVIEW QUESTIONS

1. During pregnancy, the connective tissue changes and stretch marks may form on the abdomen, breasts, and upper thighs. The stretch marks are called which of the following?
   a. Linea nigra
   b. Nevi
   c. Melasma
   d. Striae gravidarum

   The correct answer is (d).

2. The patient comes to the clinic complaining of decreased fetal movement. The nurse assesses the fetus and talks with the patient and determines that fetal movement is normal. She teaches the mother what she should be looking for while assessing fetal movement and teaches her fetal kick counts. Monitoring of fetal kick counts should begin at what gestational age?
   a. 20 weeks
   b. 22 weeks
   c. 28 weeks
   d. 30 weeks

   The correct answer is (c).

3. Evelyn presents to the clinic at 18-weeks gestation. The nurse takes her blood pressure and it is 148/98. When the nurse checks her urine, the dipstick is 4+ for protein. The nurse asks Evelyn if she has any history of high blood pressure, to which she answers no. The nurse knows that Evelyn will need close monitoring during her pregnancy because she most likely has:
   a. Gestational hypertension
   b. Chronic hypertension
   c. Preeclampsia
   d. Chronic hypertension with superimposed pre-eclampsia

   The correct answer is (d).

4. Casie comes to the clinic at 25-weeks gestation complaining of lower back pain and painful urination. The nurse taps Casie's flank area, and Casie complains of tenderness and pain. She most likely has:
   a. Interstitial cystitis
   b. Vaginal infection
   c. Pyelonephritis
   d. Chorioamnionitis

   The correct answer is (c).

5. Shamika is pregnant for the sixth time. She tells you that she has four children at home and had one ectopic pregnancy. You also discover that three of her children were preterm. How would you most accurately describe Shamika's obstetrical history?

a. G6, P3, T6, P5, A1, E1, LC4
b. G6, P5, T4, P3, A0, E1, LC5
c. G6, P3, T5, P5, A1, E0, LC5
d. G6, P5, T1, P3, A0, E1, LC4
The correct answer is (d).

6. Gail comes to her clinic visit with bruises on her arms and neck. She had a broken leg shortly before her pregnancy. She has also missed the last two appointments. You suspect abuse. What would you say to Gail?
   a. "Are you being abused? If you are, then you should have him thrown in jail."
   b. "I know you are being abused, but it will be OK. Most men stop when they realize it could hurt the baby."
   c. "You've missed your last two appointments and have bruises on your body. Is there a problem at home? I can help you get the appropriate help, if you'll let me."
   d. "Do you keep bumping into things? This can happen because your center of gravity changes during pregnancy."
   The correct answer is (c).

7. Monika presents for her first prenatal visit and tells you that she has diabetes and is on an oral medication, but she can't remember the name of it. You tell her that her medication will probably be changed since she is now pregnant. What medication will she most likely be taking instead?
   a. Methyldopa   c. Heparin
   b. Insulin   d. Hydralazine
   The correct answer is (b).

8. Susan presents to her first prenatal appointment complaining of right-sided pain. She looks very pale and complains of dizziness. On the way to the exam room, she collapses to the floor. Upon assessment, you and the other nurses discover that her pulse is fast and thready, her blood pressure is low, and she is losing consciousness. You call for immediate help because you fear she has a:
   a. Hypertensive crisis
   b. Ruptured ectopic pregnancy
   c. Severe infection
   d. Pelvic inflammatory disease
   The correct answer is (b).

9. Cheri comes to her prenatal visit complaining that she must need new contacts because her vision has become blurry. The nurse explains to her that this is a common occurrence during pregnancy because of:
   a. Excessive saliva secretion
   b. Increased mucous production
   c. Corneal thickening
   d. Increased lysozyme in tears
   The correct answer is (d).

10. Tracy is 32-weeks pregnant and presents to her prenatal visit complaining of bleeding after intercourse last night. It was just a little so she decided to wait until her appointment today to ask about it. She says this has never happened before. After ruling out any complication, you explain that during pregnancy the cervix might bleed due to increased vascularity. This is called:
    a. Friability   c. Hormonal response
    b. Chadwick's sign   d. Lightening
    The correct answer is (a).

BIBLIOGRAPHY

Aaritis, S., & Simhan, H. (2007). Management of pregnant women after inhibition of preterm labor. UpToDate®. uptodate.com

The American College of Obstetricians and Gynecologists (ACOG). (2007). *Guidelines for women's healthcare* (3rd ed.). Washington, DC: Author.

Amorim, A. R., Linné, Y., Kac, G., & Lourenco, P. M. (2008). Assessment of weight changes during and after pregnancy: Practical approaches. *Maternal Child Nutrition, 4*(1), 1–13.

Arci, A. (2006). *Myomas, an issue of obstetrics and gynecology clinics.* Philadelphia: Saunders.

Bader, T. J. (2005). *Ob/Gyn secrets* (3rd ed.). St. Louis: Mosby.

Blackburn, S. (2007). *Maternal, fetal and neonatal physiology: A clinical perspective* (3rd ed.). Philadelphia: Saunders.

Briggs, G. G., Freeman, R. K., & Yaffe, S. J. (2005). *Drugs in pregnancy & lactation: A reference guide to fetal and neonatal risk* (7th ed.). Philadelphia: Lippincott Williams & Wilkins.

Chasan-Taber, L., Evenson, K. R., Sternfeld, B., & Kengeri, S. (2007). Assessment of recreational physical activity during pregnancy in epidemiologic studies of birthweight and length of gestation: Methodologic aspects. *Women's Health, 45*(4),85–107.

Conde-Agudelo, A., Villar, J., & Lindheimer, M. (2008). Maternal infection and risk of preeclampsia: Systematic review and metaanalysis. *American Journal of Obstetrics & Gynecology, 198*(1), 7–22.

Craigo, S., & Baker, E. (2005). *Medical complications in pregnancy.* New York: McGraw-Hill.

Creasy, R. K., Resnik, R., & Iams, J. (2004). *Maternal-fetal medicine* (5th ed.). Philadelphia: Saunders.

Cunningham, F. G., Leveno, K. J., Bloom, S., Alexander, J., Hauth, J. C., Gilstrap, L.C., III, & Wenstrom, K. (2005). *Williams obstetrics* (22nd ed.). New York: McGraw-Hill.

Cunningham, S. (2006). *Williams obstetrics* (22nd ed., digital ed.). New York: McGraw-Hill.

Curtis, B., & Schuler, J. (2008). *Your pregnancy week by week* (6th ed.). Cambridge, MA: Da Capo Press.

Czeizel, A. E., Dudas, I., Fritz, G., Tecsoi, A., Hanck, A., & Kunovits, G. (1992). The effect of periconceptional multivitamin-mineral supplementation on vertigo, nausea, and vomiting in the first trimester of pregnancy. *Archives of Gynecology and Obstetrics, 251*(4), 181–185.

DeCherney, A. H., Nathan, L., & Goodwin, T. (2006). *Current obstetrics & gynecologic diagnosis & treatment* (10th ed.). New York: McGraw-Hill.

Dharan, V., Parviainen, K., Newcomb, P., & Poleshuck, V. (2006). *Psychosocial and environmental pregnancy risks.* Emedicine from WebMd.com

Dodds, L., Fell, D. B., Dooley, K. C., Armson, B. A., Allen, A. C., Nassar, B. A., Perkins, S., & Joseph, K. S. (2008). Effect of homocysteine concentration in early pregnancy on gestational hypertensive disorders and other pregnancy outcomes. *Clinical Chemistry 54*(2), 326–334.

Driggers, R. W., & Seibert, D. C. (2008). Prenatal screening: New guidelines, new challenges. *The Journal for Nurse Practitioners, 4*(5), 351–356.

Driul, L., Cacciaguerra, G., Citossi, A., Martina, M. D., Peressini, L., & Marchesoni, D. (2007). Prepregnancy body mass index and adverse pregnancy outcomes. *Archives of Gynecology and Obstetrics, 278*(1), 23–26.

Evans, A. T. (Ed.). (2007). *Manual of obstetrics* (7th ed.). Philadelphia: Lippincott Williams & Wilkins.

Fortner, K. B., Szymanski, L., Fox, H., & Wallach, E. E. (2006). *The Johns Hopkins manual of gynecology and obstetrics* (3rd ed.). Philadelphia: Lippincott Williams & Wilkins.

Freda, M. C. (2002). *Perinatal patient education.* Philadelphia: Lippincott Williams & Wilkins.

Gabbe, S. G., Simpson J. L., & Niebyl, J. R. (Eds.). (2007). *Obstetrics: Normal and problem pregnancies* (5th ed.). New York: Churchhill Livingstone.

Gilbert, E. S. (2007). *Manual of high risk pregnancy & delivery* (4th ed.). St. Louis: Mosby.

Gilbert, W. M., Young A. L., & Danielsen, B. (2007). Pregnancy outcomes in women with chronic hypertension: A population-based study. *Journal of Reproductive Medicine, 52*(11), 1046–1051.

Goldenberg, R. L., Andrews, W. W., Faye-Petersen, O., Cliver, S. P., Goepfert, A. R., & Hauth, J. C. (2008). The Alabama Preterm Birth Project: Placental histology in recurrent spontaneous and indicated preterm birth. *American Journal of Obstetrics & Gynecology, 195*(3), 792–796.

Greer, I. A., & Nelson-Piercy, C. (2007). *Maternal medicine—Medical problems in pregnancy.* New York: Churchhill Livingstone.

Gronowski, A. M. (Ed.). (2004). *Handbook of clinical laboratory testing during pregnancy.* Totowa, NJ: Humana Press.

Holmgren, C., Aagaard-Tillery, K. M., Silver, R. M., Porter, T. F., & Varner, M. (2008). Hyperemesis in pregnancy: An evaluation of treatment strategies with maternal and neonatal outcomes. *American Journal of Obstetrics & Gynecology, 198*(1), 56e1–56e4.

James, D. K., Steer, P. J., Weiner, C. P., & Gonik, B. (2005). *High risk pregnancy management options* (3rd ed.). Philadelphia: Saunders.

Johnson, R., & Taylor, W. (2006). *Skills for midwifery practice* (2nd ed.). Edinburgh: Churchhill Livingstone.

Kohn, I., Moffitt, P. L., & Wilkins, I. A. (2000). *A silent sorrow* (2nd ed.). New York: Routledge.

Lemnos, J. A., & Lockwood, C. J. (Eds.). (2007). *Guidelines for perinatal care* (6th ed.). Washington, DC: The American College of Obstetricians and Gynecologists (ACOG).

Liebschutz, J. M., Frayne, S. M., & Saxe, G. N. (Eds.). (2003). *Violence against women: A physician's guide to identification and management.* Philadelphia: American College of Physicians.

Long, V. E., & McMullen, P. (2002). *Telephone triage for obstetrics and gynecology.* Philadelphia: Lippincott Williams & Wilkins.

McKinney, E. S., James, S. R., Murray, S. S., & Ashwell, J. W. (2007). *Maternal-child nursing* (2nd ed.). Philadelphia: Saunders.

Milunsky, A., Ulcickas, M., Rothman, K. J., Willett, W., Jick, S. S., & Jick, H. (1992). Maternal heat exposure and neural tube defects. *JAMA, 268*(7), 882–885.

Morrison, J. (Ed.). (2005). *Preterm labor, prediction and treatment: An issue of obstetrics and gynecology.* Philadelphia: Saunders.

Murray, S. S., McKinney, E. S., & Gorrie, T. M. (2006). *Foundations of maternal newborn nursing* (4th ed.). Philadelphia: Saunders.

Ramsay, M. M., James, W. K., Steer, P. J., Weiner, C. P., & Gonik, B. (Eds.). (2001). *Normal values in pregnancy* (2nd ed.). London: Saunders.

Reece, E. (2008). Perspectives on obesity, pregnancy and birth outcomes in the United States: The scope of the problem. *American Journal of Obstetrics & Gynecology, 198*(1), 23–28.

Rosene-Montella, K., & Keely, E. (2008). *Medical care of the pregnant patient* (2nd ed.). Providence, RI: American College of Physicians.

Rosenfield, A. (2007). *New research on postpartum depression.* Hauppauge, NY: Nova Science Publishers.

Scott, J. R., Gibbs, R. S., Karlan, B. Y., & Haney, A. F. (Eds.). (2003). *Danforth's obstetrics & gynecology* (9th ed.). Philadelphia: Lippincott Williams & Williams.

Sharp, K., Brindle, P. M., Brown, M. W., & Turner, G. M. (1993). Memory loss during pregnancy. *British Journal of Obstetrics and Gynaecology, 100*(3), 209–215.

Shulman, L. (2007). *Yearbook of obstetrics, gynecology and women's health.* St. Louis: Mosby.

Simpson, K. R., & Creehan, P. A. (2001). *AWHONN perinatal nursing* (2nd ed.). Philadelphia: Lippincott Williams & Wilkins.

Springhouse, (Ed.). (2007). *Maternal-neonatal facts made incredibly quick* (2nd ed.). Philadelphia: Springhouse.

WEB SITES

American Academy of Pediatrics:
http://www.aap.org

The American College of Obstetricians and Gynecologists:
http://www.acog.org

Association of Women's Health, Obstetric and Neonatal Nurses:
http://www.awhonn.org

Centers for Disease Control and Prevention:
http://www.cdc.gov

eMedicine:
http://www.emedicine.com

March of Dimes:
http://www.marchofdimes.com

MD Consult:
http://www.mdconsult.com

Medline:
http://www.medline.com

PubMed:
http://www.pubmed.com

UpToDate:
http://www.uptodate.com

CHAPTER 24

The Pediatric Patient

COMPETENCIES

1. Differentiate the structural and physiological variations between pediatric patients and adults.

2. Identify personal-social, language, and fine and gross motor findings when using the Denver II.

3. Elicit a complete health history from a patient or caregiver using standard components of a pediatric health history.

4. Identify various techniques of approaching patients at different developmental levels before initiating the physical assessment.

5. Perform inspection, palpation, percussion, and auscultation in a head-to-toe assessment of a pediatric patient.

Children are unique individuals who undergo rapid changes from birth through adolescence. Physical growth, motor skills, and cognitive and social development are evidence of the numerous changes family members, friends, and health care professionals observe throughout a child's maturing years. In your assessment of the pediatric patient, you must be aware of these changes as you continually reassess what is considered within normal limits for the child.

PHYSICAL GROWTH

One important set of parameters required for pediatric health assessment is physical growth. The parameters of weight, length or height, and head circumference (dependent on age) are essential in serial physical growth measurements. (Chest circumference is of less importance.) For example, by plotting a child's growth on a chart (see Figure 24-1), you are able to determine normal or abnormal growth curves according to the child's age. Special growth charts are available for genetic syndromes such as Down or Turner syndrome.

Growth charts were revised in 2000 by the National Center for Health Statistics (NCHS), the National Center for Chronic Disease Prevention and Health Promotion (NCCDPHP), and various other experts. One addition, the Body Mass Index for Age Percentiles chart, is used to decide whether a child's weight is appropriate for his or her height. The BMI growth chart is available for use with children age 2 years and older. The charts are used to compare a child's growth to the growth of children in the United States. For example, you are plotting the growth of a 5-year-old female whose BMI is 17.3 (see Figure 24-1G). This would indicate that her BMI is higher than approximately 90% of 5-year-old girls in the United States.

For infants the average birth weight is 7.5 pounds (3.5 kg), length is 19 to 21 inches (48 to 53 cm), and head circumference is 13 to 14 inches (33 to 35.5 cm). Infants should double birth weight at 6 months and triple birth weight by 1 year of age, although it is not uncommon for infants to double birth weight at 4 months. An infant's height increases about 1 inch (2.5 cm) per month for the first 6 months, and then slows to ½ inch (1.3 cm) per month until 12 months. Growth in the toddler period (12–24 months) begins to slow. The birth weight usually quadruples by 2.5 years of age, with an average weight gain during the toddler period of 4 to 6 pounds (1.8 to 2.7 kg) per year. The toddler usually grows 3 inches (7.6 cm).

Preschoolers (2–6 years) gain an average of 5 pounds (2.3 kg) per year. Height increases between 2.5 and 3 inches (6.4 to 7.6 cm) per year. The preschooler's birth length usually is doubled by 4 years of age. In contrast, the school-age child (6–12 years) grows 1 to 2 inches (2.5 to 5 cm) per year and gains 3 to 6 pounds (1.3 to 2.7 kg) annually.

Infancy and adolescence (13–18 years) are two periods of rapid growth in the pediatric patient. Rapid growth in the adolescent is called the growth spurt. Females commonly experience this between ages 10 and 14, whereas in males, it occurs somewhat later, between 12 and 16 years of age.

ANATOMY AND PHYSIOLOGY

STRUCTURAL AND PHYSIOLOGICAL VARIATIONS

Children differ from adults and among themselves at various stages of development in their structural and physiological makeups. Following is a list of important variations that occur from birth through a child's maturation.

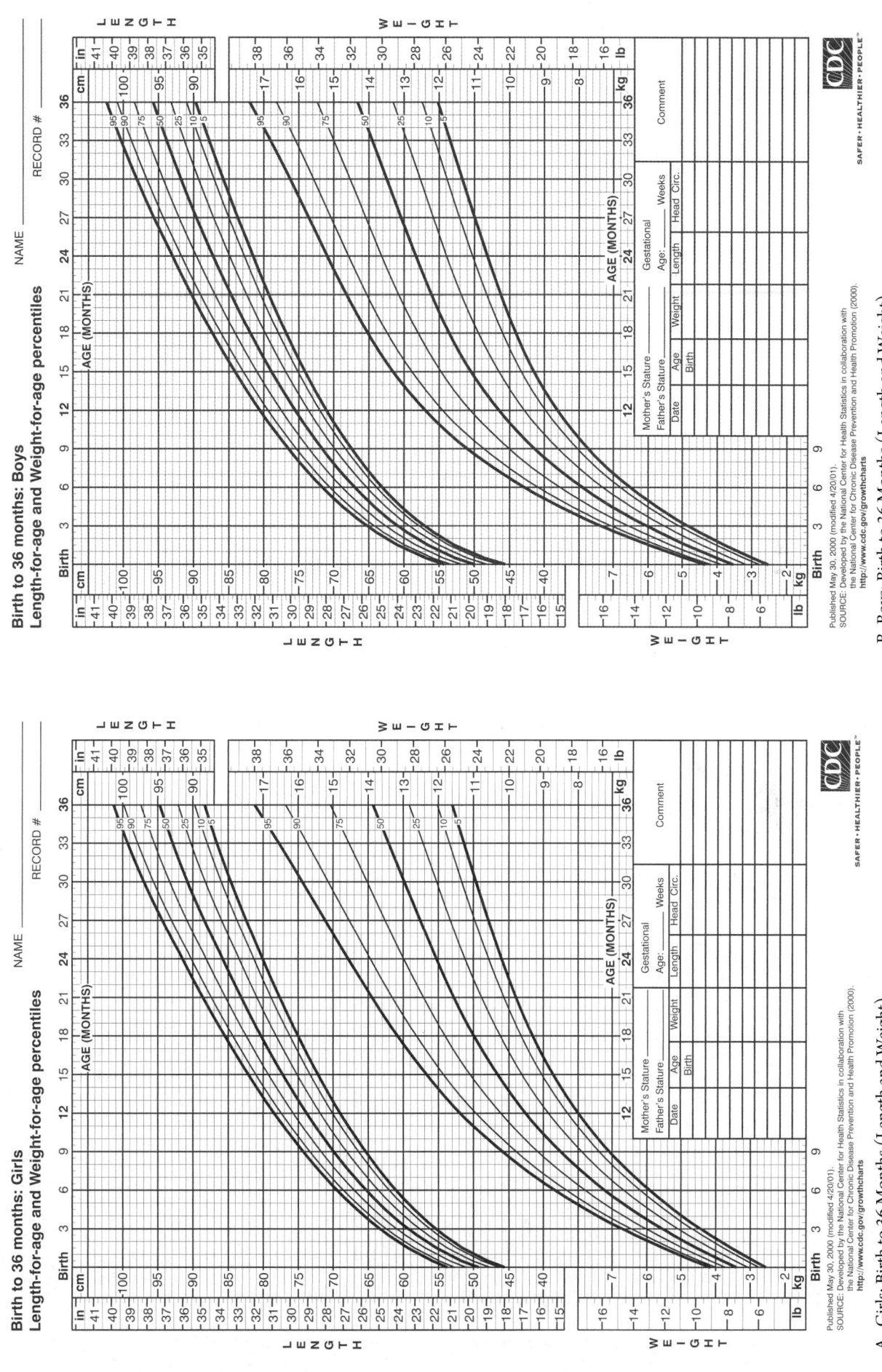

A. Girls: Birth to 36 Months (Length and Weight)

B. Boys: Birth to 36 Months (Length and Weight)

FIGURE 24-1 Physical Growth Charts. *Courtesy of National Center for Health Statistics, U.S. Centers for Disease Control and Prevention, 2001. http://cdc.gov/growthcharts. Accessed June 18, 2008.*

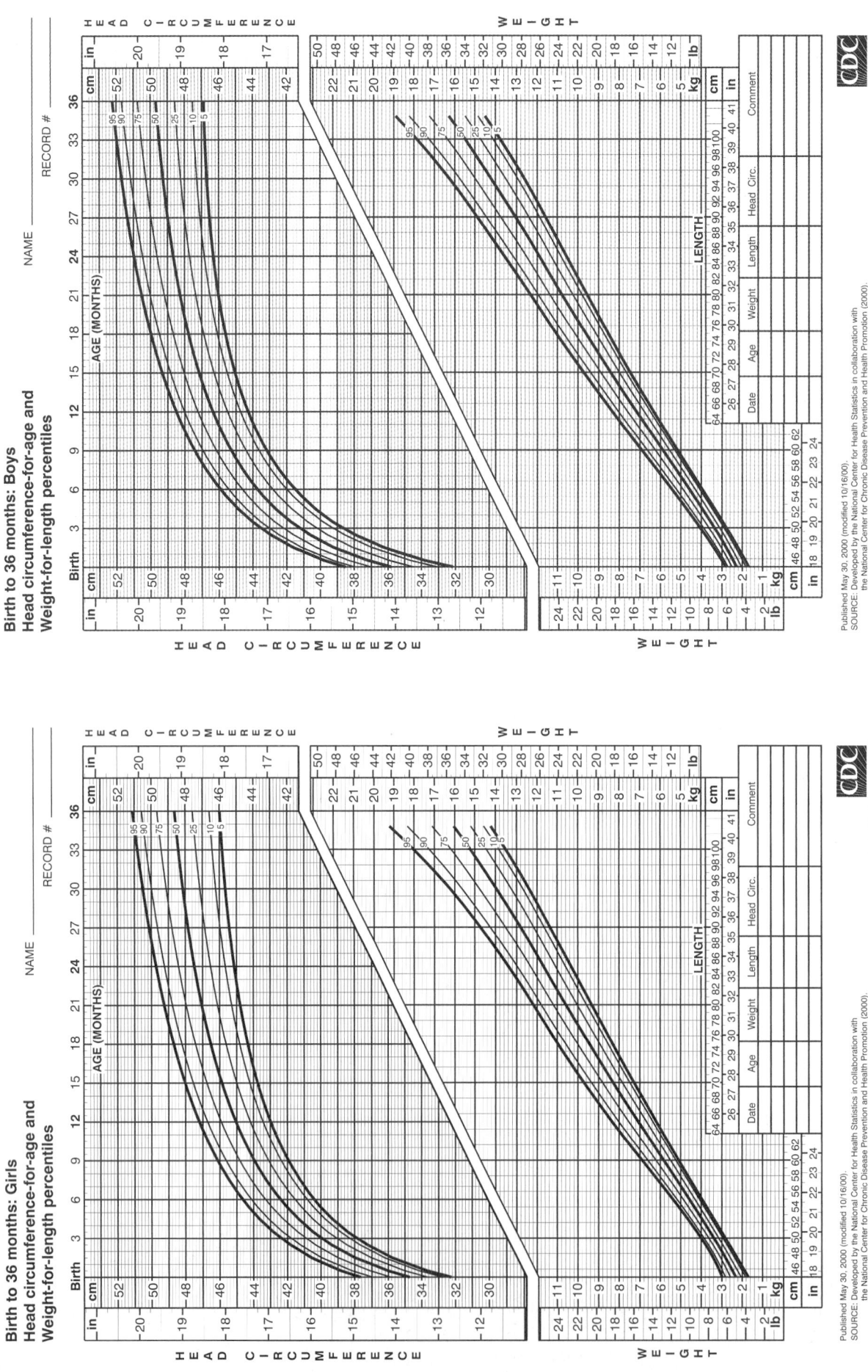

Birth to 36 months: Girls
Head circumference-for-age and
Weight-for-length percentiles

Birth to 36 months: Boys
Head circumference-for-age and
Weight-for-length percentiles

Published May 30, 2000 (modified 10/16/00).
SOURCE: Developed by the National Center for Health Statistics in collaboration with
the National Center for Chronic Disease Prevention and Health Promotion (2000).
http://www.cdc.gov/growthcharts

C. Girls: Birth to 36 Months (Head Circumference)

D. Boys: Birth to 36 Months (Head Circumference)

FIGURE 24-1 Physical Growth Charts *continues*

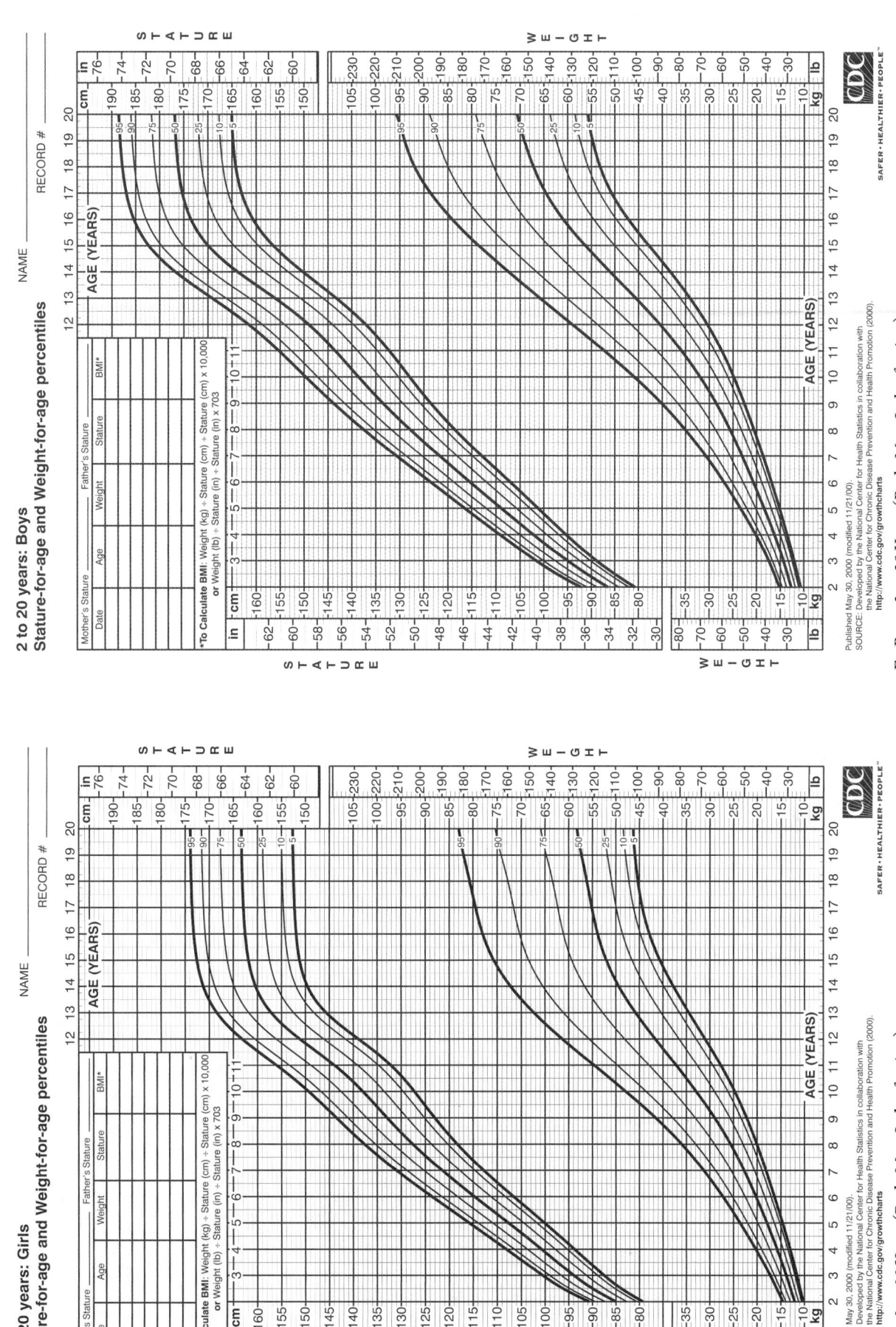

E. Girls: 2 to 20 Years (Body Mass Index for Age)

F. Boys: 2 to 20 Years (Body Mass Index for Age)

FIGURE 24-1 Physical Growth Charts *continues*

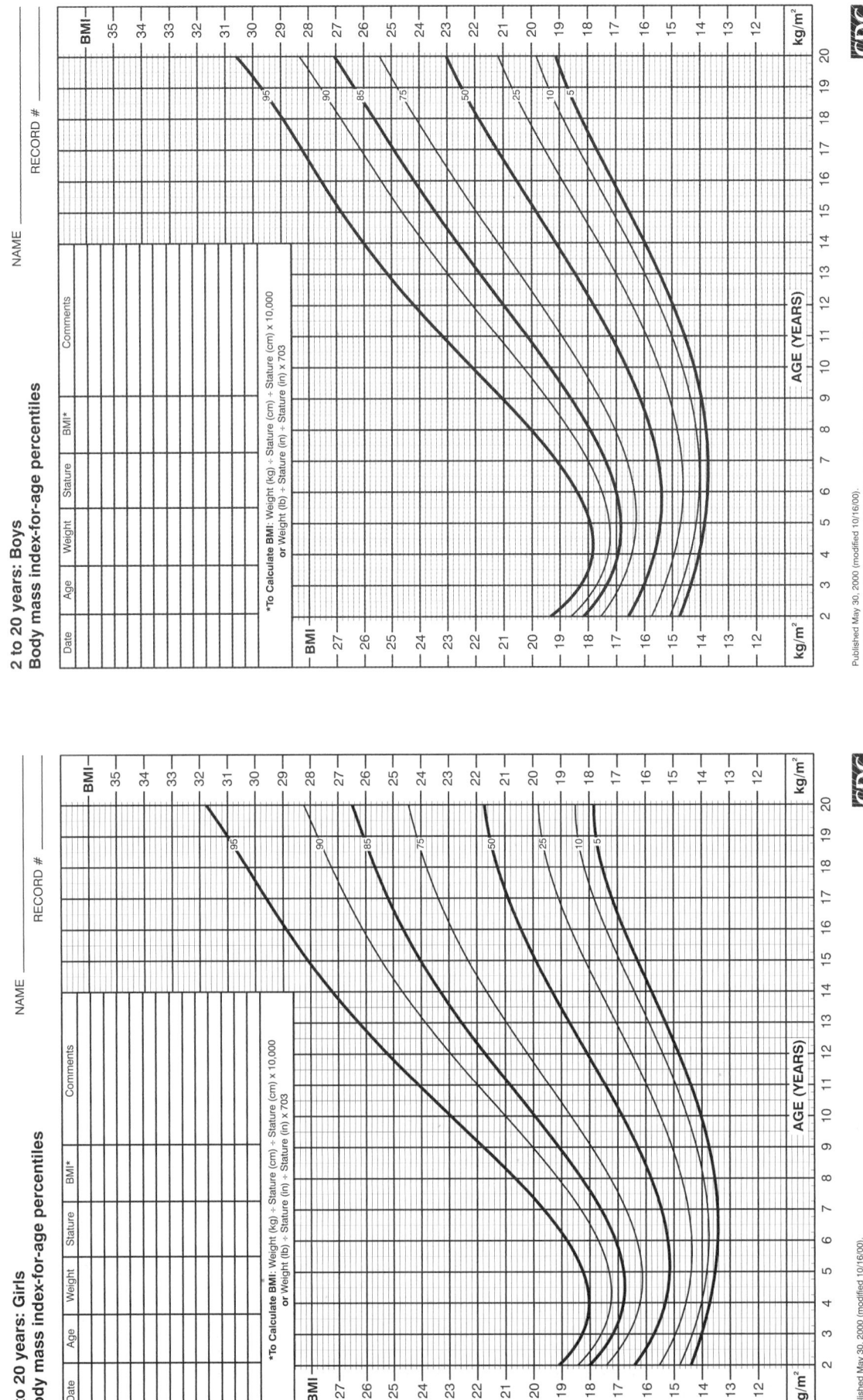

2 to 20 years: Girls
Body mass index-for-age percentiles

NAME _____

RECORD # _____

Date	Age	Weight	Stature	BMI*	Comments

*To Calculate BMI: Weight (kg) ÷ Stature (cm) ÷ Stature (cm) × 10,000
or Weight (lb) ÷ Stature (in) ÷ Stature (in) × 703

Published May 30, 2000 (modified 10/16/00).
SOURCE: Developed by the National Center for Health Statistics in collaboration with
the National Center for Chronic Disease Prevention and Health Promotion (2000).
http://www.cdc.gov/growthcharts

G. Girls: 2 to 20 Years (Stature and Weight)

2 to 20 years: Boys
Body mass index-for-age percentiles

NAME _____

RECORD # _____

Date	Age	Weight	Stature	BMI*	Comments

*To Calculate BMI: Weight (kg) ÷ Stature (cm) ÷ Stature (cm) × 10,000
or Weight (lb) ÷ Stature (in) ÷ Stature (in) × 703

Published May 30, 2000 (modified 10/16/00).
SOURCE: Developed by the National Center for Health Statistics in collaboration with
the National Center for Chronic Disease Prevention and Health Promotion (2000).
http://www.cdc.gov/growthcharts

H. Boys: 2 to 20 Years (Stature and Weight)

FIGURE 24-1 **Physical Growth Charts** *continues*

NURSING**TIP**

Allaying Childhood Fears

Throughout childhood, children exhibit various fears and behaviors in response to past and present health care encounters. The following nursing tips serve to calm fears and control behaviors children may exhibit during an examination.

Infant

The fear of parents leaving the room begins at around 6 months of age. Older infants experience a fear of strangers called stranger anxiety.

Tip: Allow parents to be present and to hold their child during the exam; speak in a calm, reassuring voice; and allow the patient to use security objects such as a pacifier, blanket, or stuffed animal during the exam.

Toddler

Fear of strangers and parents leaving the room continues in the toddler age group. Clinginess is prevalent in toddlers. They may also become upset if their parent is feeling stressed. Additionally, fear of pain and discomfort usually begins in the toddler years.

Tip: Allow parents to be present and to hold their child during the exam; speak in a calm, reassuring voice; allow use of security objects such as a pacifier, blanket, or stuffed animal during the exam; explain what is happening in simple words; and allow time for the toddler to play, explore, and express his or her feelings. Allowing choices will give the toddler a feeling of control.

Preschooler

This age group fears being left alone and experiencing pain. Behaviors exhibited include clinginess, temper tantrums, asking for help with things that were once done without help, baby talk, or thumb sucking (regression-type behaviors).

Tip: Allow parents to be present and to hold their child during the exam; speak in a calm, reassuring voice; let the child know what is going to be examined; allow manipulation of exam equipment; and be honest about what is going to happen next.

School Age

Behaviors once thought to be outgrown may often come back as mechanisms for coping with stress. Fears include separation from parents, pain, and losing control. Some behaviors seen in school-age children include asking for help with things that were once done without help, acting out by yelling or screaming, and attention seeking.

Tip: Allow parents to be present, allow time for play or manipulation of exam equipment, let the child ask questions, acknowledge feelings, allow choices, and set limits for losing control.

Adolescent

Adolescents may be skeptical concerning truth telling and think health care professionals avoid telling the truth. The fear of pain and losing control may persist during adolescence. Privacy is a big factor during adolescent exams.

Tip: Involve the adolescent in planning and decision making, allow the choice of the parent leaving during the exam, and encourage expressions of feelings.

Vital Signs

- One notable difference in the way children and adults regulate temperature is the inability of infants aged 6 months and younger to shiver in the face of lower ambient temperature. The absence of this important protective mechanism puts infants at risk for hypothermia, bradycardia, and acidosis.
- By age 4, temperature parameters are comparable to those seen in adults.
- Both pulse and respiratory rates in children tend to decline with advancing age and reach levels comparable to those found in adulthood by adolescence.
- In children 1 year of age and older, an easy rule of thumb for determining normal systolic blood pressure is:

$$\text{normal systolic BP (mm Hg)} = 80 + (2 \times \text{age in years}).$$

- Normal diastolic blood pressure is generally two-thirds of systolic blood pressure.

Skin and Hair

- **Lanugo**, a fine, downy hair, can be present on the skin of a newborn. The lanugo is most prominent over the temples of the forehead and on the upper arms, shoulders, back, and pinna of the ears. Dark-skinned newborns have an increased amount of lanugo, which is readily evident as very dark black hair.
- **Vernix caseosa**, a thick, cheesy, protective integumentary deposit that consists of sebum and shed epithelial cells, is present on the newborn's skin.
- Relative to an adult, a child has a higher ratio of body surface area to body surface mass.

Head

- Suture ridges are palpable until approximately 6 months of age, at which time unionization occurs.
- The posterior fontanel, which is triangular in shape and is formed by the junction of the sagittal and lambdoidal sutures, usually closes by 3 months of age (Figure 24-2).
- The junction of the sagittal, coronal, and frontal sutures forms the anterior fontanel. It is diamond shaped. This fontanel should close by 19 months of age.

Eyes, Ears, Nose, Mouth, and Throat

- At birth, the newborn's peripheral vision is intact. Visual acuity is approximately 20/200. The child's visual acuity is usually 20/20 at 6–8 years.
- Newborns do not produce tears until their lacrimal ducts open, at around 2 to 3 months of age.
- The external auditory canal of a child is shorter than that of an adult, and it is positioned upward.
- The eustachian tube is wider, shorter, and more horizontal than that of an adult. These factors increase the likelihood of middle ear infections caused by migration of pathogens from the nasopharynx.
- Only the ethmoid and maxillary sinuses are present at birth. At approximately 7 years of age, the frontal sinuses develop. The sphenoid sinuses do not develop until after puberty.
- Eruption of the first lower central incisors occurs between 5 and 7 months of age. By 2.5 years of age, toddlers have 20 primary, or deciduous, teeth. By puberty, permanent teeth and four molars have replaced the primary teeth. Wisdom teeth normally appear between 18 and 21 years of age (see Figure 24-3).
- Salivation starts at about 3 months, and the infant drools until the swallowing reflex is more coordinated.

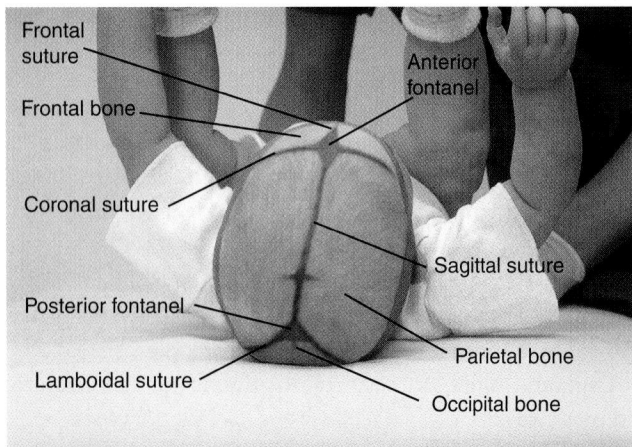

A. Superior View

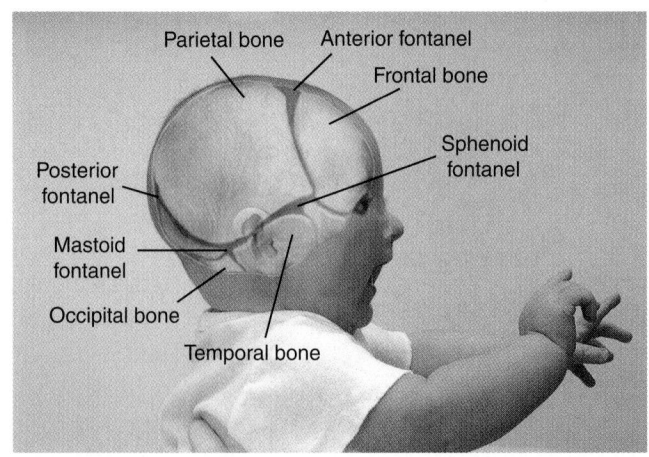

B. Lateral View

FIGURE 24-2 **Infant Head Structures**

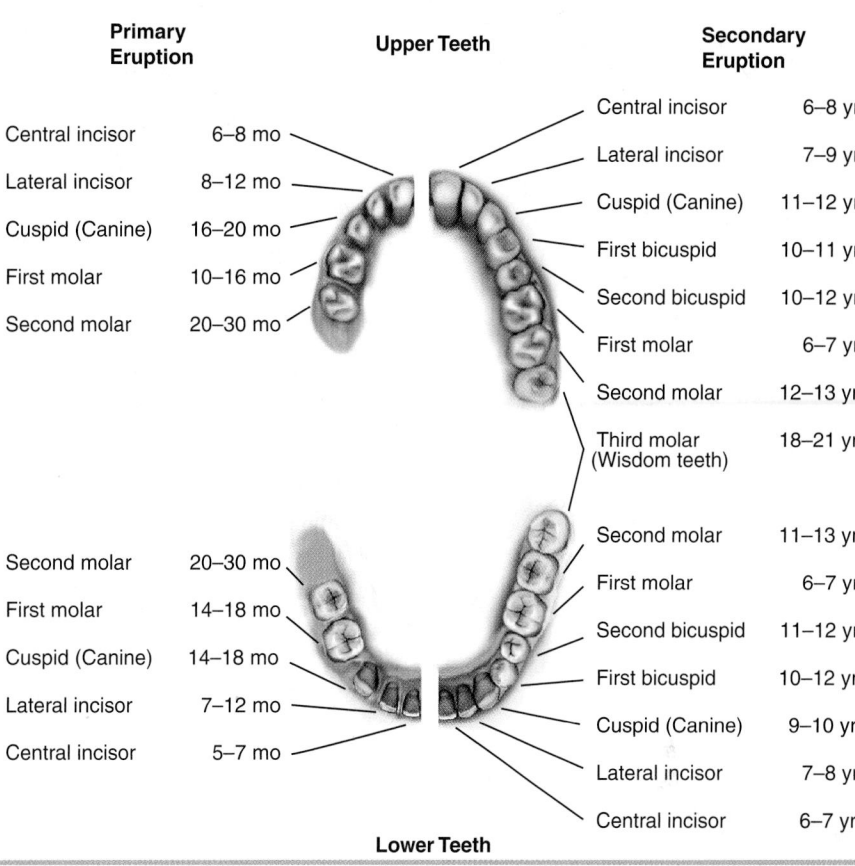

Primary Eruption		Upper Teeth	Secondary Eruption	
Central incisor	6–8 mo		Central incisor	6–8 yr
Lateral incisor	8–12 mo		Lateral incisor	7–9 yr
Cuspid (Canine)	16–20 mo		Cuspid (Canine)	11–12 yr
First molar	10–16 mo		First bicuspid	10–11 yr
Second molar	20–30 mo		Second bicuspid	10–12 yr
			First molar	6–7 yr
			Second molar	12–13 yr
			Third molar (Wisdom teeth)	18–21 yr
			Second molar	11–13 yr
			First molar	6–7 yr
Second molar	20–30 mo		Second bicuspid	11–12 yr
First molar	14–18 mo		First bicuspid	10–12 yr
Cuspid (Canine)	14–18 mo		Cuspid (Canine)	9–10 yr
Lateral incisor	7–12 mo		Lateral incisor	7–8 yr
Central incisor	5–7 mo		Central incisor	6–7 yr

Lower Teeth

FIGURE 24-3 Deciduous and Permanent Teeth

Breasts

- Breast tissue in the female starts to develop between 8 and 10 years of age. Mature adult breast tissue is achieved between 14 and 17 years of age. Refer to Table 14-1 for Tanner's Sexual Maturity Rating.

Thorax and Lungs

- A newborn's chest is circular because the anteroposterior and transverse diameters are approximately equal (Figure 24-4). By 6 years of age, the ratio of anteroposterior to lateral diameters reaches adult values.
- Decreased muscularity is responsible for the thin chest wall in infants.
- Ribs are displaced horizontally in infants.
- The trachea is short in the newborn. By 18 months of age, it has grown from the newborn length of 2 inches (5 cm) to 3 inches (7.6 cm). Toward the latter part of adolescence, the trachea has grown to adult size, normally 4 to 5 inches (10.2 to 12.7 cm).
- Until 3 to 4 months of age, infants are totally dependent on breathing through their noses.
- During infancy and the toddler period, abdominal breathing is always prevalent over thoracic expansion.

Heart and Peripheral Vasculature

- The infant's, toddler's, and preschooler's heart lies more horizontally than an adult's heart; thus the apex is higher at about the left fourth intercostal space.
- The fetal circulation changes to a pulmonary circulation when the umbilical cord is separated from the maternal circulation. Normally, the three fetal shunts (ductus venosus, foramen ovale, and ductus arteriosus) close at birth or shortly

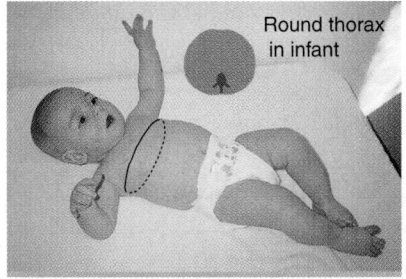

Round thorax in infant

FIGURE 24-4 Infant Chest Configuration

REFLECTIVE THINKING

Adolescent at Risk for Suicide

Sixteen-year-old Jason just moved to a small town from Chicago, Illinois. Before the interview, his mother confides in you that Jason has been acting differently, both socially and physically, since the family move. During your interview with Jason, he tells you he had so many friends before the family moved but has not been able to meet anyone to "hang out with." Jason proceeds to tell you he just mailed his coin collection and the baseball he caught at a Cubs game to a friend in Chicago.

You summarize the information Jason has given and he replies, "Life is not worth living and I just want to use my father's gun to put an end to this."

- How would you respond to Jason's last statement?
- Would you feel obligated to share this information with anyone?
- What is your institution's policy on suicide precautions?

thereafter. The ductus venosus allows blood to flow from the placenta into the right heart. Blood flows from the right side of the heart to the left through an opening called a foramen ovale. This opening is a flap valve located on the atrial septum between the septum secundum and septum primum. The ductus arteriosus, located between the left pulmonary artery and the descending aorta, allows blood to flow from the pulmonary artery to the aorta.

- The cardiac output of an infant is normally 1 liter/minute. Toward the end of the toddler period it increases to 1.5 liters/minute. At the age of 4 years it is 2.2 liters/minute. By 15 years of age cardiac output has reached the adult level of 5.5 liters/minute.
- Infants have a higher circulating blood volume (normally around 85 mL/kg) compared to that of an adult (65 mL/kg).

Abdomen

- At birth, the neonate's umbilical cord contains two arteries and one vein.
- The infant's liver is proportionately larger in the abdominal cavity than is the liver of an adult.
- Infants' and toddlers' abdomens are more protuberant, but this does not necessarily indicate pathology.

Musculoskeletal System

- Bone growth ends at age 20, when the epiphyses close.

Neurological System

- The neurological system of the infant is incompletely developed. The autonomic nervous system helps maintain homeostasis as the cerebral cortex develops.
- In the first year, the neurons become myelinated, and primitive motor reflexes are replaced by purposeful movement. The myelinization occurs in a cephalocaudal and proximodistal manner (head and neck, trunk, and extremities).
- Mylenization in the bowel and bladder allows the child to control these functions.

Urinary System

- In infancy, the urinary bladder is between the symphysis pubis and umbilicus.

Female Genitalia

- Development of pubic hair in the female begins at puberty, between 8 and 12 years of age. Within about 1 year, the pubic hair becomes dark, coarse, and curly but is not considered fully developed. Axillary hair follows 6 months later. After about age 13–15, pubic hair distribution approaches adult quantity and consistency. See Tanner's Sexual Maturity Rating in Table 20-1.

Male Genitalia

- The testes usually descend by the age of 1 year.
- Puberty usually starts between the ages of 9½ and 13½ and can last 2 to 5 years. Testicular enlargement is usually the first area of sexual development to occur. Within about 1 year, the pubic hair becomes dark, coarse, and curly but is not fully developed. Axillary hair follows 6 months later. Facial hair follows approximately 6 months after the emergence of axillary hair. See Tanner's Sexual Maturity Rating in Table 21-1 for additional information.

GROWTH AND DEVELOPMENT

Refer to Chapter 4 for a summary of motor, language, and sensory tasks that normal children from infancy through adolescence are able to accomplish.

NURSINGALERT

Risk Factors for Adolescent Suicide

1. Verbalizing about ways to commit suicide.
2. Giving personal items away to friends and family.
3. Withdrawing from friends and family.
4. Demonstrating difficulty with accepting individual failures or disappointments.
5. Exhibiting an attitude of disgust or discouragement with day-to-day living.

Source: Boynton, Dunn, Stephens, & Pulcini, 2003

NURSINGTIP

Assessing for Attention Deficit Hyperactivity Disorder (ADHD)

Pose the following questions to the caregiver if the child is having periods of inattention, impulsiveness, and hyperactivity. If the caregiver answers yes to eight or more questions and the behaviors in question have been demonstrated for at least 6 months, a referral for a more comprehensive evaluation should be made to rule out ADHD.

- Does your child fidget with his or her hands or feet or squirm in his or her seat?
- Do you notice your child having difficulty remaining seated?
- Is your child easily distracted?
- Does your child have difficulty waiting for a turn?
- Does your child blurt out answers prior to questions being completed?
- Do you have to repeatedly tell your child to do a task?
- Have you observed your child having difficulty staying focused on tasks or in play activities?
- Does your child go from one uncompleted activity to another?
- Do you notice your child having difficulty playing quietly?
- Does your child talk excessively?
- Do you notice your child interrupting others?
- Does your child have difficulty listening to what is said?
- Does your child lose items necessary for school activities or home tasks?
- Does your child take part in any activity that could be detrimental to his or her physical well-being, such as head banging?

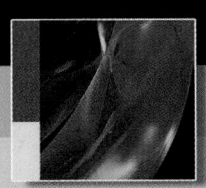

HEALTH HISTORY

The same principles that apply in obtaining an adult health history, such as questioning, listening, observing, and integrating, apply in obtaining the pediatric history. Because the historian in a pediatric history is less often the child and more likely the caregiver, it is very important to document the historian's relationship to the child. The following serves only to expand on the adult health history by providing information not previously discussed but relevant to the child.

BIOGRAPHICAL DATA

Patient Name

In addition to the patient's name, obtain the full name of the legal guardian. Occasionally, the caregiver is not the legal guardian, for example, when the child is a ward of the court or state.

Address and Phone Number

Obtain the address and phone number of the caregiver if different from those of the patient.

Source of Information

Other than the patient or caregiver, information can be obtained from medical and school records, diaries, clinic notes, and agencies such as crippled children's services, public health departments, and home health agencies. Written consent is needed to release records to a third party.

continues

CHIEF COMPLAINT

The caregiver is often the individual who seeks health care for the child and provides a description of the perceived problems, especially for infants, toddlers, and young preschoolers whose age and mental status prevent them from offering genuine descriptions of their problem. You must frequently rely on the caregiver's intuition in such cases. The caregiver is usually acutely aware of cues to the child's illness. For instance, changes in sleeping patterns (difficulty falling asleep, reversion to night waking), regression to outgrown behaviors (bedwetting, finicky eating, thumb sucking), and unusual physical complaints in an otherwise healthy child (headaches, stomachaches) are important signs that the child may be experiencing stress or illness and warrant further investigation. The older preschooler, school-age child, and adolescent are able to provide verbal descriptions of their complaints. Refer to Chapter 9 for pain rating scales that are used for children.

PAST HEALTH HISTORY

Much of the information outlined in the past health history for an adult is applicable to a child. Additional pertinent information should be elicited regarding the birth history, including prenatal, labor and delivery, and postnatal history.

Birth History

Obtaining the birth history may be one of the more sensitive topics of the past health history. You must feel comfortable and show sensitivity when inquiring whether the pregnancy was planned, the date prenatal care was first sought, and the birth order of pregnancy, taking into account miscarriages and abortions.

Prenatal

1. Did you plan your pregnancy for _____ (insert month)?

2. How many weeks after thinking that you were pregnant did you go to a health care provider for a check-up?

3. How many children have you carried to full term?

4. Were there any pregnancies that you were not able to carry to full term? What happened?

5. Did you take any prescribed or over-the-counter medications during pregnancy, including ibuprofen products?

6. Did you drink alcohol or caffeine or smoke cigarettes during pregnancy?

7. Did you take any drugs during pregnancy, such as marijuana, crack cocaine, amphetamines, or hallucinogens such as LSD and mescaline? If so, what were the amounts and frequency of use?

8. Were there any problems or illnesses that either you or your health care provider worried about during pregnancy (hypertensive disorders of pregnancy, preterm labor, gestational diabetes, group β streptococcus [GBBS], TORCH infection [toxoplasmosis, rubella, cytomegalovirus, and herpes], or an abnormal finding on a prenatal ultrasound)?

9. Was the pregnancy conceived naturally?

continues

Health History (continued)

Labor and Delivery	1. How many weeks did you carry the baby before delivering?
	2. Was the labor spontaneous or induced?
	3. How many hours was the labor?
	4. Was the baby delivered vaginally or by cesarean? If by cesarean, why?
	5. Was any analgesia or anesthetic used?
	6. Did you hold your baby immediately after delivery? (This question will provide information about the neonate's condition at delivery.)
	7. Immediately following delivery, what was the baby's color?
	8. What were the baby's Apgar scores at 1 and 5 minutes? (See later section on Apgar Scoring in this chapter.)
	9. What were the birth weight and length of the baby?
	10. Was the baby's father at the birth with you?
	11. Where was the baby born (home, hospital, automobile, or other location)?
Postnatal	1. Did you and your baby go home together? (If answered no, inquire as to the reason for separate discharges.)
	2. If hospital delivery, how long was the hospitalization for you and the baby?
	3. Did the baby have any breathing or feeding problems during the first week?
	4. To your knowledge, did your baby receive any medications during the first week?
	5. How would you describe the baby's color at 1 week? (For light-skinned babies, ask if the skin was pale, pale pink, blue, or yellow. For the dark-skinned baby, inquire about the color of the sclera, oral mucosa, and nailbeds.)
	6. Was the baby circumcised?
	7. Did you start breast- or bottle-feeding your baby?
	8. Were there any problems with your choice of feeding?
	9. Did you or the baby have a fever after delivery?
	10. How did you feel 1 to 2 weeks after delivery?
	11. Did you have anyone to help you take care of the baby in the first few weeks after delivery?
Medical History	Inquire about the circumstances and outcomes of any hospitalizations or emergency department visits. Keep in mind that some children's caregivers may use the emergency department for episodic health care and may not have a primary care provider.
Injuries and Accidents	Determine if the child has a pattern of frequent injuries or accidents. Repeat trauma may indicate abuse.
Childhood Illnesses	Document past and current exposure to measles, mumps, rubella, pertussis, chickenpox, and respiratory syncytial virus (RSV).

continues

Immunizations

Immunizations provide protection against many contagious diseases of childhood. Maternal antibodies pass through the placenta and breast milk, offering the baby limited protection from disease. Table 24-1 lists a schedule of immunizations recommended by the Advisory Committee on Immunization Practice for children aged 0–6 years. Table 24-2 shows the immunization schedule for children aged 7–18 years (CDC, 2008). Many health care providers follow the immunization schedule as a guide for well-child check-ups. A record of immunizations is often important for school admission and to avoid repeat vaccinations. Many children fall behind on their immunization schedule, while immigrants to the United States may not have received some of the recommended immunizations. See Table 24-3, which addresses immunization schedules for children and adolescents who start late or who are more than 1 month behind.

FAMILY HEALTH HISTORY

See Family Health History in Chapter 3. In addition, be sure to also ask about a family history of sudden infant death syndrome (SIDS), attention deficit hyperactivity disorder (ADHD), congenital disorders or defects, and mental retardation.

SOCIAL HISTORY

Work Environment

Day care facilities and schools are the child's equivalent of a work environment. Inquire about the number of hours the child attends a day care facility or school per week. Inquire about the child's academic performance. In addition, ask if the child is home alone before or after school.

Home Environment

Ask about potential exposure to lead in chipping paint, because lead is harmful to the developing brain and nervous system of fetuses and young children. This group is four to five times more likely to absorb lead by ingestion than are older children (Gerchufsky, 1994).

The next series of questions pertains to gun safety. Use the acronym "GUNS" to remember at-risk behaviors.

G = Are there *Guns* in your home?

U = Are there *Users* of alcohol or other drugs in the home?

N = Do you feel a *Need* to protect yourself?

S = Do any of these *Situations* apply to you?

Child's Personal Habits

1. Determine what activities the child enjoys.

2. Ask how the child copes with stress and if a security object (blanket, stuffed toy) helps calm the child.

3. Determine if the child is prone to temper tantrums and what type of discipline is used.

Domestic and Intimate Partner Violence

Adolescents are not immune to intimate partner violence (IPV). Specific questions about IPV can be asked during the Home Environment section.

1. Do you have a boyfriend or girlfriend?

2. What happens when one disagrees with the other?

3. Have you ever been hurt by someone you know?

continues

HEALTH MAINTENANCE ACTIVITIES

Sleep

1. Determine if the child takes naps and if the child shares a bedroom, because children's different sleep habits may lead to interrupted sleep.

2. Ask whether the child experiences night terrors.

3. Ask whether the child sleepwalks.

Diet

Questions concerning diet need to be tailored to the patient's developmental level. See Chapter 7 for additional information.

Safety

Childproofing the environment, especially for young children, is an essential practice. Incorporate these questions into your interview.

1. Tell me how you have childproofed your home.

2. Do you have gates on the top and bottom of the stairs?

3. Are the slats on the crib less than 2⅜ inches apart?

4. Have you taken the crib mobile down and taken out the bumper pads (applies to infants who are trying to pull themselves up)?

5. Is all sleepwear flame retardant?

6. Is the hot water thermostat turned down to 120° Fahrenheit?

7. Have you installed potty locks to keep the toilet lid down?

8. Do you keep curtain and blind strings out of reach?

9. Have you placed all sharp items such as razors and knives out of reach of the child?

10. Do you monitor your child's bath? Do you always drain the water in the tub after getting out?

11. Do you have lead paint in your living quarters?

12. Have you placed cushioned covering on the tub's water faucet and drain lever?

13. Do you use a nonskid bath mat in the tub?

14. Are there outlet covers on every outlet in the house?

15. When you are cooking, do you keep the pot or pan handles turned in?

16. Have you removed tablecloths off all tables?

17. Do you keep the phone cord out of reach?

18. Is the slack taken up on all electrical appliances and lamp cords?

19. If you have a raised hearth, have you covered it with bumpers, pads, or towels?

20. Are all of your plants out of reach?

21. Are your deck slats covered with a mesh net?

22. Are slip protectors under all rugs?

23. If you have a pool in the yard, is it fenced in or is a protective cover on the top? Is there a functional alarm system for the pool?

continues

24. Do you empty pails that contain liquid after using them?

25. Are medications, cosmetics, pesticides, gasoline, cleaning solutions, paint thinner, and all other poisonous materials out of the child's reach?

26. Do you have your local poison control center's telephone number next to each phone?

27. Do you have syrup of ipecac in the house? Do you know why it is used and its expiration date?

28. Do you have smoke detectors close to or in the child's bedroom and on each floor of the house?

29. Do you have a fire extinguisher on each floor?

30. Have you devised and practiced an escape route plan in case of fire?

31. Are you CPR trained?

32. What would you do in case of an emergency?

33. Where do you place your child's car seat—in the front or back seat, facing front or rear? Do you place your child in the car where an air bag is supplied? Do you need or use a locking clip?

34. Does your child use protective gear such as a helmet or knee or elbow pads if participating in an activity in which injuries may occur?

35. Do you keep plastic dry cleaner overwraps, latex balloons (unattended by a caregiver), plastic trash bags, and grocery bags out of the child's reach?

36. Do you have a carbon monoxide detector in the house?

37. Do you give your child nutritional supplements or herbal remedies? If so, name the type and amount given.

38. Do you have a dog? Is the dog child friendly? Do you keep the dog chained on a leash when other children are visiting your home?

LIFE ◎ 360°

Assessing Child Safety in the Home

Using the safety questions in the Health History, assess your home environment for its appropriateness for these age levels: 9-month-old, 18-month-old, 3-year-old, 6-year-old, 10-year-old, 14-year-old, 17-year-old. Bring a colleague to your house to perform the same activity. Compare your notes. Was something missed? Were any additional measures needed to ensure a child's safety?

NURSING**TIP**

$H_1E_2A_3D_4S_5$ Assessment

A valuable tool that is easily remembered during the adolescent's health history is the $H_1E_2A_3D_4S_5$ Assessment. This tool highlights vital areas of an adolescent's daily life that can impact physical and mental well-being. The letters in HEADS represent the first letter in the subject area that is to be asked, and the subscript represents the number of assessment areas that begin with this letter. The $H_1E_2A_3D_4S_5$ acronym stands for:

H_1	Home environment		Dentist
E_2	Education		Depression
	Exercise	S_5	Sleep
A_3	Alcohol		Safety
	Activities		Sexual identity and activity
	Attitudes about life		Stressors
D_4	Diet		Suicidal ideation
	Drugs		

TABLE 24-1 Recommended Immunization Schedule for Persons Aged 0 Through 6 Years — United States • 2009 *For those who fall behind or start late, see the catch-up schedule*

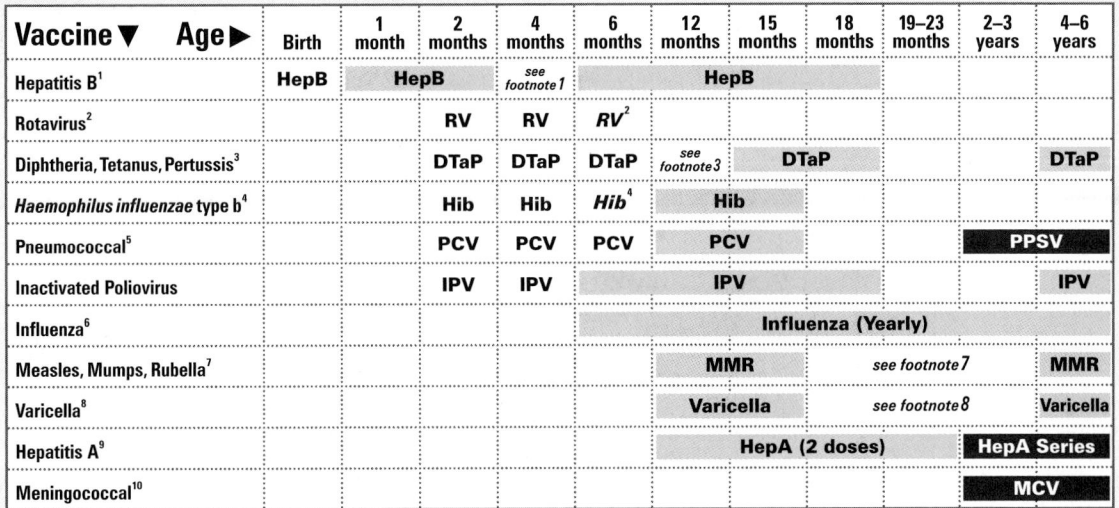

Vaccine ▼ Age ▶	Birth	1 month	2 months	4 months	6 months	12 months	15 months	18 months	19–23 months	2–3 years	4–6 years	
Hepatitis B[1]	HepB	HepB		see footnote 1		HepB						Range of recommended ages
Rotavirus[2]			RV	RV	RV[2]							
Diphtheria, Tetanus, Pertussis[3]			DTaP	DTaP	DTaP	see footnote 3	DTaP				DTaP	
Haemophilus influenzae type b[4]			Hib	Hib	Hib[4]	Hib						
Pneumococcal[5]			PCV	PCV	PCV	PCV				PPSV		Certain high-risk groups
Inactivated Poliovirus			IPV	IPV		IPV					IPV	
Influenza[6]						Influenza (Yearly)						
Measles, Mumps, Rubella[7]						MMR			see footnote 7		MMR	
Varicella[8]						Varicella			see footnote 8		Varicella	
Hepatitis A[9]						HepA (2 doses)				HepA Series		
Meningococcal[10]										MCV		

This schedule indicates the recommended ages for routine administration of currently licensed vaccines, as of December 1, 2008, for children aged 0 through 6 years. Any dose not administered at the recommended age should be administered at a subsequent visit, when indicated and feasible. Licensed combination vaccines may be used whenever any component of the combination is indicated and other components are not contraindicated and if approved by the Food and Drug Administration for that dose of the series. Providers should consult the relevant Advisory Committee on Immunization Practices statement for detailed recommendations, including high-risk conditions: http://www.cdc.gov/vaccines/pubs/acip-list.htm. Clinically significant adverse events that follow immunization should be reported to the Vaccine Adverse Event Reporting System (VAERS). Guidance about how to obtain and complete a VAERS form is available at http://www.vaers.hhs.gov or by telephone, 800-822-7967.

1. Hepatitis B vaccine (HepB). *(Minimum age: birth)*
   At birth:
   • Administer monovalent HepB to all newborns before hospital discharge.
   • If mother is hepatitis B surface antigen (HBsAg)-positive, administer HepB and 0.5 mL of hepatitis B immune globulin (HBIG) within 12 hours of birth.
   • If mother's HBsAg status is unknown, administer HepB within 12 hours of birth. Determine mother's HBsAg status as soon as possible and, if HBsAg-positive, administer HBIG (no later than age 1 week).
   After the birth dose:
   • The HepB series should be completed with either monovalent HepB or a combination vaccine containing HepB. The second dose should be administered at age 1 or 2 months. The final dose should be administered no earlier than age 24 weeks.
   • Infants born to HBsAg-positive mothers should be tested for HBsAg and antibody to HBsAg (anti-HBs) after completion of at least 3 doses of the HepB series, at age 9 through 18 months (generally at the next well-child visit).
   4-month dose:
   • Administration of 4 doses of HepB to infants is permissible when combination vaccines containing HepB are administered after the birth dose.

2. Rotavirus vaccine (RV). *(Minimum age: 6 weeks)*
   • Administer the first dose at age 6 through 14 weeks (maximum age: 14 weeks 6 days). Vaccination should not be initiated for infants aged 15 weeks or older (i.e., 15 weeks 0 days or older).
   • Administer the final dose in the series by age 8 months 0 days.
   • If Rotarix® is administered at ages 2 and 4 months, a dose at 6 months is not indicated.

3. Diphtheria and tetanus toxoids and acellular pertussis vaccine (DTaP). *(Minimum age: 6 weeks)*
   • The fourth dose may be administered as early as age 12 months, provided at least 6 months have elapsed since the third dose.
   • Administer the final dose in the series at age 4 through 6 years.

4. Haemophilus influenzae type b conjugate vaccine (Hib). *(Minimum age: 6 weeks)*
   • If PRP-OMP (PedvaxHIB® or Comvax® [HepB-Hib]) is administered at ages 2 and 4 months, a dose at age 6 months is not indicated.
   • TriHiBit® (DTaP/Hib) should not be used for doses at ages 2, 4, or 6 months but can be used as the final dose in children aged 12 months or older.

5. Pneumococcal vaccine. *(Minimum age: 6 weeks for pneumococcal conjugate vaccine [PCV]; 2 years for pneumococcal polysaccharide vaccine [PPSV])*
   • PCV is recommended for all children aged younger than 5 years. Administer 1 dose of PCV to all healthy children aged 24 through 59 months who are not completely vaccinated for their age.

   • Administer PPSV to children aged 2 years or older with certain underlying medical conditions (see *MMWR* 2000;49[No. RR-9]), including a cochlear implant.

6. Influenza vaccine. *(Minimum age: 6 months for trivalent inactivated influenza vaccine [TIV]; 2 years for live, attenuated influenza vaccine [LAIV])*
   • Administer annually to children aged 6 months through 18 years.
   • For healthy nonpregnant persons (i.e., those who do not have underlying medical conditions that predispose them to influenza complications) aged 2 through 49 years, either LAIV or TIV may be used.
   • Children receiving TIV should receive 0.25 mL if aged 6 through 35 months or 0.5 mL if aged 3 years or older.
   • Administer 2 doses (separated by at least 4 weeks) to children aged younger than 9 years who are receiving influenza vaccine for the first time or who were vaccinated for the first time during the previous influenza season but only received 1 dose.

7. Measles, mumps, and rubella vaccine (MMR). *(Minimum age: 12 months)*
   • Administer the second dose at age 4 through 6 years. However, the second dose may be administered before age 4, provided at least 28 days have elapsed since the first dose.

8. Varicella vaccine. *(Minimum age: 12 months)*
   • Administer the second dose at age 4 through 6 years. However, the second dose may be administered before age 4, provided at least 3 months have elapsed since the first dose.
   • For children aged 12 months through 12 years the minimum interval between doses is 3 months. However, if the second dose was administered at least 28 days after the first dose, it can be accepted as valid.

9. Hepatitis A vaccine (HepA). *(Minimum age: 12 months)*
   • Administer to all children aged 1 year (i.e., aged 12 through 23 months). Administer 2 doses at least 6 months apart.
   • Children not fully vaccinated by age 2 years can be vaccinated at subsequent visits.
   • HepA also is recommended for children older than 1 year who live in areas where vaccination programs target older children or who are at increased risk of infection. See *MMWR* 2006;55(No. RR-7).

10. Meningococcal vaccine. *(Minimum age: 2 years for meningococcal conjugate vaccine [MCV] and for meningococcal polysaccharide vaccine [MPSV])*
   • Administer MCV to children aged 2 through 10 years with terminal complement component deficiency, anatomic or functional asplenia, and certain other high-risk groups. See *MMWR* 2005;54(No. RR-7).
   • Persons who received MPSV 3 or more years previously and who remain at increased risk for meningococcal disease should be revaccinated with MCV.

The Recommended Immunization Schedules for Persons Aged 0 Through 18 Years are approved by the Advisory Committee on Immunization Practices (www.cdc.gov/vaccines/recs/acip), the American Academy of Pediatrics (http://www.aap.org), and the American Academy of Family Physicians (http://www.aafp.org).

DEPARTMENT OF HEALTH AND HUMAN SERVICES • CENTERS FOR DISEASE CONTROL AND PREVENTION

TABLE 24-2 Recommended Immunization Schedule for Persons Aged 7 Through 18 Years — United States • 2009 *For those who fall behind or start late, see the schedule below and the catch-up schedule*

Vaccine ▼ Age ▶	7–10 years	11–12 years	13–18 years
Tetanus, Diphtheria, Pertussis[1]	see footnote 1	Tdap	Tdap
Human Papillomavirus[2]	see footnote 2	HPV (3 doses)	HPV Series
Meningococcal[3]	MCV	MCV	MCV
Influenza[4]	Influenza (Yearly)		
Pneumococcal[5]	PPSV		
Hepatitis A[6]	HepA Series		
Hepatitis B[7]	HepB Series		
Inactivated Poliovirus[8]	IPV Series		
Measles, Mumps, Rubella[9]	MMR Series		
Varicella[10]	Varicella Series		

Range of recommended ages

Catch-up immunization

Certain high-risk groups

This schedule indicates the recommended ages for routine administration of currently licensed vaccines, as of December 1, 2008, for children aged 7 through 18 years. Any dose not administered at the recommended age should be administered at a subsequent visit, when indicated and feasible. Licensed combination vaccines may be used whenever any component of the combination is indicated and other components are not contraindicated and if approved by the Food and Drug Administration for that dose of the series. Providers should consult the relevant Advisory Committee on Immunization Practices statement for detailed recommendations, including high-risk conditions: http://www.cdc.gov/vaccines/pubs/acip-list.htm. Clinically significant adverse events that follow immunization should be reported to the Vaccine Adverse Event Reporting System (VAERS). Guidance about how to obtain and complete a VAERS form is available at http://www.vaers.hhs.gov or by telephone, 800-822-7967.

1. Tetanus and diphtheria toxoids and acellular pertussis vaccine (Tdap). *(Minimum age: 10 years for BOOSTRIX® and 11 years for ADACEL®)*
- Administer at age 11 or 12 years for those who have completed the recommended childhood DTP/DTaP vaccination series and have not received a tetanus and diphtheria toxoid (Td) booster dose.
- Persons aged 13 through 18 years who have not received Tdap should receive a dose.
- A 5-year interval from the last Td dose is encouraged when Tdap is used as a booster dose; however, a shorter interval may be used if pertussis immunity is needed.

2. Human papillomavirus vaccine (HPV). *(Minimum age: 9 years)*
- Administer the first dose to females at age 11 or 12 years.
- Administer the second dose 2 months after the first dose and the third dose 6 months after the first dose (at least 24 weeks after the first dose).
- Administer the series to females at age 13 through 18 years if not previously vaccinated.

3. Meningococcal conjugate vaccine (MCV).
- Administer at age 11 or 12 years, or at age 13 through 18 years if not previously vaccinated.
- Administer to previously unvaccinated college freshmen living in a dormitory.
- MCV is recommended for children aged 2 through 10 years with terminal complement component deficiency, anatomic or functional asplenia, and certain other groups at high risk. See *MMWR* 2005;54(No. RR-7).
- Persons who received MPSV 5 or more years previously and remain at increased risk for meningococcal disease should be revaccinated with MCV.

4. Influenza vaccine.
- Administer annually to children aged 6 months through 18 years.
- For healthy nonpregnant persons (i.e., those who do not have underlying medical conditions that predispose them to influenza complications) aged 2 through 49 years, either LAIV or TIV may be used.
- Administer 2 doses (separated by at least 4 weeks) to children aged younger than 9 years who are receiving influenza vaccine for the first time or who were vaccinated for the first time during the previous influenza season but only received 1 dose.

5. Pneumococcal polysaccharide vaccine (PPSV).
- Administer to children with certain underlying medical conditions (see *MMWR* 1997;46[No. RR-8]), including a cochlear implant. A single revaccination should be administered to children with functional or anatomic asplenia or other immunocompromising condition after 5 years.

6. Hepatitis A vaccine (HepA).
- Administer 2 doses at least 6 months apart.
- HepA is recommended for children older than 1 year who live in areas where vaccination programs target older children or who are at increased risk of infection. See *MMWR* 2006;55(No. RR-7).

7. Hepatitis B vaccine (HepB).
- Administer the 3-dose series to those not previously vaccinated.
- A 2-dose series (separated by at least 4 months) of adult formulation Recombivax HB® is licensed for children aged 11 through 15 years.

8. Inactivated poliovirus vaccine (IPV).
- For children who received an all-IPV or all-oral poliovirus (OPV) series, a fourth dose is not necessary if the third dose was administered at age 4 years or older.
- If both OPV and IPV were administered as part of a series, a total of 4 doses should be administered, regardless of the child's current age.

9. Measles, mumps, and rubella vaccine (MMR).
- If not previously vaccinated, administer 2 doses or the second dose for those who have received only 1 dose, with at least 28 days between doses.

10. Varicella vaccine.
- For persons aged 7 through 18 years without evidence of immunity (see *MMWR* 2007;56[No. RR-4]), administer 2 doses if not previously vaccinated or the second dose if they have received only 1 dose.
- For persons aged 7 through 12 years, the minimum interval between doses is 3 months. However, if the second dose was administered at least 28 days after the first dose, it can be accepted as valid.
- For persons aged 13 years and older, the minimum interval between doses is 28 days.

The Recommended Immunization Schedules for Persons Aged 0 Through 18 Years are approved by the Advisory Committee on Immunization Practices (www.cdc.gov/vaccines/recs/acip), the American Academy of Pediatrics (http://www.aap.org), and the American Academy of Family Physicians (http://www.aafp.org).
DEPARTMENT OF HEALTH AND HUMAN SERVICES • CENTERS FOR DISEASE CONTROL AND PREVENTION

TABLE 24-3 Catch-up Immunization Schedule for Persons Aged 4 Months Through 18 Years Who Start Late or Who Are More Than 1 Month Behind — United States • 2009

The table below provides catch-up schedules and minimum intervals between doses for children whose vaccinations have been delayed. A vaccine series does not need to be restarted, regardless of the time that has elapsed between doses. Use the section appropriate for the child's age.

CATCH-UP SCHEDULE FOR PERSONS AGED 4 MONTHS THROUGH 6 YEARS

Vaccine	Minimum Age for Dose 1	Minimum Interval Between Doses			
		Dose 1 to Dose 2	Dose 2 to Dose 3	Dose 3 to Dose 4	Dose 4 to Dose 5
Hepatitis B[1]	Birth	4 weeks	8 weeks (and at least 16 weeks after first dose)		
Rotavirus[2]	6 wks	4 weeks	4 weeks[2]		
Diphtheria, Tetanus, Pertussis[3]	6 wks	4 weeks	4 weeks	6 months	6 months[3]
Haemophilus influenzae type b[4]	6 wks	4 weeks if first dose administered at younger than age 12 months 8 weeks (as final dose) if first dose administered at age 12-14 months No further doses needed if first dose administered at age 15 months or older	4 weeks[4] if current age is younger than 12 months 8 weeks (as final dose)[4] if current age is 12 months or older and second dose administered at younger than age 15 months No further doses needed if previous dose administered at age 15 months or older	8 weeks (as final dose) This dose only necessary for children aged 12 months through 59 months who received 3 doses before age 12 months	
Pneumococcal[5]	6 wks	4 weeks if first dose administered at younger than age 12 months 8 weeks (as final dose for healthy children) if first dose administered at age 12 months or older or current age 24 through 59 months No further doses needed for healthy children if first dose administered at age 24 months or older	4 weeks if current age is younger than 12 months 8 weeks (as final dose for healthy children) if current age is 12 months or older No further doses needed for healthy children if previous dose administered at age 24 months or older	8 weeks (as final dose) This dose only necessary for children aged 12 months through 59 months who received 3 doses before age 12 months or for high-risk children who received 3 doses at any age	
Inactivated Poliovirus[6]	6 wks	4 weeks	4 weeks	4 weeks[6]	
Measles, Mumps, Rubella[7]	12 mos	4 weeks			
Varicella[8]	12 mos	3 months			
Hepatitis A[9]	12 mos	6 months			

CATCH-UP SCHEDULE FOR PERSONS AGED 7 THROUGH 18 YEARS

Vaccine	Minimum Age for Dose 1	Dose 1 to Dose 2	Dose 2 to Dose 3	Dose 3 to Dose 4	Dose 4 to Dose 5
Tetanus, Diphtheria/Tetanus, Diphtheria, Pertussis[10]	7 yrs[10]	4 weeks	4 weeks if first dose administered at younger than age 12 months 6 months if first dose administered at age 12 months or older	6 months if first dose administered at younger than age 12 months	
Human Papillomavirus[11]	9 yrs	Routine dosing intervals are recommended[11]			
Hepatitis A[9]	12 mos	6 months			
Hepatitis B[1]	Birth	4 weeks	8 weeks (and at least 16 weeks after first dose)		
Inactivated Poliovirus[6]	6 wks	4 weeks	4 weeks	4 weeks[6]	
Measles, Mumps, Rubella[7]	12 mos	4 weeks			
Varicella[8]	12 mos	3 months if the person is younger than age 13 years 4 weeks if the person is aged 13 years or older			

1. Hepatitis B vaccine (HepB).
- Administer the 3-dose series to those not previously vaccinated.
- A 2-dose series (separated by at least 4 months) of adult formulation Recombivax HB® is licensed for children aged 11 through 15 years.

2. Rotavirus vaccine (RV).
- The maximum age for the first dose is 14 weeks 6 days. Vaccination should not be initiated for infants aged 15 weeks or older (i.e., 15 weeks 0 days or older).
- Administer the final dose in the series by age 8 months 0 days.
- If Rotarix® was administered for the first and second doses, a third dose is not indicated.

3. Diphtheria and tetanus toxoids and acellular pertussis vaccine (DTaP).
- The fifth dose is not necessary if the fourth dose was administered at age 4 years or older.

4. *Haemophilus influenzae* type b conjugate vaccine (Hib).
- Hib vaccine is not generally recommended for persons aged 5 years or older. No efficacy data are available on which to base a recommendation concerning use of Hib vaccine for older children and adults. However, studies suggest good immunogenicity in persons who have sickle cell disease, leukemia, or HIV infection, or who have had a splenectomy; administering 1 dose of Hib vaccine to these persons is not contraindicated.
- If the first 2 doses were PRP-OMP (PedvaxHIB® or Comvax®), and administered at age 11 months or younger, the third (and final) dose should be administered at age 12 through 15 months and at least 8 weeks after the second dose.
- If the first dose was administered at age 7 through 11 months, administer 2 doses separated by 4 weeks and a final dose at age 12 through 15 months.

5. Pneumococcal vaccine.
- Administer 1 dose of pneumococcal conjugate vaccine (PCV) to all healthy children aged 24 through 59 months who have not received at least 1 dose of PCV on or after age 12 months.
- For children aged 24 through 59 months with underlying medical conditions, administer 1 dose of PCV if 3 doses were received previously or administer 2 doses of PCV at least 8 weeks apart if fewer than 3 doses were received previously.
- Administer pneumococcal polysaccharide vaccine (PPSV) to children aged 2 years or older with certain underlying medical conditions (see *MMWR* 2000;49[No. RR-9]), including a cochlear implant, at least 8 weeks after the last dose of PCV.

6. Inactivated poliovirus vaccine (IPV).
- For children who received an all-IPV or all-oral poliovirus (OPV) series, a fourth dose is not necessary if the third dose was administered at age 4 years or older.
- If both OPV and IPV were administered as part of a series, a total of 4 doses should be administered, regardless of the child's current age.

7. Measles, mumps, and rubella vaccine (MMR).
- Administer the second dose at age 4 through 6 years. However, the second dose may be administered before age 4, provided at least 28 days have elapsed since the first dose.
- If not previously vaccinated, administer 2 doses with at least 28 days between doses.

8. Varicella vaccine.
- Administer the second dose at age 4 through 6 years. However, the second dose may be administered before age 4, provided at least 3 months have elapsed since the first dose.
- For persons aged 12 months through 12 years, the minimum interval between doses is 3 months. However, if the second dose was administered at least 28 days after the first dose, it can be accepted as valid.
- For persons aged 13 years and older, the minimum interval between doses is 28 days.

9. Hepatitis A vaccine (HepA).
- HepA is recommended for children older than 1 year who live in areas where vaccination programs target older children or who are at increased risk of infection. See *MMWR* 2006;55(No. RR-7).

10. Tetanus and diphtheria toxoids vaccine (Td) and tetanus and diphtheria toxoids and acellular pertussis vaccine (Tdap).
- Doses of DTaP are counted as part of the Td/Tdap series.
- Tdap should be substituted for a single dose of Td in the catch-up series or as a booster for children aged 10 through 18 years; use Td for other doses.

11. Human papillomavirus vaccine (HPV).
- Administer the series to females at age 13 through 18 years if not previously vaccinated.
- Use recommended routine dosing intervals for series catch-up (i.e., the second and third doses should be administered at 2 and 6 months after the first dose). However, the minimum interval between the first and second doses is 4 weeks. The minimum interval between the second and third doses is 12 weeks, and the third dose should be given at least 24 weeks after the first dose.

Information about reporting reactions after immunization is available online at **http://www.vaers.hhs.gov** or by telephone, **800-822-7967**. Suspected cases of vaccine-preventable diseases should be reported to the state or local health department. Additional information, including precautions and contraindications for immunization, is available from the National Center for Immunization and Respiratory Diseases at **http://www.cdc.gov/vaccines** or telephone, **800-CDC-INFO (800-232-4636)**.

DEPARTMENT OF HEALTH AND HUMAN SERVICES • CENTERS FOR DISEASE CONTROL AND PREVENTION

EQUIPMENT

- Equipment listed in Chapters 10–22
- Scale (infant or stand-up)
- Appropriate-sized blood pressure cuff
- Snellen E and Tumbling E charts
- Allen cards
- Color vision charts
- Ophthalmoscope
- Otoscope, speculum (2.5 to 4 mm), pneumatic attachment
- Pediatric stethoscope
- Growth chart
- Peanut butter or chocolate
- Small bell
- Brightly colored object
- Denver II materials
- Clean gloves
- Disposable centimeter tape measure

DEVELOPMENTAL ASSESSMENT

A commonly used tool for assessing neuromuscular development of the child from birth through 6 years of age is the Denver II (see Figure 24-5). The test is composed of four sections: personal-social, fine motor-adaptive, language, and gross motor. There are a total of 125 items described on the test. Some items can be accomplished easily by observing the child without commands from the observer. For instance, the child may be smiling spontaneously, saying words other than "mama" or "dada," or sitting with the head held steady. Certain items can be given an automatic pass mark if the caregiver indicates that the child is able to accomplish the corresponding item, such as drinking from a cup, washing and drying hands, or dressing without help.

Before administering the test, determine the child's chronological age and draw a straight line through the four sections intersecting the age intervals on the top and bottom of the sheet. This line indicates which items are to be tested for the child's chronological age. Begin testing by assessing the item that is three items to the left of the age line. Documentation is reflected by using a "P" for pass, "F" for fail, "R" for refuses, and "NO" for no opportunity. Give up to three trials before documenting the particular item's score on the Denver II. At the end, complete the five Test Behavior questions. A normal test consists of no delays and a maximum of one caution. A caution is failure of a patient to perform an item that has been achieved by 75% to 90% of children the same age. A delay is a failure of any item to the left of the age line. A suspect test is one with one or more delays or two or more cautions; in these instances, retest the child in 1 to 2 weeks.

Keep in mind that current illness, lack of sleep, fear and anxiety, deafness, or blindness can affect a child's performance. If these or other logical rationale can explain a child's failure to successfully complete a series of Denver II items during a session, readminister the test in 1 month, providing resolution of the preexisting condition is accomplished, where appropriate. If the child does in fact have a developmental disability, early detection can lead to appropriate intervention and assistance.

PHYSICAL EXAMINATION

Many assessment techniques for the child are similar to those for the adult. Refer to the specific system chapters for detailed explanations of assessment techniques covered in those chapters.

Techniques for approaching the pediatric patient vary from one age group to the next. A basic principle during any physical assessment is building a trusting relationship; this can be done in a variety of ways. First, always explain what will be done prior to each portion of the assessment and answer questions honestly. Second, praise the patient for positive behaviors, for example, cooperating during assessment of the middle ear. Portraying a caring attitude will greatly influence both the patient's and the caregiver's sense of trust. Show respect for the patient as an individual and allow expression of feelings (whimpering, crying).

VITAL SIGNS

General Approach

1. The act of measuring vital signs is often disturbing to a young patient. Past experiences influence the degree of cooperation you will encounter.

2. Vital signs may be obtained at the beginning of the assessment or during the assessment of a certain system. Blood pressure and rectal temperature measurements are more threatening and should be performed toward the end of the assessment, preferably before using the otoscope.

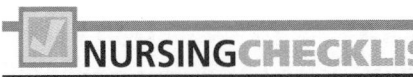

NURSINGCHECKLIST

General Approach to Pediatric Physical Assessment

1. Assess the patient in a warm, quiet room. To prevent hypothermia, always keep infants under the age of 6 months warm during the examination.
2. Use natural lighting, if available, during the assessment. Fluorescent lighting makes assessing varying degrees of cyanosis and jaundice difficult.
3. To help reduce anxiety and uncooperativeness (especially when assessing young children), have a familiar caregiver present during the assessment.
4. Talk to the child in a soothing voice; even an infant who cannot understand your words will take comfort in a calm and supportive approach.
5. Explain all procedures and allow older infants, toddlers, preschoolers, and younger school-age patients to touch or manipulate medical equipment (see Figure 24-6).
6. To promote the child's feeling of security, allow the infant who cannot sit up and the younger child to sit on the caregiver's lap for as much of the examination as possible.
7. Until the infant or toddler is comfortable, maintain eye contact with the caregiver while the assessment is taking place. Maintaining eye contact with the child who experiences anxiety in the presence of strangers can interfere with completing the examination. Maintain eye contact with caregiver if other means of alleviating the fears are not successful.
8. Interview the older school-age child or adolescent separately, without the caregiver. Talking to the individual without the caregiver present may yield important information not gained during a group interview (e.g., that the patient is using drugs).
9. Respect the patient's modesty.
10. Warm your equipment (e.g., stethoscope).
11. Avoid making abrupt movements because these may startle a child.
12. If the child is sleeping, take advantage of the situation by performing simple procedures (length, head circumference) and system assessments that require a quiet room (such as the cardiac and respiratory assessments) first.
13. Perform all invasive or uncomfortable procedures (ear inspection, hip palpation) last because they may cause discomfort, crying, fear, and increased heart rate.
14. Always provide comfort measures following pain. It is especially helpful to allow the caregiver the opportunity to provide supportive measures. This shows the child that you are genuinely concerned about his or her feelings.
15. To prevent falls, always keep one hand on any infant who is placed on the examination table.
16. Prior to completing the examination, ask the caregiver and patient what questions they have.
17. Utilize Recommendations for Preventive Pediatric Health Care (see Table 24-4) as a reference for age-specific components of the pediatric health visit.

---

3. If the child is particularly anxious, it is best to integrate the assessment of vital signs into the overall assessment.

Temperature

You need to be proficient in measuring axillary, rectal, oral, and tympanic temperatures. A rectal temperature is not appropriate in all instances, for example, in the patient who presents with a history of diarrhea, or a patient who is immunocompromised. Accurate oral temperature is difficult to obtain in most toddlers and preschoolers. Axillary temperature, while quick and painless, is often less reliable than rectal or oral temperatures.

AXILLARY.

E 1. When taking axillary temperature, have the child sit or lie on the caregiver's lap to free your hands for other observations or to prepare for the next area of assessment.

2. Explain to the patient that this type of temperature measurement does not hurt. To pass time, ask the caregiver to read the child a story.

N/A/P See Chapter 9.

| **E** Examination | **N** Normal Findings | **A** Abnormal Findings | **P** Pathophysiology |

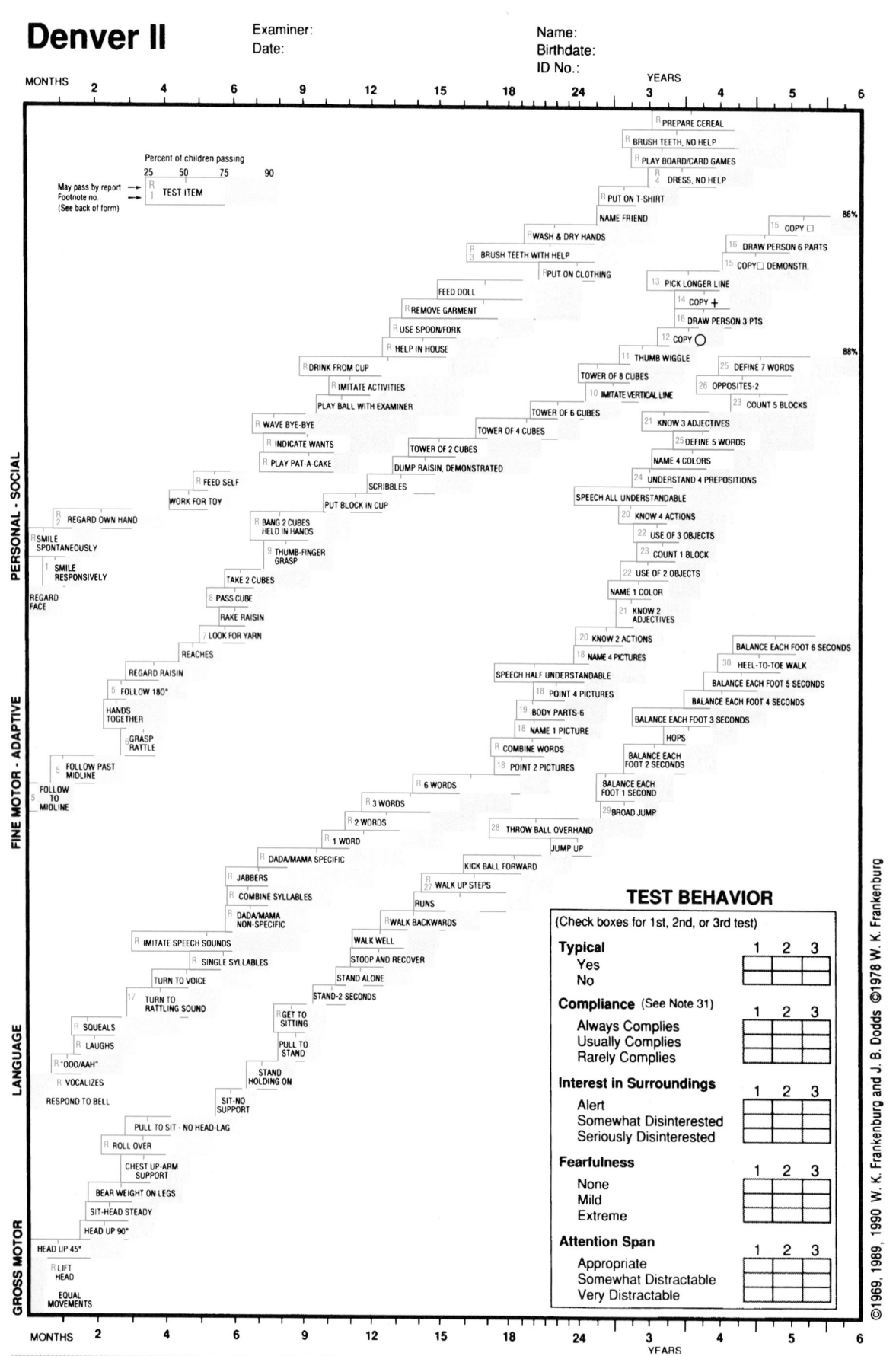

DIRECTIONS FOR ADMINISTRATION

1. Try to get child to smile by smiling, talking or waving. Do not touch him/her.
2. Child must stare at hand several seconds.
3. Parent may help guide toothbrush and put toothpaste on brush.
4. Child does not have to be able to tie shoes or button/zip in the back.
5. Move yarn slowly in an arc from one side to the other, about 8" above child's face.
6. Pass if child grasps rattle when it is touched to the backs or tips of fingers.
7. Pass if child tries to see where yarn went. Yarn should be dropped quickly from sight from tester's hand without arm movement.
8. Child must transfer cube from hand to hand without help of body, mouth, or table.
9. Pass if child picks up raisin with any part of thumb and finger.
10. Line can vary only 30 degrees or less from testers line.
11. Make a fist with thumb pointing upward and wiggle only the thumb. Pass if child imitates and does not move any fingers other than the thumb.

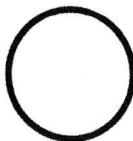   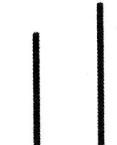   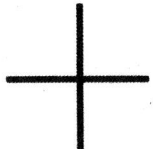   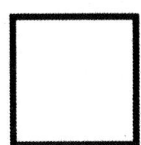

12. Pass any enclosed form. Fail continuous round motions
13. Which line is longer? (Not bigger.) Turn paper upside down and repeat. (pass 3 of 3 or 5 of 6)
14. Pass any lines crossing near midpoint.
15. Have child copy first. If failed, demonstrate

When giving items 12, 14, and 15, do not name the forms. Do not demonstrate 12 and 14.

16. When scoring, each pair (2 arms, 2 legs, etc.) counts as one part.
17. Place one cube in cup and shake gently near the child's ear, but out of sight. Repeat for other ear.
18. Point to picture and have child name it. (No credit is given for sounds only.)
    If less than 4 pictures are named correctly, have child point to picture as each is named by tester.

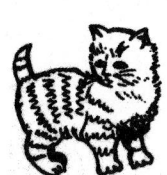   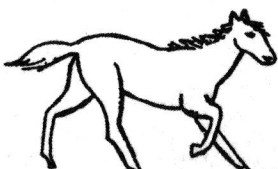   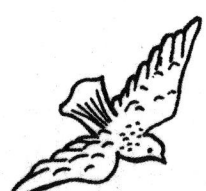   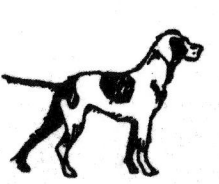   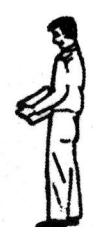

19. Using doll, tell child: Show me the nose, eyes, ears, mouth, hands, feet, tummy, hair. Pass 6 of 8.
20. Using pictures, ask child: Which one flies? . . . says meow? . . . talks? . . . barks? . . . gallops? Pass 2 of 5, 4 of 5.
21. Ask child: What do you do when you are cold? . . . tired? . . . hungry? Pass 2 of 3, 3 of 3.
22. Ask child: What do you do with a cup? What is a chair used for? What is a pencil used for?
    Action words must be included in answers.
23. Pass if child correctly placed <u>and</u> says how many blocks are on paper. (1, 5)
24. Tell child: Put block **on** table; **under** table; **in front of** me, **behind** me. Pass 4 of 4.
    (Do not help child by pointing, moving head or eyes.)
25. Ask child: What is a ball? . . . lake? . . . desk? . . . house? . . . banana? . . . curtain? . . . fence? . . . ceiling? Pass if defined in terms of use, shape, what it is made of, or general category (such as banana is fruit, not just yellow). Pass 5 of 8, 7 of 8.
26. Ask child: If a horse is big, a mouse is __? If fire is hot, ice is __? If the sun shines during the day, the moon shines during the __? Pass 2 of 3.
27. Child may use wall or rail only, not person. May not crawl.
28. Child must throw ball overhand 3 feet to within arm's reach of tester.
29. Child must perform standing broad jump over width of test sheet (8½ inches).
30. Tell child to walk forward, ⚇⚇⚇⚇➤ heel within 1 inch of toe. Tester may demonstrate.
    Child must walk 4 consecutive steps.

FIGURE 24-5 Denver II *continued*

TABLE 24-4 Recommendations for Preventive Pediatric Health Care

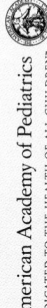

American Academy of Pediatrics
DEDICATED TO THE HEALTH OF ALL CHILDREN™

Bright Futures
Prevention and health promotion for infants, children, adolescents, and their families™

Each child and family is unique; therefore, these **Recommendations for Preventive Pediatric Health Care** are designed for the care of children who are receiving competent parenting, have no manifestations of any important health problems, and are growing and developing in satisfactory fashion. **Additional visits may become necessary** if circumstances suggest variations from normal.

Developmental, psychosocial, and chronic disease issues for children and adolescents may require frequent counseling and treatment visits separate from preventive care visits.

These guidelines represent a consensus by the American Academy of Pediatrics (AAP) and Bright Futures. The AAP continues to emphasize the great importance of **continuity of care** in comprehensive health supervision and the need to avoid **fragmentation of care.**

The recommendations in this statement do not indicate an exclusive course of treatment or standard of medical care. Variations, taking into account individual circumstances, may be appropriate.

Copyright © 2008 by the American Academy of Pediatrics.

No part of this statement may be reproduced in any form or by any means without prior written permission from the American Academy of Pediatrics except for one copy for personal use.

		INFANCY									EARLY CHILDHOOD							MIDDLE CHILDHOOD						ADOLESCENCE											
Age[a]	Prenatal[b]	Newborn[c]	3–5 d[d]	By 1 mo	2 mo	4 mo	6 mo	9 mo	12 m	15 mo	18 mo	24 mo	30 mo	3 y	4 y	5 y	6 y	7 y	8 y	9 y	10 y	11 y	12 y	13 y	14 y	15 y	16 y	17 y	18 y	19 y	20 y	21 y

HISTORY
Initial/interval

MEASUREMENTS
Length/height and weight
Head circumference
Weight for length
Body mass index
Blood pressure[e]

SENSORY SCREENING
Vision
Hearing

DEVELOPMENTAL/BEHAVIORAL ASSESSMENT
Developmental screening[f]
Autism screening[g]
Developmental surveillance[h]
Psychosocial/behavioral assessment
Alcohol and drug use assessment

PHYSICAL EXAMINATION[i]

PROCEDURES[j]
Newborn metabolic/hemoglobin screening[k]
Immunization[l]
Hematocrit or hemoglobin[m]
Lead screening[n]
Tuberculin test[o]
Dyslipidemia screening[p]
STI screening[q]
Cervical dysplasia screening[r]

ORAL HEALTH[s]

ANTICIPATORY GUIDANCE[w]

Footnotes:

a. If a child comes under care for the first time at any point on the schedule, or if any items are not accomplished at the suggested age, the schedule should be brought up to date at the earliest possible time.

b. A prenatal visit is recommended for parents who are at high risk, for first-time parents, and for those who request a conference. The prenatal visit should include anticipatory guidance, pertinent medical history, and a discussion of benefits of breastfeeding and planned method of feeding per AAP statement "The Prenatal Visit" (2001) [URL: http://aappolicy.aappublications.org/cgi/content/full/pediatrics;107/6/1456].

c. Every infant should have a newborn evaluation after birth, breastfeeding encouraged, and instruction and support offered.

d. Every infant should have an evaluation within 3 to 5 days of birth and within 48 to 72 hours after discharge from the hospital, to include evaluation for feeding and jaundice. Breastfeeding infants should receive formal breastfeeding evaluation, encouragement, and instruction as recommended in AAP statement "Breastfeeding and the Use of Human Milk" (2005) [URL: http://aappolicy.aappublications.org/cgi/content/full/pediatrics;115/2/496]. For newborns discharged in less than 48 hours after delivery, the infant must be examined within 48 hours of discharge per AAP statement "Hospital Stay for Healthy Term Newborns" (2004) [URL: http://aappolicy.aappublications.org/cgi/content/full/pediatrics;113/5/1434].

e. Blood pressure measurement in infants and children with specific risk conditions should be performed at visits before age 3 years.

f. If the patient is uncooperative, rescreen within 6 months per AAP statement "Eye Examination and Vision Screening in Infants, Children, and Young Adults" (1996) [URL: http://aappolicy.aappublications.org/cgi/content/full/pediatrics;98/1/153.pdf].

g. All newborns should be screened per AAP statement "Year 2000 Position Statement: Principles and Guidelines for Early Hearing Detection and Intervention Programs" (2000) [URL: http://aappolicy.aappublications.org/cgi/content/full/pediatrics;106/4/798]. Joint Committee on Infant Hearing. Year 2007 position statement: principles and guidelines for early hearing detection and intervention programs. Pediatrics. 2007;120:898–921.

h. AAP Council on Children With Disabilities, AAP Section on Developmental Behavioral Pediatrics, AAP Bright Futures Steering Committee, AAP Medical Home Initiatives for Children With Special Needs Project Advisory Committee. Identifying infants and young children with developmental disorders in the medical home: an algorithm for developmental surveillance and screening. Pediatrics. 2006;118:405–420 [URL: http://aappolicy.aappublications.org/cgi/content/full/pediatrics;118/1/405].

i. Gupta VB, Hyman SL, Johnson CP, et al. Identifying children with autism early? Pediatrics. 2007;119:152–153 [URL: http://pediatrics.aappublications.org/cgi/content/full/119/1/152].

j. At each visit, age-appropriate physical examination is essential, with infant totally unclothed, older child undressed and suitably draped.

k. These may be modified, depending on entry point into schedule and individual need.

l. Newborn metabolic and hemoglobin screening should be done according to state law. Results should be reviewed at visits and appropriate retesting or referral done as needed.

m. Schedules per the Committee on Infectious Diseases, published annually in the January issue of Pediatrics. Every visit should be an opportunity to update and complete a child's immunizations.

n. See AAP Pediatric Nutrition Handbook, 5th Edition (2003) for a discussion of universal and selective screening options. See also Recommendations to prevent and control iron deficiency in the United States. MMWR Recomm Rep. 1998;47(RR-3):1–36.

o. For children at risk of lead exposure, consult the AAP statement "Lead Exposure in Children: Prevention, Detection, and Management" (2005) [URL: http://aappolicy.aappublications.org/cgi/content/full/pediatrics;116/4/1036]. Additionally, screening should be done in accordance with state law where applicable.

p. Perform risk assessments or screens as appropriate, based on universal screening requirements for patients with Medicaid or high prevalence areas.

q. Tuberculosis testing per recommendations of the Committee on Infectious Diseases, published in the current edition of Red Book: Report of the Committee on Infectious Diseases. Testing should be done on recognition of high-risk factors.

r. "Third Report of the National Cholesterol Education Program (NCEP) Expert Panel on Detection, Evaluation, and Treatment of High Blood Cholesterol in Adults (Adult Treatment Panel III) Final Report" (2002) [URL: http://circ.ahajournals.org/cgi/content/full/106/25/3143] and "The Expert Committee Recommendations on the Assessment, Prevention, and Treatment of Child and Adolescent Overweight and Obesity." Supplement to Pediatrics. In press.

s. All sexually active patients should be screened for sexually transmitted infections (STIs).

t. All sexually active girls should have screening for cervical dysplasia as part of a pelvic examination beginning within 3 years of onset of sexual activity or age 21 (whichever comes first).

u. Referral to dental home, if available, otherwise, administer oral health risk assessment. If the primary water source is deficient in fluoride, consider oral fluoride supplementation.

v. At the visits for 3 years and 6 years of age, it should be determined whether the patient has a dental home. If the patient does not have a dental home, a referral should be made to one. If the primary water source is deficient in fluoride, consider oral fluoride supplementation.

w. Refer to the specific guidance by age as listed in Bright Futures Guidelines. (Hagan JF, Shaw JS, Duncan PM, eds. Bright Futures: Guidelines for Health Supervision of Infants, Children, and Adolescents. 3rd ed. Elk Grove Village, IL: American Academy of Pediatrics; 2008.)

Key:
● = to be performed ★ = risk assessment to be performed, with appropriate action to follow, if positive ● = a range during which a service may be provided, with the symbol indicating the preferred age

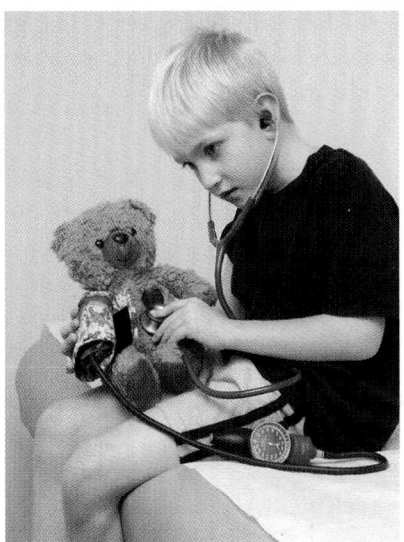

A. A preschooler listening to a teddy bear's chest will gain an understanding of the assessment that is to come.

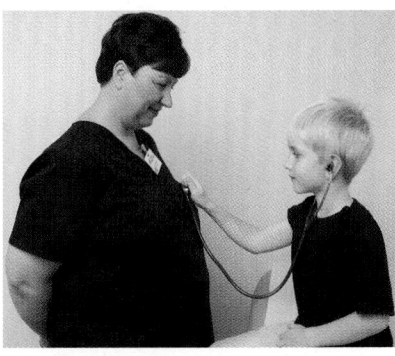

B. A child may also feel more comfortable trying his new skills on a caregiver or health care provider.

FIGURE 24-6 Allowing a child to touch and manipulate medical equipment may reduce fear and anxiety during the physical examination.

RECTAL

 1. Children dislike having rectal temperature taken, so your approach to explanation should be matter of fact: "I need to measure your temperature in your bottom. You need to hold very still while I do this. Your mommy (or other appropriate person) will be right here with you."

2. Place the patient in either a side-lying or a prone position on the caregiver's lap or place the patient on the back on the examination table and firmly grasp the feet with your nondominant hand.

3. After lubricating the stub-tipped thermometer, insert it gently into the patient's rectum: ½ inch for newborns, ¾ inch for infants, and 1 inch for preschoolers and older patients. Hold the thermometer firmly between your fingers to avoid accidentally inserting it too far.

N/A/P See Chapter 9.

Respiratory Rate

 1. Try to obtain the rate early in the assessment, when the patient is most cooperative and not crying.

2. If the patient is crying, the measurement will not be accurate and should be retaken.

3. Remember to observe the expansion of the abdomen in infants and toddlers.

N/A/P See Chapter 9.

PHYSICAL GROWTH

Weight

Use the same scale at each visit, if possible, to prevent variations in serial weight checks.

 1. If using an infant scale, cover it with a paper protector.

2. Balance or zero the scale.

3. Place infants supine and young toddlers seated on the scale (Figure 24-7). Always keep one hand on the child to prevent falls and lift your hand slightly when obtaining the actual weight reading.

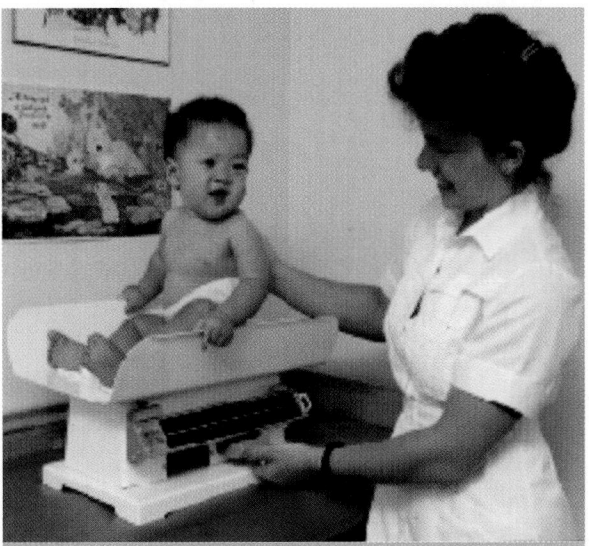

FIGURE 24-7 Measuring Weight in the Infant

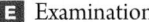 Examination   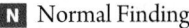 Normal Findings   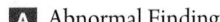 Abnormal Findings   **P** Pathophysiology

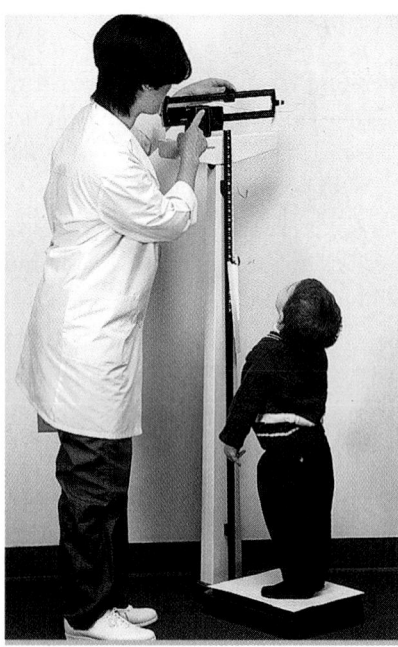

FIGURE 24-8 **Measuring Weight in the Preschooler**

4. Preschoolers and young school-age children can wear street clothes to be weighed (Figure 24-8). Have the older child undress, don a paper or cloth gown, and step on the standard platform scale.

5. Note and record weight.

N Refer to growth charts in Figures 24-1A and B and Figures 24-1E and F. Usually, neonates lose approximately 10% of birth weight by the third or fourth day after birth, then regain it by 2 weeks of age. This expected change in weight is called **physiological weight loss**, and it is due to a loss of extracellular fluid and **meconium**, a dark green, sticky, stool-like substance excreted from the rectum within the first 24 hours after birth.

A A newborn weight less than the 10th gestational age percentile is considered abnormal.

P A newborn whose growth has been retarded in utero is referred to as small for gestational age (SGA). Potential causes include alcohol, drug, or tobacco abuse by the mother, or certain genetic syndromes.

A A newborn weight greater than the 90th gestational age percentile is abnormal.

P A diabetic mother or a genetic predisposition may be responsible for producing a large for gestational age (LGA) newborn.

A A weight below the 5th or above the 95th percentiles warrants investigation, as does the patient who falls 2 standard deviations below his or her own established curve. Any such finding is abnormal.

P Possible causes include organic or nonorganic failure to thrive, congenital or cyanotic heart disease, cystic fibrosis (CF), fetal alcohol syndrome, and malabsorption diseases.

Length and Height

Recumbent length is measured for children less than 2 years old.

E 1. Position the measuring board flat on the examination table.

2. Place the child's head at the top of the board and the child's heels at the foot of the board, making sure the legs are fully extended (see Figure 24-9A).

3. Measure and record the length.

4. If a board is not available, place the child in a supine position and mark lines on the paper at the tip of the head and at the heel, making sure the legs are fully extended.

5. Measure between the lines and record.

Height for all other age groups can be measured in the same fashion as for an adult. Figure 24-9B shows a preschooler's height being measured.

N See growth charts in Figures 24-1A and B and Figures 24-1E and F.

A A height below the 5th or above the 95th percentile warrants investigation, as does the patient who falls 2 standard deviations below his or her own established curve. Any such finding is abnormal.

P Possible causes include organic or nonorganic failure to thrive, congenital or cyanotic heart disease, CF, fetal alcohol syndrome, and malabsorption diseases.

NURSING**TIP**

Obtaining Length and Height in Children under 2 Years of Age

1. If measuring a recumbent length, always plot on the birth-to-36-month chart.

2. If measuring height, plot the measurement on a birth-to-36-month growth chart and subtract 1 centimeter, or plot on a 2-to-18-year chart.

| **E** Examination | **N** Normal Findings | **A** Abnormal Findings | **P** Pathophysiology |

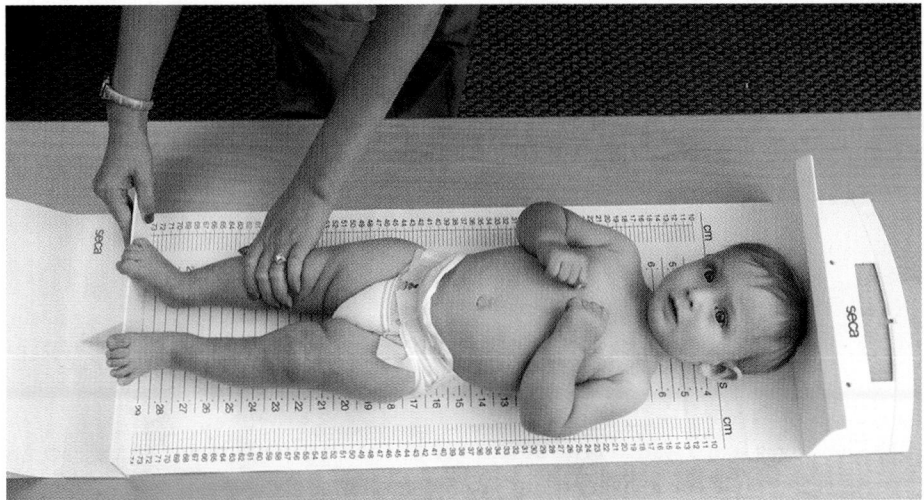

A. Recumbent Length in Infant

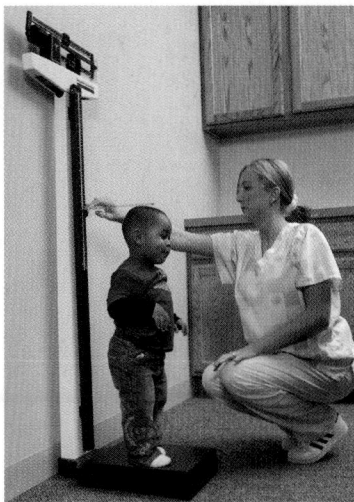

B. Height in Preschooler

FIGURE 24-9 **Measuring Length and Height in Children**

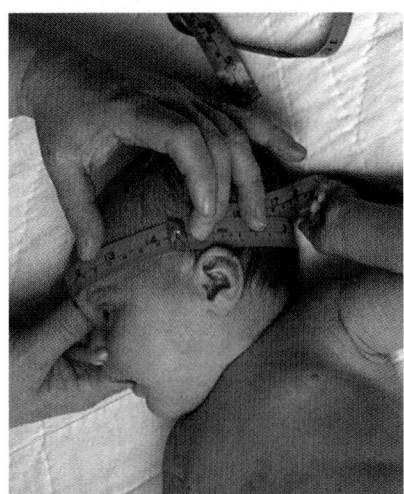

FIGURE 24-10 **Measuring Head Circumference**

Head Circumference

Head circumference is measured in all children less than 2 years of age or serially in patients with known or suspected hydrocephalus. Measuring head circumference is an invaluable tool in the infant with suspected cessation of brain growth.

E **1.** Place the patient in a sitting or supine position.

2. Using a tape measure, measure anteriorly from above the eyebrows and around posteriorly to the occipital protuberance (Figure 24-10).

N Refer to Figures 24-1C and D. Normal average head growth is 1 to 1.5 cm per month during the first year. Premature infants often have small head circumferences.

A **Microcephaly**, a condition characterized by a small brain with a resultant small head, is an abnormal finding.

P Microcephaly is a congenital finding associated with a mental deficit. Microcephaly can be caused by a variety of disorders including intrauterine infections, drug or alcohol ingestion (fetal alcohol syndrome) during pregnancy, and genetic defects.

A **Hydrocephalus** (enlarged head) is indicated when an infant's or young child's head circumference is above the 95th percentile and crosses over the patient's established percentile lines from one serial measurement to the next. Hydrocephalus is abnormal. Note if the eyes are looking downward ("setting sun" sign) and the sclera is visible above the iris.

P Hydrocephalus is characterized by an imbalance in cerebrospinal fluid (CSF) production and reabsorption. Hydrocephalus may result from embryological malformations of the nervous system. Congenital hydrocephalus can also be caused by syphilis, rubella, toxoplasmosis, or cytomegalovirus. Bacterial meningitis or tumors are acquired causes of hydrocephalus. The setting sun sign results from progressive enlargement of the lateral and third ventricles related to excessive accumulation of CSF.

Chest Circumference

Chest circumference is measured up to 1 year of age. It is a measurement that by itself provides little information but is compared to head circumference to evaluate the child's overall growth.

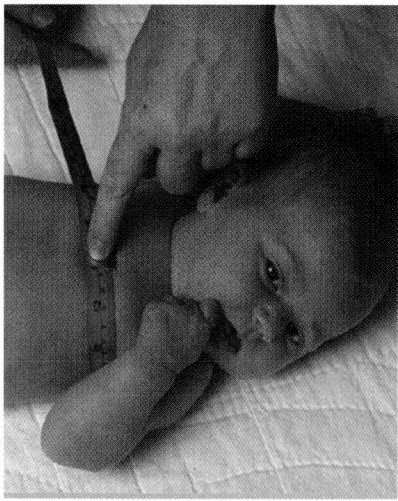

FIGURE 24-11 **Measuring Chest Circumference**

E 1. Stand in front of the supine patient.

2. Measure the chest circumference by placing the tape measure around the chest at the nipple line (Figure 24-11).

3. Measure during exhalation.

N From birth to about 1 year, the head circumference is greater than the chest circumference. After age 1, the chest circumference is greater than the head circumference.

A A measured chest circumference below normal limits is abnormal.

P A below-normal chest circumference for age can be attributed to prematurity.

Apgar Scoring

The **Apgar score** system provides a quick method to assess the need for newborn resuscitation in the delivery room. An Apgar score is given to a newborn at 1 and 5 minutes after birth. Perform steps 1 through 5 at 1 minute following birth; add the score in each category for the total. Repeat at 5 minutes following birth.

E 1. Auscultate the heart rate for 1 full minute.

2. Measure the degree of respiratory effort.

3. Evaluate muscle tone by attempting to straighten each extremity individually.

4. Evaluate the newborn's reflex irritability. Use a flicking motion of two fingers against the newborn's sole to rate reflex irritability.

5. Inspect the newborn's color.

N A score of 8 to 10 demonstrates that the newborn is in good condition. Table 24-5 outlines the scoring system for each of the five areas assessed.

A A moderately depressed newborn earns a score of 4 to 7. A score of 0 to 3 indicates that the newborn is severely depressed and needs immediate resuscitation. Either finding is abnormal.

P A low score can be the result of one or numerous problems. Prematurity, central nervous system depression, blood or meconium in the trachea, maternal history of drug abuse, certain drugs that are given to the mother in preparation for delivery and that cross over and cause fetal depression, congenital complete heart block, and congenital heart disease are some of the potential etiologies for a low Apgar score.

TABLE 24-5 Apgar Scoring

HEART RATE	RESPIRATORY RATE	TONE	REFLEX IRRITABILITY	COLOR
Absent = 0	Apnea = 0	Flaccid = 0	No response = 0	Cyanosis = 0
< 100 = 1	Slow, irregular rate = 1	Some degree of flexion = 1	Grimace = 1	Body pink, extremities acrocyanotic = 1
> 100 = 2	Crying vigorously = 2	Full flexion = 2	Crying = 2	Completely pink = 2

E Examination   **N** Normal Findings   **A** Abnormal Findings   **P** Pathophysiology

SKIN
Inspection
COLOR

E Observe the color of the body, especially at the tip of the nose, the external ear, the lips, the hands, and the feet. These areas are prominent locations for detecting cyanosis or jaundice.

N The skin of a newborn is reddish in color for the first 24 hours and then changes to varying shades of pale pink to pink to brown or black, depending on the child's race. It is normal for dark-skinned newborns to have a ruddy appearance and for light-skinned newborns to exhibit a bluish-purple color of the hands and feet while the rest of the body remains pink. This is called **acrocyanosis**. It may disappear with warming. **Mongolian spots**, deep blue pigmentation over the lumbar and sacral areas of the spine, over the buttocks, and, sometimes, over the upper back or shoulders in newborns of African, Latino, or Asian descent, are extremely common and not to be confused with ecchymosis or signs of child abuse.

A A blue hue is abnormal.

P Cyanosis in the newborn is often associated with a congenital heart defect secondary to abnormal mixing of arterial and venous blood. In the older child with unrepaired heart disease, cyanosis may be a sign of decreasing levels of oxygen saturation.

A A yellowing of the skin or sclera is abnormal.

P Physiological jaundice of the newborn occurs on the second or third day of life. This type of jaundice results from increased levels of serum bilirubin. The newborn's body is unable to remove the bilirubin, thus producing a yellow cast or hue to the skin of light-skinned infants and to the sclera of both light- and dark-skinned infants.

P Pathological jaundice of the newborn occurs within the first 24 hours of life. Possible causes of pathological jaundice include Rh/ABO incompatibility and maternal infections (rubella, herpes, syphilis, or toxoplasmosis). The pathophysiological response occurs because there is a deficiency or inactivity of bilirubin glucuronyl transferase in the newborn.

P Breast milk jaundice occurs within the first 2 weeks of life, with the onset being 4 to 5 days after birth. The etiology is not clear, but breast milk may contain an inhibitor of bilirubin conjugation.

A It is abnormal when the light-skinned newborn lies on one side and the dependent half becomes red or ruddy and the upper half turns pale in color. In dark-skinned children, the dependent half becomes a ruddy color and the upper half seems normal.

P **Harlequin color change** is a benign condition thought to be a result of poor vasomotor control; it occurs between 48 and 96 hours after birth.

A Erythema of the palms or soles, edema of the hands or feet, or periungual desquamation is found in patients presenting with Kawasaki disease (mucocutaneous lymph node syndrome). In order for a practitioner to diagnose Kawasaki disease, the child must present with fever for 5 days and with four of the five diagnostic criteria. Other than the previously mentioned signs above, other signs include bilateral, nonexudative conjunctival injection; at least one of the mucous membrane changes including injected

REFLECTIVE THINKING

Suspecting Child Abuse

A young mother of five children brings her 2-year-old child, who is wheezing and having difficulty breathing, into the emergency department. The mother tells you she was up all night with the child. On auscultation of the posterior lung fields, you note three 4 mm, rounded areas on the upper back that appear to be second-degree burns. There is erythema and tissue destruction surrounding the borders of each area.

1. What would be your first reaction?

2. How would you proceed with the assessment? What questions would you ask the mother?

3. Do you know your institution's policy and your state's laws on reporting suspected child abuse?

or fissured lips, injected pharynx, or strawberry tongue; polymorphous exanthem; and acute nonsuppurative cervical lymphadenopathy.

P The cause of Kawasaki disease is unknown. Coronary artery vasculitis is a major concern as the disease progresses.

LESIONS.

E/N See Chapter 10.

A Lesions that are usually symmetrical, scaly, erythematous patches or plaques with possible exudation and crusting are abnormal.

P Eczema or atopic dermatitis (AD) is a common abnormal skin disorder involving inflammation of the epidermis and superficial dermis. Inhaled allergens such as pollens, molds, or dust mites, or food allergens are thought to induce mast-cell responses that cause AD.

A Small, maculopapular lesions on an erythematous base, wheals, and vesicles that erupt on the newborn are abnormal.

P Erythema toxicum is a benign rash. The cause is unknown.

A Flat, deep, irregular, localized, pink areas in light-skinned children and deeper red areas in dark-skinned children are abnormal.

P **Telangiectatic nevi**, commonly known as **stork bites**, appear on the back of the neck, lower occiput, upper eyelids, and upper lip. The cause of telangiectatic nevi is capillary dilatation.

A Diffuse redness, papules, vesicles, edema, scaling, and ulcerations on the area covered by a baby's diaper are abnormal.

P Possible causes of diaper dermatitis include fecal enzymes, irritated skin, stool consistency and frequency, *Candida*, cleansing agents, sensitive skin, and poor nutrition.

A Vesicles located on the palms of hands, soles of feet, and in the mouth are abnormal. A papular erythematous rash may also be on the buttocks.

P Hand-foot-mouth disease is caused by coxsackievirus A16.

A A dark black tuft of hair or a dimple over the lumbosacral area is abnormal.

P The neural tube fails to fuse at about the fourth week of gestation and causes a vertebral defect known as spina bifida occulta.

A A myelomeningocele is an open spina bifida lesion in which there is either no skin covering or neural tissue covered only by a thin membrane.

P Myelomeningocele has been associated with maternal diabetes mellitus, obesity, fever, hyperthermia, and use of valproic acid and carbamazepine. The increased incidence of neural tube defects seen in some lower socioeconomic groups suggests that nutritional deficiencies, particularly lack of folic acid, may play a significant role in etiology. Neural tube defects are presumably caused by failure of the neural tube to close between the third and fourth week of gestation, resulting in abnormalities of the brain and spinal cord.

Palpation

TEXTURE.

E 1. Use the finger pads to palpate the skin.

2. The technique of palpating the skin of a younger child can be accomplished by playing games. For example, use the finger pads to walk up the abdomen and touch the nose.

N Skin of the pediatric patient normally is smooth and soft. **Milia**, plugged sebaceous glands, present as small, white papules in the newborn. Milia occur mainly on the head, especially the cheeks and nose. Preterm infants have vernix caseosa.

A An oily texture and appearance to the skin, particularly the face, chest, and back, can start as early as 8 to 9 years of age as puberty is beginning.

P An oily skin during puberty is caused by a surge of sex hormones called androgens. Genetics also play a role in the amount of oil that oil glands produce.

HAIR
Inspection
LESIONS.

E/N See Chapter 10.

A Yellow, greasy-appearing scales on the scalp of a light-skinned infant are abnormal. In dark-skinned infants, the scaling is light gray.

P Seborrheic dermatitis (**cradle cap**) is possibly related to increased epidermal tissue growth.

HEAD
Inspection
SHAPE AND SYMMETRY.

E With the patient sitting upright either in the caregiver's arms or on the examination table, observe the symmetry of the frontal, parietal, and occipital prominences.

N The shape of a child's head is symmetrical without depressions or protrusions. The anterior fontanel normally may pulsate with every heart beat. The Asian infant generally has a flattened occiput, more so than infants of other races.

A A flattened occipital bone with resultant hair loss over the same area is abnormal.

P A prolonged supine position places pressure on the occipital bone.

HEAD CONTROL.

E 1. Assess head control while the patient is in the position used for assessing shape and symmetry.

2. With the head unsupported, observe the patient's ability to hold the head erect.

N At 3 months of age, the infant is able to hold the head steady without lag.

A Lack of head control is evidenced by the infant who is unable to hold the head steady while in a sitting position and is abnormal. Head lag beyond 4 to 6 months of age should be further investigated.

P Documented prematurity, hydrocephalus, and illnesses causing developmental delays are possible causes of head lag.

| **E** Examination | **N** Normal Findings | **A** Abnormal Findings | **P** Pathophysiology |

Palpation

FONTANEL.

E 1. Place the child in an upright position.

2. Using the second or third finger pad, palpate the anterior fontanel at the junction of the sagittal, coronal, and frontal sutures.

3. Palpate the posterior fontanel at the junction of the sagittal and lambdoidal sutures.

4. Assess for bulging, pulsations, and size. To obtain accurate measurements, the patient should not be crying. Crying will produce a distorted, full, bulging appearance.

N The anterior fontanel is soft and flat. Size ranges from 4 to 6 centimeters at birth. The fontanel gradually closes between 9 and 19 months of age. The posterior fontanel is also soft and flat. The size ranges from 0.5 to 1.5 centimeters at birth. The posterior fontanel gradually closes between 1 and 3 months of age. It is normal to feel pulsations related to the peripheral pulse.

A Palpation reveals a bulging, tense fontanel, which is abnormal.

P Signs of increased intracranial pressure are associated with meningitis and an increased amount of CSF.

A A sunken, depressed fontanel is abnormal.

P A sunken, depressed fontanel is a sign of dehydration.

A A wide anterior fontanel in a child older than 2½ years is an abnormal finding.

P An anterior fontanel that remains open after 2½ years of age may indicate disease such as rickets. In rickets, there is a low level of vitamin D relative to decreased phosphate levels. Other causes of enlarged fontanel include congenital hypothyroidism, Down syndrome, and hydrocephalus.

SUTURE LINES.

E 1. With the finger pads, palpate the sagittal suture line. This runs from the anterior to the posterior portion of the skull in a midline position.

2. Palpate the coronal suture line. This runs along both sides of the head, starting at the anterior fontanel.

3. Palpate the lambdoidal suture. The lambdoidal suture runs along both sides of the head, starting at the posterior fontanel.

4. Ascertain if these suture lines are open, united, or overlapping.

N Grooves or ridges between sections of the skull are normally palpated up to 6 months of age.

A Suture lines that overlap or override one another, giving the head an unusual shape, warrant further investigation.

P **Craniosynostosis** is premature ossification of suture lines, whereby there is early formation and fusion of skull bones. Craniosynostosis may be caused by metabolic disorders or may be a secondary consequence of microcephaly.

SURFACE CHARACTERISTICS.

E 1. With the finger pads, palpate the skull in the same manner as the fontanels and suture lines.

2. Note surface edema and contour of the cranium.

N The skin covering the cranium is flush against the skull and without edema.

A A softening of the outer layer of the cranial bones behind and above the ears combined with a ping pong ball sensation as the area is pressed in gently with the fingers is indicative of **craniotabes**, an abnormal finding.

P Craniotabes is associated with rickets, syphilis, hydrocephaly, or hypervitaminosis A.

A A resonant or "cracked pot" sound is produced upon percussion of the skull in an older infant.

P This is Macewen's sign. It is a normal finding in young infants when the cranial sutures are open. After early infancy, hydrocephalus and other pathologies that cause increased intracranial pressure cause cranial suture separation. This is when Macewen's sign may be elicited.

A A localized, subcutaneous swelling over one of the cranial bones of a newborn is referred to as a **cephalhematoma** and is abnormal. This abnormality differs from other surface characteristics in that edema does not cross suture lines with this condition. Varying degrees of swelling can persist up to 3 months.

P Cephalhematomas acquired during forceps deliveries are due to subperiosteal bleeding and usually resolve within a couple of weeks, but may persist longer.

A Swelling over the occipitoparietal region of the skull is abnormal.

P **Caput succedaneum** results from pressure over the occipitoparietal region during a prolonged delivery. It usually resolves within 1 to 2 weeks after birth.

A **Molding** can occur in conjunction with caput succedaneum.

P The parietal bone overrides the frontal bone as a result of induced pressure during delivery. It should resolve within 1 week of delivery.

ADVANCED TECHNIQUE

Assessing for Hydrocephalus and Anencephaly: Transillumination of the Skull

Transillumination of the infant's head to rule out hydrocephalus or anencephaly can be performed as a temporary alternative to a magnetic resonance imaging (MRI) or a computerized tomography (CT) scan if head circumference is not within normal limits.

E 1. Support the child in an elevated or sitting position.
     2. Darken the room.
     3. Place a flashlight with a soft, flexible, rubber end directly against the frontal, parietal, and occipital areas of the skull.
     4. Note the size of the light over the various areas.

N A normal finding over the frontal and parietal bones is a circle of light no larger than 2 cm around the flashlight. Over the occipital area, a circle of light no larger than 1 cm is considered within normal limits. Normal findings are the same for light- and dark-skinned children.

A It is abnormal for the illuminated area to be more than 1 cm in the occipital area and 2 cm elsewhere.

P **Anencephaly** is an abnormal finding whereby the cortex or cranium does not develop. The fetal nervous system thus fails to develop normally. Between the 18th and 24th day of gestation, the neural tube fails to close, resulting in anencephaly. These patients usually do not live more than 24 hours.

P Excess fluid in the cranial vault, as in hydrocephalus, may lead to positive transillumination.

| **E** Examination | **N** Normal Findings | **A** Abnormal Findings | **P** Pathophysiology |

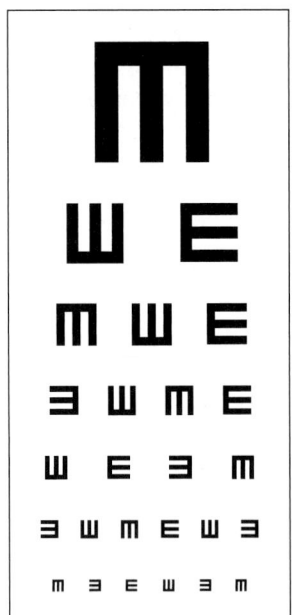

FIGURE 24-12 Tumbling E Chart

EYES

General Approach

1. From infancy through about 8 to 10 years, you should assess the eyes toward the end of the assessment, with the exception of testing vision, which should be done first. Remember that the child's attention span is short, and attentiveness decreases the longer you evaluate. Children generally are not cooperative for eyes, ears, and throat assessments.

2. Place the young infant, preschool, school-age, or adolescent patient on the examination table. The older infant or the toddler can be held by the caregiver.

3. Become proficient at performing funduscopic assessments on adults prior to assessing the pediatric patient.

Vision Screening

GENERAL APPROACH.

1. The adult Snellen chart can be used on children as young as 6 years, provided they are able to read the alphabet. The E chart is used for a patient over 3 years of age or any child who cannot read the alphabet (Figure 24-12).

2. Test every 1 to 2 years through adolescence.

3. If the child resists wearing a cover patch over the eye, make a game out of wearing the patch. For example, the young child could pretend to be a pirate exploring new territory. Use your imagination to think of a fantasy situation.

4. The Allen test (a series of seven pictures on different cards) can be used with children as young as 2 years of age.

TUMBLING E CHART.

E 1. Ask the child to point an arm in the direction the E is pointing.

2. Observe for squinting.

N Vision is 20/40 from 2 to approximately 6 years of age, when it approaches the normal 20/20 acuity. Refer the patient to an ophthalmologist if results are 20/40 or greater in a child 3 years of age or 20/30 or greater in a child 6 years or older, or if results vary by two or more lines between eyes even if in the passing range.

A/P See Chapter 12.

ALLEN TEST.

E 1. With the child's eyes both open, show each card to the child and elicit a name for each picture. Do not use any pictures with which the child is not familiar. Usually, the only pictures children have difficulty with are the 1940s vintage telephone and the Christmas tree if they belong to a cultural group that does not celebrate this holiday.

2. Place the 2- to 3-year-old child 4.5 m (15 feet) from where you will be standing. Place the 3- to 4-year-old child 6 m (20 feet) from you.

3. Ask the caregiver to help cover one of the child's eyes.

4. With the child's eye covered and the child standing at the appropriate distance, show the pictures one at a time, eliciting a response after each showing.

5. Show the same pictures in different sequence for the other eye.

6. To record findings, the denominator is always constant at 30, because a child with normal vision should see the picture on the card (target) at 9 m (30 feet). To document the numerator, determine the greatest distance at which three of the pictures are recognized by each eye, for example, right eye = 15/30, left eye = 20/30.

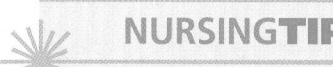
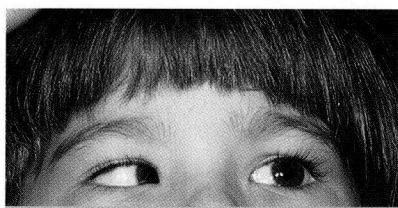

FIGURE 24-13 Infantile Esotropia.
Courtesy of the Armed Forces Institute of Pathology.

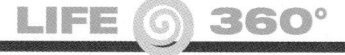

Impact of Color Blindness

Consider the developmental abilities of a 4-, 22-, 45-, and 82-year-old male who has some degree of color vision deficiency. What challenges are inherent with this condition at each of these ages? What are strategies to assist the individual when determining color matters?

N The child should correctly identify three of the cards in three trials. Two- to 3-year-old children should have 15/30 vision. Three- to 4-year-old children should be able to achieve a score of 15/30 to 20/30. Each eye should have the same score.

A/P If the scores for the patient's right and left eyes differ by 1.5 m (5 feet) or more or either or both eyes score less than 15/30, refer the patient to an ophthalmologist.

Strabismus Screening

The Hirschberg test and the cover/uncover test screen for strabismus. The latter is the more definitive test.

HIRSCHBERG TEST.

E/N See Chapter 12.

A It is abnormal for the light reflection to be displaced to the outer margin of the cornea as the eye deviates inward (Figure 24-13).

P Esotropia is thought to be congenital. Some theories suggest that neurological factors contribute to its development.

A It is abnormal for the light reflection to be displaced to the inner margin of the cornea as the eye deviates outward.

P Exotropia can result from eye muscle fatigue or can be congenital.

COVER/UNCOVER TEST.

E See Chapter 12.

N Neither eye moves when the occluder is being removed. Infants less than 6 months of age display strabismus due to poor neuromuscular control of eye muscles.

A It is abnormal for one or both eyes to move to focus on the penlight during assessment. Assume strabismus is present.

P Strabismus after 6 months of age is abnormal and indicates eye muscle weakness.

COLOR VISION.

Preschoolers aged 3–6 years old should have their ability to distinguish colors assessed during their annual well-child examination. The two most commonly used color vision assessment tools are the Ishihara color test and the Color Vision Testing Made Easy test. The Ishihara test places numbers on a pseudoisochromatic-colored background. The Color Vision Testing Made Easy tool also uses a pseudoisochromatic-colored background but uses objects that are readily recognizable to a preschooler. Objects such as a car, boat, house, and a dog are used (see Figure 24-14).

E 1. Show the child the color vision test plate.

2. Have the child identify the number or object within 3 seconds.

N The child should be able to correctly identify the number or object within 3 seconds.

A If the child is unable to correctly identify the number or object within 3 seconds, a color vision deficiency, or color blindness, should be suspected.

| **E** Examination | **N** Normal Findings | **A** Abnormal Findings | **P** Pathophysiology |

A. Car

B. House

C. Dog

D. Boat

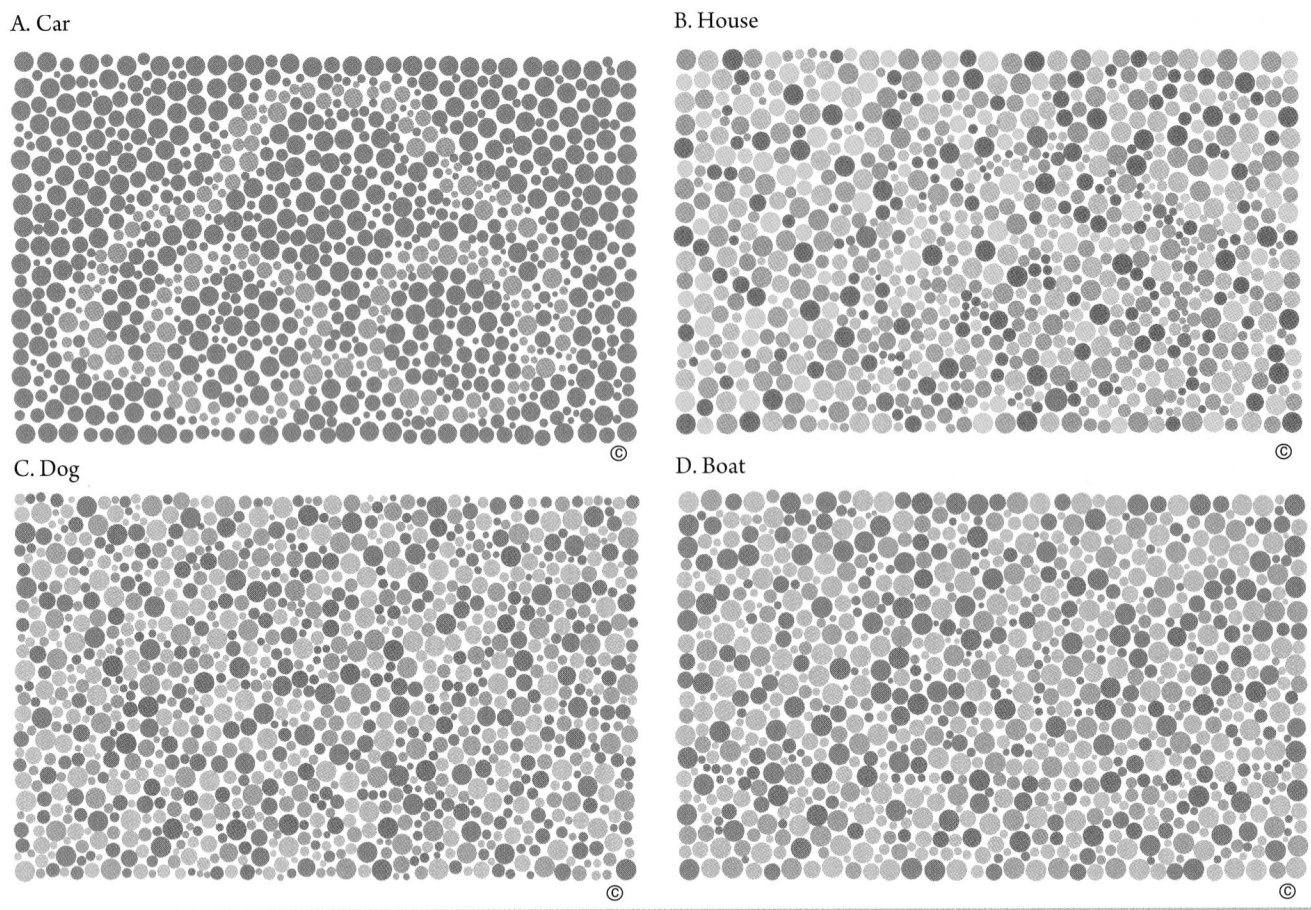

FIGURE 24-14 **Color Vision Testing. These readily recognizable objects are placed on a pseudoisochromatic background.** *Test plates reproduced from "Color Vision Testing Made Easy". Permission granted by Dr. T. L. Waggoner/www.colorvisiontesting.com.*

P This is a congenital finding in 5–8% of males and 0.5% females. A small number of individuals with color blindness acquire the condition through eye, nerve, or brain conditions.

Inspection

EYELIDS.

E 1. Sit at the patient's eye level.

2. Observe for symmetrical palpebral fissures and position of eyelids in relation to the iris.

N The palpebral fissures of both eyes are positioned symmetrically. The upper eyelid normally covers a small portion of the iris, and the lower lid meets the iris. Epicanthal folds are normally present in Asian children.

A It is abnormal for a portion of the sclera to be seen above the iris.

P The sclera is exposed above the iris in hydrocephalus. As the forehead becomes prominent, the eyebrows and eyelids are drawn up, creating a setting sun appearance of the child's eyes.

A A fold of skin covering the inner canthus and lacrimal caruncle is abnormal.

P During embryonic development, the fold of skin slants in a downward direction toward the nose. This is found in a child with Down syndrome.

E Examination   **N** Normal Findings   **A** Abnormal Findings   **P** Pathophysiology

Epicanthal folds and short palpebral fissures are seen in a child with fetal alcohol syndrome.

LACRIMAL APPARATUS.

E/N See Chapter 12.

A The patient's caregiver reports that the child is unable to produce tears, an abnormal finding.

A The lacrimal ducts should be patent by 3 months of age. Dacryocystitis results when the distal end of the membranous lacrimal duct fails to open or a blockage occurs elsewhere.

Anterior Segment Structures

SCLERA.

E See Chapter 12.

N The newborn exhibits a bluish-tinged sclera related to thinness of the fibrous tissue. The sclera is white in light-skinned children and a slightly darker color in some dark-skinned children.

A/P See Chapter 12.

IRIS.

E Conduct the examination in the same manner as for an adult.

N Up to about 6 months of age, the color of the iris is blue or slate gray in light-skinned infants and brownish in dark-skinned infants. Between 6 and 12 months of age, complete transition of iris color has occurred.

A Small white flecks, called **Brushfield's spots**, noted around the perimeter of the iris are abnormal.

P Brushfield's spots are found on the iris of the patient with Down syndrome. The spots develop during embryonic maturation.

PUPILS.

E See Chapter 12.

N When the pupils' reaction to light is assessed, a newborn will normally blink and flex the head closer to the body. This is called the optical blink reflex.

A/P See Chapter 12.

LENS.

E Examine the pediatric patient as you would the adult patient.

N The lens is transparent.

A A white or pearly gray appearance is abnormal.

P This finding can be caused by a congenital or acquired cataract (Figure 24-15).

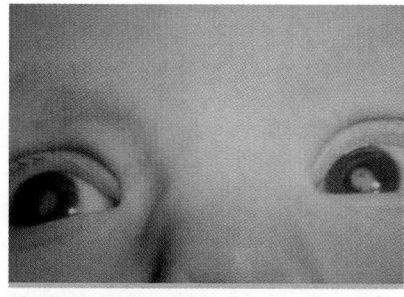

FIGURE 24-15 Pediatric Cataracts.
Courtesy of the Centers for Disease Control and Prevention (CDC).

Posterior Segment Structures

GENERAL APPROACH.

1. Observe the red reflex, retina, and optic disc.
2. The assessment is easier to accomplish if the infant or toddler is lying supine on an examination table. The assistance of another individual, such as the caregiver, to hold the patient in position is essential. The older patient may be allowed to sit, if cooperative.

Auditory Impairment in a Young Child

A mother brings her 21-month-old child to the pediatric nurse practitioner (PNP) for a suspected ear infection. The child is diagnosed with bilateral otitis media with effusion. The mother asks the PNP if the child's hearing will develop normally, as this is the child's fifth infection in 4 months. The mother starts to cry and tells the PNP that she had recurrent ear infections as a child that led to hearing impairment and subsequent language delays and speech impediments. The mother does not want her child to experience these difficulties. What response is appropriate for the PNP to make?

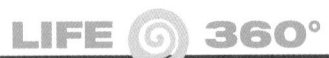

Foreign Body in the Ear

You are alerted by the Medical Technician that the toddler in Room 7 is screaming hysterically, holding her ear, and stomping her feet on the ground. As you enter the room, the mother has a look of desperation on her face and states, "I think Hannah has a bug in her ear. Before we came here, I was looking at her ear and I could hear a buzzing noise." What is your best course of action?

NURSING**TIP**

False Impression of Otitis Media

If the patient is screaming and crying, a flush or erythema on the tympanic membrane will be present. After allowing the caregiver to comfort the child, attempt to reassess. The flush or erythema can give false impressions of otitis media.

INSPECTION.

Red Reflex.

E/N See Chapter 12.

A An absent red reflex is abnormal.

P Chromosomal disorders, intrauterine infections, and ocular trauma are possible causes of cataracts in newborns.

A A yellowish or white light reflex (cat's eye reflex) is abnormal.

P Retinoblastoma is a malignant glioma located in the posterior chamber of the eye.

Retina.

E/N See Chapter 12.

A A red to dark red color is abnormal. Some areas may be rounded or flame shaped.

P Retinal hemorrhage is seen in trauma. Bleeding into the optic nerve sheath is found in children who have been physically shaken. This is called shaken baby syndrome.

Optic Disc.

E/N/A/P See Chapter 12.

EARS

Auditory Testing

GENERAL APPROACH. Hearing tests are available for newborns and even mandated in some states.

1. Prior to 3 years of age, the following are a few parameters for evaluating hearing.
   a. Does the child react to a loud noise?
   b. Does the child react to the caregiver's voice by cooing, smiling, or turning eyes and head toward the voice?
   c. Does the child try to imitate sounds?
   d. Can the child imitate words and sounds?
   e. Can the child follow directions?
   f. Does the child respond to sounds not directed at him or her?
2. Perform auditory testing at about age 3 to 4 years of age or when the child can follow directions.

External Ear

INSPECTION OF PINNA POSITION.

E/N See Chapter 13.

A The top of the ear is below the imaginary line drawn from the outer canthus to the top of the ear.

P Kidneys and ears are formed at the same time in embryonic development. If a child's ears are low set, renal anomalies must be ruled out. Low-set ears can also occur in Down syndrome.

E Examination   **N** Normal Findings   **A** Abnormal Findings   **P** Pathophysiology

Internal Ear

INSPECTION.

E 1. A cooperative patient may be allowed to sit for the assessment. A young child may be held as shown in Figure 24-16A.

2. Restrain the uncooperative young patient by placing him or her supine on a firm surface (Figure 24-16B). Instruct the caregiver or assistant to hold the patient's arms up near the head, embracing the elbow joints on both sides of either arm. Restrain the infant by having the caregiver hold the infant's hands down (Figure 24-16C).

3. With your thumb and forefinger grasping the otoscope, use the lateral side of the hand to prevent the head from jerking. Your other hand can also be used to stabilize the patient's head.

4. Pull the lower auricle down and out to straighten the canal. This technique is used in children up to about 3 years of age. Use the adult technique after age 3.

5. Insert the speculum about ¼ to ½ inch, depending on the patient's age.

6. Suspected otitis media must be evaluated with a pneumatic bulb attached to the side of the otoscope's light source.

7. Select a larger speculum to make a tight seal and prevent air from escaping from the canal.

8. Gently squeeze the bulb attachment to introduce air into the canal.

9. Observe the tympanic membrane for movement.

N/A/P See Chapter 13.

NOSE

Inspection

GENERAL APPROACH.

1. Conduct the inspection of the nose utilizing the same positioning used for the adult ear examination.

2. Observe the mucosa, nasal septum, and presence of drainage.

E 1. Gently push the patient's nose upward with one finger. Insert the speculum gently into the nare. Avoid touching the nasal septum with the speculum.

2. Note the color of the mucosa, color and consistency of drainage, presence of septal deviation, or foreign body.

N The nasal mucosa is pink or dull red. There is no evidence of polyps, foreign bodies, nasal drainage, or septal deviation.

A Nasal mucosa that is pale pink, gray, or blue may indicate allergic rhinitis.

P Allergic rhinitis is triggered by breathing in an allergen such as pollen or dust.

A A pearly gray-colored grape-like growth noted within the nasal mucosa is abnormal.

P The cause of polyps is unknown but may be attributed to several factors including allergies and rhinosinusitis. Some individuals, including those with asthma, chronic rhinosinusitis, or cystic fibrosis, are at greater risk for developing polyps.

A Persistent odor and unilateral nasal drainage in a child with a suspected foreign body warrants further evaluation by a trained clinician.

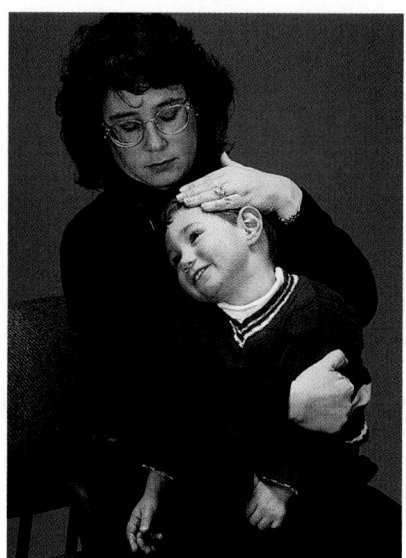

A. Preschooler in a Sitting Position

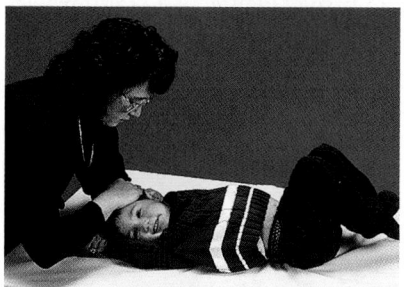

B. Preschooler in a Supine Position

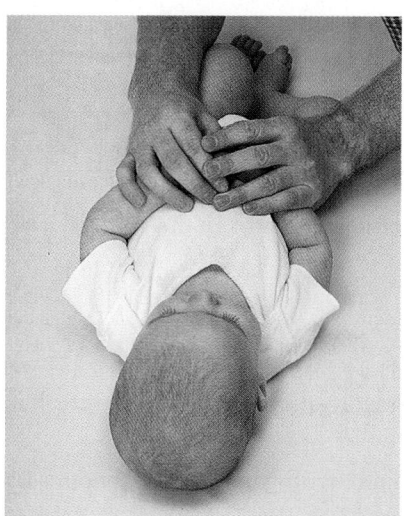

C. Infant in a Supine Position

FIGURE 24-16 **Restraining the Child for the Otoscopic Examination**

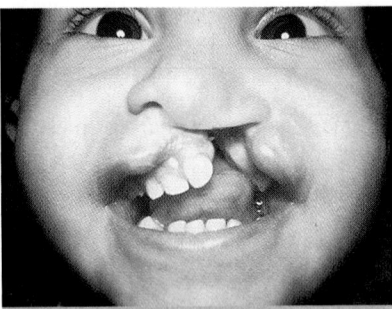

FIGURE 24-17 **Cleft Lip.** *Courtesy of Dr. Joseph Konzelman, School of Dentistry, Medical College of Georgia.*

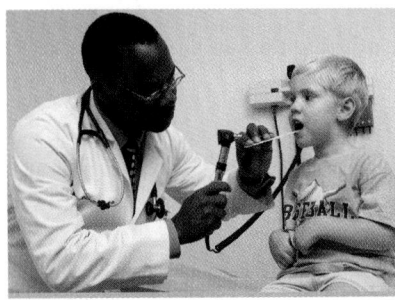

FIGURE 24-18 **The nurse gains the cooperation of the child to examine the mouth and oropharynx.**

P A foreign body lodged in a nasal cavity may need to be removed while the pediatric patient is under light sedation.

A A nasal septum that is not straight is abnormal. The septum may appear bowed into the nasal passage.

P Septal deviation may cause snoring, difficult nasal breathing, excessive nasal drainage, nosebleeds, rhinosinusitis, and headaches.

MOUTH AND THROAT

Inspection

LIPS.

E **1.** Follow the same technique described in Chapter 13.

2. Observe if the lip edges meet.

N The lip edges should meet.

A It is abnormal if the lip edges do not meet.

P Cleft lip is seen as a separated area of lip tissue (Figure 24-17). It involves the upper lip and sometimes extends into the nostril. A cleft lip is an obvious finding during a newborn assessment. It occurs mainly on the left side and is more frequently found in males. A cleft lip develops during the fifth to sixth week after fertilization. Genetics plays a small role in etiology.

A A thin upper lip is abnormal.

p A child with fetal alcohol syndrome exhibits this finding, as well as a flat and elongated philtrum.

BUCCAL MUCOSA.

E Use the same technique as for an adult (Figure 24-18). If the patient is unable to open the mouth on command, use the edge of a tongue blade to lift the upper lip and move the lower lip down.

N See Chapter 13.

A A thick, curdlike coating on the buccal mucosa or tongue is abnormal.

P Thrush can be acquired when a newborn passes through the vagina during delivery.

TEETH.

E/N See Chapter 13.

A A lack of visible teeth coupled with roentgenographic findings revealing absence of tooth buds is abnormal.

P Absence of deciduous teeth beyond 16 months of age signifies an abnormality most commonly related to genetic causes.

A It is abnormal for the teeth to turn brownish black, possibly with indentations along the surfaces of the teeth.

P Carbohydrate-rich fluid (from milk or juice) causes severe caries when a child falls asleep with a bottle in the mouth.

HARD AND SOFT PALATE.

E **1.** Observe the palate for continuity and shape.

2. For infants, you will need to use a tongue depressor to push the tongue down. Infants usually cry in response to this action, which allows visualization of the palates.

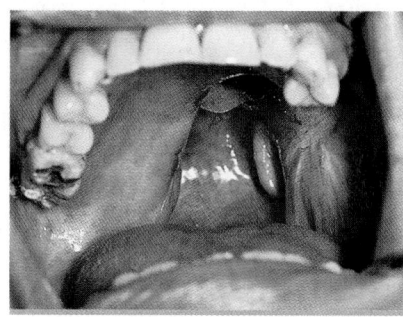

FIGURE 24-19 **Cleft Palate.** *Courtesy of Dr. Joseph Konzelman, School of Dentistry, Medical College of Georgia.*

N The roof of the mouth is continuous and has a slight arch.

A It is abnormal if the roof of the mouth is not continuous. This anomaly is called cleft palate (Figure 24-19).

P Cleft palates vary greatly in size and extent of malformation. The degree of malformation is classified into two groups. A midline malformation may involve the uvula or extend through the soft or hard palates or both. If associated with cleft lip, the malformation may extend through the palates and into the nasal cavity. Cleft palates form between the sixth and tenth week of embryonic development, during fusion of the maxillary and pre-maxillary processes. Genetics plays a small role in etiology.

A The roof of the mouth is abnormally arched. On inspection, the shape resembles an upside-down letter "V."

P High palates are usually associated with a particular syndrome. Examples include trisomy 21, trisomy 18, and Noonan syndrome.

A **Epstein's pearls** in the newborn appear on the hard palate and gum margins and are abnormal. The pearls are small white cysts that feel hard when palpated.

P These cysts result from fragments of epithelial tissue trapped during palate formation.

OROPHARYNX.

E See Chapter 13.

N Up to the age of 12 years, a tonsil grade of 2+ is considered normal. Around puberty, tonsillar tissue regresses. Tonsils should not interfere with the act of breathing.

A Excessive salivation is an early sign of a tracheoesophageal fistula (TEF). Drooling is accompanied by choking and coughing during the patient's feeding.

P The esophagus failed to develop as a continuous passage during embryonic formation.

A Exudative pharyngitis is present in infectious mononucleosis. Other symptoms include fever, sore throat, splenomegaly, petechiae on the palate, and cervical adenitis.

P Mononucleosis is caused by the Epstein-Barr virus.

A Hypertrophy of lymphoid tissue occurs in the posterior pharyngeal wall, causing a condition known as enlarged or hypertrophied adenoids.

P Excessive lymphoid tissue interferes with passage of air through the nose, resulting in snoring and apnea. Obstruction of the eustachian tubes by enlarged lymphoid tissue can lead to otitis media. Sinusitis can occur when lymphoid tissue blocks the clearance of nasal mucus.

NECK
Inspection
GENERAL APPEARANCE.

E 1. Observe the neck in a midline position while the patient is sitting upright.

2. Note shortening or thickness of the neck on both right and left sides.

3. Note any swelling.

NURSING**TIP**

Preventing Choking in Children

The infant's or toddler's airway is small, approximately the size of their "pinky" fingers. Fresh grapes, uncut hot dogs with the skin on, popcorn, and peanuts are common foods that can cause choking. These foods should not be given to young children.

| **E** Examination | **N** Normal Findings | **A** Abnormal Findings | **P** Pathophysiology |

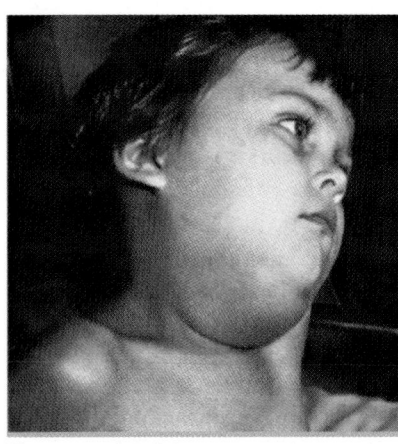

FIGURE 24-20 **Parotitis (Mumps).**
Courtesy of the Centers for Disease Control and Prevention (CDC).

N There is a reasonable amount of skin tissue on the sides of the neck. There is no swelling.

A Additional weblike tissue found bilaterally from the ear to the shoulder is abnormal.

P Webbed necks are associated with congenital syndromes. One example is Turner syndrome, noted in female children.

A Unilateral or bilateral swelling of the neck below the angle of the jaw is abnormal (Figure 24-20).

P Enlargement of the parotid gland occurs in parotitis, or mumps, an inflammation of the parotid gland. There is pain and tenderness in the affected area.

A Torticollis is observed.

P Torticollis can be congenital and acquired. An infant who is always placed on the same side when supine can develop a lateral deviation at the neck with decreased range of motion.

Palpation

THYROID.

E 1. Use the same technique as for an adult with the exception of using the first two finger pads on both hands.

2. Have the younger child who is unable to swallow on command take a drink from a bottle or cup.

N/A/P The normal findings, abnormal findings, and pathophysiology are the same as for an adult.

LYMPH NODES.

E 1. Because of the infant's short neck, you must extend the chin upward with your hand before proceeding with palpation.

2. With the finger pads, palpate the submental, submandibular, tonsillar, anterior cervical chain, posterior cervical chain, supraclavicular, preauricular, posterior auricular, and occipital lymph nodes.

3. Use a circular motion. Note location, size, shape, tenderness, mobility, and associated skin inflammation of any swollen nodes palpated.

N Lymph nodes are generally not palpable. Children often have small, movable, cool, nontender nodes referred to as "shotty" nodes. These benign nodes are related to environmental antigen exposure or residual effects of a prior illness and have no clinical significance.

A Enlargement of the anterior cervical chain is abnormal.

P This occurs in bacterial infections of the pharynx (strep throat) or viral infections (mononucleosis).

A Enlargement of the occipital nodes or posterior cervical chain nodes is abnormal.

P This can occur in infectious mononucleosis, tinea capitis, and acute otitis externa.

BREASTS

Inspection of the breasts is performed throughout childhood. Palpation is not usually performed on the patient until puberty, unless otherwise indicated.

E Examination   **N** Normal Findings   **A** Abnormal Findings   **P** Pathophysiology

Sexual Maturity Rating (SMR)

E 1. Using the Tanner stages in Table 14-1, assess the developmental stage of a female's breasts.

N Breast development usually starts between the ages of 8 and 10 and is finished after 14 to 17 years of age.

A An SMR that is less than expected for a female's age is abnormal.

P Pituitary pathology needs to be considered, as well as familial predisposition.

THORAX AND LUNGS
General Approach

1. Remove the patient's clothes or gown.
2. Keep the infant warm during the assessment by placing a blanket over the chest until ready for this portion of assessment.

Inspection

SHAPE OF THORAX.

E See Chapter 15.

N The infant has a barrel chest; by age 6, the chest attains the adult configuration.

A If a school-age child has an abnormal chest configuration, suspect pathology.

P In addition to the conditions discussed in Chapter 15, CF can lead to an altered anteroposterior-transverse diameter.

RETRACTIONS.

E 1. In children, it is important to evaluate intercostal muscles for signs of increased work of breathing.

2. If at all possible, perform this examination when the patient is quiet because forceful crying will mimic retractions.

N Retractions are not present.

A In respiratory distress, retractions are seen as an inward collapse of the chest wall. Retractions can be seen in the suprasternal, supraclavicular, subcostal, and intercostal regions of the chest wall. Other signs of respiratory distress include but are not limited to nasal flaring, stridor, expiratory grunting, and wheezing.

P Respiratory distress is a result of abnormal function or disruption of the respiratory pathway or within organs that control or influence respiration. Infants with respiratory syncytial virus (RSV) frequently present with retractions.

Palpation

TACTILE FREMITUS. Fremitus is easily felt when a child cries. If the infant or young patient is not crying, it is advisable to defer this procedure until later in the assessment, perhaps after the throat and ear examinations, which usually produce crying.

Percussion

E See Chapter 15.

N Normal diaphragmatic excursion in infants and young toddlers is one to two intercostal spaces.

A/P See Chapter 15.

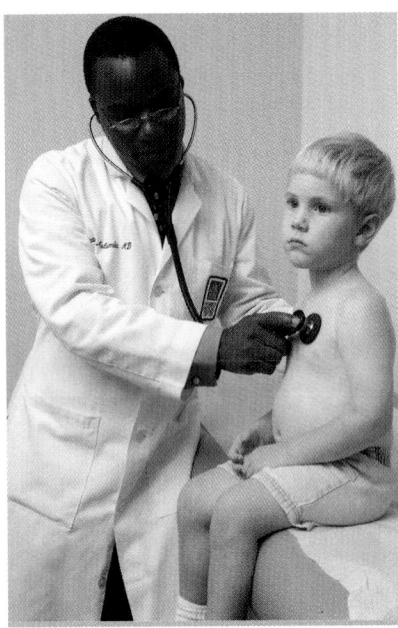

FIGURE 24-21   **The nurse auscultates the child's thorax.**

Auscultation

BREATH SOUNDS.

E   Use the same assessment techniques as for an adult (Figure 24-21). Sometimes, it is difficult to differentiate the various adventitious sounds because a child's respiratory rate is rapid; for example, differentiating expiratory wheezing from inspiratory wheezing can be difficult. Mastering the technique takes time and practice.

N   Of the three types of breath sounds—bronchial, bronchovesicular, and vesicular—the bronchovesicular are normally heard throughout the peripheral lung fields up to 5 to 6 years of age, because the chest wall is thin with decreased musculature. Lung fields are clear and equal bilaterally.

A   Crackles are abnormal.

P   Conditions such as bronchiolitis, CF, and bronchopulmonary dysplasia produce crackles.

A   Wheezing is abnormal.

P   Patients with CF and bronchiolitis may present with wheezing. Infants with RSV usually present with wheezing.

HEART AND PERIPHERAL VASCULATURE

General Approach

1. It is best to perform the cardiac assessment near the beginning of the examination, when the infant or young child is relatively calm.

2. Do not get discouraged during the assessment. The novice nurse is not expected to identify a murmur and its location within the cardiac cycle. Be patient because skill will come only with practice.

3. During the assessment, note physical signs of a syndrome such as Down's facies in a child with trisomy 21 or Down syndrome. Many children with Down syndrome have associated atrioventricular (A-V) canal malformations. These defects each involve an atrial septal defect (ASD), ventricular septal defect (VSD), and a common A-V valve.

4. Cardiac landmarks change when a child has dextrocardia. In this condition, the apex of the heart points toward the right thoracic cavity; thus heart sounds are auscultated primarily on the right side of the chest.

Inspection

APICAL IMPULSE.

E   See Chapter 16.

N   In both infants and toddlers, the apical impulse is located at the fourth intercostal space and just left of the midclavicular line. The apical impulse of a child 7 years or older is at the fifth intercostal space and to the right of the midclavicular line. The impulse may not be visible in all children, especially in those who have increased adipose tissue or muscle.

A/P   See Chapter 16.

PRECORDIUM.

E   Observe the chest wall for any movements other than the apical impulse.

N   Movements other than the apical impulse are abnormal.

| **E** Examination | **N** Normal Findings | **A** Abnormal Findings | **P** Pathophysiology |

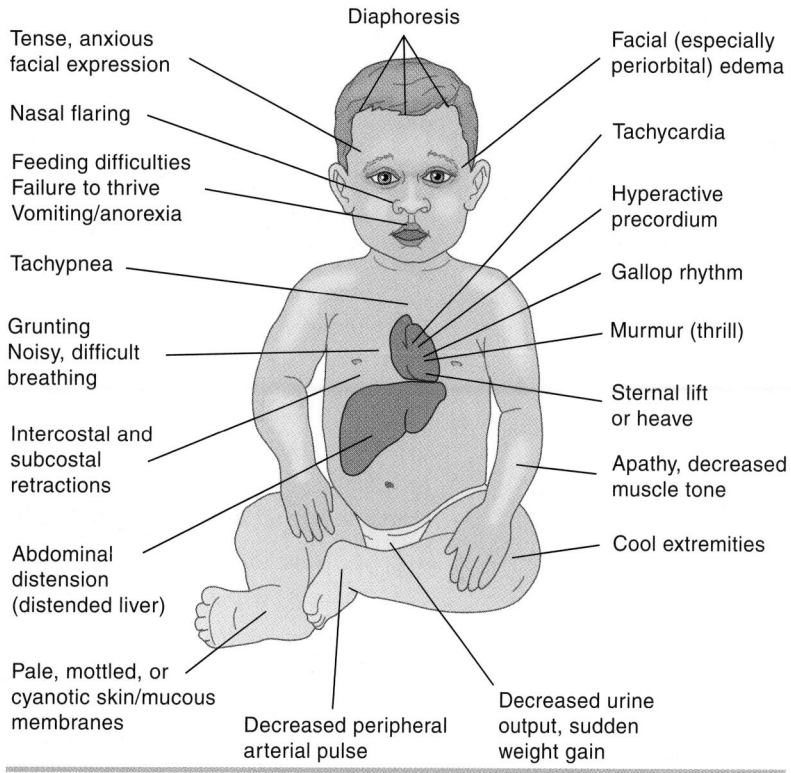

Diaphoresis

Tense, anxious facial expression

Nasal flaring

Feeding difficulties
Failure to thrive
Vomiting/anorexia

Tachypnea

Grunting
Noisy, difficult breathing

Intercostal and subcostal retractions

Abdominal distension (distended liver)

Pale, mottled, or cyanotic skin/mucous membranes

Decreased peripheral arterial pulse

Facial (especially periorbital) edema

Tachycardia

Hyperactive precordium

Gallop rhythm

Murmur (thrill)

Sternal lift or heave

Apathy, decreased muscle tone

Cool extremities

Decreased urine output, sudden weight gain

FIGURE 24-22 Infant with Congestive Heart Failure

A   Lifting of the cardiac area is abnormal.

P   Heaves are associated with volume overload. A child with congenital heart disease is at risk for developing congestive heart failure (CHF) with associated volume overload. Figure 24-22 depicts the manifestations of CHF in children. Large left-to-right shunt defects, such as a VSD, cause right ventricular volume overload.

Palpation

THRILL.

E   1. Palpate as for an adult or use the proximal one-third of each finger and the areas over the metacarpophalangeal joints. Many nurses feel the latter method yields greater sensitivity to the presence of thrills.

2. Place the hand vertically along the heart's apex and move the hand toward the sternum.

3. Place the hand horizontally along the sternum, moving up the sternal border about ½ inch to 1 inch each time.

4. When at the clavicular level, place the hand vertically and assess for a thrill at the heart's base.

5. Use the finger pads to palpate a thrill at the suprasternal notch and along the carotid arteries.

N   A thrill is not found in the healthy child.

A/P   See Chapter 16.

PERIPHERAL PULSES.

E   1. Use the same finger to assess each peripheral pulse. The sensation of one finger pad versus another can be different.

2. Use the finger pads to palpate each pair of peripheral pulses simultaneously, except for the carotid pulse.

3. Palpate the brachial and femoral pulses simultaneously.

N Pulse qualities are the same in the adult and the child.

A A brachial-femoral lag, when femoral pulses are weaker than brachial pulses when palpated simultaneously, is abnormal.

P Coarctation is due to a narrowing of the aorta before, at, or just beyond the entrance of the ductus arteriosus. Thus, blood flow to the lower body is reduced.

Auscultation

HEART SOUNDS.

Auscultating the infant's or the young pediatric patient's heart is difficult because the heart rate is rapid and breath sounds are easily transmitted through the chest wall.

E **1.** Have the child lie down. If this position is not possible, the child should be held at a 45° angle in the caregiver's arms.

2. Use the "Z" pattern to auscultate the heart. Place the stethoscope in the apical area and gradually move it toward the right lower sternal border and up the sternal border in a right diagonal line. Move gradually from the patient's left to the right upper sternal borders (Figure 24-23).

3. Perform a second evaluation with the child in a sitting position.

N Fifty percent of all children develop an innocent murmur at some time in their lives. See Table 24-6. Innocent murmurs are accentuated in high cardiac output states such as fever, stress, or pregnancy. When the patient is sitting, they are heard early in systole at the second or third intercostal space along the left sternal border and are softly musical in quality; they disappear when the patient lies down. Be aware of sinus arrhythmias during auscultation of the heart's rhythm. On inspiration, the pulse rate speeds up; the pulse rate slows with expiration. To determine if the rhythm is normal, ask the child to hold his or her breath while you auscultate the heart. If the pulse stops varying with respirations, then a sinus arrhythmia is present. S_1 is best heard at the apex of the heart, left lower sternal border. S_2 is best heard at the heart base.

A A split S_2 sound is abnormal.

P If the S_2 split is fixed with the act of respiration, you can suspect an atrial septal defect. In children, S_2 physiologically splits with inspiration and becomes single with expiration. This phenomenon is due to a greater negative pressure in the thoracic cavity.

A In children, S_3 often sounds like the three syllables of the word "Kentucky," especially when accompanied by tachycardia.

P A loud third heart sound may be present in children with CHF or VSDs. S_3 is produced by rapid filling of the ventricle.

A With tachycardia, S_4 sounds like a gallop resembling the word "Tennessee."

P S_4 is not normally heard in children. If detected, aortic stenosis may be present. The left vetricle's ability to pump blood through the stenotic valve produces a dilatation within the left ventricular muscle resulting in decreased ventricular compliance.

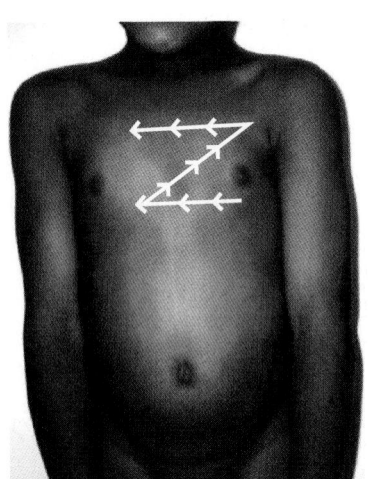

FIGURE 24-23 **Z Auscultation Pattern for Young Children**

E Examination	**N** Normal Findings	**A** Abnormal Findings	**P** Pathophysiology

TABLE 24-6 Innocent Heart Murmurs

TYPE	AGE	INTENSITY/ LOCATION	QUALITY	OTHER CHARACTERISTICS
Stills	> 2 yrs	<III/VI midsystolic located at LMSB or between LLSB and apex	Twanging, squeaking, buzzing, musical, or vibratory sound	Low frequency heard with the bell with patient in supine position, softer when the patient is standing
Pulmonary ejection	8–14 yrs	<III/VI, early midsystolic located at LUSB	Slightly grating, little radiation	Ejection-type murmur
Pulmonary flow murmur of the newborn	Low-birthweight newborn	I–II/VI with wide transmission, audible at LUSB	Rough	Disappears at 3–6 months of age
Venous hum	3–6 yrs	<III/VI continuous murmur, audible in right or left infra-clavicular and supra-clavicular areas	Humming	Originates from turbulence in jugular venous system, heard in upright position, disappears in supine position, obliterated by rotating the head or gently occluding neck veins

A A systolic ejection murmur is heard between the first and second heart sounds over the aortic or pulmonic areas.

P Ejection murmurs occur in aortic and pulmonic valvular stenosis. The murmur is the result of blood passing through stenotic valves.

A Holosystolic murmurs are heard maximally at the left lower sternal border. They begin with S_1 and continue until the second heart sound, S_2, is heard.

P Holosystolic or pansystolic murmurs are heard in children with VSDs, where blood flows from a chamber of higher pressure to one of lower pressure during systole.

A Diastolic murmurs are heard between S_2 and S_1.

P Diastolic murmurs are classified into early diastolic, mid-diastolic, and pre-systolic. Early diastolic murmurs are high-pitched and blowing. They occur in aortic regurgitation and subaortic stenosis. A mid-diastolic murmur is a low-pitched rumble. These occur in mitral stenosis or VSDs with large left-to-right shunts. A presystolic murmur is heard in patients with mitral stenosis or tricuspid stenosis.

A Continuous murmurs heard throughout the cardiac cycle are abnormal.

P Collateral blood flow murmurs are heard radiating throughout the back, such as in pulmonary atresia.

P Continuous murmurs are present in coronary artery fistulas.

P Palliative shunt murmurs are normal and should be heard; if they are not heard, there is a possibility of a clotted shunt. These murmurs are heard over the right or left upper chest in the respective area where surgically placed. A palliative shunt is created temporarily until the patient is ready for corrective surgery. A palliative shunt may be needed in a small infant with a combination of tetralogy of Fallot and pulmonary atresia or a hypoplastic pulmonary artery.

ADVANCED TECHNIQUE

Assessing for Coarctation of the Aorta

If coarctation of the aorta is suspected (as when a brachial-femoral lag is present or with upper extremity hypertension or absent or decreased pedal pulses), obtain blood pressures and compare the right upper and left lower extremity readings.

E 1. Take the upper extremity blood pressure in the right arm.

2. Because weak or absent leg pulses accompany coarctation, measurements are difficult to obtain. Use a Doppler transducer to intensify the sound of the pulse. Until you feel proficient, the Doppler technique requires two people for accurate measurement; have the caregiver hold the child's leg still while you assess the pulse.

3. Locate the right posterior tibial pulse with the Doppler transducer and make an "X" with a pen where the pulse is felt or heard.

4. Obtain the blood pressure measurement in the left leg with the cuff ½–1 inch above the pulse location. Only the systolic number is obtained with this technique.

5. Repeat the steps on the left side of body.

N Upper and lower extremity blood pressures are equal.

A If the systolic blood pressure in the leg is lower than that in the arm and femoral, popliteal, posterior tibial, or dorsalis pedis pulses are weak or absent, you can assume coarctation of the aorta is present. If undiagnosed, as the child becomes older, the upper extremity pulses are bounding.

P During the fifth or sixth week of embryonic development, the aorta may form abnormally.

ABDOMEN

General Approach

1. If possible, ask the caregiver to refrain from feeding the infant prior to the assessment because palpation of a full stomach may induce vomiting.

2. Children who are physically able should be encouraged to empty the bladder prior to the assessment.

3. The young infant, school-age child, or adolescent should lie on the examination table. For the toddler or preschooler, have the caregiver hold the child supine on the lap, with the lower extremities bent at the knees and dangling.

4. If the child is crying, encourage the caregiver to help calm the child before you proceed with the assessment.

5. Observe nonverbal communication in children who are not able to verbally express feelings. During palpation, listen for a high-pitched cry and look for a change in facial expression (Figure 24-24) or for sudden protective movements that may indicate a painful or tender area.

Inspection

CONTOUR.

E See Chapter 17.

N The young child may have a "potbelly."

PERISTALTIC WAVE.

E/N See Chapter 17.

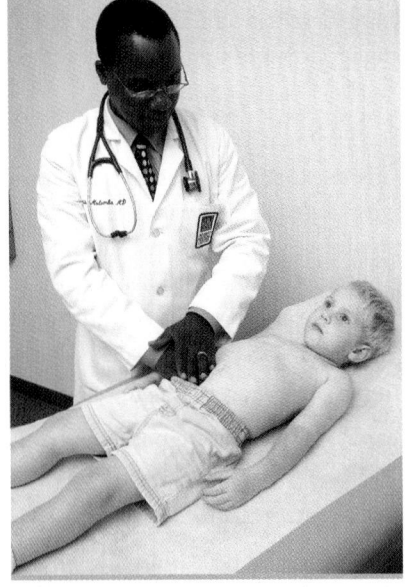

FIGURE 24-24 During palpation of the child's abdomen the nurse observes for facial grimacing or other signs of discomfort.

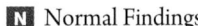

E Examination   **N** Normal Findings   **A** Abnormal Findings   **P** Pathophysiology

NURSING**TIP**

Assessing for Umbilical Hernias in Children

If the child is upset and crying, assess the umbilicus for an outward projection, which is indicative of an umbilical hernia. If an umbilical hernia is present, palpate the area to determine if the hernia reduces easily. Approximate the size of the inner ring (the diameter of the hernia).

NURSING**TIP**

Measuring the Abdomen in Children

If abdominal distension is seen during inspection, evaluate its circumference. Place the tape measure around the abdomen at the level of the umbilicus. Use a marking pen to indicate the location where the tape measure was placed, if serial abdominal circumference measurements are to be taken.

A Visible peristaltic waves seen moving across the epigastrium from left to right are abnormal.

P Obstruction at the pyloric sphincter causes a condition called pyloric stenosis. The pyloric muscle hypertrophies, causing obstruction during embryonic development.

Auscultation

After performing auscultation of the lungs, it is helpful to proceed to auscultating the abdomen because doing so allows you to complete a good portion of auscultation all at once. If the child is not cooperating, a simple distracting phrase such as "I can hear your breakfast in there" is helpful during auscultation.

Palpation

GENERAL PALPATION.

E/N See Chapter 17.

A On palpation, an olive-shaped mass felt in the epigastric area and to the upper right of the umbilicus is abnormal.

P This is indicative of pyloric stenosis.

A Abdominal distension coupled with palpable stool over the abdomen and the absence of stool in the rectum is abnormal.

P An aganglionic segment of the colon is responsible for Hirschsprung's disease, which produces abnormal gastrointestinal findings.

A A sausage-shaped mass that produces intermittent pain when palpated in the upper abdomen is abnormal.

P Administration of the rotavirus vaccine (RotaShield) is thought to be responsible for numerous cases of **intussusception**. Most commonly, the ileocecal region of the intestine telescopes down into the ileum itself. Classic symptoms are vomiting and currant jelly stools. RotaShield has been taken off the market. Rota has taken its place in standard pediatric immunizations.

A Bowel sounds heard in the thoracic cavity, a scaphoid abdomen, an upwardly displaced apical impulse, and signs of respiratory distress are abnormal findings in the newborn.

P Approximately in the eighth week of embryonic development, the diaphragm fails to fuse, creating a **diaphragmatic hernia**. This condition results in protrusion of the intestines into the thoracic cavity.

LIVER PALPATION.

E For infants and toddlers, use the outer edge of your right thumb to press down and scoop up at the right upper quadrant. For the remaining age groups, use the same technique as for an adult.

N The liver is not normally palpated, although the liver edge can be found 1 cm below the right costal margin in a normal, healthy child. The liver edge is soft and regular.

A It is abnormal for the liver edge to be palpated more than 1 cm below the right costal margin and be full with a firm, sharp border.

P Hepatomegaly occurs in several disease states such as viral or bacterial illnesses, tumors, congestive heart failure, and fat and glycogen storage diseases. Viral and bacterial illnesses and tumors cause liver cells to multiply in number, creating an enlarged liver. In heart failure, the hepatic veins and sinusoids enlarge from congestion, resulting in hemorrhage and fibrosis of the liver. In fat and glycogen storage diseases, fat and glycogen accumulate within the liver, and fibrosis ensues.

MUSCULOSKELETAL SYSTEM

General Approach

1. The extent or degree of assessment depends greatly on the patient's or caregiver's complaints of musculoskeletal problems. Be aware that during periods of rapid growth, children complain of normal muscle aches.

2. Try to incorporate musculoskeletal assessment techniques into other system assessments. For instance, while inspecting the integument, inspect the muscles and joints.

3. Inspecting the musculoskeletal system in the ambulatory child is accomplished by allowing the child to move freely about and play in the examination room while you inquire about the health history. Your observations of the child enable you to assess posture, muscle symmetry, and range of motion of muscles and joints.

4. Do not rush through the assessment. Throughout the assessment, incorporate game playing that facilitates evaluation of the musculoskeletal system.

5. Observe range of motion and joint flexibility as the child undresses.

Inspection

MUSCLES.

E 1. Have the child disrobe down to a diaper or underwear.

2. To evaluate the small infant's shoulder muscles, place your hands under the axillae and pull the infant into a standing position. The infant should not slip through your hands. Be prepared to catch the infant if needed.

3. Evaluate the infant's leg strength in a semistanding position. Lower the infant to the examination table so the infant's legs touch the table.

4. Place the infant older than 4 months in a prone position. Observe the infant's ability to lift the upper body off the examination table using the upper extremities.

N Degree of joint flexibility and range of motion are the same for the child as for the adult.

A Increased muscle tone (spasticity) is abnormal.

P Cerebral palsy (CP) results from a nonprogressive abnormality in the pyramidal motor tract. One of the more common contributing factors, perinatal asphyxia, causes abnormal posture and gross motor development and varying degrees of abnormal muscle tone.

A The inability to rise from a sitting to a standing position is abnormal. In attempting to rise from a supine position, the child first turns over onto the abdomen and raises the trunk to a crawling position. Then, with the aid of the arms, the child places the feet firmly on the floor and gradually elevates the upper part of the body by climbing up the legs with the arms.

P   This is called Gower's sign. Gower's sign occurs in Duchenne's muscular dystrophy (MD) early in childhood. Genetics is responsible for the abnormality in the short arm of the X chromosome.

JOINTS.

E   See Chapter 18.

N   The infant's spine is C-shaped. Head control and standing create the normal S-shaped spine of the adult. Lordosis is normal as the child begins to walk. A toddler's protruding abdomen is counterbalanced by an inward deviation of the lumbar spine.

A   Extra fingers or toes are abnormal.

P   Supernumerary digits, or polydactyly, may be found in certain congenital syndromes such as Carpenter, fetal hydantoin, orofaciodigital, Smith-Lemli-Opitz, trisomy 13, and VATER.

A   A fusion between two or more digits is abnormal.

P   Syndactylism is also associated with certain congenital syndromes such as Aarskog, Apert, Carpenter, orofaciodigital, Russell-Silver, and acrocephalosyndactyly. Look for other physical signs of a syndrome if either syndactyly or polydactyly is present.

A   It is abnormal for a young male (usually 2 to 12 years old) to present with a painless limp from the affected hip. The limp is accompanied by limited abduction and internal rotation, muscle spasm, and proximal thigh atrophy.

P   Legg-Calvé-Perthes disease, also called coxa plana, is caused by an interruption in the blood supply to the capital femoral epiphysis. Avascular necrosis of the femoral head results.

A   The affected hip has loss of flexion. The patient is unable to rotate the hip inward. The affected leg turns outward and may appear shorter compared to the other leg while in a standing position. The adolescent often presents with a limp.

P   These findings occur in slipped capital femoral epiphysis. The ball at the upper end of the femur slips from its normal position in a backward direction. This is due to weakness of the growth plate. It commonly develops during periods of accelerated growth, shortly after the onset of puberty. Slipped capital femoral epiphysis occurs with greater frequency in males and children who are overweight.

A   An exaggerated lumbar curvature of the spine is abnormal after 6 years of age.

P   Lordosis can be attributed to bilateral developmental dislocation of the hip or postural factors such as progression of congenital kyphosis, or can occur secondary to contractures of hip flexors.

TIBIOFEMORAL BONES.

E   1. Instruct the child to stand on the examination table with the medial condyles together.

2. Stand at eye level of the patient's knees.

3. Measure the distance between the two medial malleoli.

4. Measure the distance between the two medial condyles.

N The distance between the medial malleoli is less than 2 inches (5 cm). The distance between the medial condyles is less than 1 inch (2.5 cm). Knock-knee, or genu valgum, is common between 2 and 4 years of age. Bowleg, or genu varum, is normally present in many infants up to 12 months of age.

A Genu valgum persisting after 6 years of age is abnormal. The distance between the medial condyles is less than 1 inch (2.5 cm) and the distance between the medial malleoli is more than 2 inches (5 cm).

P The cause of genu valgum is usually physiological.

A The measured distance between the two medial condyles is greater than 2.5–5 cm (1 to 2 inches).

P Genu varum persisting after 2 years of age is abnormal and may be caused by rickets.

Palpation

JOINTS.

E/N See Chapter 18.

A Knee pain aggravated by any motion or activity that puts undue pressure on the joint is abnormal. Palpation of a slight elevation of the tibial tuberosity is abnormal.

P The deformed tubercle in Osgood-Schlatter disease is caused by repetitive stress on the area. A fibrocartilage microfracture may cause joint pain.

A Swollen, inflamed, painful joints are abnormal.

P Juvenile rheumatoid arthritis causes synovial inflammation and degeneration of the joint. Its cause is unknown.

FEET.

E 1. Place the patient on the examination table or caregiver's lap.

2. Stand in front of the child.

3. Hold the right heel immobile with one hand while pushing the forefoot (medial base of great toe) toward a midline position with the other hand.

4. Observe for toe and forefoot adduction and inversion.

5. Repeat on the left foot.

N The toes and forefoot are not deviated.

A Toes or forefeet that are deviated are abnormal.

P **Metatarsus varus** is a medial forefoot malignment. In **talipes equinovarus** (clubfoot), there is heel inversion, forefoot adduction, and plantar flexion of the foot. Heredity plays a role in the etiology as well as abnormal intrauterine position of the fetal foot.

HIP AND FEMUR.
Ortolani's maneuver is always performed at the very end of the assessment because it may produce crying. The test is performed on one hip at a time. Evaluate the hips up until 18 months of age or until the child is an established walker.

E 1. Place the infant supine on an examination table with the feet facing you.

2. Stand directly in front of the infant.

| **E** Examination | **N** Normal Findings | **A** Abnormal Findings | **P** Pathophysiology |

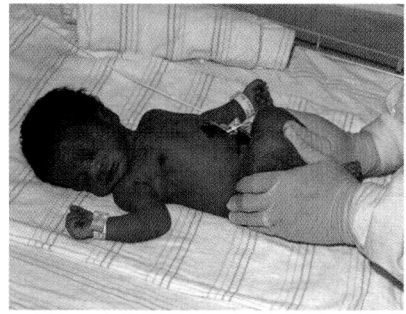

A. Hand Placement

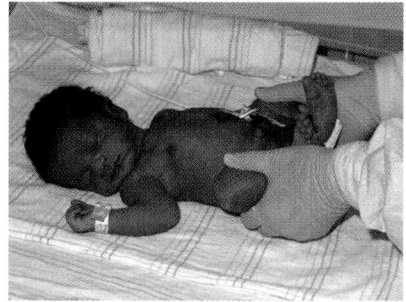

B. Hip Abduction

FIGURE 24-25 **Ortolani Maneuver**

3. With the thumb, hold the inner thigh of the femur and with the index and middle fingers, hold the greater trochanter (Figure 24-25A). These two fingers should rest over the hip joint.

4. Slowly press outward and abduct until the lateral aspects of the knees nearly touch the table (Figure 24-25B). The tips of the fingers should palpate each femora's head as it rotates outward.

5. Listen for an audible clunk (Ortolani's sign).

6. With the fingers in the same locations, adduct the hips to elicit a palpable clunk (Ortolani's sign). As each hip is adducted, it is lifted anteriorly into the acetabulum.

7. Place both of the infant's feet flat on the examination table with the knees together.

8. Observe the height of the knees. This is called Allis sign.

9. Turn the infant to a prone position and observe the levels of the gluteal folds.

N A clunk is not audible or palpated. The knees should be at the same height with the feet on the examination table. The gluteal folds are approximately at the same level.

A Abnormal findings include a positive Ortolani's sign; a sudden, painful cry during the test; asymmetrical thigh skin folds; uneven knee level; and limited hip abduction.

P Epidemiology of **developmental dislocation of the hip** (DDH) is related to familial factors, maternal hormones associated with pelvic laxity, firstborn children, oligohydramnios, and breech presentations.

A Knees that are not at the same level are abnormal.

P This is another technique that can potentially detect DDH.

A Unequal gluteal folds are abnormal.

P This also can lead to a finding of DDH.

NEUROLOGICAL SYSTEM

General Approach

1. Some aspects of the neurological assessment are different for the infant and the young child as compared to the adult. An infant functions mainly at the subcortical level. Memory and motor coordination are about three-fourths developed by 2 years of age, when cortical functioning is acquiring dominance.

2. Incorporate findings for fine and gross motor skills previously tested during the musculoskeletal assessment. In addition, use the Denver II to assess personal-social and language skills. Refer to normal developmental milestones (see Chapter 4) and extrapolate warning signs of neurological development lag.

3. Because the infant cannot verbally express level of consciousness, instead assess the newborn's ability to cry, level of activity, positioning, and general appearance.

4. Only reflex mechanisms and cranial nerve testing are described in this section. Refer to the adult neurological assessment for all other testing.

Reflex Mechanisms of the Infant

Neonatal reflexes must be lost before motor development can proceed.

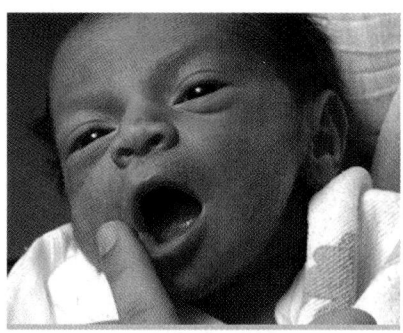

FIGURE 24-26 Rooting Reflex

ROOTING REFLEX.

E 1. Place the infant supine with the head in a midline position.

2. With your forefinger, stroke the skin located at one corner of the mouth (Figure 24-26).

3. Observe movement of the head.

N Up until 3 or 4 months of age, the infant will turn the head toward the side that was stroked. In the sleeping infant, the rooting reflex can be present normally until 6 months of age.

A An absent rooting reflex from birth through 3 to 4 months is abnormal.

P Central nervous system disease such as frontal lobe lesions accounts for an absent rooting reflex.

SUCKING REFLEX.

E 1. Place the infant in a supine position.

2. With your forefinger, touch the infant's lips to stimulate a response (Figure 24-27).

3. Observe for a sucking motion.

N The sucking reflex occurs up to approximately 10 months.

A Absence of the sucking reflex is abnormal.

P A premature infant or a breast-fed infant of a mother who ingests barbiturates does not exhibit the reflex secondary to CNS depression.

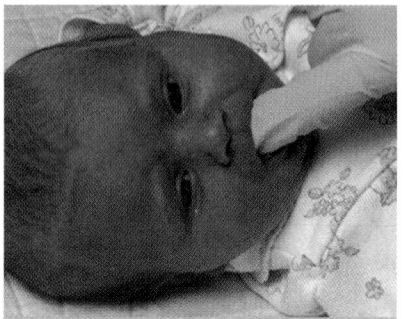

FIGURE 24-27 Sucking Reflex

PALMAR GRASP REFLEX.

E 1. Place the infant supine with the head in a midline position.

2. Place the ulnar sides of both index fingers into the infant's hands while the infant's arms are in a semiflexed position (Figure 24-28).

3. Press your fingers into the infant's palmar surfaces.

N Normally, the infant grasps your fingers in flexion.

A Presence of the palmar grasp reflex after 4 months of age is abnormal.

P The etiology is attributed to frontal lobe lesions.

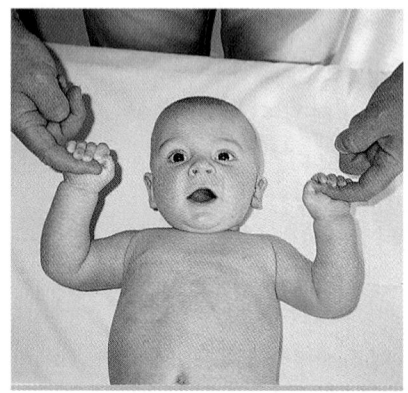

FIGURE 24-28 Palmar Reflex

TONIC NECK REFLEX.

E 1. Place the infant in a supine position on the examination table.

2. Rotate the head to one side and hold the jaw area parallel to the shoulder.

3. Observe for movement of the extremities.

N The upper and lower extremities on the side to which the jaw is turned extend, and the opposite arm and leg flex (Figure 24-29). Sometimes, this reflex does not show up until 6 to 8 weeks of age.

A After 6 months of age, the tonic neck reflex is abnormal.

P Cerebral damage is suspected if the tonic neck reflex is seen after 6 months of age.

STEPPING REFLEX.

E 1. Stand behind the infant, grasp the infant under the axillae, and bring the body to a standing position on a flat surface. Use the thumbs to support the back of the head if needed.

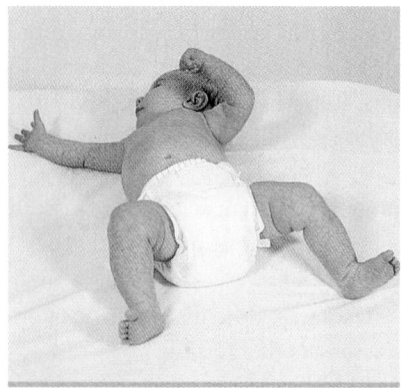

FIGURE 24-29 Tonic Neck Reflex

| **E** Examination | **N** Normal Findings | **A** Abnormal Findings | **P** Pathophysiology |

2. Push the infant's feet toward a flat surface and simultaneously lean the infant's body forward (Figure 24-30).

3. Observe the legs and feet for stepping movements.

N Stepping movements are made by flexing one leg and moving the other leg forward. This reflex disappears at about 3 months of age.

A Presence of the stepping reflex beyond 3 months of age is abnormal.

P Patients with CP demonstrate a stepping reflex beyond 3 months of age.

PLANTAR GRASP REFLEX.

E 1. Position the infant supine on the examination table.

2. Elevate the foot to be examined.

3. Touch the infant's foot on the plantar surface beneath the toes (Figure 24-31).

4. Repeat on the other side.

N The toes curl down until 8 months of age.

A It is abnormal for the plantar grasp reflex to be absent on one or both feet.

P An obstructive lesion such as an abscess or tumor can cause the plantar grasp reflex to be absent on the affected side. Bilateral absence can occur in CP.

BABINSKI REFLEX.

E 1. Position the infant supine on the examination table.

2. Elevate the foot to be examined.

3. Stroke the plantar surface of the foot from the lateral heel upward with the tip of the thumbnail.

N A child less than 15 to 18 months of age normally fans the toes outward and dorsiflexes the great toe (Figure 24-32).

A After the child masters walking, presence of the Babinski reflex is abnormal.

P Presence of the Babinski reflex after 18 months of age can be indicative of a perinatal insult such as cerebral palsy.

MORO (STARTLE) REFLEX.

E 1. Place the infant supine on the examination table.

2. Make a sudden, loud noise such as hitting your hand on the examination table.

3. Another technique is to brace the infant's neck and back on the undersurface of your arm while holding the undersurface of the buttocks with the other hand and then mimicking a falling motion by quickly lowering the infant.

N The infant under 4 months of age quickly extends, then flexes the arms and fingers while the maneuver is performed. The thumb and index fingers form a C shape (see Figure 24-33).

A Presence of the startle reflex after 4 to 6 months of age is abnormal.

P Neurological disease such as CP can be a cause of a positive response after the normal age of disappearance.

GALANT REFLEX.

E 1. Place the infant prone, with the infant's hands under the abdomen.

2. Use your index finger to stroke the skin along the side of the spine (see Figure 24-34).

3. Observe the stimulated side for any movement.

N An infant less than 1 to 2 months of age will turn the pelvis and shoulders toward the stimulated side.

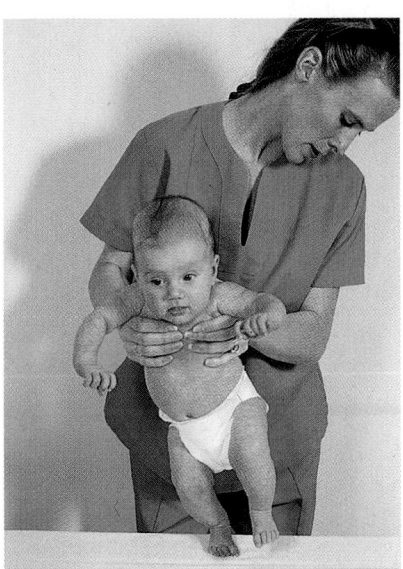

FIGURE 24-30 Stepping Reflex

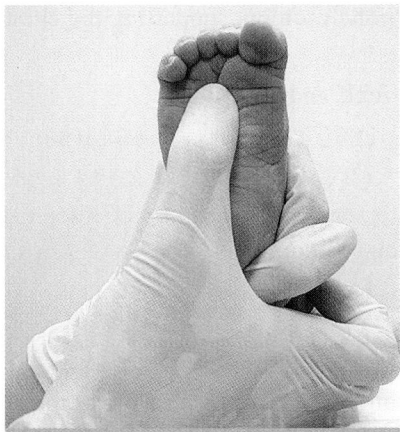

FIGURE 24-31 Plantar Grasp Reflex

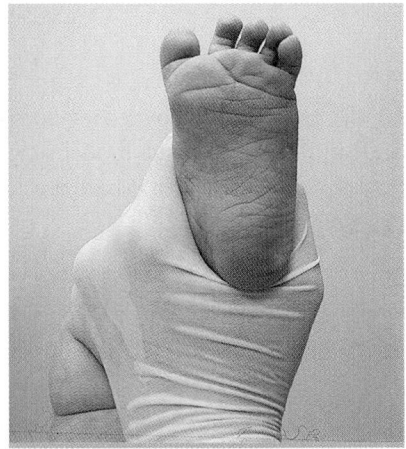

FIGURE 24-32 Babinski Reflex

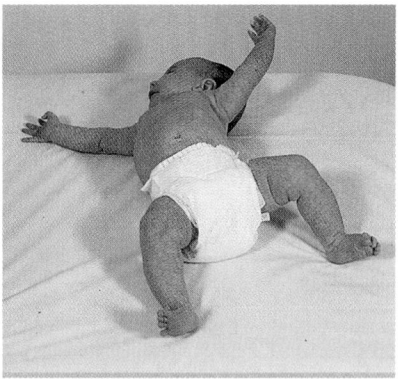

FIGURE 24-33   **Moro Reflex**

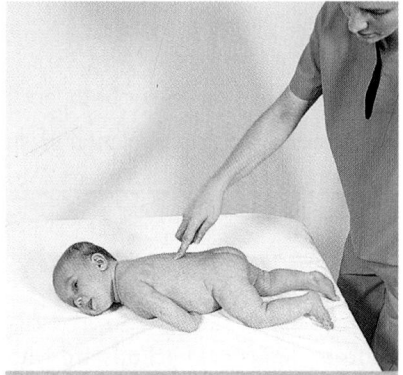

FIGURE 24-34   **Galant Reflex**

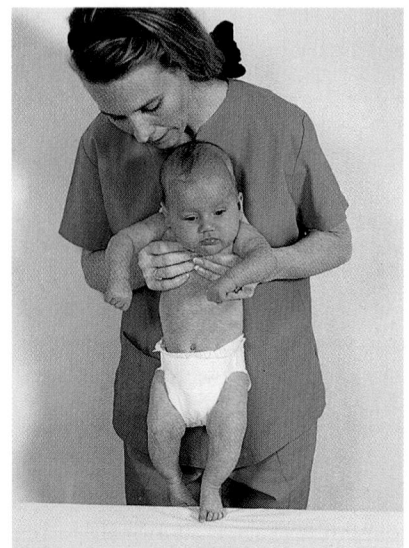

FIGURE 24-35   **Placing Reflex**

A   Lack of response from an infant less than 2 months of age is abnormal.

P   A spinal cord lesion is suspected.

PLACING REFLEX.

Do not test the placing and stepping reflexes at the same time because they are two different reflexes.

E   1. Grasp the infant under the axillae from behind and bring the body to a standing position. Use the thumbs to support the back of the head if needed.

   2. Touch the dorsum of one foot to the edge of the examination table (Figure 24-35).

   3. Observe the tested leg for movement.

N   The infant's tested leg will flex and lift onto the examination table.

A   Lack of response is abnormal.

P   It is difficult to elicit this reflex in breech-born babies and in those with paralysis or cerebral cortex abnormalities.

LANDAU REFLEX.

E   1. Carefully suspend the infant in a prone position, supporting the chest with your hand.

   2. Observe for extension of the head, trunk, and hips.

N   The arms and legs extend during the reflex. The reflex appears at about 3 months of age.

A   Presence of the Landau reflex beyond 2 years of age is abnormal. Also, it is abnormal for the infant to assume a limp position.

P   Mental retardation may account for an abnormality.

Cranial Nerve Function

A thorough assessment of cranial nerve function is difficult to perform on the infant less than 1 year old. Difficulty is also encountered with toddlers and preschoolers because they often cannot follow directions or are not willing to cooperate. Testing for the school-age child or the adolescent is carried out in the same manner as for an adult.

INFANT (BIRTH TO 12 MONTHS).

E   1. To test cranial nerves (CNs) III, IV, and VI, move a brightly colored toy along the infant's line of vision. An infant older than 1 month responds by following the object. Also evaluate the pupillary response to a bright light in each eye.

   2. CN V is tested by assessing the rooting or sucking reflexes.

   3. CN VII is tested up until 2 months by assessng the sucking reflex and by observing symmetrical sucking movements. After 2 months of age, an infant will smile, allowing assessment of symmetry of facial expressions.

   4. A positive Moro reflex in an infant less than 6 months old is evidence of normal functioning of CN VIII.

   5. CNs IX and X are examined by using a tongue blade to produce a gag reflex. Do not test if a positive response was already elicited by using a tongue blade to view the posterior pharynx.

| **E** Examination | **N** Normal Findings | **A** Abnormal Findings | **P** Pathophysiology |

6. To test CN XI, evaluate the infant's ability to lift the head up while in a prone position.

7. CN XII is assessed by allowing the infant to suck on a pacifier or a bottle, abruptly removing the pacifier or bottle from the infant's mouth, and observing for lingering sucking movements.

N/A/P See Chapter 19.

TODDLER AND PRESCHOOLER (1 TO 5 YEARS).

E 1. The older preschooler is able to identify familiar odors. Most children readily identify the smells of peanut butter and chocolate. Test CN I one side at a time by asking the child to close the eyes and to identify the smells of peanut butter and chocolate. Test each nostril with different substances while occluding the other nostril with your finger.

2. Test vision (CN II) using Allen cards.

3. CNs III, IV, and VI are tested in the same fashion as for the infant.

4. CN V is tested by giving the child something to eat and evaluating chewing movements. Sensory responses to light and sharp touch are still not easily interpreted in these age groups.

5. Observe facial weakness or paralysis (CN VII) by making the child smile or laugh. An older preschooler may cooperate by raising the eyebrows, frowning, puffing the cheeks out, and closing the eyes tightly on command.

6. To evaluate CN VIII, ring a small bell out of the child's vision and observe the response to unseen sounds.

7. Test CNs IX and X in the same manner as for the infant.

8. CN XII is difficult to assess in this particular age group.

N/A/P See Chapter 19.

FEMALE GENITALIA

General Approach

1. Place the up-to-preschool-age child on the caregiver's lap or examination table. Ask the caregiver to assist by holding the child's legs in a froglike position. Place the child older than 4 years on the examination table in a semilithotomy position, without the feet in stirrups. Reserve the lithotomy position with the feet in stirrups for the older adolescent.

2. Explain the procedure prior to the assessment. Never ask the caregiver of the infant or young school-age child to leave the room during this portion of the examination because the caregiver is a source of comfort to the child.

3. The child should be told before the genitalia exam that it is all right for the provider to touch the genitals with the parent present but not for anyone else to do so for any reason.

4. Drape the older-than-preschool-age child.

5. A vaginal and pelvic exam is not routinely performed on young females. A vaginal assessment is warranted, however, when signs of possible sexual abuse are present. See the Nursing Alert on Signs of Sexual Abuse in Children later in this chapter. The assessment is undertaken by a health care provider who is trained to perform pediatric vaginal examinations and can evaluate these problems.

6. Any female who has reached menarche needs to be evaluated for a pregnant uterus, when dictated by the health history.

Inspection

SEXUAL MATURITY RATING.

E 1. Using the Tanner stages in Table 20-1, assess the developmental stage of the pubic hair.

2. Determine the SMR.

N Adolescents usually start developing pubic hair by 8 to 12 years of age. Females usually reach the adult stage by age 15.

A An SMR that is less than expected for a female's age is abnormal.

P Delayed puberty may be familial, genetic, or caused by chronic illnesses.

PERINEAL AREA.

E See Chapter 20.

N The infant's labia minora are sometimes larger than the labia majora. The hymen is sometimes intact up until the point of sexual activity.

A It is abnormal for the female infant to display a rudimentary penis in the clitoral area.

P Genital ambiguity occurs during embryonic development as a consequence of genetic causes, androgens, or androgen inhibitors that reverse genital characteristics.

A A bloody discharge noted at the vaginal opening or on the diaper is abnormal.

P It is not uncommon to note pseudomenstruation in an infant under 2 weeks of age. Maternal hormones such as estrogen are the cause.

MALE GENITALIA

General Approach

1. Female nurses may encounter difficulty assessing a reluctant adolescent. Be firm when explaining that this portion of the assessment is a required part of his examination. Infants and toddlers do not object to the assessment.
2. In case the infant or toddler urinates during the examination, have a diaper or disposable cloth available to catch the stream of urine.
3. The older school-age child and the adolescent should be draped in order to maintain modesty.

Inspection

SEXUAL MATURITY RATING.

E 1. Using the Tanner stages in Table 21-1, assess the developmental stage of the pubic hair, penis, and scrotum.

2. Determine the SMR.

N Males usually begin puberty between the ages of 9½ and 13½. The average male proceeds through puberty in about 3 years, with a possible range of 2 to 5 years.

A An SMR that is less than expected for a male's age is abnormal.

P Delayed puberty may be familial or caused by chronic illnesses.

A A normally formed but diminutive penis is abnormal. There is a discrepancy between the penile size and the age of the individual.

E Examination   **N** Normal Findings   **A** Abnormal Findings   **P** Pathophysiology

P A **microphallus** penis can result from a disorder in the hypothalamus or pituitary gland. It may be secondary to primary testicular failure due to partial androgen insensitivity. Maternal DES exposure has teratogenic effects caused by defects in nonandrogen-dependent regulatory agents. Microphallus can also be idiopathic in nature.

A It is abnormal when the penis appears larger than what is generally expected for the stated age. This condition is usually evident only before the age of normal puberty.

P Hormonal influence of tumors of the pineal gland or hypothalamus, tumors of the Leydig cells of the testes, tumors of the adrenal gland, or precocious genital maturity may cause penile hyperplasia.

A A testicle that is smaller and softer than normal (less in the fully developed male) is abnormal.

P An atrophic testicle may be the result of Klinefelter's syndrome (hypogonadism), hypopituitarism, estrogen therapy, or orchitis.

PENIS.

E 1. Note the appearance of the penis. If you are not able to determine circumcision status, ask the caregiver if the child was circumcised.

2. Note the position of the urethral meatus.

N The meatus is normally found on the tip of the penis. A disappearing penis phenomenon occurs normally in infants with increased adipose tissue in the area surrounding the penis. Reassure the caregiver that this is normal and will resolve after adipose tissue is lost.

A It is abnormal for the urethral meatus to be located behind or along the ventral side of the penis.

P During the third month of fetal development, the urethral meatus fails to move toward the glans penis, creating a condition known as hypospadias. Children at greater risk for hypospadias are those whose mothers were on hydantoin for epilepsy during pregnancy.

A It is abnormal for the meatal opening to be on the dorsal surface of the penis.

P During the third month of fetal development, the urethral meatus fails to move toward the glans penis, causing an epispadias deformity.

SCROTUM.

E 1. Evaluate scrotal size and color.

2. Note if the testes are seen in the scrotal sac.

N The scrotum appears proportionately large in size when compared to the penis. The sac color is brown or black in dark-skinned children and pink in light-skinned children. Two testes should be present, but, in infants, they may retract into the inguinal canal or abdomen due to various stimuli, including cold and palpation.

A/P See Chapter 21.

Palpation

SCROTUM.

E 1. Place the infant in a supine position on the examination table. Instruct the young child to sit cross-legged to inhibit the cremasteric reflex from occurring. The older child may be allowed to stand for this portion of the exam.

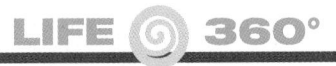

Sexual Maturity Concerns of Adolescent Males

You are the pediatric nurse practitioner performing physical examinations on middle school-age males. While performing a hernia check, you inspect the genitalia and assess the Tanner stage of sexual development in 13-year-old Harry. After the examination, you ask Harry if he has any questions. Sheepishly he asks you why he is not as big down there as his friends. How would you answer Harry? What anticipatory guidance would you provide?

2. Locate each testis within the scrotal sac by using the fingers of one hand in a milking motion to cause the testes to descend.

3. Palpate and note the size, shape, and mobility of each testis.

N See Chapter 21.

A It is abnormal to be unable to palpate the testes.

P **Cryptorchidism** is a failure of a testis to descend into the scrotal sac. One or both testes failing to descend within the inguinal canal occurs during embryonic development.

A An enlargement of the scrotum is abnormal.

P A congenital hydrocele results from failure of the male reproductive tract to develop properly while the fetus is in utero. This mass will transilluminate.

HERNIA.

E **1.** For the infant who is unable to stand, place him supine on the examination table. All other children should stand during the examination.

2. Use the little finger for the infant's and the index finger for the younger child's examination.

3. Follow the inguinal canal as is done on an adult male.

4. If possible, perform the assessment on a crying infant.

5. Have preschoolers and early school-age children attempt to blow up a balloon while you palpate the inguinal areas.

6. Palpate the inguinal areas while the older school-age child or adolescent coughs.

N/A/P See Chapter 21.

ANUS

As a rule, rectal assessments are not performed on children unless you detect a problem or suspect abuse; in these cases, refer children for further evaluation if you are not trained specifically for this procedure and follow your institution's guidelines.

Inspection

E **1.** Ask the child to lie on the abdomen.

2. Gently separate the buttocks to allow direct visualization of the anal opening.

3. Observe for bleeding, fissures, prolapse, skin tags, hemorrhoids, lesions, and pinworms.

4. During separation of the buttocks, observe any movement of the anus.

5. Stroke the perianal area with your finger and note any movement. This is called the anal reflex or anal wink.

N No bleeding, fissures, prolapse, skin tags, hemorrhoids, lesions, or pinworms should be present. An anal reflex is observed.

A An absent anal reflex is abnormal.

P Conditions such as a spinal cord lesion, trauma, and tumors that interrupt nervous innervation to the anal sphincter cause this finding.

E Examination   **N** Normal Findings   **A** Abnormal Findings   **P** Pathophysiology

The Patient with Accidental Ingestion of Kerosene

This case study illustrates the application and objective documentation of the pediatric assessment.
Pei Nguyen is a 20-month-old Asian female transported by ambulance from the pediatrician's office. The mother is present on the child's arrival to the emergency department.

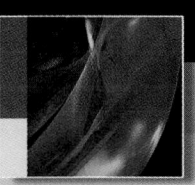

HEALTH HISTORY

LEGAL GUARDIAN	Mr. and Mrs. Tuan Nguyen
SOURCE OF INFORMATION	Mrs. My Hanh Nguyen (mother)
PATIENT PROFILE	20-month-old Asian female
CHIEF COMPLAINT	"Pei got into some kerosene her grandfather stored in the garage." (per mother's report)
HISTORY OF PRESENT ILLNESS	Mom and siblings were visiting grandparents for lunch. After lunch the children were taken outside by the grandfather to play while mom and grandmother cleaned up the kitchen. Grandfather had kerosene stored in a glass soft drink bottle in the garage. Mom states grandfather walked up to Pei just as she swallowed a "mouthful" of the liquid substance. Mom rushed child to Dr. Jink's office about ½ mile from the grandparents' house. Upon arrival, Pei vomited twice, nonbloody emesis. Dr. Jink's office staff called for an ambulance. Within minutes Pei began grunting with an ↑ RR and shortness of breath.

PAST HEALTH HISTORY

Birth History

Prenatal	Mother has 4 children carried full term. All were planned pregnancies. Prenatal care started at 10 wks. Denies drug, alcohol, tobacco, caffeine, or ibuprofen use during pregnancy.
Labor and Delivery	Pt full term at 39 weeks gestation, spontaneous vaginal delivery after a 6 hr labor; father cut cord in delivery room, newborn put to breast immediately, Apgar scores were 7 and 9; birth wt was 3.8 kg (8.4 lbs), length was 54.0 cm (21.3 in.)
Postnatal	Mom and baby home after 48 hours, no feeding or breathing problems; hepatitis B vaccine administered in hospital, breastfed without difficulty, dad able to take 1 wk off following birth.
Medical History	No reported health problems
Surgical History	No reported past surgery
Allergies	No known allergies
Medications	None per mother's report

continues

CASE STUDY (Continued)
The Patient with Accidental Ingestion of Kerosene

Communicable Diseases	No known exposures
Injuries and Accidents	None
Blood Transfusions	None
Immunizations	Up-to-date per mother's report, no records available

FAMILY HEALTH HISTORY

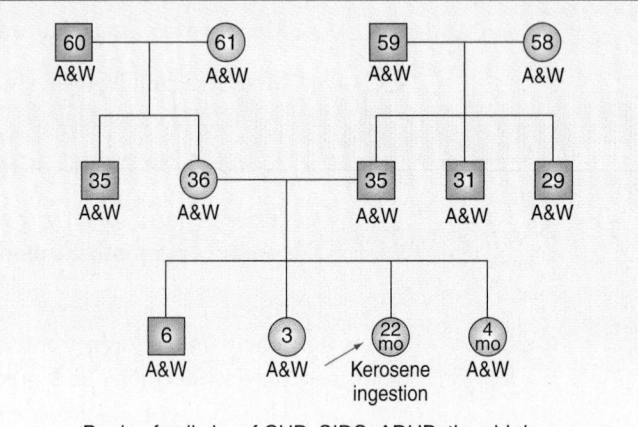

LEGEND
- ○ Living female
- □ Living male
- ⊗ Deceased female
- ⊠ Deceased male
- ╱ Points to patient

A&W = Alive and well
ADHD = Attention-deficit hyperactivity disorder
CHD = Childhood diseases
dz = Disease
SIDS = Sudden infant death syndrome

Denies family hx of CHD, SIDS, ADHD, thyroid dz.

SOCIAL HISTORY

Alcohol, Tobacco, and Drug Use, Sexual Practice	N/A
Domestic and Intimate Partner Violence	Denies
Travel History	Family has not traveled more than 50 miles from home since Pei's birth.
School Performance	N/A
Home Environment	Family lives in a 5-BR home built in 1999; no guns in home; caregivers deny use of alcohol or drugs; one outside dog; two turtles in a cage in the kitchen
Hobbies, Leisure Activities, Stress, Education	N/A
Economic Status	Pei's parents carry health insurance with a $1 million cap through the father's employer.
Military Service	N/A
Religion	Church of Jesus Christ of Latter-Day Saints; family converted 5 yrs ago; My Hahn stays home to care for the 4 children; has wkly gathering with other women from her LDS community; Tuan involved with outreach in LDS

continues

CASE STUDY (Continued)
The Patient with Accidental Ingestion of Kerosene

Ethnic Background	Pei's grandparents originally from Vietnam; family celebrates some Vietnamese holidays
Roles and Relationships	Parents married; mom is sole caregiver for children, dad works as an engineer at a chemical company
Child's Personal Habits	Pei likes a pacifier at naptime and bedtime
Characteristic Patterns of Daily Living	"Pei does what every toddler does… sleeps, plays, eats, gets into everything!" states mother.
HEALTH MAINTENANCE ACTIVITIES	
Sleep	Takes 1 nap per day from 12:30 PM to 2:30 PM, sleeps at night from 8 PM to 8 AM. Shares bedroom with 3 yo female sibling
Diet	Takes variety of table foods including meats, vegetables, fruits, and grains. Eats 3 meals per day plus 2 snacks. Total intake of whole milk = 24 oz/day, 8 oz of water/day, does not drink juice
Exercise	Plays with siblings, runs around backyard and playground daily
Use of Safety Devices	Car seat used at all times, forward-facing middle seat of van
Safety	House childproofed with outlet covers, gates on stairs leading to basement, all poisons locked on high shelf of kitchen cabinet, medications locked in same cabinet, poison control center's number posted next to phone, smoke and carbon monoxide detectors on first floor and basement, fire extinguisher located under sink in kitchen, mother is CPR certified for infant and child CPR
Health Check-ups	Up-to-date on all well-child checks
DEVELOPMENT	
Gross Motor and Fine Motor-Adaptive	All milestones met, walks, runs, able to walk up stairs, able to throw ball overhand, able to build tower of 6 blocks, holds crayon in Ⓡ hand and scribbles
Language	Speech understandable, combines 2 words, able to point to 6 body parts
Personal-Social	Able to undress self, puts on shirt and pull-up shorts, brushes teeth with help, washes and dries hands
PHYSICAL ASSESSMENT	
Vital Signs	T: 98.7°F axillary; pulse: 184; resp: 36; B/P: 122/90; SpO_2: 100%
Physical Growth	Wt: 13.2 kg (29 lbs) (75th–90th %); length: 84.0 cm (33 in.) (50th %); head circumference: 48 cm (18.9 in.) (50th %)

continues

Skin

Inspection

No erythema, papules, vesicles, scaling, ulcerations, or edema; pale skin

Palpation

Soft, smooth $\bar{s}$ roughness, dryness, scaliness, or keratic areas; turgor WNL, no diaphoresis; extremities cool to touch $\bar{c}$ 3-second capillary refill in all 4 extremities

Hair and Nails

Inspection and Palpation

Hair soft, nails clean

Head

Inspection

Symmetrical, round, no bulges or prominences of forehead, no involuntary movements, face symmetrical

Palpation

Anterior and posterior fontanel closed

Eyes

Vision Screening

N/A

Inspection

No ptosis, sclera white, positive optical blink response, conjunctiva nonerythematous, cornea smooth and transparent, iris blue, PERRLA, $\oplus$ red reflex, optic disc creamy $\bar{s}$ hemorrhages

Ears

Auditory Testing

Reacts to loud noises, follows simple commands

Inspection (External Ear)

Top of pinna positioned at level of eyebrows bilaterally, pinna $\bar{s}$ lesions or masses

Palpation (External Ear)

No pain $\bar{c}$ movement

Inspection (Internal Ear)

No erythema or cerumen in canal, bilateral TMs pearly $\bar{s}$ retraction, bulging, perforation, fluid, or air bubbles; TMs move well, landmarks intact, $\oplus$ light reflex

Nose

Inspection

Patent nares $\bar{c}$ mild flaring, mucosa pink, septum midline, no edema of turbinates

Mouth and Throat

Inspection

Lips pink, no fissures/cracking, edges meet, buccal mucosa pink $\bar{s}$ lesions, 16 teeth present and in good condition $\bar{s}$ visible caries, tongue pink and midline, normal positioned palate, both hard and soft palates intact $\bar{s}$ lesions, tonsils 1+/4+, no erythema or exudates, uvula midline

continues

CASE STUDY (Continued)
The Patient with Accidental Ingestion of Kerosene

Neck

Inspection — Symmetrical, no edema noted

Palpation — Thyroid nonpalpable, trachea midline, no lymphadenopathy

Breasts and Regional Lymphatics

Inspection — Tanner stage 1, no retractions, erythema, venous distention, edema; areolas circular and even bilaterally, negative masses/ulcerations, nipples circular s̄ retractions/inversions, erythema, discharge, ulceration, or supernumerary nipples

Palpation — Negative for nodes, glands, masses, or tenderness; axillary area: nonpalpable nodes, negative tenderness or masses

Thorax and Lungs

Inspection — Thorax round, mild subcostal and intercostal retractions

Palpation — ⊕ tactile fremitus bilaterally

Percussion — Diaphragmatic excursion 1 ICS bilaterally

Auscultation — Breath sounds equal bilaterally, bronchial sounds over trachea, bronchovesicular breath sounds throughout peripheral lung fields, coarse rales throughout

Heart and Peripheral Vasculature

Inspection — Apical impulse at 4th ICS Ⓛ of MCL, no heaves, precordial lifts, no digital clubbing, negative JVD

Palpation — Negative thrill, no brachial/femoral lag, pulses 2+/4+ bilaterally

Auscultation — Apical HR even and regular, normal S_1 and S_2, no S_3 or S_4 audible, no M/G/R

Abdomen

Inspection — Rounded and symmetrical, abdominal musculature continuous, no visible peristalsis

Auscultation — ⊕ bowel sounds in all 4 quadrants, no venous hums, no bruits at femoral, iliac, renal, or aortic areas; no peritoneal friction rub

Percussion — Tympanic

Palpation — No pain or tenderness, no masses, no HSM, kidneys nonpalpable

Musculoskeletal

Inspection — AROM in all 4 extremities

continues

CASE STUDY   (Continued)
The Patient with Accidental Ingestion of Kerosene

Palpation	WNL for age
Neurological	
Inspection	Cranial nerves II–XII grossly intact
Female Genitalia	
Inspection	Tanner stage 1, labia s̄ hypertrophy, no rashes, perineum smooth s̄ lacerations, hymen intact
Rectum and Anus	
Inspection	Anal area s̄ lesions, bleeding, fissures, prolapse, or hemorrhoids

ASSESSMENT IN BRIEF

Pediatric Patient Assessment*

Developmental Assessment
- Denver II

Physical Growth
- Weight
- Length and height
- Head circumference
- Chest circumference
- Body mass index

Physical Assessment
- Apgar scoring
- Head
  - Inspection
    Head control
  - Palpation
    Anterior fontanel
    Posterior fontanel
    Suture lines
    Surface characteristics
- Eyes
  - Vision screening
    Allen test
    Color vision screening

- Musculoskeletal system
  - Inspection
    Tibiofemoral bones
  - Palpation
    Feet (metatarsus varus)
    Hip and femur (Ortolani's maneuver)
- Neurological System
  - Rooting reflex
  - Sucking reflex
  - Palmar grasp reflex
  - Tonic neck reflex
  - Stepping reflex
  - Plantar grasp reflex
  - Babinski reflex
  - Moro (startle) reflex
  - Galant reflex
  - Placing reflex
  - Landau reflex

Advanced Techniques
- Assessing for hydrocephalus and anencephaly: Transillumination of the skull
- Assessing for coarctation of the aorta

Only pediatric-specific tests are listed.

REVIEW QUESTIONS

1. Hannah, a 13-year-old female patient, is at her primary care provider's office for a well-child check. Dr. Hall is concerned about a weight gain of 10 kilograms over the past year. Which of the following pieces of information is most important?
   a. Family history of obesity
   b. BMI
   c. Vital signs
   d. School adaptation
   The correct answer is (b).

2. Julia's mother called the nurse referral line of the local children's hospital, stating she is concerned about her daughter's recent withdrawn behavior. Which of the following behavior warrants immediate evaluation?
   a. Wanting to be alone in her room
   b. Ignoring her siblings and parents at the dinner table
   c. Giving her friend a prized rabbit's foot
   d. Ignoring curfew rules
   The correct answer is (c).

3. In the 2008 recommendations for Preventive Pediatric Health Care policy statement by the American Academy of Pediatrics, the measurement of head circumference is recommended up to which age?
   a. 2 months   c. 18 months
   b. 9 months   d. 24 months
   The correct answer is (d).

4. The nurse caring for Jacob in Room 2135 suspects child abuse. Which of the following observations led the nurse to suspect abuse?
   a. Constant crying despite consoling measures
   b. Scratch mark near the ankle where the identification band is placed
   c. Bruising noted on the patient's back near the left shoulder
   d. Circumferential erythema at the antecubital area where the previous nurse had started an IV
   The correct answer is (c).

5. Sean, a 2-year-old toddler, comes into the clinic for his yearly well-child check. He is extremely upset when approached. Which of the following measures would help Sean?
   a. Allowing the mother to reschedule Sean's appointment
   b. Allowing Sean's mother to hold him during the examination
   c. Allowing Sean's mother to step out of the room while you take his vital signs

   d. Allowing Sean to take a walk outside with his mother while he calms down
   The correct answer is (b).

6. A 7-month-old patient is admitted to the hospital for dehydration. As the health care provider for this patient, you are assessing reflex mechanisms. You note that the rooting reflex is absent. At what age does the rooting reflex disappear in the nonsleeping infant?
   a. 2 months   c. 6 months
   b. 4 months   d. 8 months
   The correct answer is (b).

7. You are educating a new mother on safety guidelines for her newborn infant. Which of the following information should you give when discussing SIDS prevention?
   a. Allow the newborn to sleep in the parent's bed.
   b. Place the newborn on his/her back when sleeping.
   c. Prop the newborn on a pillow when sleeping.
   d. Burp the newborn before putting him/her down to sleep.
   The correct answer is (b).

8. Rota, the rotavirus vaccine, must be started before what age?
   a. 6 weeks   c. 10 weeks
   b. 8 weeks   d. 12 weeks
   The correct answer is (d).

9. At birth, a Caucasian infant has a heart rate of 112, a respiratory rate that is slow and irregular, and full flexion of the limbs; is crying; and has acrocyanotic limbs with a pink torso. What is the Apgar score of this infant?
   a. 7   c. 9
   b. 8   d. 10
   The correct answer is (b).

10. Which of the following is an expected finding in a 3-year-old toddler in a vision screening assessment?
    a. Tumbling E chart: right eye 20/30
    b. Hirschberg test: light reflection located on the inner margin of the left cornea as the eye deviates outward
    c. Cover/uncover test: both eyes move to focus on the penlight
    d. Snellen chart: left eye 20/50
    The correct answer is (a).

Visit the Estes online companion resource at
www.delmar.cengage.com
for additional content and study aids.
Click on Online Companions, and then
select the Nursing discipline.

REFERENCES

Boynton, R. W., Dunn, E. S., Stephens, G. R., & Pulcini, J. (2003). *Manual of ambulatory pediatrics* (5th ed.). Philadelphia: Lippincott.

Centers for Disease Control and Prevention. (2008). Catch-up immunization schedule for persons aged 4 months–18 years who start late or who are more than 1 month behind. Retrieved March 10, 2008, from http://www.cdc.gov/vaccines/recs/acip/default.htm

Centers for Disease Control and Prevention. (2008). Recommended immunization schedule for persons aged 0–6 years. Retrieved March 10, 2008, from http://www.cdc.gov/vaccines/recs/acip/default.htm

Centers for Disease Control and Prevention. (2008). Recommended immunization schedule for persons aged 7–18 years. Retrieved March 10, 2008, from http://www.cdc.gov/vaccines/recs/acip/default.htm

Committee on Practice and Ambulatory Medicine and Bright Futures Steering Committee. (2007). Recommendations for preventive pediatric health care. *Pediatrics, 120*(6), 1376.

Frankenburg, W. K. (1990). *Denver II screening manual.* Denver, CO: Denver Developmental Materials, Inc.

Gerchufsky, M. (1994). Lead poisoning. *Advance for Nurse Practitioners, 2*(11), 19–37.

BIBLIOGRAPHY

American Academy of Pediatrics. (2008). *Pediatric clinical practice guidelines & policies* (8th ed.). Elk Grove Village, IL: Author.

Anderson, C. A. (2000). Revisiting the parenting profile assessment to screen for child abuse. *Journal of Nursing Scholarship, 31*(1), 53.

Blackmon, L. R., Patton, D. G., Bell, E. F., Engle, W. A., Kanto, W. P., Martin, G. J., et al. (2003). Apnea, sudden infant death syndrome, and home monitoring. *Pediatrics, 111*, 914–917.

Custer, J. W., Rau, R. E., & Lee, C. K. (2008). *The Harriet Lane handbook: A manual for pediatric house officers* (18th ed.). Philadelphia: Elsevier.

Doshi, N. R., & Rodriguez, M. L. F. (2007). Amblyopia. *American Family Physician, 75*(3), 361–367.

Fleisher, G. R., Ludwig, S., & Henretig, F. M. (2006). *Textbook of pediatric emergency medicine* (5th ed.). Philadelphia: Lippincott, Williams & Wilkins.

Fonseca, H., & Greydanus, D. E. (2007). Sexuality in the child, teen, and young adult: Concepts for the clinician. *Primary Care: Clinics in Office Practice, 34*(2), 275–292.

Hayes, D. N., & Sege, R. (2003). FiGHTS: A preliminary screening tool for adolescent firearms-carrying. *Annals of Emergency Medicine, 42*(6), 798–807.

Kleigman, R., Marcdante, K., Jenson, H., & Behrman, R. (2006). *Nelson essentials of pediatrics* (5th ed.). Philadelphia: W. B. Saunders.

Mitchell, K. J., Finkelhor, D., & Wolak, J. (2007). Youth Internet users at risk for the most serious online sexual solicitations. *American Journal of Preventive Medicine, 32*(6), 532–537.

National High Blood Pressure Education Program Working Group on High Blood Pressure in Children and Adolescents. (2004). The fourth report on the diagnosis, evaluation, and treatment of high blood pressure in children and adolescents. *Pediatrics, 114*, 555–576.

Pearce, P. F., Harrell, J. S., & McMurray, R. G. (2008). Middle-school children's understanding of physical activity: "If you're moving, you're doing physical activity." *Journal of Pediatric Nursing, 23*(3), 169–182.

Potts, N. L., & Mandleco, B. L. (2007). *Pediatric nursing, caring for children and their families* (2nd ed.). Clifton Park, NY: Delmar Cengage Learning.

Pruitt, B. (2005). Keeping respiratory syncytial virus at bay. *Nursing 2005, 35*(11), 62–64.

Rebeschi, L. M., & Brown, M. L. H. (2007). *Pediatric nurse's survival guide* (3rd ed.). Clifton Park, NY: Delmar Cengage Learning.

Ricciardi, R. (2008). The first pelvic examination in the adolescent: An update. *The Journal for Nurse Practitioners, 4*(5), 377–383.

Sampson, H. A. (2005). Food allergy—accurately identifying clinical reactivity. *Allergy, 60*(s79), 19–24.

Spragud, L. J., Piira, T., & von Baeyer, C. L. (2003). Children's self-report of pain intensity—The FACES pain scale revised. *American Journal of Nursing, 103*(12), 62–64.

Steinmann, R. (2007). Pediatric diabetic ketoacidosis. *American Journal of Nursing, 107*(3), 72 cc–72 kk.

Tingen, M. S., Waller, J. L., Smith, T. M., Baker, R. R., Reyes, J., & Treiber, F. A. (2006). Tobacco prevention in children and cessation in family members. *Journal of the American Academy of Nurse Practitioners, 18*(4), 169–179.

Von Sadovszky, V., Kovar, C. K., Brown, C., & Armbuster, M. (2006). The need for sexual health information: Perceptions and desires of young adults. *The American Journal of Maternal/Child Nursing, 31*(6), 373–380.

Zitelli, B., & Davis, H. (2007). *Atlas of pediatric physical diagnosis* (5th ed.). Philadelphia: Elsevier.

WEB SITES

Alcohol and Drug Information, U.S. Department of Health and Human Services:
http://www.health.org

American Academy of Pediatrics:
http://www.aap.org

Anabolic Steroid Abuse, NIDA:
http://www.steroidabuse.gov

Bright Futures:
http://www.brightfutures.org

Centers for Disease Control and Prevention:
http://www.cdc.gov

ClubDrugs.gov, NIDA:
http://www.clubdrugs.gov

The Congenital Heart Information Network:
http://www.tchin.org

KidsHealth:
http://www.kidshealth.org

National Association of Pediatric Nurse Practitioners:
http://www.napnap.org

CHAPTER 25
The Elderly Patient

COMPETENCIES

1. Describe the structural and physiological variations of the older adult compared with a nongeriatric patient.

2. Discuss techniques that facilitate the health history interview of the older adult.

3. Discuss various tools that can be used to assess functional status and cognition in the older adult.

4. Describe modifications of the physical assessment techniques for use within the older adult population.

5. Perform inspection, palpation, percussion, and auscultation in a head-to-toe assessment of the older adult.

6. Document a complete health history and physical examination of the older adult.

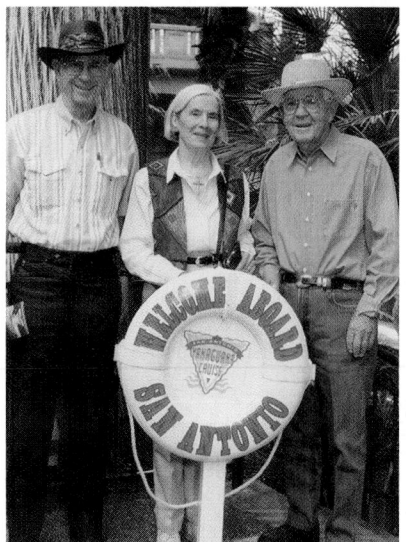

FIGURE 25-1 **Older adults are the population group increasing at the fastest rate. Every adult ages in different ways and at different paces.**

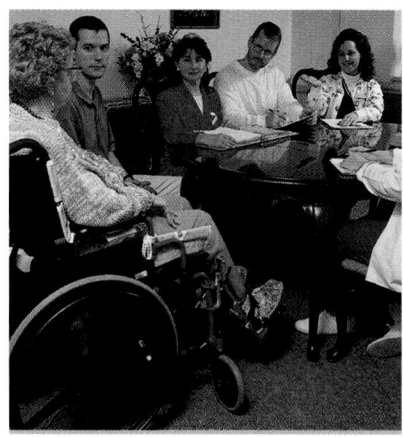

FIGURE 25-2 **Quality care of the older adult occurs best in an interdisciplinary setting.**

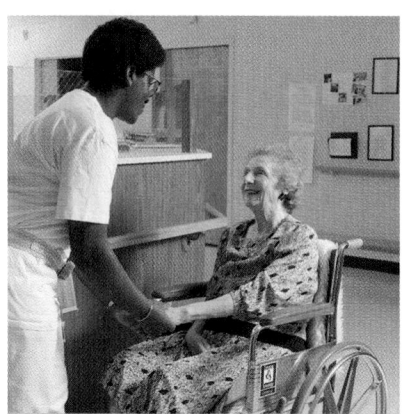

FIGURE 25-3 **Care is delivered to older adults in a variety of settings.**

An overview of the examination of the older adult will be presented in this chapter. Many of the assessment techniques used are the same ones used in the younger adult population. The nurse will need to modify the approach and individualize the assessment of the older adult. It is, however, essential that the nurse understand the differences both within this special population and compared to the younger adult population.

EPIDEMIOLOGY

The number of older adults is increasing exponentially, according to the U.S. Census Bureau (He, Sengupta, Velkoff, & DeBarros, 2005). The National Institute on Aging in 2005 released the report "65+ in the United States: 2005" (He, Sengupta, Velkoff, & DeBarros, 2005). While the group most rapidly increasing in numbers is individuals over age 85, older adults are usually grouped as young-old, which is 65–75 years; old, which is 75–85 years; and old-old, which are those individuals 85 and older. Older individuals will be seen at all levels of the health care system, and nurses must address their unique health care needs, keeping in mind that people living to an older age may have one or more chronic conditions that may impact their ability to function. While disability increases with the increased number of chronic conditions, much of the aging population remains highly functional.

Older adults are a unique population who experience specific changes in their bodies related to age (Figure 25-1). As a consequence, they will have different and unique presentations in their healthy, normal, and disease states. The older an individual is, the more differences among individuals will be seen, as well as differences in rates of decline related to disease. The nurse must be able to differentiate between the normal changes of aging and pathologic processes in order to correctly care for the individual. It is essential to identify how the changes of aging have affected the individual so that care can be modified appropriately. It is vital that the nurse be acutely aware of these changes and incorporate them into the assessment and care planning of each elderly patient. Optimal care for this population is most effectively delivered in an interdisciplinary setting (Figure 25-2), after a carefully organized, methodical exam.

Deterioration of the human organism begins around the fourth decade. This deterioration, while significant, is usually not detectable clinically; while one may notice graying hair and decreasing visual acuity, overall function is not affected. All presentations and complaints should be addressed and assessed and not automatically attributed to age. Failure of the health care provider to recognize a treatable condition may result in long-term pain, suffering, and loss of function and a decreased quality of life for the patient.

ISSUES IN PRESENTATION

The older population resides in a variety of venues. They may live independently in their own homes, with a caregiver (spouse, son or daughter, other family member, or paid assistant), or in an organized setting. These range from senior congregate living with no assistance offered, to senior living where there are some services, to assisted living with varying levels of assistance, to long-term nursing home residence. Older individuals may also spend short periods in skilled nursing facilities receiving rehabilitative services post-illness or post-hospitalization (Figure 25-3). The majority of older persons live in homes and not in skilled long term care. They may have more than one comorbid condition and some limitations on their functioning.

Disease and disability are not automatic consequences of the aging process. The number of chronic or comorbid diseases and conditions one has does increase with age; generally, however, the older adult's functional abilities remain intact,

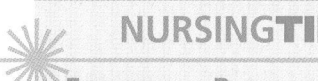

NURSINGTIP

Emergency Response System

Many older adults wear an electronic device that is used to activate emergency care when warranted. Frequently this device is worn on a chain around the patient's neck and is activated by pushing a button. Depending on the company, some type of response is initiated when the patient activates the device. You need to note the presence of such a device and validate that the patient knows how to use it.

although his or her vulnerability to functional decline increases. Increasing age results in extreme variability of that decline when it occurs. The incidence of vague complaints or symptoms—and neglect by patients, family, and health care providers—also place the older adult at increased risk of functional decline and frailty. Decreased organ function and declining homeostatic mechanisms further increase the older adult's susceptibility to disease and disability.

Frequently, presentation of disease in the older patient is not attributable to a specific pathology. Poor management of chronic conditions as well as nonspecific presentations predispose the older person to an even higher risk of disability. The older population, having lived through a number of hardships and life experiences, may also erroneously attribute specific symptoms to normal aging and delay seeking treatment. Older adults do not present with the same signs and symptoms as younger persons. The most common complaints tend to be somewhat nonspecific and vague, frequently general lethargy or weakness, loss of appetite, or generalized fatigue.

Issues compromising the recognition of disease are, in some cases, the gradual onset and vague symptomatology with which diseases present. Many caregivers see symptoms of disease as normal changes of aging. Stoicism of the older adult and misperception of normal aging by the patient are impediments to reporting developing symptoms, as is the worry of testing and fear of bad news. Fears of possible expense, physical discomfort, and loss of independence are all concerns expressed by older adults. Reporting may also be hampered by cognitive impairment, inability to verbalize symptoms, and concerns of not being taken seriously by the health care provider.

ANATOMY AND PHYSIOLOGY

STRUCTURAL AND PHYSIOLOGICAL VARIATIONS

Every cell, tissue, organ, and organism is affected by the process of aging. Most systems have specific changes, while a few systems have vague, deregulatory changes. These changes are due to a combination of factors, among them genetics, environment, nutrition, and activity. Changes of aging are not harmful in isolation, but physiologic resilience is compromised primarily due to loss of reserves. Homeostasis becomes more difficult to maintain in times of stress such as injury, illness, or surgery. These changes are more commonly seen in the very old or frail older adult. While most changes seen in the older adult are part of the normal aging process, many can also indicate underlying systemic or localized disease. Therefore, it is prudent not to generalize changes as routine.

Vital Signs

RESPIRATIONS. The normal respiratory rate is between 12 and 24 breaths per minute. An elevated respiratory rate frequently precedes usual symptoms of upper respiratory infection or a developing illness.

PULSE. In the older adult, the resting heart rate remains constant but the maximum heart rate declines. Reflex tachycardia is delayed due to a blunted baroreceptor reflex.

TEMPERATURE. The elderly may have an abnormally low body temperature and greater variations in temperature. Diurnal variations are not affected by age. Frail elderly may present with an infective process with the absence of fever.

BLOOD PRESSURE. Both diastolic and systolic blood pressure rise due to the loss of elasticity in the vasculature of the older adult. Emergence of new diastolic hypertension in an older person usually has a secondary etiology, which should be explored. In addition, approximately 20% of older individuals exhibit postural hypotension. Postprandial hypotension is more commonly seen in older adults than in younger adults. A widening of the pulse pressure also occurs.

Skin, Hair, and Nails

The most visible signs of aging are manifested in the skin and hair. These signs include wrinkles, sagging skin folds, graying hair, and hair loss. Light-skinned individuals appear to manifest the changes of aging more rapidly than do dark-skinned individuals, and these changes are accelerated by sun exposure. Skin disorders are also more likely to occur as a person ages.

With aging, the epidermis thins and elastic fibers that provide support to the dermis degenerate and lead to sagging skin folds. The vascularity of the skin declines, which can lead to senile purpura. Because the number of sweat and sebaceous glands diminishes, a disruption in the body's thermoregulation occurs. There is also an increased incidence of hypothermia due to vasodilation and vasoconstriction of the dermal arterioles and loss of subcutaneous fat. The loss of subcutaneous tissue over bony prominences increases the risk of skin breakdown in the older adult.

In elderly individuals, a diminished inflammatory response and a diminished perception of pain increase the risk of adverse effects from noxious stimuli. The elderly are thus at a greater risk for frostbite and burns because of their diminished pain perception, and their injuries are more serious because of the thinning of the epidermis and prolonged wound healing. Reepithelialization takes approximately twice as long in patients over the age of 75 as in those who are 25 years of age (Bolognia, 1995).

Wrinkling is the change most associated with aging. Wrinkles are most prominent on the face and neck because these areas have the greatest sun exposure. Other factors leading to wrinkling are loss of subcutaneous fat and diminished elasticity of the skin.

Senile pruritus is the most common skin affliction in elderly individuals. Pruritus is due to a decrease in water content of the skin, a decrease in the number of sebaceous glands, and atrophy of the eccrine glands. The latter contributes to the risk of hyperthermia in the older adult. Dryness and itching are exacerbated during the winter months because humidity is low, indoor temperatures are high, and drying winds are present. The condition is aggravated by frequent bathing in hot water, which robs the skin of moisture. Generalized itching is also associated with systemic diseases such as diabetes mellitus, atherosclerosis, and liver disease.

The number and thickness of terminal hairs generally diminish, and there is a conversion of vellus hair to terminal hair in areas such as the rims of the ears and nose in men, and on the upper lip and chin in women. Decreased melanin production decreases the melanocytes at the hair follicles and leads to hair pigment loss manifested as graying hair.

The nails in the older adult may thicken, split, and become more yellow and dull. There may be an overcurvature of the toenails if tight shoes were worn for a large portion of the adult's life.

Head, Neck, and Regional Lymphatics

Loss of subcutaneous fat and musculoskeletal changes due to the aging process affect the appearance and function of the head and neck. Wrinkles are more prominent. Facial symmetry may be altered because of the presence of dentures or loss of teeth. Due to reabsorption of mandibular bone, a change in facial appearance is expected. Neck veins may be more prominent due to loss of fat.

The head, neck, and lower jaw may be thrust forward, especially with a kyphotic posture. A "buffalo hump" may appear as an accumulation of fat over the posterior cervical vertebrae. This is seen in patients with osteoporosis or a kyphotic posture. Range of motion of the head may be limited, painful, or possible only with a jerking or "cogwheel" motion. Dizziness accompanying movement of the head may create safety problems. All of these changes may affect the older adult's ability to maintain normal activities of daily living.

Eyes

Visual impairments are among the most prevalent chronic conditions in the older adult. Sight provides information to enable people to function in the environment. Thus prevention of sensory impairment and resulting handicaps are challenges for the individual and health care providers.

During the aging process, the eye undergoes significant changes. First, by the age of 42, the lens cortex becomes more dense, compromising its ability to change shape and focus. This condition, **presbyopia**, is responsible for farsightedness and the need for bifocals. A decrease in aqueous humor secretion and increased vitreous gel debris lead to decreased cleansing of the lens and cornea as well. Next, there is a tendency for the lens to yellow and become cloudy. This change impairs a person's ability to discern colors, especially blues and greens. In addition, pupils become smaller, causing the amount of light reaching the retina to be reduced. As a consequence, older adults need more light to see and their eyes take longer to accommodate to darkness and glare. Peripheral vision is decreased and an upward gaze may be limited, which can create safety issues for driving and other activities.

Externally, the older adult has a loss of pigment in the iris, decreased orbital fat, and a thinning of the eyelid tissue. Decreased corneal sensitivity and a decreased corneal reflex, in conjunction with the presence of entropion, ectropion, or ptosis, can result in corneal abrasion or infection. The globe appears to be deeper in the eye socket, and the lacrimal gland may be visible because of the loss of subcutaneous fat around the eye.

Ears

Hearing loss, presbycusis, is a common condition among older adults. Conductive hearing loss occurs in the outer or middle ear and usually makes things sound softer. High-pitched tones are lost first. However, the more common age-related hearing loss is sensorineural, which involves the inner ear. Ossicular joint deterioration occurs, there is a degeneration of hair cells in the inner ear, and vestibular structures, the cochlea, and organ of Corti, all atrophy. These bilateral ear changes can also result in an increased risk of balance and equilibrium deficits.

Externally, the pinna increases in length and width in the older adult and cerumen production decreases. This can lead to ear dryness and cerumen impaction. Otoscopic assessment may reveal more pronounced landmarks if atrophic or sclerotic changes have occurred.

Nose

Nasal hairs are coarser, and less efficient filtration occurs as a person ages. This can lead to sinus and respiratory problems. In addition, the sense of smell declines rapidly after age 50. The smaller number of smell receptors is less efficient, and smells must be more intense to be perceived. This diminished smell may result in decreased appetite.

Mouth and Throat

Common alterations in the mouth of an older adult are precancerous and cancerous lesions; untreated caries (due to decreased saliva production, lack of funds to obtain dental care, and neglect of oral hygiene); periodontal disease (i.e., receding gum lines, gingivitis); tooth loss, which can affect closure of the mouth; worn tooth surfaces; and orofacial pain. Swallowing problems increase in part due to a decreased saliva production. In addition, side effects from medications (e.g., xerostomia from anticholinergic medications and antihistamines, possible oral candidiasis from inhaled steroids) can alter the normal anatomy of the mouth.

Taste may not diminish with age, but it may become less reliable due to a decreased number of taste buds and a decline in their function. Specifically, the older adult has a more difficult time discriminating the tastes of sweet, sour, salt, and bitter.

There is a higher incidence of loss of teeth and periodontal disease in the older population than in the younger age groups. Those wearing dentures may not realize that their dentures may need adjusting every year or two due to changing mandibular bone structure. Oral hygiene practices should be assessed on each comprehensive visit. Frequently heard symptoms with which the older patient may present are foul breath and sensitivity to extremes of temperature. Periodontal disease may be the cause and should always be evaluated, as this is a major cause of tooth loss. The same symptoms, however, can be presentations of sinusitis or a pulmonary infection.

Breasts and Regional Nodes

The adipose tissue of the breast atrophies with age and is replaced with connective tissue. The glandular tissue gradually decreases, causing the breasts to feel granular instead of lobular. Breast tissue mass decreases with age and becomes pendulous and wrinkled. The nipples become smaller and flatter. Ductal tissue becomes more palpable, especially around the nipples, and may become firm and stringy. In addition, the musculature around the breasts tends to atrophy, which contributes to the overall droopiness of the breasts.

There is an increased incidence of breast cancer after the age of 50. In women, it is the second major cause of cancer death, exceeded only by lung cancer (What Are the Key Statistics for Breast Cancer, 2007).

Thorax and Lungs

The older adult undergoes changes that involve the external and internal anatomy of the thorax and lungs. As a result, the physiology of the respiratory system becomes altered. The resulting state of the patient depends on the extent of the changes and the presence of comorbid conditions. Variations of the respiratory system include four broad areas:

1. Anatomic changes
2. Alveolar gas exchange
3. Regulation of ventilation
4. Lung defense mechanisms

Older adults experience degeneration of the intervertebral discs, stiffening of ligaments and joints, and calcification of the costochondral cartilage. These changes limit chest wall expansion during the respiratory cycle. Muscles atrophy and become weaker and the diaphragm flattens out, leading to decreased respiratory endurance for the older adult. Strenuous exercise is taxing secondary to the decrease in oxygen uptake and decreased elastic recoil of the lung parenchyma. Most older adults will have some degree of a barrel chest and some kyphosis.

Forced vital capacity decreases, residual volume and functional residual capacity increase, and the total lung capacity remains unchanged.

The second major change in the older adult is the alveolar gas exchange. The lung's decreased elastic recoil causes the closure of airways for a portion of the respiratory cycle. This occurs particularly in the lower lobes of the lungs. As a result, the apices and the bases of the lungs have a ventilation-perfusion mismatch. Other contributing factors to this loss of alveolar gas exchange are the loss of lung tissue and alveolar capillaries and pulmonary wall thickening. In essence, this creates a situation in which there is less surface area for diffusion, and this surface area is thicker. In addition, hemoglobin's affinity for oxygen decreases, which leads to a decrease in the partial pressure of oxygen.

The aging adult experiences changes in the regulation of ventilation. The medulla is less sensitive to changes in carbon dioxide and oxygen levels, which normally trigger the respiratory drive. There is a compromised acid-base balance. Neural output to respiratory muscles is decreased. Both peripheral and central chemoreceptors are affected.

The last area of change in the older adult is in lung defense mechanisms. There is less ciliary and macrophage activity, which increases susceptibility to infection. The cough reflex decreases, and the risk of aspiration increases.

Heart and Peripheral Vasculature

As adults age, their cardiovascular systems undergo physiologic changes that in many instances are complicated by disease processes. In the older adult, the size of the cardiac muscle decreases with age. As fibrotic and sclerotic changes take place in the atria and the ventricles, cardiac output can fall by as much as 35% at rest after the age of 70. Skeletal changes such as osteoporosis, kyphosis, or collapsed vertebrae can alter the position of the heart within the thoracic cavity, giving rise to changes in the electrocardiogram. Obesity leads to increased abdominal girth and diaphragm elevation, which can also displace the heart within the chest.

With the aging process, cardiac valves may develop calcifications or fibrosis, which results in systolic or diastolic murmurs. A systolic ejection murmur commonly found at the left lower sternal border is of no diagnostic significance. If the left ventricle has thickened or enlarged, thus losing its compliance, an S_4 heart sound can be auscultated. Changes in the conduction system resulting from electrolyte imbalance, pharmacotherapy, debilitating states, or thickened myocardial fibers can cause cardiac irritability, leading to a variety of dysrhythmias. The aging adult also has a reduced beta adrenergic response.

Vascular integrity is also affected in the aging process. The arterial system becomes increasingly rigid as the blood vessels become fibrotic. If a pathological process such as atherosclerosis is present, the insult to the vasculature becomes even greater. Elasticity is lost, the vessel lumen is narrowed, and peripheral vascular resistance is increased, thus impeding blood flow. Conditions such as smoking, which cause vascular spasm, contribute to a decrease in vascular flow. In the venous system, there is intimal thickening with dilation and loss of valve competency. Venous return to the heart is affected, and edema or varicosities may develop. The baroreceptors located in the aortic arch and the carotid sinuses are also affected by vascular integrity. In the presence of impaired compliance, these structures are altered in their abilities to respond to blood pressure changes. A dilated aorta and cool extremities are commonly found with decreased peripheral pulses.

Abdomen

In the process of aging, the abdominal musculature diminishes in mass and loses much of its tone. At the same time, the fat content of the body increases, leading

NURSINGTIP

Gastrointestinal Complaints

Gastrointestinal complaints such as flatus, dyspepsia, or heartburn constitute many of the reasons the older adult seeks health care. Although many of theses complaints may be functional in nature, other cues should be investigated. Gastric irritation can result from an increased consumption of alcohol, aspirin, or nonsteroidal anti-inflammatory drugs. Occult bleeding may go undetected until a GI bleed occurs or anemia is detected.

In addition, constipation is a frequent complaint. Changes in bowel habits may be benign manifestations of diet, medications, a loss of sphincter tone, or lack of exercise. However, in the older adult, these symptoms might signify the presence of gastric or colon malignancies.

to increased fat deposition in the abdominal area. The mucosal lining of the gastrointestinal tract becomes less elastic, and changes in gastric motility result in alterations in digestion and absorption.

Decreased esophageal motility and lower esophageal sphincter pressure can lead to complaints of GERD symptoms. Pancreatic, enzymatic, and hormonal secretions decrease, and there is an atrophy of antral cells, causing a decreased secretion of hydrochloric acid and intrinsic factor. These can cause malabsorption, altered digestion, and a cobalamin deficiency. A decrease in intestinal motility can lead to constipation, one of the most frequent complaints of the older adult.

As the intestinal wall weakens, diverticuli increase. These can progress to inflammation and obstruction.

There is little evidence that liver function changes significantly with age. However, hepatic weight, blood flow, and regenerative capacity decrease progressively with age. The decrease in liver mass and blood flow alters the pharmacokinetics of medications.

Musculoskeletal System

Bone density decreases in the older adult due to an increased rate of reabsorption, which exceeds the rate of bone replenishment. Both cortical and trabecular bone mass decrease. These changes lead to a weaker bone that is more susceptible to fracture. Bone density loss is accentuated in the postmenopausal female due to an estrogen deficiency. Other manifestations of the bone density loss are thoracic kyphosis and a reduction in height. Thoracic kyphosis will cause a change in the older adult's center of gravity, making the individual more prone to loss of balance and to falls. Refer to Chapter 18 for risk factors for osteoporosis.

With age, muscle fibers deteriorate and are replaced by fibrous connective tissue. Muscle atrophy is accompanied by a reduction in muscle mass, a loss of muscle strength against resistance, and a reduction in overall body mass. The fat content of the body increases, with particular distribution around the waistline.

There is a decrease in the water content of cartilage, which leads to a narrowing of joint spaces, intervertebral discs, possibly pain, crepitus, and decreased movement of the affected area. There is also a reduction in the ability of cartilage to repair itself following trauma or surgery. Articulating cartilage will deteriorate due to a lifetime of wear and tear.

Mental Status and Neurological System

Neuronal changes occur with aging. The myelin sheath surrounding each nerve begins to degenerate, decreasing impulse transmissions and nerve conduction rates. This can lead to a decreased reaction time manifested in slowed DTRs and decreased vibratory sense. The axons of the neuron become smaller. Biochemically, the amount of neurotransmitter produced in the neuron is diminished, and the activity of the enzymes that degrade the neurotransmitter increases. Changes in neurotransmitters are known to affect sleep, temperature control, and mood. Depression, for example, is associated with decreased levels of norepinephrine.

Total brain weight, the number of synapses, and the number of neurons diminish with aging, beginning at age 50. Most of the loss occurs in the cerebral cortex and the cerebellum, and less so in the brain stem. The brain atrophies, causing a widening of the sulci and gyri, especially in the frontal lobes. The tendency of the brain to atrophy increases the size of the subdural space, leaving the cortical bridging veins vulnerable to trauma, bleeding, and the formation of a chronic subdural hematoma. The ventricles increase in size and the amount of cerebrospinal fluid increases to fill the space.

Cognitive changes characteristic of aging include a decline in mental flexibility, abstract thinking, recall, and visual-spatial ability. However, recognition, attention, and language skills remain unchanged. The older adult typically has an extended learning and word retrieval time. Short-term memory may slightly decrease, but this must be evaluated because it may not be due to a decline in neurological function. In addition, changes in affect, mood, and orientation need to be investigated, as they may be signs of dementia, delirium, or acute mental confusion, especially in the older adult suffering from infection, dehydration, or CNS damage. Cognitive screening should be a part of each interaction with the older patient and any abnormal findings investigated.

Urinary System

RENAL. In the older adult the kidney shrinks. Renal function can be altered due to glomerular degeneration, thickening of glomerular and tubular basement membranes, decreased length of proximal and distal tubes, and decreased renal blood flow. As a result, the glomerular filtration rate decreases by 60–70% by age 75. The kidney does not respond as efficiently to vasopressin, and the ability to dilute, concentrate, and acidify urine is compromised. Impaired sodium regulation can also occur.

BLADDER. The bladder becomes less elastic because of reduced muscle tone from the aging process. Because the older adult has a bladder with a smaller capacity and delayed perception of voiding signals, urinary incontinence is a frequent occurrence. In addition, the bladder has increased detrusor muscle instability, a weakened urinary sphincter, and involuntary contractions. Increased nocturnal production of urine leads to nocturia in both men and women.

Female Genitalia

The older female adult undergoes definite physical changes in her internal and external genitalia and her reproductive organs. These changes begin with menopause, which usually occurs between the ages of 45 and 55. Menopause is characterized by low estrogen levels, which cause the cessation of menses. As aging progresses, a generalized atrophy of the external and internal female reproductive organs evolves.

Atrophy of the internal reproductive organs causes the ovaries and fallopian tubes to diminish in size so that they are rarely palpable. The uterus atrophies so that it may be difficult to palpate. Also, a delayed and reduced production of vaginal secretions may cause alterations in sexual response. These changes in the vagina may cause the female to complain of dyspareunia. An increase in the pH of the vaginal secretions and a decrease in the normal vaginal flora lead to an increase in vaginal infections in elderly women. However, the older female adult experiences no change in sexual desire or pleasure or in the ability to experience orgasm.

The pelvic muscles also atrophy, causing a decrease in the support of the pelvic organs. These muscles are often already weakened by trauma from childbirth; thus, prolapse of the uterus and vaginal walls is common.

Male Genitalia

Testicular degeneration seems to occur in patchy distribution, which allows normal spermatogenesis to be present in the majority of men until 70 years of age, when sperm count and motility decline. Sperm output may be slightly decreased.

Typically, the older male adult has no change in sexual desire or satisfaction, but the ability to obtain or maintain an erection is affected. Also, erection is often not as complete. Testosterone levels decline slightly with age but are related to impotence in only a small minority of men who have low hormone levels. An absence or marked reduction of ejaculatory fluid emission is often seen in the older adult male. The refractory period before rearousal, after a cycle of erection and ejaculation, lengthens with age. This physiologic change in what used to be an almost automatic erection is often perceived by men as the onset of impotence. Anxiety levels rise, thus further triggering erectile dysfunction. Physiologic impotence can be caused by vascular disease, diabetes mellitus, and hypogonadism.

Anus, Rectum, and Prostate

Anorectal function changes in the older adult due to the loss of muscle elasticity in the rectum. Older adults have reduced maximum tolerated volumes in the rectum, with higher rectal pressures in response to distension. Rectal prolapse is most commonly seen in elderly women. Constipation commonly occurs due to a decline in large bowel transit and decreased fecal water excretion.

Fecal incontinence may develop due to denervation associated with an increase in the motor unit fiber density and the rectal wall's afferent neuron degeneration. This interferes with the ability to detect changes in pressure and creates a decrease in internal sphincter tone. Fecal incontinence in the older adult is usually the result of impairment of more than one of the factors that ordinarily maintain continence. Table 25-1 lists some of the causes of fecal incontinence in this population.

The prostate begins to enlarge after the age of 40 and often leads to the development of benign prostatic hypertrophy. The prostate capsule may contract and prostatic urethral tone may increase, resulting in urinary obstruction. There are lower levels of zinc in the prostatic fluid of older men, which appear to reduce the amount of prostatic antibacterial factor, therefore making the older man more susceptible to urinary tract infections.

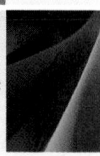

TABLE 25-1 Causes of Fecal Incontinence in Elderly Patients

- Diarrhea
- Fecal impaction
- Irritable bowel syndrome
- Anorectal carcinoma
- Rectal trauma
- Stroke
- Diabetes mellitus
- Dementia
- Multiple sclerosis
- Rectal prolapse

INTERVIEW OF THE OLDER ADULT

The older adult ranges from age 65 years on up; however, this population spans a lengthy time period. Chronological age should not be the major factor considered in the approach to the patient. Ability to function and interact will be as diverse as the individual regardless of age. Those young-old adults, ages 65–75, in most cases will be highly functional, independent individuals, and the examiner's approach will need minimal modification. However, the true elderly, those 85 and up, may have limitations that will call for modification of both the interview and the examination itself (Figure 25-4). The presence of frailty may mandate multiple appointments in order to complete a comprehensive exam. Additional time should be incorporated into the interview to allow for accurate interpretation of the information needed and the responses.

The health history of the older adult encompasses the same major areas as the health history for a younger patient; however, there are some basic differences. Reasons for seeking care may be a chronic condition or a new issue or problem. Issues of depression, weakness, or self-care deficits may be more difficult to identify but will emerge from a thorough, skilled assessment. New pains or discomfort should never be attributed to "getting old," and patient teaching should emphasize this point. Past health history for the older patient is similar to that for the younger adult. The length of time covered is extended, however, and therefore the interview may take more time to complete. Medication should always be carefully evaluated and, if possible, the patient should bring all prescription medications, OTC medications, and vitamins to the appointment (Figure 25-5). Multiple providers can result in multiple medications treating similar conditions, which can increase the risk of drug interactions and adverse drug effects. Family history may

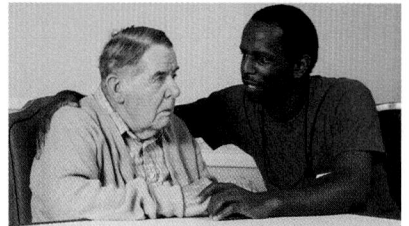

FIGURE 25-4 The health history interview of the frail elderly poses a unique challenge to nurses.

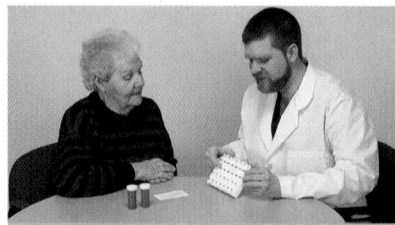

FIGURE 25-5 Older adults should be encouraged to bring all their prescription and nonprescription medications with them to each health care appointment.

be less helpful in the older adult, and its utility is especially questionable in the very old patient because the main purpose of collecting it is to identify those conditions that may cause premature illness and death, concerns that are no longer applicable in such a patient. Table 25-2 identifies strategies to enhance the health history interview and examination of the older adult.

The psychosocial aspect of the interview is similar to that for the younger adult, with some areas receiving increased focus. Current living situation and the older

TABLE 25-2 Guide to Enhanced Interview and Examination

POTENTIAL DEFICIT	GOAL	INTERVENTION
Vision	Maximize visual component of communication	Sit facing patient to ensure clear view of your face.
		Avoid light behind you.
		Provide bright, indirect light without glare.
		Ensure patient has clean glasses (clean as needed).
		Provide written material in 14-point font on matte paper with clear contrast between text and background.
Hearing	Maximize auditory component of communication and enhance information gathering	Provide quiet environment with no background noise.
		Ask if there is a hearing deficit and which ear is better. Speak directly to the good ear.
		Address the patient by the correct title and last name at the initiation of new or returning conversation.
		Assist with the use of working hearing aids.
		If needed, use alternate mechanisms for communication such as writing, signing, or using a stethoscope as an assistive device.
		Validate that information is understood.
Mobility	Promote independence and autonomy	Explain what parts of the exam will be done.
		Plan to reinforce the explanation during the exam.
		Allow extra time for the patient to prepare for the exam.
		Ask if the patient would like assistance in preparation.
		Ask who the patient would like present during the exam, if anyone.
Fatigue	Enhance quality of information and accuracy and efficacy of exam	Allow flexibility in scheduling so patient can select his or her best time of day.
		May need to break comprehensive exam into sections and allow for rest periods as needed or schedule on separate days.
		Ensure positioning is not adding to fatigue. Patient may have less fatigue if exam is done in semirecumbent position.
Eliciting minimal information	Enhance quality of information and accuracy and efficacy of exam	Ensure issues above are addressed adequately.
		Ask open-ended questions that cannot be answered yes/no.
Difficulty with focus	Enhance quality of information and accuracy and efficacy of exam	Limit questions with essential subjective information to closed-ended questions.
		Organize reminiscences to enhance data gathering.
Pain	Promote comfort and enhance quality of information	Allow patient to assume position of most comfort.
		Provide patient with available interventions to enhance comfort.

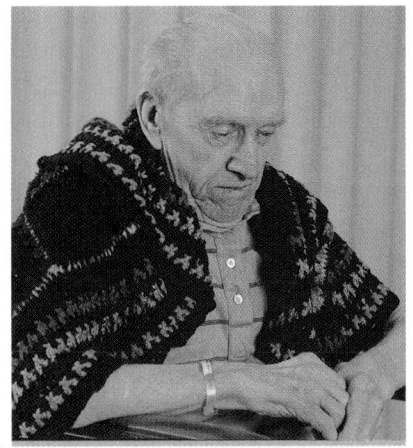

FIGURE 25-6 Assessing for cognitive changes and depression in the older adult should occur at each nursing visit.

adult's satisfaction with the living arrangements should be elicited. Engagement with friends and family should be explored as should spousal issues that may present.

Older adults experience many life changes and these changes may accelerate with age. Their ability to cope with the stressors associated with aging, such as retirement, moving, illness, or deaths of significant others, should be assessed. The nurse should also be assessing for depression, personality changes, or other signs of cognitive issues (Figure 25-6). Cognitive issues may result from medical issues and will be amenable to treatment. The normal exam findings should be emphasized, and patient teaching should occur regarding commonly experienced issues of aging.

SPECIAL ASSESSMENTS

DEVELOPMENTAL ASSESSMENT

Many older adults fear the aging process. It is often seen as a time of uselessness and decline. However, older adults are not useless and they have their own developmental tasks to accomplish. Older adults demonstrate tremendous flexibility in their thinking, learning, and adaptive ability. They have to be resilient to incorporate the aging process into their self-image (Figure 25-7). Growing old is a time of enormous individual growth. Coping with the losses of spouse, family, and friends through death, illness, or relocation; adjusting to altered living arrangements; retiring; and adjusting to changing sexual and physical function are just a few examples of the developmental work that older adults accomplish. Refer to Chapter 4 for a summary of developmental tasks of the older adult.

Assessment of the older adult's functioning may allow the health care provider to assist the patient in adapting to these changes or in compensating and planning for the future (see Figure 25-8). Assessing functionality, nutrition, sleep, and caregiver strain will improve the quality of life and adaptation of the older patient. Reliable and valid tools for use with the older population may be found at http://www.hartfordign.org. These tools include the Mini-Cog, the CAM

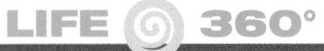

Physical Changes in the Older Adult

An 84-year-old woman is seen for her osteoarthritis. She tells you that she can no longer knit sweaters for her grandchildren. This is very upsetting to the patient. How should you proceed with the physical examination? What recommendations can you make to the patient?

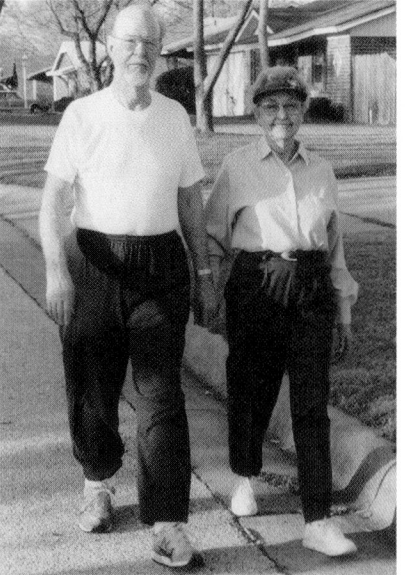

A. This couple is enjoying a brisk walk together. They are spending time together as a couple and maintaining their physical endurance.

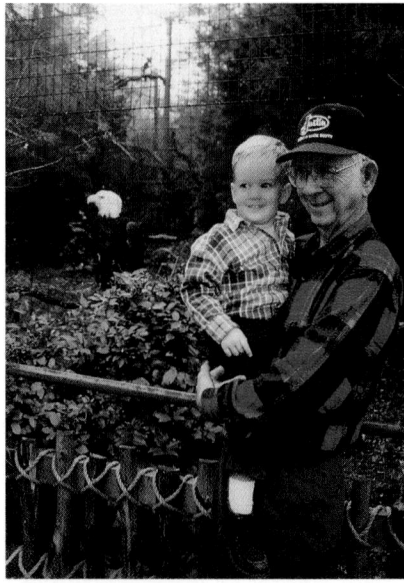

B. The oldest and youngest members of the family are enjoying their time together.

FIGURE 25-7 Developmental Tasks of the Older Adult

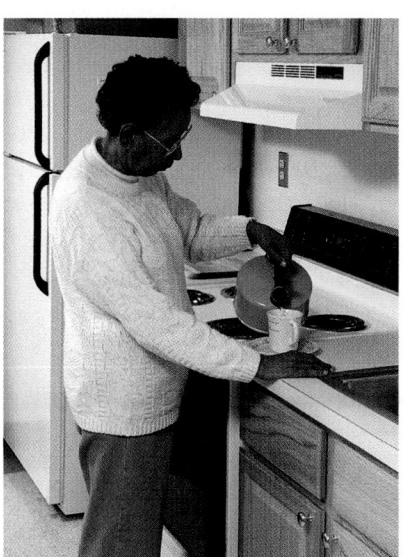

FIGURE 25-8 Preparing meals is one of the functional abilities that is assessed in older adults.

(Confusion Assessment Method), the Katz Index of Independence in Activities of Daily Living (ADL), the Lawton Instrumental Activities of Daily Living Scale (IADL), Mini-Nutritional Assessment (MNA), the Pittsburgh Sleep Quality Index (PSQI), and the Modified Caregiver Strain Index (CSI).

CULTURAL ASSESSMENT

The number of minority elders is increasing at a rate similar to the increase in the population as a whole. Some ethnic groups suffer a higher rate of specific disorders. For example, African American and Hispanic elders have a higher rate of dementias than Caucasian elders (Mouton & Esparza, 2000). Just as older patients present with great variation, there is a large amount of variety among ethnic groups. Older individuals with cultural origins elsewhere may have differing health practices and beliefs.

Assessment may be complicated further by the lack of a common language between the nurse and the non-English-speaking older adult. As a sign of respect, all older adults should be addressed by title and last name. Validation of understanding of answers to questions in addition to instructions is essential. Many cultures nod "yes" without understanding. When addressing topics that are private in other cultures, the assessor should explain that it is necessary to discuss these topics to deliver appropriate care.

Attempts should be made to assess and honor individual beliefs and attitudes to health and illness. This will facilitate the development of respect and rapport with the older patient. Cognitive examination instruments have been found to be affected by ethnicity, education, and language (Mouton & Esparza, 2000). Refer to Chapter 5 for additional information.

SPIRITUAL ASSESSMENT

Investigators have found a strong link between faith and health. This is also true for the older adult. When older adults are questioned, the majority believe in the healing power of prayer, that faith can facilitate recovery, and that their faith and religious practices are an important means of coping with illness and disability. Just as faith is an individual perception and practice at the younger age, so it is with the older adult. Older adults do not become more religious as they age. Rather, they maintain the same support and belief system that has supported them throughout their lives.

A spiritual history is the same as for the younger adult and should include the key concepts of the older adult's idea of a higher power, the meaning of illness, the mechanisms used to maintain hope, and his or her support system. Chapter 6 provides a comprehensive spiritual assessment tool.

NUTRITIONAL ASSESSMENT

Nutritional assessments are performed for a number of reasons. Specific, identified nutritional deficits, risk factors placing the individual at risk for nutritional deficiencies, and weight loss are the main stimuli. The older adult faces unique challenges in attempting to maintain good nutritional intake (Figure 25-9). For instance, caloric requirements decline with age, and older adults have decreased or blunted taste perception in addition to less efficient intestinal absorption. Chewing and swallowing issues are the most prevalent in this age group, and disabilities may impair actual food preparation. Financial constraints in shopping and food-buying habits are frequently seen in the elderly living on a fixed income, and loss of partners, friends, and spouses decreases the many social aspects of eating.

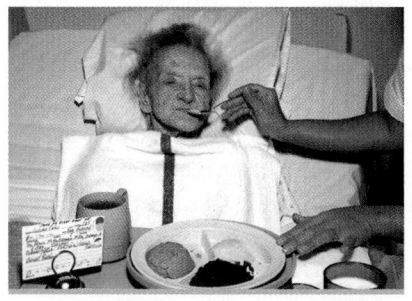

FIGURE 25-9 Assessing an older adult's nutritional status is important to helping him or her maintain a healthy lifestyle.

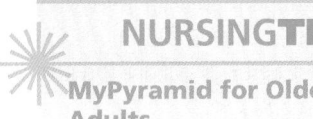

EQUIPMENT

- Equipment listed in Chapters 10–22
- Equipment/forms needed to conduct cognition and functional assessments

The nutritional assessment should be performed as for the younger adult, with additional information on medications, social interactions, living arrangements, and functional ability elicited. Food and drug interactions are more common in this age group. Single living, loneliness, and loss of spouse are major risk factors for inadequate nutrition. Assessment may be standardized using an evidence-based tool such as the Mini-Nutritional Assessment (MNA), which may be found at http://www.hartfordign.org. Refer to Chapter 7 for the comprehensive nutritional assessment.

PAIN ASSESSMENT

Always ask the older patient about pain. Many older patients assume that pain is an inevitable part of aging. Older adults may use other words such as *discomfort, soreness,* or *achiness* when describing their pain to you.

Assessment of pain should include:

- How long has the pain been a problem?
- Is this new pain or have you had it before?
- Where is the pain? Does it radiate? Where is it the worst?
- How severe is the pain? (Ask the person to rate the pain using the Visual Analog Scale.)
- Is the pain sharp, stabbing, dull, or aching?
- Is there any numbness or tingling associated with the pain?
- Has the pain interfered with any activities?
- What makes the pain worse or better?
- What have you tried to relieve the pain? Did it work?

Use of a valid and reliable pain assessment instrument will improve the rating of the pain and the evaluation of the effectiveness of treatment. Examples of tools that can be used may be found at http://www.hartfordign.org.

Severely cognitively impaired patients may not be able to communicate or describe their pain. There are specific pain assessment instruments available for use with this population. Two are the Checklist of Non-Verbal Pain Indicators (CNPI) and PAINAD. They can be found at http://painconsortium.nih.gov and http://amda.com, respectively.

Pain should be reassessed at regular intervals to evaluate the effectiveness of interventions.

PHYSICAL ASSESSMENT

The older adult population is an extremely heterogeneous group. The older the patients, the less likely there will be obvious similarity. Life experiences coupled with genetics, exposures, lifestyles, and diverse culture, diet, recreation, education, environmental influences, and work types all impact an individual's health and wellness status. Key to the assessment of older individuals is their functional ability within their own environment and community.

There is no specific age at which the aging process routinely warrants screening. The older adult may have unique concerns and requirements secondary to disability, comorbid conditions, normal changes of aging, and personal coping strategies.

An essential facet of the care of the older adult is incorporating the caregiver into the assessment. Care should be taken to defer to the wishes of the older adult in the need to involve another individual in assessment and care. Communication should always be directed toward the patient while still attending to caregiver or family input.

Functional testing and cognitive testing should be conducted at each visit with the older adult. In addition, Table 25-3 offers a quick screening tool to assess the health of the older adult.

TABLE 25-3	Quick Screen
ASSESSMENT	**SCREEN**
Function	Positive response to one or more questions, when asked, "Do you need help with:"
	Shopping?
	Doing light housework?
	Walking across a room?
	Washing in shower or bath?
	Doing finances?
Mobility	Perform "Timed Get Up and Go Test" (should be completed in < 20 sec)
Nutrition	Weight loss of more than 10 pounds in the past 6 months without trying (or)
	Body mass index < 20
Vision	Check ability to read newspaper headline and one sentence with correction. If unable, check each eye with Snellen chart.
Hearing	Unable to hear fingertip friction at 6 inches both ears (or)
	If audioscope available, check for 40 dB at 1,000–2,000 Hz in one or both ears or either in one ear.
Cognition	Mini-Cog test: three-item recall, clock drawing, and recheck recall without reminder.
	Patients recalling none of the three words are classified as demented (Score = 0). Patients recalling all three words are classified as nondemented (Score = 3). Patients with intermediate word recall of 1–2 words are classified based on the Clock Drawing Test (CDT) (Abnormal = demented; Normal = nondemented).
Depression	Positive answer to "Do you often feel sad or depressed?"

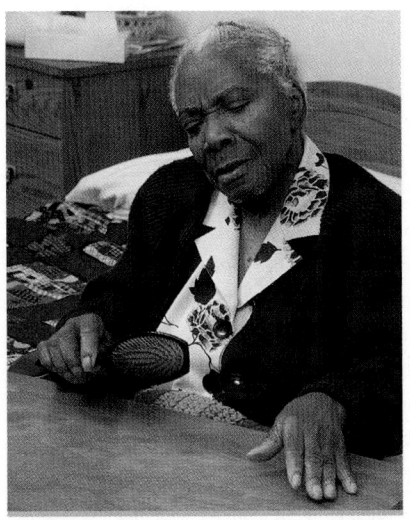

FIGURE 25-10 The nurse needs to assess the older adult's cognitive status at each encounter.

FUNCTIONAL TESTING

Functional testing may be accomplished using any of a number of valid and reliable tools. The tool selected should be specific to the older population and to the older adult's situation. If the older adult is living independently, the Lawton IADL scale should be used, as it covers all activities needed to maintain oneself at home and maintain independence safely. If the older adult resides in an institution offering assistance or resides with and receives assistance from caregivers, the Katz ADL index's narrower focus may be more appropriate. These tests may be accessed at http://www.hartfordign.org. If the individual resides in a facility with a high level of care and the major concern is safety, the "Get Up and Go" Test allows evaluation of the older adult's ability to be mobile safely. This test can be accessed at: www.aan.com.

COGNITION

Safety is impacted by cognitive function. Early identification of cognitive impairment has a significant influence on quality of life, and many etiologies of impairment can be treated (Figure 25-10). New developments in the treatment and delay of the progression of dementias are emerging and driving initiatives aimed at earlier recognition. Once recognition is established, the etiology of the cognitive disorder must be established, as each disorder is treated differently. The major etiologies to be considered are depression, dementia, and delirium. Their contrasting characteristics are found in Table 19-8.

Cognition may be assessed using a number of reliable and valid tools specific to the older adult. The Folstein Mini Mental State Exam is the gold standard of cognitive tests for all ages even though it is susceptible to educational and cultural bias. It is now copyrighted, and information on obtaining this tool is in Chapter 19.

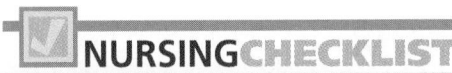

NURSINGCHECKLIST

General Approach to Assessment of the Older Adult

1. Assess the older adult in an environment that is warm, comfortable, and welcoming.
2. Always address questions to the older adult even in the presence of the caregiver. If the caregiver is not giving the patient the opportunity to speak, assure the patient that his or her concerns will be addressed.
3. Use bright, indirect light to enhance the patient's ability to function. Ensure a quiet environment with minimal background noise.
4. Minimize interruptions in the interview and examination.
5. Allow adequate time for the exam. A comprehensive exam of the frail older individual may require an extended visit with rest periods, or multiple visits.
6. Allow the older adult to maintain independence in all activities related to the exam even if it increases the time needed.
7. Ask prior to assisting him or her whether the older patient would like assistance preparing for the exam.
8. Instruct the older adult to remove all items of clothing for a full examination and provide a gown with instructions for its use. Always respect patient modesty.
9. Provide a warmer temperature or, if unadjustable, offer blankets to the older adult.
10. Ascertain that the older adult has clean glasses (clean as needed) and working hearing aids if needed. If a hearing aid would enhance the exam, offer a temporary amplification device. If no amplification is wanted or available, ask which is the older adult's better ear. Use low-pitched, normal-volume speech. Validate that all information presented to the patient has been heard correctly.
11. Ask if the frail older adult would like the caregiver to remain during the exam.
12. Allow the older adult to select a position of comfort. Frail older adults may be less fatigued and more comfortable if examined in a semirecumbent position.
13. Maximize the visual cues the older adult can use by ensuring a clear view of your face without bright background glare.
14. Ask open-ended questions and avoid "yes/no" questions to ensure completeness of interview and examination.
15. At the conclusion of the exam, elicit essential subjective information related to answers to the closed-ended questions to validate findings.
16. Utilize evidence-based tools specific to the older adult to ensure accuracy of information.
17. Always conclude the examination by asking if there are other concerns that have not been addressed or if the patient has questions about anything discussed.

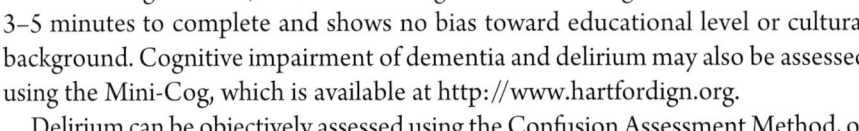

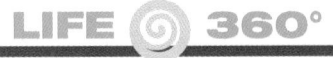

Maintaining Health of Older Adults

Research what resources are available in your community for aging adults. What resources are available for aging adults with physical and cognitive special needs?

The Mini-Cog is a valid, reliable screening tool to assess cognitive status that takes 3–5 minutes to complete and shows no bias toward educational level or cultural background. Cognitive impairment of dementia and delirium may also be assessed using the Mini-Cog, which is available at http://www.hartfordign.org.

Delirium can be objectively assessed using the Confusion Assessment Method, or CAM. Delirious older adults will have a labile level of consciousness, drifting in and out during the exam; they may be able to perform cognitive testing well during lucid periods but still demonstrate impairment on testing. The etiology may be infection, metabolic abnormalities, CNS damage, cranial lesions, or the addition of new medications. Withdrawal from medicines, prescribed and OTC, must also be considered. Older adults exhibiting signs of delirium should be questioned about alcohol use. A complete workup is indicated to determine the etiology. Secondary treatment includes assessment and maintenance of patient safety and symptomatic treatment.

Depression may be easily screened for using the Geriatric Depression Scale. Refer to Table 25-4. Adults obtaining a score of 5 or greater should have further evaluation and treatment. The presence of depression necessitates the nurse to always ask about suicidal ideation prior to the older adult's departure. Older white males have the highest successful suicide rates of all age groups. Geriatric depression responds as well to treatment as depression in a younger population does. The patient's safety is paramount and must be ensured.

TABLE 25-4 Geriatric Depression Scale

Directions: Have the patient reflect over the last week and choose the best answer for how he or she has felt. Score 1 point for each shaded answer.

1. Are you basically satisfied with your life?	YES	**NO**
2. Have you dropped many of your activities and interests?	**YES**	NO
3. Do you feel that your life is empty?	**YES**	NO
4. Do you often get bored?	**YES**	NO
5. Are you in good spirits most of the time?	YES	**NO**
6. Are you afraid that something bad is going to happen to you?	**YES**	NO
7. Do you feel happy most of the time?	YES	**NO**
8. Do you often feel helpless?	**YES**	NO
9. Do you prefer to stay at home rather than going out and doing new things?	**YES**	NO
10. Do you feel you have more problems with memory than most?	**YES**	NO
11. Do you think it is wonderful to be alive now?	YES	**NO**
12. Do you feel pretty worthless the way you are now?	**YES**	NO
13. Do you feel full of energy?	YES	**NO**
14. Do you feel that your situation is hopeless?	**YES**	NO
15. Do you think that most people are better off than you are?	**YES**	NO

5 points indicates that the patient is depressed and further evaluation is indicated.

Adapted from Development of a Comprehensive Assessment Toolbox for Stroke, by P. W. Duncan, 1999, *Clinics in Geriatric Medicine, 15*(4), pp. 885–894.

VITAL SIGNS

Vital signs should be assessed in the manner one would use with the younger adult patient. Usually performed at the initiation of the exam, vital sign assessment is an introduction to the exam almost universally accepted and expected by the older adult. This allows the examiner to introduce personal touch and establish rapport. Refer to Chapter 9 for a complete discussion of vital signs.

Pulse

As in the younger patient, the radial artery is used for heart rate assessment. If the patient has an irregular heart rate, accuracy of assessment will be better if an apical pulse is assessed. Heart rate normals are the same as in younger adults.

Temperature

An older adult with severe cognitive impairment may be unable to comprehend the instruction to hold the thermometer under the tongue. An axillary or tympanic temperature may thus be easier to obtain (Figure 25-11).

N The older adult may normally have a lower body temperature, down to 96°F.

Blood Pressure

Blood pressure should be measured in the supine and standing postures, especially if the patient is taking antihypertensive medication.

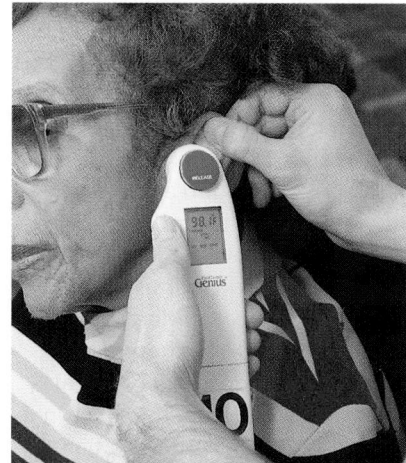

FIGURE 25-11 The tympanic thermometer can be used with ease in the older adult.

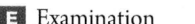 **E** Examination   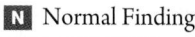 **N** Normal Findings   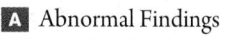 **A** Abnormal Findings   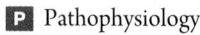 **P** Pathophysiology

N Increased systolic and diastolic pressures may be seen. Widening of pulse pressure is common.

A A fall in diastolic blood pressure is seen more frequently in older adults with risk factors for hypotension. Decreases may range from 20 to 40 mm Hg.

A Bilateral differences in blood pressure from each arm may be present.

A Isolated systolic hypertension is a blood pressure of greater than 160 mm Hg (systolic) over less than 90 mm Hg (diastolic).

P These changes can occur due to the consequences of atherosclerosis and arteriosclerosis.

HEIGHT AND WEIGHT

The frail or weak older adult may require assistance with getting weighed. A modified standing or sitting scale may be necessary. Adults may note that their height is decreasing as they age, and this is due to osteoporosis. Older adults may also lose weight. Weight should be assessed at each patient interaction and carefully documented and monitored. Unexplained weight loss should be investigated.

SKIN

Skin assessment in the older adult should be performed as presented in Chapter 10.

N The following changes can be observed in the older adult:

- Skin may be drier and may or may not be accompanied by less perspiration.
- A thin, parchment-like appearance of the skin with wrinkles and sagging skin folds may be present.
- Liver spots, or solar lentigo, are irregular, flat, deeply pigmented macules that appear in sun-exposed areas (Figure 25-12). They result from the inability of melanocytes to produce an even pigmentation of the skin. Larger areas, called lentigines, are generally seen on the backs of the hands and wrists of light-skinned people and are related to the degree of sun exposure.

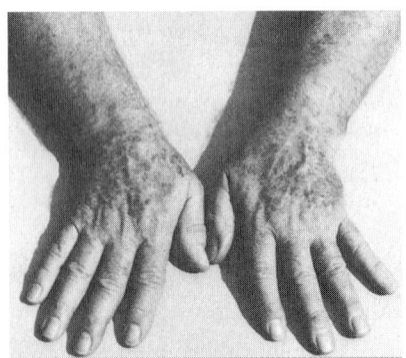

FIGURE 25-12 Senile Lentigo

NURSING**TIP**

Skin Changes in the Older Adult

Hypothermia and hyperthermia occur more frequently in the older patient. The older adult has a decreased ability to compensate for changes in temperature because of impaired vasoconstriction or vasodilation and the normal loss of subcutaneous fat. Decreased dermatome activity, inflammatory response, and pain perception increase the risk of frostbite and burns.

Skin should be monitored for hydration status, lesions, bruising, and changes in temperature, turgor, color, and pigmentation. Intertriginous areas should be cleaned, dried, and regularly assessed for fungal infections. Monitor feet for the need for podiatry interventions. Older patients should be assessed regularly for skin breakdown and the risk of skin breakdown. Appropriate interventions need to be implemented. Patients and families may be following the usual norms of daily hot showers, which may not be indicated for aging skin.

E Examination   **N** Normal Findings   **A** Abnormal Findings   **P** Pathophysiology

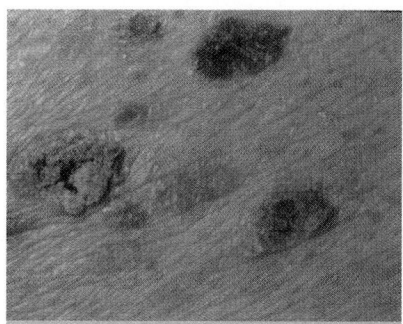

FIGURE 25-13 **Seborrheic Keratoses.**
Courtesy of Robert A. Silverman, M.D., Clinical Associate Professor, Department of Pediatrics, Georgetown University.

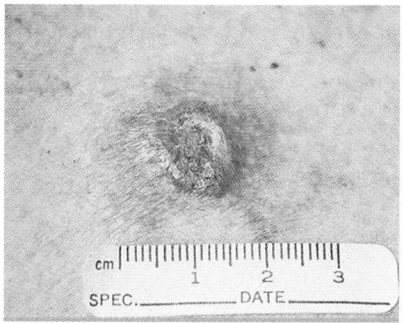

FIGURE 25-14 **Basal Cell Carcinoma.**
Courtesy of Robert A. Silverman, M.D., Clinical Associate Professor, Department of Pediatrics, Georgetown University.

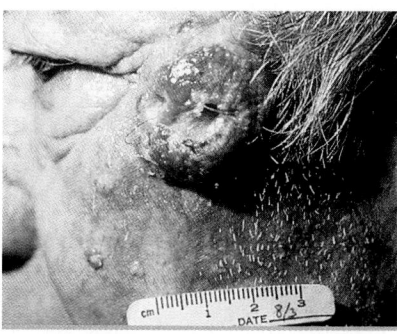

FIGURE 25-15 **Squamous Cell Carcinoma.** *Courtesy of Robert A. Silverman, M.D., Clinical Associate Professor, Department of Pediatrics, Georgetown University.*

- Sebaceous hyperplasia are flattened papules with a central depression and are usually yellowish.
- Sebaceous keratoses are characterized by overgrowth of the horny layer. Lesions are raised but flattened growths with a wart-like appearance (Figure 25-13). They commonly appear somewhat greasy and as though they could easily be scraped from the skin surface. They may be scaly and dry in presentation and range from pale white to brownish in color. They are usually not premalignant.
- Senile purpura is a bluish-purple spot that develops on the older adult's skin, especially in areas of trauma, even slight trauma.

A Actinic keratosis, or solar keratosis, is seen in areas of the greatest sun exposure and is premalignant to squamous cell carcinoma (SCC). These lesions are superficial, flattened papules covered by dry scales, which may be irregular in shape and pink or tan in color.

A Basal cell carcinoma (BCC), is more common among the older adult population but is usually not life threatening (Figure 25-14). The majority of instances occur on the head and neck. Caucasian males are at highest risk, especially those with prolonged exposure to the sun and tanning salons, and previous therapy with ionizing radiation. The lesions can be pigmented or pearly white or pink, and they frequently bleed or scab.

A Squamous cell carcinoma (Figure 25-15) is also more common in older adults but is far less common than BCC. Unlike BCC, SCC tends to occur on the backs of the hands, scalp, and top of the pinna. The SCC lesion often appears red and has an inflamed base. The lesion is mobile with well-defined borders.

P These lesions are associated with sun exposure. UVB radiation is a risk factor for SCC as is damage from thermal burns or chronic inflammation.

HAIR

Assess the hair as described in Chapter 10.

N The hair becomes thinner and coarser, possibly with some degree of alopecia, in the older adult. Facial hair may be seen on women.

NURSING**TIP**

Safety Tips to Help the Elderly Patient Avoid Integumentary Damage

1. Assist elderly patients in identifying hazards in the home that could cause trauma (e.g., loose rugs, sharp table edges, glass items in the bathroom, stoves, electric appliances, and the like). Assist them in finding avenues to decrease the risk of trauma.
2. Remind elderly patients that sensation to temperature diminishes with age and that they may therefore wish to check their bath water with a thermometer (should not be warmer than 105°F).
3. Advise elderly patients to wear multiple layers of clothing in cooler temperatures and gloves and socks to protect the distal extremities from hypothermia and frostbite.
4. Remind elderly patients to keep electric blankets and heating pads on a medium setting to prevent burns.
5. Advise elderly patients to apply emollient lotions to decrease xerosis and pruritus but to avoid lotions with a high alcohol content, which can cause further drying of the skin.
6. Warn elderly patients that their skin will tear more easily and be prone to shearing because their epidermal layers are thinner and that because the integumentary system is slower to recover from trauma, healing from such injuries will take longer.

NAILS

Assess the nails as detailed in Chapter 10.

N Nails commonly become thicker, harder, and yellowish in the older adult. Nails may develop ridges and split into layers.

HEAD AND NECK

Refer to Chapter 11 for complete information on assessing the head and neck.

E In the older adult, range of motion of the neck should be assessed using a single motion at a time to diminish the possibility of dizziness. Monitor for pain, crepitus, and dizziness in addition to range of motion.

N There should be a full range of motion. In addition, there may be an altered appearance of the face due to tooth loss and the absence or presence of dentures.

A Range of motion may be limited. A stiff neck may indicate the presence of cervical arthritis.

P Cartilage and ligaments become less elastic and may be prone to calcification as a person ages. Tendons and muscles lose elasticity and tone. Cervical intervertebral discs lose water and disc space narrows.

EYES

Assess the eyes as described in Chapter 12.

Inspection

N The following changes can occur in the older adult's eyes as part of the normal aging process and may be noted on inspection:

- Graying of eyebrows and eyelashes
- Diminished tearing
- Loss of pigment in the iris
- Diminished or absent corneal reflex
- Decreased peripheral vision
- Altered color perception; difficulty discriminating blue, green, and violet colors
- Arcus senilis, a grayish or whitish arc or circle around the limbus not associated with an underlying condition

A The lower eyelid can drop away from the eye (ectropion) in the older adult.

P Genetic predisposition, lid muscle dysgenesis, trauma, infection, and autoimmune causes can lead to ectropion.

A The lower lid can turn inward (entropion) in the older adult.

P Laxity of medial and lateral muscles, CN III or VII paralysis, Bell's palsy, herpes zoster, or cranial nerve lesions—in addition to trauma, infection, and autoimmune disorders—are etiologies of entropion.

A Decreased central vision can occur in the older adult. This can occur in conjunction with the older adult looking forward when addressing someone who is standing to the side.

P Macular degeneration is commonly age-related and is a common visual problem affecting the older adult. The older adult will require significant

---

E Examination   **N** Normal Findings   **A** Abnormal Findings   **P** Pathophysiology

magnification to compensate for the central loss. An altered head position maximizes available vision.

Anterior Chamber and Lens

A The pupil may have a pearly gray appearance.

P This may indicate cataract formation.

P Acute-angle glaucoma occurs in the elderly at a higher rate than in the younger adult. It may be caused by an inhibition of the flow of fluid from the posterior to the anterior chamber or by "plateau iris syndrome" with iris laxity, which comes into close proximity to the angle. Other causes are anterior uveal displacement, posterior segment inflammation, or tumors.

Pupil

N The older adult may have a decreased pupil size with slow accommodation.

A An irregularly shaped pupil, either bilaterally or unilaterally, is abnormal.

P Cataract repair will alter the shape of the surgical pupil.

Posterior Segment Structures

N The older adult's posterior segment structures may have the following changes:

- **Dullness of retinal structures**
- **Pale blood vessels**
- **Narrower light reflex of arterioles**
- **Straighter and narrower retinal vessels**

EARS

During the examination, the older patient's ears should be assessed for wax buildup and impaction, which can be removed by irrigation and curette. Ensure that any hearing aids are functional, with working batteries and correct placement. If impairment is noted and the patient has not had an audiological examination, one should be encouraged. Face the older individual to whom you are speaking. Make sure there is no background glare obscuring the older patient's view. Speak slowly, in a low-pitched voice, and avoid raising your voice or yelling. Eliminate as much background noise as possible. Monitor balance and equilibrium and assess the risk for falls. Arrange to have the home environment assessed and educate the patient and caregiver on modifications to enhance safety. Review Chapter 13 for a complete description of the ear examination.

Auditory Testing

Ask the older adult about hearing problems. Consider using standardized tools to assess the individual's perception of hearing, such as the Brief Hearing Loss Screener (which may be found at http://www.hartfordign.org).

A Some hearing loss or presbycusis is common in the older adult.

P Conductive hearing loss occurs in the outer ear (because of obstruction or loss of elastic tissue in the tympanic membrane) and middle ear (because of rigidity of movable bones in the inner ear) and mutes sound.

P Sensorineural loss is common in the older adult and involves the inner ear.

NURSING**TIP**

Communicating with the Older Adult Who Has Changes in Hearing

Changes in auditory function are highly probable as an adult ages and will continue to worsen over time. Hearing impairment has the potential to isolate an older individual. If the patient cannot benefit from or use a hearing aid, use a portable amplifier with headphones if available. A "Pocket Talker" is one example of a device that enhances social interactions and improves independence and functioning. If temporary assistive technology is not available, a stethoscope can serve the same purpose. Place the earpieces into the patient's ears and speak quietly into the diaphragm. Allow the older person adequate time to process and respond to interactions. These individuals are hearing impaired, not cognitively impaired. Speak to the hearing-impaired patient with the same respect you would give to a nonimpaired individual. Older adults found to have hearing loss that interferes with their functioning and quality of life should be referred for an audiology exam and fitted with hearing aids if indicated.

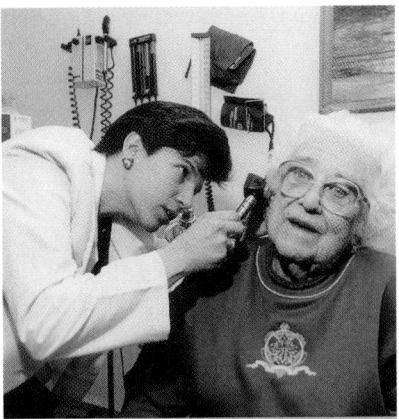

FIGURE 25-16 The nurse may find a slightly altered appearance to the tympanic membrane in the older adult.

External Ear

N Pendulous earlobes that are wrinkled can develop normally in the older adult. Wiry hair protruding from the auditory canal is normal. Cerumen is dry, which leads to an increased incidence of impaction.

A Skin lesions on the external ear may be malignant (SCC or BCC) or premalignant and need to be evaluated.

P The external ear receives a significant amount of sun exposure, especially in men.

Internal Ear

N The aging adult's normal ear may have pronounced landmarks if atrophic or sclerotic changes have occurred (Figure 25-16). The tympanic membrane may appear white, opaque, and thickened. It is also less resilient.

NOSE

Chapter 13 should be consulted for complete information on nasal assessment.

N The following are changes in the nose of an older adult:

- The nose increases in size due to increased cartilage formation.
- Nasal hairs are coarser.
- There is a decrease in the sense of smell because the number of sensory cells in the nasal lining decreases.

MOUTH AND THROAT

If the older adult has dentures, the mouth and oral cavity should be examined both with dentures and without. Chapter 13 provides additional information.

N The following changes occur in the older adult:

- Lip surface develops deep wrinkling, with an increase in granular lining on the lips and cheeks.
- The buccal mucosa thins, with a decrease in its vascularity.
- Gums are more pale in color with recession.
- Saliva production decreases (may be partly due to medications).
- Fissuring of the tongue increases with atrophy of papilla.
- Taste sensation diminishes due to atrophy and loss of taste buds.
- Gingival tissue has less elasticity.
- Dental roots become exposed.

A Fissures may develop at the corners of the mouth.

P This may be due to a vitamin deficiency or yeast (due to impaired immunity).

A Lesions on the lips, especially on smokers, are abnormal and should always be investigated.

P Lips are exposed to the elements and sun damage. Tobacco use increases the risk of oral cancer.

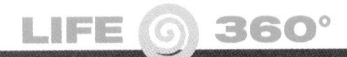

LIFE 360°

Diminished Sense of Taste

If a patient is experiencing some loss of taste, you can suggest adding seasonings to the diet such as garlic, pepper, and curry. Heavy use of salt should be avoided. You can also suggest preparing aromatic foods that first stimulate the olfactory sense to enhance appetite.

E Examination   **N** Normal Findings   **A** Abnormal Findings   **P** Pathophysiology

BREASTS

Breast exams should continue throughout the lifespan. The major risk factor for breast cancer is advancing age. Refer to Chapter 14.

N The following are breast changes in the older adult female:

- Breasts may appear flattened and elongated due to relaxation of suspensory ligaments.
- The nipples may be smaller and flatter.
- Cystic breasts may feel smoother as the woman ages and glandular tissue decreases.
- The inframammary ridge thickness increases in prominence.

A Masses or lesions should be evaluated.

P Increased incidence of breast cancer occurs with advancing age.

THORAX AND LUNGS

This examination may necessitate frequent breaks for the older adult to avoid fatigue and hyperventilation (Figure 25-17). Refer to Chapter 15.

N Expansion of the chest wall decreases with increased inspiratory effort in the older adult.

HEART AND PERIPHERAL VASCULATURE

The aging heart functions without compromise under normal stress. However, it has reduced reserve and may not be able to compensate for stress, blood loss, extreme exertion, or high fever. Chapter 16 provides comprehensive assessment information.

N The apical impulse may be displaced due to a decrease in the size of the heart in the older adult. A systolic ejection murmur may be auscultated at the left lower sternal border due to stiffening of the musculature and valvular leaflets.

A An S_4 heart sound is a common finding.

P Left ventricular thickening and/or enlargement resulting in loss of compliance result in the S_4.

A Decreased pulse volume may be present. Limbs may be cool.

P This can be due to arteriosclerosis and atherosclerosis.

ABDOMEN

Chapter 17 provides comprehensive information on the abdominal assessment.

N Abdominal musculature diminishes in mass and tone in the older adult. The fat content of the body increases with age, leading to increasing deposits in the abdomen. The liver decreases in size.

A Increased incidence of urinary and fecal incontinence commonly occurs but is not a normal change of aging and should be evaluated.

P Incontinence is secondary to changes of aging such as thinning of perineal tissues secondary to loss of estrogen, damage from childbirth, surgery, prostate problems, neurological disorders, and functional disability. Refer to Table 17-4.

MUSCULOSKELETAL SYSTEM

Health of the musculoskeletal system can impact the quality of life of the older adult dramatically. Assessment should include mobility, fine and gross motor skills,

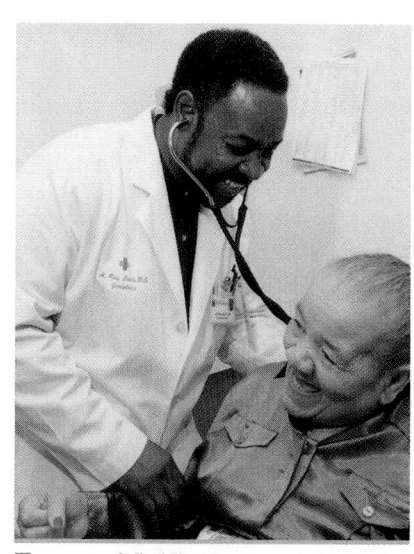

FIGURE 25-17 The nurse may need to give the older adult frequent rest periods when assessing the lungs.

and activities of daily living (ADL). Examination should be carefully performed to ensure joint stabilization. Slow, gentle, passive movements should be used to assess range of motion (ROM). Regular exercise should be encouraged, and information regarding the components of a program should be discussed. Maximal benefit will occur when the patient includes aerobic exercise in addition to muscle strengthening and balance. The older patient garners significant benefit from physical or occupational therapy consultation and information on environmental modifications to maximize function. Consult Chapter 18 for detailed information.

Inspection

N The following changes occur in the musculoskeletal system with the aging process:

- Posture changes to a more flexed position, which changes the center of gravity.
- Steps tend to be smaller, with a wider base in men while women maintain a narrow standing base. The step height is reduced.
- The gait has a higher risk for unsteadiness due to changes in the center of gravity and changes in the ear cochlea that result in a decreased ability to compensate.
- Transfers in and out of a sitting position will be more difficult for the older adult because of vertebral inflexibility and reduced muscle strength.

A A reduction in height occurs with the aging adult. Kyphosis may be present.

P Intervertebral discs lose water, causing narrowing of the disc space and a resultant loss of 1.5 to 3 inches in height.

A The lordotic curve of the back flattens, and both flexion and extension of the back decrease.

P Bone mass loss, bone density loss due to increased rate of bone reabsorption, and slowed bone cell replacement lead to these variations.

MUSCLES.

N Reduced muscle mass and loss of strength, especially against resistance, occur in the muscles of the older adult.

JOINTS.

A Decreased range of motion of individual joints and pain at rest and with range of motion can occur with the aging process. Crepitus may be present with joint movement.

P There is a decrease in the water content of cartilage and a narrowing of joint space with age. A lifetime of wear and tear results in deterioration.

MENTAL STATUS AND NEUROLOGICAL TECHNIQUES

Changes of aging affect the nervous system in a gradual fashion. The changes are both structural and functional. Chapter 19 provides comprehensive information.

Mental Status

N A slight decline in short-term memory is normal in the aging adult. There is minimal cognitive decline in normal aging.

| **E** Examination | **N** Normal Findings | **A** Abnormal Findings | **P** Pathophysiology |

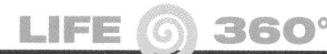

Recognizing Possible Elder Abuse and Neglect

A 78-year-old female with Alzheimer's disease is admitted through the emergency department with a diagnosis of probable aspiration pneumonia. Chest X-ray reveals pulmonary infiltrates consistent with the diagnosis of pneumonia but also multiple old rib fractures. Further assessment of the patient indicates cachexia, poor general hygiene, urinary and fecal incontinence, fecal impaction, decubiti of the sacral area, bruising of both arms in a "grip" fashion, and multiple bruises and abrasions of the buttocks and lower legs. The patient moans in pain frequently during the physical assessment. Follow-up limb X-rays reveal an old healed fracture of the left humerus. The patient is a widow and has been living with her divorced daughter for the last year. The daughter is the patient's only child as well as the patient's primary caregiver. During the day, the daughter works full time and the patient is cared for by hired help. The hired caregiver claims that the patient "falls frequently during the day."

- What is your initial reaction to these clinical findings?
- Do the findings of the physical assessment indicate possible physical abuse or neglect? Explain.
- What would you say to the patient's daughter?
- What questions would you ask the patient?

A There is an increased incidence of depression in the older adult.

P Decreases in the neurotransmitters norepinephrine and serotonin caused by changes in dendrite distribution and decreased enzymatic activity can lead to depression.

Sensory Assessment

N The following changes occur in the sensory assessment of the older adult:

- Reduced sensation of vibrations
- Reduced sensation of cold/heat
- Reduced sensation of touch discrimination, especially fine touch; some older adults develop an increased sensitivity to light touch due to thinner skin
- Decline in proprioception

Cranial Nerves

Refer to Chapter 19.

Cerebellar Function

N The older adult commonly has some balance impairment and may have an altered gait. There may be a decline in coordination.

A Abnormal gait accompanied by new incontinence or confusion is abnormal.

P Normal pressure hydrocephalus is more frequently seen in the older adult.

DTRs

N In the older adult there may be a decline in deep tendon reflexes, and the Achilles reflex may extinguish.

FEMALE GENITALIA

Examination of the pelvis should not be avoided in the older adult. The focus of the exam changes to evaluation for the problems of incontinence, pelvic relaxation, irritation, dryness, or rectal problems. Always screen for cancer if intact reproductive organs remain, if consistent with the goals of care. A smaller speculum may be needed. See Chapter 20.

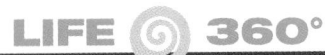

Inspection

N These changes may be found during inspection of the older adult female's genitalia:
- The clitoris and labia become smaller.
- The labia become flatter and lose pigmentation.
- The labial skin becomes thin, shiny, avascular, and dry.
- Pubic subcutaneous fat is lost.
- Pubic hair becomes sparse and turns gray or white.

Palpation

N These changes may be found during palpation of the older adult female's genitalia:
- The ovaries and fallopian tubes may not be palpable due to shrinkage.
- The uterus atrophies and may be difficult to palpate.
- The cervix becomes smaller, paler, and less mobile.
- The cervical os becomes smaller but remains palpable.
- The vagina shortens, narrows, and thins.
- The introitus constricts due to atrophy.
- The vaginal wall loses rugae and elasticity.
- Vaginal secretions are delayed, and production is reduced.

A The risk of a prolapsed uterus and vagina increases with age.

P This is caused by the atrophy of pelvic muscles, which leads to a decrease in pelvic organ support. Ligaments and connective tissue of the pelvis also lose muscle tone.

A Uterine enlargement, nodularity, irregularity, or induration should be investigated.

P Advancing age is a risk factor for malignancies such as ovarian, cervical, and endometrial cancers.

MALE GENITALIA

Inspection

See Chapter 21 for more information.

N The following changes may be found during the inspection of the older adult male's genitalia:
- The pubic hair thins and turns white or gray.
- The penis atrophies.
- The scrotal sac loses elasticity and elongates.
- The testicles may be smaller.

Palpation

N The testicles are smaller and atrophic.

ANUS, RECTUM, AND PROSTATE

Chapter 22 contains additional information.

| **E** Examination | **N** Normal Findings | **A** Abnormal Findings | **P** Pathophysiology |

Palpation

 The older male adult typically has a smooth and rubbery prostate that is enlarged.

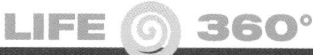

Rectal Incontinence in the Elderly

Rabin is an 87-year-old man who has been in the hospital for 10 days. Initially, he was admitted with a diagnosis of pneumonia. He was placed on intravenous antibiotics. On day five of his therapy Rabin developed persistent diarrhea, having 8 to 12 stools per day. His perianal skin is excoriated. You assist him in cleaning up after another stool, and he starts to cry. Rabin tells you that this is no way for a man of his age to live. He expresses his wish to die. How would you respond to this man?

CASE STUDY

The Older Adult with Leg Pain and Cognitive Impairment

This case study illustrates the application and objective documentation of the elderly patient assessment.
Eimear is a 75-year-old woman brought to the clinic by her daughter to have her leg pain evaluated.

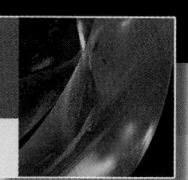

HEALTH HISTORY

PATIENT PROFILE	75 yo MWF
CHIEF COMPLAINT	"My right leg hurt all wk."
HISTORY OF PRESENT ILLNESS	Patient was in usual state of hl until 2 wks ago, when she c/o pain in the ℞ knee and ℞ upper leg. Pt said it improved and she canceled last wk's appt. Daughter reports that patient never really stopped c/o leg pain despite canceling her appointment. Per daughter, pt limping while shopping at mall past wk. Reported some improvement while seated, but discomfort resumed upon rising. Patient took no OTC analgesics. Daughter reports worsening of cognitive status for years. Patient is becoming more forgetful, suspicious at times, and tearful at other times. ⊕ nasal congestion/nasal discharge. ⊖ sinus pressure, ear pain, throat pain, cough. Denies SOB, CP, N/V/D, fever, H/A, decrease in LOC, or falls.
PAST HEALTH HISTORY	
Medical History	Frequent strep throat infections in her 20s–40s; chronic allergic rhinitis for which the patient continues to medicate with Actifed (OTC); chronic insomnia, self-medicated with Unisom (OTC); dementia, probably Alzheimer's type first noted 1997 in her medical record

continues

CASE STUDY (Continued)

The Older Adult with Leg Pain and Cognitive Impairment

Surgical History	Pterygium removal from eyes × 3 (once ℝ eye and twice 𝕃 eye) age late 20s–30s; TAH at age 39; anterior/posterior bladder repair age 57 yrs; left breast biopsy age 73 yrs (benign cyst)
Reproductive History	G: 4, P: 4, T: 4, P: 0, A: 0, E: 0, LC: 4, vaginal deliveries × 4 without complications
Allergies	NKDA, ⊕ seasonal (mostly spring), environmental (never tested). Gets runny nose, nasal and sinus congestion, and sniffles. OTC Actifed prn
Medications	Donepezil 10 mg qhs po, memantine 10 mg bid po, conjugated estrogen 0.625 mg daily po; OTC Actifed 1 tab po q 4 h prn, and Unisom 1 tab po hs prn
Communicable Diseases	None reported, denies HSV, STD, hepatitis, HIV
Injuries and Accidents	Denies
Special Needs	Denies; however, pt has cognitive impairment progressing rapidly per daughter
Blood Transfusions	None
Childhood Illnesses	Presumed UCHD
Immunizations	Pneumovax 1998; flu shot annually; diphtheria/tetanus 2003; neg for zostavax immunization

FAMILY HEALTH HISTORY

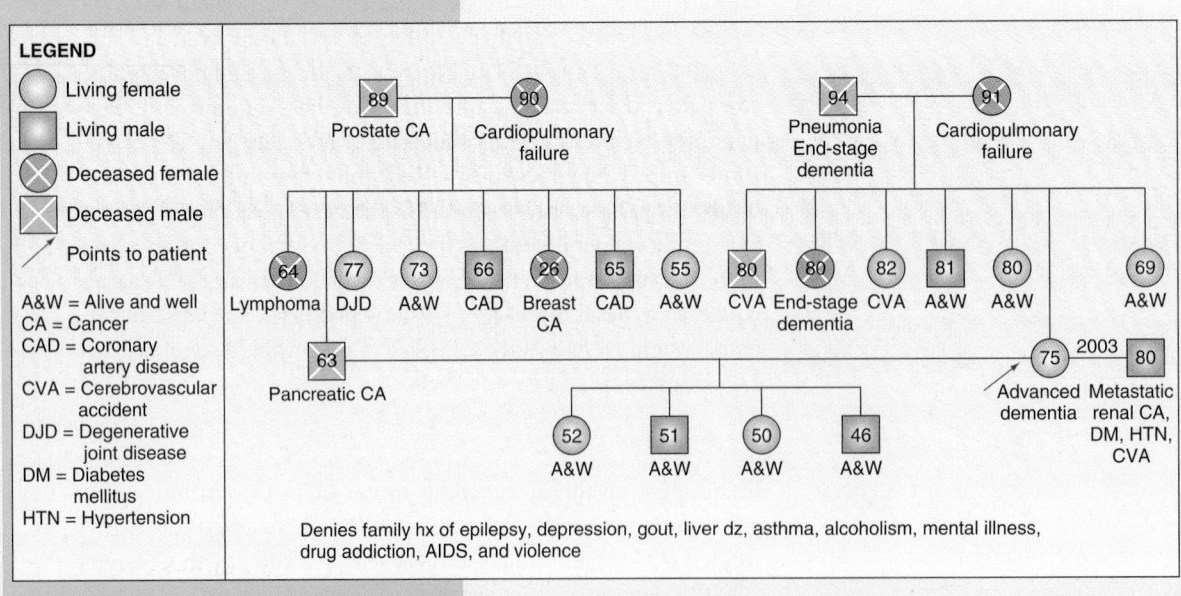

LEGEND

- ◯ Living female
- ▢ Living male
- ⊗ Deceased female
- ⊠ Deceased male
- ⤢ Points to patient

A&W = Alive and well
CA = Cancer
CAD = Coronary artery disease
CVA = Cerebrovascular accident
DJD = Degenerative joint disease
DM = Diabetes mellitus
HTN = Hypertension

Denies family hx of epilepsy, depression, gout, liver dz, asthma, alcoholism, mental illness, drug addiction, AIDS, and violence

continues

SOCIAL HISTORY	
Alcohol Use	Denies alcohol abuse; 1 glass of red wine with dinner 4 times a wk
Tobacco Use	20 pack/yr history; quit in 1989
Drug Use	Denies illicit use
Domestic and Intimate Partner Violence	Denies
Sexual Practice	Married, monogamous
Travel History	Travels to Ireland yearly
Work Environment	Retired secretary/administrative assistant
Home Environment	Lives in 3-bedroom condo with 2nd husband. Receives assistance from children with care, doctor visits, prescriptions, and activities
Hobbies and Leisure Activities	Enjoys dancing, church activities, bowling, and reading but is limited due to physical limitations of husband and access
Stress	None presently due to memory impairment; does remember son is in Iraq and becomes concerned and distressed but is easily redirected/distracted
Education	Completed BA degree in English literature 1986 as adult after getting GED
Economic Status	Upper middle class; no financial concerns
Military Service	Denies
Religion	Practicing Roman Catholic
Ethnic Background	Born and raised in Ireland; immigrated to United States in 1954
Roles and Relationships	Lives with husband, who is obese, has diabetes, HTN, peripheral neuropathy, and old CVA, and cannot walk more than 20 ft without resting. Pt has 4 surviving siblings who phone weekly; 4 children: one daughter in Georgia, who is very involved, and pt likes to visit there; one daughter in Virginia who is primary caregiver with husband; son in Iraq; son in Virginia with 3 grandchildren whom pt frequently visits. Pt's friends call daughter but pt unable to maintain contact with them due to cognitive status. Pt does not drive.
Characteristic Patterns of Daily Living	Awakens early and waits for husband to get up. Eats breakfast prepared by husband. Washes and dresses with cuing. Goes out for lunch, goes for drives (husband is driver), out for shopping, and dinner most days.

continues

HEALTH MAINTENANCE ACTIVITIES	
Sleep	Sleeps poorly, with frequent awakening. Awakens early. Naps some during the day. Takes OTC as sleep aid against PCP advice.
Diet	Regular diet without restriction. Needs to have food cut up outside of her view and then be reminded to eat.
Exercise	No exercise
Stress Management	Denies stress
Use of Safety Devices	Uses seat belt only when it is applied to her; wanders; wears Alzheimer's ID bracelet
Health Check-ups	Every 6 months visits PCP; sees ophthalmologist and dentist annually. Last mammogram 10 yrs ago.
REVIEW OF SYSTEMS	
General	Usually healthy
Skin	Denies rashes, ⊕ spots that occasionally itch on legs, ⊕ age spots on hands, does not use sunblock or wear hat when outside
Hair	Denies alopecia, hirsutism, or itching
Nails	Has acrylic nails, manicure, and pedicure q 3 wks, nails without splitting, breaking, or Δ in texture
Eyes	Denies photophobia, tearing, diplopia, drainage, bloodshot eyes, pain, spots, lights, or halos; sees ophthalmologist annually, daughter reports beginning cataracts
Ears	Denies hearing deficits, no hearing aids, pain, discharge, vertigo, earaches, tinnitus, or infection
Nose and Sinuses	Allergies per PHH; ⊕ postnasal drip, stuffiness; denies URI, discharge, itching, polyps, obstruction, Δ in smell, nosebleeds
Mouth	Brushes teeth bid, ⊕ gum recession, ⊖ flossing, ⊖ bleeding, denies swelling, difficulty chewing, soreness; denies Δ in taste, lesions; Δ in salivation, bad breath; sees dentist annually
Throat/Neck	Denies hoarseness, Δ in voice, difficulty swallowing, pain/stiffness, or goiter
Breasts	Denies pain, tenderness, discharge, lumps, dimpling; neg BSE
Respiratory	Denies SOB, DOE, cough, sputum, wheezing, hemoptysis, asthma; medical record shows PPD neg 1 yr ago

continues

Cardiovascular	Denies PND, CP, orthopnea, murmur, palpitations, syncope, edema, cold hands/feet, anemia; $\oplus$ MI at some point in past per daughter, $\oplus$ nocturnal leg cramps
Gastrointestinal	Hard brown stool q wk; denies Δ in appetite, N/V/D, melena, hematemesis, Δ in stool color, flatulence, belching, regurgitation, heartburn, dysphagia, abd pain, jaundice, hemorrhoids, hepatitis, PUD, gallstones; colonoscopy age 55 yr and refused to repeat
Musculoskeletal	Denies back pain, redness, swelling, bone deformity, weakness, broken bones, dislocations, sprains, gout, arthritis, herniated disc. Of note: pt denies joint pain or leg pain.
Neurological	Denies Δ in balance, coordination, loss of movement, Δ in sensation/perception, Δ in speech, Δ in smell, loss of memory, tremors, involuntary movement, Δ LOC, sz, weakness; daughter reports pt walking more tentatively as though she can't see doors, curbs, and steps. Frequently misses chairs unless guided down. Significant memory loss continues to worsen per daughter.
Psychological	Denies irritability, nervousness, tension, stress, difficulty concentrating, mood changes, suicidal thoughts, depression. Per daughter: Pt becomes quite irritable when she can't remember or is told by husband that she is wrong about an event. Cannot concentrate more than 2 minutes on any activity.
Urinary	Denies dysuria, Δ in urine color, hesitancy, reduced force of stream, bedwetting, incontinence, suprapubic pain, kidney stones, UTI. Per daughter: Pt smells of urine frequently, panties are soiled.
Female Reproductive	Menarche age 16, TAH age 39, has taken HRT since sgy, sexually active, denies discharge or bleeding
Nutrition	Denies weight loss, difficulty eating. Per daughter: Has regained weight lost (25 lbs) while living alone several years: regained 15 lbs upon moving in with spouse, gained 10 lbs more in past 3 months. Usual weight 125–130 lbs and now 143 lbs; eats well when food cut up and reminded to continue eating.
Endocrine	Denies bulging eyes, fatigue, Δ in size of head/hands/feet, heat/cold intolerance, sweating, thirst, hunger, Δ in hair distribution, swelling ant neck, diabetes
Lymph Nodes	Denies tenderness or enlargement
Hematological	$\oplus$ bruises easily, bleeds for long time when injures self, denies anemia, thinks she is A+ blood type

continues

CASE STUDY   (Continued)

The Older Adult with Leg Pain and Cognitive Impairment

FUNCTIONAL ASSESSMENT

Katz ADL: Pt scored 3/6. Needs cuing to bathe, dress, and eat.
Lawton IADL: Pt scored 2/8. Patient able only to answer phone and direct housekeeping.
Get Up and Go Test: Gait steady, hesitant at changes in tile color, then tentative stepping. Able to complete test in 10 seconds.

COGNITIVE ASSESSMENT

General Discussion

Pt pleasant with appropriate social skills. Can't recall children's names. Confused about which son is overseas. Daughter reports pt becomes suspicious, especially about money. Can usually be distracted. Occasionally becomes quite angry and belligerent without specific precipitant. Monitoring pt from a distance for safety and wandering usually most effective at that time. After a half hour to an hour can usually be distracted.

Mini Mental State Examination: 10/30; could not state day of the week, date, month, or year; named the proper season. Pt knew she was in office of some sort in the correct city and state. 1/3 word immediate recall, 0/3 recall at 1 minute; could not spell "world" backward; ⊕ identification of watch and "writing thing," could not explain proverb, could not perform 3-part command, could follow written command, and abnormal intersecting pentagon diagram copy.

Clock Drawing Test: Abnormal

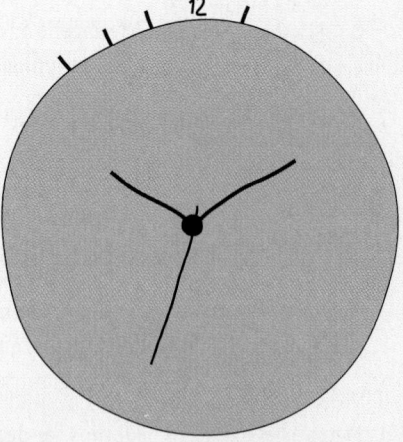

Geriatric Depression Scale: 0/15 with no positive questions answered, which possibly indicates depression

continues

CASE STUDY (Continued)

The Older Adult with Leg Pain and Cognitive Impairment

PHYSICAL EXAMINATION

General Survey and Vital Signs	WDWNWF who looks stated age in NAD or pain
	HT: 5'2" (150 cm)
	Wt: 143 lbs (65 kg)
	T: 98.8°F (37°C), oral
	P: 78
	R: 14
	B/P: 122/68 mm Hg (Ⓛ arm sitting)
	       122/70 mm Hg (Ⓛ arm supine)
	       124/70 mm Hg (Ⓡ arm sitting)
	
	Posture upright and erect. Poor attention to hygiene in areas of pt responsibility. Slight body odor from pt and clothing.

Skin, Hair, and Nails	Thinning hair on legs, 2 inch ecchymosis on Ⓡ lower arm, scrape on Ⓛ shin, without rashes, edema; skin warm to touch without diaphoresis, smooth texture, ↓ turgor; hair gray, clean, and long, without infestations; nails manicured, without clubbing
Head	Normocephalic without lesions, masses, depressions, or tenderness; face symmetrical, without involuntary mvt or swelling; scalp shiny and intact, without lesions or masses; TMJ articulates smoothly, without clicking or creptitus
Eyes	Acuity by Snellen chart: right eye 20/40, left eye 20/30 with glasses; able to read letters on newspaper without difficulty, color vision intact, visual fields by confrontation intact; eyebrows gray, full, coarse, and symmetrical; eyelashes evenly distributed and without inflammation, no ptosis or lid lag; lacrimal apparatus without inflammation; corneal light reflex symmetrical without strabismus; cover/uncover test without deviation, EOMI, no nystagmus, conjunctiva pink, no foreign bodies, no tearing, sclera white without exudate, ⊕ arcus senilis, PERRLA at 3 mm Funduscopic: ⊕ red reflex, Ⓡ lens whitened and semitransparent, Ⓛ lens clear, discs flat with sharp margins, vessels in A-V ratio of 2:3, background uniformly pink without hemorrhages or exudate
Ears	Gross hearing intact by watch-tick test; pinna without masses, lesions, nodules, inflammation, or tenderness; EAC with dry wax, without inflammation; TMs shiny, ⊕ light reflex; Weber midline; Rinne: AC greater than BC
Nose and Sinuses	No deformities, bleeding, lesions, masses, swelling; nares patent, nontender; septum midline without perforation; mucosa pale; maxillary sinuses tender to palpation, dull; frontal sinuses nontender, resonant

continues

Mouth and Throat	$\oplus$ halitosis, lips pink, without swelling, 2 mm dry ulcer on $\circledR$ lower lip, gums and mucosa pink and moist, teeth in good repair, gingival recession throughout, tongue midline, well papillated, and without fasciculation, lesions, swelling, or bleeding; hard and soft palates intact without lesions or masses; pharynx pink nonedematous, uvula midline and rises with phonation; $\oplus$ gag reflex; no exudates
Neck	Supple without masses or spasms and with FROM, neck symmetrical without masses or tenderness, no lymphadenopathy, trachea midline, thyroid nontender without enlargement or masses, no bruits, no JVD at 90°, 45°, and supine
Breasts	Old ¾" scar on right upper outer quadrant of $\textcircled{L}$ breast, no thickening, edema, vascularity, erosion, fissures, lesions, masses, retraction, discharge; areola and nipples dark in pigmentation; nonpalpable lymph nodes
Thorax and Lungs	AP: transverse diameter = 1:2; chest wall symmetrical, costal angle less than 90°, angle of ribs with sternum = 45°, no bulging of ICS or retractions, no use of accessory muscles, respirations regular, thoracic expansion 3 cm ant and 3 cm post, $\oplus$ tactile fremitus bilat, lungs resonant, diaphragmatic excursion 4 cm bilat, clear breath sounds; no adventitious breath sounds
Heart	Precordium without pulsations/heaves/thrills, apical pulse 74, apical impulse 1 cm at 5th ICS at $\textcircled{L}$ MCL, S_1 and S_2 present, SEM II/VI at LLSB, no radiation
Abdomen	Round with striae, no dilated veins, scars, incisions; $\oplus$ bowel sounds in 4 quads, no bruits, venous hum, friction rub; tympanic throughout except dullness superior to symphysis pubis for 2 cm; abd soft, no masses/tenderness to light/deep palpation; liver span 6 cm in $\circledR$ MCL; negative bilat CVAT
Peripheral Vasculature	No edema or ulcerations, neg Homan's sign, pulse regular and strong, no pulsus paradoxus, no bruits

	CAROTID	BRACHIAL	RADIAL	FEMORAL	POPLITEAL	DORSALIS PEDIS	POSTERIOR TIBIAL
Right	3+	3+	3+	3+	3+	3+	3+
Left	3+	3+	3+	3+	3+	3+	3+

Scale: 0–3+

Musculoskeletal	Refer to "Get up and Go" Test. No new injury on legs. Has healing old shin lesions as noted earlier. Pt not sure how she got them; however, they were present when seen last month and are healing well. Hips, knees, and ankles have FROM. Knees in

continues

CASE STUDY (Continued)

The Older Adult with Leg Pain and Cognitive Impairment

	alignment bilat without erythema, joint swelling, or tenderness; suprapatellar pouch and bursa without swelling, pain, or tenderness
Advanced Techniques	Bulge Sign: Neg Patellar Ballottement: Neg Apley's Grinding Sign: Neg
	McMurray's Sign: Neg Drawer Test: Neg Lachman's Test: Neg Varus and Valgus Stress: Neg
Neurological	

Mental Status: Refer to Cognitive Assessment.

Sensory: Light touch, superficial pain, 2-point discrimination and extinction intact; position: unable to verbalize finger or leg position, motion intact; vibration not detectable below ankles bilaterally; stereognosis—unable to identify 2 objects; graphesthesia—unable to identify 3 different letters

Cranial Nerves: CN II–XII intact, CN I deferred

Motor: Size = bilaterally; tone: firm and supple throughout; strength: strong and equal LUE 5/5, RUE 5/5, LLE 5/5, RLE 5/5; involuntary movements: none; pronator drift: none

Cerebellar Function: Coordination: finger to nose intact but slow with eyes open, cannot perform with eyes closed; unable to perform (understand?) rapid alternating movements or heel slide bilaterally; station: posture erect; Romberg: unable to perform; gait: cannot perform tiptoe or heel walking; cannot perform heel-to-toe walking or hopping on one leg bilaterally

Reflexes:

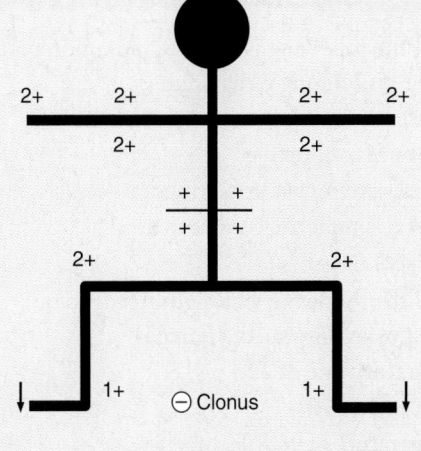

Scale = 4+

continues

CASE STUDY (Continued)

The Older Adult with Leg Pain and Cognitive Impairment

Genitalia and Rectum	Rectum without masses or lesions, occult blood negative. Pt refused additional exam.
DIAGNOSTIC DATA	

	PT'S RESULTS	NORMAL RESULTS
CT scan of the head without contrast	Diffuse white matter changes. Greater than age-related atrophy, no acute process	Age-appropriate atrophy

ASSESSMENT IN BRIEF

Elderly Patient Assessment

Special Assessments
- Developmental assessment
- Cultural assessment
- Spiritual assessment
- Nutritional assessment
- Pain assessment

*Physical Examination**
- Quick screen
- Functional testing
- Cognition

* All other assessment skills are performed as described in Chapters 10–22.

REVIEW QUESTIONS

1. Which of the following is the most common pattern of hearing loss among older adults?
   a. Unilateral sensorineural
   b. Unilateral conductive
   c. Bilateral symmetric sensorineural
   d. Bilateral symmetric conductive
   The correct answer is (c).

2. Which of the following vital signs needs to be addressed in an 85-year-old female?
   a. Respiratory rate of 22
   b. Heart rate of 96
   c. Temperature of 96.8°F
   d. Blood pressure of 142/98
   The correct answer is (d).

3. An older adult may complain of difficulty driving at night. Which physiological change in the eyes may explain this?
   a. Accommodation is increased.
   b. Peripheral vision widens.
   c. The ability to discern the colors red and green is impaired.
   d. The pupils become smaller.
   The correct answer is (d).

4. Which functional testing tool is most appropriate for an older adult who is living independently?

a. The Lawton Instrumental Activities of Daily Living

b. The Katz Independence in Activities of Daily Living

c. The Elder Assessment

d. The Get Up and Go Test

The correct answer is (a).

Questions 5–7 refer to the following situation:

You are conducting an admission interview on a 92-year-old man at an assisted living facility. He tells you that he used to work in road construction. He is wearing glasses and a hearing aid. The patient is scratching lesions on his hands.

5. You note that this man has a pearly white lesion on his left cheek. The patient tells you that the lesion has become itchy and it bleeds. What lesion do you suspect this patient has?

a. Actinic keratosis

b. Basal cell carcinoma

c. Squamous cell carcinoma

d. Melanoma

The correct answer is (b).

6. During the admission interview you note that the patient looks straight ahead while addressing his son, who is seated to his right. The older man should be further evaluated for which of the following conditions?

a. Presbycusis

b. Macular degeneration

c. Hearing aid malfunction

d. Cranial nerve III palsy

The correct answer is (b).

7. Bluish-purple lesions are noted on the patient's hands and arms. You identify these lesions as most likely being:

a. Seborrheic keratoses c. Senile purpura

b. Solar lentigo   d. Sebaceous hyperplasia

The correct answer is (c).

8. Which of the following reasons best describes why the S_4 heart sound is a common finding in the older adult?

a. The increase in the incidence of congestive heart failure

b. Decreased compliance of the left ventricle

c. Sclerosis of the mitral and aortic valves

d. Turbulent blood flow from the vena cava into the right atrium

The correct answer is (b).

9. A patient takes 25 seconds to complete the Get Up and Go Test. What information does this tell us about the patient?

a. The patient has a high level of independence.

b. The patient is capable of performing transfers without assistance.

c. The patient requires a walker for additional ambulation.

d. The patient has an increased risk of falls.

The correct answer is (d).

10. Mrs. Dunlop is an 87-year-old nursing home resident who has been hospitalized for pneumonia. On admission she is pleasant, alert, and oriented to person, place, and time. The next day Mrs. Dunlop awakens when her name is called but then closes her eyes during the conversation. She is distracted by voices in the hallway, and questions must be repeated. She is now slurring her words and having difficulty with word finding. Which condition best explains Mrs. Dunlop's symptoms?

a. Alzheimer's disease   c. Depression

b. Dementia   d. Delirium

The correct answer is (d).

REFERENCES

Bolognia, J. L. (1995). Aging skin. *American Journal of Medicine, 98*(1A), 99S.

He, W., Sengupta, S., Velkoff, V., & DeBarros, K. (2005). 65+ in the United States: 2005. Retrieved January 3, 2008, from http://www.census.gov/prod/2006pubs/p23-209.pdf

Duncan, P. W. (1999). Development of a comprehensive assessment toolbox for stroke. *Clinics in Geriatric Medicine, 15*(4), 885–894.

Mouton, C., & Esparza, Y. (2000). Ethnicity and geriatric assessment. In J. Gallo, T. Fulmer, G. Paveza, & W. Reichel (Eds.), *Handbook of geriatric assessment* (3rd ed., pp. 13–27). Gaithersburg, MD: Aspen Publishers, Inc.

Reno, B. (2001). Urinary and reproductive problems. In A. Luggen & S. Meiner (Eds.), *NGNA curriculum for gerontological nursing* (2nd ed., pp. 84–87). Philadelphia: Mosby Publishing.

What are the key statistics for breast cancer. (2007). Retrieved July 29, 2008, from http://www.cancer.org/docroot/CRI/content/CRI_2_4_1X_What_are_the_key_statistics_for_breast_cancer_5.asp

BIBLIOGRAPHY

Alzheimer's disease. (2006). Retrieved May 25, 2007, from http://www.cdc.gov/nchs/fastats/alzheimr.htm

Alzheimer's disease statistics. (2007). Retrieved May 25, 2007, from http://www.alz.org/grtrcinc/aaWhatStatistics.htm

Amella, E. J. (2004). Presentation of illness in older adults. *American Journal of Nursing, 104*(10), 40–51.

Amella, E. J. (2006). Presentation of illness in older adults. If you think you know what you're looking for, think again. *AORN Journal, 83*(2), 372–374.

Amella, E. J. (2007). TRY THIS: Assessing nutrition in older adults. Retrieved January 12, 2008, from http://www.hartfordign.org/publications/trythis/issue_9.pdf

Bloom, H., & Edelberg, H. (2008). Preventative care. Retrieved January 2, 2008, from http://www.frycomm.com/ags/teachingslides/slides.asp

Borson, S., Scanlan, J., Brush, M., Vitaliano, P., & Dokmak, A. (2000). The Mini-Cog: A cognitive "vital signs" measure for dementia screening in multi-lingual elderly. *International Journal of Geriatric Psychiatry, 15*(11), 1021–1027.

Borson, S., Scanlan, J., Chen, P., & Ganguli, M. (2003). The mini-cog as a screen for dementia: Validation in a population-based sample. *Journal of the American Geriatrics Society, 51*, 1451–1454.

Borson, S., Scanlan, J., Watanabe, J., Tu, S. P., & Lessig, M. (2005). Simplifying detection of cognitive impairment: Comparison of mini-cog and mini-mental state examination in a multiethnic sample. *Journal of the American Geriatrics Society, 53*, 871–874.

Borson, S., Scanlan, J. M., Watanabe, J., Tu, S. P., & Lessig, M. (2006). Improving identification of cognitive impairment in primary care. *International Journal of Geriatric Psychiatry, 21*(4), 349–355.

Carolan Doerflinger, D. (2007). TRY THIS: Mental status assessment of older adults: The mini-cog. Retrieved January 19, 2008, from http://www.hartfordign.org/publications/trythis/issue03.pdf

Cassel, C. K. (Ed.). (2003). *Geriatric medicine: An evidence-based approach* (4th ed.). New York: Springer Publishing.

Changes with aging. (2004). Retrieved March 18, 2007, from http://www.ageworks.com/information_on_aging/changeswithaging/index.shtml

Cotter, V., & Smith, C. (2006). Normal aging changes. Retrieved March 10, 2007, from http://www.geronurseonline.org/index.cfm?section_id=31&geriatric_topic_id=11&sub_section_id=77&page_id=166&tab=2

Demers, K. (2007). TRY THIS: Hearing screening in older adults: A brief hearing loss screener. Retrieved January 14, 2008, from http://www.hartfordign.org/publications/trythis/issue_12.pdf

Dowling-Castronovo, A. (2007). TRY THIS: Urinary incontinence assessment in older adults. Retrieved January 14, 2008, from http://www.hartfordign.org/publications/trythis/issue11-1.pdf

Dramatic changes in U.S. aging highlighted in new census, NIH report. (2006). Retrieved January 3, 2008, from http://www.census.gov/Press-Release/www/releases/archives/aging_population/006544.html

Flaherty, E., & Zwicker, D. (2006). Atypical presentations in the elderly. Retrieved March 10, 2007, from http://www.geronurseonline.org/index.cfm?section_id=36&geriatric_topic_id=16&sub_section_id=101&page_id=234&tab=2

Folstein, M., Folstein, S., & McHugh, P. (1975). "Mini-mental state": A practical method for grading the cognitive state of patients for the clinician. *Journal of Psychiatric Research, 12*, 189–198.

Gill, T. (2008). Assessment of the older adult. Retrieved January 2, 2008, from http://www.frycomm.com/ags/teachingslides/slides.asp

Gomolin, I. H., Aung, M. M., WolfKlein, G., & Auerbach, C. (2005). Older is colder: Temperature range and variation in older people. *Journal of the American Geriatrics Society, 53*(12), 2170–2172.

Graf, C. (2007). TRY THIS: The Lawton instrumental activities of daily living (IADL) scale. Retrieved January 13, 2008, from http://www.hartfordign.org/publications/trythis/issue23.pdf

Ham, R., J. Sloane, P. D., & Warshaw, G. Bernard, M. A., & Flaherty E. (2006). *Primary care geriatrics: A case based approach (5th ed.)*. St. Louis: Mosby.

Lopez, M. N., Charter, R. A., Mostafavi, B., Nibut, L. P., & Smith, W. E. (2005). Psychometric properties of the Folstein mini-mental state examination. *Assessment, 12*(2), 137–144.

Mokdad, A. H., Giles, W. H., Bowman B. A., Mensah, G. A., Ford, E. S., Smith, S. M., & Marks, J. S. (2004). Changes in health behaviors among older Americans, 1990 to 2000. *Public Health Reports, 119*(3), 356–361.

Ouslander, J., Abrass, I., & Kane, R. (Eds.). (2004). *Essentials of clinical geriatrics* (5th ed.). New York: McGraw Hill Publishing.

Roth Maguire, S. (2006). Gerontologic assessment. In S. Meiner & A. Lueckenotte (Eds.), *Gerontologic nursing* (3rd ed., pp. 65–83). St. Louis: Mosby Elsevier.

U.S. Bureau of the Census and the National Center for Health Statistics. Retrieved March 17, 2007, from http://www.aoa.gov/PROF/Statistics/profile/2005/3.asp

Wallace, M., & Grossman, S. (Eds.). (2008). *Gerontological nurse certification review*. New York: Springer Publishing.

Wallace, M., & Shelkey, M. (2007). TRY THIS: Katz index of independence in activities of daily living (ADL). Retrieved January 14, 2008, from http://www.hartfordign.org/publications/trythis/issue02.pdf

Waszinski, C. (2007). TRY THIS: The confusion assessment method CAM. Retrieved January 14, 2008, from http://www.hartfordign.org/publications/trythis/issue13.pdf

What are the key statistics for breast cancer. (2007). Retrieved July 29, 2008, from http://www.cancer.org/docroot/CRI/content/CRI_2_4_1X_What_are_the_key_statistics_for_breast_cancer_5.asp

What is normal aging? Retrieved March 10, 2007, from http://www.agingcarefl.org/aging/normalAging

WEB SITES

AARP [American Association of Retired Persons]:
   http://www.aarp.org

The AGS Foundation for Health in Aging:
   http://www.healthinaging.org

Alzheimer's Disease Education and Referral Center:
   http://www.alzheimers.org

American Geriatrics Society:
   http://www.americangeriatrics.org

Building Academic Geriatric Nursing Capacity:
   http://www.geriatricnursing.org

Canadian Gerontological Nursing Association:
   http://www.cgna.net

Geriatric Nursing:
   http://www.gnjournal.com

The Gerontological Society of America:
   http://www.geron.org

Hartford Institute for Geriatric Nursing:
   http://www.hartfordign.org

Hospice and Palliative Nurses Association:
   http://www.hpna.org

Hospice Foundation of America:
   http://www.hospicefoundation.org

Institute for Geriatric Nursing:
   http://www.consultGeriRN.org

National Association for Home Care & Hospice:
   http://www.nahc.org

National Conference of Gerontological Nurse Practitioners:
   http://www.ncgnp.org

National Council on Aging:
   http://www.ncoa.org

National Gerontological Nursing Association:
   http://www.ngna.org

National Institute on Aging:
   http://www.nia.nih.gov

Nurse Assist:
   http://www.rnplus.com

University of Iowa College of Nursing Areas of Excellence:
   http://www.nursing.uiowa.edu

University of Iowa College of Nursing: The John A.
Hartford Center of Geriatric Nursing Excellence:
   http://www.nursing.uiowa.edu

U.S. Administration on Aging:
   http://www.aoa.dhhs.gov

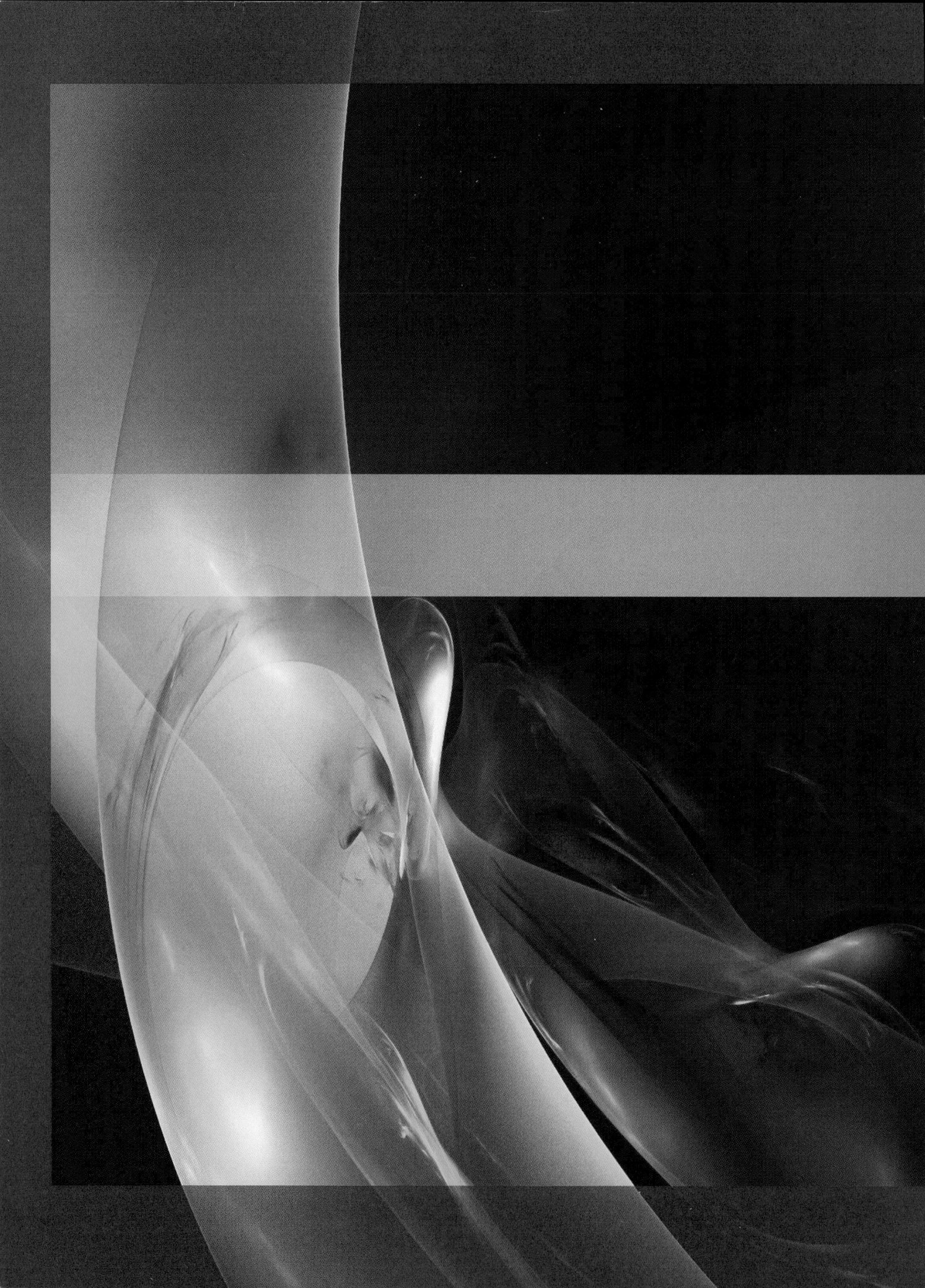

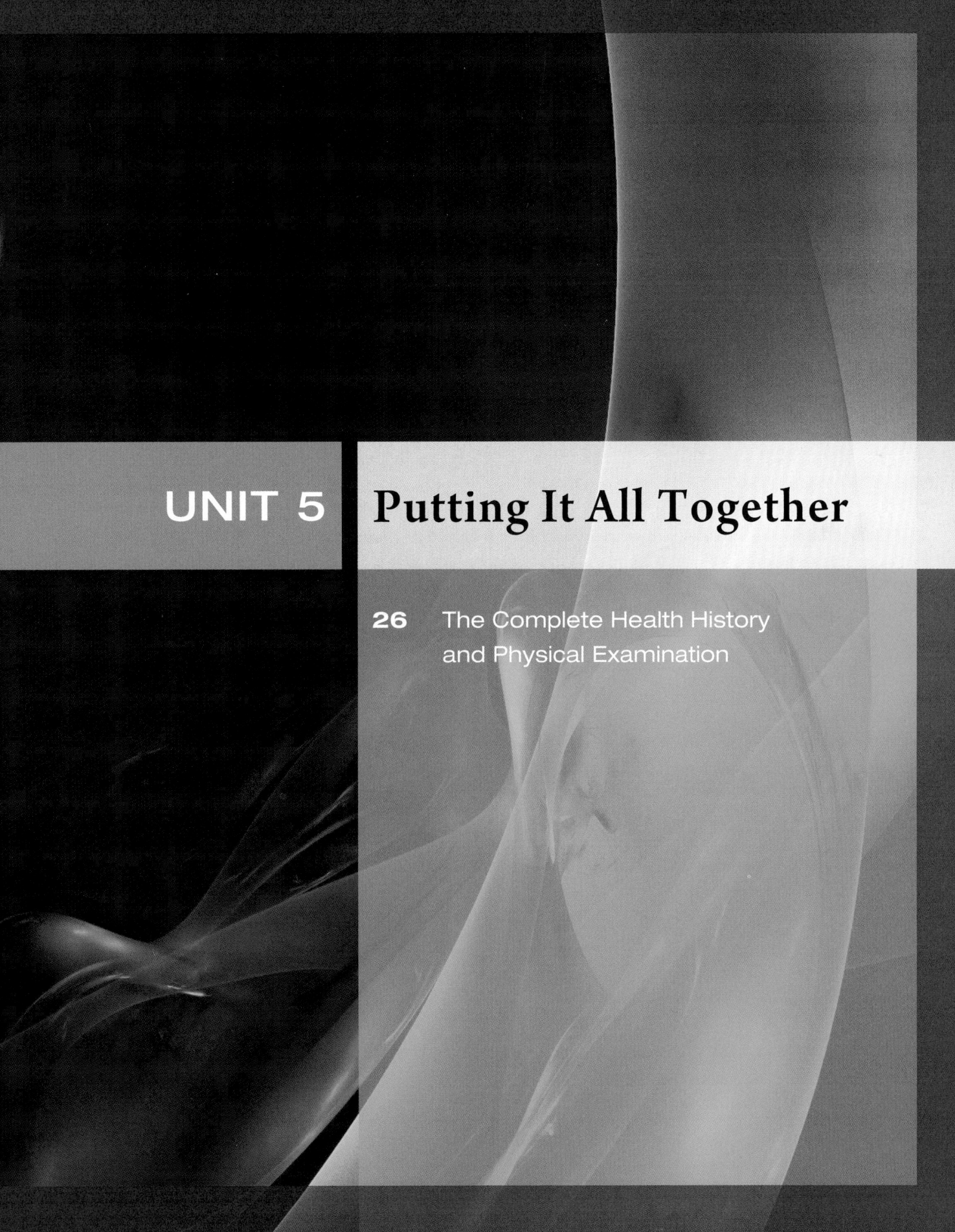

UNIT 5 | Putting It All Together

26 The Complete Health History
and Physical Examination

Every day ... knowledge of nursing ... of how to put the constitution in such a state as that it will have no disease, or that it can recover from disease, takes a higher place.

—Florence Nightingale

CHAPTER 26

The Complete Health History and Physical Examination

COMPETENCIES

1. Identify ethical and legal considerations for the health history and physical examination.

2. Identify the components of the complete health history and physical examination.

3. Conduct a complete health history and physical examination on a patient.

4. Document a complete health history and physical examination.

NURSING**TIP**

Fostering Patient Cooperation

The success of any health history and physical examination rests, in part, with obtaining and maintaining the patient's cooperation. Guidelines to assist you in this endeavor are:

- Have the patient wait as little as possible prior to the examination; explain any delays that occur.
- Greet the patient first, shake hands, and put the patient at ease (Figure 26-1).
- Proceed in an efficient and organized manner.
- Encourage the patient to actively participate in the assessment process (e.g., provide information, ask questions, teach).
- Use terms the patient will understand.
- Ask the patient to repeat home care or self-examination instructions and to demonstrate learned skills when appropriate to verify patient understanding.
- Be honest; do not offer false reassurance or jump to conclusions.
- Discuss findings first without diagnosing; validate findings when indicated.
- Arrange for the presence of a third party if requested.

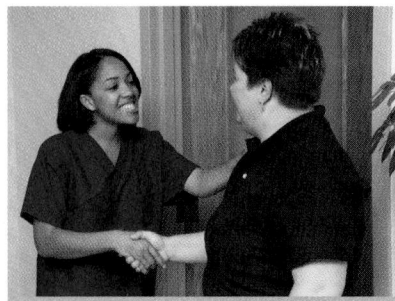

FIGURE 26-1 A friendly greeting will help to get the examination off to a successful start.

Performing a complete health history and physical examination is a skill that takes time and practice to develop. You must concentrate on perfecting interviewing techniques and assessment skills. You must be able to accurately recognize normal findings in order to appreciate abnormal and pathological findings. Practicing in an academic laboratory setting or on a volunteer patient is a crucial step leading to skill mastery. Learning the assessment techniques system by system, as described in this text, helps you to gradually build on previously developed skills.

Keep in mind that as assessment skills are perfected, the amount of time it takes to perform them will decrease. Plan on spending between 30 and 90 minutes conducting the complete health history and physical examination. If the patient's chief complaint is not of an urgent or critical nature, the patient's first visit to the health care facility is the ideal time to perform a comprehensive assessment. Interval or follow-up visits frequently require partial assessments that document changes from the initial database; these visits require substantially less time.

It is important to develop a routine that is comfortable so that steps in the assessment process will not be overlooked. The patient's physical, emotional, or mental state may necessitate a change in the usual progression of the assessment. Clinical judgment and experience will dictate when specific steps should be omitted, deferred, or repeated.

Once the content of Chapters 9 to 22 is learned and you are comfortable performing each assessment, it is time to integrate the entire health assessment and physical examination. This chapter provides a step-by-step approach to guide you through the entire process for an adult patient. With time, you will develop a personal rhythm.

Advanced techniques are normally inserted in the assessment process at different phases, depending on the techniques to be performed and the patient's condition. Experience will guide you in determining when these advanced techniques are warranted. They are omitted from the following assessment sequence, which illustrates a "typical" head-to-toe assessment.

☑ NURSING**CHECKLIST**

General Assessment Reminders

- Understand illness in human terms, not just scientific terms.
- Approach the patient from a holistic viewpoint and try to understand the patient's perspective.
- Remember that nursing is both art and science.
- Follow your judgment; critical thinking incorporates the consideration of objective and subjective data. Always ask, "Why?"
- Act unhurried.
- Act in a professional manner at all times; remember that the patient is simultaneously examining you (mannerisms, facial expressions, hesitations in speech).
- Recognize both the patient's and your potential stressors (work, home environment, schedules) and try to account for them.
- Acknowledge emotional reactions to illness (anger, fear, anxiety, disbelief, confusion, guilt, shame, blame, hurt, and betrayal).
- Embrace sensitivity to cultural and spiritual issues.
- Show respect for the patient and his or her circumstances.
- Possess a sense of self-awareness to guide your actions.

LEGAL CONSIDERATIONS

The increasingly litigious nature of society has not bypassed the nursing profession. More and more nurses are being named as codefendants in lawsuits. What is legally expected of the nurse is to conduct himself or herself in a reasonably prudent manner at all times. Some specific guidelines are:

- Document all patient interactions (face-to-face, telephone, letters, faxes).
- Respect the patient's confidentiality. Do not discuss any patient's case in a public area or with colleagues who are not on that patient's care team; keep discussions at a strictly professional level.
- Report any disease that is considered a public health concern (according to local, state, and federal regulations).
- Respect a patient's right to privacy.
- Respect a patient's right to refuse treatment or assessments (document thoroughly).
- When appropriate, ask the patient for permission to perform various assessments, especially those that may be uncomfortable (breast, thorax, genitalia). If the patient denies permission, explain the importance of the assessment and repeat the request. If the patient still denies permission, omit the assessment and document the patient's refusal.
- Know your institution's policies and standards of practice, and practice within those guidelines.
- Know your state's Nurse Practice Act and practice within that scope.
- Consult with your nurse manager, risk manager, or institutional attorney when indicated.

These guidelines are neither foolproof nor comprehensive. When in doubt, use your professional judgment.

ETHICAL CONSIDERATIONS

It is helpful to keep in mind the following ethical principles to guide your critical thinking within an ethical framework:

- Autonomy: a patient's right to self-determination; the duty to respect a patient's thoughts and actions as to what she or he thinks is best for herself or himself
- Beneficence: to do what is "good" for the patient
- Nonmaleficence: to do no harm to the patient
- Justice: to be fair and impartial to the patient
- Fidelity: the duty to be faithful to the patient
- Veracity: to be truthful to the patient
- Utilitarianism: the duty to perform the greatest good for the greatest number of people

These principles may create challenges for you and the patient when an ethical dilemma presents itself in the clinical setting. The principles are not foolproof nor are they always easy to practice. Having an awareness of them helps to guard the rights of a patient, which is ultimately one of the key roles of the nurse.

Many institutions have a multidisciplinary ethics committee. Some institutions employ an ethicist. Many professional nursing organizations issue ethics statements, both general and specific in nature, to help guide nursing actions. For example, in 2001 the ANA developed a new code of ethics to guide nurses' actions as they face unprecedented challenges with the evolving role of nurses in the 21st century. Use these or whatever resources are available to you when presented with ethical dilemmas or questions.

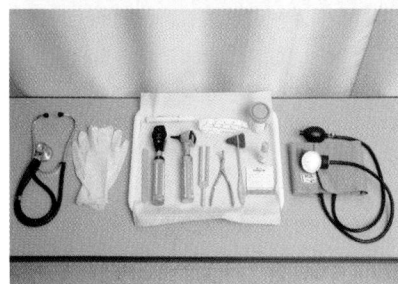

FIGURE 26-2 All equipment required for the examination should be neatly organized and readily available.

HEALTH HISTORY

Conduct the health history (see Figure 26-3). Depending on the patient's reason for the visit, this can be the complete, episodic, interval (follow-up), or emergency health history. The patient can be dressed in street clothes for this interview.

Components of the developmental, cultural, and spiritual assessments are continually evaluated during the course of the patient interaction. Thorough assessments of any or all of these special assessments can be completed if dictated by the patient's situation. The inspection component of the nutrition assessment is noted during the health history. See Chapters 4 to 7.

NURSING**CHECKLIST**

General Approach to the Physical Examination

- Develop an approach that is logical but allows flexibility.
- Use clinical judgment to modify the examination sequence and adapt it to circumstances.
- Allow time at the conclusion of the examination to discuss relevant findings and to allow the patient to ask questions.
- Assist older or disabled patients to focus on how well they can meet the demands of daily life rather than on their limitations.
- Remember that a physical examination can be tiring, both for you and for the patient.

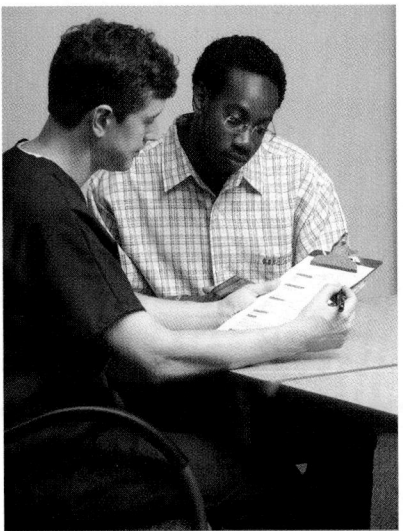

FIGURE 26-3 The nurse and patient review health history information during the initial interview.

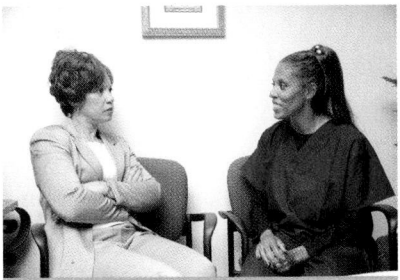

FIGURE 26-4 Observe the patient's overall appearance and demeanor during the interview.

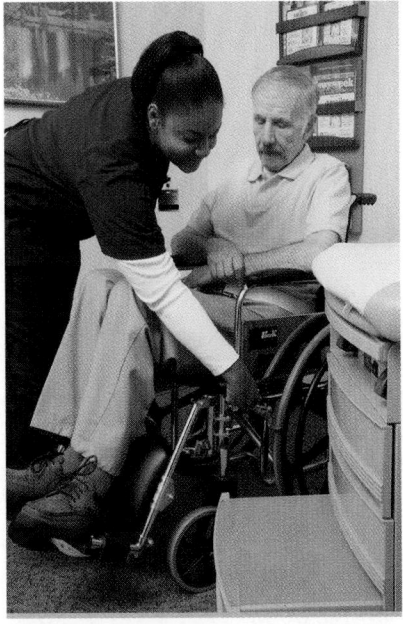

FIGURE 26-5 It may be necessary to assist the patient with certain tasks, such as moving onto the examination table or donning an examination gown.

PHYSICAL EXAMINATION

This text has provided a head-to-toe assessment format in order to discuss body systems in their entirety. However, in practice, a head-to-toe assessment combines systems when assessing most body parts. For example, when assessing the hands, you combine components of the skin, musculoskeletal, and neurological assessments. For this reason, the complete physical examination, which demonstrates how to put it all together, reflects this clinical approach. The sample case study at the end of this chapter documents a standard format of the complete physical assessment.

GENERAL SURVEY

The patient's general appearance is assessed during the health history (Figure 26-4). Incorporate the following into this assessment:

1. Physical Presence
   Age: stated age versus apparent age
   General appearance
   Body fat
   Stature: posture, proportion of body limbs to trunk
   Motor activity: gait, speed, and effort of movement; weight bearing; absence or presence of movement in different body areas
   Body and breath odors
2. Psychological Presence
   Dress, grooming, and personal hygiene
   Mood and manner
   Speech
   Facial expressions
3. Distress
   Physical
   Psychological
   Emotional
4. Pain

NEUROLOGICAL SYSTEM

1. Assess mental status: facial expression, affect, level of consciousness, fund of information, attention span, memory, judgment, insight, spatial perception, calculations, abstract reasoning, thought processes, and content.

After the mental status examination, ask the patient to undress and don an examination gown; underwear may be worn (Figure 26-5). Ask the patient to empty the bladder prior to commencing the assessment process. The urine may be collected for a specimen. Ask the patient to sit on the examination table with the legs hanging over the front. A second drape can be provided to cover the lap and legs. Stand in front of the patient.

MEASUREMENTS

Record the patient's (see Figure 26-6):

1. Height
2. Weight
3. Temperature
4. Pulse (radial preferred site in adult)

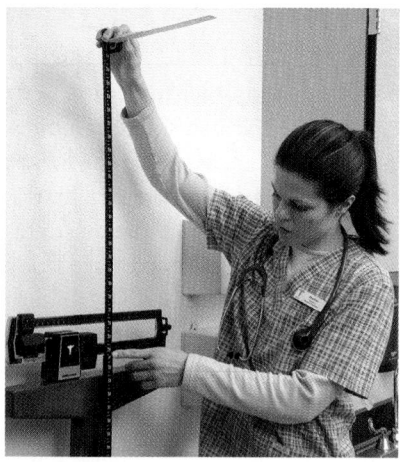

A. Measuring Height

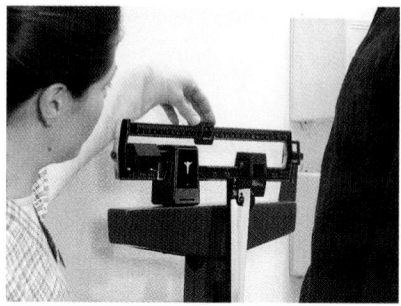

B. Weighing the Patient

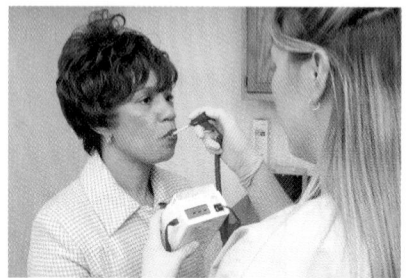

C. Taking Temperature

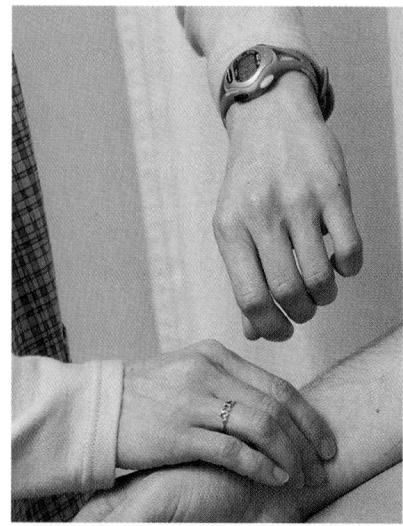

D. Pulse Determination

FIGURE 26-6 General Measurements

5. Respirations
6. Blood pressure (both arms)
7. Anthropometric measurements (if indicated)

SKIN

Throughout the entire head-to-toe assessment, inspect the skin for the following characteristics (see Figure 26-7):

1. Color
2. Bleeding
3. Ecchymosis
4. Vascularity
5. Lesions

Throughout the entire head-to-toe assessment, palpate the skin for:
1. Moisture
2. Temperature
3. Texture
4. Turgor
5. Edema

HEAD AND FACE

1. Inspect the shape of the head.
2. Inspect and palpate the head and scalp.
3. Inspect the color and distribution of the hair. Note any infestations; palpate the hair.
4. Inspect the face for expression, shape, symmetry (CN VII), symmetry of eyes, eyebrows, ears, nose, and mouth.
5. Instruct the patient to raise the eyebrows, frown, smile, wrinkle the forehead, show the teeth, purse the lips, puff the cheeks, and whistle (CN VII).
6. Palpate the temporal pulses. Palpate the temporalis muscles (CN V).
7. Palpate and auscultate the temporomandibular joints.
8. Palpate the masseter muscles (CN V).

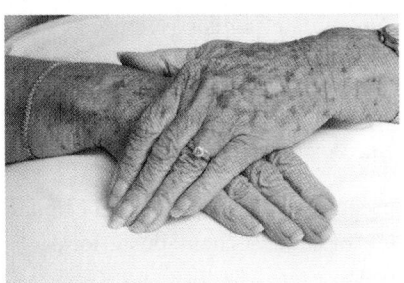

FIGURE 26-7 Inspect the characteristics of the skin such as color, vascularity, and presence of lesions.

Eyes

1. Test distance vision and near vision (Figure 26-8A) (CN II).
2. Test color vision (Figure 26-8B).
3. Test visual fields via confrontation (CN II).
4. Assess extraocular muscle mobility: cover/uncover test, corneal light reflex, and six cardinal fields of gaze (CNs III, IV, VI).
5. Assess direct and consensual light reflexes and accommodation (CN III).
6. Inspect the eyelids, eyebrows, palpebral fissures, and position of eyes.
7. Inspect and palpate the lacrimal apparatus.
8. Inspect the conjunctiva, sclera, cornea, iris, pupils, and lenses.
9. Assess the corneal reflex.
10. Conduct funduscopic assessment: retinal structures, macula.

Ears

1. Test gross hearing: voice-whisper test or watch-tick test (CN VIII).
2. Inspect and palpate the external ear.
3. Assess ear alignment.
4. Conduct otoscopic assessment: EAC and tympanic membrane (Figure 26-9).
5. Perform Weber and Rinne tests.

Nose and Sinuses

1. Inspect the external surface of the nose.
2. Assess nostril patency bilaterally.
3. Test olfactory sense (CN I).
4. Conduct internal assessment with nasal speculum: mucosa, turbinates, and septum.
5. Inspect, percuss, and palpate frontal and maxillary sinuses.

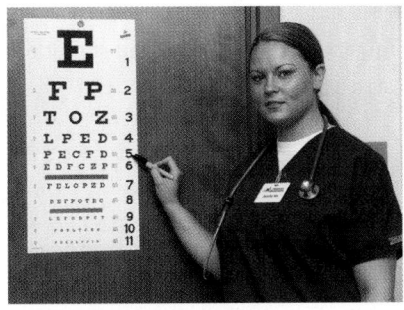

A. Test distance vision.

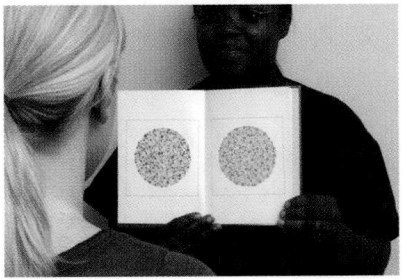

B. Test color vision.

FIGURE 26-8 Vision Assessment

Mouth and Throat

1. Note breath odor.
2. Inspect the lips, buccal mucosa, gums, and hard and soft palates.
3. Inspect the teeth; count the teeth.
4. Inspect the tongue; ask the patient to stick out the tongue (CN XII).
5. Inspect the uvula; note movement when the patient says "ah" (CNs IX, X).
6. Inspect the tonsils; note grade.
7. Inspect the oropharynx.
8. Test gag reflex (CNs IX, X).
9. Test taste (CN VII).
10. Palpate the lips and mouth if indicated.

Neck

1. Inspect the musculature of the neck.
2. Inspect range of motion, shoulder shrug, and strength of sternocleidomastoid and trapezius muscles (CN XI).
3. Palpate the musculature of the neck.
4. Inspect and palpate the trachea.
5. Palpate the carotid arteries (one at a time).

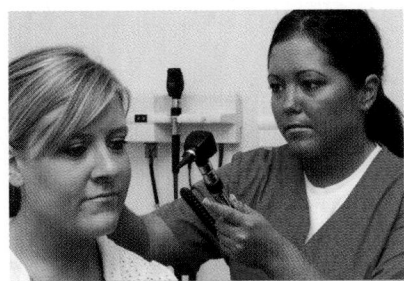

FIGURE 26-9 Perform the otoscopic examination.

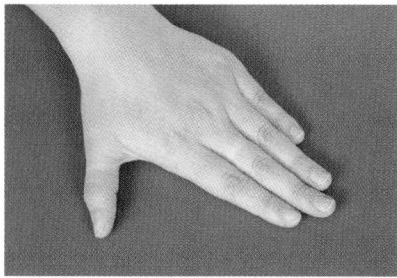

A. Inspect the nailbeds.

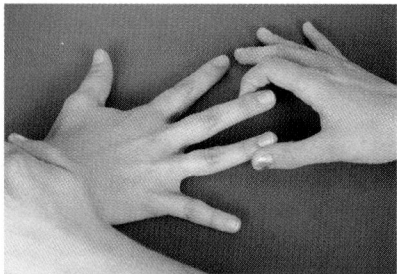

B. Assess range of motion and strength of the fingers.

FIGURE 26-10 Upper Extremity Assessment

6. Inspect the jugular veins for distension; estimate jugular venous pressure (JVP) if indicated.
7. Inspect and palpate the thyroid (use only one approach, either anterior or posterior).
8. Auscultate the thyroid and carotid arteries.
9. Inspect and palpate the lymph nodes: preauricular, postauricular, occipital, submental, submandibular, tonsillar, anterior cervical chain, posterior cervical chain, supraclavicular, and infraclavicular.

UPPER EXTREMITIES

1. Inspect nailbed color, shape, and configuration; (Figure 26-10A) palpate nailbed texture.
2. Assess capillary refill on nailbed.
3. Inspect muscle size and palpate muscle tone of hands, arms, and shoulders.
4. Palpate the joints of fingers, wrists, elbows, and shoulders.
5. Assess range of motion and strength of fingers, wrists, elbows, and shoulders (Figure 26-10B).
6. Test position sense.
7. Palpate radial and brachial pulses.
8. Palpate the epitrochlear node.

Move behind the patient. Untie the gown so that the entire back is exposed. The gown should cover the shoulders and the anterior chest.

BACK, POSTERIOR AND LATERAL THORAXES

1. Palpate the thyroid (posterior approach).
2. Inspect and palpate the spinous processes; inspect range of motion of the cervical spine.
3. Note thoracic configuration, symmetry of shoulders, and position of scapula.
4. Palpate the posterior thorax and lateral thorax.
5. Perform posterior thoracic expansion.
6. Perform tactile fremitus on the posterior thorax and lateral thorax.
7. Percuss the posterior thorax (Figure 26-11A) and lateral thorax.
8. Perform diaphragmatic excursion.
9. Palpate the costovertebral angle (CVA); percuss the CVA with your fist.
10. Auscultate the posterior thorax and lateral thorax; perform voice sounds if indicated (Figure 26-11B).

Move in front of the patient. Drape the patient's gown at waist level (females may cover their breasts).

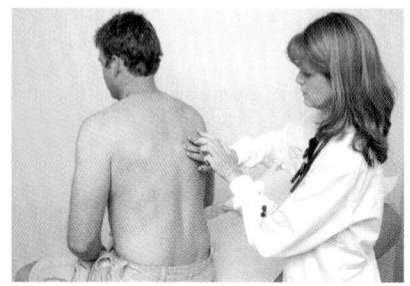

A. Percuss the posterior thorax.

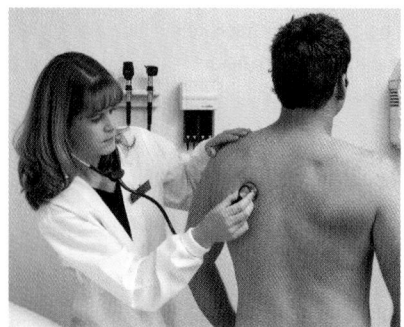

B. Auscultate the posterior thorax.

FIGURE 26-11 Posterior Thorax Assessment

ANTERIOR THORAX

1. Inspect shape of the thorax, symmetry of the chest wall, presence of superficial veins, costal angle, angle of ribs, intercostal spaces, muscles of respiration, respirations, and sputum (see Figure 26-12).
2. Palpate the anterior thorax.
3. Perform anterior thoracic expansion.
4. Perform tactile fremitus.
5. Percuss the anterior thorax.
6. Auscultate the anterior thorax; perform voice sounds if indicated.

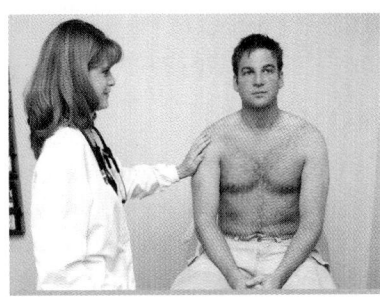

FIGURE 26-12 Inspect the anterior thorax for shape and symmetry.

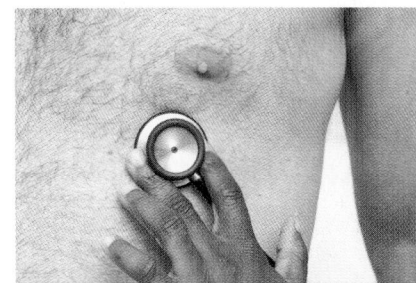

FIGURE 26-13 Auscultate the cardiac landmarks.

HEART

1. Auscultate cardiac landmarks: aortic, pulmonic, mitral, and tricuspid areas and Erb's point (Figure 26-13).

Ask the female patient to uncover her breasts.

FEMALE BREASTS

1. Inspect the breasts for color, vascularity, thickening or edema, size, symmetry, contour, lesions or masses, and discharge with the patient in these positions: arms at side, arms raised over the head, hands pressed into hips, hands in front and patient leaning forward (Figure 26-14).
2. Palpate the breasts with the patient's arms first at her side and then raised over her head.
3. Palpate the brachial, central axillary, pectoral, and subscapular lymph nodes.
4. Teach breast self-examination.

MALE BREASTS

1. Repeat the sequence used for female breasts. Having the patient lean forward is usually unnecessary unless gynecomastia is present.
2. Assist the patient into a supine position with the chest uncovered. Drape the abdomen and legs. Stand on the right side of the patient.

JUGULAR VEINS

As the patient changes from a sitting to a supine position for the remainder of the breast assessment, observe the jugular veins when the patient is at a 45° angle. Assess again when the patient is supine.

1. Inspect the jugular veins for distension; estimate JVP if indicated.

FEMALE AND MALE BREASTS

1. Palpate each breast. The arm on the same side of the assessed breast should be raised over the head.
2. Compress the nipple to express any discharge.

HEART

1. Inspect cardiac landmarks for pulsations.
2. Palpate cardiac landmarks for pulsations, thrills, and heaves.
3. Palpate the apical impulse.
4. With the diaphragm of the stethoscope, auscultate the cardiac landmarks; count the apical pulse.
5. With the bell of the stethoscope, auscultate the cardiac landmarks.
6. Turn the patient on the left side and repeat auscultation of cardiac landmarks.

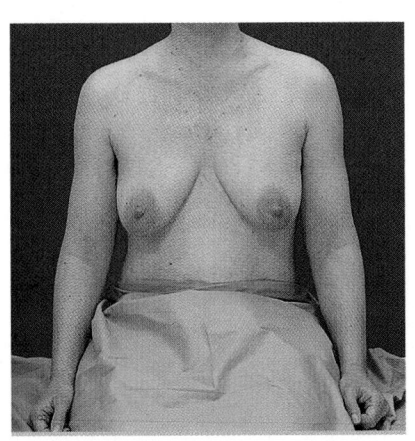

FIGURE 26-14 Inspect the breasts with the patient in a sitting position.

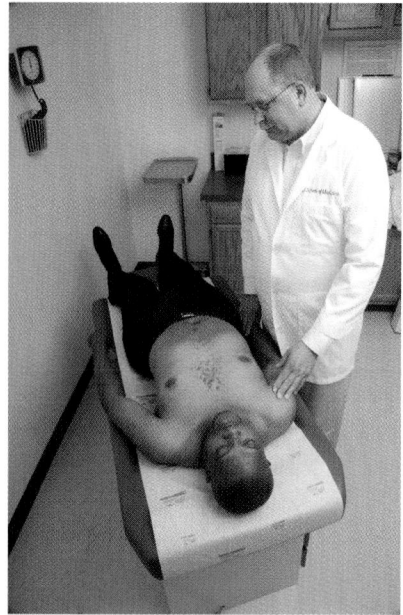

A. Inspect the abdomen.

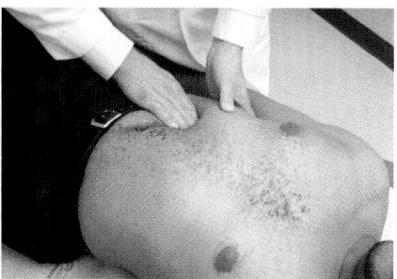

B. Palpate the abdominal quadrants.

FIGURE 26-15 Inspection and Palpation of the Abdomen

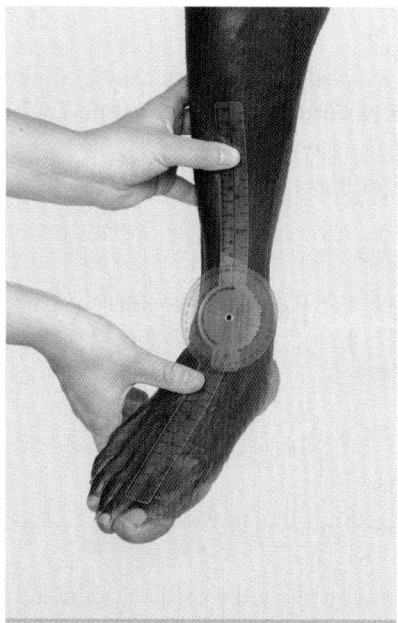

FIGURE 26-16 Inspect the lower extremities and determine range of motion.

Return the patient to a supine position. Cover the patient's anterior thorax with the gown. Uncover the abdomen from the symphysis pubis to the costal margin.

Abdomen

1. Inspect contour, symmetry, pigmentation, and color (Figure 26-15A).
2. Note scars, striae, visible peristalsis, masses, and pulsations.
3. Inspect the rectus abdominis muscles (supine and with head raised) and respiratory movement of the abdomen.
4. Inspect the umbilicus.
5. Auscultate bowel sounds.
6. Auscultate for bruits, venous hum, and friction rub.
7. Percuss all four quadrants.
8. Percuss liver span and liver descent; percuss liver with fist if indicated.
9. Percuss the spleen, stomach, and bladder.
10. Lightly palpate all four quadrants.
11. Note any muscle guarding.
12. Deeply palpate all four quadrants (Figure 26-15B).
13. Palpate the liver, spleen, kidney, aorta, and bladder.
14. Assess superficial abdominal reflexes.
15. Perform hepatojugular reflux if indicated.

Inguinal Area

1. Inspect and palpate the inguinal lymph nodes.
2. Inspect for inguinal hernias.
3. Palpate the femoral pulses.
4. Auscultate the femoral pulses for bruits.

Cover the exposed abdomen with the gown. Lift the drape from the bottom to expose the lower extremities.

Lower Extremities

1. Inspect for color, capillary refill, edema, ulcerations, hair distribution, and varicose veins.
2. Palpate for temperature, edema, and texture.
3. Palpate the popliteal, dorsalis pedis, and posterior tibial pulses.
4. Inspect muscle size and palpate muscle tone of the legs and feet.
5. Palpate the joints of the hips, knees, ankles, and feet.
6. Assess range of motion (Figure 26-16) and strength of the hips, knees, ankles, and feet.
7. Test position sense.
8. Assess for clonus.

Drape the lower extremities. Assist the patient to a sitting position and note the ease with which the patient sits up. Have the patient dangle the legs over the edge of the examination table.

Neurological System

1. Assess light touch: face (CN V), hands, lower arms, abdomen, feet, and legs.
2. Assess superficial pain (sharp and dull): face (CN V), hands, lower arms, abdomen, feet, and legs.
3. Assess two-point discrimination: tongue, lips, fingers, dorsum of hand, torso, and feet.

4. Assess vibration sense: fingers and toes.

5. Assess stereognosis, graphesthesia, and extinction.

6. Assess cerebellar function: finger to nose, rapid alternating hand movements, touching thumb to each finger, running heel down shin, and foot tapping.

7. Assess deep tendon reflexes: biceps, triceps, brachioradialis, patellar, and Achilles.

8. Assess plantar reflex and Babinski reflex.

Ask the patient to stand barefoot on the floor. If the patient is unsteady, use caution when performing the next few tests. Remain physically close to the patient at all times.

Musculoskeletal System

1. Assess mobility: casual walk, heel walk, toe walk, tandem walk, backward walk, stepping to the right and left, and deep knee bends (one knee at a time). Note any indications of discomfort.

Stand behind the patient.

2. Assess range of motion of the spine.

Open the patient's gown to expose the back. Ask the patient to bend forward at the waist.

3. Inspect the spine for scoliosis.

Close the patient's gown. Stand in front of the patient.

Neurological System

1. Perform the Romberg test; assess pronator drift.

2. Assess the ability to hop on one foot, run heel down shin, and draw a figure 8 with foot.

Assist the female patient back to the examination table. Ask her to assume the lithotomy position. Drape the patient (Figure 26-17). Sit on a stool in front of the patient's legs.

Female Genitalia, Anus, and Rectum

1. Inspect pubic hair and skin color and condition: mons pubis, vulva, clitoris, urethral meatus, vaginal introitus, sacrococcygeal area, perineum, and anal mucosa.

2. Palpate the labia, urethral meatus, Skene's glands, vaginal introitus, and perineum.

3. Insert the vaginal speculum.

4. Inspect the cervix: color, position, size, surface characteristics, discharge, and shape of cervical os; inspect the vagina.

5. Collect specimens for cytological smears and cultures.

Stand in front of the patient's legs.

6. Perform bimanual assessment of the vagina, cervix, fornices, uterus, and adnexa.

7. Perform rectovaginal assessment.

8. Palpate the anus and rectum.

9. If stool is on the glove, save it to test for occult blood.

Assist the patient to a sitting position. Offer her some tissues to wipe the perineal area. Ask her to redress. You can answer her questions when she is dressed.

Ask the male patient to stand. Sit on a stool in front of the patient. Have the patient lift the gown to expose the genitalia.

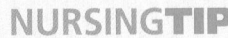

NURSING**TIP**

Assessing the Comatose Patient

For the comatose patient, the family and prior health care records can provide valuable information for the health history. Do not let the patient's condition deter you from conducting a thorough physical assessment. Omit components of the assessment that require volition and patient cooperation; complete the remainder of the assessment as indicated. Remember to assess neurological status thoroughly. Consider assessing: doll's eyes phenomenon, corneal reflex, Babinski reflex, clonus, and superficial and deep pain response.

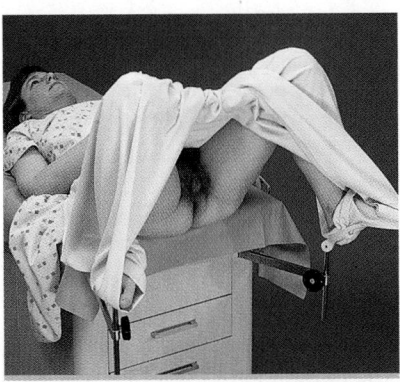

Figure 26-17 Assist the female patient into the lithotomy position and drape the abdomen and legs for the genital exam.

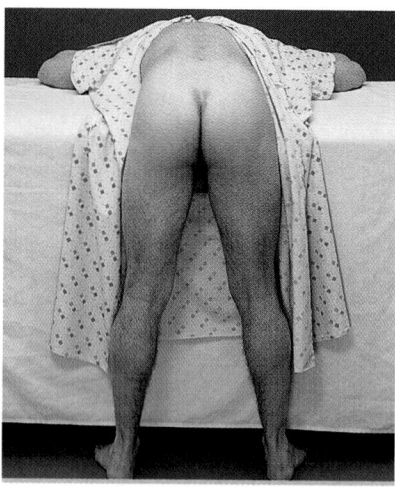

FIGURE 26-18 Ask the male patient to bend over the examination table for the rectal exam.

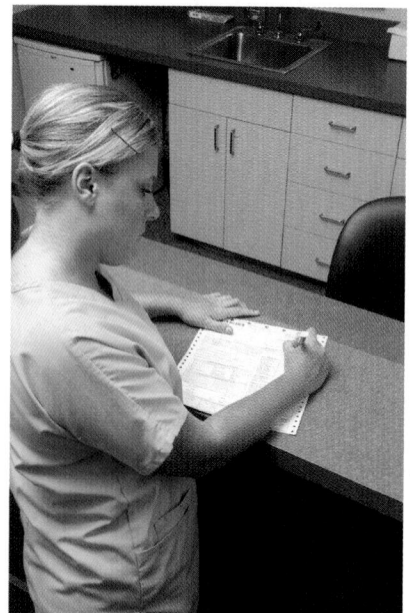

FIGURE 26-19 Be certain to carefully document all assessment findings and patient responses.

MALE GENITALIA

1. Inspect hair distribution, penis, scrotum, and urethral meatus.
2. Palpate the penis, urethral meatus, and scrotum.
3. Palpate the inguinal area for hernias.
4. Auscultate the scrotum if indicated.
5. Teach testicular self-examination.

Ask the patient to bend over the examination table (Figure 26-18). If the patient is bedridden, the knee-chest or left lateral position may be used. Expose the buttocks. Stand behind the patient.

MALE ANUS, RECTUM, AND PROSTATE

1. Inspect the perineum, sacrococcygeal area, and anal mucosa.
2. Palpate the anus and rectum.
3. Palpate the prostate.
4. If stool is on the glove, save it to test for occult blood.

Re-cover the buttocks. Ask the patient to stand up and redress. Offer him tissues to wipe the rectal area. You can answer his questions when he is dressed.

The patient has the opportunity to regain composure and formulate questions about the assessment while getting redressed. It is often difficult for patients to discuss future plans when wearing an examination gown. For this reason, give the patient a few minutes to redress in privacy before you proceed with the assessment. Always thank the patient for his or her time and explain what can be expected next.

When completing the assessment, ensure that you return the patient to the state in which you found him or her at the beginning of the assessment. For example, for the bedridden patient, ensure that the side rails are up (if appropriate) and that the call bell is readily accessible. Ask the patient if there is anything else that can be done to make him or her comfortable.

Now that you have all of this information, what do you do with it and how do you make sense of it? (See Figure 26-19.) Refer back to Chapter 1, which discussed how to make the leap from assessment data to formulating a nursing diagnosis and nursing care plan.

NURSING**TIP**

Assessing the Bedridden Patient

The bedridden patient is usually capable of cooperating for the health history and physical assessment. Components of the physical assessment that require the patient to be out of bed can be omitted. Cerebellar function of the lower extremities can still be assessed by having the patient run the heel of each foot down each shin and draw a figure 8 with each foot on the bed or in the air.

Frequently, assessing the bedridden patient requires the assistance of a second person to help hold the patient in a side-lying position while a posterior assessment is conducted. If the patient can tolerate a sitting position, the second person can help hold the patient in this position while an assessment of the head, face, neck, and anterior thorax is conducted. Always use extra caution to protect the patient against falls.

NURSINGTIP

Communicating Bad News

Be sensitive when communicating bad or unexpected news to the patient, significant other(s), or caregiver. Talk to the patient in a quiet, private room. Be specific and straightforward. Speak in terms that will be understood. Give the patient time to process the information, alone if desired. Convey the same high level of respect that you have shown throughout the interview and assessment process. Finally, allow time for questions.

LABORATORY AND DIAGNOSTIC DATA

The laboratory and diagnostic data that are obtained from the patient vary according to presenting symptoms and clinical assessment. Order only those tests that are necessary. Consider the risks, time, discomfort, cost, limitations, and contraindications of each test. Actively involve the patient in preparing for each test and incorporate clinical teaching when appropriate. Remember that technology can never replace the art of listening to what your patient is saying and the skill with which you perform physical examinations.

PROBLEM LIST

The health history, physical examination, and laboratory and diagnostic data provide the database on which clinical action is taken. As described in Chapter 1, similar signs, symptoms, and findings are clustered together in a meaningful way. These clusters are then named. Some nurses may use nursing diagnoses to name the clusters of meaningful information. Other nurses may use a medical model approach and formulate a problem list. The problem list is a provider-generated list of active and inactive health problems. Each problem is numbered and referred to in the patient record by number. The onset date of each problem is noted, as is the date of problem resolution. An example of a problem list is seen below:

ONSET DATE	PROBLEM #	ACTIVE PROBLEM	INACTIVE PROBLEM
1963	1		Pneumonia
1964	2		ITP
1984	3	Bilat ovarian cysts	
1989	4	Allergic rhinitis	
1990	5	Reactive airway disease	
1997	6	Ⓛ plantar fasciitis	
2000	7	Cystocele	

From this problem list, a care plan is developed to address each active problem. The implementation and evaluation of the care plan then ensue. A SOAP note is one method that can be used to document this process.

REFLECTIVE THINKING

Evaluating Children for Sports Participation

Being a middle school nurse, you are asked to evaluate a 12-year-old for his ability to play in the school's intramural basketball program. This male is 62 inches tall and weighs 154 lbs. You read from his school file that he has exertional asthma. His blood pressure today was 152/85. What would you tell this child? What interventions would you plan?

PREPARTICIPATION ATHLETIC EVALUATION

Nurses frequently evaluate school-age and adolescent children for their ability to participate in athletic activities. The purpose is to assess whether a child can safely participate in a desired activity, and if that is not possible, to suggest other activities that can safely provide a physical outlet. The evaluation encompasses both a thorough family and personal health history (especially cardiovascular and musculoskeletal) and a physical examination (emphasis also on cardiovascular and musculoskeletal health).

It is important to remember those conditions that contraindicate participation in sporting events: atlantoaxial instability, carditis, hypertrophic cardiomyopathy, uncontrolled severe hypertension, suspected coronary artery disease, specific EKG abnormalities (e.g., long QT interval), absence of a paired organ, poorly controlled seizure disorder, and hepatosplenomegaly. There are many relative contraindications that need to be evaluated on a case-by-case basis, taking into consideration the child's history and the intended sport. Organizations such as the American Academy of Pediatrics, American Academy of Family Physicians, American Society for Sports Medicine, and American Orthopaedic Society for Sports Medicine publish standard athletic evaluation forms that can be used to guide the preparticipation athletic evaluation. They should be consulted to guide your evaluative process.

HEALTHY PEOPLE 2010

The U.S. government established measurable health goals for its people in the document *Healthy People 2000: National Health Promotion and Disease Prevention Objectives* (U.S. Department of Health and Human Services, 1990). The main goals of this document were to increase the span of healthy life, to reduce health disparities among people living in the United States, and to enable people to obtain access to preventive services. *Healthy People 2000* contained over 300 specific objectives based on 22 priority areas. The priority areas were centered around health promotion, health protection, preventive services, and surveillance and data systems. This initiative was to be achieved by the cooperative efforts of government, families, individuals, communities, health professionals, and the media.

Healthy People 2000 and the 1979 Surgeon General's report *Healthy People* were used as the basis for *Healthy People 2010*. This document lists 28 focus areas that target the people of the United States in the first decade of the new millennium. The two main goals of *Healthy People 2010* are to increase the quality of life and the number of years of healthy life and to eliminate health disparities. *Healthy People 2010* contains 467 science-based objectives that are meshed with 10 leading health indicators (LHI). The LHI highlight high-priority public health issues. It is vital that nurses be aware of these public health initiatives as they are major forces that contribute to health promotion and disease prevention. Whether a bedside nurse, school nurse, home health nurse, nurse practitioner, nurse anesthetist, or other advanced practice nurse, we all are responsible for improving the health of our patients and our community. These documents provide information on where to start.

ROLE OF TECHNOLOGY

Technology is changing the way we interface with the health care arena. Computers are used at the bedside to document assessment findings and patient care. Patients are providing health history on computers, scheduling appointments and obtaining test results via e-mail, and querying their health care providers about treatment issues using e-mail. Health care providers are using computers to link directly to pharmacies when prescribing medications and are soliciting patients' health histories, signs, and symptoms; diagnosing patients; and implementing treatment plans all via e-mail and the Internet. Technology can readily put the patient in direct contact with a health care provider, but the privacy and legal issues are complex and still evolving.

Electronic medical records (EMRs) create a paperless system that can reduce charting/documentation time once the clinician is familiar with the system. EMRs enable the nurse to use voice recognition, narrative writing, and/or check boxes with drop-down menus to record patients' histories and assessment findings. Other advantages of EMRs are their legibility, easy accessibility, ability to be

NURSING**TIP**

Joint Commission and ISMP's Do Not Use List

The Joint Commission and the Institute for Safe Medication Practices (ISMP) issued a list of abbreviations, symbols, and dose designations that have frequently contributed to medication errors that compromised patient safety. See Appendix C.

NURSING**TIP**

Personal Health Record

Another use of technology that is patient-centered and used to assist in accurate relaying of patient information is the personal health record (PHR). The PHR is a digital medical record of a patient that is secured on a Web page. The PHR contains basic patient information, current clinical diagnoses, medications taken, test results, and progress notes. The patient frequently wears a bracelet or necklace that provides the Web address of the PHR with the password so that it can be accessed in an emergency situation.

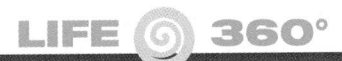

Starting an EMR System

You are the nurse educator and head clinician in an outpatient setting. You are told that your clinic will adopt an EMR system in 6 months and that you will be responsible for coordinating the transition. None of the facility's nurses, including yourself, has ever worked with an EMR system. Devise a teaching plan to educate the staff on the new system and establish a time line. What problems can you anticipate? How will you convince the staff of the system's need? What support will you need?

accessed by multiple users simultaneously at different work stations in different areas in real time, and capability of accessing real-time laboratory and diagnostic studies.

In recent years, personal digital assistants (PDAs) or palm pilots have found their way into daily clinical life. PDAs are used as warehouses of clinical data on patients and as reference tools for easily accessible data. Some nursing schools have formally incorporated PDAs into their curriculum as a technology that is required in various courses. Nurses need to be comfortable with these technologies in order to remain leaders in the health care environment.

CONCLUSION

Today's nurse is a sophisticated professional prepared to meet the demands of the health care market. Hospitalized patients have a greater acuity and are being discharged at a faster rate to the home environment. The home health nurse is therefore seeing a greater variety of patients who are sicker. Nurses in advanced practice settings are providing care to patients who are positioned at different points on the health-illness continuum. Because the entire plan of care is based on patient assessment, all nurses must possess expert assessment skills. This text has supplied the information to assist the novice and the experienced nurse in acquiring, refining, and perfecting health history and physical examination skills. The pathophysiological basis for the physical assessment findings empowers the nurse to fully understand the patient's clinical state and make appropriate clinical decisions. Ultimately, the patients are the benefactors of your knowledge, wisdom, and experience.

CASE STUDY

The Patient with Multisystem Problems

HEALTH HISTORY

TODAY'S DATE	April 5, 2009
BIOGRAPHICAL DATA	
Patient Name	Eduarado Rodriguez
Address	6748 Blue Ridge Lane Lincoln, NE 68516
Phone Number	(402) 420-9858
Date of Birth	February 5, 1948
Birthplace	Santiago, Chile

continues

CASE STUDY (Continued)

The Patient with Multisystem Problems

Social Security Number	987-65-4321
Occupation	Architect (currently on disability)
Work Address	Not employed
Work Phone Number	N/A
Insurance	Blue Cross/Blue Shield
Usual Source of Health Care	Dr. Larry Grimm (stopped going to practice 8 mos ago due to distance from home)
Source of Referral	Wife's coworker
Emergency Contact	Carmen Rodriguez (wife)
Source and Reliability of Information	Pt ≠ always remember circumstances of events and dates; some info given contradicts info given earlier in interview
PATIENT PROFILE	61 yo married Hispanic male
REASON FOR SEEKING HEALTH CARE	"I have not seen any medical person for 8 mos. I decided that I needed to get back on track."
PRESENT HEALTH	Pt has not been seen by a hl care provider in over 8 mos despite his long and complex medical hx. He decided that he has been feeling sorry for himself and is now ready to assume responsibility for his hl. Pt does not want to die ā age 62 (age at which his father died). Pt would like refills on all meds. Can't recall which he already ran out of and which he still has.
PAST HEALTH HISTORY	(Pt has hl hx info written down by wife but is unable to elaborate on it)
Medical History	Brainstem CVA '93 HTN '93 Hypothyroidism '94 WPW, complete heart block c̄ pacemaker insertion '94 MI c̄ cardiomyopathy '98 (ejection fraction on echocardiogram 40% c̄ global hypokinesia and mild LVH) Hyperlipidemia '98 Gout '99 Open-angle glaucoma '01 BPH '03 Rectal bleeding '04 (colonoscopy WNL)
Surgical History	EPS mapping and pacemaker insertion '94
Allergies	Codeine (GI upset and rash); denies allergies to foods, insect bites/bee stings, environmental/seasonal allergens

continues

CASE STUDY (Continued)

The Patient with Multisystem Problems

Medications	Warfarin 3 mg po at bedtime Carvedilol 6.25 mg po BID Enalapril 2.5 mg po daily Atorvastatin 10 mg po daily Furosemide 40 mg po BID Potassium chloride 20 mEq 2 po daily Levothyroxine 0.088 mg po Q AM Finasteride 5 mg po daily Doxazosin 4 mg po daily Latanoprost 0.005% ophth soln 1 gtt in both eyes every evening Indomethacin 50 mg po TID prn Colchicine 0.6 mg po BID prn
Communicable Diseases	Denies HSV, STDs, hepatitis, ⊕ HIV
Injuries and Accidents	Denies
Special Needs	On disability since '98; has some income from disability insurance; walks c̄ cane prn
Blood Transfusions	Denies
Childhood Illnesses	Recalls chickenpox as a child
Immunizations	Not sure; nothing in the past 8 mos
FAMILY HEALTH HISTORY	

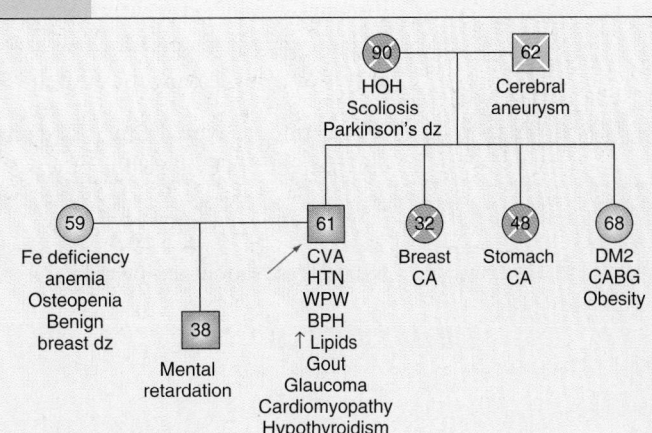

LEGEND

◯ Living female
▢ Living male
⊗ Deceased female
⊠ Deceased male
╱ Points to patient

BPH = Benign prostatic hypertrophy
CA = Cancer
CABG = Coronary artery bypass graft
CVA = Cerebrovascular accident
DM = Diabetes mellitus
dz = Disease
Fe = Iron
HOH = Hard of hearing
HTN = Hypertension
WPW = Wolff-Parkinson-White Syndrome

90 — HOH Scoliosis Parkinson's dz
62 — Cerebral aneurysm

59 — Fe deficiency anemia Osteopenia Benign breast dz
61 — CVA HTN WPW BPH ↑ Lipids Gout Glaucoma Cardiomyopathy Hypothyroidism
32 — Breast CA
48 — Stomach CA
68 — DM2 CABG Obesity
38 — Mental retardation

Denies FHH of kidney dz, epilepsy, liver dz, asthma, alcoholism, mental illness, drug addiction, allergic disorders, ulcerative colitis, celiac dz, Crohn's dz, muscular disorders

Note: Pt provided above information. Refused to discuss it further.

continues

CASE STUDY (Continued)

The Patient with Multisystem Problems

SOCIAL HISTORY	
Alcohol Use	Nothing since CVA
Tobacco Use	Denies
Drug Use	Denies
Domestic and Intimate Partner Violence	Denies
Sexual Practice	Monogamous relationship × 35 yrs
Travel History	Born in Chile; family moved to U.S. age 5; growing up went to Chile q few yrs; no travel since CVA
Work Environment	Not currently employed
Home Environment	After CVA moved to house c̄ all necessities on 1st floor; wife takes care of the house
Hobbies and Leisure Activities	Watches sports on TV
Stress	Current hl status; has 38 yo son c̄ mental retardation who lives in a group home—worries about him
Education	Finished college, employed as architect until CVA
Economic Status	"It's tough."
Military Service	Denies
Religion	Roman Catholic; currently nonpracticing but is thinking about becoming part of a parish ("my parents must be rolling in their graves over my leaving the church 15 yrs ago")
Ethnic Background	"I'm proud of who I am"; 1st-generation American; parents emigrated from Chile when pt was 5 yo
Roles and Relationships	Depends on wife for everything
Characteristic Patterns of Daily Living	No pattern, sedentary lifestyle
HEALTH MAINTENANCE ACTIVITIES	
Sleep	5½–6½ hrs q PM; feels tired much of the day; has difficulty falling asleep; naps frequently during the day
Diet	"I eat what I want."
Exercise	None
Stress Management	Nothing
Use of Safety Devices	Denies

continues

CASE STUDY (Continued)

The Patient with Multisystem Problems

Health Check-ups	Has not sought med care in 8 mos; prior to this he saw someone when he needed it; no recent blood work/scans
REVIEW OF SYSTEMS	
General	"I have no energy, I feel lousy . . . I am a mess!"
Skin	Denies rashes, itching, Δ in skin pigmentation, ecchymoses, Δ in skin texture, sores, lumps, odors, sweating, acne, denies sunbathing, ≠ use sunblock
Hair	Occasional dandruff and itchy scalp; losing some hair on top of head; denies hirsutism
Nails	Denies Δ in texture, splitting, breaking, onychomycosis
Eyes	Wears glasses, some blurred vision; has difficulty seeing at night; denies diplopia, eye pain, and halos around objects; thinks he saw ophth 2 yrs ago
Ears	Denies discharge, vertigo, otalgia, tinnitus, hearing aid, hearing problems
Nose and Sinuses	Denies epistaxis, Δ in sense of smell, allergies, sinusitis, PND; admits to snoring
Mouth	Denies halitosis, toothache, tooth abscess, bleeding/swollen gums, difficulty chewing, Δ in taste; brushes teeth bid, no flossing, can't recall when he saw dentist last
Throat and Neck	Denies hoarseness, dysphagia, goiter, Δ in voice
Breasts	Denies pain, tenderness, discharge, lumps, dimpling
Respiratory	⊕ SOB if forgets to take diuretic; has had many chest X-rays c̄ all his medical problems in past 15 yrs; denies asthma, pneumonia
Cardiovascular and Peripheral Vasculature	See PHH; currently no chest pain, orthopnea, palpitations, syncope; feet/ankle edema if he is on his feet a lot or is late in taking diuretic
Gastrointestinal	Rectal bleeding started again last wk, notes it c̄ straining; denies hemorrhoids, BMs regular and soft, denies hematochezia; denies N/V/D, GERD, abd pain
Musculoskeletal	Generalized weakness since CVA; had PT for many mos p̄ CVA; walks c̄ cane prn; gout attacks c̄ ↑ in red meat consumption; denies LBP, sprains, fx
Neurological	Can't remember things as well as in past yrs; denies tremors, involuntary mvt, Δ LOC, sz
Psychological	Difficulty concentrating, unable to balance checkbook; denies depression, irritability, sleep disturbances, suicidal ideation

continues

CASE STUDY (Continued)

The Patient with Multisystem Problems

Urinary	Per PHH; nocturia 2–3×Q night, ↓ force of stream, ⊕ hesitancy; denies incontinence, UTI, nephrolothiasis; can't recall when he last saw urologist
Male Reproductive	Refuses to discuss
Nutrition	Does not know wt, has noticed that his clothes are getting tighter in past 4 wks, snacks on chips, pretzels, and chocolate candy; wife cooks or he eats a frozen dinner; few vegetables
Endocrine	⊕ fatigue; denies exophthalmos, heat/cold intolerance, ↑ sweating, ↑ thirst, ↑ hunger, swelling in ant neck, DM
Lymph Nodes	Denies enlargement, tenderness
Hematological	⊕ bruising, even c̄ little force; denies h/o anemia
PHYSICAL EXAMINATION	
General Survey and Vital Signs	WDWN Hispanic ♂ in NAD or pain who looks older than his stated age No obvious deformity, speech is occasionally slurred HT: 5′9″ (175 cm) WT: 242 lbs (110 kg) T: 98.6°F (37°C) P: 72 R: 22 BP: 152/89 mm Hg (Ⓛ arm sitting) 148/87 mm Hg (Ⓛ arm supine) 160/90 mm Hg (Ⓡ arm sitting)
Skin, Hair, and Nails	2⁺ edema feet and ankles, s̄ lesions, rashes, ecchymoses, bleeding; warm to touch s̄ diaphoresis, smooth texture, ↓ turgor; hair s̄ infestations; patches of scattered seborrhea; nailbeds pink, firm c̄ 1 sec cap refill, no clubbing
Head	Normocephalic s̄ lesions, masses, depressions, or tenderness; face symmetrical s̄ involuntary mvt or swelling; scalp shiny and intact s̄ lesions or masses; TMJ articulates smoothly s̄ clicking or crepitus
Eyes	Acuity by Snellen chart c̄ glasses: right eye: 20/40, left eye 20/40; s̄ glasses both eyes 20/70; has difficulty reading magazine at 14″; color vision intact, visual fields by confrontation intact, eyebrows full and symmetrical, eyelashes evenly distributed and s̄ inflammation, Ø ptosis or lid lag, raised, yellow plaque on upper Ⓛ lid, nonpainful; lacrimal apparatus s̄ inflammation or discharge, corneal light reflex symmetrical s̄ strabismus,

continues

	cover-uncover test s̄ deviation, EOM mvt intact, Ø nystagmus, conjunctiva pink, Ø foreign bodies, Ø tearing, sclera white s̄ exudate, PERRLA (3 mm) Funduscopic: ⊕ red reflex, discs flat c̄ sharp margins, ⊕ cotton wool spots
Ears	Gross hearing intact by watch-tick test; pinna s̄ masses, lesions, nodules, inflammation, or tenderness; EAC clear s̄ inflammation; TMs shiny c̄ visible light reflex; Ø bulging or perforation; Weber midline; Rinne AC greater than BC
Nose and Sinuses	Ø deformities, bleeding, lesions, masses, swelling; nares patent, nontender; septum midline s̄ perforation; mucosa pale and boggy; sinuses nontender, resonant
Mouth and Throat	⊕ halitosis; lips pink s̄ swelling or lesions; gums and mucosa pink and moist; 30 teeth in good repair; tongue midline, well papillated, and s̄ fasciculations, lesions, swelling, or bleeding; hard and soft palates intact s̄ lesions or masses; pharynx erythematous; uvula midline and rises c̄ phonation; 2+/4+ tonsils; ⊕ gag reflex
Neck	Supple s̄ masses or spasms, neck symmetrical s̄ masses or tenderness, Ø lymphadenopathy, trachea midline, thyroid nontender s̄ enlargement/mass/goiter, Ø bruits, Ø JVD at 90°, 45°, and supine
Breasts	Ø thickening, edema, vascularity, erosion, fissures, lesions, masses, retraction, discharge; areola and nipples dark in pigmentation; nonpalpable lymph nodes
Thorax and Lungs	AP: transverse diameter = 1:2, chest wall symmetrical, costal angle less than 90°, angle of the ribs c̄ sternum = 45°, Ø bulging of ICS or retractions, no use of accessory muscles, resp reg, thoracic expansion 3 cm ant and 3 cm post, tactile fremitus = bilaterally, lungs resonant, diaphragmatic excursion 2 cm bilat, clear breath sounds; Ø adventitious breath sounds
Heart	Precordium s̄ pulsations/heaves/thrills, apical pulse 72, apical impulse 2 cm at 5th ICS 3 cm to Ⓛ of MCL, S_1 and S_2 present, s̄ MGR
Abdomen	Protuberant c̄ striae, Ø dilated veins, scars, incisions; ⊕ bowel sounds in 4 quads, Ø bruits, venous hum, friction rub; tympanic abd soft, Ø masses/tenderness to light/deep palpation; liver span 8 cm in Ⓡ MCL; neg CVA tenderness

continues

CASE STUDY (Continued)

The Patient with Multisystem Problems

Peripheral Vasculature	2+/4+ nonpitting edema in feet and ankles, Ø ulcerations, ⊖ Homan's sign, pulse reg and strong, Ø pulsus paradoxus, Ø bruits	

	CAROTID	BRACHIAL	RADIAL	FEMORAL	POPLITEAL	DORSALIS PEDIS	POSTERIOR TIBIAL
R	2+	2+	2+	2+	2+	2+	2+
L	2+	2+	2+	2+	2+	2+	2+

Scale: 0–4+

Musculoskeletal	Obese male sitting in chair c̄ cane in Ⓛ hand, stands c̄ difficulty c̄ wide stance; mild kyphosis; gait is slow and rhythmic; has difficulty going from ♀ to ↻ position; joints s̄ erythema, swelling, bruising, nodules, deformities, masses; Ø crepitus; muscle strength UE and LE 4/5 bilaterally; Ø involuntary mvt; bilat hallux valgus; ROM deferred 2° pt's fatigue
Neurological	Mental status: pt demanding refill on meds despite being new pt to practice and no recent labs; A, A, and O × 3, thought processes intact; recent memory intact, short-term and long-term memories not always consistent c̄ written information that pt's wife typed up for today's visit
	Remainder of neuro exam deferred 2° to pt's complaint of not getting Rx immediately and agitation
Genitalia and Rectum	Bleeding, nonthrombosed ext hemorrhoid; pt refused internal exam and threatened lawsuit if it was attempted
LABORATORY DATA	(From last set of labs in December 2007)

Metabolic Panel (Serum)

	PT'S VALUES	NORMAL VALUES
Glucose (fasting)	150 mg/dL	(70–110 mg/dL)
BUN	35 mg/dL	(8–25 mg/dL)
Creatinine	1.7 mg/dL	(0.6–1.5 mg/dL)
Sodium	142 mEq/L	(135–145 mEq/L)
Potassium	4.8 mEq/L	(3.5–5.0 mEq/L)
Chloride	105 mEq/L	(100–108 mEq/L)
Carbon dioxide	23 mEq/L	(24–30 mEq/L)
Calcium	8.9 mg/dL	(8.5–10.5 g/dL)
Protein, total	6.8 g/dL	(6.0–8.5 g/dL)
Albumin	4.1 g/dL	(3.5–5.0 g/dL)
Globulin	2.7 g/dL	(1.5–4.5 g/dL)

continues

The Patient with Multisystem Problems

	PT'S VALUES	NORMAL VALUES
Bilirubin, total	0.3 mg/dL	(0.1–1.2 mg/dL)
Alkaline phosphatase	73 International Units/L	(25–150 International Units/L)
AST	26 International Units/L	(0–40 International Units/L)
ALT	17 International Units/L	(0–55 International Units/L)
Cholesterol, total	245 mg/dL	(< 200 mg/dL)
Triglycerides	247 mg/dL	(< 150 mg/dL)
HDL	38 mg/dL	(> 40 mg/dL)
LDL	178 mg/dL	(< 100 mg/dL)
HbA1c	7.9%	(4.0–6.0 %)
INR	4.1	(2–3)
PSA	4.5 ng/mL	(0.0–4.0 ng/mL)
TSH	6.80 International Units/mL	(0.50–5.0 International Units/mL)
Creatinine kinase, total	88 units/L	(24–204 U/L)

PROBLEM LIST

ONSET DATE	PROBLEM #	ACTIVE PROBLEM	INACTIVE PROBLEM
1993	1		Brainstem CVA
1993	2	High-risk medication (warfarin)	
1993	3	HTN	
1994	4	Hypothyroidism	
1994	5		WPW c̄ cardiomyopathy
1998	6	Hyperlipidemia	
1999	7		Gout
2001	8	Open-angle glaucoma	
2003	9	BPH	
2004	10	Rectal bleeding	
2009	11	Pedal edema	

REVIEW QUESTIONS

1. Advanced physical examination techniques are performed in which of the following situations?
   a. Preparticipation sports physicals
   b. Episodic visits
   c. Every health care visit
   d. When warranted by the patient's condition
   The correct answer is (d).

2. Which ethical principle represents the duty to be faithful to a patient?
   a. Autonomy   c. Fidelity
   b. Beneficence   d. Justice
   The correct answer is (c).

3. Which of the following situations exemplifies the nurse practicing in a legally advisable manner?
   a. Documenting an office visit 1 week after the event
   b. Discussing a patient's medical condition outside the patient's room
   c. Insisting that a patient have a pelvic exam because of vaginal discharge
   d. Reporting a patient with a condition that is a public health concern
   The correct answer is (d).

4. Which of the following statements is accurate regarding special assessments?
   a. The spiritual assessment is conducted on all hospitalized patients upon admission.
   b. The developmental assessment is performed on children at discharge.
   c. The nutritional assessment is conducted on all patients over the age of 25.
   d. The cultural assessment can provide clues as to whether a patient may follow health care recommendations.
   The correct answer is (d).

5. The problem list is:
   a. Generated after the patient's health history
   b. The basis for the diagnostic code for billing purposes
   c. Deleted when a patient's health status improves
   d. Used to develop a care plan for a patient
   The correct answer is (d).

6. For which of the following teenagers would it be inadvisable to play high school soccer?
   a. A 16-year-old female with an uncontrolled seizure disorder
   b. A 17-year-old male with prehypertension
   c. A 15-year old female with bulimia
   d. A 14-year-old male with exercise-induced asthma
   The correct answer is (a).

7. One of the primary goals of *Healthy People 2010* is to:
   a. Stop chronic disease in the United States
   b. Eliminate health disparities in the United States
   c. Reduce the mortality of infectious diseases
   d. Increase surveillance of biological weapons
   The correct answer is (b).

8. Which of the following assessment techniques is performed correctly?
   a. Palpating the thyroid via a posterior approach
   b. Percussing the cardiac silhouette while the patient is in the right-side-lying position
   c. Palpating the carotid arteries simultaneously and comparing amplitude
   d. Percussing the sternal angle in a patient with pyelonephritis
   The correct answer is (a).

9. Which of the following neurological assessments can be performed on a comatose patient?
   a. Cerebellar function
   b. Romberg test
   c. Pronator drift
   d. Deep pain response
   The correct answer is (d).

10. The Preparticipation Athletic Evaluation stresses the importance of clinical safety primarily in which body systems?
    a. Neurological and respiratory
    b. Musculoskeletal and cardiovascular
    c. Head and neck and lymphatic
    d. Skin and peripheral vasculature
    The correct answer is (b).

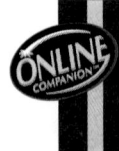 Visit the Estes online companion resource at **www.delmar.cengage.com** for additional content and study aids. Click on Online Companions and then select the Nursing discipline.

REFERENCE

U.S. Department of Health and Human Services. (1990). *Healthy People 2000: National health promotion and disease prevention objectives* (PHS Publication No. 91-50213). Washington, DC: Author.

BIBLIOGRAPHY

Aiken, T. D. (2002). *Legal and ethical issues in health occupations.* Philadelphia: Saunders.

American Nurses Association. (2001). *Code of ethics for nurses with interpretive statements.* Washington, DC: Author.

Anderson, H. J. (2006). With shortage of nurses, instructional technology becomes more essential. *Health Data Management, 14*(7), 4.

Austin, S. (2006). Ladies & gentlemen of the jury, I present . . . the nursing documentation. *Nursing 2006, 36*(1), 57062.

Back, A. L., Arnild, R. M., Baile, W. F., Fryer-Edwards, K. A., Alexander, S. C., Barley, G. E., Gooley, T. A., & Tulsky, J. A. (2007). Efficacy of communication skills training for giving bad news and discussing transitions to palliative care. *Archives of Internal Medicine, 167*(5), 453–460.

Bandman, E., & Bandman, B. (2002). *Nursing ethics through the life span* (4th ed.). Upper Saddle River, NJ: Prentice Hall.

Bauchner, H., Adams, W., & Burstin, H. (2002). "You've got mail": Issues in communicating with patients and their families by e-mail. *Pediatrics, 109*(5), 954–956.

Boulware, L. E., Marinopoulos, S., Phillips, K. A., Hwang, C. W., Maynor, K., Merenstein, D., Wilson, R. F., Barnes, G. J., Bass, E. B., Powe, N. R., & Daumit, G. L. (2007). Systematic review: The value of the periodic health evaluation. *Annals of Internal Medicine, 146*(4), 289–300.

Burkhardt, M., & Nathaniel, A. (2002). *Ethics & issues in contemporary nursing* (2nd ed.). Clifton Park, NY: Delmar Thomson Learning.

Carson-Smith, W., & Klein, C. (2003). Legal file: NP errors lead to litigation. *The Nurse Practitioner: The Journal of Primary Health Care, 28*(3), 52–56.

Catalano, J. T. (2006). *Nursing now! Today's issues, tomorrow's trends* (4th ed.). Philadelphia: F. A. Davis.

Doyle, M. (2006). Promoting standardized nursing language using an electronic medical record system. *AORN Journal, 83*(6), 1336–1342.

Edelman, C. L., & Mandle, C. L. (2006). *Health promotion throughout the life span* (6th ed.). St. Louis: Mosby.

Giese, E. A., O'Connor, F. G., Brennan, F. H., Depenbrock, P. J., & Oriscello, R. G. (2007). The athletic preparticipation evaluation: Cardiovascular assessment. *American Family Physician, 75*(7), 1008–1014.

Griswold, D. P., & Griswold, D. B. (2000). Minors' rights to refuse medical treatment requested by their parents: Remaining issues. *Journal of the American Academy of Nurse Practitioners, 12*(8), 325–328.

Guido, G. W. (2006). *Legal & ethical issues in nursing* (4th ed.). Upper Saddle River, NJ: Pearson Prentice Hall.

Hall, J. K. (2003). Legal consequences of the moral duty to report errors. *JONA's Healthcare Law, Ethics, and Regulation, 5*(3), 60–64.

Karch, A. M., & Karch, F. E. (2003). Looks can be deceiving: Use caution when using abbreviations. *American Journal of Nursing, 103*(10), 73.

Killion, S. W., & Dempski, K. M. (2001). *Quick look nursing: Legal and ethical issues.* Clifton Park, NY: Delmar Thomson Learning.

Monarch, K. (2002). *Nursing & the law: Trends and issues.* Washington, DC: American Nurses Association.

Murphy, D. P., Radwany, S., & Bhatnagar, M. (2008). End-of-life discussions: The art of delivering bad news. *Consultant, 48*(2), 156–162.

Pelliccia, A., Maron, B. J., Culasso, F., et al. (2000). Clinical significance of abnormal electrocardiographic patterns in trained athletes. *Circulation, 102*, 278–284.

Roberts, R. (2007). Strategies to lower your malpractice risk. *The Clinical Advisor, 10*(4), 39–45.

Segal-Isaacson, A. E. (2003). Jump on the PDA bandwagon. *The Nurse Practitioner: The Journal of Primary Health Care, 28*(Suppl. 1), 24–26.

Spiotta, V. L. (2003). Legal concerns surrounding e-mail use in a medical practice. *JONA's Healthcare Law, Ethics, and Regulation, 5*(3), 53–57.

Thompson, I. E., Melia, K. M., Boyd, K. M., & Horsburgh, D. (2006). *Nursing ethics* (5th ed.). Edinburgh: Churchill Livingstone.

Tschudin, V. (2003). *Approaches to ethics—nursing beyond borders.* London: Butterworth-Heinemann.

White, G. (2001). The code of ethics for nurses. *American Journal of Nursing, 101*(10), 73–75.

WEB SITES

American Association of Legal Nurse Consultants:
http://www.aalnc.org

The American Association of Nurse Attorneys:
http://www.taana.org

Centers for Disease Control and Prevention:
http://www.cdc.gov

Healthy People 2010:
http://www.healthypeople.gov

The Joint Commission:
http://www.jointcommission.org

Portal to U.S. Government Health Programs:
http://www.health.gov

APPENDIX A
NANDA International Nursing Diagnoses 2009–2011

Activity Intolerance
Ineffective Activity Planning
Risk for Activity Intolerance
Ineffective Airway Clearance
Latex Allergy Response
Risk for Latex Allergy Response
Anxiety
Death Anxiety
Risk for Aspiration
Risk for Impaired Attachment
Autonomic Dysreflexia
Risk for Autonomic Dysreflexia
Risk-Prone Health Behavior
Risk for Bleeding
Risk for Unstable Blood Glucose Level
Disturbed Body Image
Risk for Imbalanced Body Temperature
Effective Breastfeeding
Ineffective Breastfeeding
Interrupted Breastfeeding
Ineffective Breathing Pattern
Decreased Cardiac Output
Caregiver Role Strain
Risk for Caregiver Role Strain
Readiness for Enhanced Childbearing
    Process
Impaired Comfort
Readiness for Enhanced Comfort
Impaired Verbal Communication
Readiness for Enhanced
    Communication
Decisional Conflict (Specify)
Parental Role Conflict

Acute Confusion
Chronic Confusion
Risk for Acute Confusion
Constipation
Perceived Constipation
Risk for Constipation
Contamination
Risk for Contamination
Defensive Coping
Ineffective Coping
Readiness for Enhanced Coping
Ineffective Community Coping
Readiness for Enhanced Community
    Coping
Compromised Family Coping
Disabled Family Coping
Readiness for Enhanced Family Coping
Risk for Sudden Infant Death Syndrome
Readiness for Enhanced Decision Making
Ineffective Denial
Impaired Dentition
Risk for Delayed Development
Diarrhea
Risk for Compromised Human Dignity
Risk for Disuse Syndrome
Deficient Diversional Activity
Risk for Electrolyte Imbalance
Impaired Urinary Elimination
Readiness for Enhanced Urinary
    Elimination
Disturbed Energy Field
Impaired Environmental Interpretation
    Syndrome

Adult Failure to Thrive
Risk for Falls
Dysfunctional Family Processes
Interrupted Family Processes
Readiness for Enhanced Family
    Processes
Fatigue
Fear
Readiness for Enhanced Fluid Balance
Deficient Fluid Volume
Excess Fluid Volume
Risk for Deficient Fluid Volume
Risk for Imbalanced Fluid Volume
Impaired Gas Exchange
Grieving
Complicated Grieving
Risk for Complicated Grieving
Delayed Growth and Development
Risk for Disproportionate Growth
Ineffective Health Maintenance
Impaired Home Maintenance
Readiness for Enhanced Hope
Hopelessness
Hyperthermia
Hypothermia
Disturbed Personal Identity
Readiness for Enhanced Immunization
    Status
Bowel Incontinence
Functional Urinary Incontinence
Overflow Urinary Incontinence
Reflex Urinary Incontinence
Stress Urinary Incontinence

Urge Urinary Incontinence

Risk for Urge Urinary Incontinence

Disorganized Infant Behavior

Risk for Disorganized Infant Behavior

Readiness for Enhanced Organized Infant Behavior

Ineffective Infant Feeding Pattern

Risk for Infection

Risk for Injury

Risk for Perioperative-Positioning Injury

Insomnia

Decreased Intracranial Adaptive Capacity

Neonatal Jaundice

Deficient Knowledge

Readiness for Enhanced Knowledge (Specify)

Sedentary Lifestyle

Risk for Impaired Liver Function

Risk for Loneliness

Risk for disturbed Maternal/Fetal Dyad

Impaired Memory

Impaired Bed Mobility

Impaired Physical Mobility

Impaired Wheelchair Mobility

Moral Distress

Dysfunctional Gastrointestinal Motility

Risk for Dysfunctional Gastrointestinal Motility

Nausea

Unilateral Neglect

Noncompliance

Imbalanced Nutrition: Less than Body Requirements

Imbalanced Nutrition: More than Body Requirements

Readiness for Enhanced Nutrition

Risk for Imbalanced Nutrition: More than Body Requirements

Impaired Oral Mucous Membrane

Acute Pain

Chronic Pain

Readiness for Enhanced Parenting

Impaired Parenting

Risk for Impaired Parenting

Ineffective Peripheral Tissue Perfusion

Risk for Decreased Cardiac Tissue Perfusion

Risk for Ineffective Cerebral Tissue Perfusion

Risk for Ineffective Gastrointestinal Perfusion

Risk for Ineffective Renal Perfusion

Risk for Peripheral Neurovascular Dysfunction

Risk for Poisoning

Post-Trauma Syndrome

Risk for Post-Trauma Syndrome

Readiness for Enhanced Power

Powerlessness

Risk for Powerlessness

Ineffective Protection

Rape-Trauma Syndrome

Readiness for Enhanced Relationship

Impaired Religiosity

Readiness for Enhanced Religiosity

Risk for Impaired Religiosity

Relocation Stress Syndrome

Risk for Relocation Stress Syndrome

Impaired Individual Resilience

Readiness for Enhanced Resilience

Risk for Compromised Resilience

Urinary Retention

Ineffective Role Performance

Bathing Self-Care Deficit

Dressing Self-Care Deficit

Feeding Self-Care Deficit

Readiness for Enhanced Self-Care

Toileting Self-Care Deficit

Readiness for Enhanced Self-Concept

Chronic Low Self-Esteem

Situational Low Self-Esteem

Risk for Situational Low Self-Esteem

Ineffective Self Health Management

Readiness for Enhanced Self Health Management

Self-Mutilation

Risk for Self-Mutilation

Self Neglect

Disturbed Sensory Perception (Specify: Visual, Auditory, Kinesthetic, Gustatory, Tactile, Olfactory)

Sexual Dysfunction

Ineffective Sexuality Pattern

Risk for Shock

Impaired Skin Integrity

Risk for Impaired Skin Integrity

Sleep Deprivation

Disturbed Sleep Pattern

Readiness for Enhanced Sleep

Impaired Social Interaction

Social Isolation

Chronic Sorrow

Spiritual Distress

Risk for Spiritual Distress

Readiness for Enhanced Spiritual Well-Being

Stress Overload

Risk for Suffocation

Risk for Suicide

Delayed Surgical Recovery

Impaired Swallowing

Ineffective Family Therapeutic Regimen Management

Ineffective Thermoregulation

Impaired Tissue Integrity

Ineffective Peripheral Tissue Perfusion

Impaired Transfer Ability

Risk for Trauma

Risk for Vascular Trauma

Impaired Spontaneous Ventilation

Dysfunctional Ventilatory Weaning Response

Risk for Other-Directed Violence

Risk for Self-Directed Violence

Impaired Walking

Wandering

APPENDIX B
Functional Assessments:
Instrumental Activities of Daily Living (IADLs) and Physical Self-Maintenance Activities

I. Instrumental Activities of Daily Living
A. Ability to use telephone
1. Operates telephone independently—looks up and dials numbers
2. Dials a few well-known numbers
3. Answers phone but does not dial or use touch tone
4. Does not use telephone at all

B. Housekeeping
1. Maintains house independently or with occasional assistance for "heavy work"
2. Performs light tasks such as bedmaking and dishwashing
3. Performs light daily tasks but cannot maintain adequate level of cleanliness
4. Needs assistance with all home maintenance tasks
5. Does not participate in any tasks

C. Laundry
1. Does personal laundry completely
2. Launders small items such as socks and stockings
3. All laundry must be done by others

D. Mode of transportation
1. Independently drives own car or uses public transportation
2. Arranges own travel via taxi or special transportation services, but does not use public transportation and does not drive
3. Travels on public transportation when assisted or with others
4. Travel limited to taxi or auto with assistance
5. Does not travel at all

E. Responsibility for medications
1. Takes medication in correct dosages at correct time independently
2. Takes medication if medication is prepared in advance in separate doses
3. Not capable of dispensing own medications

F. Ability to handle finances
1. Independently manages finances—writes checks, pays bills, keeps track of income
2. Manages own finances with assistance
3. Not capable of managing own finances

G. Shopping
1. Does all of the shopping independently
2. Shops for small purchases independently
3. Not able to go shopping without assistance
4. Unable to shop for any purchase

H. Food preparation
1. Able to prepare and serve food without assistance
2. Prepares adequate meals if supplied with food
3. Able to heat and serve prepared meals
4. Unable to prepare and serve meals

Adapted from "Assessment of Older People: Self-Maintaining and Instrumental Activities of Daily Living" by M. Lawton and E. Brody, 1969, The Gerontologist, 9, pp. 179–186.

II. Physical Self-Maintenance Activities
A. Feeding
1. Eats without assistance
2. Eats with minor assistance at meal times and helps in cleaning up
3. Feeds self with moderate assistance
4. Requires extensive assistance—all meals
5. Does not feed self at all and resists efforts of others to feed him or her

B. Toilet
1. Cares for self completely, no incontinence
2. Needs to be reminded or needs help in cleaning self

3. Soils the bed while asleep—more than once a week
4. Soils clothing while awake—more than once a week
5. No control of bladder or bowel

C. Grooming (hairs, nails, hands, face)
   1. Able to care for self
   2. Occasional minor assistance needed (e.g., with shaving)
   3. Moderate and regular assistance needed
   4. Needs total grooming care, but accepts some
   5. Actively negates efforts of others to maintain grooming

D. Bathing
   1. Bathes self without help
   2. Bathes self with help into and out of tub or shower
   3. Can wash face and hands only
   4. Does not wash self but is cooperative
   5. Does not try to wash self and resists efforts of others to help

E. Dressing
   1. Dresses, undresses, and selects clothes from wardrobe
   2. Dresses and undresses with minor assistance

3. Needs moderate assistance in dressing or selection of clothes
4. Needs major assistance
5. Completely unable to dress self and resists efforts of others to help

F. Ambulation
   1. Ambulates about grounds or city without assistance
   2. Ambulates within residence or nearby
   3. Ambulates with assistance of
      a. another person
      b. a railing
      c. cane
      d. walker
      e. wheelchair
   4. Sits unsupported in chair or wheelchair but cannot propel self
   5. Bedridden more than half the time

APPENDIX C
ISMP List of Error-Prone Abbreviations, Symbols, and Dose Designations

Abbreviations	Intended Meaning	Misinterpretation	Correction
μg	Microgram	Mistaken as "mg"	Use "mcg"
AD, AS, AU	Right ear, left ear, each ear	Mistaken as OD, OS, OU (right eye, left eye, each eye)	Use "right ear," "left ear," or "each ear"
OD, OS, OU	Right eye, left eye, each eye	Mistaken as AD, AS, AU (right ear, left ear, each ear)	Use "right eye," "left eye," or "each eye"
BT	Bedtime	Mistaken as "BID" (twice daily)	Use "bedtime"
cc	Cubic centimeters	Mistaken as "u" (units)	Use "mL"
D/C	Discharge or discontinue	Premature discontinuation of medications if D/C (intended to mean "discharge") has been misinterpreted as "discontinued" when followed by a list of discharge medications	Use "discharge" and "discontinue"
IJ	Injection	Mistaken as "IV" or "intrajugular"	Use "injection"
IN	Intranasal	Mistaken as "IM" or "IV"	Use "intranasal" or "NAS"
HS	Half-strength	Mistaken as bedtime	Use "half-strength" or "bedtime"
hs	At bedtime, hours of sleep	Mistaken as half-strength	
IU**	International unit	Mistaken as IV (intravenous) or 10 (ten)	Use "units"
o.d. or OD	Once daily	Mistaken as "right eye" (OD-oculus dexter), leading to oral liquid medications administered in the eye	Use "daily"
OJ	Orange juice	Mistaken as OD or OS (right or left eye); drugs meant to be diluted in orange juice may be given in the eye	Use "orange juice"
Per os	By mouth, orally	The "os" can be mistaken as "left eye" (OS-oculus sinister)	Use "PO," "by mouth," or "orally"
q.d. or QD**	Every day	Mistaken as q.i.d., especially if the period after the "q" or the tail of the "q" is misunderstood as an "i"	Use "daily"
qhs	At bedtime	Mistaken as "qhr" or every hour	Use "at bedtime"
qn	Nightly	Mistaken as "qh" (every hour)	Use "nightly"
q.o.d. or QOD**	Every other day	Mistaken as "q.d." (daily) or "q.i.d. (four times daily) if the "o" is poorly written	Use "every other day"
q1d	Daily	Mistaken as q.i.d. (four times daily)	Use "daily"
q6PM, etc.	Every evening at 6 PM	Mistaken as every 6 hours	Use "6 PM nightly" or "6 PM daily"
SC, SQ, sub q	Subcutaneous	SC mistaken as SL (sublingual); SQ mistaken as "5 every"; the "q" in "sub q" has been mistaken as "every" (e.g., a heparin dose ordered "sub q 2 hours before surgery" misunderstood as every 2 hours before surgery)	Use "subcut" or "subcutaneously"
ss	Sliding scale (insulin) or ½ (apothecary)	Mistaken as "55"	Spell out "sliding scale"; use "one-half" or "½"
SSRI	Sliding scale regular insulin	Mistaken as selective-serotonin reuptake inhibitor	Spell out "sliding scale (insulin)"
SSI	Sliding scale insulin	Mistaken as Strong Solution of Iodine (Lugol's)	

continues

Abbreviations	Intended Meaning	Misinterpretation	Correction
1/d	One daily	Mistaken as "tid"	Use "1 daily"
TIW or tiw	3 times a week	Mistaken as "3 times a day" or "twice in a week"	Use "3 times weekly"
U or u**	Unit	Mistaken as the number 0 or 4, causing a 10-fold overdose or greater (e.g., 4U seen as "40" or 4u seen as "44"); mistaken as "cc" so dose given in volume instead of units (e.g., 4u seen as 4cc)	Use "unit"

Dose Designations and Other Information	Intended Meaning	Misinterpretation	Correction
Trailing zero after decimal point (e.g., 1.0 mg)**	1 mg	Mistaken as 10 mg if the decimal point is not seen	Do not use trailing zeros for doses expressed in whole numbers
No leading zero before a decimal dose (e.g., .5 mg)**	0.5 mg	Mistaken as 5 mg if the decimal point is not seen	Use zero before a decimal point when the dose is less than a whole unit
Drug name and dose run together (especially problematic for drug names that end in "L" such as Inderal40 mg; Tegretol300 mg)	Inderal 40 mg Tegretol 300 mg	Mistaken as Inderal 140 mg Mistaken as Tegretol 1300 mg	Place adequate space between the drug name, dose, and unit of measure
Numerical dose and unit of measure run together (e.g., 10mg, 100mL)	10 mg 100 mL	The "m" is sometimes mistaken as a zero or two zeros, risking a 10- to 100-fold overdose	Place adequate space between the dose and unit of measure
Abbreviations such as mg. or mL. with a period following the abbreviation	mg mL	The period is unnecessary and could be mistaken as the number 1 if written poorly	Use mg, mL, etc., without a terminal period
Large doses without properly placed commas (e.g., 100000 units; 1000000 units)	100,000 units 1,000,000 units	100000 has been mistaken as 10,000 or 1,000,000; 1000000 has been mistaken as 100,000	Use commas for dosing units at or above 1,000, or use words such as 100 "thousand" or 1 "million" to improve readability

Drug Name Abbreviations	Intended Meaning	Misinterpretation	Correction
ARA A	vidarabine	Mistaken as cytarabine (ARA C)	Use complete drug name
AZT	zidovudine (Retrovir)	Mistaken as azathioprine or aztreonam	Use complete drug name
CPZ	Compazine (prochlorperazine)	Mistaken as chlorpromazine	Use complete drug name
DPT	Demerol-Phenergan-Thorazine	Mistaken as diphtheria-pertussis-tetanus (vaccine)	Use complete drug name
DTO	Diluted tincture of opium, or deodorized tincture of opium (Paregoric)	Mistaken as tincture of opium	Use complete drug name
HCl	hydrochloric acid or hydrochloride	Mistaken as potassium chloride (The "H" is misinterpreted as "K")	Use complete drug name unless expressed as a salt of a drug
HCT	hydrocortisone	Mistaken as hydrochlorothiazide	Use complete drug name
HCTZ	hydrochlorothiazide	Mistaken as hydrocortisone (seen as HCT250 mg)	Use complete drug name
MgSO4**	magnesium sulfate	Mistaken as morphine sulfate	Use complete drug name
MS, MSO4**	morphine sulfate	Mistaken as magnesium sulfate	Use complete drug name
MTX	methotrexate	Mistaken as mitoxantrone	Use complete drug name
PCA	procainamide	Mistaken as Patient Controlled Analgesia	Use complete drug name
PTU	propylthiouracil	Mistaken as mercaptopurine	Use complete drug name
T3	Tylenol with codeine No. 3	Mistaken as liothyronine	Use complete drug name
TAC	triamcinolone	Mistaken as tetracaine, Adrenalin, cocaine	Use complete drug name
TNK	TNKase	Mistaken as "TPA"	Use complete drug name
ZnSO4	zinc sulfate	Mistaken as morphine sulfate	Use complete drug name

Stemmed Drug Names	Intended Meaning	Misinterpretation	Correction
"Nitro" drip	nitroglycerin infusion	Mistaken as sodium nitroprusside infusion	Use complete drug name
"Norflox"	norfloxacin	Mistaken as Norflex	Use complete drug name
"IV Vanc"	intravenous vancomycin	Mistaken as Invanz	Use complete drug name

continues

Symbols	Intended Meaning	Misinterpretation	Correction
ℨ	Dram	Symbol for dram mistaken as "3"	Use the metric system
℥	Minim	Symbol for minim mistaken as "mL"	
x3d	For three days	Mistaken as "3 doses"	Use "for three days"
> and <	Greater than and less than	Mistaken as opposite of intended; mistakenly use incorrect symbol; "< 10" mistaken as "40"	Use "greater than" or "less than"
/ (slash mark)	Separates two doses or indicates "per"	Mistaken as the number 1 (e.g., "25 units/10 units" misread as "25 units and 110" units)	Use "per" rather than a slash mark to separate doses
@	At	Mistaken as "2"	Use "at"
&	And	Mistaken as "2"	Use "and"
+	Plus or and	Mistaken as "4"	Use "and"
°	Hour	Mistaken as a zero (e.g., q2° seen as q 20)	Use "hr," "h," or "hour"

**These abbreviations are included on The Joint Commission's "minimum list" of dangerous abbreviations, acronyms and symbols that must be included on an organization's "Do Not Use" list, effective January 1, 2004. Visit www.jointcommission.org for more information about this Joint Commission requirement.

GLOSSARY

A

Abruptio Placenta Separation of the placenta from the uterine wall, which may cause significant internal (and perhaps external) bleeding, pain, and fetal compromise.

Accommodation Visual focusing from a far to a near point as pupils constrict and eyes converge.

Acculturation Informal process of adaptation through which the beliefs, values, norms, and practices of a dominant culture are learned by a new member born into a different culture.

Acini *See* **Alveoli (of the Breast)**.

Acrocyanosis Normal phenomenon in light-skinned newborns whereby the hands and feet are blue and the rest of the body is pink.

Acromegaly Abnormal enlargement of the skull, bony facial structures, and bones of the extremities, caused by excessive secretion of growth hormone.

Action Response Attempt to stimulate patients to make some change in their thinking and behavior.

Active Listening Act of perceiving what is said both verbally and nonverbally.

Actual Nursing Diagnosis Statement describing human responses that have been validated by the nurse.

Adnexa Fallopian tubes, ovaries, and their supporting ligaments.

Advance Directive Document (living will or durable medical power of attorney) outlining what should be done if a patient is too ill to self-direct medical care.

Adventitious Breath Sound Added breath sound that is superimposed on normal breath sounds.

Afterload Initial resistance that the ventricles must overcome in order to open the semilunar valves to propel the blood into both the systemic and the pulmonary circulation.

Ages and Stages Developmental Theory Belief that individuals experience much the same sequential physical, cognitive, socioemotional, and moral changes during the same age periods, each of which is termed a developmental stage.

Ageusia Loss of the sense of taste.

Aggravating Factors Events that worsen the severity of the patient's chief complaint.

Agnosia Inability to recognize the form and nature of objects or persons.

Agnostic Person who is unsure if God exists.

Agonal Respirations Irregularly irregular respirations that signal impending death.

Agraphia Loss of the ability to write.

Air Trapping Abnormal respiratory pattern with rapid, shallow respirations and forced expirations; the lungs have insufficient time to fully exhale and air becomes trapped, leading to overexpansion of the lungs.

Albinism A generalized whiteness of the skin, hair, and eyebrows, which is caused by a congenital inability to form melanin.

Albumin Substance that transports nutrients, blood, and hormones and helps maintain osmotic pressure.

Alexia Loss of the ability to grasp the meaning of written words and sentences; also known as word blindness.

Allen Test Test used to assess for the patency of the radial and ulnar arteries.

Alleviating Factors Events that decrease the severity of the patient's chief complaint.

Alogia Inability to express oneself through speech.

Alopecia   Partial or complete loss of hair.

Alveoli (of the Breast)   Milk-producing glands located in the lobules; also called acini.

Alveoli (of the Lung)   Smallest functional unit of the respiratory system; where gas exchange occurs.

Amblyopia   Permanent loss of visual acuity resulting from certain uncorrected medical conditions.

Amenorrhea   Absence of menses.

Anal Canal   Terminal 3 to 4 cm of the large intestine.

Anal Columns   Longitudinal folds of mucosa in the superior portion of the anal canal.

Anal Fissure   Linear tear in the epidermis of the anal canal.

Anal Incontinence   Involuntary release of rectal contents.

Anal Orifice   Exit to the gastrointestinal tract; located at the seam of the gluteal folds.

Anal Sinuses   Pockets in the anal canal that lie superior to the anal valves; they secrete mucus when compressed by feces.

Anal Valves   Folds in the anal canal that are formed by joining anal columns.

Analgesia   Absence of normal sense of pain.

Anemia   Decreased number of red blood cells.

Anencephaly   Condition where the cerebral cortex or cranium does not develop.

Anergy   Diminished reaction to antigens.

Aneroid Manometer   Blood pressure measurement equipment with a calibrated dial and indicator that points to numbers representing blood pressure.

Anesthesia   Absence of touch sensation.

Angina   Myocardial ischemia that manifests as chest, neck, or arm pain.

Angle of Louis (Manubriosternal Junction or Sternal Angle)   Junction of the manubrium and the sternum.

Animism   Belief that all things in nature have souls.

Anisocoria   Difference in pupil sizes.

Anoderm   Epithelial tissue that lies in the lower 2 cm of the anal canal.

Anorectal Abscess   Undrained collection of perianal pus of the tissue spaces in and adjacent to the anorectum.

Anorectal Fistula   Hollow, fibrous tract lined by granulation tissue and filled with purulent or serosanguineous discharge; it has an opening inside the anal canal or rectum, and one or more orifices in the perianal skin.

Anorectum   Area where the anal canal fuses with the rectum.

Anosmia   Loss of the sense of smell.

Anterior Axillary Line   Vertical line drawn from the origin of the anterior axillary fold along the anterolateral aspect of the thorax.

Anterior Chamber   Space anterior to the pupil and iris.

Anterior Triangle   Area of the neck formed by the mandible, the trachea, and the sternocleidomastoid muscle; contains the anterior cervical lymph nodes, the trachea, and the thyroid gland.

Anthropometric Measurements   Measurements of the human body, including height, weight, and body proportions.

Anticipatory Guidance   Approach covering health promotion and education; designed to inform at-risk individuals of physical, cognitive, psychological, and social changes that occur and what their nutritional needs are.

Antigen Skin Testing   Test of immune function.

Apex (of the Heart)   Lower portion of the heart.

Apex (of the Lung)   Top of the lung.

Apgar Score   A system for evaluating the newborn at 1 and 5 minutes of age, giving 0–2 points for heart rate, respiratory effort, muscle tone, reflex irritability, and color.

Aphasia   Impairment or absence of language function.

Aphonia   Total loss of voice.

Apnea   Lack of spontaneous respirations for 10 or more seconds.

Apneustic Respirations   Prolonged gasping in inspiration followed by a very short, inefficient pause that can last 30 to 60 seconds.

Apocrine Glands   Sweat glands that are associated with hair follicles.

Appendicular Skeleton   Peripheral skeleton including the limbs, pelvis, scapula, and clavicle.

Apraxia   Inability to convert intended speech into the motor act of speech; inability to perform purposeful acts or to manipulate objects.

Arcus Senilis   Hazy, gray ring about 2 mm in size and located just inside the limbus; most commonly found in older individuals.

Areola   Pigmented area approximately 2.5 to 10 cm in diameter that surrounds the nipple.

Arrector Pili Muscle   Muscle that causes contraction of the skin and hair, resulting in "goose bumps."

Arrhythmia   Irregular heart rhythm; also known as dysrhythmia.

Ascites   Excess accumulation of fluid in the abdominal cavity.

Assessment   First step of the nursing process; the orderly collection of objective and subjective data on the patient's health status.

Associated Manifestations   Signs and symptoms that accompany a patient's chief complaint.

Astereognosis   Inability to recognize the nature of objects by touch.

Asystole   Absence of cardiac activity, flat line on EKG.

Ataxic Respirations   *See* **Biot's Respirations**.

Atheist   Person who does not believe in God.

Atherosclerosis   Development of lipid plaques along the coronary arteries.

Atlas   First cervical vertebra.

Atrial Kick   Final phase of ventricular diastole, when the atria contract to complete the final 20% to 30% of ventricular filling.

Atrioventricular (A-V) Node   One of the heart's pacemakers that delays the impulse from the atria before it goes to the ventricles; inherent rate is 40 to 60 beats per minute.

Atrioventricular (A-V) Valves   Valves that prevent blood from entering the ventricles until diastole and prevent retrograde blood flow during systole; composed of the tricuspid and mitral valves.

Atrophy   Reduction in muscle size.

Augmentation Mammoplasty   Surgical breast augmentation.

Auricle   External flap of the ear; also called the pinna.

Auscultation   Process of active listening to sounds within the body to gather information on a patient's health status.

Auscultatory Gap   A silent interval that may be heard between the systolic and diastolic blood pressures that can occur in hypertensive patients; this can lead to a falsely elevated high diastolic or falsely low systolic blood pressure measurement.

Avolition   Lack of motivation for work or other goal-directed activity.

Axial Skeleton   Central skeleton, including the facial bones, skull, auditory ossicles, hyoid bone, ribs, sternum, and vertebrae.

Axillary Nodes   Nodes composed of four groups: brachial (lateral) central axillary (mid axillary), pectoral (anterior), subscapular (posterior).

Axis   Second cervical vertebra.

B

Balanitis   Inflammation of the glans penis.

Ballottement   Palpation technique to identify an organ or fluid.

Baroreceptors   Receptors located in the walls of most of the great arteries that sense hypotension and initiate reflex vasoconstriction and tachycardia to bring the blood pressure back to normal.

Barrel Chest   Abnormal thorax configuration where the ratio of the anteroposterior diameter to the transverse diameter of the chest is approximately 1:1.

Bartholin's Glands (Greater Vestibular Glands)   Located in the cleft between the labia minora and the hymenal ring; these glands secrete a clear, viscid, odorless, alkaline mucus that improves the viability and motility of sperm along the female reproductive tract.

Base (of the Heart)   Uppermost portion of the heart.

Base (of the Lung)   Bottom of the lung.

Bell's Palsy   Idiopathic facial palsy of CN VII resulting in asymmetry of the palpebral fissures, nasolabial folds, mouth, and facial expression on the affected side.

Bilingualism   Habitual use of two different languages, particularly when speaking.

Biot's (or Ataxic) Respirations   Irregularly irregular respiratory pattern caused by damage to the medulla.

Blepharitis   Inflamed, scaly, red-rimmed eyelids, sometimes with loss of the eyelashes.

Blood Pressure   Vital sign collected to assess cardiac output and vascular resistance; it measures the force exerted by the flow of blood pumped into the large arteries.

Body Mass Index (BMI)   Measurement that indicates body composition based on a person's height and weight; an increased BMI indicates obesity and a decreased BMI indicates possible malnutrition.

Borborygmi   Loud, audible, gurgling bowel sounds.

Bouchard's Node   Bony enlargement of the proximal interphalangeal joint of the finger.

Bow Legs   *See* **Genu Varum**.

Bradycardia   Pulse rate under 60 beats per minute in a resting adult.

Bradypnea   Respiratory rate under 12 breaths per minute in a resting adult.

Braxton Hicks Contractions   A pattern of intermittent, painless uterine contractions that occurs more frequently at the end of pregnancy (every 10–20 minutes or even more frequently). These are not true labor pains.

Breasts   Pair of mammary glands located on the anterior chest wall and extending vertically from the second to the sixth rib and laterally from the sternal border to the axillae.

Bregma   Junction of the coronal and sagittal sutures.

Bronchial (or Tubular) Breath Sound   Breath sound that is high in pitch and loud in intensity and that is heard best over the trachea; has a blowing or hollow quality; heard longer in expiration than inspiration.

Bronchophony   Voice sound where the patient says the words "ninety-nine" or "one, two, three" to determine if the lung is filled with air, fluid, or a solid.

Bronchovesicular Breath Sound   Breath sound that is moderate in pitch and intensity and that is heard best between the scapula and the first and second intercostal spaces lateral to the sternum; its quality is a combination of bronchial and vesicular breath sounds; heard equally in inspiration and expiration.

Bruit   Blowing sound that can be auscultated when the blood flow becomes turbulent because blood is rushing past an obstruction.

Brushfield's Spots   Small, white flecks located around the perimeter of the iris, associated with Down syndrome.

Bulbar Conjunctiva   Covering of the anterior surface of the sclera.

Bulbourethral Glands   Pea-sized glands located below the prostate; secretions are emptied from here at the time of ejaculation.

Bursae   Sacs filled with fluids.

C

Cachexia   Extreme malnutrition in which the patient exhibits wasting.

Callus   Thickening of the skin due to prolonged pressure.

Canthus   Nasal or temporal angle where the eyelids meet.

Caput Medusae   Venous pattern of congested veins around the umbilicus; attributed to obstruction of the portal vein and seen in liver dysfunction.

Caput Succedaneum   Swelling over the occipitoparietal region of the skull that occurs during delivery of the newborn.

Carbohydrate   Major source of energy for various functions of the body; supplies fiber and assists in the utilization of fat.

Cardiomegaly   Enlargement of the heart.

Carotenemia   Orange-yellow coloration of palmar and plantar surfaces caused by elevated levels of serum carotene.

Carpal Tunnel Syndrome   Pressure on the median nerve at the carpal tunnel of the wrist, causing numbness, tingling, weakness, and pain.

Caruncle   Round, red structure in the inner canthus; contains sebaceous glands.

Castration Anxiety   Young boys' fear of having the penis cut off or mutilated.

Cataract   Opacity in the lens of the eye that gives the pupil a pearly gray appearance.

Cephalhematoma   Localized subcutaneous swelling over one cranial bone that occurs during delivery of the newborn.

Cephalocaudal   Head-to-toe approach.

Cerumen   Waxlike substance produced in the ear canal.

Cervix   Inferior aspect of the uterus.

Chadwick's Sign   A blue, soft cervix, normally during pregnancy.

Chalazion   Chronic inflammation of the meibomian gland in the upper or lower eyelid.

Chancre   Reddish, round ulcer or small papular lesion with a depressed center and raised, indurated edges.

Chancroid   Tender, ulcerated, exudative, papular lesion with an erythematous halo, surrounding edema, and a friable base.

Chandelier's Sign   Cervical motion tenderness on palpation.

Characteristic Patterns of Daily Living   Patient's normal daily routines; includes meal, work, and sleeping schedules and patterns of social interactions.

Chemosis   Swelling of the palpebral conjunctiva.

Cherry Angioma   Bright red, circumscribed area that may be flat or raised and that darkens with age.

Cheyne-Stokes Respirations   Crescendo or decrescendo respiratory pattern interspersed between periods of apnea.

Chief Complaint   Symptom or problem that causes the patient to seek health care.

Chloasma   *See* **Melasma**.

Cholelithiasis   Presence or formation of bile stone or calculi in the gallbladder or duct.

Cholestasis   Arrest of bile excretion.

Cholesterol   Lipid found only in animal products; it is transported in the body by high-density lipoproteins (HDLs) and low-density lipoproteins (LDLs).

Chorionic Villi Sampling (CVS)   Intracervical (or less commonly, intra-abdominal) sampling of the chorionic villi for chromosome analysis. It is an alternative to traditional or early amniocentesis and is typically performed at approximately 9–10 weeks.

Choroid   Vascular tissue of the posterior uveal tract lining the inner surface of the globe of the eye, beneath the retina; provides nutrition to the retina and helps absorb excess light.

Ciliary Body   Extension of the uveal tract that produces aqueous humor.

Circadian Rhythm   Normal fluctuation of body temperature, pulse, and blood pressure during a 24-hour period.

Click   Extrasystolic heart sound that is high-pitched and can radiate in the chest wall.

Clinical Reasoning   A disciplined, creative, and reflective thinking used with critical thinking to establish potential strategies for patients to reach their health goals.

Clitoris   Cylindrical, erectile body located at the superior aspect of the vulva, between the labia minora; it contains erectile tissue and has a significant supply of nerve endings.

Clonus   Rhythmic oscillation of involuntary muscle contraction.

Clustering   Placing similar or related data into meaningful groups.

Cochlea   Snail-shaped structure in the bony labyrinth of the inner ear.

Code of Ethics   Codified beliefs and lists of mandatory or prohibited acts.

Collaborative Intervention   Physician-prescribed orders that are implemented by nurses.

Collaborative Problem   Patient problem for which the nurse works jointly with the physician and other health care workers to monitor, plan, and implement treatment.

Colloquialism   Word or phrase particular to a community and used in informal conversation and writing.

Coloboma   Defect of the choroid and retina resulting when development in utero is interrupted.

Colostrum   A thin, milky secretion expressed by the breast during pregnancy and for a few days after parturition; it is rich in antibodies and colostrum corpuscles.

Complete Health History   Comprehensive history of the patient's past and present health status; includes physical, emotional, psychological, developmental, cultural, and spiritual data.

Condyloma Acuminatum   Genital wart.

Cones   Retinal structures in the macular region that are responsible for color vision.

Confabulation   Fabrication of answers, experiences, or situations unrelated to facts.

Conservation   The understanding that altering the physical state of an object does not change the basic properties of that object.

Constructional Apraxia   Inability to reproduce figures on paper.

Cooper's Ligaments   Ligaments that extend vertically from the deep fascia through the breast to the inner layer of the skin and provide support for the breast tissue.

Corn   Conical area of thickened skin.

Cornea   Transparent covering of the iris.

Costal Angle   Angle formed by the intersection of the costal margins at the sternum.

Costal Margin   Medial border created by the articulation of the false ribs.

Cradle Cap   Seborrheic dermatitis manifesting as greasy-appearing scales on an infant's scalp.

Craniosynostosis   Abnormal shape of the skull due to premature ossification of one or more suture lines before brain growth is complete.

Craniotabes   Softening of the skull.

Creatinine   Substance found in muscle and excreted in the urine.

Crepitus   Subcutaneous emphysema; beads of air escape from the lungs and create a crackling sound when palpated. A grating or crackling sound that can be felt/heard with joint movement.

Crescendo   Heart murmur configuration that proceeds from soft to loud.

Critical Pathway   Map in the case management patient care delivery system that shows the outcome of predetermined patient goals over a period of time.

Critical Thinking   A purposeful, goal-directed thinking process that strives to problem solve patient care issues through clinical reasoning.

Cross-Cultural Nursing Care   Nursing care that is provided within the cultural context of a patient who is a member of a culture or subculture other than that of the nurse.

Cryptorchidism   Condition in which a testicle has not descended into the scrotum.

Cullen's Sign   Bluish discoloration encircling the umbilicus and indicative of blood in the peritoneal cavity.

Cult   Organized group centered around religious devotion to a set of beliefs or to a person.

Cultural Beliefs   Explanatory ideas and knowledge about various aspects of the world in which members of a given culture place their faith and confidence.

Cultural Diversity   State of different combinations of cultural and subcultural minorities (e.g., ethnic, racial, national, religious, generational, marital status, socioeconomic, occupational, health status, and preference in life partner orientations) coexisting in a given location.

Cultural Identity   Subjective sense of cultural definition or cultural orientation with which an individual self-identifies.

Cultural Norms   Often unwritten but generally understood prescriptions for acceptable behavior by members of a cultural group.

Cultural Relativism   Belief that no culture is either inferior or superior to another; that behavior must be evaluated in relation to the cultural context in which it occurs; and that respect, equality, and justice are basic rights for all racial, ethnic, subcultural, and cultural groups.

Cultural Rituals   Highly structured and prescribed patterns of behavior used by a cultural group to respond to or in anticipation of specific life events such as birth, death, illness, healing, marriage, and worship.

Cultural Values   Fundamental, often unshakable and unchanging, set of principles on which the cultural beliefs, behaviors, and customs of all members of the culture are based.

Culturally Competent Nursing Care   Nursing care that is provided by nurses who use cross-cultural nursing models and research to identify health care needs and to plan and evaluate the care provided within the cultural context of their patients.

Culture   Learned and socially transmitted orientation and way of life of a group of people that is based on shared values, beliefs, customs, and norms of behavior and that determines how members of the group think, act, and relate to and with others as well as how they perceive and respond to all aspects of their lives.

Culture Shock Disorientation and uncertainty that results from the expenditure of mental, emotional, and physical energy during the process of adjusting to a new cultural group; it can lead to frustration, anger, alienation, or depression.

Custom Frequent or common practice carried out by tradition; culturally learned behaviors associated with a specific culture, including communication patterns, family and kinship relations, work patterns, dietary and religious practices, and health behaviors and practices.

Cutaneous Hypersensitivity Stimulus detecting specific zones of peritoneal irritation.

Cyanosis Blue coloration of the skin or nails that occurs when more than 5 g/dL of hemoglobin is deoxygenated in the blood.

Cystocele Bulging of the anterior vaginal wall.

Cystourethrocele Bulging of the anterior vaginal wall, bladder, and urethra into the vaginal introitus.

D

Dacryoadenitis Acute inflammation of the lacrimal gland.

Dacryocystitis Inflammation of the lacrimal duct.

Decerebrate Rigidity Rigidity and sustained contraction of the extensor muscle.

Decorticate Rigidity Hyperflexion of the arms, hyperextension and internal rotation of the legs, and plantar flexion.

Decrescendo Heart murmur configuration that proceeds from loud to soft.

Deep Palpation Palpating the body's internal structures to a depth of 4 to 5 cm to elicit information on organs and masses, including position, size, shape, mobility, consistency, and areas of discomfort.

Defecation Expulsion of feces from the rectum.

Defining Characteristics Signs, symptoms, or statements made by the patient that validate the existence of the health problem or situation.

Dehydration Lack of fluid in the tissues.

Dermatome Skin area innervated by afferent spinal nerves from a specific nerve root.

Dermis Corium, or the second layer of the skin.

Descriptor or Qualifier Adjective that describes or qualifies the human response.

Desquamation Shedding of old skin cells as new cells are pushed up from the lower layers of the epidermis.

Development Patterned and predictable increases in the physical, cognitive, socioemotional, and moral capacities of individuals that enable them to successfully adapt to their environments.

Developmental Dislocation of the Hip Dislocated hip found in newborns and young infants and related to familial factors, maternal hormones, firstborn children, and breech presentations.

Developmental Stage One of multiple sequential age periods during which individuals experience the same physical, cognitive, socioemotional, and moral changes.

Developmental Task Specific physical or psychosocial skill that must be achieved during each developmental stage.

Diaphragmatic Excursion Technique used to assess the patient's depth of ventilation.

Diaphragmatic Hernia Protrusion of intestines into the thoracic cavity.

Diaphysis Central shaft of the long bone.

Diastasis Recti Separation of the rectus muscle of the abdominal wall.

Diastole Phase in the cardiac cycle when the heart is at rest.

Dietary Reference Intakes Nutrient reference values developed by the Institute of Medicine that are used to assess a person's diet; comprised of three components: Adequate Intake, Tolerable Upper Intake Level, and Recommended Dietary Allowances.

Direct Fist Percussion Using the ulnar aspect of a closed fist to strike the patient's body to elicit tenderness over specific body areas.

Direct Inguinal Hernia Protrusion of the bowel and/or omentum directly through the external inguinal ring.

Direct (or Immediate) Auscultation Active listening to body sounds via the unaided ear.

Direct (or Immediate) Percussion Striking of an area of the body directly with the index or middle finger pad or fist to elicit sound.

Dislocation Complete dislodgement of a bone from its joint cavity.

Distress Negative stress that is harmful and unpleasant.

Disuse Atrophy Decrease in muscle mass and strength as a result of immobility.

Dogma Beliefs that are essential to the identity of a religion.

Doppler Device that emits ultrasound waves and senses shifts in frequency as the ultrasound waves are reflected from fetal heart valves.

Down Syndrome Congenital chromosomal aberration marked by slanted eyes with inner epicanthal folds; a short, flat nose; a protruding, thick tongue; and mental retardation.

Ductus (Vas) Deferens Tube that permits sperm to exit from the epididymis and pass from the scrotal sac upward into the abdominal cavity.

Dullness Descriptor for a percussable sound that is moderate in intensity, moderate in duration, of high pitch, thudlike, and normally located over organs.

Duration (of Percussion)   Time period over which a sound is heard.

Dysarthria   Disturbance in muscular control of speech.

Dyscalculia   Inability to perform calculations.

Dysdiadochokinesia   Inability to perform rapid alternating movements.

Dysesthesia   Abnormal interpretation of a stimulus such as burning or tingling from a stimulus such as touch or superficial pain.

Dysmenorrhea   Pain or cramping during menses.

Dysmetria   Impairment of judgment of distance, range, speed, and force of movement.

Dyspareunia   Painful sexual intercourse.

Dysphagia   Difficulty swallowing.

Dysphonia   Difficulty in making laryngeal speech sounds.

Dyspnea   Subjective feeling of shortness of breath.

Dysrhythmia   *See* **Arrhythmia**.

Dyssynergy   Lack of coordinated action of the muscle groups.

E

Ecchymosis   A red-purple discoloration of varying size caused by extravasation of blood into the skin; a black-and-blue mark.

Eccrine glands   Sweat glands that are not associated with hair follicles.

Echolalia   Involuntary repetition of a word or sentence that was uttered by another person.

Eclampsia   Seizure associated with hypertensive disorder of pregnancy.

Ecomap   A diagram depicting a person's relationship with his or her family as well as significant friends, peers, neighbors, and work associates.

Ectodermal Galactic Band   *See* **Milk Line**.

Ectopic pregnancy   A pregnancy other than intrauterine; nonviable, and often leading to surgical intervention.

Ectropion (or Eversion, of the Cervix)   A red, inflamed appearance of the cervix as the columnar epithelium extends from the os past the normal squamocolumnar junction.

Ectropion (of the Eye)   Turning outward or eversion of the eyelid, usually the lower.

Edema   Accumulation of fluid in the intercellular spaces, leading to swelling of the extremities, usually the feet and hands.

Ego   Personality component that is conscious, rational, emerges during the first year of life, and seeks realistic and acceptable ways to meet needs.

Egocentrism   Viewing the world in terms of only the self and interpreting one's own actions and all other events in terms of the consequences for the self.

Egophony   Voice sound where the patient says the sound "ee" to determine if the lungs are filled with air, fluid, or a solid.

Ejaculatory Ducts   Ducts located posterior to the urinary bladder; they eject sperm into the prostatic urethra prior to ejaculation.

Electrocardiogram (EKG)   Record of the electrical activity of the heart.

Eleidin   Translucent substance that aids in the formation of keratin.

Emergency Health History   History taken from the patient or other sources when the patient is experiencing a life-threatening state.

Enculturation   Informal process through which the beliefs, values, norms, and practices of a culture are learned by members born into that culture.

Enophthalmos   Backward displacement of the globe of the eye.

Entropion   Turning inward or inversion of the eyelid, usually the lower.

Epidermis   Multilayered outer covering of the skin, consisting of four layers throughout the body, except for the palms of the hands and soles of the feet, where there are five layers.

Epididymis   Comma-shaped organ that lies along the posterior border of each testis; consists of a tightly coiled tube where sperm maturation occurs.

Epimysium   Connective tissue sheath covering the muscle belly.

Epiphyses   Ends of the long bone.

Episodic Health History   History taken from the patient for a specific problem or need.

Epispadias   Congenital abnormality in which the urethral meatus lies on the dorsal surface of the penis.

Epistaxis   Nosebleed.

Epstein's Pearls   Small, hard, white cysts found on a newborn's hard palate and gum margins.

Eructation   Belching.

Erythema   An inflammatory redness of the skin.

Escutcheon   Characteristic triangular pattern of coarse, curly hair that develops over the mons pubis at puberty.

Esophoria   Latent misalignment of the eye; nasal, or inward, drift.

Esotropia   Inward deviation of the eye.

Ethnic Group   Classification of individuals based on their unique national or regional origin and social, cultural, and linguistic heritage.

Ethnic Identity   Subjective sense of ethnic definition or social orientation with which an individual self-identifies.

Ethnocentrism   Condition that occurs when individuals or groups of people perceive their own cultural group and cultural values, beliefs, norms, and customs to be superior to all others and have disdain for the expression of any way of life but their own.

Eupnea   Normal breathing; respirations are 12 to 20 per minute for the resting adult.

Eustachian Tube   Auditory tube that serves as an air channel connecting the middle ear to the nasopharynx to allow equalization between the air pressure in the ear and in the atmosphere.

Eustress   Positive stress that challenges, provides motivation, and prevents stagnation.

Evaluation   Last step of the nursing process; the patient's progress in achieving the outcomes is determined.

Evidence-Based Practice   Uses the outcomes of well-designed and executed scientific studies to guide clinical decision making and clinical care.

Exophoria   Latent misalignment of the eye; temporal, or outward, drift.

Exophthalmos   Abnormal protrusion of the globe of the eye.

Exotropia   Outward deviation of the eye.

F

Faith   Orientation to a belief structure.

Fallopian Tubes   Site of fertilization; they extend from the cornu of the uterus to the ovaries and are supported by the broad ligaments.

False Ribs   Rib pairs 8–10.

Fat-Soluble Vitamins   Vitamins stored in dietary fat and absorbed in the fat portions of the body's cells.

Fats   Substances that supply essential fatty acids, which form a part of the structure of all cells.

Femoral Hernia   Protrusion of the omentum or bowel through the femoral wall.

Fetal Alcohol Syndrome (FAS)   A pattern of craniofacial, cardiovascular, and limb defects, with prenatal and postnatal growth retardation associated with maternal alcohol use.

Fetoscope   Special stethoscope for hearing fetal heart beats.

Fibroma   Fibrous, encapsulated tumor of connective tissue, often called fibroid or myoma.

Fissure   Groove separating the different lobes of the lungs.

Flatness   Descriptor for a percussible sound that is soft in intensity, short in duration, of high pitch, and normally located over muscle or bone.

Flatulence   Passage of excess gas via the rectum.

Floating Ribs   Rib pairs 11 and 12; they do not articulate at their anterior ends.

Folk Illness   Illness believed to be caused by disharmony, an imbalance, or a punishment.

Folk Practitioner   Healer or other individual who is not part of the scientific care system but is believed to have special knowledge or power to prevent, treat, or provide resources needed to heal folk illnesses.

Follow-Up Health History   *See* **Interval Health History**.

Fornices   Pouchlike recesses around the cervix.

Fourchette   Transverse fold of skin of the posterior aspect of the labia minora; also known as a frenulum.

Fovea Centralis   Center of the macula; the area of sharpest vision.

Frenulum (of the Mouth)   Tissue that connects the tongue to the floor of the mouth.

Friability   Susceptibility to bleeding from the cervix.

Functional Health Assessment   Documents a person's ability to perform instrumental activities of daily living and physical self-maintenance activities.

Functional Health Patterns   Groups of human behavior that facilitate nursing care; there are 11 patterns.

Fundus   Superior aspect of the uterus.

G

Gallop   Extra heart sound; an S_3 is a ventricular gallop, whereas an S_4 is an atrial gallop.

Ganglion   Benign, cystic growth.

Genogram   Pictorial representation of a patient's family health history.

Genomics   The study of the genetic makeup of the human cell.

Genu Valgum   Inward deviation toward the midline at the level of the knees; also known as knock-knees.

Genu Varum   Outward deviation away from the midline at the level of the knees; also known as bow legs.

Glans Penis   Bulbous end of the penis.

Glasgow Coma Scale   International scale used in grading neurological response.

Glaucoma   Disease in which intraocular pressure is elevated.

Glycosuria   Glucose in the urine.

God   Concept of a deity or personal, present being.

Goiter   Enlargement of the thyroid gland.

Goniometer   Device used to measure the angle of the skeletal joint during range of motion; it is a protractor with two movable arms.

Granulation Tissue   Inflamed tissue, new vessels, and white blood cells at the base of a wound in the process of healing.

Granulomatous Reaction (in the Breast)   Development of small, nodular, inflammatory lesions and capsular membranes over the breasts.

Graphanesthesia   Inability to identify numbers, letters, or shapes drawn on the skin.

Graphesthesia   Ability to identify numbers, letters, or shapes drawn on the skin.

Growth   Increase in body size and function to the point of optimum maturity.

Gynecomastia   Enlargement of male breast tissue; may occur normally in adolescent and elderly males.

H

Hallux Valgus   Lateral deviation of the big toe and medial deviation of the first metatarsal; also known as a bunion.

Hammer Toe   Flexion of the proximal interphalangeal joint and hyperextension of the distal metatarsophalangeal joint.

Harlequin Color Change   Condition in which one-half of a newborn's body is red or ruddy and the other half appears pale.

Health Maintenance Activities   Practices that a person incorporates into a lifestyle that can promote healthy living.

Heave   Lifting of the cardiac area secondary to an increased workload and force of left ventricular contraction; also known as a lift.

Heaven   Blissful resting place for souls after death, according to Christianity.

Heberden's Node   Bony enlargement of the distal interphalangeal joint of the finger.

HELLP Syndrome   Complication of hypertensive disorder of pregnancy; the acronym represents hemolysis, elevated liver enzymes, and low platelets.

Hematemesis   Vomiting of blood.

Hematocrit   Measurement to determine the percentage of red blood cells in the volume of whole blood.

Hemiparesis   Unilateral weakness or paralysis; also known as hemiplegia.

Hemiplegia   *See* **Hemiparesis**.

Hemoglobin   Measurement of the iron component that transports oxygen in the blood.

Hemorrhoids   Dilatation of hemorrhoidal veins in the anorectum.

Heretic   Person who rejects the official teachings or dogma of a religion or belief system.

High-Density Lipoprotein   Substance that carries cholesterol away from the heart and arteries and toward the liver.

Hirsutism   Excessive body hair.

History of the Present Illness   Chronological account of the patient's chief complaint and the events surrounding it.

Holistic Nursing   A form of nursing that addresses all aspects of a patient's health and well-being, including spirituality and religion.

Holosystolic   Murmur that is heard throughout all of systole; also known as pansystolic.

Homan's Sign   Pain in the calf when the foot is dorsiflexed; sign of venous thrombosis of the deep veins of the calf.

Hordeolum   Infection of a sebaceous gland in the eyelid.

Human Response Patterns   Groups of human behavior that facilitate nursing care; there are nine patterns.

Hydatidiform Mole   Molar or trophoblastic pregnancy. Often requires careful monitoring of HCG after dilation and curettage of the uterus. If HCG remains elevated, chemotherapy may be indicated.

Hydrocele   Fluid collection within the tunica vaginalis of the testis.

Hydrocephalus   Enlargement of the head without enlargement of the facial structures; it is due to increased accumulation of cerebrospinal fluid within the ventricles of the brain.

Hymen   Avascular, thin fold of connective tissue surrounding the vaginal introitus; it may be annular or crescentic in shape.

Hypalgesia   Diminished sensitivity to pain.

Hyperalgesia   Increased sensitivity to pain.

Hyperemesis Gravidarum   Excessive nausea and vomiting during pregnancy.

Hyperesthesia   Abnormal acuteness to the sensitivity of touch.

Hyperglycemia   Increase in serum glucose.

Hyperkinetic   Increased movement.

Hyperopia   Farsightedness.

Hyperpnea   Breath that is greater in volume than the resting tidal volume.

Hyperresonance   Descriptor for a percussable sound that is very loud in intensity, long in duration, of very low pitch, boomlike, and normally not found in the healthy adult.

Hypertelorism   Abnormal width between the eyes.

Hypertension   Blood pressure remaining consistently above 140 mm Hg systolic or 90 mm Hg diastolic in an adult.

Hyperthermia   Generalized or localized excessive warming of the skin; body temperature that exceeds 38.5°C or 101.5°F.

Hypertrophy   Increase in muscle size due to an increase in the bulk of muscle fibers.

Hypesthesia   Diminished sense of touch; also known as hypoesthesia.

Hyphema   Condition in which there is blood in the anterior chamber of the eye.

Hypoesthesia   *See* **Hypesthesia**.

Hypogeusia   Diminution of taste.

Hypoglycemia   Decrease in serum glucose.

Hypokinetic   Decreased movement.

Hypospadias Congenital abnormality in which the urethral meatus lies on the ventral surface of the penis.

Hypotension Blood pressure that is lower than what is needed to maintain adequate tissue perfusion and oxygenation.

Hypothermia Generalized or localized cooling of the skin; body temperature that is below 34°C or 93.2°F.

Hypotonicity Decrease in normal muscle tone (flaccidity).

I

Id Personality component that is inborn, unconscious, and driven by biological instincts and urges to seek immediate gratification of needs such as hunger, thirst, and physical comfort.

Iliopsoas Muscle Test Technique used to assess for an inflamed appendix.

Immediate Auscultation *See* **Direct Auscultation**.

Immediate Percussion *See* **Direct Percussion**.

Implementation Fifth step of the nursing process; the execution of the nursing interventions that were devised during the planning stage to help the patient meet predetermined outcomes.

Impotence Inability to achieve or maintain an erection.

Independent Nursing Interventions Actions that the nurse is legally capable of implementing based on education and experience.

Indirect Fist Percussion Using the closed ulnar aspect of the fist of the dominant hand to strike the nondominant hand to elicit tenderness over specific body areas.

Indirect Inguinal Hernia Portions of the bowel or omentum that enter the inguinal canal through the internal inguinal ring and exit at the external inguinal ring.

Indirect (or Mediate) Auscultation Active listening to body sounds via some amplification or mechanical device, such as a stethoscope or Doppler transducer.

Indirect (or Mediate) Percussion Using the plexor to strike the pleximeter to elicit sound.

Infarction (Myocardial) Necrosis of cardiac muscle due to decreased blood supply.

Injection Redness around the cornea.

Inspection Use of one's senses to consciously observe the patient; in physical assessment, vision, hearing, smell, and touch are used.

Insufficiency *See* **Regurgitation**.

Integumentary System Skin, or cutaneous tissue.

Intensity (of Percussion) Relative loudness or softness of sound; amplitude.

Intercostal Space Area between the ribs.

Intermediary Individual who serves to assist with communication between the patient and another individual, usually a member of the health care team.

Interpleural Space *See* **Mediastinum**.

Interval (or Follow-Up) Health History History that builds on the patient's last health care visit and documents resolution or nonresolution of a problem or health care need.

Intervention Nursing action designed to achieve patient outcomes.

Intussusception Formation of a sausage-shaped mass in the upper abdomen that results when the ileocecal region of the intestine telescopes into the ileum.

Iris Most anterior portion of the uveal tract; provides a distinctive color for the eye.

Ischemia (Myocardial) Local and temporary lack of blood supply to the heart; may progress to an infarction if left untreated.

Isoelectric Line Electrical resting period after the T-wave on the EKG.

Iso-immunization Most common Rh hemolytic disease, now almost completely eliminated by the antepartum administration of Rh gamma globulin to Rh-negative mothers, and readministration after delivery if newborn is Rh positive.

Isthmus (of the Thyroid) Narrow portion of the thyroid gland that connects the two lobes and lies over the tracheal rings.

Isthmus (of the Uterus) Constricted area between the body of the uterus and the cervix.

J

Jaundice Yellow-green to orange cast or coloration of skin, sclera, or mucous membranes; caused by an elevated bilirubin level.

Joining Stage Introduction or first stage of the interview process, during which the nurse and patient establish rapport.

Joint Union between two bones.

K

Keratosis Lesions on the epidermis characterized by overgrowth of the horny layer.

Kilocalorie Amount of heat required to raise 1 gram of water 1 degree Celsius; also called calorie.

Knock-Knees *See* **Genu Valgum**.

Korotkoff Sounds Sounds generated when the flow of blood through an artery is altered by the inflation of a blood pressure cuff around an extremity.

Kussmaul's Respirations Respirations characterized by extreme increased rate and depth, as in diabetic ketoacidosis.

Kwashiorkor Severe deficiency of protein.

Kyphosis Excessive convexity of the thoracic spine; known as "humpback."

L

Labia Majora   Two longitudinal folds of adipose and connective tissue that extend from the clitoris anteriorly and gradually narrow to merge and form the commissure of the perineum posteriorly.

Labia Minora   Two thin folds of skin that enclose the vulval vestibule and extend to form the prepuce, or hood, of the clitoris anteriorly and a transverse fold of skin that forms the fourchette posteriorly.

Labyrinth   Bony and membranous system of interconnecting tubes in the inner ear; essential for hearing and equilibrium.

Lacrimal Apparatus   Lacrimal gland and ducts.

Lactiferous Ducts   Openings at the nipple through which milk and colostrum are excreted.

Lagophthalmos   Condition in which the patient is unable to completely close the eyelid.

Lanugo   Fine, downy hair present during gestational life and that gradually disappears toward the end of pregnancy; it remains in smaller quantities over the temples, back, shoulders, and upper arms after birth.

Lens   Crystalline structure of the eye that changes shape to refract light from various focusing distances.

Lentigo   Areas of hyperpigmentation resulting from the inability of melanocytes to produce even pigmentation of the skin; known as "liver spots."

Lesion   Circumscribed, pathological change in tissue.

Lichenification   Localized thickening, hardening, and roughness of the skin; can be a result of chronic pruritus.

Life Event or Transitional Developmental Theory   Belief that development occurs in response to specific events, such as new roles (e.g., parenthood), and life transitions (e.g., career changes).

Life Review   Reflection on the experiences, relationships, and events of one's life as a whole, viewing successes and failures from the perspective of age, and accepting one's life and accompanying life choices and outcomes in their entirety.

Lift   *See* **Heave.**

Ligament   Strong, fibrous, connective tissue that connects bones to each other at a joint.

Light Palpation   Superficial palpation; depressing the skin 1 cm to elicit information on skin texture and moisture, masses, fluid, muscle guarding, and tenderness.

Lightening   Descent of the presenting fetal part into the pelvis.

Limbus   Junction of the sclera and cornea.

Linea Alba   Tendinous tissue that extends from the sternum to the symphysis pubis in the middle of the abdomen.

Linea Nigra   Darkening of the abdominal linea alba during pregnancy.

Linear Raphe   Linear ridge in the middle of the hard palate.

Lipoma   Nonmobile, fatty mass with a smooth, circular edge.

List   Leaning of the spine.

Listening Response   Attempt made by the nurse to accurately receive, process, and respond to the patient's messages.

Lobes (of the Breast)   Glandular breast tissue arranged radially in the form of 12 to 20 spokes.

Lobules (of the Breast)   Grapelike bunches that are clustered around several lactiferous ducts; each lobe is composed of 20 to 40 lobules that contain milk-producing glands called alveoli or acini.

Long-Term Outcome   Goal that a patient strives to achieve and having a time frame of weeks or months.

Lordosis   Excessive concavity of the lumbar spine.

Low-Density Lipoprotein   Substance that carries cholesterol toward the heart.

Lunula   White, crescent-shaped area at the proximal end of each nail.

Lymphatic Drainage   Yellow, alkaline drainage originating in the lymph vessels and composed primarily of lymphocytes.

M

Macromineral   Major mineral needed by the body in large amounts.

Macrosomia   Newborn weighing more than 4,000 grams.

Macula   Tiny, darker area in the temporal area of the retina.

Major Defining Characteristics   Signs and symptoms that must be present in the patient for the nurse to use a specific NANDA-I approved diagnostic label.

Manubriosternal Junction   *See* **Angle of Louis.**

Manubrium   Upper bone of the sternum; it articulates with the clavicles and the first pair of ribs.

Marasmus   Form of protein calorie malnutrition.

Mast Cells   Body's major source of tissue histamine, which triggers the body's reaction to invasive allergens.

Mastectomy   Excision, or surgical removal, of the breast.

Maternal Serum Alpha-Fetal Protein (MSAFP)   A blood test to screen for certain fetal abnormalities.

Matrix   Undifferentiated epithelial tissue from which keratinized cells arise to form the nail plate.

McBurney's Point   Anatomic location that is approximately at the normal location of the appendix in the right lower quadrant; point of increased tenderness in appendicitis.

Meconium   Dark green, sticky, stool-like material excreted from the rectum of the newborn within the first 24 hours after birth.

Mediastinum (Interpleural Space)   Area between the lungs.

Mediate Auscultation   *See* **Indirect Auscultation**.

Mediate Percussion   *See* **Indirect Percussion**.

Medullary Cavity   Interior of the diaphysis; contains the bone marrow.

Melanocytes   Cells that produce pigmented substances that provide color to the hair, skin, and choroid of the eye.

Melasma   Irregular pigmentation on the face due to pregnancy; also known as chloasma.

Melena   Black, tarry stool.

Menarche   Onset of menstruation.

Menopause   Cessation of menstruation.

Menorrhagia   Heavy menses.

Mercury Manometer   Blood pressure measurement equipment that uses a calibrated column of mercury that corresponds to blood pressure values.

Metatarsus Varus   Medial forefoot misalignment

Microcephaly   Small brain with a resultant small head.

Micromineral   Trace mineral needed by the body in small amounts.

Microphallus   Small penis for developmental stage.

Mid-Arm Circumference (MAC)   Anthropometric measurement that provides information on skeletal muscle mass and adipose tissue.

Mid-Arm Muscle Circumference (MMAC)   Anthropometric measurement derived from mid-arm circumference; provides information on skeletal muscle mass and adipose tissue.

Midaxillary Line   Vertical line drawn from the apex of the axilla; it lies midway between the anterior and the posterior axillary lines.

Midclavicular Line   Vertical line drawn from the midpoint of the clavicle.

Midspinal (or Vertebral) Line   Vertical line drawn from the midpoint of the spinous processes.

Midsternal Line   Vertical line drawn from the midpoint of the sternum.

Milia   Plugged sebaceous glands manifesting as small, white papules and appearing on the infant's head, especially on the cheeks and nose.

Milk Line   Ectodermal galactic band that develops from the axilla to the groin during the fifth week of fetal development.

Mineral   Inorganic element that regulates body processes and builds body tissue; classified into macrominerals and microminerals.

Minor Defining Characteristics   Signs and symptoms that need not be present in the patient for the nurse to use a specific NANDA-I approved diagnostic label, but that add validity to the diagnosis.

Minority Group Members   Individuals who are considered by themselves and others to be members of a minority because they have a different racial, ethnic, cultural, gender, socioeconomic, or sexual orientation than the members of the dominant cultural group.

Molding   Condition in which the newborn's parietal bone overrides the frontal bone as a result of increased pressure during delivery.

Mongolian Spots   Various irregularly sized areas of deep bluish pigmentation on the upper back, shoulders, buttocks, and lumbosacral area of newborns of African, Latino, and Asian descent.

Monotheism   Belief in one all-powerful, omnipresent, and omnipotent god.

Monounsaturated Fats   Fatty acids that contain one double bond between carbon atoms.

Mons Pubis   Pad of subcutaneous fatty tissue lying over the anterior symphysis pubis.

Montgomery's Tubercles   Sebaceous glands present on the surface of the areola.

Multicultural Identity   Unique combination of cultural influences that result from membership in a variety of subcultures within the primary culture.

Multiculturalism   The act of living and functioning in two or more cultures simultaneously.

Multiparous   Any number of prior deliveries.

Murphy's Sign   Abnormal finding elicited during abdominal palpation in the right upper quadrant and revealing gallbladder inflammation; characteristically, the patient will abruptly stop inspiration and complain of sharp pain with palpation.

Myopia   Nearsightedness.

N

Nabothian Cysts   Small, round, yellow lesions on the cervical surface.

Nail Plate   Tissue that covers and protects the distal portion of the fingers and toes.

Nail Root   Nail portion that is posterior to the cuticle and attached to the matrix.

Nailbed   Vascular bed located beneath the nail plate.

NANDA   North American Nursing Diagnosis Association; the professional nursing organization that sets the standards for the development, clinical testing, and approval of nursing diagnoses.

Naturalistic Illness   Illness believed to be caused by an imbalance or disequilibrium between essentially impersonal factors, for example, hot and cold.

Neologism   Word coined by a patient that is meaningful only to the patient.

Nevi   Pigmented moles that may be flat or elevated.

New Age   A popular, heterogeneous, free-flowing spiritual movement that has no holy book, organization, membership, clergy, geographic center, dogma, or creed, but includes a cluster of common beliefs that may be grafted onto an existing religion.

Nipple   A round, hairless, pigmented protrusion of erectile tissue approximately 0.5 to 1.5 cm in diameter located in the center of the breast.

Nirvana   Buddhist belief of the perfect blessedness and peace of the soul.

Nitrogen   Component of amino acids.

Nociception   A multistep process that involves the nervous system and other body systems in perceiving pain.

Nociceptors   Receptive neurons of pain sensation that are located in the skin and various viscera.

Nocturia   Excessive urination at night.

Nonverbal Communication   Communicating a message without using words.

Nulliparous   Descriptor for a woman who has not given birth.

Nursing Care Plan   Patient care record that uses the nursing process as its framework.

Nursing Diagnosis   "A clinical judgment about individual, family, or community responses to actual or potential health problems/life processes" (NANDA-I, 2009, p. 4.

Nursing Process   Dynamic, six-step process that incorporates information in a meaningful way in the use of problem-solving strategies to place the patient, family, or community in an optimal health state; includes assessment, nursing diagnosis, planning, outcome identification, implementation, and evaluation.

Nutrient   Substance found in food that is nourishing or useful to the body.

Nutrition   Processes of the human body that metabolize and utilize nutrients.

Nystagmus   Involuntary oscillation of the eye.

O

Obesity   Weight greater than 120% of ideal body weight.

Object Permanence   Ability to form a mental image of an object and to recognize that, although removed from view, the object still exists.

Objective Data   Data that are tangible or visible and can be corroborated by others; unbiased data not based on opinion or feeling.

Obturator Sign   Differential technique for assessing appendicitis; indicative of an irritated obturator internus muscle.

Oedipus Complex   Boys' sexual attraction toward their mothers and feelings of rivalry toward their fathers.

Oogenesis   Development and formation of an ovum.

Optic Disc   Round area on the nasal side of the retina, where retinal fibers join to form the optic nerve.

Orchitis   Acute onset of testicular swelling.

Orthopnea   Difficulty breathing except in an upright position.

Orthostatic Hypotension   Hypotension that occurs when changing from a supine to an upright position.

Ossicles   Three tiny bones in the middle ear that play a crucial role in the transmission of sound: the malleus, the incus, and the stapes.

Osteoporosis   Disease characterized by reduced bone mass.

Otitis Media   Inflammation or infection of the middle ear.

Outcome Identification   The fourth step of the nursing process.

Ovaries   Pair of almond-shaped glands, approximately 3 to 4 cm in length, in the upper pelvic cavity; oogenesis and hormonal production are the ovaries' principal functions.

P

Pack/Year History   Term used to describe the quantity of cigarettes smoked over a period of time.

Pagan   A person who does not belong to a monotheistic religion, or a person whose principles reflect an animistic, and usually polytheistic, spirit-filled belief system.

Paget's Disease   Malignant breast neoplasm that is usually unilateral in its involvement and presents as persistent eczematous dermatitis of the areola and nipple.

Pain   An unpleasant sensory or emotional experience associated with actual or potential tissue damage, or described in terms of such damage.

Pallor   Lack of color.

Palpation   Touching the patient in a diagnostic manner to elicit specific information.

Palpebral Conjunctiva   Mucous membrane covering the interior surface of the eyelid.

Palpebral Fissure   Opening between the eyelids.

Palpitation   Irregular and rapid heart beat, or sensation of fluttering of the heart.

Pansystolic   *See* **Holosystolic**.

Pantheism   A religion in which God is believed to be in everything that exists, reincarnation, auras, energy fields, ecology, personal transformation, and evolution toward a "new age" in which wars and discrimination will not exist, and all will be peace and harmony.

Papilla   Small projection on the dorsal surface of the tongue and containing openings to taste buds.

Papillary Layer   Upper layer of the dermis; composed primarily of loose connective tissue, small elastic fibers, and an extensive network of capillaries that serve to nourish the epidermis.

Papule   Red, solid, circumscribed, elevated area of the skin.

Paranasal Sinuses   Air-filled cavities in the cranial bones that are lined with mucous membranes.

Paraphimosis   Condition in which the retracted foreskin develops a fixed constriction proximal to the glans penis.

Paresthesia   An abnormal sensation such as numbness, pricking, or tingling.

Parietal Pericardium   Pericardial layer that lies close to the fibrous tissues.

Parietal Pleura   Lining of the chest wall and the superior surface of the lungs.

Parish Nursing   A movement in which nurses work within worship communities to promote spiritual and physical health.

Parous   Descriptor for a woman who has given birth to one or more neonates.

Past Health History   History that covers the patient's health from birth to the present.

Pastoral Care   Care and response needed when a person is in spiritual crisis.

Patient Goal   Broad, unmeasurable statement directed toward removal of related factors or patient response to an adverse condition.

Patient Outcome   Measureable statement of the expected change in patient behavior.

Patient Profile   Demographics that may be linked to health status.

Peau d'Orange   Thickening or edema of the breast tissue or nipple; may present itself as enlarged skin pores that give the appearance of an orange rind.

Pectus Carinatum   Abnormal thorax configuration in which there is a marked protrusion of the sternum; known as "pigeon chest."

Pectus Excavatum   Abnormal thorax configuration in which there is a depression in the lower body of the sternum; known as "funnel chest."

Penis   Cylindrical male organ of copulation and urination.

Penis Envy   Young girls' desire to have a penis.

Percussion   Striking one object against another to cause vibrations that produce sound.

Pericarditis   Inflammation of the pericardium.

Perineum   External surface located between the fourchette and the anus.

Peripheral Vascular Resistance   Opposing force against which the left ventricle must contract to pump blood into the aorta; also known as systemic vascular resistance.

Periungual Tissue   Tissue that surrounds the nail plate and the free edge of the nail.

Personalistic Illness   Illness that is believed to occur either because an individual committed some offense and is being punished, or because of acts of aggression (sometimes unintentional) by other individuals.

Pertinent Negatives   Manifestations that are expected in the patient with a suspected pathology but that are denied or absent.

Pes Cavus   Foot with an exaggerated height to the arch.

PES Method   Acronym for problem, etiology, and signs or symptoms; the nursing diagnosis comprises these elements.

Pes Planus   Foot with a low, longitudinal arch; also known as "flatfoot."

Pes Valgus   Foot that is turned laterally away from the midline.

Pes Varus   Foot that is turned inward toward the midline.

Petechiae   Reddish-purple skin discoloration that is less than 0.5 cm in diameter and does not blanch.

Phimosis   Constriction of the distal penile foreskin that prevents normal retraction over the glans.

Phoria   Latent misalignment of an eye.

Physiologic Cup   Pale, central area of the optic disc.

Physiological Weight Loss   Tendency of a neonate to lose approximately 10% of birth weight within a few days to after birth and regain it by 2 weeks of age.

Pica   Craving for substances other than food (e.g., dirt, clay, starch, ice cubes).

Pinguecula   Yellow nodule on the nasal, or temporal, side of the bulbar conjunctiva.

Pinna   External flap of the ear; also called the auricle.

Pitch (of Percussion)   Highness or lowness of a sound.

Placenta Previa   Placenta implantation partially (partial previa) or totally (complete previa) covering the cervical os.

Planning   Third step of the nursing process; involves the prioritization of nursing diagnoses, formulation of patient goals, and selection of nursing interventions.

Pleura   Serous sac that encases the lung.

Pleural Friction Fremitus   Palpable grating that feels more pronounced on inspiration when there is an inflammatory process between the pleura.

Pleural Friction Rub   Continuous adventitious breath sound caused by inflamed parietal and visceral pleura; it resembles a creaking or grating sound.

Pleximeter   Stationary finger of the nondominant hand used in indirect percussion.

Plexor   Middle finger of the dominant hand used to strike the pleximeter to elicit sound in indirect percussion.

Polycythemia   Elevated number of red blood cells.

Polydactyly   Extra digits on the hand or foot.

Polytheism   Belief in many gods of different levels of power and status.

Posterior Axillary Line   Vertical line drawn from the posterior axillary fold.

Posterior Chamber   Space immediately posterior to the iris.

Posterior Triangle   Area of the neck between the sternocleidomastoid and the trapezius muscles, with the clavicle at the base; contains the posterior cervical lymph nodes.

Prayer Communication with a higher, spiritual power.

Prealbumin (also called thyroxine-binding prealbumin) The transport protein for thyroxine and retinol-binding protein.

Precordium Anterior area of the body that lies over the heart, its great vessels, the pericardium, and some pulmonary tissue.

Preload Resting force on the myocardium as determined by the pressure in the ventricles at the end of diastole.

Prepuce Foreskin covering the glans penis.

Presbycusis Hearing loss commonly found in older individuals.

Presbyopia Impaired near vision occurring in middle-aged or older individuals.

Priapism Abnormal prolonged penile erection unrelated to sexual desire.

Prioritize Ranking the patient's nursing diagnoses; the most critical concerns should be dealt with first.

Proprioception Position sense.

Prostate Glandular organ that lies anterior to the wall of the rectum and encircles the urethra; an accessory male sex organ.

Protein Group of complex nitrogenous compounds, each containing amino acids.

Proteinuria Presence of protein in the urine.

Prurigo Itchy skin eruptions of unknown cause.

Pruritus Severe itching.

Pterygium Triangular, yellow thickening of the bulbar conjunctiva, extending from the nasal side of the cornea to the pupil.

Ptosis Drooping of the eyelid.

Ptyalism Excessive secretion of saliva.

Puddle Sign Percussion technique that identifies an ascitic abdomen.

Pulse Palpable expansion of an artery in response to cardiac functioning; used to determine heart rate, rhythm, and estimated volume of blood being pumped by the heart.

Pulse Deficit Apical pulse rate greater than radial pulse rate; occurs when some heart contractions are too weak to produce a palpable pulse at the radial site.

Pulse Pressure Difference between systolic and diastolic blood pressures.

Pulsus Paradoxus Pathological decrease in systolic blood pressure by 10 mm Hg or more on inspiration.

Puncta Opening at the inner canthus of the eye through which tears drain.

Pupil Opening in the center of the iris; regulates the amount of light entering the eye.

Purpura Condition characterized by the presence of confluent petechiae or confluent ecchymosis over any part of the body.

Pyelonephritis Kidney infection or inflammation.

Q

Qualifier *See* **Descriptor**.

Quality (of Percussion) Timbre; how a sound is perceived musically.

Quickening First fetal movements felt by a pregnant woman.

R

Race Classification of individuals based on shared inherited biological traits such as skin color, facial features, and body build.

Rash Cutaneous skin eruption that may be localized or generalized.

Reason for Seeking Health Care Problem or health care need that brought the patient to seek health care.

Rebound Tenderness Pain elicited during deep palpation, frequently associated with peritoneal inflammation or appendicitis.

Recommended Dietary Allowance Recommended amount of nutrients to be eaten daily; recommendations differ according to sex, age, and pregnancy or lactation status.

Rectal Prolapse Protrusion of the rectum through the anal orifice.

Rectocele Bulging of the posterior vaginal wall with a portion of the rectum.

Rectouterine Pouch Deep recess formed by the outer layer of the peritoneum; the lowest point in the pelvic cavity, encompassing the lower posterior wall of the uterus, the upper portion of the vagina, and the intestinal surface of the rectum.

Rectovaginal Septum Surface that separates the rectum from the posterior aspect of the vagina.

Rectum Lower portion of the large intestine; passes downward in front of the sacrum.

Reepithelialization Reformation of epithelium over denuded skin.

Regurgitation Backward flow of blood through a diseased heart valve; also known as insufficiency.

Reincarnation Belief that, after death, a person lives another life on earth in another body.

Related Factors "Factors that appear to show some type of patterned relationship with the nursing diagnosis" (NANDA-I, 2009, p. 420).

Religion Organized system of beliefs that is usually centered around the worship of a supernatural force or being and that, in turn, defines the self and the self's purpose in life.

Resonance Descriptor for a percussable sound that is loud in intensity, moderate to long in duration, low in pitch, hollow, and normally located in healthy lungs.

Respiration   Breathing act that supplies oxygen to the body and occurs in response to changes in the concentration of oxygen, carbon dioxide, and hydrogen in the arterial blood.

Reticular Layer   Lower layer of the dermis that is formed by a dense bed of vascular connective tissue; it also includes nerves and lymphatic tissue.

Retina   Innermost layer of the eye.

Retroflexed Uterus   A condition in which the main body of the uterus is tipped back at the cervix.

Retromammary Adipose Tissue   Tissue that composes the bulk of the breast.

Retroverted Uterus   A uterus that is displaced backward, with the cervix pointing upward toward the symphysis pubis.

Reversibility   The understanding that an action does not need to be experienced before one can anticipate the results or consequences of the action.

Review of Systems   The patient's subjective responses to a series of body system–related questions; serves as a double-check that vital information is not overlooked.

Rhonchal Fremitus   Coarse, palpable vibration produced by the passage of air through thick exudate in the large bronchi or the trachea.

Rinne Test   Method of evaluating hearing loss by comparing air and bone conduction of tuning fork vibrations.

Risk Nursing Diagnosis   "Describes human responses to health conditions/life processes that may develop in a vulnerable individual, family, or community" (NANDA-I, 2009, p. 419).

Ritual   Solemn, ceremonial act that reinforces faith.

Rod   Retinal structure responsible for peripheral vision and dark or light discrimination.

Rovsing's Sign   Technique to elicit referred pain indicative of peritoneal inflammation.

S

Saturated Fats   Lipids derived from animal or vegetable sources.

Scapular Line   Vertical line drawn from the inferior angle of the scapula.

Schismatic   Person who shares the essential beliefs or dogma of a religion but who is separated from the group because of political or other disagreements.

Scientific Illness   Illness in which the presence of pathology is the defining characteristic.

Sclera   Opaque covering of the eye; appears white.

Scoliosis   Lateral curvature of the thoracic or lumbar vertebrae.

Scrotum   Pouchlike supporting structure of the testes.

Sebaceous Glands   Sebum-producing glands that are found almost everywhere in the dermis except the palmar and plantar surfaces.

Seborrhea   Dandruff.

Sebum   Oily secretion that is thought to retard evaporation and water loss from the epidermal surface.

Seizure   Transient disturbance of cerebral function caused by an excessive discharge of neurons.

Semicircular Canals   Anterior, posterior, and lateral canals in the bony labyrinth of the inner ear that provide balance and equilibrium.

Seminal Vesicles   Paired pouches located posteriorly to and at the base of the bladder; fluid from here forms 60% of the volume of semen.

Septum (of the Heart)   Wall that divides the left side of the heart from the right side.

Sequelae   Aftermath.

Serum Iron   Amount of transferrin-bound iron.

Shifting Dullness   Abnormal finding elicited during percussion and corresponding to positive identification of ascites.

Short-Term Outcome   Goal that a patient strives to achieve in a relatively brief time frame (hour, day, or week).

Sighing   Normal respiration interrupted by a deep inspiration and followed by a deep expiration.

Sign   Objective finding.

Sin   Deliberate and conscious act against the teachings of a belief system.

Sinoatrial (S-A) Node   Normal pacemaker of the heart; intrinsic adult rate is approximately 70 beats per minute.

Skene's Glands (Paraurethral Glands)   Glands that open in a posterolateral position to the urethral meatus and provide lubrication to protect the skin.

Skinfold Thickness   Anthropometric measurement to determine body fat stores and nutritional status.

Smegma   White, cottage cheese-type substance sometimes found under the female labia minora or the male foreskin.

Snap   High-pitched sound that is heard in early diastole; usually occurs in mitral stenosis.

Snellen Chart   Chart used for testing distance vision; contains letters of various sizes with standardized visual acuity numbers at the end of each line of letters.

Social History   Information related to the patient's lifestyle that can have an impact on his or her health.

Soul   Essential, spiritual part of a person; thought to continue after physical death.

Spasticity   Increase in muscle tension on passive stretching, especially rapid or forced stretching of a muscle.

Spermatic Cord   Connective tissue sheath made up of arteries, nerves, veins, lymphatic vessels, and the cremaster muscle.

Spermatocele   Well-defined cystic mass on the superior testes.

Spermatogenesis   Production of sperm.

Sphygmomanometer   Gauge used to measure blood pressure; consists of a blood pressure cuff with an inflatable bladder, connecting tubes, bulb air pump, and a manometer.

Spider Angioma   Bright red, star-shaped vascular marking that often has a central pulsation; it blanches in the extensions when pressure is applied.

Spinnbarkeit   Elasticity of cervical mucus during ovulation.

Spirit   Soul, being, or supernatural force.

Spiritual Distress   State in which a person feels that the belief system, or her or his place within it, is threatened.

Spirituality   A person's concern for the meaning and purpose of life.

Sputum   Substance that is produced by the respiratory tract and can be expectorated or swallowed; it is composed of mucus, blood, purulent material, microorganisms, cellular debris, and, occasionally, foreign objects.

Squamocolumnar Junction   Cervical area between the squamous epithelial surface and the columnar epithelial surface.

Standard Precautions   Practices health care providers use to prevent the exchange of blood and body fluids when coming into contact with a patient; outlined by the Centers for Disease Control and Prevention (CDC).

Steatorrhea   Pale yellow, greasy, fatty stool.

Stenosis   Narrowing or constriction (e.g., diseased heart valve).

Stensen's Ducts   Openings from the parotid glands; located just opposite the upper second molars.

Stereognosis   Ability to identify objects by manipulating and touching them.

Sternal Angle   *See* **Angle of Louis**.

Stork Bites   *See* **Telangiectatic Nevi**.

Strabismus   True deviation of gaze due to extraocular muscle dysfunction.

Stratum Corneum   Horny layer, or outer layer of the epidermis.

Stratum Germinativum   Basal cell layer, or deepest layer of the epidermis.

Stratum Granulosum   Epidermal layer where skin cell death occurs; it overlays the stratum spinosum.

Stratum Lucidum   Additional skin layer found exclusively on the palmar and plantar surfaces.

Stratum Spinosum   Epidermal layer that overlays the stratum germinativum and consists of layers of polyhedral cells.

Stress   Physiologically defined response to changes that disrupt the resting equilibrium of an individual.

Striae   Atrophic lines or scars commonly found on the abdomen, breasts, thighs, or buttocks.

Striae Gravidarum   Stretch marks that occur in pregnancy.

Subculture   Within a larger cultural group, a smaller group whose members share most of the beliefs and ways of life of the larger cultural group but differ on others.

Subcutaneous Tissue   Superficial fascia composed of loose areolar connective tissue or adipose tissue, depending on its location in the body; it lies below the dermis.

Subjective Data   Information perceived by the patient to be real; such data cannot always be verified by an independent observer.

Subluxation   Partial dislodgement of a bone from its place in the joint cavity.

Sulcus Terminalis   Midline depression separating the anterior two-thirds from the posterior one-third of the tongue.

Superego   Personality component that represents the internalization of the moral values formed as children interact with their parents and significant others.

Supernumerary Nipples   Extra nipples or breast tissue along the milk line resulting from incomplete atrophy of the galactic band.

Suprasternal Notch   Visible and palpable depression in the midsternal line superior to the manubrium.

Sutures   Immovable joints connecting the cranial bones.

Sweat Glands   Glands that produce perspiration; composed of two types: eccrine and apocrine glands.

Symptom   Subjective finding.

Syncope   Fainting; transient loss of consciousness due to decreased oxygen or glucose supply to the brain.

Syndactyly   Fusion between two or more digits on the hand or foot.

Synovial Effusion   Excessive synovial joint fluid.

Systemic Vascular Resistance   *See* **Peripheral Vascular Resistance**.

Systole   Phase in the cardiac cycle during which the myocardial fibers contract and tighten to eject blood from the ventricles; correlates with the first Korotkoff sound.

T

Tachycardia   Pulse rate greater than 100 beats per minute in an adult.

Tachypnea   Respiratory rate greater than 20 breaths per minute in an adult.

Tactile (or Vocal) Fremitus   Palpable vibration of the chest wall that is produced by the spoken word.

Tail of Spence   Upper outer quadrant of the breast that extends into the axilla.

Talipes equinovarus (clubfoot)   Medially adducted and inverted toes and forefoot.

Tangential Lighting   Light that is shone at an angle on the patient to accentuate shadows and highlight subtle findings.

Tarsal Plates   Connective tissue that gives shape to the upper eyelid.

Taxonomy   Classification system.

Telangiectatic Nevi   Marks appearing on the back of the neck, lower occiput, upper eyelids, and upper lip of the newborn that are flat, deep, irregular, and pink in light-skinned children and deep red in dark-skinned children; also known as "stork bites."

Temperature   Vital sign collected to assess core body heat.

Tendons   Epimysium ends that attach a muscle to a bone.

Terminal Hair   Coarse body hair in the axillary and pubic areas as well as the eyebrows, eyelashes, scalp, and, in men, the chest and face.

Termination Stage   Last segment of the interview process, during which information is summarized and validated.

Testes   Pair of ovoid glands located in the scrotum.

Thenar Eminence   Rounded prominence at the base of the thumb.

Thoracic Expansion   The extent and symmetry of chest wall expansion.

Thrill   Vibrations related to turbulent blood flow that feel similar to what one feels when a hand is placed on a purring cat.

Tilts   Set of blood pressures taken in supine, sitting, and standing positions.

Torticollis   Lateral deviation of the neck; intermittent or sustained dystonic contraction of the muscles on one side of the neck.

Total Iron-Binding Capacity (TIBC)   Amount of iron with which transferrin can bind.

Transferrin   Protein that regulates iron absorption.

Transmission-Based Precautions   Infection control practices involving contact, droplet, and airborne transmission of microorganisms that are known to exist in a patient or are suspected in a patient. They are practiced in conjunction with Standard Precautions.

Triceps Skinfold   Anthropometric measurement used to determine body fat stores and nutritional status.

Triglyceride   Substance that accounts for most of the fat stored in the body's tissues.

True Ribs   *See* **Vertebrosternal Ribs**.

Tubular Breath Sound   *See* **Bronchial Breath Sound**.

Turbinate (or Concha)   Projection from the lateral wall of the nose and covered with mucous membranes that greatly increase the surface area within the nose.

Turgor   Elasticity of the skin; it reflects the skin's state of hydration.

Tussive Fremitus   Palpable vibration produced by coughing.

Tympany   Descriptor for a percussable sound that is loud in intensity, long in duration, of high pitch, drumlike, and normally located over a gastric air bubble.

U

Urethra   Duct from the urinary bladder to the urethral meatus; carries urine and, in the male, semen.

Uterus   Inverted, pear-shaped, hollow, muscular organ in which the impregnated ovum develops into a fetus.

Uvula   Fingerlike projection hanging down from the center of the soft palate.

V

Vagina   Pink, hollow, muscular tube extending from the cervix to the vulva, located posterior to the bladder and anterior to the rectum.

Vaginal Introitus   Entrance to the vagina, situated at the inferior aspect of the vulval vestibule.

Value Orientation   Patterned principles (about time, human nature, activity, relations, and people-to-nature) that provide order and give direction to an individual's thoughts and behaviors related to the solution of commonly occurring human problems.

Varicocele   Bluish mass resulting from abnormal dilatation of the veins of the pampiniform plexus of the spermatic cord.

Vellus Hair   Fine, faint hair that covers most of the body.

Venous Hum   Continuous, medium-pitched sound originating in the inferior vena cava and associated with obstructed portal circulation.

Venous Star   Linear or irregularly shaped, blue vascular pattern on the skin; does not blanch when pressure is applied.

Vernix Caseosa   Protective integumentary mechanism of the newborn; consists of sebum and shed epithelial cells.

Vertebra Prominens   The long spinous process of the seventh cervical vertebra.

Vertebrosternal (or True) Ribs   Rib pairs 1–7; they articulate via the costal cartilage to the sternum.

Vertigo   Dizziness or lightheadedness.

Vesicular Breath Sound   Breath sound that is low in pitch and soft in intensity and is heard best over the peripheral lung; has a breezy, gentle, rustling quality; heard longer on inspiration than expiration.

Vestibule   Boat-shaped area between the labia minora and containing the urethral meatus, the openings of Skene's glands, the hymen, the openings of Bartholin's glands, and the vaginal introitus.

Vestibule (of the Ear)   Part of the inner ear located between the cochlea and the semicircular canals.

Visceral Pericardium   Pericardial layer that lies against the actual heart muscle.

Visceral Pleura   Lining of the external surface of the lungs.

Visual Analog Scale   Numerical scale used to rate pain from 0 to 10.

Vital Signs   Measurements, including temperature, pulse, respirations, and blood pressure, that provide an index of a patient's physiological status.

Vitamin   Organic substance needed to maintain the function of the body.

Vitiligo   Patchy, symmetrical areas of white on the skin.

Vitreous Humor   Gelatinous material that fills the center cavity of the eye and helps maintain the shape of the eye and the position of the internal structures.

Vocal Fremitus   *See* **Tactile Fremitus**

Voice Sounds   Techniques used to assess whether the lungs are filled with air, fluid, or a solid.

W

Water-Soluble Vitamin   Vitamin soluble in water; is not stored in the body but is excreted in the urine.

Weber Test   Tuning fork test to evaluate hearing loss and determine whether the loss is conductive or sensorineural.

Wellness Nursing Diagnosis   "Describes human responses to levels of wellness in an individual, family, or community that have a readiness for enhancement" (NANDA-I, 2009, p. 420).

Wharton's Ducts   Openings from the submaxillary glands; located on either side of the frenulum.

Whispered Pectoriloquy   Voice sound where the patient whispers the words "ninety-nine" or "one, two, three" to determine if the lungs are filled with air, fluid, or a solid.

Working Stage   That segment of the interview process during which the majority of data are collected.

X

Xanthelasma   Creamy, yellow plaque on the eyelid and secondary to hypercholesterolemia.

Xerosis   Excessive dryness of the skin.

Xiphoid Process   Cartilaginous process at the base of the sternum; it does not articulate with the ribs.

INDEX

Note: Page numbers in italics reference figures, page numbers followed by "t" reference tables, and page numbers followed by "b" indicate boxed text.

I

N

Q

IMPORTANT! READ CAREFULLY: This End User License Agreement ("Agreement") sets forth the conditions by which Cengage Learning will make electronic access to the Cengage Learning-owned licensed content and associated media, software, documentation, printed materials, and electronic documentation contained in this package and/or made available to you via this product (the "Licensed Content"), available to you (the "End User"). BY CLICKING THE "I ACCEPT" BUTTON AND/OR OPENING THIS PACKAGE, YOU ACKNOWLEDGE THAT YOU HAVE READ ALL OF THE TERMS AND CONDITIONS, AND THAT YOU AGREE TO BE BOUND BY ITS TERMS, CONDITIONS, AND ALL APPLICABLE LAWS AND REGULATIONS GOVERNING THE USE OF THE LICENSED CONTENT.

1.0 SCOPE OF LICENSE

1.1 *Licensed Content.* The Licensed Content may contain portions of modifiable content ("Modifiable Content") and content which may not be modified or otherwise altered by the End User ("Non-Modifiable Content"). For purposes of this Agreement, Modifiable Content and Non-Modifiable Content may be collectively referred to herein as the "Licensed Content." All Licensed Content shall be considered Non-Modifiable Content, unless such Licensed Content is presented to the End User in a modifiable format and it is clearly indicated that modification of the Licensed Content is permitted.

1.2 Subject to the End User's compliance with the terms and conditions of this Agreement, Cengage Learning hereby grants the End User, a nontransferable, nonexclusive, limited right to access and view a single copy of the Licensed Content on a single personal computer system for noncommercial, internal, personal use only. The End User shall not (i) reproduce, copy, modify (except in the case of Modifiable Content), distribute, display, transfer, sublicense, prepare derivative work(s) based on, sell, exchange, barter or transfer, rent, lease, loan, resell, or in any other manner exploit the Licensed Content; (ii) remove, obscure, or alter any notice of Cengage Learning's intellectual property rights present on or in the Licensed Content, including, but not limited to, copyright, trademark, and/or patent notices; or (iii) disassemble, decompile, translate, reverse engineer, or otherwise reduce the Licensed Content.

2.0 TERMINATION

2.1 Cengage Learning may at any time (without prejudice to its other rights or remedies) immediately terminate this Agreement and/or suspend access to some or all of the Licensed Content, in the event that the End User does not comply with any of the terms and conditions of this Agreement. In the event of such termination by Cengage Learning, the End User shall immediately return any and all copies of the Licensed Content to Cengage Learning.

3.0 PROPRIETARY RIGHTS

3.1 The End User acknowledges that Cengage Learning owns all rights, title and interest, including, but not limited to all copyright rights therein, in and to the Licensed Content, and that the End User shall not take any action inconsistent with such ownership. The Licensed Content is protected by U.S., Canadian and other applicable copyright laws and by international treaties, including the Berne Convention and the Universal Copyright Convention. Nothing contained in this Agreement shall be construed as granting the End User any ownership rights in or to the Licensed Content.

3.2 Cengage Learning reserves the right at any time to withdraw from the Licensed Content any item or part of an item for which it no longer retains the right to publish, or which it has reasonable grounds to believe infringes copyright or is defamatory, unlawful, or otherwise objectionable.

4.0 PROTECTION AND SECURITY

4.1 The End User shall use its best efforts and take all reasonable steps to safeguard its copy of the Licensed Content to ensure that no unauthorized reproduction, publication, disclosure, modification, or distribution of the Licensed Content, in whole or in part, is made. To the extent that the End User becomes aware of any such unauthorized use of the Licensed Content, the End User shall immediately notify Cengage Learning. Notification of such violations may be made by sending an e-mail to infringement@cengage.com.

5.0 MISUSE OF THE LICENSED PRODUCT

5.1 In the event that the End User uses the Licensed Content in violation of this Agreement, Cengage Learning shall have the option of electing liquidated damages, which shall include all profits generated by the End User's use of the Licensed Content plus interest computed at the maximum rate permitted by law and all legal fees and other expenses incurred by Cengage Learning in enforcing its rights, plus penalties.

6.0 FEDERAL GOVERNMENT CLIENTS

6.1 Except as expressly authorized by Cengage Learning, Federal Government clients obtain only the rights specified in this Agreement and no other rights. The Government acknowledges that (i) all software and related documentation incorporated in the Licensed Content is existing commercial computer software within the meaning of FAR 27.405(b)(2); and (ii) all other data delivered in whatever form, is limited rights data within the meaning of FAR 27.401. The restrictions in this section are acceptable as consistent with the Government's need for software and other data under this Agreement.

7.0 DISCLAIMER OF WARRANTIES AND LIABILITIES

7.1 Although Cengage Learning believes the Licensed Content to be reliable, Cengage Learning does not guarantee or warrant (i) any information or materials contained in or produced by the Licensed Content, (ii) the accuracy, completeness or reliability of the Licensed Content, or (iii) that the Licensed Content is free from errors or other material defects. THE LICENSED PRODUCT IS PROVIDED "AS IS," WITHOUT ANY WARRANTY OF ANY KIND AND CENGAGE LEARNING DISCLAIMS ANY AND ALL WARRANTIES, EXPRESSED OR IMPLIED, INCLUDING, WITHOUT LIMITATION, WARRANTIES OF MERCHANTABILITY OR FITNESS FOR A PARTICULAR PURPOSE. IN NO EVENT SHALL CENGAGE LEARNING BE LIABLE FOR: INDIRECT, SPECIAL, PUNITIVE OR CONSEQUENTIAL DAMAGES INCLUDING FOR LOST PROFITS, LOST DATA, OR OTHERWISE. IN NO EVENT SHALL CENGAGE LEARNING'S AGGREGATE LIABILITY HEREUNDER, WHETHER ARISING IN CONTRACT, TORT, STRICT LIABILITY OR OTHERWISE, EXCEED THE AMOUNT OF FEES PAID BY THE END USER HEREUNDER FOR THE LICENSE OF THE LICENSED CONTENT.

8.0 GENERAL

8.1 *Entire Agreement.* This Agreement shall constitute the entire Agreement between the Parties and supercedes all prior Agreements and understandings oral or written relating to the subject matter hereof.

8.2 *Enhancements/Modifications of Licensed Content.* From time to time, and in Cengage Learning's sole discretion, Cengage Learning may advise the End User of updates, upgrades, enhancements and/or improvements to the Licensed Content, and may permit the End User to access and use, subject to the terms and conditions of this Agreement, such modifications, upon payment of prices as may be established by Cengage Learning.

8.3 *No Export.* The End User shall use the Licensed Content solely in the United States and shall not transfer or export, directly or indirectly, the Licensed Content outside the United States.

8.4 *Severability.* If any provision of this Agreement is invalid, illegal, or unenforceable under any applicable statute or rule of law, the provision shall be deemed omitted to the extent that it is invalid, illegal, or unenforceable. In such a case, the remainder of the Agreement shall be construed in a manner as to give greatest effect to the original intention of the parties hereto.

8.5 *Waiver.* The waiver of any right or failure of either party to exercise in any respect any right provided in this Agreement in any instance shall not be deemed to be a waiver of such right in the future or a waiver of any other right under this Agreement.

8.6 *Choice of Law/Venue.* This Agreement shall be interpreted, construed, and governed by and in accordance with the laws of the State of New York, applicable to contracts executed and to be wholly preformed therein, without regard to its principles governing conflicts of law. Each party agrees that any proceeding arising out of or relating to this Agreement or the breach or threatened breach of this Agreement may be commenced and prosecuted in a court in the State and County of New York. Each party consents and submits to the nonexclusive personal jurisdiction of any court in the State and County of New York in respect of any such proceeding.

8.7 *Acknowledgment.* By opening this package and/or by accessing the Licensed Content on this Web site, THE END USER ACKNOWLEDGES THAT IT HAS READ THIS AGREEMENT, UNDERSTANDS IT, AND AGREES TO BE BOUND BY ITS TERMS AND CONDITIONS. IF YOU DO NOT ACCEPT THESE TERMS AND CONDITIONS, YOU MUST NOT ACCESS THE LICENSED CONTENT AND RETURN THE LICENSED PRODUCT TO CENGAGE LEARNING (WITHIN 30 CALENDAR DAYS OF THE END USER'S PURCHASE) WITH PROOF OF PAYMENT ACCEPTABLE TO CENGAGE LEARNING, FOR A CREDIT OR A REFUND. Should the End User have any questions/comments regarding this Agreement, please contact Cengage Learning at Delmar.help@cengage.com.

STUDYWARE™ TO ACCOMPANY *DELMAR'S* HEALTH ASSESSMENT & PHYSICAL EXAMINATION, *FOURTH EDITION*

MINIMUM SYSTEM REQUIREMENTS

- Operating systems: Microsoft Windows 2000 w/SP 4, Windows XP w/SP 2, Windows Vista w/SP 1
- Processor: Minimum required by Operating System
- Memory: Minimum required by Operating System
- Hard Drive Space: 500 MB
- Screen resolution: 800 x 600 pixels
- CD-ROM drive
- Sound card and listening device required for audio features
- Flash Player 9. The Adobe Flash Player is free, and can be downloaded from http://www.adobe.com/products/flashplayer/

SETUP INSTRUCTIONS

1. Insert disc into CD-ROM drive. The StudyWare™ installation program should start automatically. If it does not, go to step 2.
2. From My Computer, double-click the icon for the CD drive.
3. Double-click the *setup.exe* file to start the program.

TECHNICAL SUPPORT

Telephone: 1-800-648-7450
8:30 A.M.–6:30 P.M. Eastern Time
E-mail: delmar.help@cengage.com
StudyWare™ is a trademark used herein under license.
Microsoft® and Windows® are registered trademarks of the Microsoft Corporation.
Pentium® is a registered trademark of the Intel Corporation.

ASSESSMENT IN BRIEF

CRITICAL THINKING AND NURSING PROCESS REVIEW

- Critical thinking and clinical reasoning are incorporated into all aspects of patient care.
- The quality of critical thinking can be evaluated by applying the seven Universal Intellectual Standards.
- Nurses frame their critical thinking by using the nursing process.
- Apply all six phases of the nursing process to address different patient problems.
- Begin with a thorough assessment of the patient, using a health history, physical assessment, and laboratory data and diagnostic procedures. Document findings.
- Formulate and prioritize nursing diagnoses according to the patient's status. Record on the patient's clinical record.
- Work with the patient to develop mutually agreeable and achievable outcomes and interventions.
- Implement actions in conjunction with other members of the health care team.
- Evaluate the patient's progress toward achieving outcomes.
- Continually reassess and reprioritize diagnoses and outcomes as the patient's status changes in order to provide the best patient care.
- Document the patient's progress toward outcomes.

ASSESSMENT IN BRIEF

GENERAL APPROACH TO THE HEALTH HISTORY

- Present with a professional appearance. Avoid extremes in dress so that your appearance does not become a hindrance to information gathering.
- Ensure an appropriate environment, e.g., good lighting, comfortable temperature, lack of noise and distractions, and adequate privacy.
- Sit facing the patient at eye level, with the patient in a chair or on a bed. Ensure that the patient is as comfortable as possible because obtaining the health history can be a lengthy process.
- Ask the patient whether there are any questions about the interview before it is started.
- Avoid the use of medical jargon. Use terms the patient can understand.
- Reserve asking intimate and personal questions for after rapport has been established.
- Remain flexible in obtaining the health history. It does not have to be obtained in the exact order it is presented in this chapter or on institutional forms.
- Remind the patient that all information will be treated confidentially.

ASSESSMENT IN BRIEF

DEVELOPMENTAL ASSESSMENT

- Note the patient's stated chronological age.
- Tailor your questions to the patient's expected level of ability according to developmental parameters until you can accurately assess the actual developmental level.
- When assessing small children, verify information with the caregiver.
- If a third party is assisting in the interview (for an elderly or special needs patient), address all questions to the patient, not the intermediary.

ASSESSMENT IN BRIEF

FUNDAMENTAL CULTURAL VALUES

- What are the values and beliefs that most characterize each culture and subculture to which you belong, and with which do you agree?
- Do any of your values and beliefs that are derived from membership in one culture or subculture conflict with those from any other?
- If there is any conflict between the values of two or more of the cultures or subcultures with which you identify (e.g., health care professional subculture, religious subculture, socioeconomic subculture, political party subculture), have you resolved these conflicts, and if so, how have you done this and what helped you to reconcile these conflicts?
- What is your time orientation?
- What do you believe about the basic nature of human beings?
- What do you believe is your basic nature?
- What do you believe is your primary purpose in life?
- What do you believe about the purpose of human relations?
- What do you believe your relation is to nature and the supernatural?

EFFECTIVE INTERVIEWING

- Be aware of personal beliefs and how these were acquired. Avoid imposing your beliefs on those you interview.
- Listen and observe. Attend to verbal and affective content as well as to nonverbal cues.
- Keep your attention focused on the patient. Do not listen with "half an ear." Do not think about other things when you are interviewing.
- Maintain eye contact with the patient as is appropriate for the patient's culture.
- Notice the patient's speech patterns and any recurring themes. Note any extra emphasis that the patient places on certain words or topics.
- Do not assume that you understand the meaning of all patient communications. Clarify frequently.
- Paraphrase and summarize occasionally to help patients organize their thinking, clarify issues, and begin to explore specific concerns more deeply.
- Allow for periods of silence.
- Remember that attitudes and feelings may be conveyed nonverbally.
- Consistently monitor your reactions to the patient's verbal and nonverbal messages.
- Avoid being judgmental or critical. Avoid preaching.
- Avoid the use of nontherapeutic interviewing techniques.

ASSESSMENT IN BRIEF

GENERAL APPROACH TO SPIRITUAL ASSESSMENT

- If possible, choose a quiet, private room that will be free from interruptions.
- Ensure that the room's light is sufficiently bright to observe the patient's verbal and nonverbal reactions.
- Greet the patient, introduce yourself, and explain that you will be taking a health history.
- Position yourself at eye level with the patient.
- Portray an interested, nonjudgmental manner throughout the interview. Respect silence and diversity.
- Use a spiritual assessment tool like FICA to engage the patient:
  Faith and Belief
  Importance
  Community
  Address

ASSESSMENT IN BRIEF

NUTRITIONAL ASSESSMENT

Nutritional History
Physical Assessment
Anthropometric Measurements

- Height
- Weight
- Body mass index
- Waist circumference and waist to hip ratio
- Skinfold thickness
- Mid-arm and mid-arm muscle circumferences

Laboratory Data

- Hematocrit and hemoglobin
- Lipids
- Transferrin, total iron-binding capacity, and iron
- Total lymphocyte count
- Antigen skin testing
- Prealbumin
- Albumin
- Glucose
- HbA1c
- Creatinine height index
- Nitrogen balance
- Vitamin D

Diagnostic Data

- X-rays
- DEXA scan

ASSESSMENT IN BRIEF

COMPREHENSIVE NUTRITIONAL ASSESSMENT

Nutritional History
Physical Assessment

- General appearance
- Skin
- Hair
- Nails
- Eyes
- Mouth
- Head and neck
- Heart and peripheral vasculature
- Abdomen
- Musculoskeletal system
- Neurological system
- Female genitalia

Anthropometric Measurements

- Height: _____ in or cm
- Weight: _____ lbs or kg
- % Ideal body weight: _____
- % Usual body weight: _____
- % Weight Change: _____
- Body Mass Index: _____
- Waist circumference: _____ in or cm
- Waist to hip ratio: _____
- Triceps Skinfold: _____ mm
- Mid-arm circumference: _____ cm
- Mid-arm muscle circumference: _____ cm

 continues

ASSESSMENT IN BRIEF

DIET HISTORY

Part 1: General Diet Information

- Do you follow a particular diet?
- What are your food likes and dislikes?
- Do you have any especially strong cravings?
- How often do you eat fast foods?
- How often do you eat at restaurants?
- Do you have adequate financial resources to purchase your food?
- How do you obtain, store, and prepare your food?
- Do you eat alone or with a family member or other person?
- Do you consume any food supplements (e.g., high-caloric beverages)?
- In the last 12 months have you
  - Experienced any change in weight?
  - Had a change in your appetite?
  - Had a change in your diet?
  - Experienced nausea, vomiting, or diarrhea from your diet?
  - Changed your diet because of difficulty in feeding yourself, eating, chewing, or swallowing?

 continues

QUESTIONS FOR ASCERTAINING A PATIENT'S SPIRITUAL BELIEFS

- What kind of faith do you have?
- Are you a person of faith?
- Do you attend worship services regularly?
- What is the most important thing in your life?
- What do you depend on when things go wrong?
- Do you pray?
- What do you believe in?
- Why do you think you have become ill now?
- Is there anything more important to you than regaining your health?

Diet History continued (2 of 2)

Part 2: Food Intake History
(24-hour recall, three-day diary, direct observation)

Time	Food/Drink	Amount	Method of Preparation	Eating Location

Comprehensive Nutritional Assessment continued (2 of 2)

Laboratory Data

- Hematocrit (Hct): _____%
- Hemoglobin (Hgb): _____ g/dL
- Cholesterol: _____ mg/dL
- HDL: _____ mg/dL
- LDL: _____ mg/dL
- Triglycerides: _____ mg/dL
- Transferrin: _____ mg/dL
- TIBC: _____ μg/dL
- Iron: _____ μg/dL
- Total lymphocyte count: _____ cells/mm^3
- Antigen skin testing: _____
- Prealbumin: _____ mg/dL
- Albumin: _____ g/dL
- Glucose: _____ mg/dL
- HbA1c _____ %
- CHI: _____
- Nitrogen balance: _____ g
- Vitamin D: _____ ng/mL

Diagnostic Data

- X-rays _____
- DEXA Scan _____

ASSESSMENT IN BRIEF

PHYSICAL ASSESSMENT TECHNIQUES

Inspection
- Vision
- Smell

Palpation
- Light palpation
- Deep palpation

Percussion
- Direct, or immediate percussion
- Indirect, or mediate percussion
- Direct fist percussion
- Indirect fist percussion

Auscultation
- Direct, or immediate auscultation
- Indirect, or mediate auscultation

ASSESSMENT IN BRIEF

GENERAL SURVEY, VITAL SIGNS, AND PAIN

General Survey
- Physical presence
  - Stated age versus apparent age
  - General appearance
  - Body fat
  - Stature
  - Motor activity
  - Body and breath odors
- Psychological presence
  - Dress, grooming, and personal hygiene
  - Mood and manner
  - Speech
  - Facial expression
- Distress

Vital Signs
- Respiration
- Pulse
- Temperature
- Blood pressure

Pain

ASSESSMENT IN BRIEF

SKIN, HAIR, AND NAILS ASSESSMENT

Inspection of the Skin
- Color
- Bleeding, ecchymosis, and vascularity
- Lesions

Palpation of the Skin
- Moisture
- Temperature
- Tenderness
- Texture
- Turgor
- Edema

Inspection of the Hair
- Color
- Distribution
- Lesions

Palpation of the Hair
- Texture

Inspection of the Nails
- Color
- Shape and configuration

Palpation of the Nails
- Texture

Advanced Technique
- Skin scraping for scabies

ASSESSMENT IN BRIEF

HEAD, NECK, AND REGIONAL LYMPHATICS ASSESSMENT

Inspection
- Shape of the head
- Scalp
- Face
  - Symmetry
  - Shape and features
- Neck
- Thyroid gland
- Lymph nodes

Palpation
- Head
- Scalp
- Mandible
- Neck
- Thyroid gland
  - Posterior approach
  - Anterior approach
- Lymph nodes

Auscultation
- Mandible
- Thyroid gland

Eye Assessment

Visual Acuity
- Distance vision
- Near vision
- Color vision

Visual Fields

External Eye and Lacrimal Apparatus
- Eyelids, eyebrows, and eyelashes
- Lacrimal apparatus
  - Inspection
  - Palpation

Extraocular Muscle Function
- Corneal light reflex
- Cover/uncover test
- Cardinal fields of gaze

Anterior Segment Structures
- Conjunctiva
- Sclera
- Cornea
- Anterior chamber
- Iris
- Pupil
- Lens

Posterior Segment Structures
- Retinal structures
- Macula

Ears, Nose, Mouth, and Throat Assessment

Ears
- Auditory screening
  - Voice-whisper test
  - Tuning fork tests
    Weber test
    Rinne test
- External ear
  - Inspection
  - Palpation
- Otoscopic Assessment

Nose
- External inspection
- Patency
- Internal inspection

Sinuses
- Inspection
- Palpation and percussion

Mouth and Throat
- Mouth
  - Breath
  - Lips
    Inspection
    Palpation
  - Tongue
  - Buccal mucosa
  - Gums
  - Teeth
  - Palate
- Throat

Advanced Technique
- Transillumination of the sinuses

Breasts and Regional Nodes Assessment

Inspection
- Color
- Vascularity
- Thickening or edema
- Size and symmetry
- Contour
- Lesions or masses
- Discharge

Palpation
- Supraclavicular and infraclavicular lymph nodes
- Breasts: Patient in sitting position
- Axillary lymph node region
- Breasts: Patient in supine position

Thorax and Lung Assessment

Inspection
- Shape of thorax
- Symmetry of chest wall
- Presence of superficial veins
- Costal angle
- Angle of the ribs
- Intercostal spaces
- Muscles of respiration
- Respirations
  - Rate
  - Pattern
  - Depth
  - Symmetry
  - Audibility
  - Patient position
  - Mode of breathing
- Sputum

Palpation
- General palpation
  - Pulsations
  - Masses
  - Thoracic tenderness
  - Crepitus
- Thoracic expansion

continues

- Tactile fremitus
- Tracheal position

Percussion
- General percussion
- Diaphragmatic excursion

Auscultation
- Breath sounds
- Adventitious sounds
- Voice sounds

Advanced Techniques
- Locating the site of a fractured rib
- Forced expiratory time

Assistive Devices
- Oxygen
- Incentive spirometer
- Endotracheal tube
- Tracheostomy tube
- Mechanical ventilation
- Pulse oximeter
- Peak flow meter

ASSESSMENT IN BRIEF

HEART AND PERIPHERAL VASCULATURE ASSESSMENT

Assessment of the Precordium
- Inspection
  - Aortic area
  - Pulmonic area
  - Midprecordial area
  - Tricuspid area
  - Mitral area
- Palpation
  - Aortic area
  - Pulmonic area
  - Midprecordial area
  - Tricuspid area
  - Mitral area
- Auscultation
  - Aortic area
  - Pulmonic area
  - Midprecordial area
  - Tricuspid area
  - Mitral area
  - Mitral and tricuspid areas (S_3)
  - Mitral and tricuspid areas (S_4)
  - Murmurs
  - Pericardial friction rub
  - Prosthetic heart valves

continues

ASSESSMENT IN BRIEF

ABDOMINAL ASSESSMENT

Inspection
- Contour
- Symmetry
- Rectus abdominis muscles
- Pigmentation and color
- Scars
- Striae
- Respiratory movement
- Masses or nodules
- Visible peristalsis
- Pulsation
- Umbilicus

Auscultation
- Bowel sounds
- Vascular sounds
- Venous hum
- Friction rub

Percussion
- General percussion
- Liver span
- Liver descent
- Spleen
- Stomach
- Fist percussion
  - Kidney
  - Liver
- Bladder

Palpation
- Light palpation
- Abdominal muscle guarding
- Deep palpation
- Liver
  - Bimanual method
  - Hook method
- Spleen
- Kidneys
- Aorta
- Bladder
- Inguinal lymph nodes

continues

ASSESSMENT IN BRIEF

MUSCULOSKELETAL ASSESSMENT

General Assessment
- Overall appearance
- Posture
- Gait and mobility

Inspection
- Muscle size and shape
- Joint contour and periarticular tissue

Palpation
- Muscle tone
- Joints

Range of Motion

Muscle Strength

Examination of Joints
- Temporomandibular joint
- Cervical spine
- Shoulders
- Elbows
- Wrists and hands
- Hips
- Knees
- Ankles and feet
- Spine

Advanced Techniques
- Measuring limb circumference
- Using a goniometer
- Chvostek's sign (assessing for neuroexcitability)

continues

ASSESSMENT IN BRIEF

MENTAL STATUS ASSESSMENT AND NEUROLOGICAL TECHNIQUES

Mental Status Assessment
- Physical appearance and behavior
  - Posture and movements
  - Dress, grooming, and personal hygiene
  - Facial expression
  - Affect
- Communication
- Level of consciousness
- Cognitive abilities and mentation
  - Attention
  - Memory
  - Judgment
  - Insight
  - Spatial perception
  - Calculation
  - Abstract reasoning
  - Thought process and content
  - Suicidal ideation

Sensory Assessment
- Exteroceptive sensation
  - Light touch
  - Superficial pain
  - Temperature
- Proprioceptive sensation
  - Motion and position
  - Vibration sense
- Cortical sensation
  - Stereognosis
  - Graphesthesia
  - Two-point discrimination
  - Extinction

continues

Advanced Techniques

- Liver scratch test
- Assessing for ascites
  - Shifting dullness
  - Puddle sign
- Fluid wave
- Murphy's sign
- Rebound tenderness
- Rovsing's sign
- Cutaneous hypersensitivity
- Iliopsoas muscle test
- Obturator muscle test
- Ballottement

Abdominal Tubes and Drains

- Tubes
  - Enteral tube
  - Nasogastric suction tube
  - Intestinal tube
  - Gastrostomy
- Drains
  - Abdominal cavity drain
  - Biliary drain
- Intestinal diversions
  - Colostomy
  - Ileostomy
- Urinary diversions
  - Ileal conduit
  - Ureteral stent
  - Indwelling catheter

Assessment of the Peripheral Vasculature

- Inspection of the jugular venous pressure
- Inspection of the hepatojugular reflux
- Palpation and auscultation of arterial pulses
- Inspection and palpation of peripheral perfusion
  - Peripheral pulse
  - Color
  - Clubbing
  - Capillary refill
  - Skin temperature
  - Edema
  - Ulcerations
  - Skin texture
  - Hair distribution
- Palpation of the epitrochlear node

Advanced Techniques

- Orthostatic hypotension assessment
- Assessing for pulsus paradoxus
- Assessing the venous system
  - Homan's sign
  - Manual compression
  - Retrograde filling or Trendelenburg test
- Assessing the arterial system
  - Pallor
  - Color return and venous filling time
  - Allen test
  - Ankle-Brachial Index

Assistive Devices

- Artificial cardiac pacemakers
- Hemodynamic monitor
- Antiembolic stockings
- Chest tubes
- EKG monitor
- Intravenous catheters
- Pneumatic compression stockings

Cranial Nerves Assessment

- Olfactory nerve (CN I)
- Optic nerve (CN II)
  - Visual acuity
  - Visual fields
  - Funduscopic examination
- Oculomotor nerve (CN III)
  - Cardinal fields of gaze
  - Eyelid elevation
  - Pupil reactions
- Trochlear nerve (CN IV)
  - Cardinal fields of gaze
- Trigeminal nerve (CN V)
  - Motor component
  - Sensory component
- Abducens nerve (CN VI)
  - Cardinal fields of gaze
- Facial nerve (CN VII)
  - Motor component
  - Sensory component
- Acoustic nerve (CN VIII)
  - Cochlear division
    Hearing
    Weber test
    Rinne test
  - Vestibular division
- Glossopharyngeal nerve (CN IX)
- Vagus nerve (CN X)
- Spinal accessory nerve (CN XI)
- Hypoglossal nerve (CN XII)

Motor System Assessment

- Muscle size
- Muscle tone
- Muscle strength
- Involuntary movements
- Pronator drift

Cerebellar Function

- Coordination
- Station
- Gait

continues

- Drop arm test (assessing for rotator cuff damage)
- Trousseau's sign (assessing for neuroexcitability)
- Assessing grip strength using a blood pressure cuff
- Tinel's sign (assessing for carpal tunnel syndrome)
- Phalen's sign (assessing for carpal tunnel syndrome)
- Trendelenburg test (assessing for hip dislocation)
- Measuring limb length
- Bulge sign (assessing for small effusions)
- Patellar ballottement (assessing for large effusions)
- Apley's grinding sign (assessing for meniscal tears)
- McMurray's sign (assessing for meniscal tears)
- Drawer test (assessing the cruciate ligaments)
- Lachman's test (assessing the anterior cruciate ligament)
- Varus stress test (assessing the lateral collateral ligament)
- Valgus stress test (assessing the medial collateral ligament)
- Anterior drawer test (assessing for ankle sprain)
- Talar tilt test (assessing for ankle sprain)
- Assessing status of distal limbs and digits
- Thompson squeeze test (assessing for ruptured Achilles tendon)
- Adams forward bend test (assessing for scoliosis) and use of the scoliometer
- Straight leg raising test (Lasègue's test) (assessing for herniated disc)
- Milgram test (assessing for herniated disc)

Assistive Devices

- Crutches
- Cane
- Walker
- Brace, splint, immobilizer
- Cast

Reflexes

- Deep tendon reflexes
  - Brachioradialis
  - Biceps
  - Triceps
  - Patellar
  - Achilles
- Superficial reflexes
  - Abdominal
  - Plantar
  - Cremasteric
  - Bulbocavernosus
- Pathological reflexes
  - Glabellar
  - Clonus
  - Babinski

Advanced Techniques

- Doll's eyes phenomenon
- Romberg test
- Meningeal irritation
  - Nuchal rigidity
  - Kernig's sign
  - Brudzinski's sign

ASSESSMENT IN BRIEF

FEMALE GENITALIA ASSESSMENT

Inspection of the External Genitalia

- Pubic hair
- Skin color and condition
  - Mons pubis and vulva
  - Clitoris
  - Urethral meatus
  - Vaginal introitus
  - Perineum and anus

Palpation of the External Genitalia

- Labia
- Urethral meatus and Skene's glands
- Vaginal introitus
- Perineum

Speculum Examination of the Internal Genitalia

- Cervix
  - Color
  - Position
  - Size
  - Surface characteristics
  - Discharge
  - Shape of the cervical os

continues

ASSESSMENT IN BRIEF

MALE GENITALIA ASSESSMENT

Inspection

- Sexual maturity rating
- Hair distribution
- Penis
- Scrotum
- Urethral meatus
- Inguinal area

Palpation

- Penis
- Urethral meatus
- Scrotum
- Inguinal area

Auscultation

- Scrotum

Advanced Techniques

- Acetowhitening: Assessing for HPV
- Urethral culture: Identifying penile pathogens
- Prehn's sign: Assessing for testicular torsion
- Transillumination of the scrotum: Assessing for a scrotal mass

ASSESSMENT IN BRIEF

ANUS, RECTUM, AND PROSTATE ASSESSMENT

Inspection

- Perineum and sacrococcygeal area
- Anal mucosa

Palpation

- Anus and rectum
- Prostate

Advanced Technique

- Anal Pap collection

Collecting Specimens for Cytological Smears and Cultures

- Pap smear
  - Endocervical smear
  - Cervical smear
- Chlamydia culture specimen
- Gonococcal culture specimen
- Saline mount or "wet prep"
- KOH prep
- Five percent acetic acid wash
- Anal culture

Inspection of the Vaginal Wall

Bimanual Examination

- Vagina
- Cervix
- Fornices
- Uterus
- Adnexa

Rectovaginal Examination

ASSESSMENT IN BRIEF

PREGNANT PATIENT ASSESSMENT*

Fundal Height

Fetal Heart Rate

Leopold's Maneuvers
- First maneuver
- Second maneuver
- Third maneuver
- Fourth maneuver

Only pregnancy-specific assessments are listed.

ASSESSMENT IN BRIEF

PEDIATRIC PATIENT ASSESSMENT*

Developmental Assessment
- Denver II

Physical Growth
- Weight
- Length and height
- Head circumference
- Chest circumference
- Body mass index

Physical Assessment
- Apgar scoring
- Head
  - Inspection
    Head control
  - Palpation
    Anterior fontanel
    Posterior fontanel
    Suture lines
    Surface characteristics
- Eyes
  - Vision screening
    Allen test
    Color vision screening

Only pediatric-specific tests are listed.

 continues

ASSESSMENT IN BRIEF

ELDERLY PATIENT ASSESSMENT

Special Assessments
- Developmental assessment
- Cultural assessment
- Spiritual assessment
- Nutritional assessment
- Pain assessment

Physical Examination*
- Quick screen
- Functional testing
- Cognition

All other assessment skills are performed as described in Chapters 10–22.

ASSESSMENT IN BRIEF

REVIEW OF SYSTEMS

General
- Patient's perception of general state of health at the present, difference from usual state, vitality and energy levels, body odors, fever, chills, night sweats

Skin
- Rashes, itching, changes in skin pigmentation, ecchymoses, change in color or size of mole, sores, lumps, dry or moist skin, pruritus, change in skin texture, odors, excessive sweating, acne, warts, eczema, psoriasis, amount of time spent in the sun, use of sunscreen, skin cancer

Hair
- Alopecia, excessive growth of hair or growth of hair in unusual locations (hirsutism), use of chemicals on hair, dandruff, pediculosis, scalp lesions

Nails
- Change in nails, splitting, breaking, thickened, texture change, onychomycosis, use of chemicals, false nails

Eyes
- Blurred vision, visual acuity, glasses, contacts, photophobia, excessive tearing, night blindness, diplopia, drainage, bloodshot eyes, pain, blind spots, flashing lights, halos around objects, floaters, glaucoma, cataracts, use of sunglasses, use of protective eyewear

 continues

Pediatric Patient Assessment continued (2 of 2)

- Musculoskeletal system
  - Inspection
    Tibiofemoral bones
  - Palpation
    Feet (metatarsus varus)
    Hip and femur (Ortolani's maneuver)
- Neurological System
  - Rooting reflex
  - Sucking reflex
  - Palmar grasp reflex
  - Tonic neck reflex
  - Stepping reflex
  - Plantar grasp reflex
  - Babinski reflex
  - Moro (startle) reflex
  - Galant reflex
  - Placing reflex
  - Landau reflex

Advanced Techniques

- Assessing for hydrocephalus and anencephaly: Transillumination of the skull
- Assessing for coarctation of the aorta

Review of Systems continued (2 of 5)

Ears

- Cleaning method, hearing deficits, hearing aid, pain, phonophobia, discharge, lightheadedness (vertigo), ringing in the ears (tinnitus), usual noise level, earaches, infection, piercings, use of ear protection, amount of cerumen

Nose and Sinuses

- Number of colds per year, discharge, itching, hay fever, postnasal drip, stuffiness, sinus pain, sinusitis, polyps, obstruction, epistaxis, change in sense of smell, allergies, snoring

Mouth

- Dental habits (brushing, flossing, mouth rinses), toothache, tooth abscess, dentures, bleeding or swollen gums, difficulty chewing, sore tongue, change in taste, lesions, change in salivation, bad breath, caries, teeth extractions, orthodontics

Throat and Neck

- Hoarseness, change in voice, frequent sore throats, dysphagia, pain or stiffness, enlarged thyroid (goiter), lymphadenopathy, tonsillectomy, adenoidectomy

Breasts and Axilla

- Pain, tenderness, discharge, lumps, change in size, dimpling, rash, benign breast disease, breast cancer, results of recent mammogram, breast self-examination

Respiratory

- Dyspnea on exertion, shortness of breath, sputum, cough, sneezing, wheezing, hemoptysis, frequent upper respiratory tract infections, pneumonia, emphysema, asthma, tuberculosis, tuberculosis exposure, result of last chest X-ray or PPD

Cardiovascular and Peripheral Vasculature

- Paroxysmal nocturnal dyspnea, chest pain, cyanosis, heart murmur, palpitations, syncope, orthopnea (state number of pillows used), edema, cold or discolored hands or feet, leg cramps, myocardial infarction, hypertension, valvular disease, intermittent claudication, varicose veins, thrombophlebitis, deep vein thrombosis, use of support hose, anemia, result of last EKG

Gastrointestinal

- Change in appetite, nausea, vomiting, diarrhea, constipation, usual bowel habits, melena, rectal bleeding, hematemesis, change in stool color, flatulence, belching, regurgitation, heartburn, dysphagia, abdominal pain, jaundice, ascites, hemorrhoids, hepatitis, peptic ulcers, gallstones, gastroesophageal reflux disease, appendicitis, ulcerative colitis, Crohn's disease, diverticulitis, hernia

Urinary

- Change in urine color, voiding habits, dysuria, hesitancy, urgency, frequency, nocturia, polyuria, dribbling, loss in force of stream, bedwetting, change in urine volume, incontinence, urinary retention, suprapubic pain, flank pain, kidney stones, urinary tract infections

Musculoskeletal

- Joint stiffness, muscle pain, cramps, back pain, limitation of movement, redness, swelling, weakness, bony deformity, broken bones, dislocations, sprains, crepitus, gout, arthritis, osteoporosis, herniated disc

 continues

ASSESSMENT IN BRIEF

COMPLETE HEALTH HISTORY

- Today's date

Biographical Data

- Patient's name
- Address
- Phone number
- Date of birth
- Birthplace
- Social Security Number
- Occupation
- Insurance
- Usual source of health care
- Source of referral
- Emergency contact
- Work address and phone number
- Source and reliability of information

Patient Profile

- Age
- Gender
- Race
- Marital status

Reason for seeking health care and chief complaint

Present health and history of the present illness

Past Health History

- Medical history
- Surgical history
- Medications
  - Prescription
  - OTC
- Communicable diseases
- Allergies
- Injuries and accidents
- Special needs
- Blood transfusions
- Childhood illnesses
- Immunizations

Family Health History

Social History

- Alcohol use
- Tobacco use

 continues

ASSESSMENT IN BRIEF

FAMILY HEALTH HISTORY

The family health history records the health status of the patient as well as immediate blood relatives. At a minimum, the history needs to contain the age and health status of the patient, spouse, children, siblings, and the patient's parents. Ideally, the patient's grandparents, aunts, and uncles should be incorporated into the history as well. Documentation of this information is done in two parts: the genogram, or family tree, and a list of familial diseases.

The second component of the family health history is the report of occurrences of familial or genetic diseases. Such information is crucial to the patient's health and may not have been revealed previously because some familial illnesses do not occur in every generation. The pertinent negative findings are documented in the family health history below the genogram.

Nutrition

- Present weight, usual weight, desired weight, food intolerances, food likes and dislikes, where meals are eaten, caffeine intake, vitamin supplements

Endocrine

- Exophthalmos, fatigue, change in size of head, hands, or feet, weight change, heat and cold intolerances, excessive sweating, polydipsia, polyphagia, polyuria, increased hunger, change in body hair distribution, goiter, diabetes mellitus

Lymph Nodes

- Enlargement, tenderness

Hematological

- Easy bruising or bleeding, anemia, sickle cell anemia, blood type, exposure to radiation

 continues

- Drug use
- Domestic and intimate partner violence
- Sexual practice
- Travel history
- Work environment
- Home environment
  – Physical environment
  – Psychosocial environment
- Hobbies and leisure activities
- Stress
- Education
- Economic status
- Military service
- Religion
- Ethnic background
- Roles and relationships
- Characteristic patterns of daily living

Health Maintenance Activities

- Sleep
- Diet
- Exercise
- Stress management
- Use of safety devices
- Health check-ups

Review of Systems

- General
- Skin
- Hair
- Nails
- Eyes
- Ears
- Nose and sinuses
- Mouth
- Throat and neck
- Breasts and axilla
- Respiratory
- Cardiovascular and peripheral vasculature
- Gastrointestinal
- Urinary
- Musculoskeletal
- Neurological
- Psychological
- Reproductive
- Nutrition
- Endocrine
- Lymph nodes
- Hematological

Neurological

- Headache, change in balance, incoordination, loss of movement, change in sensory perception or feeling in an extremity, change in speech, change in smell, syncope, loss of memory, tremors, involuntary movement, loss of consciousness, seizures, weakness, head injury, vertigo, tremor, tic, paralysis, stroke, spasm

Psychological

- Irritability, nervousness, tension, increased stress, difficulty concentrating, mood changes, suicidal thoughts, depression, anxiety, sleep disturbances

Female Reproductive

- Vaginal discharge, change in libido, infertility, sterility, pelvic pain, pain during intercourse, postcoital bleeding; menses: last menstrual period (LMP), menarche, regularity, duration, amount of bleeding, premenstrual symptoms, intermenstrual bleeding, dysmenorrhea, menorrhagia, fibroids; menopause: age of onset, duration, symptoms, bleeding; obstetrical: number of pregnancies, number of miscarriages or abortions, number of children, type of delivery, complications; type of birth control, hormone replacement therapy

Male Reproductive

- Change in libido, infertility, sterility, impotence, pain during intercourse, age at onset of puberty, testicular or penile pain, penile discharge, erections, emissions, hernias, enlarged prostate, type of birth control, testicular self-examination

Family Health History continued (2 of 2)

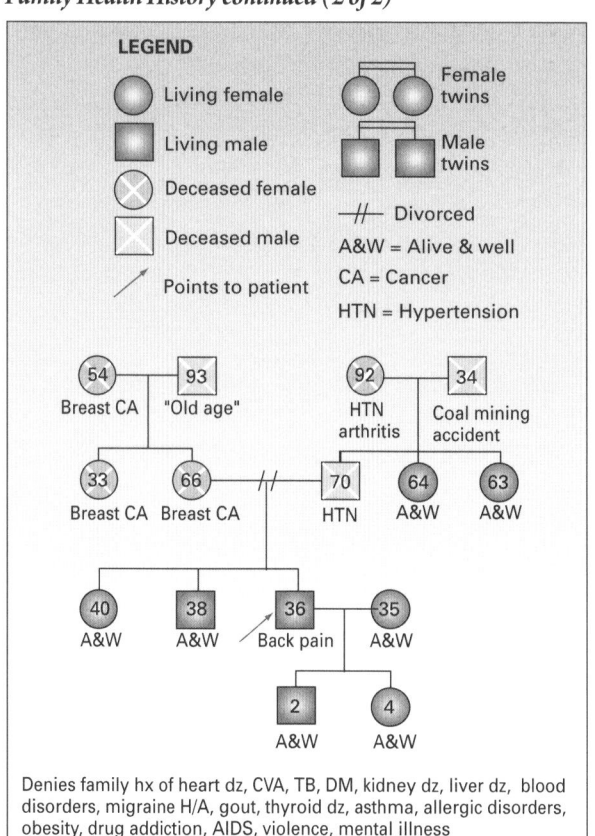

Family Health History and Genogram

ABBREVIATIONS

ā	before
A, A, & O × 3	awake, alert, and oriented times three (to person, place, and time)
AB	abortion
abd	abdomen; abdominal
ABG	arterial blood gas
a̅c	before meals
ACL	anterior cruciate ligament
ADL	activities of daily living
AEB	as evidenced by
AFI	amniotic fluid index
AGA	appropriate for gestational age
AIDS	acquired immune deficiency syndrome
ALS	amyotrophic lateral sclerosis
ANA	American Nurses Association
ant	anterior
AOM	acute otitis media
AP	apical pulse; anteroposterior
A&P	anterior and posterior; auscultation and percussion; anatomy and physiology
AR	allergic rhinitis
AROM	active range of motion; artificial rupture of membranes
AS	aortic stenosis
ASA	acetylsalicylic acid
ASD	atrial septal defect
Atb	antibiotic
AV	arteriovenous
A-V	atrioventricular
A&W	alive and well
ax	axillary
BCC	basal cell carcinoma
BCG	Bacille Calmette-Guérin vaccine
BCP	birth control pills
BF	black female
bid	twice a day
bilat	bilateral
BM	black male; breast milk; bowel movement
BP	blood pressure
BPH	benign prostatic hypertrophy
BPM	beats per minute
BS	bowel sounds; breath sounds
BSE	breast self-examination
b/t	between
bx	biopsy
C	Celsius, centigrade
c̅	with
CA	cancer
CABG	coronary artery bypass graft
CAD	coronary artery disease
CC	chief complaint
CCD	congenital cardiovascular defect
CDC	Centers for Disease Control and Prevention
CHD	childhood diseases; congenital heart disease
CHF	congestive heart failure
CHI	closed head injury; creatinine height index
CMT	cervical motion tenderness
CMV	cytomegalovirus
CN I–XII	cranial nerves I–XII
CNS	central nervous system
c/o	complaining of; complaints of
CO	carbon monoxide; cardiac output
CO₂	carbon dioxide
COA	coarctation of the aorta
COPD	chronic obstructive pulmonary disease
CP	chest pain; cerebral palsy
CPD	cephalopelvic disproportion
CT	computerized tomography
CV	cardiovascular
CVA	costovertebral angle; cerebrovascular accident
CVAT	costovertebral angle tenderness
CVP	central venous pressure
CVS	chorionic villi sampling
cx	cervix
CX-ray	chest X-ray
DBP	diastolic blood pressure
D&C	dilation and curettage
DDST II	Denver Developmental Screening Test II
DES	diethylstilbestrol
DJD	degenerative joint disease
DM	diabetes mellitus
DOA	dead on arrival
DOB	date of birth
DOE	dyspnea on exertion
dT	diphtheria, tetanus (vaccine)
DTR	deep tendon reflex
DUB	dysfunctional uterine bleeding
DVT	deep vein thrombosis
DWM	divorced white male (DWF, DBM, DBF are variations of this)
dx	diagnosis
dz	disease
EAC	external auricular canal
ED	emergency department; erectile dysfunction
EDC	expected date of confinement (delivery date)
EDD	estimated date of delivery
EEG	electroencephalogram
EENT	eyes, ears, nose, throat
EFM	electronic fetal monitoring
EKG	electrocardiogram
EMR	electronic medical record
ENAP	examination, normal findings, abnormal findings, pathophysiology
ENT	ears, nose, and throat
EOMI	extraocular muscles intact
ER	emergency room
ETOH	ethyl alcohol
F	Fahrenheit
FAS	fetal alcohol syndrome
FHH	family health history
FHR	fetal heart rate
FHT	fetal heart tone
FIT	fecal immunochemical test
FLM	fetal lung maturity
FM	fetal movement
FOB	father of baby
FOBT	fecal occult blood test
FROM	full range of motion
FSH	follicle-stimulating hormone
FTT	failure to thrive
fx	fracture
Ⓖ	gallop
GC	gonorrhea and chlamydia
GCS	Glasgow Coma Scale
GDM	gestational diabetes mellitus
GERD	gastroesophageal reflux disease
GI	gastrointestinal
GSW	gunshot wound
gtt	drop
GU	genitourinary
GYN	gynecologic
H/A	headache
HCG	human chorionic gonadotropin
HDL	high-density lipoprotein
HDP	hypertensive disorders of pregnancy
HEENT	head, eyes, ears, nose, throat
HELLP	hemolysis, elevated liver enzymes, low platelets
Hib	Haemophilus influenza b
HIV	human immunodeficiency virus
hl	health
h/o	history of
HOB	head of bed
HPI	history of present illness
HPV	human papillomavirus
HR	heart rate
hr(s)	hour(s)
HRT	hormone replacement therapy
HSM	hepatosplenomegaly
HSV	herpes simplex virus
ht	height
HTN	hypertension
hx	history
IADL	instrumental activities of daily living
IBW	ideal body weight
ICP	intracranial pressure
ICS	intercostal space
IDDM	insulin-dependent diabetes mellitus
IDM	infant of diabetic mother
IOP	intraocular pressure
IPPA	inspection, palpation, percussion, auscultation
IPV	intimate partner violence
ITP	idiopathic thrombocytopenia purpura
IUD	intrauterine device
IUGR	intrauterine growth retardation
IUP	intrauterine pregnancy
IV	intravenous
JVD	jugular venous distension
JVP	jugular venous pressure
KOH	potassium hydroxide
KUB	kidneys, ureters, bladder
L	liter
Ⓛ	left
LAD	left anterior descending (coronary artery)
lat	lateral
LBP	low back pain
lbs	pounds
LCM	left costal margin
LDL	low-density lipoprotein
LE	lower extremity
lg	large
LGA	large for gestational age
LGBT	lesbian, gay, bisexual, and transgender
LH	leutinizing hormone
LLE	left lower extremity
LLL	left lower lobe (of lung)
LLQ	left lower quadrant (of abdomen)
LLSB	left lower sternal border
LMP	last menstrual period
LOC	level of/loss of consciousness
LSB	left sternal border
LUE	left upper extremity
LUL	left upper lobe (of lung)
LUQ	left upper quadrant (of abdomen)
LVH	left ventricular hypertrophy
Ⓜ	murmur
MAC	mid-arm circumference
MAL	midaxillary line
MAMC	mid-arm muscle circumference
MCL	midclavicular line; medial collateral ligament
MD	muscular dystrophy; medical doctor